D1753037

CURRENT TECHNIQUES IN SPINAL STABILIZATION

NOTICE

Medicine is an ever-changing science. As new research and clinical experience broaden our knowledge, changes in treatment and drug therapy are required. The editors and the publisher of this work have checked with sources believed to be reliable in their efforts to provide information that is complete and generally in accord with the standards accepted at the time of publication. However, in view of the possibility of human error or changes in medical sciences, neither the editors nor the publisher nor any other party who has been involved in the preparation or publication of this work warrants that the information contained herein is in every respect accurate or complete, and they are not responsible for any errors or omissions or for the results obtained from use of such information. Readers are encouraged to confirm the information contained herein with other sources. For example and in particular, readers are advised to check the product information sheet included in the package of each drug they plan to administer to be certain that the information contained in this book is accurate and that changes have not been made in the recommended dose or in the contraindications for administration. This recommendation is of particular importance in connection with new or infrequently used drugs.

CURRENT TECHNIQUES IN SPINAL STABILIZATION

Editor-in-Chief
RICHARD G. FESSLER, M.D., Ph.D.
Department of Neurological Surgery
University of Florida
Gainesville, Florida

Associate Editor
Regis W. Haid, M.D.
Associate Professor
Department of Surgery, Emory Clinic
Atlanta, Georgia

McGRAW-HILL
Health Professions Division

New York St. Louis San Francisco Auckland Bogotá Caracas Lisbon London Madrid
Mexico City Milan Montreal New Delhi San Juan Singapore Sydney Tokyo Toronto

McGraw-Hill
A Division of The McGraw·Hill Companies

Copyright 1996 by The McGraw-Hill Companies, Inc. All rights reserved. Printed in the United States of America. Except as permitted under the United States Copyright Act of 1976, no part of this publication may be reproduced or distributed in any form or by any means, or stored in a data base or retrieval system, without the prior written permission of the publisher.

1234567890 DOCDOC 9876

ISBN 0-07-020645-7

This book was set in Times Roman by York Graphic Services, Inc.

The editors were James T. Morgan and Peter McCurdy; the production supervisor was Clare Stanley; the project was managed by York Production Services; the cover designer was Karen Quigley. R. R. Donnelley & Sons was printer and binder.

This book is printed on acid-free paper.

To our wives and children for their enduring patience and also to our secretaries and nurses for their devoted assistance in the completion of this textbook.

Contents

Contributors   xi
Preface   xv

PART I.
Anterior Cervical Instrumentation

1. **Odontoid Screw Fixation**   3
   Curtis A. Dickman
   Volker K.H. Sonntag

2. **Caspar System for Anterior Cervical Fusion and Interbody Stabilization**   13
   Peter M. Klara

3. **The Anterior Cervical Spine Locking Plate: A Technique for Surgical Decompression and Stabilization**   25
   Iain H. Kalfas

4. **Stabilization of the Cervical Spine Utilizing the Orion Anterior Cervical Plate System**   35
   Gary L. Lowery

PART II.
Posterior Cervical Instrumentation

SECTION A.
Occipitocervical and C1-2 Instrumentation

5. **Wiring Techniques for Occipitocervical and Atlantoaxial Pathology**   45
   Curtis A. Dickman
   Volker K.H. Sonntag

6. **Posterior Cervical Arthrodesis Using the Songer Cable System**   57
   Matthew N. Songer

7. **Interlaminar Fixation of the Posterior Cervical Spine for Atlantoaxial Instability**   77
   Regis W. Haid
   Cargill H. Alleyne, Jr.

8. **Application of the Luque Rectangle Fixation for Occipital-Cervical and Atlantoaxial Instability**   89
   Brian Pikul
   Gary L. Rea

9. **Application of the Posterior Interfacet Screw for Atlantoaxial Pathology**   93
   Andreas Weidner

10. **Application of the Occipitocervical Plate for Occipitocervical and Atlantoaxial Pathology**   101
    Dieter Grob

SECTION B.
Lower Cervical Spine

11 Wiring Techniques of the Lower Cervical Spine — 107
Andrew Cappuccino
Paul C. McAfee

12 Application of the Codman Sof'wire System for Stabilization of the Lower Cervical Spine — 113
Michael MacMillan

13 Application of the Halifax Clamp for Pathology of the Lower Cervical Spine — 123
Michael G. O'Sullivan
Patrick Statham
Thomas Russell

14 Use of Lateral Mass Plates for Stabilization of the Lower Cervical Spine — 129
Paul R. Cooper

15 AXIS Fixation System Surgical Technique — 139
Chester E. Sutterlin, III
David E. Jenkins

16 Application of the Roy-Camille Posterior Screw Plate Fixation System for Stabilization of the Cervical Spine — 147
R. Roy-Camille
Claude Laville

PART III.
Anterior Thoracolumbar Instrumentation

17 Application of the Kaneda Anterior Spinal Stabilization System — 159
Terry J. Coyne
Michael G. Fehlings

18 Anterior Kostuik-Harrington Distraction Systems for the Treatment of Acute and Chronic Kyphotic Deformities — 171
John P. Kostuik

19 Application of the Rezaian Anterior Fixation System for the Management of Fractures of Thoracolumbar Spine — 193
S.M. Rezaian

20 Use of the Syracuse I-Plate and Anterior Locking Plate System (ALPS) for Anterior Spinal Fixation — 201
John D. Schlegel
Rand L. Schleusener
Hansen Yuan

21 Z-Plate Anterior Thoracolumbar Instrumentation — 211
Thomas A. Zdeblick

22 Application of the AO Titanium Anterior Thoracolumbar Locking Plate System — 225
John S. Thalgott
Mark B. Kabins
Marcus Timlin
Kay Fritts
James M. Giuffre

23 Methylmethacrylate and Steinmann Pin Stabilization of the Anterior Thoracolumbar Spine — 235
John Shiau
Narayan Sundaresan
Frank Moore
Alfred A. Steinberger

PART IV.
Posterior Thoracolumbar Instrumentation

24 Application of Harrington Rods and the Harri-Luque System for Stabilization of the Thoracolumbar Spine — 251
Brian G. Cuddy
Wade M. Mueller

25 Application of Luque Rods and Luque Rectangles for Stabilization of the Thoracolumbar Spine — 257
James P. Hollowell
Dennis J. Maiman

26 Utilization of the Texas Scottish Rite Hospital Universal System for Stabilization of the Thoracic and Lumbar Spine — 273
Richard G. Fessler
Michael Sturgill

27 Utilization of the Cotrel-Dubousset Instrumentation System for Stabilization of the Thoracolumbar and Lumbosacral Spine — 287
Paul C. McCormick

28 Utilization of the Compact Cotrel-Dubousset System for Stabilization of the Thoracolumbar and Lumbar Spine — 297
Phillippe Gillet

29 Dynalok Fixation System — 309
Stephen E. Heim
Douglas L. Johnson

30 **Utilization of the Simmons Plating System for Stabilization of the Spine** 325
James W. Simmons

31 **Utilization of the Rogozinski Spinal Rod System for Stabilization of the Lumbosacral and Thoracolumbar Spine** 333
Chaim Rogozinski
Abraham Rogozinski
William C. Watters, III

32 **The AMS Reduction Fixation System** 357
Mark N. Hadley
Benjamin H. Fulmer

33 **Segmental Fixation of the Lumbosacral Spine Using the Isola/VSP System** 367
Setti S. Rengachary
Eric Flores

34 **Fixateur Interne** 379
Ronald W. Lindsey
Markus Rittmeister

35 **Application of the Louis System for Thoracolumbar and Lumbosacral Spine Stabilization** 399
René Louis

36 **Puno-Winter-Byrd (PWB) Transpedicular Spine Fixation System** 409
J. Abbott Byrd, III
Ronald M. Puno

37 **Correction of Spinal Deformity and Instability Using the Edwards Modular System** 421
Charles C. Edwards

Index 455

Contributors*

Cargill H. Alleyne, Jr. [7]
Department of Neurosurgery
Emory Clinic
Atlanta, Georgia

J. Abbott Byrd, III, M.D. [36]
Department of Orthopedic Surgery
Eastern Virginia Medical School and Vann Orthopedic Specialists, P.C.
Norfolk, Virginia

Andrew Cappuccino, M.D. [11]
Lockport, New York

Paul R. Cooper, M.D. [14]
Department of Neurosurgery
New York University Medical Center
New York, New York

Terry J. Coyne, F.R.C.S. [17]
Department of Neurosurgery
New York University Medical Center
New York, New York

Brian G. Cuddy, M.D. [24]
Department of Neurosurgery
College of Medicine
Medical University of South Carolina
Charleston, South Carolina

Curtis A. Dickman, M.D. [1, 5]
Associate Chief, Spine Section
Director, Spinal Research
Division of Neurological Surgery
St. Joseph's Hospital and Medical Center
Phoenix, Arizona

Charles C. Edwards, M.D. [37]
Baltimore, Maryland

Michael G. Fehlings, M.D., Ph.D., FRCS [17]
Division of Neurosurgery
The Toronto Hospital, Toronto Western Division
Toronto, Ontario

Richard G. Fessler, M.D., Ph.D. [26]
Dunspaugh Dalton Chair in Brain and Spinal Surgery
Department of Neurological Surgery
College of Medicine
University of Florida
Gainesville, Florida

*The numbers in brackets following the contributor name refer to chapter(s) authored or co-authored by the contributor.

Eric Flores, M.D. [33]
Department of Neurosurgery
Minnesota Medical School
Minneapolis, Minnesota

Kay Fritts, R.N. [22]
International Spinal Development Research Foundation
Las Vegas, Nevada

Benjamin H. Fulmer, M.D. [32]
The Division of Neurological Surgery
The University of Alabama
Birmingham, Alabama

Phillippe Gillet, M.D. [28]
Orthopedic Department
University Hospital (CHU)
Liege, Belgium

James M. Giuffre, B.A. [22]
International Spinal Development Research Foundation
Las Vegas, Nevada

Dieter Grob, M.D. [10]
Schulthess Hospital
Spine Unit
Neumunsteralle 3
Zurich, Switzerland

Mark N. Hadley, M.D. [32]
Associate Professor
The Division of Neurological Surgery
The University of Alabama
Birmingham, Alabama

Regis W. Haid, M.D. [7]
Associate Professor
Department of Neurosurgery
Emory Clinic
Atlanta, Georgia

Stephen E. Heim, M.D. [29]
Orthopedic Association
Mona Kea Medical Park
Carol Stream, Illinois

James P. Hollowell, M.D. [25]
Froedtert Memorial
Lutheran Hospital
Milwaukee, Wisconsin

David E. Jenkins, CST, CFA [15]
Gainesville, Florida

Douglas L. Johnson, M.D., Ph.D. [29]
Department of Neurology
Glenn Ellen Clinic
Glenn Ellen, Illinois

Mark B. Kabins, M.D. [22]
International Spinal Development Research Foundation
Las Vegas, Nevada

Iain H. Kalfas, M.D. [3]
Department of Neurosurgery
The Cleveland Clinic Foundation
Cleveland, Ohio

Peter M. Klara, M.D., Ph.D. [2]
Neurosurgery Consult, Inc.
Norfolk, Virginia

John P. Kostuik, M.D. [18]
Professor of Orthopedics Neurosurgery
Chief Spinal Division–Orthopedics
Johns Hopkins Hospital
Johns Hopkins University
Baltimore, Maryland

Claude Laville [16]
Groupe Hospitalier
Pitie Salpetriere
Paris, France

Ronald W. Lindsey, M.D. [34]
Associate Professor
Baylor College of Medicine
Department of Orthopedic Medicine
Houston, Texas

René Louis, M.D. [35]
Hospital de la Conception
Universite de Marseille
Marseille, France

Gary L. Lowery, M.D., Ph.D. [4]
Medical Director
Research Institute International, Inc.
Gainesville, Florida

Michael MacMillan, M.D. [12]
Department of Orthopedics
Gainesville, Florida

Dennis J. Maiman, M.D., Ph.D. [25]
Froedtert Memorial
Lutheran Hospital
Milwaukee, Wisconsin

Paul C. McAfee, M.D. [11]
Chief, Spine and Scoliosis Center
Towson, Maryland

Paul C. McCormick, M.D. [27]
Assistant Professor of Neurological Surgery
Columbia Presbyterian Medical Center
The Neurological Institute
New York, New York

Frank Moore, M.D. [23]
New York, New York

Wade M. Mueller, M.D. [24]
Department of Neurosurgery
College of Medicine
Medical University of South Carolina
Charleston, South Carolina

Michael G. O'Sullivan, M.D. [13]
Department of Clinical Neuroscience
Western General Hospital
Crewe Road
Edinburgh, Scotland

Brian Pikul, M.D. [8]
Ohio State University Hospital
Division of Neurological Surgery
Columbus, Ohio

Rolando M. Puno, M.D. [36]
Department of Orthopedic Surgery
University of Louisville and Kenton D. Leatherman Spine Center
Louisville, Kentucky

Gary L. Rea, M.D., Ph.D. [8]
Ohio State University Hospital
Division of Neurological Surgery
Columbus, Ohio

Setti S. Rengachary, M.D. [33]
Department of Neurosurgery
Minnesota Medical School
Minneapolis, Minnesota

S.M. Rezaian, M.D., F.R.C.S., Ph.D. [19]
Orthopedic and Spine Surgeon
California Orthopedic Clinic, Inc.
Beverly Hills, California

Markus Rittmeister, M.D. [34]
Department of Orthopedic Medicine
Baylor College of Medicine
Houston, Texas

Abraham Rogozinski, M.D. [31]
Rogozinski Orthopedic Clinic
Jacksonville, Florida

Chiam Rogozinski, M.D. [31]
Rogozinski Orthopedic Clinic
Jacksonville, Florida

R. Roy-Camille* [16]
Group Hospitalier
Pitie Salpetriere
Paris, France

Thomas Russell, M.D. [13]
Department of Clinical Neuroscience
Western General Hospital
Crewe Road
Edinburgh, Scotland

John D. Schlegel, M.D. [20]
Associate Professor
Division of Orthopedic Surgery
University of Utah School of Medicine
Salt Lake City, Utah

Rand L. Schleusener, M.D. [20]
Salt Lake City, Utah

John Shiau, M.D. [23]
New York, New York

James W. Simmons, M.D. FACS [30]
Alamo Bone and Joint Clinic
San Antonio, Texas

Matthew N. Songer, M.D. [6]
Orthopedic Surgery Associates of Marquette, P.C.
Marquette Medical Center
Marquette, Michigan

Volker K.H. Sonntag, M.D. [1, 5]
Chief, Spine Section
Division of Neurological Surgery
Barrow Neurological Institute
St. Joseph's Hospital and Medical Center
Phoenix, Arizona

Patrick Statham, M.D. [13]
Department of Clinical Neuroscience
Western General Hospital
Crewe Road
Edinburgh, Scotland

Alfred A. Steinberger, M.D. [23]
New York, New York

Michael Sturgill, M.D. [26]
Department of Neurological Surgery
University of Florida
Gainesville, Florida

Narayan Sundaresan, M.D., Ph.D. [23]
New York, New York

Chester E. Sutterlin, III, M.D., P.A. [15]
Gainesville, Florida

John S. Thalgott, M.D. [22]
International Spinal Development Research Foundation
Las Vegas, Nevada

Marcus Timlin, M.D. [22]
International Spinal Development Research Foundation
Las Vegas, Nevada

*Deceased.

William C. Watters, III, M.D. [31]
Rogozinski Orthopedic Clinic
Jacksonville, Florida

Andreas Weidner, M.D. [9]
Director of Spine Center
Rengericher Landstrabe 19 b
Professor of Neurosurgery
Osnabruck, Germany

Hansen Yuan, M.D. [20]
Department of Orthoepdic Surgery
State University of New York
Syracuse, New York

Thomas A. Zdeblick, M.D. [21]
Assistant Professor
Division of Orthopedic Surgery
Madison, Wisconsin

PREFACE

Instrumentation of the spine has undergone revolutionary changes over the past decade. As our understanding of spinal biomechanics improved, available instrumentation systems have evolved from the use of wires, to wires holding rods, to rods with hooks on each end, to universal systems in which a series of hooks and screws can be combined with a contoured rod to enable segmental control of individual vertebrae. At the same time, plate systems have evolved from simple stainless steel plates and screws to contoured titanium alloy systems in which screws are "locked" to plates to provide easy-to-apply, stable systems for anterior spinal application. The net result of this expansion of knowledge and advancement in technology has been a clear improvement in our ability to treat a variety of disease processes that affect the spine. This has influenced our treatment not only of spinal trauma, but also congenital lesions, cancer, infections, and degenerative disease. In many cases it has enabled the skilled surgeon to effectively treat disease processes that were previously untreatable. Overall, hospitalization time is reduced, patients are mobilized more rapidly, rehabilitation is begun earlier, and substantial data suggest improved outcomes and decreased pain.

On the other hand, this rapid advancement in knowledge and technology has created several problems. A large number of practicing surgeons have found themselves inadequately trained in the appropriate use of these systems. This is true not only in regard to their physical application, but also in relation to the decision-making process regarding their use. Second, many training programs suddenly have found themselves not offering strong training in this important and rapidly expanding area of surgery. Finally, both novice and experienced "instrumentation" surgeons are presented with a bewildering variety of instrumentation systems, with very little opportunity to compare and contrast them. Therefore, a rational decision regarding which system is easiest to use and the most versatile is very difficult to make. Furthermore, which system is best for specific problems is nearly impossible to decide.

It is the goal of this textbook to be a modest part of the solution to these problems. The chapters that follow are organized to cover the systems available for anterior and posterior stabilization of each level of the spine. Because there is an inevitable delay between writing and publication, some very new systems may not be represented. Systems represented cover posterior occipitocervical stabilization, anterior and posterior cervical stabilization, anterior and posterior thoracic and lumbar stabilization, and posterior sacral stabilization. Multiple systems are represented at each level of the spine. Although this introduces some redundancy, it allows the reader to compare directly each of the systems. Each chapter is written by the system's inventor or another surgeon experienced in the use of the system. Therefore, instructions on each system's use are specific and based on broad experience. Hints and "pearls of wisdom" from each chapter may prove very helpful.

This book is intended for surgeons, fellows, residents, and students who are interested in pursuing knowledge and experience in spinal instrumentation. It will be most useful to those with moderate experience in instrumentation but may be helpful as a teaching adjunct for even experienced surgeons. Each chapter is organized to provide a brief introduction to the system to be discussed and the procedure of its intended use. The equipment is described, and its application is described in detail. Tables are provided in each chapter with the author's indications and contraindications for use of each system. In addition, these tables will provide the reader with a rapid means of comparing alternative systems that could be used for the same procedure. Finally, the author's experience is summarized in the discussion and conclusions.

This book can be efficiently used in several ways. First, a surgeon who knows which system he or she wishes to use can review the indications, contraindications, advantages, disadvantages, and technique for that specific system by going directly to that chapter. Second, a surgeon who wishes to compare several alternative systems can rapidly do so by refering to the highlighted tables or can compare them in detail by reading the appropriate sections of each chapter. This could help with decisions regarding which system may work better for specific problems, or which system may be the best to purchase and have available on a permanent basis. Finally, surgeons who wish to survey a variety of opinions and suggestions regarding techniques for instrumentation of specific regions of the spine can do so by reading the various authors represented within each section.

Therefore, depending on the individual reader's goal, this book can be used in any of several ways. Through this approach and organization, it will be useful both as a teaching tool for fellows, residents, and students and as a reference for experienced spinal surgeons.

CURRENT TECHNIQUES IN SPINAL STABILIZATION

PART 1

Anterior Cervical Instrumentation

CHAPTER 1

Odontoid Screw Fixation

Curtis A. Dickman
Volker K.H. Sonntag

HIGHLIGHTS

Anterior screw fixation of the odontoid process has become popular to treat patients with unstable odontoid fractures. Although a variety of methods have been used to fuse C1 and C2 posteriorly, atlantoaxial fixations sacrifice C1-2 motion. The major advantage of the odontoid screw technique is that it fixes the odontoid fracture directly, yet completely preserves all normal cervical motion. This chapter reviews the clinical indications, surgical techniques, biomechanics, and merits and limitations of odontoid screw fixation.

INDICATIONS

Anderson and D'Alonzo (1974) proposed a classification system for odontoid fractures that has been used to guide treatment (Fig. 1-1). Type I fractures are through the tip of the dens. Type II fractures occur across the base of the dens. Type III fractures extend from the base of the dens into the body of C2.

Odontoid screw fixation is designed primarily for treating patients with Type II dens fractures (Table 1-1). With the exception of widely displaced Type II odontoid fractures, most odontoid fractures heal satisfactorily with an external cervical orthosis. (Anderson & D'Alonzo, 1974; Apuzzo, Heiden, & Weiss, 1978; Clark & White, 1985; Hadley, Dickman, Brown, et al., 1989). The fracture morphology and predisposition for nonunion make displaced Type II dens fractures well suited for screw fixation. In comparison, Type III dens fractures rarely develop nonunion and are poorly suited to screw fixation because the screw can lever out of the weakened C2 body.

The indications for treating Type II fractures surgically depends on the clinical circumstances. The probability of a Type II fracture uniting when treated with an orthosis depends primarily on the extent of bone displacement. (Anderson & D'Alonzo, 1974; Apuzzo et al., 1978; Clark & White, 1985; Dunn & Seljeskog, 1986; Hadley et al., 1989). Nondisplaced fractures or fractures displaced less than 6 mm have a 90% chance of healing with an orthosis (Hadley et al., 1989). In comparison, Type II fractures displaced 6 mm or more have a 78% chance of nonunion when treated with an orthosis (Hadley et al., 1989).

Surgery for screw fixation can be considered an initial treatment for patients with fractures that have a high risk of nonunion (≥6 mm displacement). Surgery may also be indicated for patients with a displaced dens fracture who object to wearing a halo brace, who cannot tolerate a halo brace (i.e., because of psychological concerns or multiple skull fractures), or who prefer to have surgery rather than wear a halo brace.

Odontoid fractures that fail treatment with an orthosis (i.e., recurrent subluxations of the dens, inability to restore satisfactory C1-2 alignment or nonunions) require surgery. If the dens heals in a malaligned position, spinal stenosis, chronic compression, and neurologic deficits may develop. When the alignment of the dens cannot be restored with traction or maintained with a halo brace, surgical fixation should be considered.

In patients treated with an orthosis, meticulous follow-up is needed to detect nonunion and persistent atlantoaxial instability. Nonunions can be treated with odontoid screw fixation; however, to promote bone healing one needs to curette the fibrous tissue from the fracture surfaces.

OPERATIVE TECHNIQUES

Preparation and Positioning

Preoperative computerized tomograms are required to evaluate the bone architecture and to assess abnormalities that

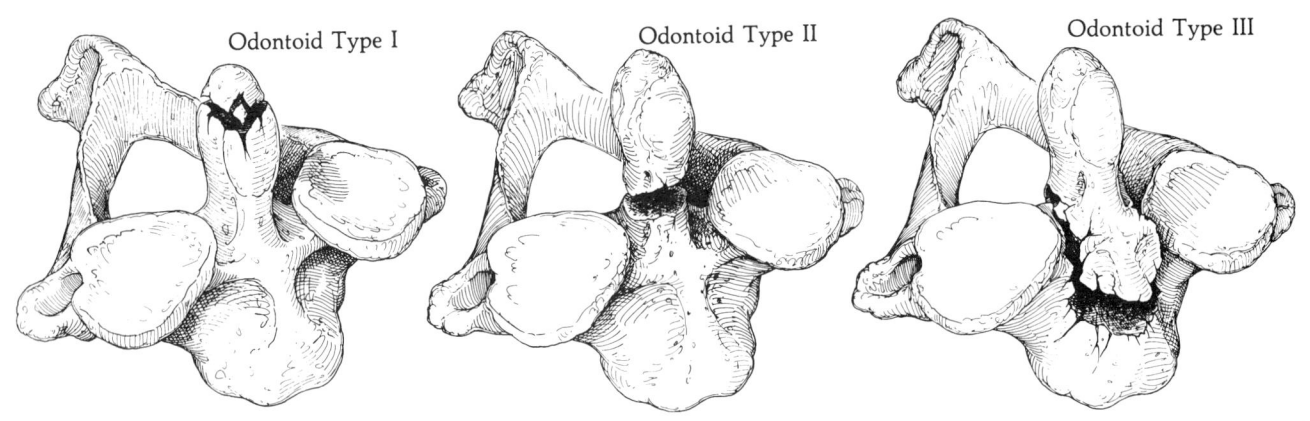

FIG. 1-1. Anderson and D'Alonzo's classification of odontoid fractures. Type I fractures are at the apex of the dens. Type II fractures are across the base of the dens. Type III fractures extend into the body of C2. With permission of Barrow Neurological Institute.

may preclude screw placement (e.g., an aberrant course of the vertebral artery or extensive concurrent cervical fractures). Magnetic resonance (MR) imaging of the cervical ligaments can also help preoperatively (Dickman, Mamourian, & Sonntag). When the transverse atlantal ligament is disrupted, odontoid screw fixation is contraindicated because the screw will not restore atlantoaxial stability.

Odontoid screw fixation is performed through an anterior approach to the cervical spine. Somatosensory evoked potentials are monitored. Anteroposterior (AP) open-mouth and lateral plane fluoroscopy are mandatory to visualize C2 intraoperatively in order to guide the screw trajectory accurately. This is best achieved with two C-arms but can be performed with one C-arm.

The fracture must be reduced with head positioning or intraoperative manipulation prior to screw placement. The screws generate a lag effect to compress the fractured bone surfaces together. The screws will not restore alignment if C1 and the dens are horizontally subluxed. A malaligned fixation can result in neural compression from canal stenosis and must be avoided.

Odontoid screw fixation is performed using an anterior cervical operative exposure with the patient in the supine position. The head is extended to provide the proper screw trajectory into the tip of the dens (Fig. 1-2). To avoid distraction or subluxation of the fracture, neck extension is performed under fluoroscopic guidance. The drill and screw trajectory are positioned parallel to the anterior surface of the cervical spine in order to aim the screw into the tip of the dens. Barrel-shaped large chests and short necks hinder the correct screw trajectory and are contraindications to odontoid screw fixation. Instead, a posterior C1-2 fixation should be performed in these patients.

Fixation of the head can be achieved with a Mayfield skull clamp or with a Caspar head/neck rest. Alternatively, the patient can be kept in a halo brace until screw fixation is achieved. The mouth is propped open to allow AP open-mouth fluoroscopy. Cloth, gauze, or other radiolucent materials are used to keep the patient's mouth open intraoperatively. Positioning of the patient and setup of the C-arms are critical for the success of this procedure. These maneuvers often take longer than the surgical insertion of the screw. The AP C-arm is positioned above the head of the operating table. The lateral C-arm is brought in from the patient's left side. The anesthesia machines are positioned on the patient's left, near the thorax. The surgeon is positioned on the right side of the patient's neck (Fig. 1-3).

SURGICAL PROCEDURE

Exposure

A transversely oriented cervical incision is made in the neck at the level of the cricothyroid junction. This low-neck incision facilitates a drill trajectory parallel to the anterior border of the cervical spine. The platysma muscle is widely undermined to allow adequate soft-tissue retraction. The deep cervical fascia is dissected with blunt and sharp techniques, separating the carotid sheath from the strap muscles, trachea, and esophagus. Hand-held soft-tissue retractors aid in the initial exposure. The dissection is deepened to the level of the prevertebral fascia over the anterior cervical vertebrae. Care must be taken to avoid the laryngeal nerves.

Kittner dissectors are used to dissect the prevertebral fascia bluntly from the anterior C2-3 level. The longus colli

Table 1-1
Indications and Contraindications for Use of Odontoid Screw Fixation System

Indications
   Type II dens fractures with ≥6 mm of displacement
   Type II dens fractures in patients who:
     (1) cannot or will not tolerate a halo brace
     (2) prefer to have surgery rather than wear a halo brace
   Odontoid fractures that fail to fuse with an orthosis
   Odontoid fractures which cannot adequately be aligned in a halo

Contraindications
   Severe osteoporosis
   Non-union over 3 months from time of fracture
   Transverse ligament rupture
   Large patients with "barrel-shaped" chests or short necks

CHAPTER 1 / ODONTOID SCREW FIXATION 5

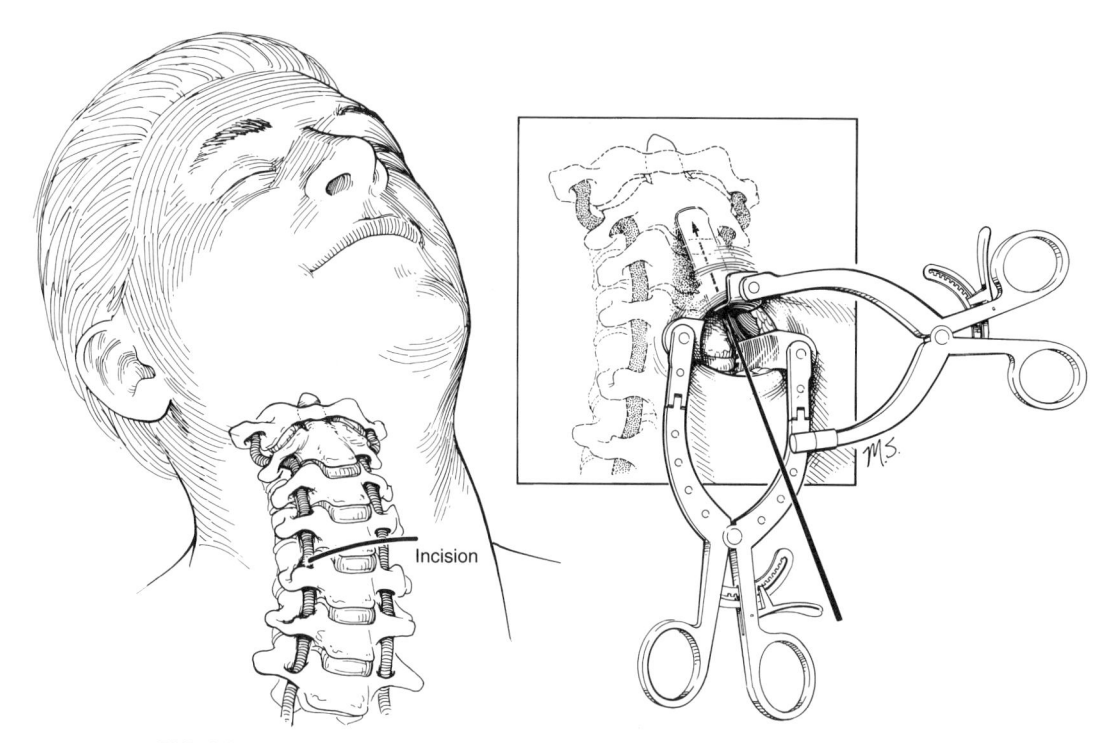

FIG. 1-2. Patients should be in the supine position, with the head and neck extended to facilitate placing the screw into the tip of the dens. A transverse incision is made over the C4-5 interspace to facilitate a trajectory parallel to the anterior surface of the spine. *(Insert)* The Apfelbaum retraction system and the screw trajectory are depicted. *[From Dickman, C.A., Sonntag, V.K.H., & Marcotte, P.J. (1992). Techniques of screw fixation of the cervical spine. Barrow Neurological Institute Quarterly 8(2):9–26.]* With permission.

FIG. 1-3. (a) Illustration of surgical suite demonstrating relative positioning of patient, personnel, and equipment. (b) The anteroposterior C-arm is positioned to provide an open-mouth view of the dens. With permission of Barrow Neurological Institute.

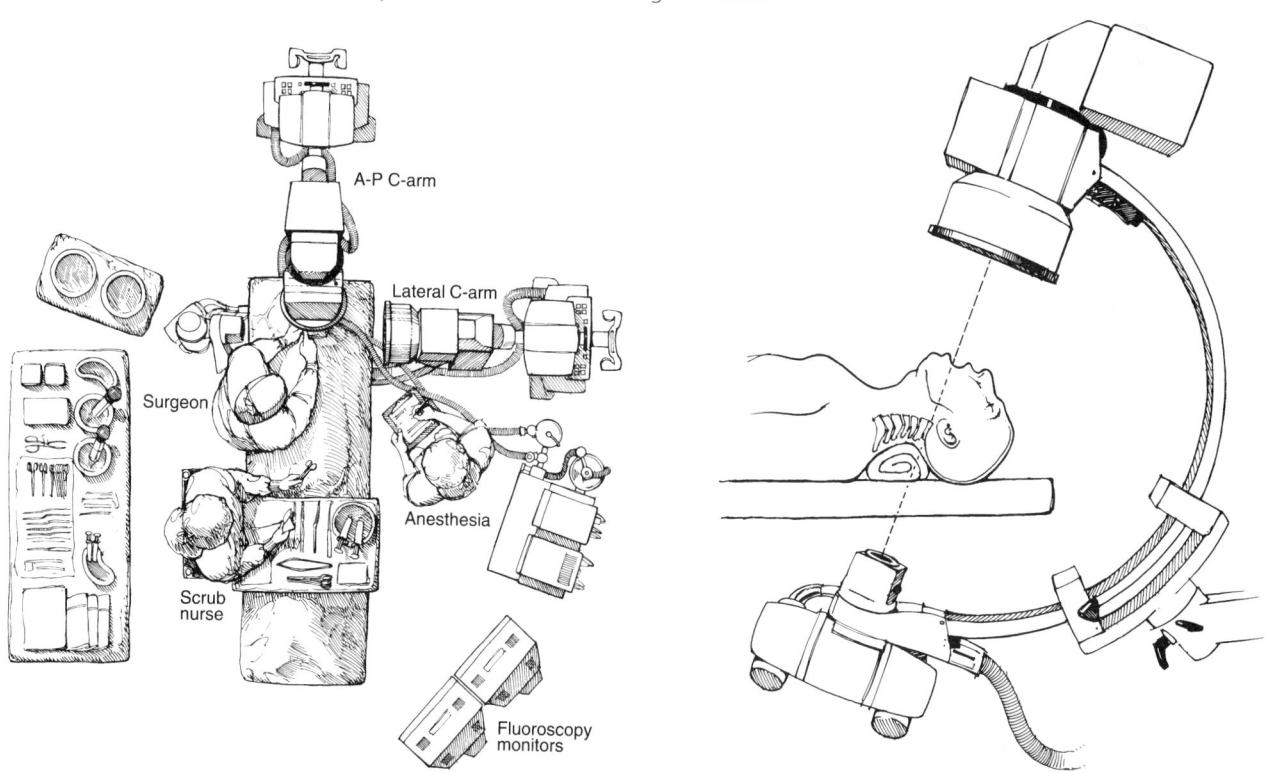

muscles are coagulated at their medial borders and are elevated from the surface of the bone at the C2-3 interspace. Self-retaining retractors are inserted.

Ronald Apfelbaum developed retractors and instrumentation to facilitate odontoid screw fixation (Aesculap; San Francisco, CA) (Fig. 1-4) (Apfelbaum, 1992). Self-retaining retractor blades maintain soft-tissue retraction medially and laterally. An angled blade is attached to a post in the retractor. The angled blade maintains soft-tissue retraction superiorly in the midline to provide access for drilling and screwing. If the Apfelbaum retractor system is unavailable, retraction can be provided with other types of self-retaining retractors, hand-held retractors, or malleable blade retractors. Radiolucent retractors are recommended to facilitate intraoperative radiographic imaging.

SCREW INSERTION TECHNIQUES

The entry points for drill and screw insertion are selected. When one screw is placed, a midline entry point is used. When two screws are placed, each screw enters 5 mm lateral to the midline and is directed 5 to 10 degrees medially into the tip of the dens (Fig. 1-5). Preoperatively the surgeon should decide whether to place one or two screws in the dens. If two screws are planned, the dens must be wide enough to accommodate both screws.

A trough is cut into the anterior-superior edge of the C3 vertebral body and the C2-3 annulus with a rongeur or drill to attain a flat screw trajectory into the tip of the dens (Fig. 1-6). The drill and screw should enter the C2 body at the anterior edge of the inferior C2 end plate. The cortical bone at the entry point for insertion of the drill should be penetrated with a bone awl, Kirschner wire (K-wire), or high-speed drill, which will allow the cylindrical drill bit to engage the bone securely as the pilot hole is drilled. Ideally, the dens should be realigned preoperatively, and the alignment should be verified after positioning the patient on the operating table. However, it is not always possible to restore C1-2 alignment preoperatively. When the dens is posteriorly displaced, alignment may be restored intraoperatively by pushing the C2 body posteriorly. When the dens is anteriorly displaced, alignment can sometimes be restored by pushing C1 and the dens posteriorly; however, this is difficult to achieve.

Apfelbaum System

The Apfelbaum (1992) instrumentation system uses noncannulated, partially threaded titanium screws. A K-wire is placed into the inferior end plate of C2 with a mallet. A hand drill is threaded over the K-wire to remove the anterior lip of C3 and a portion of the C2-3 annulus. A drill guide is subsequently threaded over the K-wire. The drill guide has spikes that seat into the C3 vertebral body. The inner sleeve of the

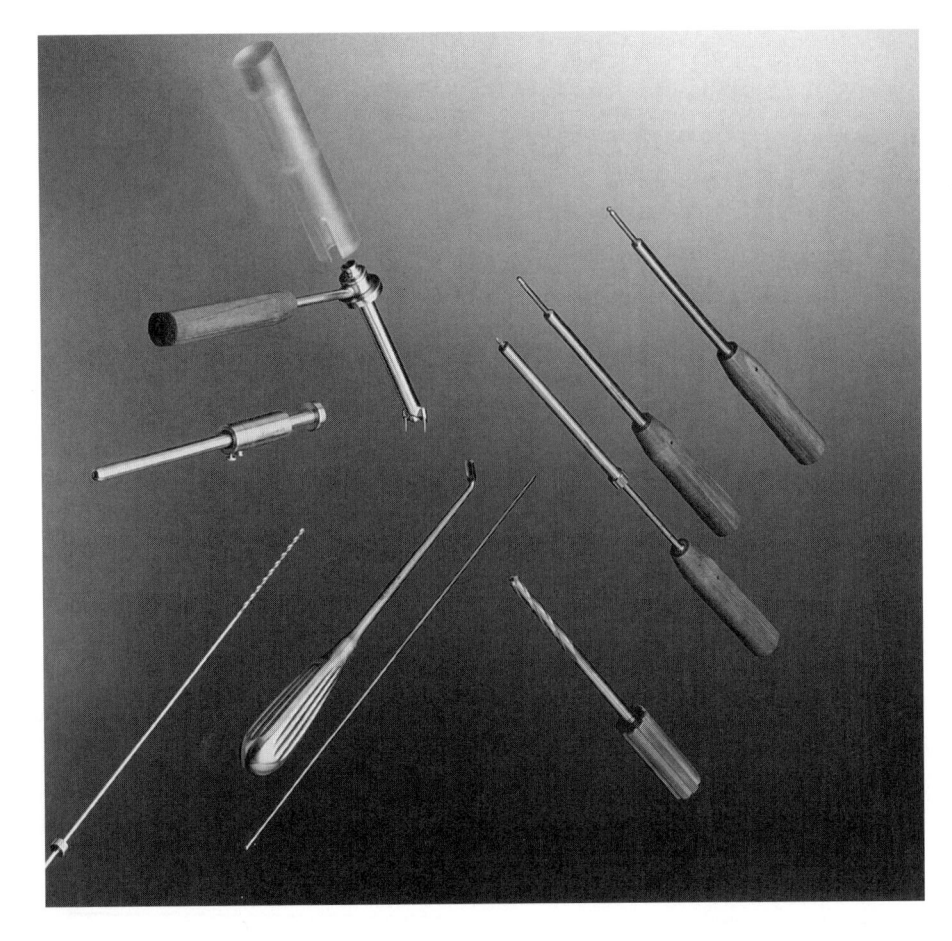

FIG. 1-4. Photographs of the Apfelbaum instrumentation (Aesculap). *Clockwise:* screw drivers, tap, hand drill, Kirschner wire, double-edged curette, drill bit, inner drill guide, outer drill guide. [*Provided courtesy of Aesculap, Inc.*]

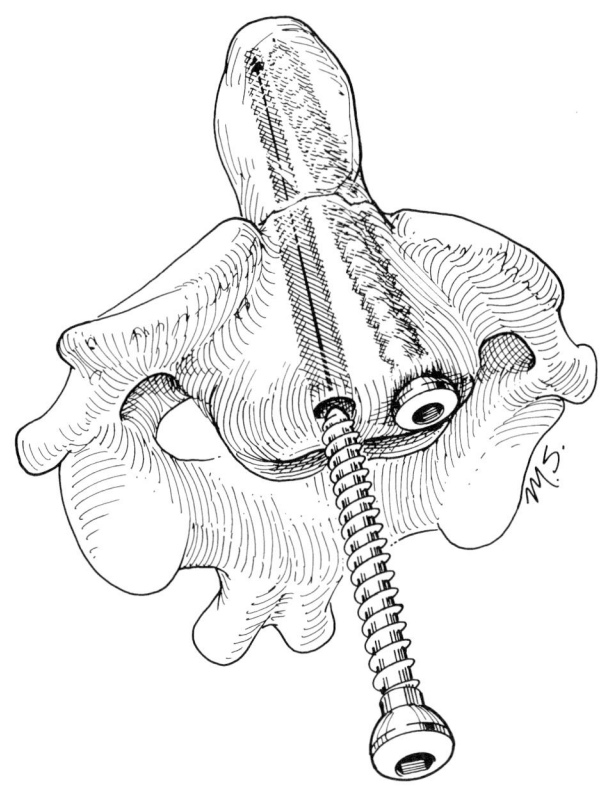

FIG. 1-5. When two screws are placed into the dens, the screws are angled 5 to 10 degrees medially. [From Dickman, C.A., Sonntag, V.K.H., & Marcotte, P.J. (1992). Techniques of screw fixation of the cervical spine. Barrow Neurological Institute Quarterly 8(2):9–26.] With permission.

drill guide is advanced until its tip touches the inferior end plate of C2 and then the K-wire is removed (Fig. 1-7).

A 2.5-mm diameter drill bit is used to drill a pilot hole into the dens. The drill should just barely penetrate the tip of the dens. Intradural drill penetration is avoided by drilling carefully and by closely monitoring intraoperative maneuvers with fluoroscopy. The drill is removed, the inner sleeve of the drill guide is removed, and the pilot hole is tapped with a tool to cut the screw thread profile into the bone.

An end-threaded titanium screw is inserted into the pilot hole. The screw length is measured from calibrated markers on the drill bit or on the tap. A variable angle Allen screwdriver is used to drive the screw into the bone.

The screw tip should barely penetrate the tip of the dens. If the odontoid fragment is widely separated from the C2 body, a screw shorter than the distance measured on the drill is needed because the gap will be obliterated as the bone fragments become reduced. The screw head should be flush against the C2 body so that it does not protrude into the C2-3 interspace. If the screw extends into the interspace, a lever effect may occur that can cause screw loosening or screw breakage.

Cannulated Screw Systems

Cannulated screw systems use a thin K-wire to drill the initial pilot hole into the bone (Fig. 1-8) (Dickman, Sonntag,

FIG. 1-6. A trough is cut into the edge of the C3 body and C2-3 annulus using a drill, curette or rongeur. [Provided courtesy of Aesculap, Inc.] [Reprinted with permission from Apfelbaum R. (1992). Anterior screw fixation of odontoid fractures. In S.S. Rengachary & R.H. Wilkins (Eds.), Neurosurgical Operative Atlas (Vol. 2) (pp. 189–199), Baltimore: Williams & Wilkins.]

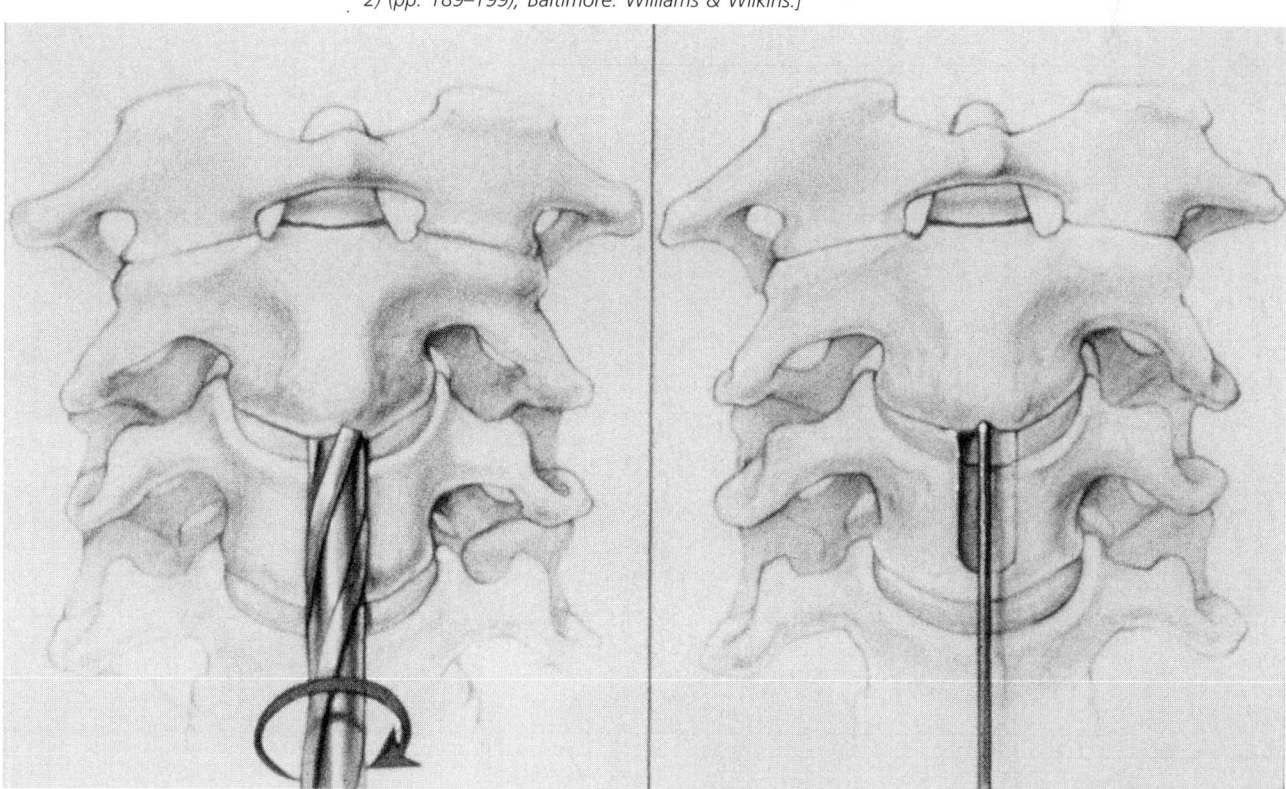

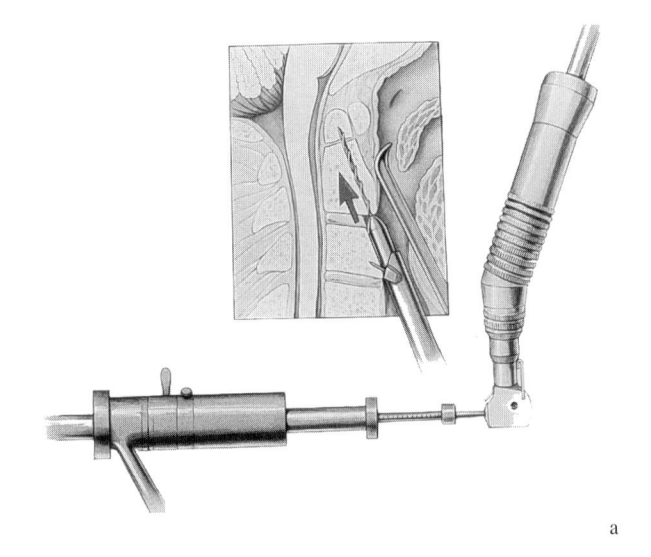

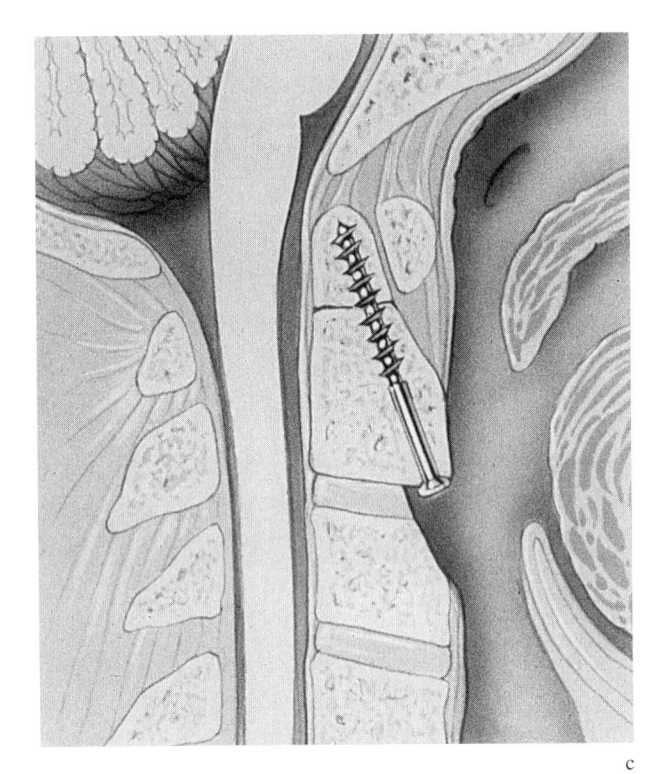

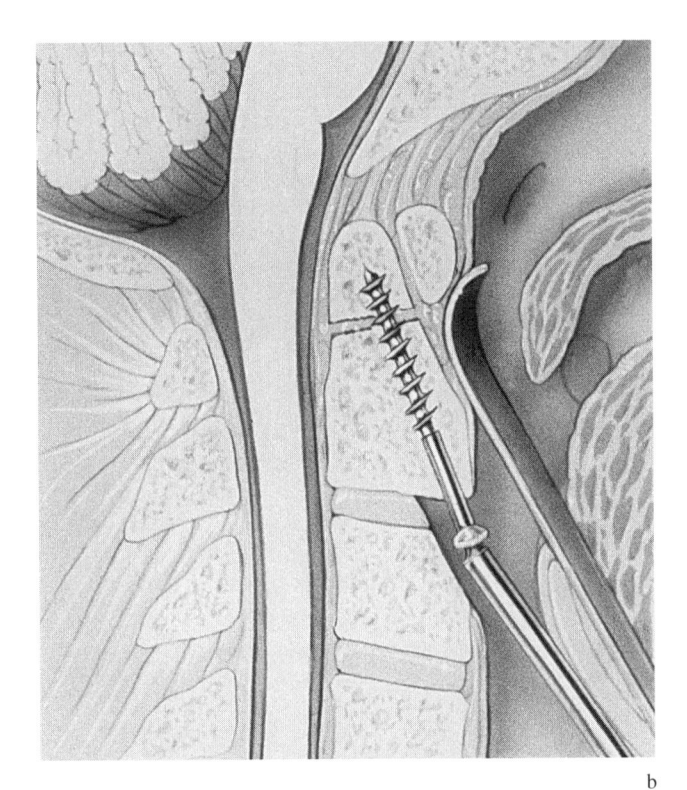

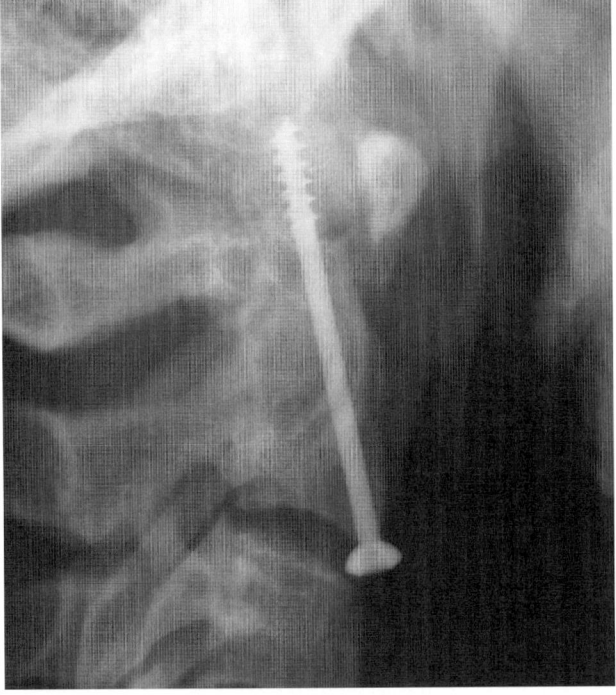

FIG. 1-7. (a) The Apfelbaum drill guide has sharp spikes that anchor it to the C3 vertebral body. It has an inner sheath through which the pilot hole is drilled. The length of the screw needed can be measured from calibrated markings on the proximal drill bit. The pilot hole is subsequently tapped with a bone tap. [Provided courtesy of Aesculap, Inc.] [Reprinted with permission from Apfelbaum R. (1992). Anterior screw fixation of odontoid fractures. In S.S. Rengachary & R.H. Wilkins (Eds.). Neurosurgical Operative Atlas (Vol. 2) (pp. 189–199). Baltimore: Williams & Wilkins.] (b and c) The screw is inserted into the bone using an Allen screwdriver. [Provided courtesy of Aesculap, Inc.] [Reprinted with permission from Apfelbaum R. (1992). Anterior screw fixation of odontoid fractures. In S.S. Rengachary & R.H. Wilkins, (Eds.), Neurosurgical Operative Atlas (Vol. 2) (pp. 189–199). Baltimore: Williams & Wilkins.] (d) Postoperative lateral cervical radiograph of an odontoid screw fixation.

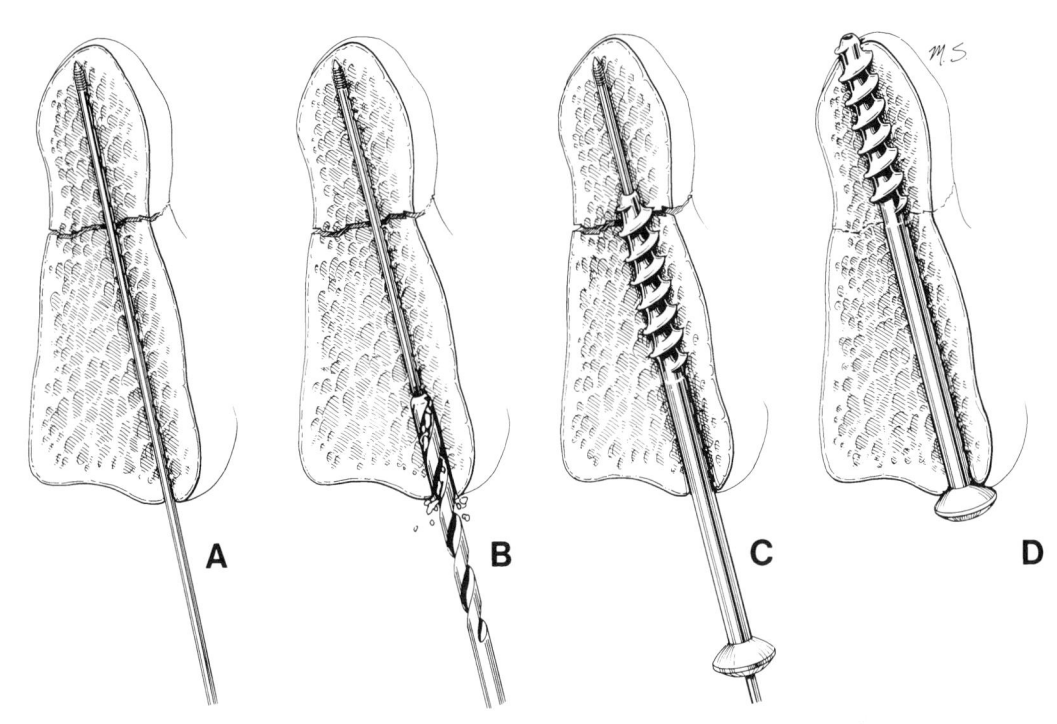

FIG. 1-8. Cannulated screws use a Kirschner wire (K-wire) to direct the insertion of hollow tools and hollow screws into the bone. (a) The K-wire is inserted. (b) A 5-mm deep pilot hole is drilled in the proximal bone to allow the screw threads to purchase the bone. (c) A self-tapping screw is inserted. (d) The K-wire is removed. *[From Dickman, C.A., Sonntag, V.K.H., & Marcotte, P.J. (1992). Techniques of screw fixation of the cervical spine. Barrow Neurological Institute Quarterly 8(2):9–26.]* With permission.

& Marcotte, 1992; Etter, Cosica, & Jaberg, et al., 1991). Hollow drills, hollow taps, and hollow screws are sequentially threaded over the K-wire in order to maintain the intended trajectory into the bone. Cannulated screw systems have an advantage: if the K-wire trajectory is not ideal, the wire can be repositioned without destroying the bone. In comparison, if wide drill bits or wide screws are malpositioned, the screws often cannot be repositioned in the adjacent bone because of a wide bone defect. Cannulated screws have the disadvantage of possible intradural advancement of the K-wire during drilling, tapping, and screw insertion. Maneuvers should be performed under fluoroscopic guidance to avoid K-wire displacement.

Noncannulated Screws

Noncannulated bone screws can also be used for odontoid fixation (Apfelbaum, 1992; Barbour, 1971; Borne, Bedou, & Pinadeau, 1988; Bohler, 1982; Dickman et al., 1992; Donovan, 1979; Geisler, Cheng, Poka, et al., 1989; Knoringer, 1987). A pilot hole is drilled with a drill bit that matches the core diameter of the screw (i.e., a 2.5-mm bit for a 3.5-mm diameter screw). Self-tapping screws have sharp threads and can be inserted directly into the bone without previously cutting the thread profile into the pilot hole. In comparison, non-self-tapping screws have a dull thread profile and require tapping prior to screw insertion.

A lag effect is required regardless of the screw type used (Dickman et al., 1992). Lag screws compress bone fragments together to facilitate bone healing. The lag effect is achieved when the screw threads purchase only the distal bone fragment but not the proximal bone. This is provided by an end-threaded screw, or by a fully threaded screw after drilling a wide gliding hole in the proximal bone (Fig. 1-9) (Dickman et al., 1992).

Postoperative Care

A Philadelphia collar or semirigid cervical orthosis is worn postoperatively until the bone unites satisfactorily. The immediate fixation strength of an odontoid screw is only one half the strength of the normal odontoid (Doherty, Heggeness, & Esses, 1993; Sasso, Doherty, Crawford, et al., 1993). Therefore, excessive loads placed on the screw prior to bone healing may cause the screw to bend or to lever out of the anterior C2 vertebral body. An orthosis is needed until the bone heals satisfactorily, usually within 10 to 12 weeks. Meticulous follow-up with flexion-extension radiographs is needed to detect nonunion, late screw failure, screw backout, or delayed instability.

DISCUSSION

Odontoid screw fixation is ideal for fixating acute, widely displaced Type II odontoid fractures. Unlike other methods

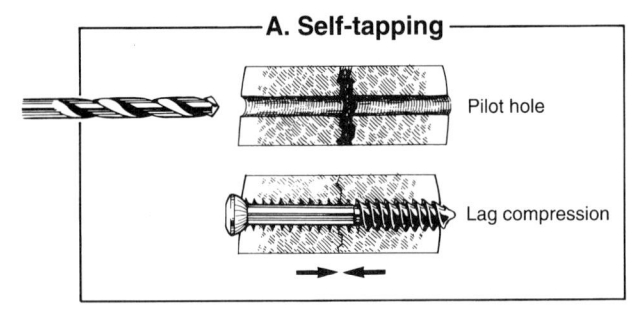

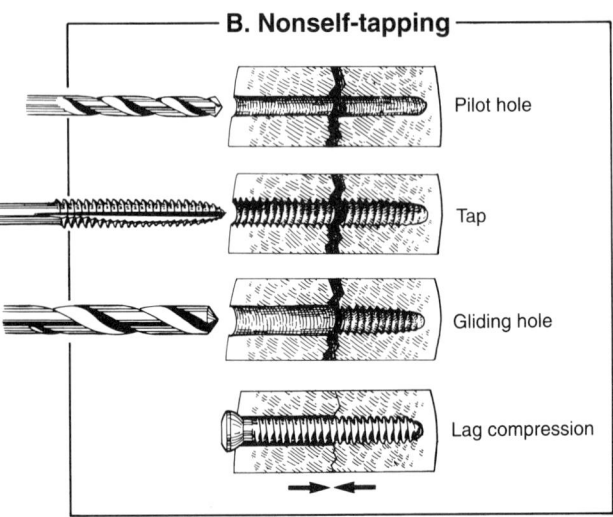

FIG. 1-9. Lag screws compress bone fragments together. A lag effect is achieved by several methods. (a) An end-threaded screw engages only the distal fragment of bone. If the threads purchase the proximal bone, a lag effect (i.e., compression) will not be generated. (b) A lag effect can be achieved with a fully threaded screw by drilling a wide gliding hole in the proximal bone so that the proximal threads of the screw do not engage the bone. [From Dickman, C.A., Sonntag, V.K.H., & Marcotte, P.J. (1992). Techniques of screw fixation of the cervical spine. Barrow Neurological Institute Quarterly 8(2):9–26.] With permission.

of cervical fixation, odontoid screws fixate the fracture, yet completely preserve normal cervical motion. Patients with chronic nonunions are more difficult to treat with this technique because fibrous scar tissue must be removed from the bone surfaces with a curette (Fig. 1-10). In this case the bone surface must be thoroughly denuded with a double-edged curette to promote fusion.

Patients with irreducible fractures, a large chest, a short neck, or severe osteoporosis are ineligible for an odontoid screw. Screws will easily fracture out of soft, weak bone. In these patients a posterior fusion should be performed.

The biomechanics of odontoid screw fixation needs to be considered. Oblique Type II dens fractures can be difficult. If a displaced oblique dens fracture is fixed with a lag screw, shearing forces are generated as the screw is tightened, which can cause the bone fragments to shift and a malaligned fixation to occur (Fig. 1-11). When odontoid screws are excessively loaded and fail, the screws either bend across the fracture site or a lever effect occurs, causing the proximal screw shaft to fracture through the anterior C2 vertebral body (Fig. 1-12) (Doherty et al., 1993; Sasso et al., 1993).

Odontoid screws do not restore normal strength to the dens immediately (Doherty et al., 1993; Sasso et al., 1993), and until the fracture heals, restore only half of the original mechanical strength to the dens. Therefore, screws should not be relied on as the only source of mechanical fixation needed during the immediate postoperative phase. An orthosis should also be used.

There is no mechanical difference in the immediate fixation strength, whether one or two screws are used (Sasso et al., 1993). Theoretically, two screws provide some rotational control of the dens; however, the risk of inserting a second screw must be weighed against its potential benefit.

SUMMARY

Odontoid screw fixation is unique compared with other methods of spinal stabilization because it stabilizes the fracture directly and completely preserves all normal cervical motion (Table 1-2). Normal motion at C1-2 is particularly important because of the prominent axial rotation at this level. More than 80 degrees of axial rotation (more than half of all cervical axial rotation) occurs at C1-2.

Acute displaced Type II dens fractures are best suited for an odontoid screw. Chronic nonunions have scar tissue that can

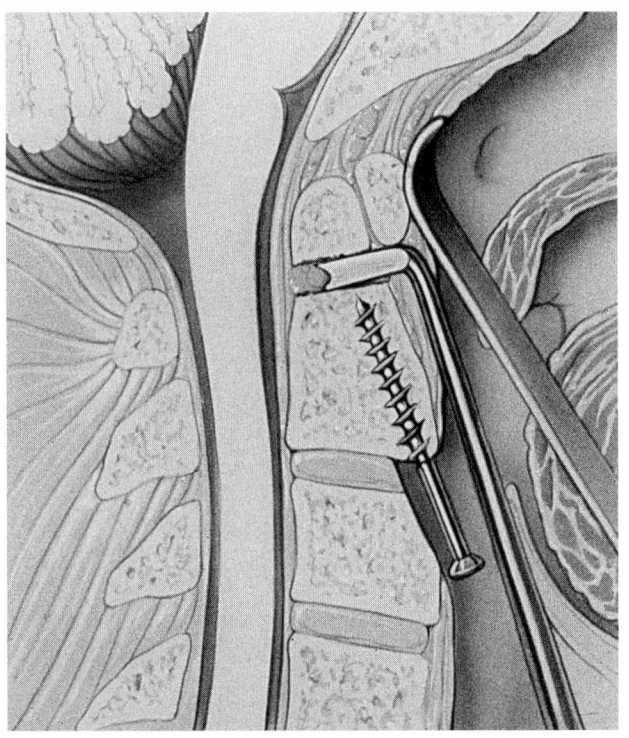

FIG. 1-10. A double-edged curette can be used to remove soft tissue from the bone surfaces in chronic nonunions. [Provided courtesy of Aesculap, Inc.] [Reprinted with permission from Apfelbaum R. (1992). Anterior screw fixation of odontoid fractures. In S.S. Rengachary & R.H. Wilkins (Eds.), Neurosurgical Operative Atlas (Vol. 2) (pp. 189–199). Baltimore: Williams & Wilkins.]

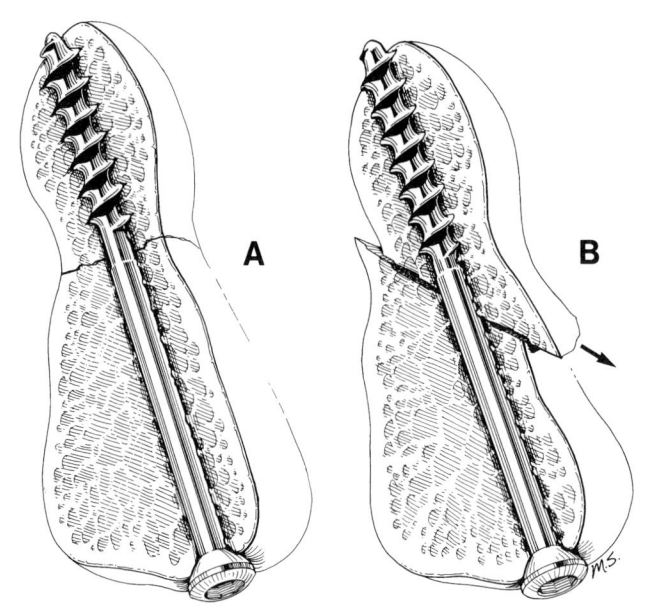

FIG. 1-11. When a lag screw is used to reduce an oblique dens fracture, shearing forces may occur that cause the bone fragments to shift as the bones are compressed together. (a) Transverse Type II fracture. (b) Oblique, malaligned Type II fracture. [From Dickman, C.A., Sonntag, V.K.H., & Marcotte, P.J. (1992). Techniques of screw fixation of the cervical spine. *Barrow Neurological Institute Quarterly 8(2):9–26.*] With permission.

be difficult to remove in an attempt to promote fusion. Os odontoideum should not be treated with odontoid screws because the bone surfaces cannot be prepared properly to ensure fusion.

Odontoid screws are contraindicated when the bone will not hold a screw securely (e.g., if the bone is soft or excessively fractured) or when the screws cannot be properly inserted (irreducible fractures or an unsuitable body habitus). In these patients a different method of C1-2 fixation should be performed.

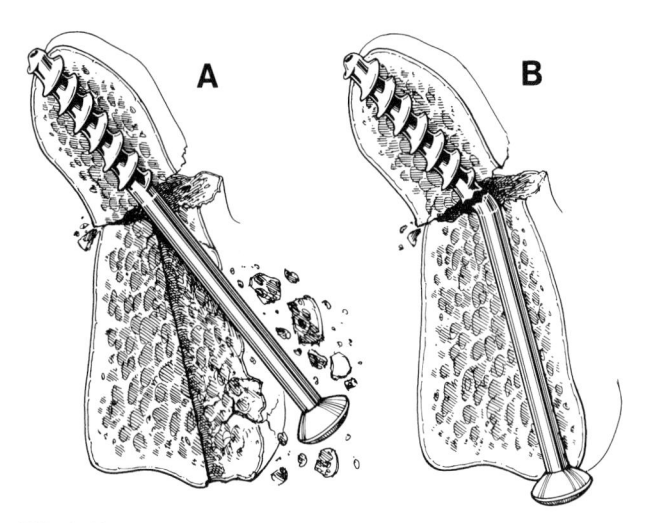

FIG. 1-12. Mechanisms of odontoid screw failure. (a) The proximal shaft of the screw can break through the anterior vertebral body of C2, or (b) The screws can bend or break across the fracture site. With permission of Barrow Neurological Institute.

Table 1-2
Advantages and Disadvantages of the Odontoid Screw Fixation System

Advantages
  Preserves normal cervical motion
  Relatively small surgical procedure

Disadvantages
  Limited indications
  Difficult to perform in patients with "barrel" chests or short necks

Odontoid screws are reasonably strong, but they do not immediately restore normal strength to the dens. An orthosis is suggested as a postoperative load-sharing device in order to minimize stress on the fixation until bone healing occurs.

ACKNOWLEDGMENTS

The authors wish to thank Mark Schornak, medical illustrator, and the editorial staff at the Barrow Neurological Institute for their assistance in the preparation of this manuscript.

REFERENCES

Anderson, L.D., & D'Alonzo, R.T. (1974). Fracture of the odontoid process of the axis. *Journal of Bone and Joint Surgery, American Volume, 56,* 1663–1674.

Apfelbaum R. (1992). Anterior screw fixation of odontoid fractures. In S.S. Rengachary & R.H. Wilkins (Eds.), *Neurosurgical Operative Atlas* (Vol. 2) (pp. 189–199). Baltimore: Williams & Wilkins.

Apuzzo, M.L.J., Heiden, J.S., Weiss, M.H., et al. (1978). Acute fractures of the odontoid process: An analysis of 45 cases. *Journal of Neurosurgery, 48,* 85–91.

Barbour, J.R. (1971). Screw fixation in fracture of the odontoid process. *Southern Australian Clinics, 5,* 20–24.

Bohler, J. (1982). Anterior stabilization for acute fractures and non-unions of the dens. *Journal of Bone and Joint Surgery, American Volume, 64,* 18–27.

Borne, G.M., Bedou, G.L., Pinadeau, M., et al. (1988). Odontoid process fracture osteosynthesis with a direct screw fixation technique in nine consecutive cases. *Journal of Neurosurgery, 68,* 223–226.

Clark, C.R., & White, A.A., III. (1985). Fractures of the dens: A multicenter study. *Journal of Bone and Joint Surgery, American Volume, 67,* 1340–1348.

Dickman, C.A., Mamourian, A., Sonntag, V.K.H., et al. (1991). Magnetic resonance imaging of the transverse atlantal ligament for the evaluation of atlantoaxial instability. *Journal of Neurosurgery, 75,* 221–227.

Dickman, C.A., Sonntag, V.K.H. & Marcotte, P.J. (1992). Techniques of screw fixation of the cervical spine. *Barrow Neurological Institute Quarterly, 8(2),* 9–26.

Donovan, M.M. (1979). Efficacy of rigid fixation of fractures of the odontoid process: Retrospective analysis of fifty-four cases. *Orthopedic Transactions, 3,* 309.

Doherty, B.J., Heggeness, M.H., Esses, S.I. (1993). A biomechanical study of odontoid fractures and fracture fixation. *Spine, 18(2),* 178–184.

Dunn, M.E., & Seljeskog, E.L. (1986). Experience in the management of odontoid process injuries: An analysis of 128 cases. *Neurosurgery, 18,* 306–310.

Etter, C., Coscia, M., Jaberg, H., et al. (1991). Direct anterior fixation of dens fractures with a cannulated screw system. *Spine, 16,* 525–531.

Geisler, F.H., Cheng, C., Poka, A., et al. (1989). Anterior screw fixation of posteriorly displaced Type II odontoid fractures. *Neurosurgery, 25,* 30–38.

Hadley, M.N., Dickman, C.A., Browner, C.A., et al. (1989). Acute axis fractures: A review of 229 cases. *Journal of Neurosurgery, 71,* 642–647.

Knoringer, P. (1987). Double-threaded compression screws for osteosynthesis of acute fractures of the odontoid process. In D. Voth, & P. Glees (Eds.), *Diseases in the Cranio-Cervical Junction: Anatomical and Pathological Aspects and Detailed Clinical Accounts* (pp. 127–136). Berlin: de Gruyter.

Sasso, R.C., Doherty, B.J., Crawford, M.J., et al. (1993). Biomechanics of odontoid fracture fixation: Comparison of the one- and two-screw technique. *Spine, 18*(4), 1950–1953.

CHAPTER 2

Caspar System for Anterior Cervical Fusion and Interbody Stabilization

Peter M. Klara

HIGHLIGHTS

The Caspar System for anterior cervical fusion and interbody stabilization was developed by Wolfhard Caspar, at the Department of Neurosurgery, Medical School, University of Saarland, Homburg/Saar, Germany. It is manufactured by Aesculap, South San Francisco, CA. The set consists of instrumentation organized into three functional categories (Fig. 2-1): (1) soft-tissue exposure, (2) spinal realignment, decompression, and fusion, and (3) osteosynthetic stabilization of the diseased or injured spinal segments. The instrumentation as well as the standardized method developed by Caspar has proven utility and safety when used appropriately by trained surgeons and with the assistance of fluoroscopy. Instability is the main indication for plating. Restoration of stability by the plate is temporary and designed to provide stability until fusion occurs. The plating technique is therefore an adjunct to fusion and can be used in clinical situations in which fusion is desirable (Tables 2-1 and 2-2).

POSITIONING

Patients undergoing anterior cervical surgery are put in the supine position, with a slight break at the knees and the back to relieve stress. This chaise lounge position can be enhanced by utilizing the Caspar head holder (Fig. 2-2, *a*). This device attaches to the operating table much as a Mayfield adapter and allows the surgeon close access to the patient's neck. The device supports the head and the nape of the neck and has attachments for an elastic chin strap that assists in maintaining midline position. The head holder also comes equipped with attachments for supporting weights for cervical tong traction. The design of the head holder allows for both lateral and anteroposterior (AP) fluoroscopy.

SOFT-TISSUE RETRACTORS AND BASIC EXPOSURE

With proper technique, horizontal skin incisions may be employed to perform even three-level corpectomies. This is generally the case, but individual patients and anatomy are a consideration. Short necks or minimal ability to flex or extend the cervical spine may present problems. A longitudinal incision is an acceptable alternative. The basic horizontal incision is made at the appropriate level as demonstrated by intraoperative x-ray film. The skin incision should extend from the medial border of the sternocleidomastoid muscle to slightly past the midline. The platysma is identified and transected and a substantial subplatysmal dissection should be performed so that the sternocleidomastoid and the investing cervical fascia is released. The fascial release should be taken superiorly and inferiorly. Ultimately, a plane between the trachea and esophagus medially and the carotid artery laterally can be developed. Fascial release is directly proportional to the vertebral levels to be exposed. Hand-held retractors can be used initially until the insertions of the longus colli muscle are exposed and separated from the vertebral bodies. Retractor blades should be inserted under the longus colli muscle so that distractive forces are applied to the muscle rather than associated soft-tissue structures, such as the carotid artery or esophagus. The soft-tissue retractors are designed so they can accommodate the patient's anatomy. Eventually, a cylinder is formed with equal exposure at the top and the bottom. This minimizes force transmission to soft tissues and possible associated injuries. It should be noted that retractor blades come in large-toothed, small-toothed, and smooth varieties. Either the large-toothed or small-toothed can be used for retraction against the insertions of the longus colli muscle, while the smooth blades are used in a retractor placed at 90 degrees to the lateral retractor. This retractor can obtain additional superior and inferior exposure. The soft-tissue retractors are hinged so that the handles can be rotated in a convenient position to afford the operating surgeon unimpeded access to the surgical field.

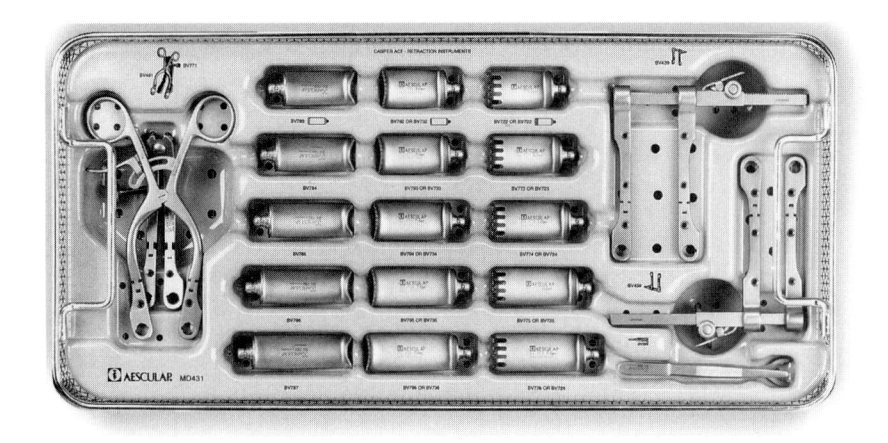

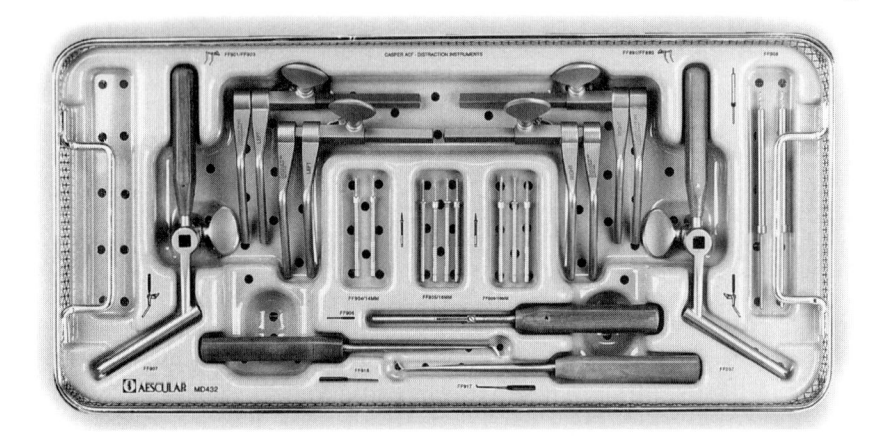

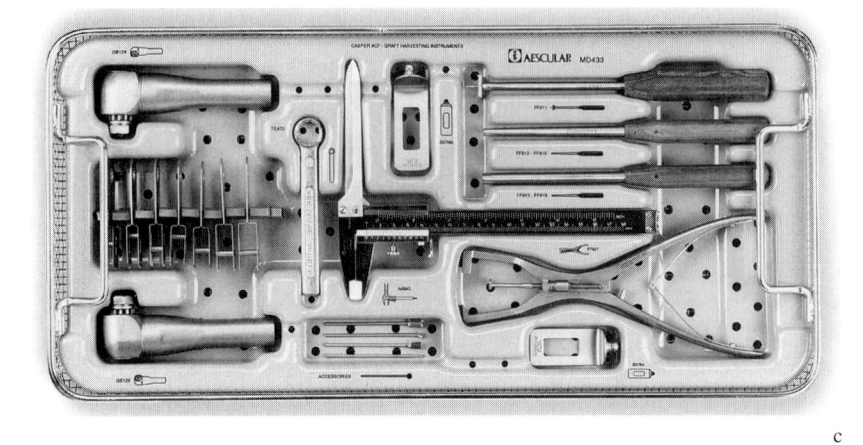

Table 2-1
Indications for Plating

Traumatic instability
Degenerative disease (hard and soft disks)
Iatrogenic instability (Postoperative instability, e.g., body resection for tumor, swan neck, etc.)
Pseudarthrosis (anterior or posterior)
Adjunct to posterior fusions

VERTEBRAL-BODY DISTRACTOR

This critical instrument has been a major contribution. By placing screws in the vertebral bodies and applying distraction, excellent bilateral exposure to the disk space is

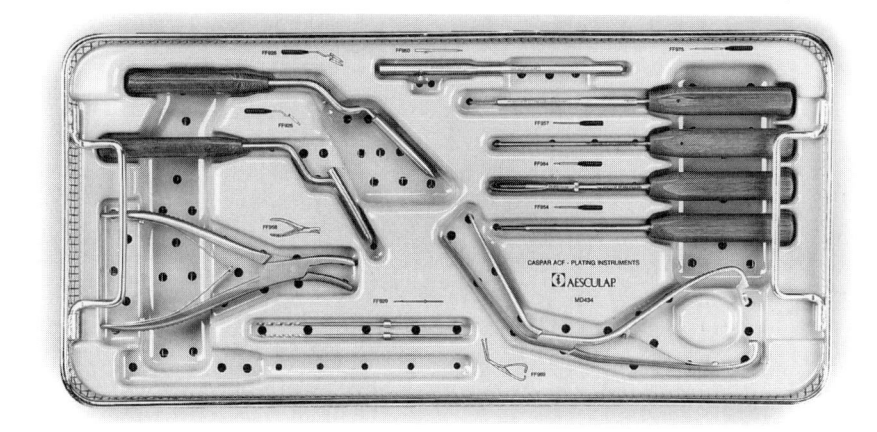

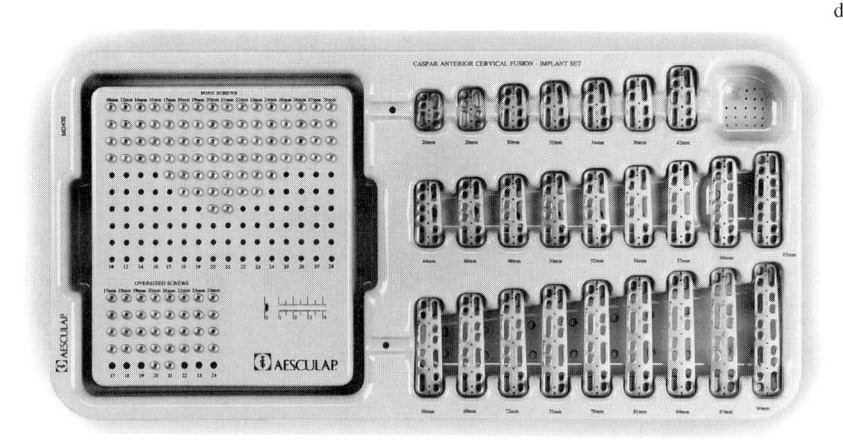

FIG. 2-1. Instrumentation. (a) Soft tissue retractors for exposure. (b) Distractor instrumentation. (c) Graft harvesting instrumentation. (d) Plating instrumentation. (e) Plates and screws.

obtained. Also, damage to the cortical end plates is eliminated. Insertion of the distractor pins can be accomplished as outlined in Figs. 2-3 through 2-5.

Once the anterior aspects of the appropriate vertebral bodies have been exposed, distractor pins are placed in the appropriate vertebral bodies. This is accomplished by placing the distractor drill guide in the middle third of the inferior-most vertebral body. Using the drill to make a pilot hole will prevent inadvertent enlargement that can occur with manual insertion of the distractor pins. It is critical to use the distraction drill bit, which has a preset stop to limit the pilot hole to 8 mm. This prevents inadvertent penetration into the canal. Intraoperative fluoroscopy can be used to ensure a slight caudal inclination of the pilot hole so that distractor pin placement is parallel to vertebral end plates. After drilling, the self-tapping distractor screw can be placed through the drill guide and tightened so that the base plate contacts the vertebral body. A construct is then fashioned, consisting of one half the vertebral body distractor and the distractor drill guide (Fig. 2-4). This construct will allow for drilling of the next pilot hole in a superior vertebral body, and for the parallel placement of the next pilot hole and distractor screw.

Moving superiorally, this operation can be repeated on as many segments as necessary (Fig. 2-5). Once the distractor pins have been placed, the vertebral body distractor is inserted over the shafts of the distractor pins and distraction is applied after incising the annulus. It is important to remember that distraction should not be applied on segments with an intact annulus. Distraction should be applied in a slow, incremental fashion, allowing soft tissues time to relax. The vertebral body distractors come in right and left

Table 2-2
Advantages of Plating

Improved bone healing	Improved patient care	More cost effective
Anatomical alignment	Early patient mobilization	Decreased hospital stay
Internal immobilization	Minimized use of external orthosis	Decreased failure rate
Graft under compression	Decreased pain	
Increased bone-to-bone contact	Increased rate of recovery	

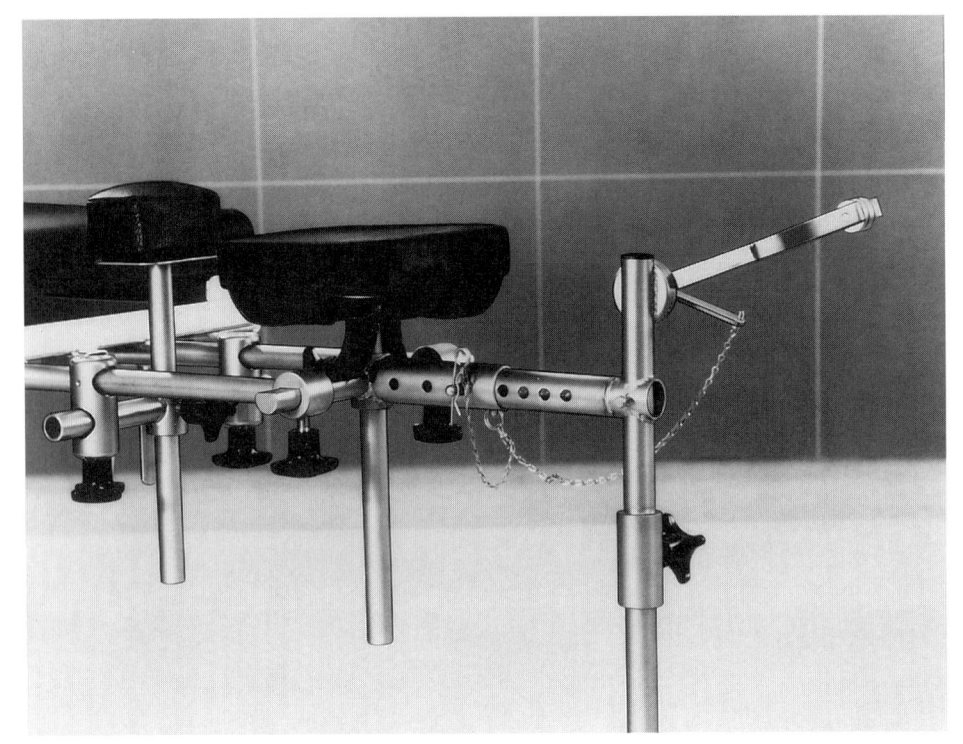

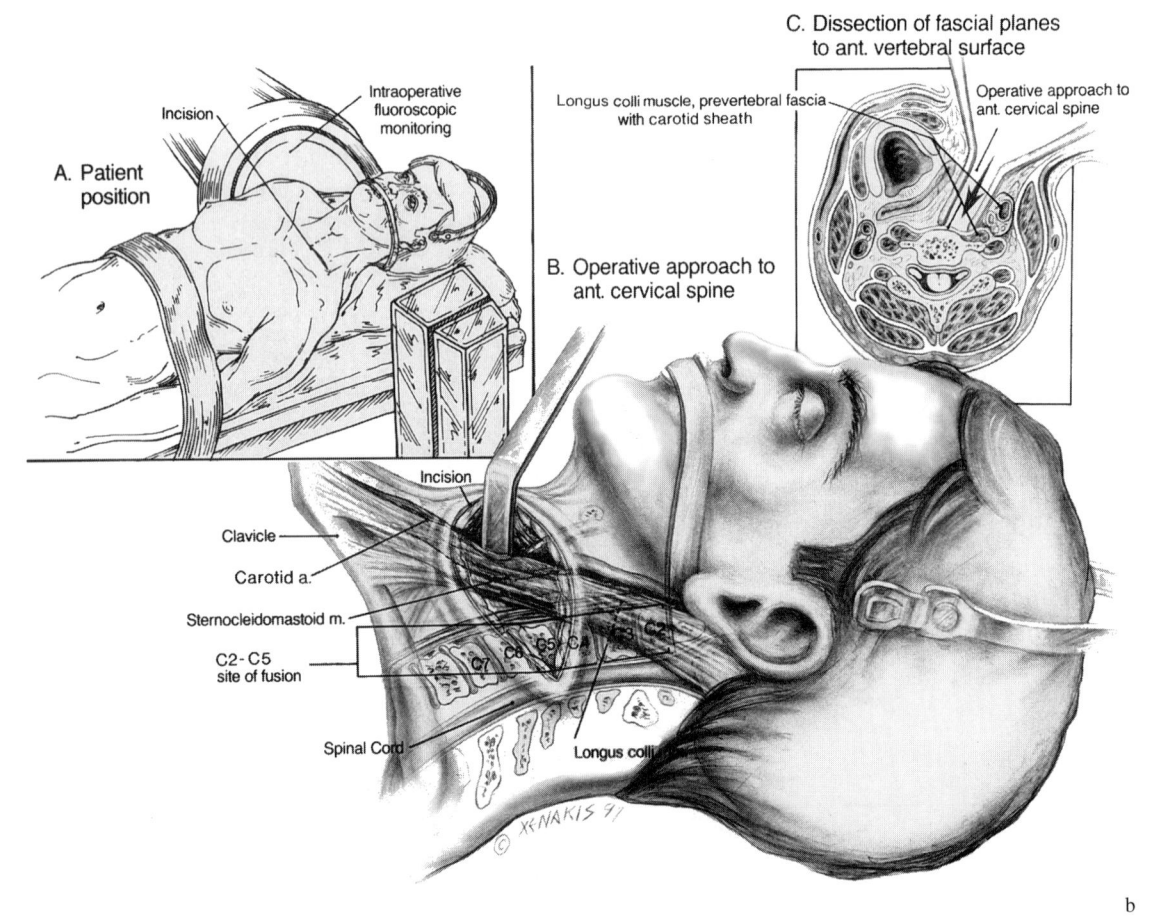

FIG. 2-2. Positioning. (a) Caspar head holder. (b) Fluoroscopy setup and surgical incision.

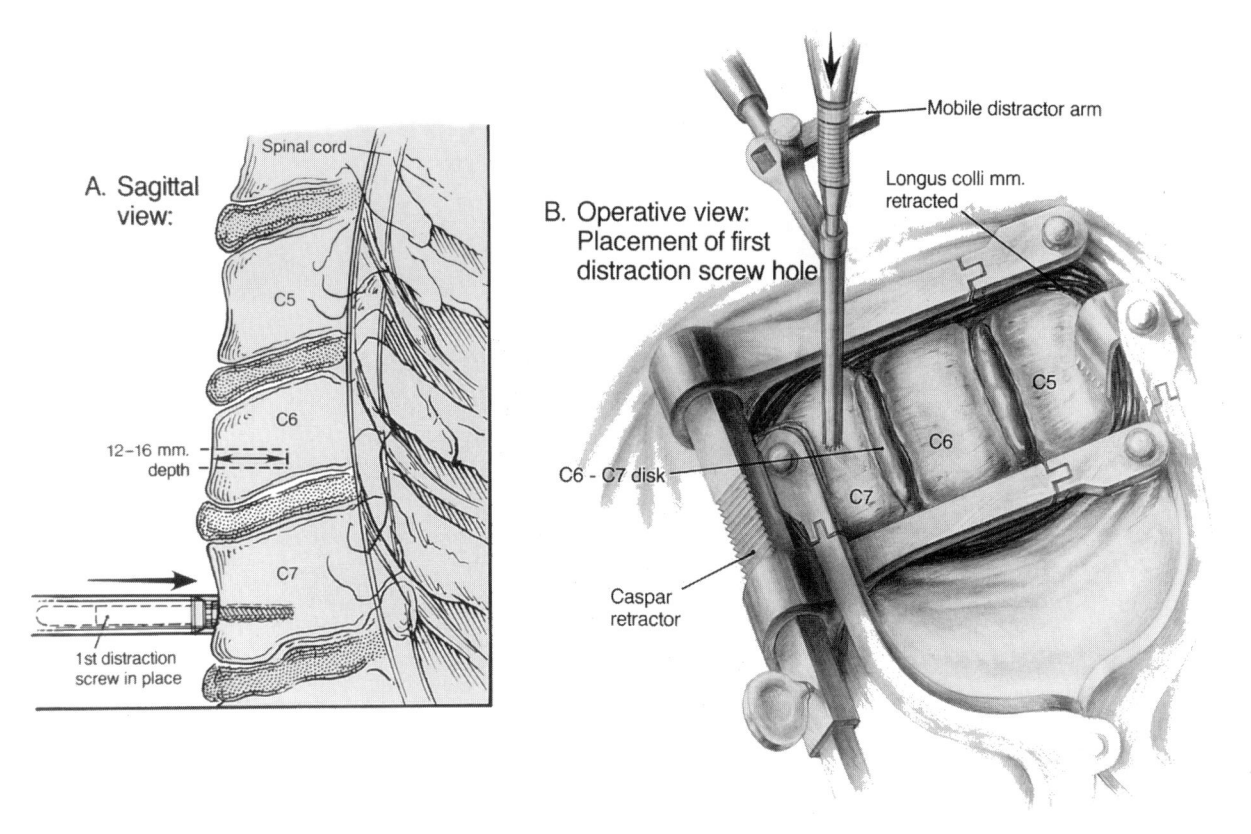

FIG. 2-3. Vertebral-body distractor, with initial distractor screw placement.

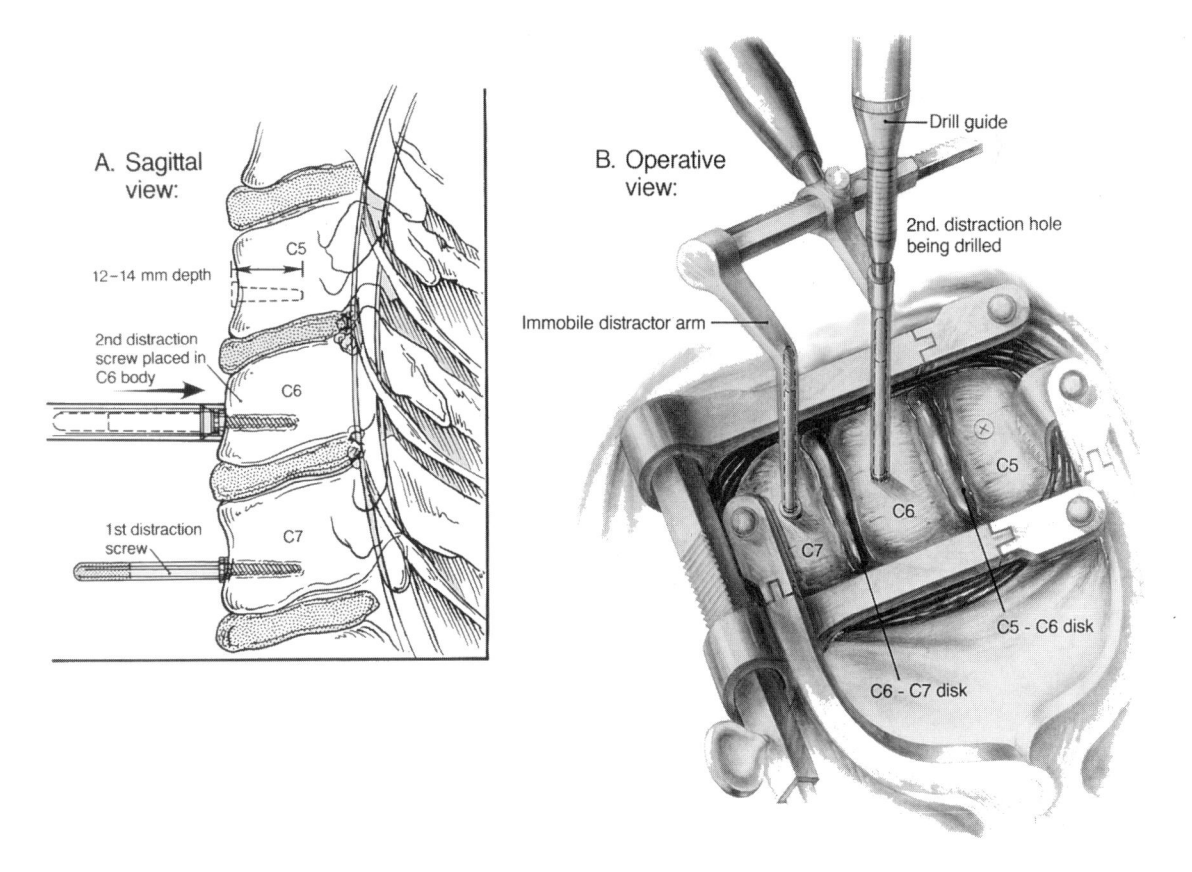

FIG. 2-4. Vertbral-body distractor, with parallel placement of distractor screw.

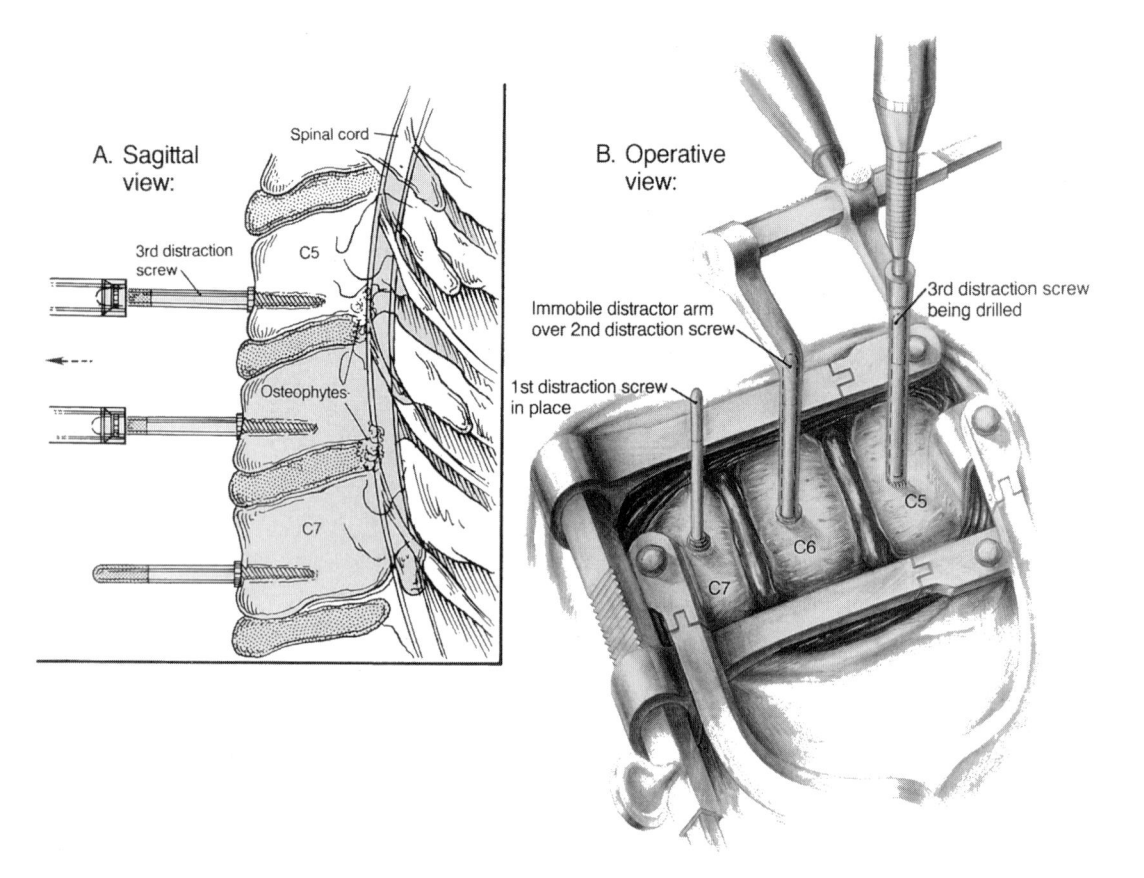

FIG. 2-5. Vertebral-body distractor, multi-level.

angles, with standard and extended shafts. This variety accommodates patient anatomy as well as multiple-level surgeries. If the high cervical area is being addressed, the vertebral body distractor should be placed so that the crossbar is directed inferiorally away from the patient's mandible. If the lower cervical spine is being addressed, the distractor crossbar should be directed superiorly away from the clavicle. Because the distractors are available in left and right models, the upper and lower cervical spine can be optimally addressed from either a right- or left-sided approach. Application of distraction provides optimal visualization of the disk space and facilitates diskectomy.

GRAFT-SITE PREPARATION

Once diskectomy or corpectomy has been completed, removal of the cartilaginous end plates is mandatory to optimize fusion. It is then desirable to establish parallelism of the vertebral-body cortical end plates. This can be accomplished by using burrs to remove anterior and posterior osteophytic lipping. Parallelism of the vertebral end plates will minimize or eliminate the "ramp effect." Nonparallel vertebral end spaces may promote graft extrusion by this mechanism. Furthermore, parallel end spaces allow maximum bone-to-bone contact, which promotes fusion.

SIZING THE GRAFT

Once the diskectomy is completed and parallelism has been established, distraction should be released. The undistracted end space can then be carefully measured. This is facilitated by using the Caspar caliper (Fig. 2-6). The graft ultimately taken should be approximately 2 mm greater in height than the measurement of the undistracted disk space in the case of diskectomy. In the case of corpectomy, more variability exists but usually an additional 4 mm of graft length is required (as compared with undistracted space).

HARVESTING THE GRAFT

If autologous graft is to be used, exposure of the iliac crest is performed in the usual fashion. Harvesting graft from the crest has been facilitated by the development of a double saw blade and graft cutter. The double saw blades are available in widths from 6 to 12 mm in 1-mm increments. Once the oscillating double saw blade has created its parallel cuts, the graft cutter, which has been adjusted to the appropriate depth, is inserted and cuts the base of the graft. This reliably produces an appropriately sized graft and avoids inadvertent fracturing that can sometimes occur if an osteotome or other device is used to obtain the graft. Graft height should

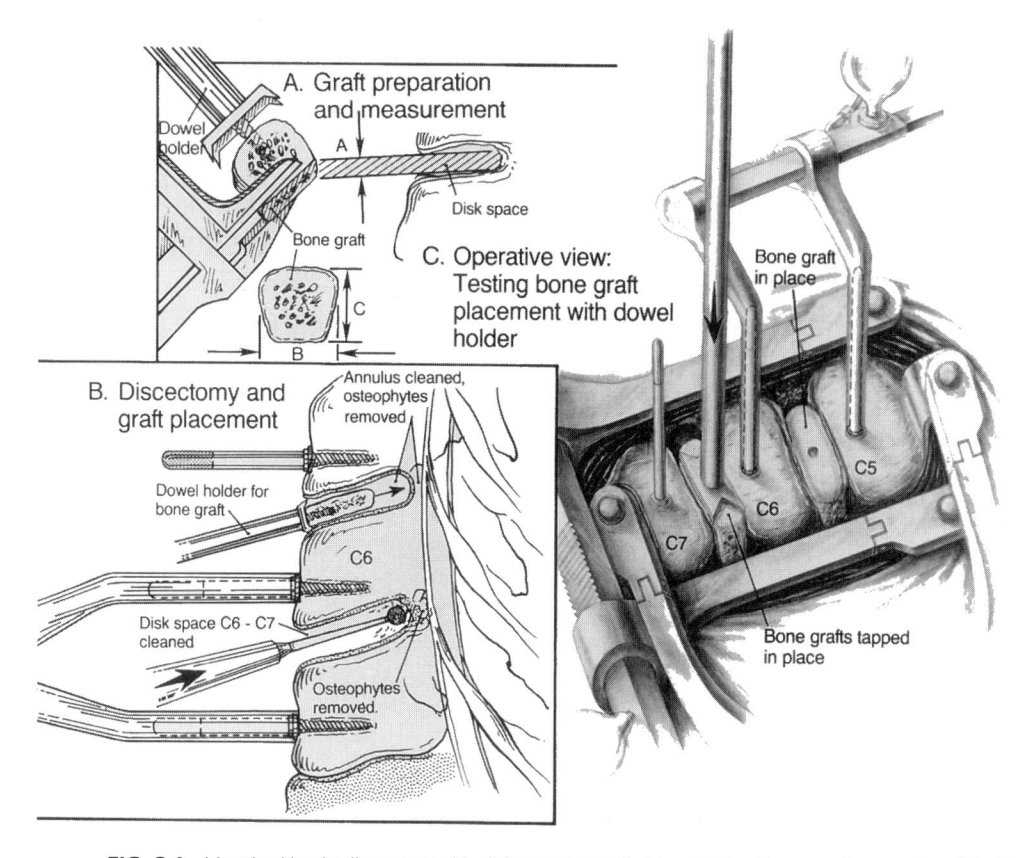

FIG. 2-6. Vertebral-body distractor, with diskectomy and fusion. (a) The Caspar caliper and graft holder assists in fashioning the graft for a precise fit. This maximizes bone-to-bone contact and promotes fusion. (b) The Caspar distractor facilitates diskectomy and allows for direct visualization of the disk space without damaging vertebral end plates. (c) The Caspar distractor is used in reverse to apply compression to the graft after positioning.

average 6 to 8 mm for a single interspace and the average AP depth should be 15 mm. The width of the graft is determined by the individual anatomy of the iliac crest and the region of the crest used to harvest the graft.

Once the graft has been obtained, distraction can be applied and the graft inserted. Minor adjustments of the graft's size can be made using a cylinder burr as needed prior to insertion. After graft insertion, the vertebral body distractor can be used as a compressor to seat the graft. Since the graft has been slightly oversized, the resulting compression should enhance fusion.

PLATING

If the surgeon elects internal fixation, four basic constructs are available: (1) single-level diskectomy and plating (Fig. 2-7); (2) multiple-level diskectomy and plating (Fig. 2-8); (3) partial corpectomy and plating (Fig. 2-9); and (4) corpectomy and plating (Fig. 2-10).

Single-Level Diskectomy and Plating

This consists of a diskectomy and interbody graft with a plate extending over two vertebral bodies, fusing a single motion segment.

Multiple-Level Diskectomy and Plating

This is essentially an extension of a single-level diskectomy and plating, and involves fusion across multiple motion segments.

Partial Corpectomy and Plating

Multiple diskectomies are performed; however, if the posterior third of the vertebral body is intact, trough corpectomy is not necessary. The anterior half to two thirds of the affected vertebral body can be removed following diskectomy at the levels above and below. A graft can then be placed across multiple motion segments and secured with screws placed through the plate into the posterior cortex of the remaining vertebral body. This results in the most stable construct possible.

Corpectomy

Diskectomies are performed on at least two levels, with removal of the midportion of the vertebral body. Similarly, multiple trough corpectomies can be performed; however, it is essential that diskectomies be performed at all levels of intended fusion. In this construct, the plate is affixed to intact vertebral bodies above and below the extent of corpectomy.

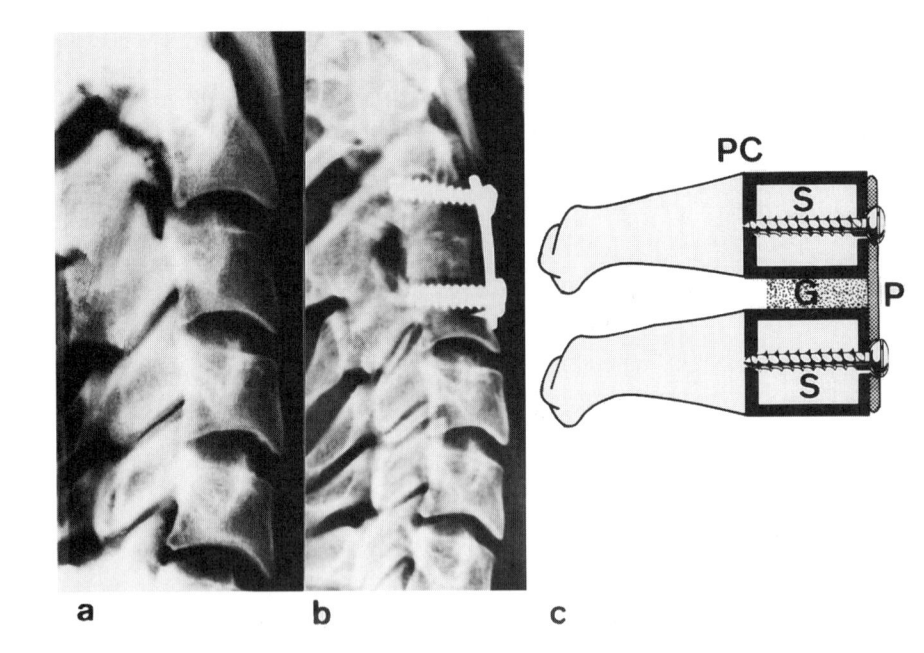

FIG. 2-7. Single-level fusion and plates. (a) Preoperative plain film of C2 fracture. (b) Postoperative plain film of single-level fusion and plating. (c) Diagrammatic illustration of single-level fusion and plating. G = graft; P = plate; PC = posterior cortex; S = screw.

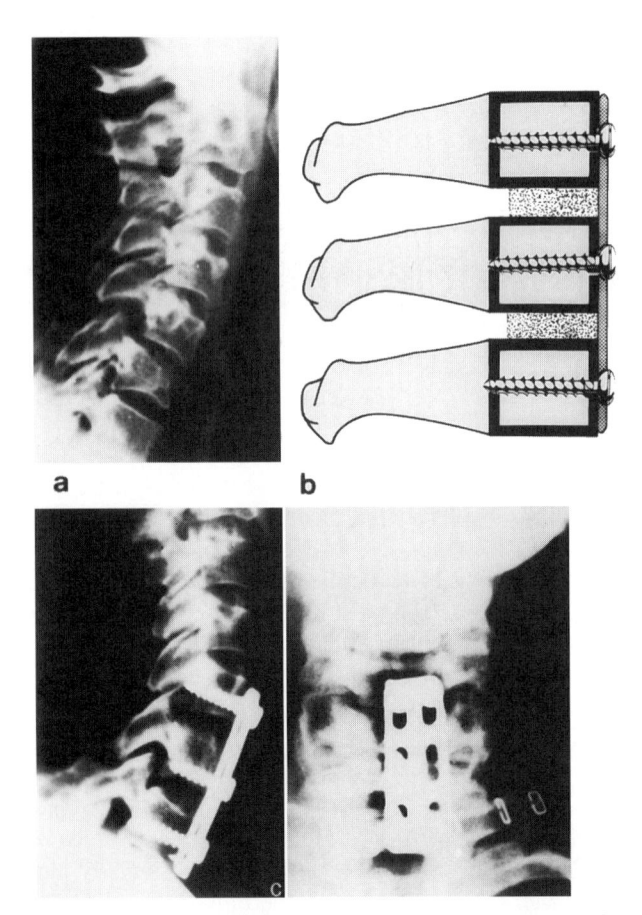

FIG. 2-8. Multiple-level fusion and plating. (a) Preoperative plain film. (b) Diagrammatic illustration of multiple-level fusion and plating. (c) Postoperative lateral plain film of multiple-level fusion and plating. (d) Postoperative AP plain film of multiple-level fusion and plating.

Plating Technique

Ideally, a plate must be chosen to extend from the top of the vertebral body above to the bottom of the vertebral body below the levels of concern. Care should be taken to prevent impingement of the plate on a healthy disk space (Fig. 2-11, *a*). Such impingement may cause premature degeneration of a healthy disk. Interoperative fluoroscopy assists the surgeon in plate positioning and ensures against extension onto healthy disks. Occasionally, the lower cervical or upper thoracic levels cannot be visualized. Careful preoperative measurements on plain x-ray films (taking into account magnification in nonstandard distances) may assist in choosing the correct plate. Once the appropriate size plate has been selected and contoured, it must be secured with bicortical screw fixation (Fig. 2-11, *b*). The plate can be held in place with the plate holder. Either the single or the dual drill guide is set to a predetermined measurement and the pilot hole is drilled under fluoroscopic guidance (Fig. 2-11, *c*). Placement of the pilot hole is in the middle third of the vertebral body parallel to the disk space in the sagittal plane, and angled 10 to 20 degrees medially in the axial plane.

Alternative angulation of the screw may be employed; however, this is acceptable only if the posterior cortex is engaged and the screw does not violate the disk space. The first pilot hole is drilled into the slot at the base of the Caspar plate. Surgeons experienced in drilling can differentiate the tactile sensation of cortical versus cancellous bone. In addition, the pitch of the drill motor changes as the transition is made from cancellous to cortical bone. The surgeon can actually "feel" the drill bit just penetrate the posterior vertebral body cortex. Of course, careful fluoroscopic monitoring during the drilling process is also used to prevent inadvertent penetration into the spinal canal.

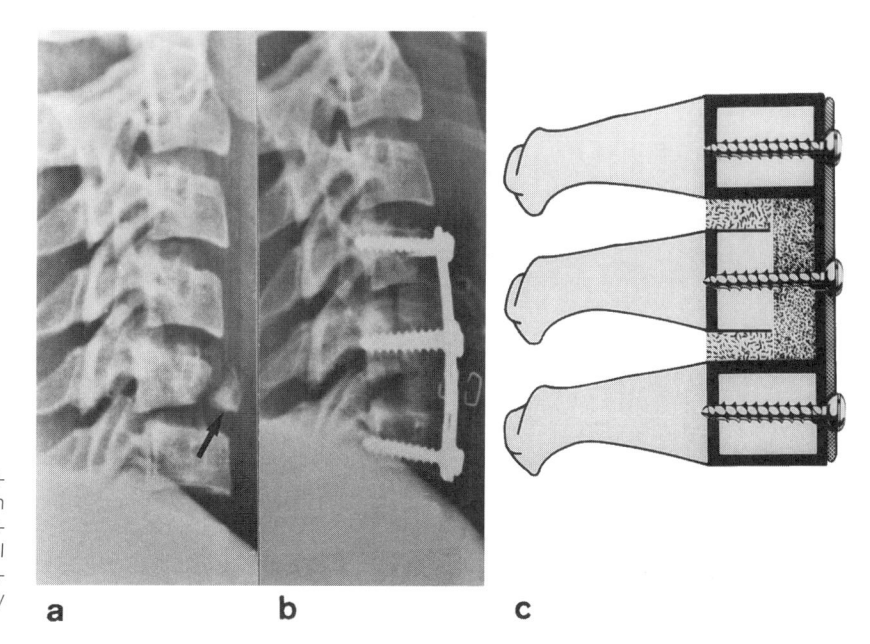

CHAPTER 2 / CASPAR SYSTEM FOR ANTERIOR CERVICAL FUSION AND INTERBODY STABILIZATION   **21**

FIG. 2-9. Partial corpectomy and plating. (a) Preoperative lateral plain film showing teardrop fracture. (b) Postoperative lateral plain film of partial corpectomy and plating. (c) Diagrammatic illustration of partial corpectomy and plating.

FIG. 2-10. Corpectomy and plating. (a) Preoperative lateral plain film. (b) Preoperative lateral tomogram. (c) Preoperative myelogram. (d) Postoperative lateral plain film of corpectomy and plating. (e) Diagrammatic illustration of corpectomy and plating.

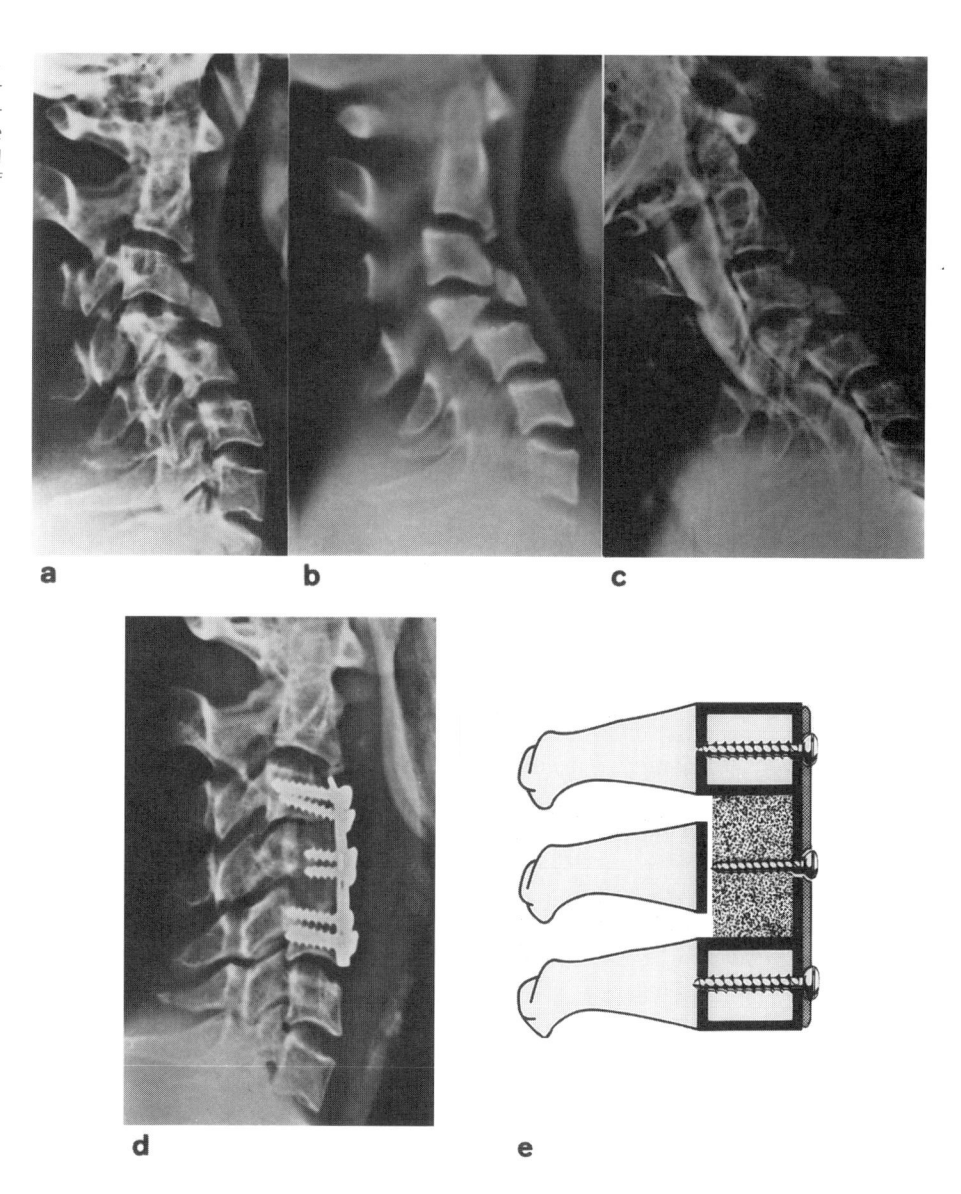

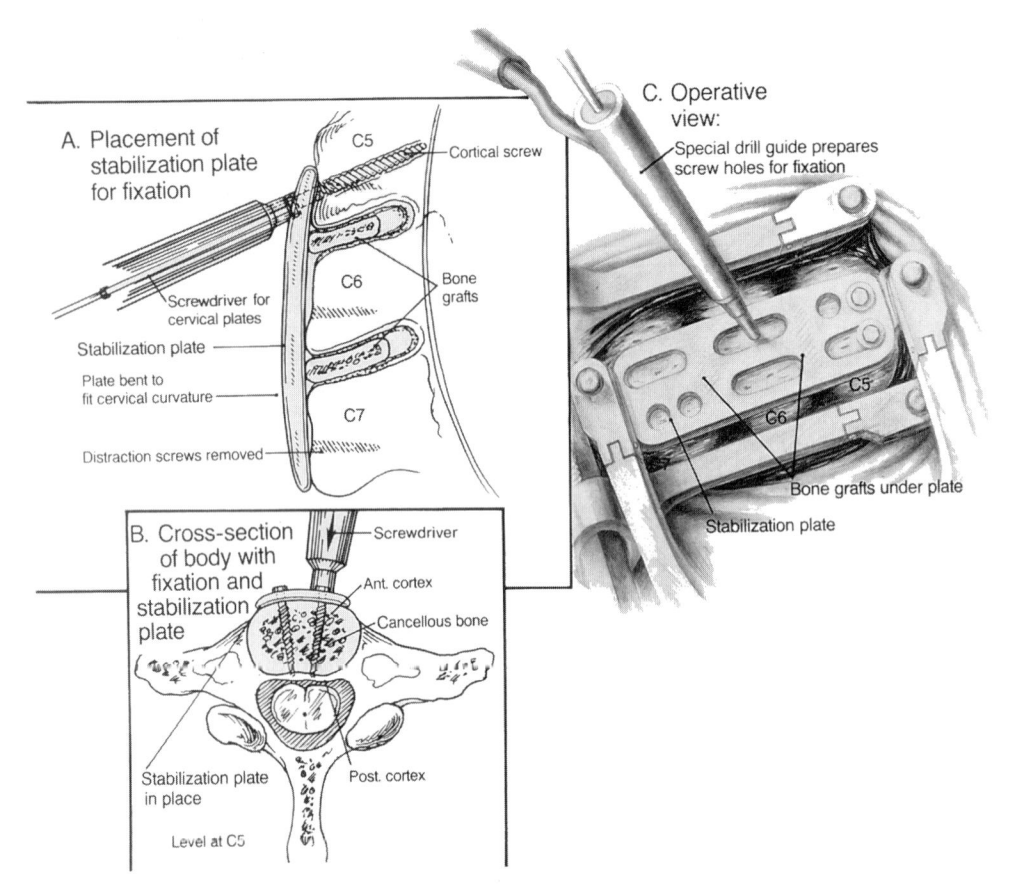

FIG. 2-11. Caspar plate osteosynthes and stabilization. (a) Fixation of plate to vertebral body. (b) Bicortical penetration. (c) Operative view.

A technique for safe, progressive drilling has been developed. This involves intentionally setting the micrometer drill guide short of the predetermined penetration. Once this pilot hole has been drilled, the drill can be removed and a blunt K-wire inserted to palpate the depth of the pilot hole carefully. As incomplete penetration is identified, the micrometer drill guide can be advanced one full turn, which translates into an additional millimeter of drill exposure. The K-wire is then removed and the drill guide, with the drill in place, reinserted. If these steps are repeated, one can actually advance the drill in 1-mm increments. This procedure safely allows penetration of the posterior cortical surface without inadvertent plunging of the drill. The anterior cortex of the pilot hole is then tapped prior to screw insertion. Routinely, a 3.5-mm screw that measures 1 to 2 mm longer than the final drill guide micrometer setting is selected. This compensates for the screw head and thickness of the plate. The screw is then inserted and secured into the posterior cortex. A second pilot hole is drilled into the slot at the apex of the Caspar plate, diagonal to the first pilot hole. Prior to drilling this hole, the plate should assume its final position (and can be rotated and translated about the yet-not-fully-tightened first screw). Screw length selection follows the same process as outlined above. These two screws can then be tightened, using the thumb, index, and middle fingers only (two-finger tightness). In this manner, at least two screws should be placed in each available vertebral body (Fig. 2-12). Should situations warrant, additional screws can be placed as deemed necessary.

Adequate screw purchase should be obtained on all screws. Should a screw fail to obtain two-finger tightness, a screw of larger diameter (rescue screws) can be used. Alternatively, methylmethacrylate can be used to secure loose screws. This is accomplished by placing a small amount of methylmethacrylate in the pilot hole with a K-wire and applying it to the walls of the pilot hole. Only a small amount of plastic should be used to ensure that excess plastic does not extend through the posterior cortex and possibly impinge on the canal. Screws can be placed into the pilot hole after the application of plastic and should be allowed to sit for several minutes. Substantially increased torque is obtained once the plastic has set. All screws should be rechecked for torque prior to closure. The wound is irrigated and closed in the usual fashion. A drain is optional, and it is unusual for patients to require intensive care monitoring after this procedure. Neurologic examination should be conducted immediately on reversal of anesthesia. The patient is fitted with a cervical collar or equivalent and allowed to recover. Most

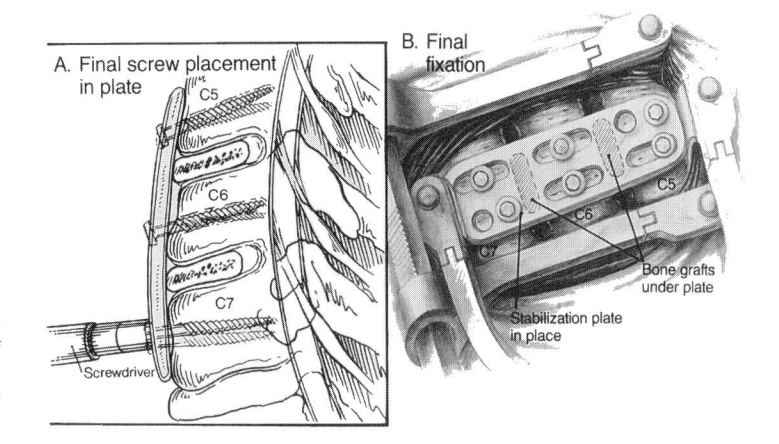

FIG. 2-12. Multiple-level fusion and plating. (a) Diagrammatic illustration of multiple-level fusion and plating. (b) Diagrammatic illustration of operative view.

patients are ambulatory on the first postoperative day and are able to tolerate liquids by the evening of surgery. It is recommended that patients continue to wear the cervical collar for 30 days to minimize the possibility of screw loosening. Patients with severely osteoporotic bone may require additional external support. This may be accomplished with prolonged use of a cervical collar or application of a halo. White-collar work may be resumed in 2 to 4 weeks, and fusion is usually obtained by 12 weeks.

BIOMECHANICS

Biomechanical evaluation of Caspar plates has been conducted in both a calf spine model (Sutterlin, McAfee, Warden, Rey, & Farey, 1988) and human cadavers (Coe, Warden, Sutterlin, et al., 1989). Early evaluation suggested that the Caspar plates provided less stiffness than other available techniques (lateral mass plates and posterior wiring techniques). These authors concluded that Caspar plates should not be used in the presence of posterior instability. Significant clinical experience by numerous surgeons indicated that the plate could be used safely and effectively in spite of posterior instability.

The seeming discrepancy may result from the fact that both calf spine model and the human cadaver model are imperfect simulators of the clinical situation. Furthermore, the failure of the plate to provide increased stiffness, as compared with other techniques, does not preclude the possibility that it provides adequate stiffness to improve healing and promote fusion.

More recent biomechanical studies (Traynelis, Donaher, Roach, Kojimoto, & Goel, 1993) in a cadaver corpectomy model demonstrate that anterior plating provides more stability in extension and lateral bending than does posterior wiring. While further biomechanical evaluation is warranted, this study supports the continued use of bicortical anterior plate fixation for the treatment of traumatic instability.

CLINICAL RESULTS

Numerous reports are currently available demonstrating the safety and effectiveness of the Caspar plate when applied by trained surgeons, following correct methods, for appropriate indications (Caspar, Barbier, & Klara, 1989; Garvey, Eismont, & Roberti, 1992; Tippets & Apfelbaum, 1988; Goffin, Plets, & Van den Bergh, 1989; Randle, Wolf, Levi, et al., 1991). The utility of anterior cervical decompression, arthrodesis and stabilization with plates is documented in the literature by Illgner (1991), Aebi (1991), and Bohlman (1993). The disadvantages of plating are summarized in Table 2-3.

COMPARISON TO ALTERNATIVE SYSTEM

Alternatives to the Caspar plate include the Acroplate (Acromed) and the Synthes plate. The Acroplate is similar to the Caspar plate, however, little published clinical data is available at present. The Synthes plate requires only unicortical penetration and the screws are coupled (locked) to the plate.

Advantages

Caspar

1. Ability to vary screw angle; especially helpful when plating upper or lower cervical segments.
2. Variable screw placement; helpful to reestablish cervical lordosis. Multiple screws may be placed with single segment (redirection of screws possible after initial drilling).

Synthes

1. Easier to apply in midcervical area. Less potential for neural injury (unicortical).
2. Minimal use of fluoroscopy required.
3. Minimal learning curve (user-friendly).
4. Screw loosening decreased (locking plate).

Table 2-3
Disadvantages of Plating

Instrumentation (learning curve)
Hardware failure (screw loosening, etc.)
Risk of neural injury (related to bicortical drilling)
Slightly increased operating time
Foreign body
Impaired postoperative imaging (minimal with titanium)
Increased initial cost

Disadvantages

Caspar

1. Bicortical penetration required (potential for increased risk of neural injury).
2. Fluoroscopic control required during surgery.
3. Significant learning curve.

Synthes

1. Fixed screw plate angle complicates application to upper (C2) and lower (C2, T1) segments.
2. Bendability of plate limited. If done through screw hole, screw plate locking mechanism may be disabled.
3. Limited to two screws per segment. Repositioning difficult after initial drilling.

COMPLICATIONS

Complications associated with Caspar anterior cervical plating can be separated into two categories: complications associated with the surgical approach (soft-tissue) and bone or disk work (diskectomy/corpectomy) and complications directly associated with hardware failure (loose or broken screws and plates).

In an attempt to evaluate complication rates associated with Caspar instrumentation, five different reports employing this technique are summarized in Table 2-4. Five different groups of surgeons performed 197 procedures. All surgeries used Caspar plates and the recommended techniques to include posterior cortical purchase. While overall morbidity from complications was high (>20%) this was related to the treatment of acute spinal injuries and not a direct result of surgery. Surgical complications were not unusual in any of the reports. Hardware failure consisted of screw loosening or breakage and averaged 4.0%. Only 4/197 (2%) of hardware failures required surgical reoperation. None of these five studies reported additional neurologic deficits that could be attributed to the plating procedure. The conclusion of all five reports was that the Caspar technique was safe and useful in the hands of trained surgeons who follow the recommended technique.

Table 2-4
Results with Caspar Instrumentation

Author	Hardware failure/ patients (%)	Reoperation/cause
Caspar (1989)	1/60 (1.6)	1/Loose screw
Garvey (1992)	2/15 (13.0)	0
Goffin (1989)	2/41 (5.0)	0
Randle (1991)	2/54 (3.7)	2/1 Infection, 1 loose screw
Tippets (1988)	1/28 (3.0)	1/Infection

REFERENCES

Caspar Technique

Caspar, W., Barbier, D.D., & Klara, P.M. (1989). Anterior cervical fusion and Caspar plate stabilization for cervical trauma. *Neurosurgery, 25,* 491–502.

Garvey, T.A., Eismont, F.J., & Roberti, L.J. (1992). Anterior decompression, structural bone grafting, and Caspar plate stabilization for unstable cervical spine fractures and/or dislocations. *Spine, 17,* (10S), S431–S435.

Goffin, J., Plets, C., & Van den Bergh, R. (1989). Anterior cervical fusion and osteosynthetic stabilization according to Caspar: A prospective study of 41 patients with fractures and/or dislocations of the cervical spine. *Neurosurgery, 25,* 865–871.

Randle, M.J., Wolf, A., Levi, L., Rigamonti, D., et al. (1991). The use of anterior Caspar plate fixation in acute cervical spine injury. *Surgical Neurology, 36,* 181–189.

Tippets, R.H., & Apfelbaum, R.I. (1988). Anterior cervical fusion with the Caspar instrumentation system. *Neurosurgery, 22,* 1008–1013.

Biomechanics

Coe, J.D., Warden, K.E., & Sutterlin, C.E., III, et al. (1989). Biomechanical evaluation of cervical spinal stabilization methods in a human cadaveric model. *Spine, 14,* 1122–1131.

Schulte, K., Clark, C.R. & Goel, V.K. (1989). Kinematics of the cervical spine followng discectomy and stabilization. *Spine, 14,* 1116–1121.

Sutterlin, C.E., III, McAfee, P.C., Warden, K.E., Rey, R.M., & Farey, I.D. (1988). A biomechanical evaluation of cervical spinal stabilization methods in a bovine model. *Spine, 13,* 795–802.

Traynelis, V.C., Donaher, P.A., Roach, R.M., Kojimoto, H., & Goel, V.K. (1993). Biomechanical comparison of anterior Caspar plate and three-level posterior fixation techniques in a human cadaveric model. *Journal of Neurosurgery, 79,* 96–103.

Anterior Plating (General)

Aebi, M., Zuber, K., & Marchesi, D. (1991) Treatment of cervical spine injuries with anterior plating: Indications, techniques, and results. *Spine, 16,* (3S), S38–S45.

Bohlman, H.H., Emery, S.E., Goodfellow, D.B., & Jones, P.K. (1993). Robinson anterior cervical discectomy and arthordesis for cervical radiculopathy. *Journal of Bone and Joint Surgery, American Volume, 75,* 1298–1307.

Illgner, A., Haas, N., & Tscherne, H. (1991). A review of the therapeutic concept and results of operative treatment in acute and chronic lesions of the cervical spine: The Hannover experience. *Journal of Orthopedic Trauma, 5,* 100–113.

CHAPTER 3

The Anterior Cervical Spine Locking Plate: A Technique for Surgical Decompression and Stabilization

Iain H. Kalfas

HIGHLIGHTS

The use of anterior decompression and stabilization techniques to manage cervical spine disorders has steadily gained acceptance in the neurosurgical and orthopedic communities (Cloward, 1958; Smith & Robinson, 1958). Initially devised for the management of cervical disk disease, the anterior approach is now used for more complex decompressive procedures involving the removal of one or more vertebrae. In addition to managing degenerative disorders, the anterior approach is also effective in managing a variety of conditions, including cervical trauma, posttraumatic or postlaminectomy kyphosis, neoplastic disorders, and osteomyelitis involving the vertebrae.

Most anterior cervical decompressive procedures are combined with the insertion of a bone graft to provide long-term spinal stability. Success rates of anterior cervical fusion in cases of spondylosis have ranged from 74 to 98%, with graft dislodgment occurring at a rate of 2 to 5% (Gore & Sepic, 1986; Riley, Robinson, Johnson, & Walker, 1969; Simmons & Bhalla, 1969; White, Southwick, DePonte, et al., 1973). In multiple-level fusions, pseudoarthrosis can occur at a rate as high as 33% (White et al., 1973). In cases of cervical trauma, graft extrusion rates range from 10 to 29%, and persistent postoperative deformity rates range from 38 to 64% (Bell & Bailey, 1977; Capen, Garland, & Waters, 1985; Van Peteghem & Schweigel, 1979). These rates of fusion failure, graft dislodgment and postoperative cervical deformity have stimulated the development of plate fixation devices for the cervical spine to optimize the fusion process.

For several decades, orthopedic surgeons have applied metal plates and screws to hold two bone fragments in approximate alignment (Lane, 1914). Studies of fracture healing using plate osteosynthesis have shown that optimal results are achieved by absolute immobilization and compression of the fracture fragments. The rigid plate, coupled with screws that insert into the vertebral bodies adjacent to the bone graft, provides a construct that resists a variety of potential distortional forces, including flexion, extension, rotational and lateral forces. In addition, when a bone graft underneath the plate is held in contact under load, the plate becomes part of the load-bearing cross-sectional area, thus adding to the stability of the construct (Cochran, 1982).

In 1975, Herrmann first described the application of a metal plate to the anterior cervical spine. Others reported variations of this approach, but acceptance of the technique was minimal because of the difficulty of plate application, the risk of neurologic injury, and the potential for screw loosening and subsequent fixation failure (Bohler & Gaudermak, 1980; Brown, Havel, Ebraheim, Greenblott, & Jackson, 1988; Goodman & Seligson, 1983).

Anterior cervical plate fixation advanced with the introduction of a plating system designed by Caspar (1986). This system consists of a standardized and universal set of instruments, retractors, distractors, and osteosynthetic plates of various lengths with fixation screws. The Caspar system, when coupled with intervertebral-body bone grafting, provides immediate cervical stabilization without the need for postoperative halo immobilization. It meets all the criteria for optimal fracture healing and graft incorporation—specifically, anatomical realignment, absolute immobilization, bone-to-bone contact, and compression of the fracture fragments or the bone graft. The single disadvantage is that the system requires that the screws used for plate fixation ideally engage both the anterior and posterior vertebral-body cortex. This specification introduces the potential for neurologic injury if a drill bit or screw passes beyond the posterior vertebral body cortex into the spinal canal. The incidence of this complication is low, but the necessary precautions to avoid neurologic injury do add to the difficulty and length of the procedure.

Morscher recently introduced an anterior cervical plating system that maintains the mechanical advantage of internal fixation but reduces the neurologic injury risk associated with screw fixation of the posterior vertebral body cortex (Morscher, Sutter, Jennis, & Olerud, 1986; Raveh, Stesh, Sutter, & Greiner, 1984). The cervical spine locking plate (CSLP) system is based on a unique two-screw fixation system that enhances screw-plate fixation and minimizes the risk of screw backout. This enhanced screw-plate fixation also eliminates the need for screw engagement in the posterior cortex of the vertebral body and minimizes the need for intraoperative fluoroscopy required by the Caspar system. The risk of neurologic injury, the degree of technical difficulty, and the length of the procedure are all reduced. This chapter describes the CSLP system and technique as well as patient outcome in the author's experience.

DESCRIPTION OF THE CERVICAL SPINE LOCKING PLATE SYSTEM

The CSLP system (Synthes, Paoli, PA) consists of plates of various lengths that are 2 mm thick and have five-hole or eight-hole configurations (Fig. 3-1). The primary set of plates has 15 different-sized plates 24 to 63 mm in length. A supplementary set of eight slightly thicker plates 66 to 92 mm in length has recently been added to the system, expanding its application to larger decompressive and stabilization procedures.

The plates are secured to the anterior cervical spine using two different types of screws. The anchor screw is 4.0 mm in diameter and 14 mm long; it is placed through the plate holes into the vertebral body or bone graft. The anchor screw has a hollow head surrounded by a segmented, expandable collar. Once the anchor screw has been positioned, a shorter locking screw 1.8 mm in diameter is inserted in the head of the anchor screw, forcing the collar of the anchor screw against the inner walls of that plate hole. This effectively locks the screw to the plate minimizing the potential for the anchor screw to back out (Fig. 3-2).

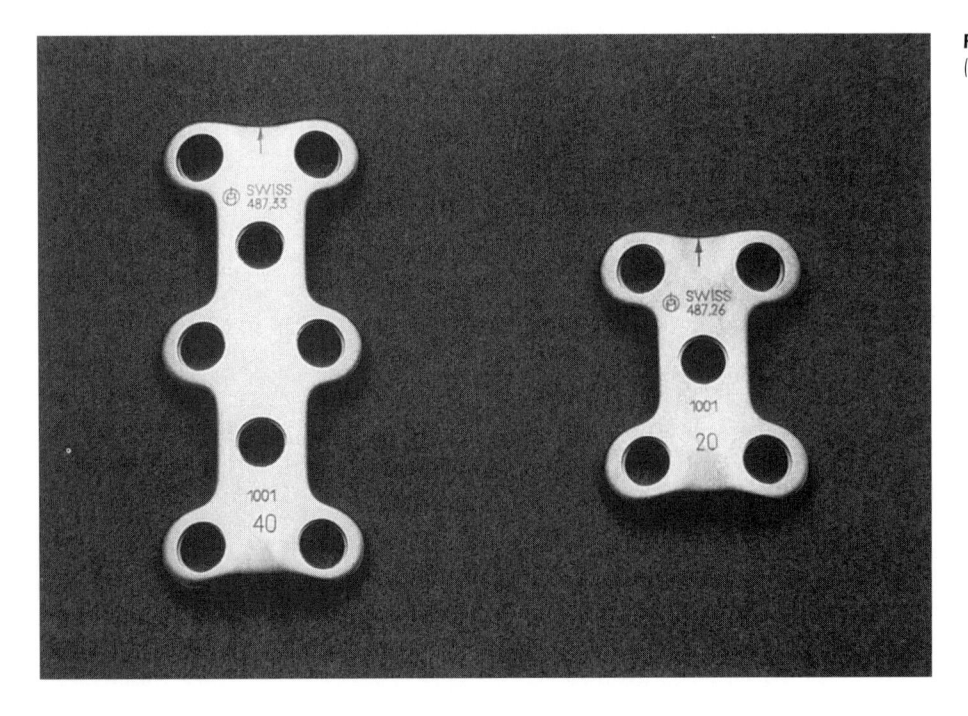

FIG. 3-1. Cervical spine locking plates (8-hole and 5-hole configurations).

CHAPTER 3 / THE ANTERIOR CERVICAL SPINE LOCKING PLATE: A TECHNIQUE FOR SURGICAL DECOMPRESSION AND STABILIZATION 27

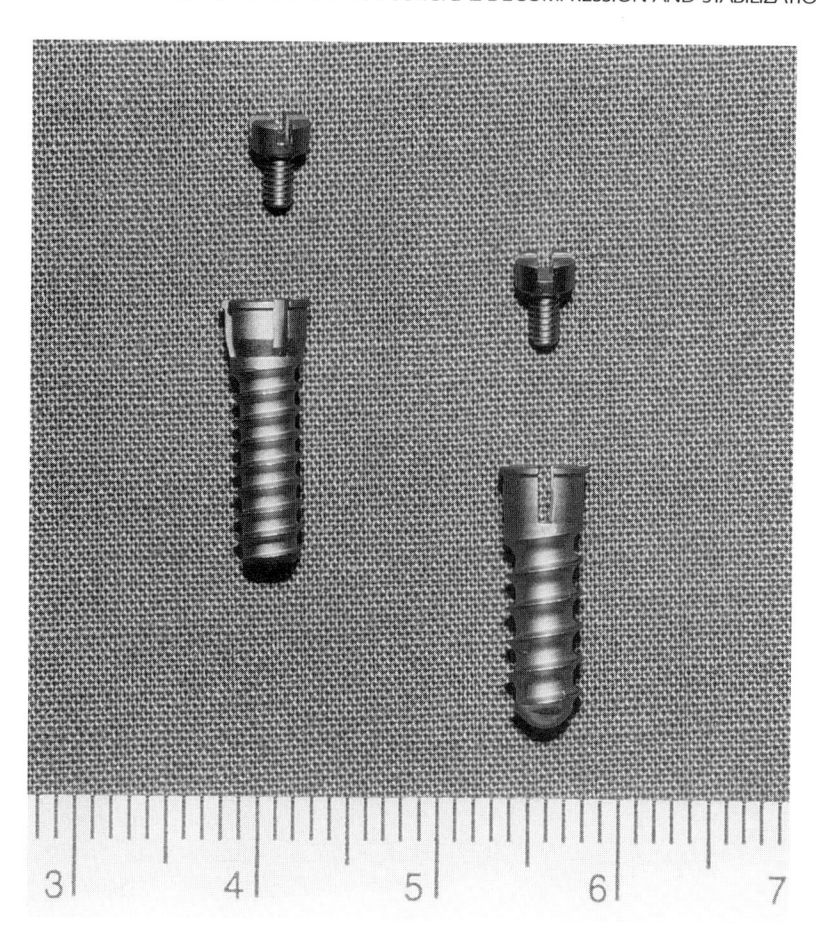

FIG. 3-2. Two sizes of anchor screws: 4.0 mm diameter on the left and 4.35 mm diameter on the right. The larger anchor screw is used with the set of longer plates. The smaller locking screws insert into the head of the anchor screws.

A second stabilizing feature of the CSLP system involves the angulation of the anchor screws when positioned. The rostral end of each plate is marked by an arrow imprinted on the plate. The two screw holes at the rostral end are specifically designed so that screws passed through these holes are inclined rostrally and medially. The two caudal screw holes are angled medially in a plane perpendicular to the plate. This screw configuration reduces the potential for failure at the screw-bone interface and reduces the potential for screw-plate backout.

In addition to the plates and screws, a standardized set of instruments is provided (Table 3-1). These include a plate holder, a 3.0-mm drill bit and drill guide, a bond tap for setting screw threads into the drilled holes, and two screwdrivers for the anchor and locking screws (Fig. 3-3). A drill is not included, but any battery or compressed air drill with a standard Jacobs chuck to receive the drill bit will suffice.

An additional advantage of the CSLP system is that the screws and plates are composed of titanium. Titanium is highly biocompatible with minimal risk for metal sensitivity. Furthermore, the titanium composition allows for better postoperative radiographic imaging with minimal distortion, particularly with magnetic resonance imaging (Fig. 3-4).

Table 3-1
System Components of the Cervical Spine Locking Plate

Plates
    Standard set (24 to 63 mm)
    Long plate set (66 to 92 mm)

Screws
    Anchor screw
    Locking nut

Drill guide and bit
Plate holder
Tap
Screwdriver

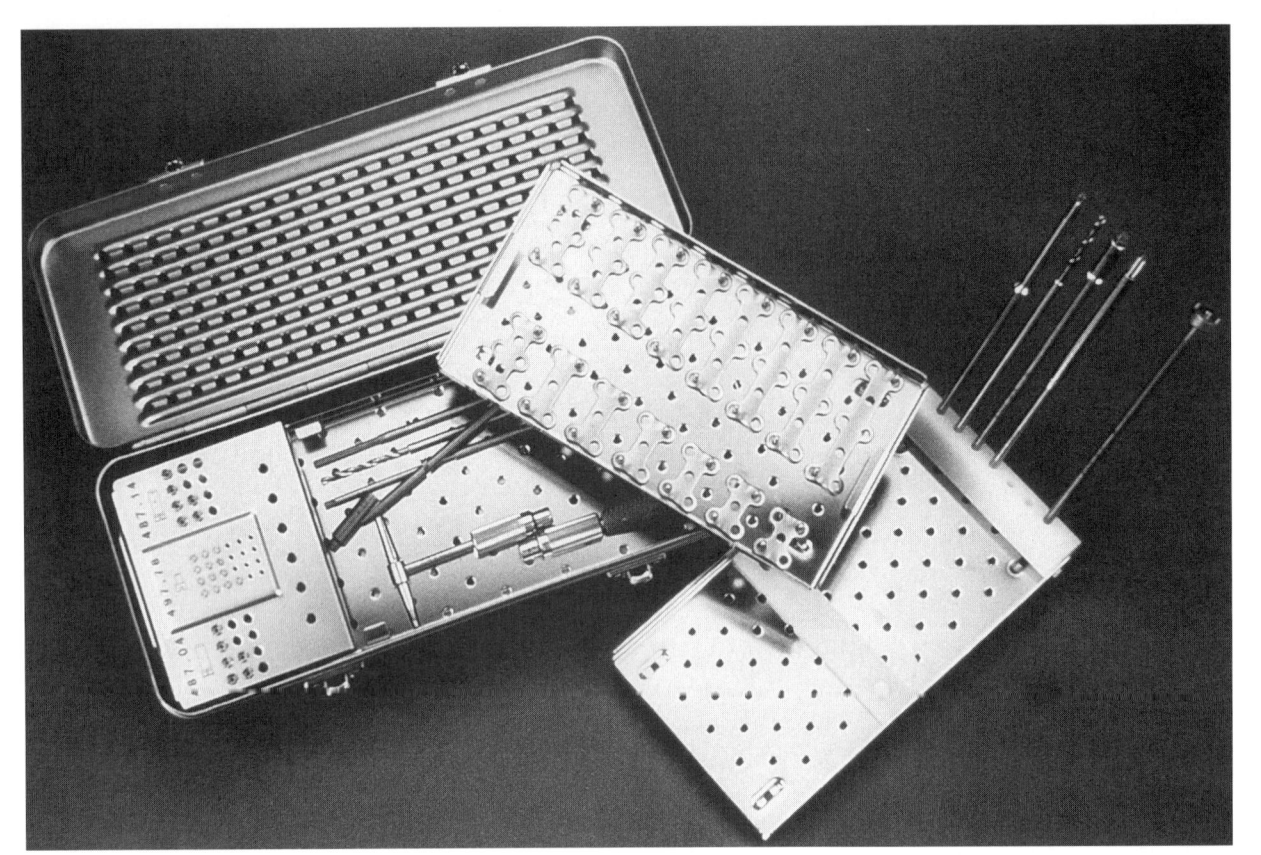

FIG. 3-3. Cervical spine locking plate system.

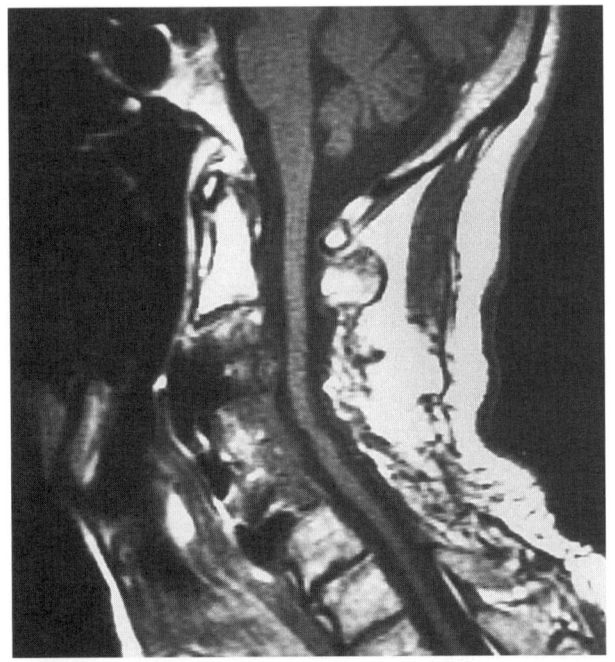

FIG. 3-4. Postoperative magnetic resonance imaging scan following a C5 and C6 corpectomy and application of plate and graft from C4 to C7.

Indications and Contraindications

The CSLP system is indicated for the management of complex spinal disorders requiring anterior stabilization (Table 3-2). Specifically, it can promote an anterior cervical fusion following a single- or multiple-level corpectomy performed in cases of fractures or neoplasms of the cervical vertebrae, spondylosis, or postlaminectomy kyphosis (Figs. 3-5 and 3-6).

Table 3-2
Indications for Anterior Cervical Plate Instrumentation

Following corpectomy for:
   Spondylosis
   Trauma
   Vertebral neoplasm
   Kyphotic deformity

Following diskectomy:
   Multiple-level
   Prior posterior decompression

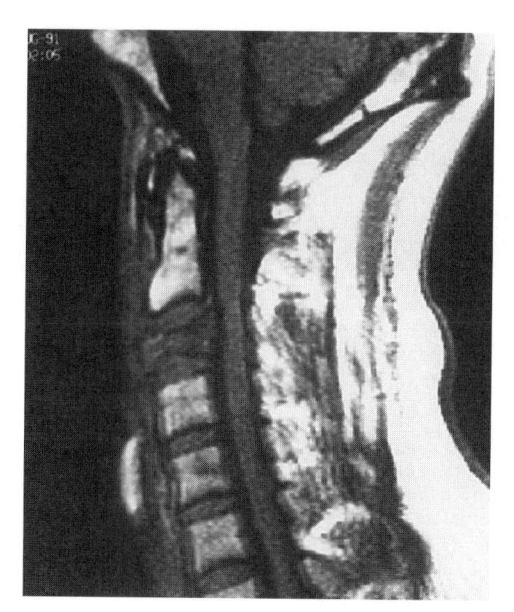

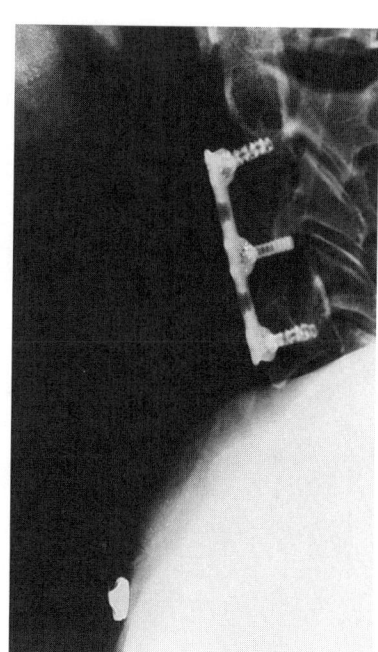

FIG. 3-5. *Left,* Preoperative magnetic resonance imaging scan demonstrating a C3 metastatic neoplasm. *Right,* Postoperative lateral radiograph following a C3 corpectomy with graft and CSLP plate reconstruction.

Its use is not advocated following a single-level anterior diskectomy and interbody fusion. However, the system may be beneficial after multiple-level anterior diskectomy with interbody fusion or after a single-level anterior diskectomy and interbody fusion when that level has previously undergone a posterior decompression (laminectomy or foraminotomy) (Fig. 3-7).

Contraindications for CSLP use in the cervical spine include suboptimal bone for screw fixation (i.e., osteoporosis) or infection (i.e., vertebral osteomyelitis) (Table 3-3). Its use in cases of cervical trauma has several restrictions. Although the plating technique can be used to manage vertebral body fractures or traumatic disk herniations, it must be coupled to a posterior stabilization procedure when posterior element

FIG. 3-6. *Left,* Preoperative computed tomographic/myelographic scan demonstrates marked ventral cord compression resulting from an ossified posterior longitudinal ligament. *Right,* Postoperative lateral radiograph following a C6 corpectomy with graft and CSLP plate reconstruction.

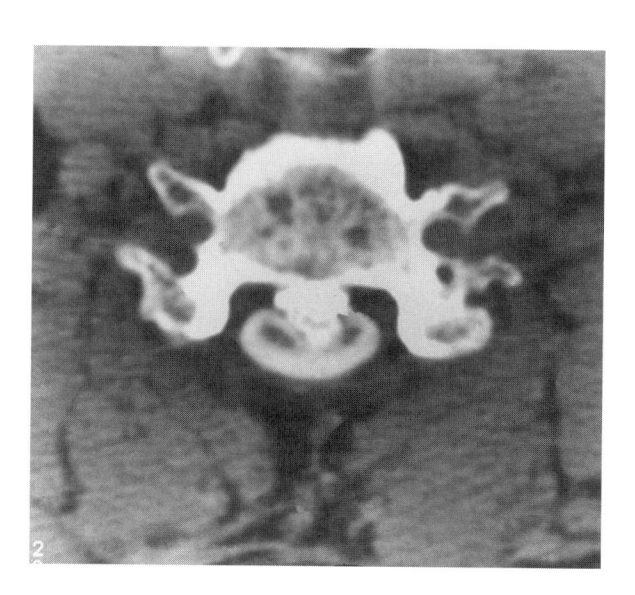

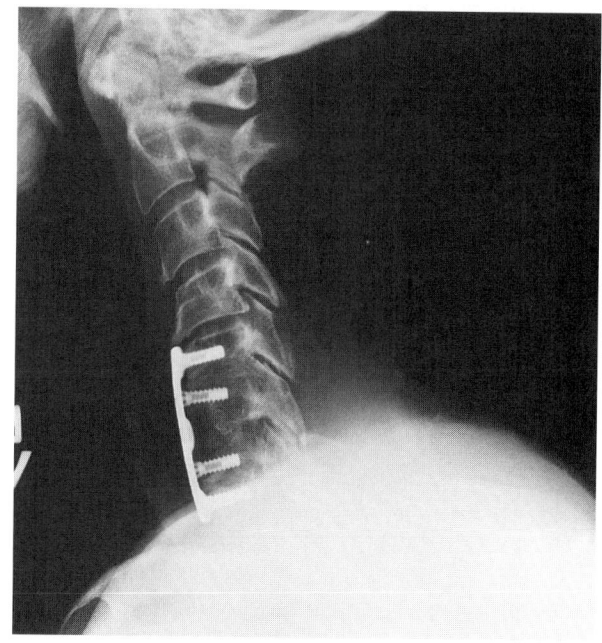

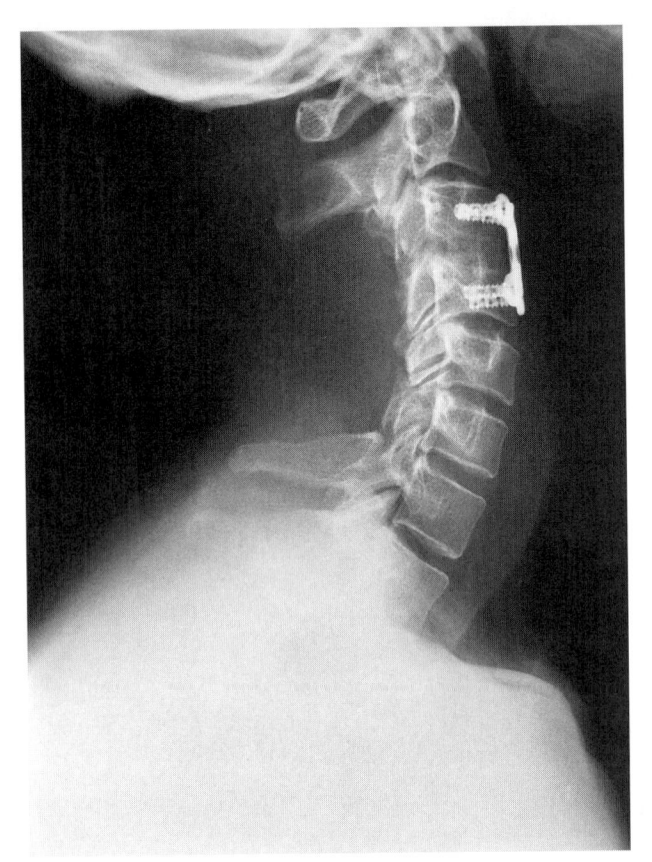

FIG. 3-7. Postoperative cervical spine film demonstrating plate application in conjunction with an interbody fusion in a patient with a prior laminectomy at the same level.

disruption is significant (Fig. 3-8). Furthermore, it does not effectively stabilize a cervical subluxation injury. This injury is best treated with a posterior stabilization procedure alone.

TECHNIQUE

The supine patient is placed with the head and neck in a neutral or slightly extended position. The fluoroscope, if used, is positioned to provide a lateral image of the cervical spine at the appropriate levels. However, the procedure can be performed without fluoroscopy because the anchor screws of the CSLP system do not need to engage the posterior cortex of the vertebral body.

The standard exposure to the anterior cervical spine through a unilateral oblique or transverse incision is performed. The oblique incision along the medial border of the sternocleidomastoid muscle provides greater exposure for

Table 3-3
Contraindications for Anterior Cervical Plate Instrumentation

Vertebral osteomyelitis
Vertebral osteoporosis
Flexion-dislocation injury (without posterior fixation)

multiple-level corpectomy procedures but is less cosmetically attractive than the transverse incision. After radiographic localization of the appropriate spinal level, self-retaining retractor blades are inserted. The appropriate disks and vertebrae are resected to approximately 15 mm in width. This width ensures a satisfactory decompression across the spinal canal and epidural space. A premeasured cotton pad placed in the corpectomy site can serve as a measurement guide.

Bone is removed with a high-speed drill. A larger cylindrical drill bit can be used for the initial bone resection. When the posterior vertebral body cortex is reached, the drill bit is exchanged for one with a smaller, rounded head. This drill head permits finer bone removal near the posterior longitudinal ligament and epidural space.

After satisfactory bone resection, the posterior longitudinal ligament and any remaining compressive osteophytes are resected with a Kerrison rongeur. Excessive bleeding from the bone can be controlled with the intermittent application of a thin layer of bone wax. Bleeding from the epidural veins can be controlled with bipolar electrocautery or Gelfoam pledgets. If a cerebrospinal fluid leak occurs, a layer of Gelfoam or fibrin glue can be placed over the dural opening.

Following a satisfactory decompression of the epidural space, the corpectomy site is measured for insertion of a bone graft. A caliper can accurately determine the length, width, and depth of the graft to be inserted.

The optimal source for an anterior cervical bone graft is either the iliac crest or the fibula. While a fibular graft has a higher cortical bone content for structural support, it lacks the cancellous bone present in iliac crest grafts that facilitates rapid graft incorporation. Although an allograft may be used, early experience with cervical plating techniques has primarily been with autogenous bone grafts.

Once the graft is obtained, it is cut to the appropriate size and shape with an oscillating saw. The anteroposterior height of the bone graft should measure approximately two-thirds the depth of the corpectomy site. The graft should not be so long as to produce excessive distraction on the cervical spine when positioned because this may be a source of postoperative cervical discomfort.

Before graft insertion, the corpectomy site is prepared. Several options exist for preparing this site. A small hole can be drilled in the end plates of the two vertebrae that will lie adjacent to each end of the graft. The ends of the graft can then be fashioned so that a small prong of bone fits tightly into these two holes. This "keystone" approach minimizes the risk of graft dislodgment, but insertion of the graft can be technically difficult and time-consuming.

A second approach involves leaving a shelf of bone along the posterior margins of the two end plates that will lie adjacent to the graft. Although this technique prevents posterior graft migration into the epidural space, it does not prevent anterior graft dislodgment and limits the extent of the

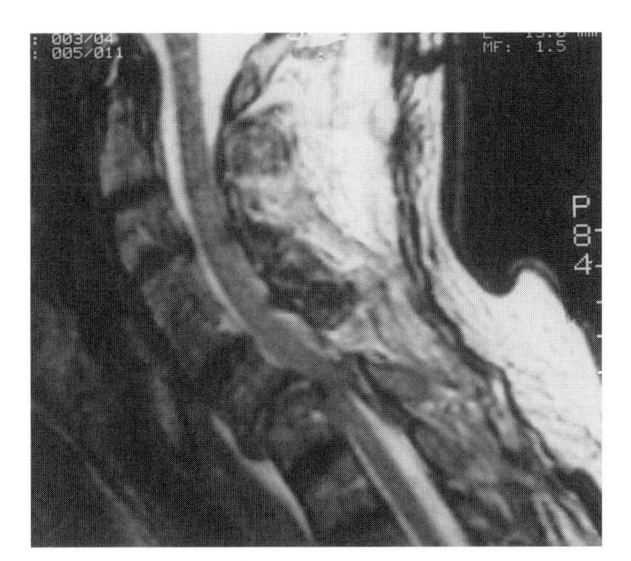

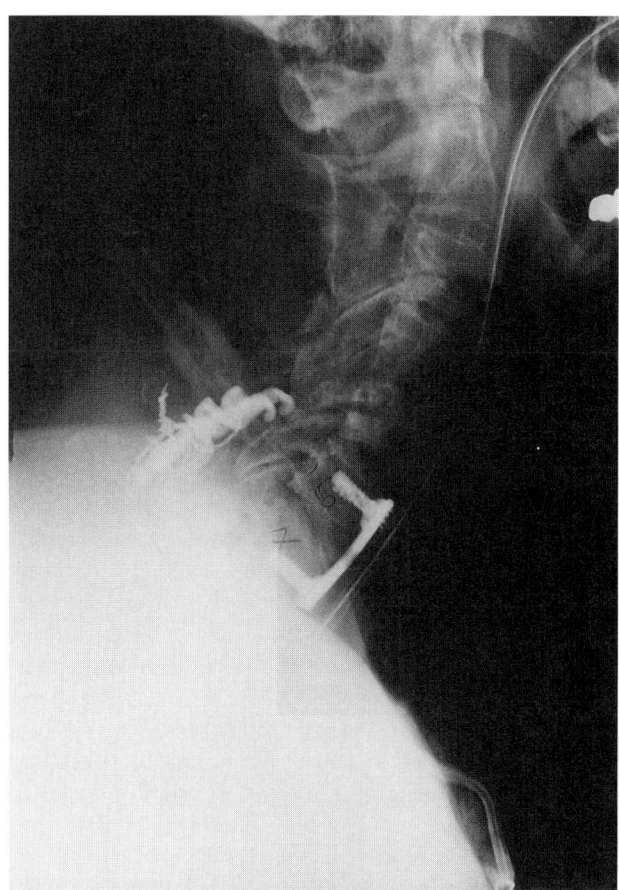

FIG. 3-8. *Left,* Preoperative magnetic resonance imaging scan demonstrating a C6-7 subluxation with marked ventral cord compression. *Right,* Postoperative lateral cervical radiograph demonstrating combined anterior and posterior stabilization following anterior C6-7 diskectomy and interbody fusion.

decompression of the epidural space. Osteophytes compressing the ventral epidural space may extend rostrally or caudally beyond the ends of the corpectomy site. These osteophytes can be removed by undercutting the vertebrae with a bone rongeur. If a bony ledge is to be maintained, however, these osteophytes cannot be removed, and a satisfactory decompression may not be achieved.

The third and preferred option for preparing the corpectomy site is to prepare each vertebral end plate by removing only the cartilaginous surface and the anterior bony margin of the upper end plate. The two end plates are fashioned so that they are parallel to one another. This process leaves a broad, flat surface of cortical bone to accept a graft in which each end is also broad and flat. The increased surface area of bone-to-bone contact facilitates the fusion process. In addition, there is less risk for "telescoping" of the graft, which can occur with the keystone technique if the rigid cortical bone of the graft migrates superiorly into the softer cancellous bone of the vertebral body. Although the end plates are not contoured to prevent graft dislodgment, the risk of dislodgment is minimized with the screw fixation of the overlying plate to the graft.

After preparation of the graft and corpectomy site, halter traction or manual in-line traction is applied to the patient's cervical spine and the graft is tapped into position. The graft is oriented so that one of its cortical surfaces is directed anteriorly. This will permit screw fixation of the overlying plate to the graft. If a satisfactory fit is not achieved on initial placement, the graft is removed, appropriately contoured, and reinserted.

The appropriate length plate is then selected and positioned. The arrow on the rostral end aids in positioning the plate. If the plate length is correct, the two pairs of holes on either end of the plate should lie just beyond the ends of the bone graft and over the adjacent vertebrae. This length permits the anchor screws to be positioned optimally in the center of the vertebrae. The plate should not overlap with an intact disk space, as this overlap increases the risk of screw loosening and fixation failure. If the plate must be bent to conform better to the curvature of the anterior cervical spine, a slightly longer plate should be selected because any bending will reduce the plate length. The underlying bone surface should be inspected for elevated bony ridges that prevent the plate from sitting flush on the graft and adjacent vertebral bodies. If present, these ridges are removed with a drill or rongeur and the plate is bent to fit the spine and graft contours better. Excessive bending of the plate should be avoided because bending can fatigue the metal and compromise its structural integrity. Furthermore, excessive bending may cause the plate center to ride too high over the underlying bone graft, compromising fixation of the plate to the graft.

When the plate and underlying bony surface have been satisfactorily contoured, the plate is positioned. The drill guide is placed in the superior lateral hole of the plate. When the drill guide is positioned properly in the rostral holes, it is directed superiorly and medially. The 3-mm drill bit is then passed through the drill guide and the hole is drilled. The guide limits the depth of drill insertion to 14 mm. In most individuals, this limits the depth of the hole to the anterior two thirds of the vertebrae. However, in children, a 14-mm depth may traverse the entire vertebrae and require intraoperative fluoroscopy to monitor the drill and screw position closely. The hole is then tapped to set the threads into the bone, and the anchor screw is inserted. The screw should not be excessively tightened because too much force may strip the threads in the bone and compromise screw-to-bone fixation. The proper amount of torque can be gauged approximately by using only the thumb and two fingers to tighten the screw.

The drill guide is then positioned in the inferior plate hole closest to the surgeon. Any final adjustment of the medial-lateral alignment of the plate needs to be made at this point. Alignment in this plane can best be approximated by using the patient's sternal notch and nasion as reference marks. Insertion of the anchor screw through this hole will limit any further plate movement.

The two remaining holes at either end of the plate on the side of the plate furthest from the surgeon are then drilled in a similar manner. These holes are more difficult to drill because the trachea and esophagus must be retracted. If these holes are drilled before securing the plate, the chance that the plate will slip out of position during the drilling is greater.

An alternative to plate and screw positioning may be required when the system is used at the cervicothoracic junction. Because of the overlying soft-tissue structures and the curvature of the anterior surface of the spinal column at this level, it may be difficult to position the two lower screws in the vertebral body in a direction perpendicular to the plane of the plate. In this case, the plate may be turned 180 degrees so that the arrow on the plate points caudally. This position permits the drill to be directed in a more favorable angle at the caudal end of the plate. The remainder of the technique is unchanged.

After placing the four screws at the two ends of the plate, the remaining plate holes overlying the graft are located. One or two of the holes closest to the graft and away from either end plate are selected. These holes are used to secure the plate to the graft. A hole is drilled, taking care to avoid excessive pressure on the graft. Excessive pressure may result in posterior dislodgment of the graft and the need to remove the screws and plate rapidly for graft removal and repositioning. If the space between either lateral corpectomy margin and the graft is large enough, a small dural guide or nerve hook can be placed so that the distal end lies underneath the graft and permits gentle, upward pressure during the drilling procedure. Once made, the hole is tapped and the anchor screw and locking nut are inserted. At this point, the CSLP procedure is complete.

If a screw hole in either the vertebrae or bone graft is stripped, two options exist. The screw can be removed and the hole filled with a small amount of methylmethacrylate. The screw is then reinserted before the methylmethacrylate sets. Alternatively, the anchor screws used for the ancillary set of extra long plates have a slightly larger diameter (4.35 mm) and can be used to replace the smaller screws in the 4.0-mm diameter hole. If firm screw fixation still is not achieved, a shorter or longer plate should be selected and new holes drilled if space allows. If sufficient space does not exist for a different size plate, the system should not be applied. The patient can be placed in a halo or suboccipital-mandibular-immobilization (SOMI) brace instead.

After satisfactory plate application, the wound is closed, and a hard cervical collar is worn for 8 to 12 weeks. Halo brace immobilization is rarely needed. Postoperative cervical spine radiographs are obtained immediately after surgery and at 2, 6, and 12 months postoperatively.

CLINICAL RESULTS

A preliminary report of anterior cervical plate fixation using the CSLP system has indicated favorable results (Table 3-4) (Suh, Kostuik, & Esses, 1990). No incidents of pseudoarthrosis or iatrogenic neurologic injury resulting from screw insertion have been reported, and the incidence of postoperative screw migration has been minimal.

Table 3-4
Indications and Contraindications for Use of Anterior Cervical Spine Locking Plate System

Indications
   Cervical instability
     Tumor
     Trauma
     Remote infection
     Disk disruption
     Ligament disruption
   Decompression corpectomy for stenosis
   Maintain cervical lordosis

Contraindications
   Absolute
     Infection
     Metal sensitivity
   Relative
     Osteoporosis
     Subacute infection
     Rheumatoid arthritis
     Diabetes

The author's experience with the CSLP system includes 43 patients. Thirty-three patients underwent a single- or multiple-level corpectomy followed by plate fixation. In 10 patients, a plate was applied after a single- or multiple-level diskectomy and interbody fusion. All patients in whom the system was placed after a diskectomy had previously undergone a posterior decompressive procedure at the same level.

There were no incidents of pseudoarthrosis, iatrogenic neurologic injury, or isolated screw backout. Two patients who had each undergone plate fixation following a two-level corpectomy required a second operation for plate dislodgment. One plate was dislodged inferiorly during urgent reintubation of the patient 4 days after the initial surgery. The first plate was removed and a slightly longer plate inserted.

The second patient's plate dislodged after the vertebrae in which the caudal pair of screws had been inserted collapsed. This collapse necessitated removing the initial plate and graft construct, in addition to the collapsed vertebrae. A longer plate and graft construct was then inserted, and the patient was placed in a halo brace postoperatively. Both patients subsequently obtained satisfactory cervical fusion.

SUMMARY

The CSLP is an easy, safe, and effective means of internally stabilizing the cervical spine and facilitating a solid arthrodesis. It minimizes the complications associated with graft dislodgment and virtually eliminates the need for a halo brace. When properly applied to the appropriate patient, the incidence of system failure is minimal. If a system failure does occur (i.e., screw or plate breakage or dislodgment), the variety of plate lengths permits revision in most cases. If a solid arthrodesis is achieved before a system failure, the plate and screws can be removed because the objective of their use is achieved. Although the technique of plate and screw insertion is relatively straightforward, it does require care and attention to detail in preparing the plating site, selecting a plate of the proper length, and applying the plate and screws to the spinal column.

REFERENCES

Bell, G.D., & Bailey, S.I. (1977). Anterior cervical fusion for trauma. *Clinical Orthopaedics and Related Research, 128,* 155–158.

Bohler, J., & Gaudermak, T. (1980). Anterior plate stabilization for fracture dislocations of the lower cervical spine. *Journal of Trauma, 20,* 203–205.

Brown, J.A., Havel, P., Ebraheim, N., Greenblott, S.M., Jackson, W.T. (1988). Cervical stabilization by plate and bone fusion. *Spine, 13,* 236–240.

Capen, D.A., Garland, D.E., & Waters, R.L. (1985). Surgical stabilization of the cervical spine. *Clinical Orthopaedics and Related Research, 196,* 229–237.

Caspar, W. (1986). Anterior cervical fusion and interbody stabilization with the trapezial osteosynthetic plate technique. Aesculap Scientific Information Leaflet S-039. Burlingame, CA: Aesculap Instruments Corporation.

Cloward, R.B. (1958). The anterior approach for removal of ruptured cervical discs. *Journal of Neurosurgery, 15,* 602–614.

Cochran, G. (1982). *A Primer of Orthopaedic Biomechanics* (pp. 180–198). New York: Churchill Livingstone.

Goodman, J., & Seligson, D. (1983). The anterior cervical plate. *Spine, 8,* 700–706.

Gore, D.R., Sepic, S.B. (1986). Anterior cervical fusion for degenerated or protruded discs. *Spine, 9,* 667–671.

Herrmann, H.D. (1975). Metal plate fixation after anterior fusion of unstable fracture dislocation of the cervical spine. *Acta Neurochirurgica, 32,* 101–111.

Lane, A.W. (1914). *The operative treatment of fractures.* London: Medical Publishing, 1914.

Morscher, E., Sutter, F., Jennis, M., & Olerud, S. (1986). Die vordere Verplattung der Halswirbelsaule mit dem Hohlschraubenplattensystem. *Der Chirurg, 57,* 702–707.

Raveh, J., Stesh, M., Sutter, F., & Greiner, R. (1984). Use of titanium-coated hollow screw and reconstruction plate system in bridging of lower jaw defects. *Journal of Oral and Maxillofacial Surgery, 42,* 281–294.

Riley, L.H., Robinson, R.A., Johnson, K.A., & Walker, A.E. (1969). The results of anterior interbody fusion of the cervical spine. *Journal of Neurosurgery, 30,* 127–133.

Simmons, E.H., & Bhalla, S.K. (1969). Anterior cervical discectomy and fusion. *Journal of Bone and Joint Surgery, British Volume, 51,* 225–236.

Smith, G.W., & Robinson, R.A. (1958). The treatment of cervical spine disorders by anterior removal of the intervertebral disc and interbody fusion. *Journal of Bone and Joint Surgery, American Volume, 40,* 607–624.

Suh, P.B., Kostuik, J.P., & Esses, S.I. (1990). Anterior cervical plate fixation with the titanium hollow screw plate system: A preliminary report. *Spine, 15,* 1079–1081.

Van Peteghem, P.K., & Schweigel, J.F. (1979). The fractured cervical spine rendered unstable by anterior cervical fusion. *Journal of Trauma, 19,* 110–114.

White, A.A., III, Southwick, W.O., DePonte, R.J., et al. (1973). Relief of pain by cervical spine fusion for spondylosis. *Journal of Bone and Joint Surgery, American Volume, 55,* 525–534.

CHAPTER 4

Stabilization of the Cervical Spine Utilizing the Orion Anterior Cervical Plate System

Gary L. Lowery

HIGHLIGHTS

The Orion Anterior Cervical Plate System was developed in accordance with several important biomechanical and biologic principles. The author's philosophy for stabilization of the anterior cervical spine led to a specific design rationale. Implementation of the design and subsequent manufacturing of the Orion system was carried out through Sofamor-Danek Group, Inc. (Memphis, TN).

Several anterior cervical implants that are currently available and widely used have uniformly met with good clinical success, both in the author's experience and in the literature. This experience led to modifications that form the basis of the features and benefits of the Orion system (Table 4-1).

The primary indication for use of the Orion plate in the cervical spine is to reestablish stability. Instability can be from anterior column deficiencies such as trauma, tumor, and remote infection or from diskal and ligamentous disruption as in facet dislocations. Decompressive corpectomy for stenosis (i.e., multiple-level osteophytosis or OPLL) with strut reconstruction also benefits from the added stability of internal fixation. The author believes that multiple-level interbody grafting requires the additional stability provided by selective vertebral immobilization through anterior plate and screws. This selective immobilization cannot be achieved through the use of a halo.

Internal fixation can help to maintain a lordotic posture of the cervical spine and may improve the percentage of successful fusions for difficult reconstructions. Posterior column deficiencies, such as facet dislocation, can be stabilized via an anterior approach provided the interspace is not overdistracted by the anterior graft. Placement of a lordotically wedged graft is helpful. Iatrogenic posterior column deficiencies, such as postlaminectomy kyphosis, present a bigger challenge for anterior fixation alone. These cases may require anteroposterior procedures. However, if the facets are intact and one can insert lordotic interbody grafts, then anterior fixation alone may be sufficient. Lordotic positioning of the spine as well as multiple vertebral body screws are mandatory.

Acute infections and metal sensitivity are two strong contraindications for anterior plate fixation. Relative contraindications for any anterior plate fixation are osteoporotic bone, subacute period of infection, and poor constitutional factors such as diabetes and rheumatoid arthritis that may be associated with a higher incidence of postoperative infection. Inability or unwillingness to cooperate with postoperative instructions would also be a relative contraindication for metallic implantation anteriorly (Table 4-2).

Advantages and disadvantages of the Orion Anterior Cervical Plate System can best be viewed from the concept of features and benefits (Table 4-1). An important feature of the Orion plate is the predetermined lordotic curvature of the plate. A series of lateral radiographs (flexion/neutral/extension) were reviewed to determine an appropriate neutral lordotic attitude (C3-7) of the cervical spine. The Orion plate can, therefore, be used to obtain and maintain cervical lordosis. This posture allows for a more normal physiologic functioning of the posterior cervical musculature postoperatively. Posterior musculature fatigue in the postoperative period should be minimized if the spine is not in a relative kyphotic position. This is obviously more significant when multiple levels are being stabilized. Whether this helps prevent the advanced degeneration of adjacent levels is theoretical, and long-term follow-up is required to answer these questions. Although the plate can be contoured further, the surgeon has to remember that the cephalad and caudad screw angulations will then change relative to the vertebral body when the plate contour is altered.

The next important feature of the Orion plate is the locked cephalad and caudad screws. These provide a secure constrained construct of the plate and screws with the bone. If the screw breaks, the locking mechanism prevents screw migration, ensuring both surgeon and patient that the risk of tracheoesophageal or neurovascular injuries is minimized. The screws can be locked whether placement is unicortical or bicortical.

The current plate design allows for screws to be placed convergent into the cervical vertebrae. The screws converge in a 6-degree medial direction, providing ultimate safety from injury to the vertebral artery and, if placed unicortically, posing no threat to the spinal cord or nerve roots. The screws also are directed 15 degrees cephalad and 15 degrees caudad at the ends of the construct. When the screws are locked, this feature provides additional stability for pullout, especially for flexion and extension forces on the longer plate-graft constructs.

Variable-length 4.0-mm cancellous screws are available from 10 to 26 mm in 1.0-mm increments. Although a 13-mm screw (actual thread under plate and in bone) will uniformly be safe to insert, longer screws provide additional stability. The cancellous thread design provides excellent purchase in the vertebral body, and biomechanical data have substantiated that longer screws are superior in pullout. The variable length of the screws gives the surgeon the ability to purchase the "posterior vertebral cortex" if desired. The screws can be locked or nonlocked, depending on the surgeon's preference.

An extensive range of plates are available. Plate sizes progress in 2.5-mm increments for the 25-to-90-mm plates and in 5.0-mm increments for longer plates (90 to 100 mm). This extensive plate range allows for multiple-level interbody fusions and most any anterior strut reconstruction. Again, the plate can be contoured, for example, to reverse the curvature across the cervicothoracic junction.

The Orion plate has intervening diagonal slots that enable variable positioning of the screws to the vertebral body. Selective vertebral immobilization is important to control forces (especially torsion) acting on the cervical spine. This variable access also aids in obtaining and maintaining cervical lordosis. The intervening screws are nonlocked. Care should be taken to use the longest screw that can be safely inserted to increase pullout strength. Angling the screws (not straight ahead) will also aid in obtaining lordosis and decreasing pullout. If the bone is osteoporotic or there is insecurity in the purchase of the screw, a 4.35-mm screw can be used. This screw is designed only for use at the intervening slots and must be directed straight ahead (90 degrees to the plate). This 4.35-mm screw will effectively be locked into the slots through interference fit and should not back out (specialized screw-retrieval instruments are available if the screws need to be removed). The intervening screws (4.0 and 4.35 mm) are also available in a variety of lengths.

One last important feature of the Orion plate is its metallic makeup. Titanium makes this plate biocompatible and allows for less image artifact on both computed tomographic (CT) and magnetic resonance imaging (MRI) scans than stainless steel implants. Excellent values have been achieved in the biomechanical testing of the Orion plate, which is made of a titanium alloy (Ti 6 Al-4V) with a tiodized surface coating. This provides 56% more tensile strength, 65% more yield strength, and 70% more fatigue strength than commercially pure (CP) titanium. The tiodized processing increases the surface resistance to galling and fretting wear as well as improving the fatigue life.

Table 4-1
Advantages and Disadvantages of Use of the Orion Anterior Cervical Plate System

Feature	Advantages	Disadvantages
Predetermined lordotic curvature	Obtain and maintain appropriate cervical lordosis Prevent kyphosis: stabilize grafts from fragmentation and collapse	
Locked cephalad and caudad screws	Secure constrained construct Prevent screw loosening 6-degree convergence: surgeon familiarity and unicortical safety 15-degree cephalad/caudad: more stable construct in pullout	Some decrease in flexibility at upper and lower ends of cervical spine Limited overlap of plate with cephalad and caudad vertebrae make revision of "poor screw purchase" problematic
Intervening diagonal slots	Multiple and variable screw access Selective vertebral immobilization Obtain and maintain lordosis 4.35-mm constrained intervening screws	
Cancellous screws	Improved vertebral purchase Variable lengths (10–26 mm) in 1.0-mm increments Unicortical or bicortical Locked ends of construct and intervening slots	
Extensive range of plate lengths	25–90 mm in 2.5-mm increments 90–110 mm in 5.0-mm increments	
Titanium with tiodized surface coating	Biocompatible Less image artifact with CT and MRI Can be easily contoured further Improved tensile strength, yield strength, and fatigue strength Increased surface resistance to galling and fretting	

Table 4-2
Indications and Contraindications for Anterior Plate

Indications
    Cervical instability
        Tumor
        Trauma
        Remote infection
        Disk disruption
        Ligament disruption
    Decompressing corpectomy for stenosis
    Maintain cervical lordosis
Contraindications
    Absolute
        Infection
        Metal sensitivity
    Relative
        Osteoporosis
        Subacute infection
        Rheumatoid arthritis
        Diabetes

SURGICAL TECHNIQUE

Many constrained systems require precise angles to be drilled for screw insertion. Although the flexibility for screw placement is taken out of the hands of the surgeon, a safety factor is added for precise and safe angulation of the screws. A three- or four-level corpectomy, reconstruction, and anterior plating can easily be performed through a transverse incision by performing extensive subcutaneous and fascial dissection without additional morbidity. In difficult dissections or reconstructions, a carotid incision may be better. To date, the Orion plate has been successfully inserted across the occipitocervical junction and cervicothoracic junction through expansile approaches. However, most standard procedures from C2 to T1 can be performed without an expansile approach.

Preliminary Steps

- Position the head in a stable supine position (head rest or traction) with slight extension of the neck. Confirm positioning and vertebral levels to be visualized via fluoroscopy. Traction on the arms is often helpful.
- A standard transverse incision can be made for one- or two-level corpectomies. It is important to dissect the fascial planes fully for longer constructs. Occasionally a carotid incision is necessary for difficult exposures and long reconstructions.
- Perform corpectomy or prepare interbody fusion receptor sites.
- Obtain cervical lordosis and/or distraction if necessary.
- Prepare trapezoidal strut construct or trapezoidal interbody fusion wedge(s).
- Carefully position and impact strut or interbody fusion construct(s).
- Release distraction (promoting compression) and check stability of construct.
- Again, be sure that levels to be instrumented can be easily identified on fluoroscopy.
- Ensure that all anterior osteophytes are removed for proper plate positioning.

Step 1: Determine Appropriate Plate Length

Position the convergent plate screw holes close to the graft receptor site at both cephalad and caudad ends (Fig. 4-1, *a*).

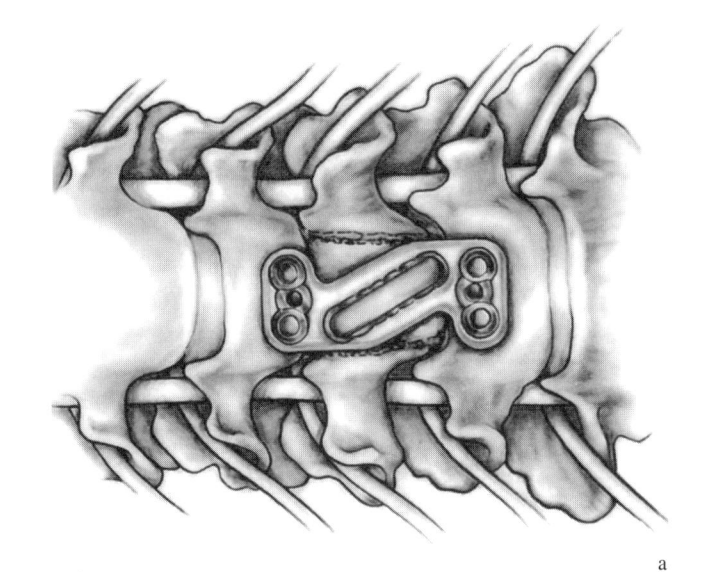

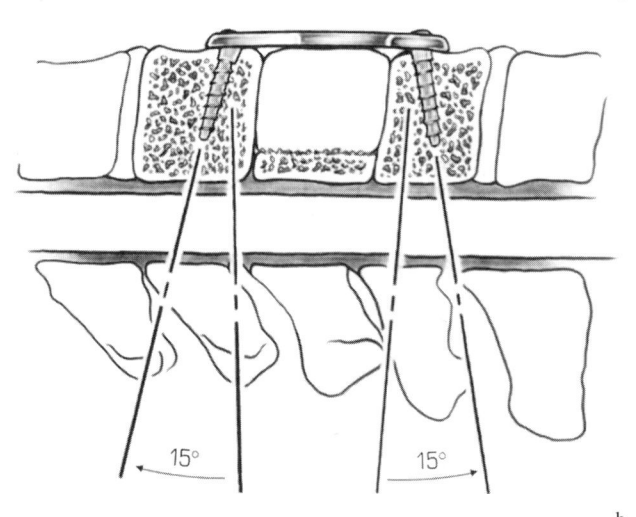

FIG. 4-1. (*a*) Bone graft and plate position. (*b*) Cephalad/caudad screw angulation.

This allows for the 15-degree cephalad and caudad screw angulation (Fig. 4-1, *b*) and helps ensure that the plate does not extend over the adjacent disk spaces.

Step 2: Adjust Lordotic Curvature of Plate if Necessary

The amount of lordosis designed into the Orion anterior cervical plate is acceptable in most cases. If required, changes can be made to the standard machined lordotic curve by using the Orion plate bender. A gentle bend should be made over the entire length of the plate, and sharp angulations must be avoided. It is important to note that plate contouring will alter the standard cephalad and caudad angulation of the end screws.

Step 3: Secure the Orion Plate to the Plate Holder

Two options are available for holding the Orion plate. One design locks within the central slots of the various plates (except for the smallest plates less than 30 mm) (Fig. 4-2, *a*). To attach the plate holder to the plate, slide the sleeve toward the handle and engage the feet into the plate's diago-

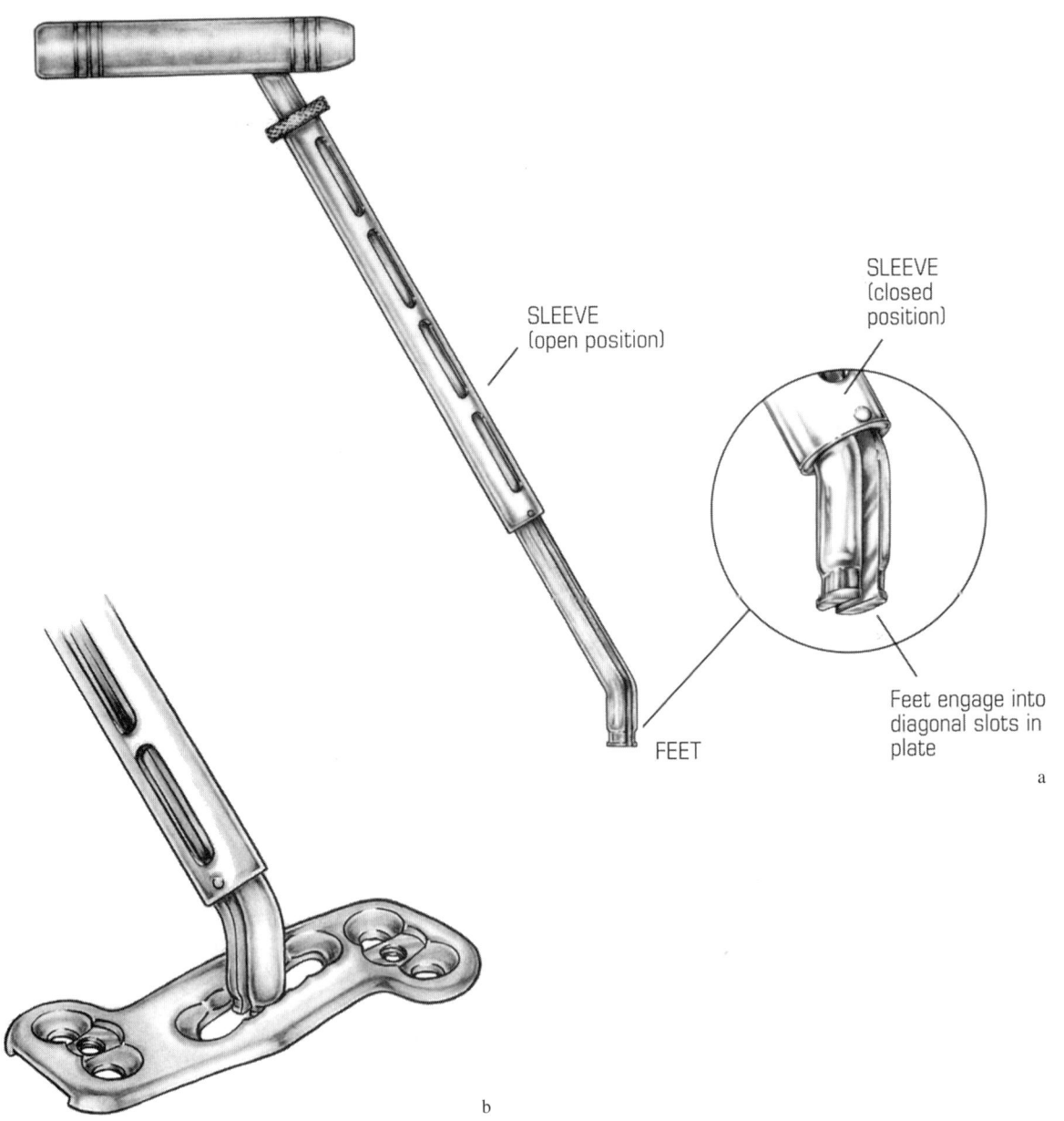

FIG. 4-2. (a) Orion plate holder. (b) Plate holder locked into plate.

nal slot. Slide the sleeve down toward the plate to lock the holder to the plate (Fig. 4-2, b). The second plate holder clamps down to the side of the plate and is currently being manufactured for use especially with the smaller plates.

Step 4: Position the Orion Plate on the Anterior Surface of the Spine

Review landmarks to ensure that the plate is centered medially/laterally on the spine. The uncinate processes serve as excellent reference points.

Step 5: Insert the Drill Guide

Seat the drill guide into the plate at the correct 15-degree cephalad/caudad angle (Fig. 4-3, a) and 6-degree convergent angle (Fig. 4-3, b). Once the drill guide is correctly seated in the plate, it can then be securely locked into the plate by applying light downward pressure on the drill guide handle, making sure to align the handle along the longitudinal axis of the plate.

Step 6: Drill Holes for Taps/Screws

Insert the appropriate drill bit into the drill guide. Drill the screw holes using either the 13-mm drill bit (Fig. 4-4, a) or the adjustable drill bit and adjustable drill stop (Fig. 4-4, b). Screw length is determined by the depth of bone purchase required.

For standard unicortical screw purchase, the 13-mm drill bit is used. For screws other than 13 mm in length, the adjustable drill bit (10 to 26 mm depth) and adjustable drill stop are used (Fig. 4-4, b). If required, controlled penetration of the posterior cortex may be achieved by setting the

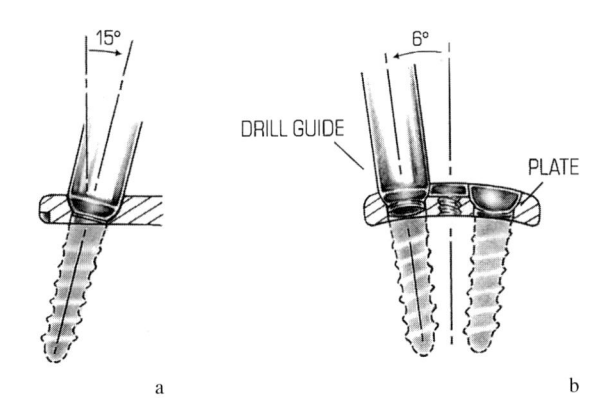

FIG. 4-3. (a) Angulation of drill guide in cephalad/caudad direction. (b) Angulation of drill guide toward midline.

adjustable drill stop at the appropriate depth. The adjustable drill stop provides for 1-mm increments and an additional safety factor during the drilling procedure as well as fluoroscopic visualization.

Step 7: Tap the Vertebral Bodies

Remove the drill guide, insert the appropriate tap into the predrilled hole at the same angulation, and tap the vertebral bodies using the tap that corresponds to the drill-bit length determined in Step 6. Taps are available in the same configuration as the drill bits—13-mm screw tap (Fig. 4-5, a) and adjustable screw tap and adjustable tap stop for 10 to 26 mm (Fig. 4-5, b).

Step 8: Implant Screws

A depth gauge may be required to confirm the depth of the hole for proper screw length. The depth gauge works either through the plate (Fig. 4-6, a) or against the bone (Fig. 4-6, b) and is accurate for both unicortical and bicortical techniques. The appropriate-length screw can be verified using the screw/plate gauge (Fig. 4-6, c). Insert the appropriate-length screw through the plate, using the screwdriver (tapered, self-holding tip) and tighten the screw securely (not final tightening) (Fig. 4-6, d).

The preferred method of screw insertion is as follows: (1) Drill, tap, and place one screw securely through the plate (if concerns requiring mediolateral tilt or positioning arise, obtain an anteroposterior (AP) radiograph prior to drilling the screw hole). (2) Drill, tap, and place one screw securely at the opposite end of the plate diagonally from the first screw position. (3) Drill the remaining two screw implant sites and tap until the screws are securely inserted.

Step 9: Final Tightening of Bone Screws

Normally, the plate holder is not required after the first one or two screws have been implanted. However, it can be used throughout the entire procedure and can also be easily repositioned during implantation.

Tighten the screws to ensure screw seating below the surface of the plate. Obtain radiographs to ensure that screw length and screw position are appropriate. Although plate malposition may be determined from a lateral radiograph

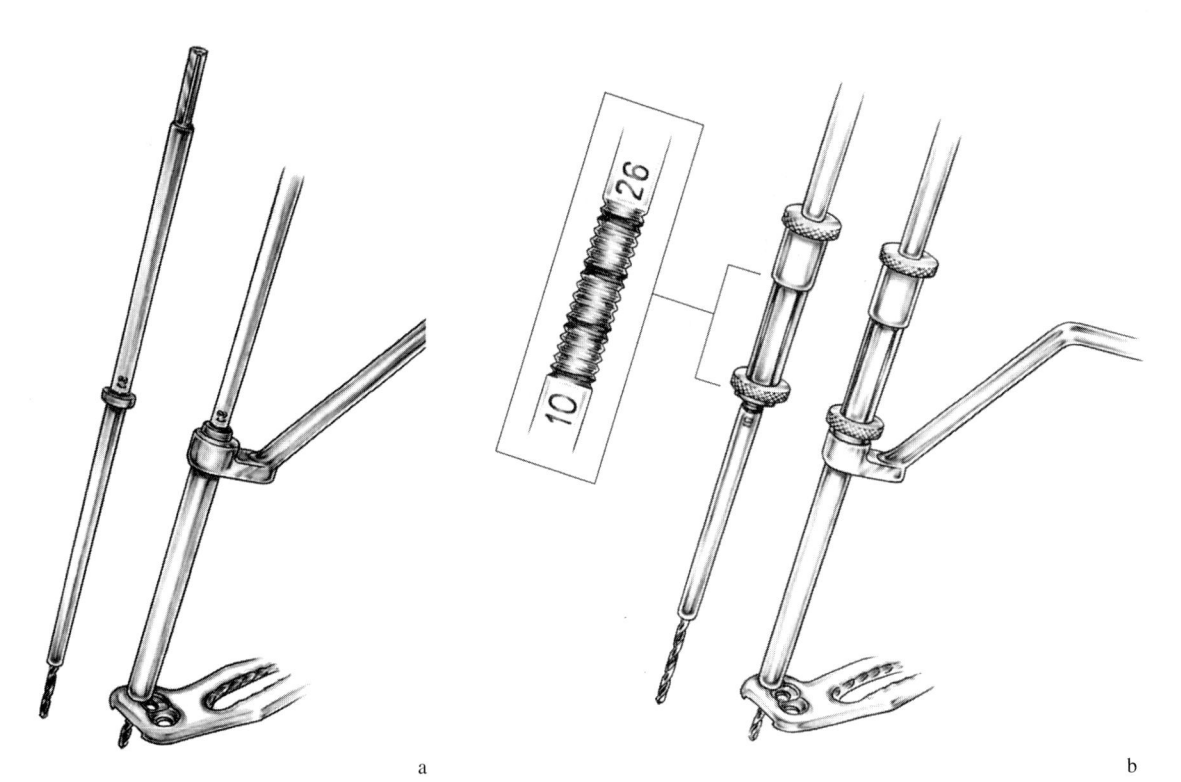

FIG. 4-4. (a) Drill guide and 13-mm drill bit. (b) Drill guide with adjustable drill bit and adjustable drill stop.

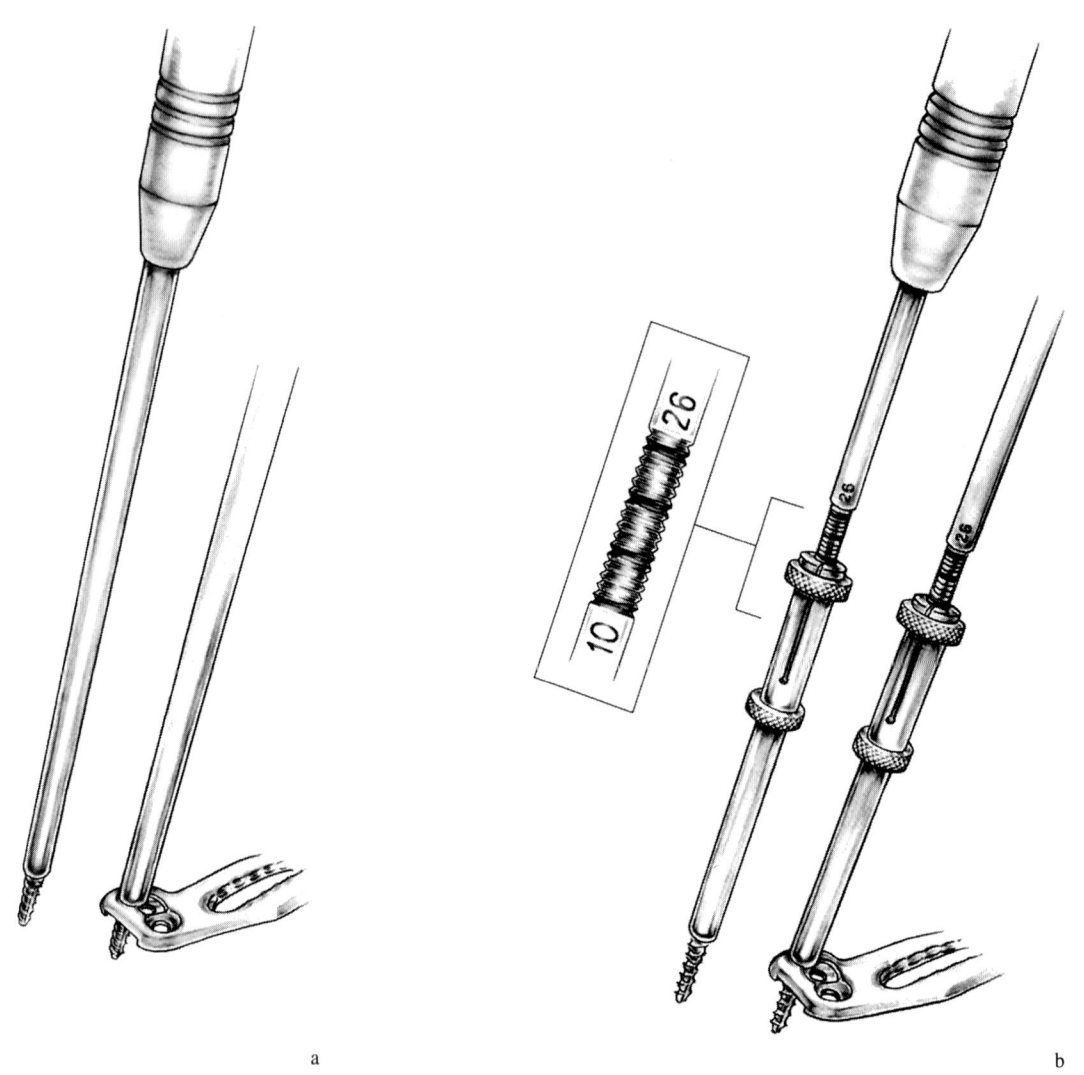

FIG. 4-5. (a) 13-mm screw tap. (b) Adjustable screw tap and adjustable tap stop.

(i.e., screws not aligned in the same plane), an AP radiograph provides additional information regarding verification of implant position.

Screws (4.0 mm) can now be placed in the diagonal slot if necessary (i.e., multiple-level interbody fusions or long strut graft reconstructions). If the bone is osteoporotic or there is insecurity in screw purchase, the gold-colored 4.35-mm diameter central slot screws (11-, 13-, or 15-mm lengths) are recommended for use in the diagonal slots. The drill guide is positioned in the center slot of the plate, and the hole is drilled to either an 11-, 13-, or 15-mm depth. These holes should be drilled in a "straight ahead" manner (90 degrees) into the bone. The gold-colored 4.35-mm tap and adjustable tap stop are then used to tap the hole to the appropriate depth. The 4.35-mm screws are then inserted using the screwdriver and firmly tightened.

Step 10: Insert the Locking Screws

Attach the lock screw holder to the lock screw by gently squeezing the prongs and then engage the holder in the lock screw (Fig. 4-7, *a*). Slide the sleeve down toward the end of the holder. After the lock screw is initially threaded into the plate (Fig. 4-7, *b*), detach the lock screw holder by pulling the sleeve up and tilting the holder to release from the lock screw. (*Note:* **Do not attempt to tighten the lock screw with the lock screw holder. Doing so will damage the instrument.**) Final tightening of the lock screw is accomplished through the use of the lock screwdriver (Fig. 4-7, *c*). Once the lock screwdriver is firmly placed into the slot, turn the lock screw clockwise while maintaining axial pressure until the screwdriver slips out of the slot (this is a self-limiting device). The lock screw is now firmly secured.

Step 11: Irrigate Wound and Close Wound over a Drain.

A summary of technical hints appears in Table 4-3.

EARLY CLINICAL RESULTS

Eighty-six procedures using the Orion plate have been performed at five initial centers. All but two (98%) are avail-

CHAPTER 4 / STABILIZATION OF THE CERVICAL SPINE UTILIZING THE ORION ANTERIOR CERVICAL PLATE SYSTEM

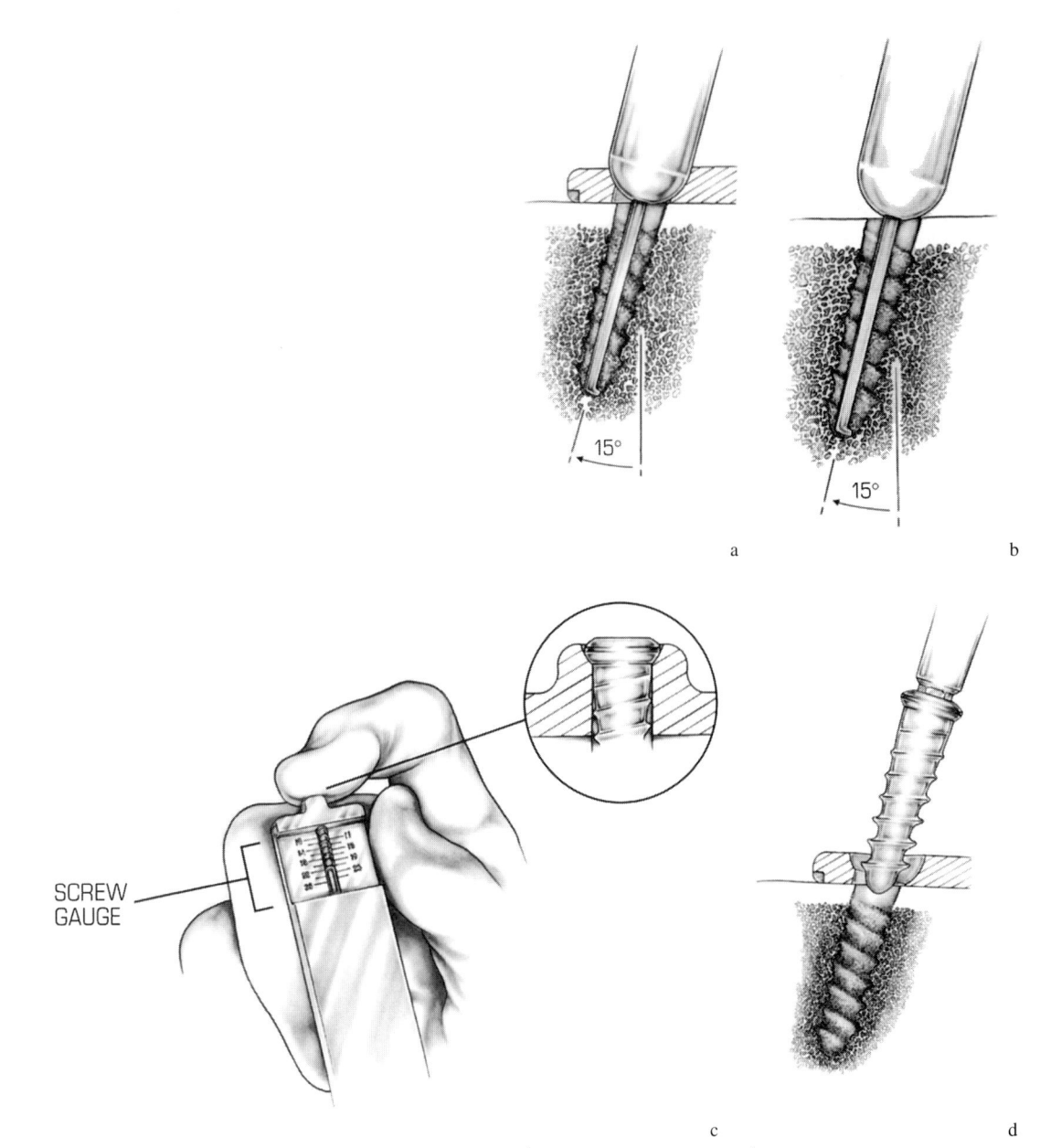

FIG. 4-6. (a) Depth gauge through plate. (b) Depth gauge on bone. (c) Verifying screw length. (d) Screw insertion.

Table 4-3
Orion Anterior Cervical Plate System—Technical Hints

Use the longest unicortical screw for ultimate safety and improved stability (routinely 16 mm).
Go bicortical for longer, more difficult reconstructions.
If the screws are loose, go bicortical or redirect them.
Start screws (and Orion plate) just past the graft receptor site.
Use 4.35-mm central slot screws for intervening diagonal slot if screws are not secure.
Angle 4.0-mm intervening screws. Do not place "straight ahead."
Position lordotic interbody grafts or lordotic strut reconstruction.
Use intervening slots to obtain and maintain lordosis.

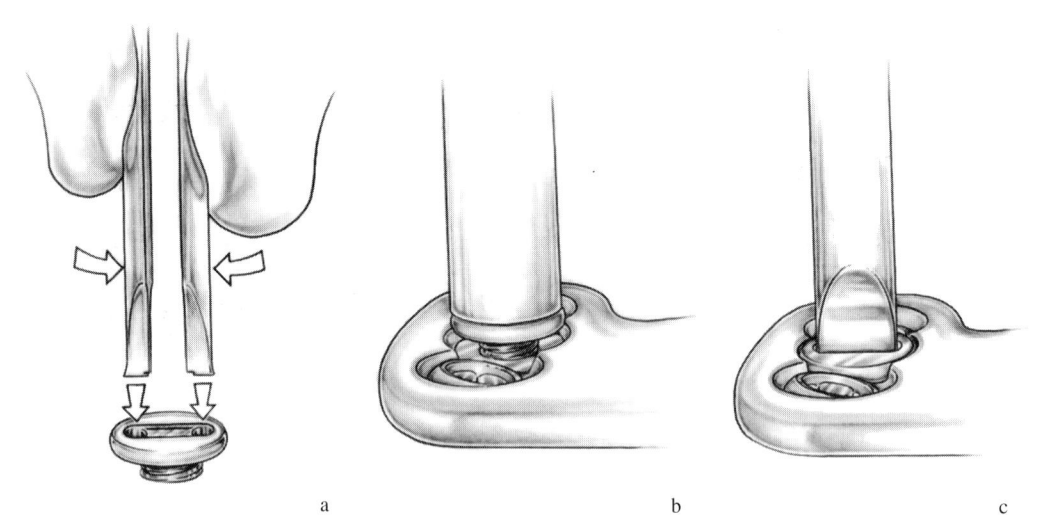

FIG. 4-7. (a) Attaching the lock screw holder to the lock screw. (b) Initial threading of the lock screw into plate. (c) Final tightening of the lock screw with the lock screwdriver.

able for follow-up. The average follow-up is 9 months (range, 6–16 months). Sixty-nine patients underwent anterior cervical diskectomy and interbody fusions (ACDF), and 15 patients underwent corpectomy and strut reconstruction. The indication for surgery was cervical spondylosis in all but two cases. Allograft bone was used in 40% of the vertebral-body reconstructions and 52% of the ACDF patients.

The procedures in three patients (4%) were revised because of early dislodgment of the plate/graft construct. Eighty of the remaining 81 patients (99%) have gone on to solid fusions; one patient had a surgically confirmed nonunion, which was successfully revised. One patient (1%) was noted to have an insignificant broken screw. Two patients (2%) initially had a slight (2-mm) pullout of the inferior end of the plate without further migration. Three patients (4%) were noted to have intervening screws that were loosened slightly (2 mm) and have not changed on later examination. There were no other hardware failures.

PART 2

Posterior Cervical Instrumentation

Section A
Occipitocervical and C1-2 Instrumentation

CHAPTER 5

Wiring Techniques for Occipitocervical and Atlantoaxial Pathology

Curtis A. Dickman
Volker K.H. Sonntag

HIGHLIGHTS

Wire was one of the first methods available to fixate the vertebral column surgically (Peek & Wiltse, 1992). Posterior cervical fixation wires provide a tension band or a method to secure bone grafts or metal implants to the vertebrae.

Stainless steel wires were first developed in the 1930s and have been the principal alloy used for spinal wires (Furgeson & Allen, 1992; Peek & Wiltse, 1992). Titanium, vitallium and other materials have been used for surgical wire; however, alloys other than stainless steel are stiff, weak, susceptible to fatigue and breakage, or are difficult to manipulate (Furgeson & Allen, 1992; Geisler, Mirvis, Zrebeet, et al., 1989; Scuderi, Greenberg, Latta, et al., 1992; White & Panjabi, 1978).

This chapter describes the surgical techniques for occipitocervical and atlantoaxial stabilization using monofilament steel wire. The special features of handling and applying monofilament wires are reviewed. Many of the fixation constructs can also be performed with braided wire cables (Huhn, Wolf, Meyer, et al., 1991; Songer, Spencer, Meyer, et al., 1991). However, monofilament wire has the advantages of being inexpensive, and relatively strong, safe, and easy to apply.

GENERAL CONSIDERATIONS

Wire is usually produced by forced extrusion of metal through a series of dies (Boerre & Dove, 1993). The wire is subsequently treated with an annealing process to make it less stiff and more fatigue-resistant. Steel wires are usually made of 316L or MP 35N grade steel, which is an iron-based chromium alloy (Boerre & Dove, 1993; Furgeson & Allen, 1992; White & Panjabi, 1978).

The goal of wiring is to fixate the spine until solid bone fusion develops (Fielding, 1988; Kaufmann & Jones, 1989). The strength of fixation of a wire construct is determined by (1) the way that the wire is handled; (2) the methods of wire application; (3) the integrity of the bone structure; (4) the strength of the wire-bone interface; (5) the fatigue characteristics of the wire; and (6) the extent of injury to the spine (Furgeson & Allen, 1992; Grob, Crisco, Panjabi, et al., 1992; Ulrich, Woersdoerfer, Kaliff, et al., 1991; White & Panjabi, 1978). If the bone is soft and osteoporotic, if the wire is improperly handled, or if the spine is excessively loaded, a wire fixation will fail. The ways in which wire can fail include the wire cutting through bone or the wire breaking. With repetitive loading, all wire can become fatigued and break.

Monofilament stainless steel wire is the most common type of wire used for spinal fixation and is available in various diameters (Table 5-1). Because it is flexible and is relatively strong, 20-gauge wire is the most convenient for fixating the cervical spine. Although 18-gauge wire is stronger than 20-gauge wire, it is stiff and therefore difficult to twist, contour, and manipulate. Twenty-two-gauge wire is more flexible than 20-gauge wire, but it is also weaker and is more likely to fatigue and break. For the cervical spine, 20-gauge wire is usually used to fixate the occiput, spinous processes, and laminae. Bone struts or the facets are fixated with either 20- or 22-gauge wire; however, depending on the patient's needs, these applications are modified.

Double-stranded, twisted, 24-gauge wire can be used as an alternative to 20-gauge monofilament wire with the advantage of being strong, yet flexible. If two strands of monofilament wires are twisted with 2.5 turns per centimeter, the wires become stronger. Taitsman and Saha (1977) discovered that the tensile strength of double-stranded wire increased when up to eight turns per inch were placed in the wires (2.5 turns per centimeter) and decreased when this was exceeded. Double-stranded wires can be prepared intraoperatively using a hand drill or a wire twister. To do this, the end of a pair of wires is held by the wire twister, or the end

Table 5-1
Wire Size Comparisons*

Wire Gauge	Diameter (mm)	Diameter (in.)
28	0.3	0.0126
26	0.4	0.0159
24	0.5	0.0201
22	0.6	0.0254
20	0.8	0.032
18	1.0	0.04
16	1.2	0.05

*Wire gauge varies depending upon the manufacturer.
Modified from Stauffer (1988). Reprinted with permission.

is inserted into the shaft of the twist drill, and the free ends of the wires are held with a Kocher clamp. The wires are then pulled taut and twisted uniformly, and the number of turns per inch is measured with a ruler.

Twisting the ends of the wire together is the preferred method to set wire tension progressively in order to fixate wires to bone surfaces. Wire can be twisted with a heavy needle holder or with a Robinson wire twister (Fig. 5-1). The wires are crossed 1 to 2 in. from the bone surface and one or two twists are started in the wire. The intersection of the wires is grasped with a wire twister. While the wire is being twisted, the force is directed away from the bone surface in order to distribute uniform tension in the wire. Monofilament wire is usually twisted unilaterally to remove slack from the wire. However, the wire can also be twisted bilaterally to distribute the wire tension evenly (Fig. 5-2).

Acute bends, kinks, notches in the wire, or excessive twisting of wire increase the risk of fatigue and breakage. Twisted wire should have a uniform, even twisting. Excessive twisting causes a local change in wire color and also causes secondary turns to appear in the wire.

OPERATIVE TECHNIQUES

Atlantoaxial or occipitocervical fixation can be achieved using various wire constructs. The spinous processes, the laminae, the facets, the C1 ring, and the occiput can be secured with wire. In the section below, each technique is described in detail.

Spinous Process Wiring

Spinous process wires can be used to fixate single or multiple cervical motion segments (Abdu & Bohlman, 1992; Geisler et al., 1989; Rogers, 1957; Stauffer, 1988). A hole is made in the center of the base of the spinous process with a drill or a bone awl (Fig. 5-3). The hole is positioned at the junction of the spinous processes and laminae, preserving a wide margin of bone adjacent to the hole in order to resist wire pullout. The hole is completed with a towel clip or a Lewin clamp (Fig. 5-3, *a* and *b*). The wire is passed through this hole and looped beneath the inferior adjacent spinous process or passed through a similar hole in the adjacent spinous process.

Spinous process wires provide a tension band that is safe and easy to apply. Although using spinous process wires avoids risks associated with sublaminar instrumentation (Geremia, Kim, Cerullo, et al., 1985), spinous process wires do not resist extension, weakly inhibit rotation and lateral

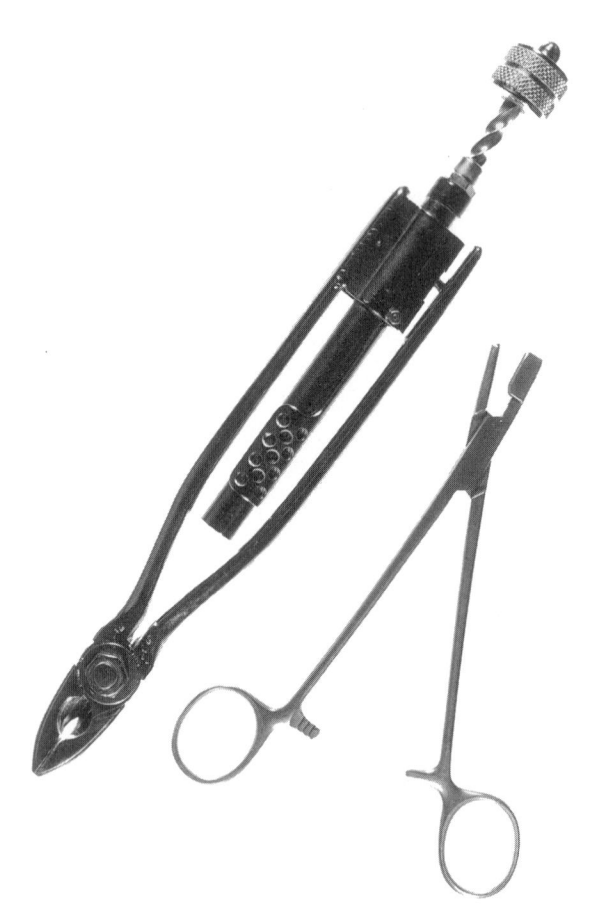

FIG. 5-1. Wire-twisting devices for monofilament wire. *Left,* Robinson wire twister; *right,* wire-holding forceps.

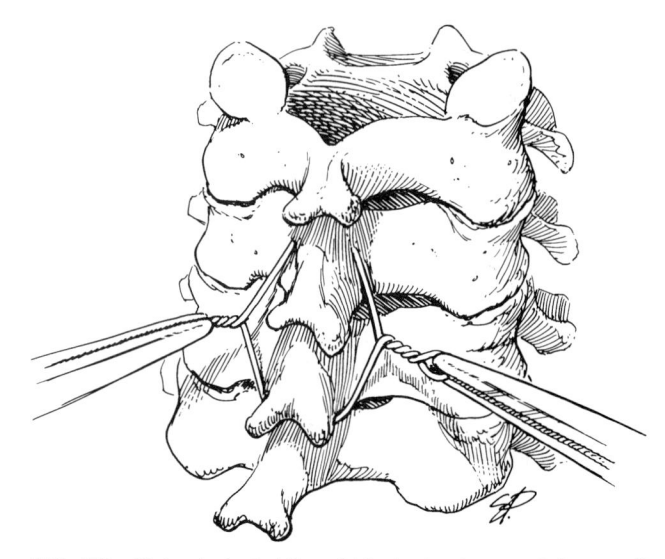

FIG. 5-2. Bilateral wire twisting distributes tension evenly in monofilament wire.

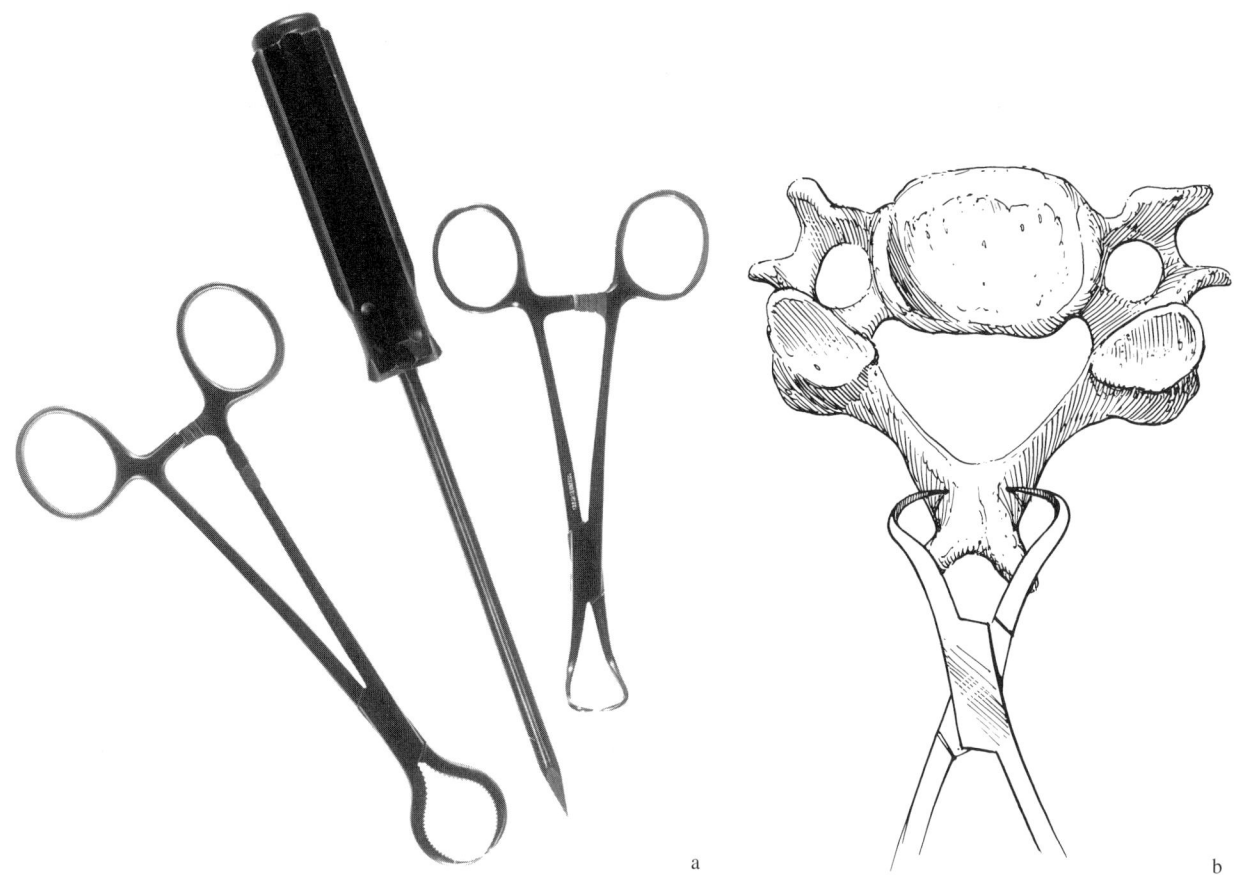

FIG. 5-3. (a) A bone awl (*center*) or a drill is used to penetrate the cortical bone in order to create a hole for spinous process wires. A Lewin clamp (*left*) or towel clip (*right*) are used to complete the hole through the bone. (b) Spinous process wires are passed through holes in the base of the spinous process. The holes are tunneled with a Lewin clamp or towel clip. With permission of Barrow Neurological Institute.

bending, and cannot be used after a laminectomy (Abdu & Bohlman, 1992; Furgeson & Allen, 1992; Stauffer, 1988; Ulrich et al., 1991; White & Panjabi, 1978).

Facet Wiring

Facet wires are placed into the inferior articular facets of the cervical vertebrae (Abdu & Bohlman, 1992; Callahan, Johnson, Margolis, et al., 1977; Furgeson & Allen, 1992; Garfin, Moore, & Marshall, 1988; Stauffer, 1988). The facet joint is opened with a small curette and is held open with a Penfield dissector (Fig. 5-4). A drill hole is placed through the middle of the inferior facet into the facet joint, and 20- or 22-gauge wires are passed through the holes. The facet wires can then be used to attach bone struts or metal implants to the vertebrae.

Because facets are relatively thin, wires can pull out of the facets if sufficient force is applied, if the wires are overtightened, or if the bone is osteoporotic. Facet wires are an excellent alternative after a laminectomy; however, facet wires are weaker than sublaminar or spinous process wires (Ulrich et al., 1991; White & Panjabi, 1978). If facet wires are used, a rigid or semirigid orthosis may be needed to supplement the wiring until bone healing occurs.

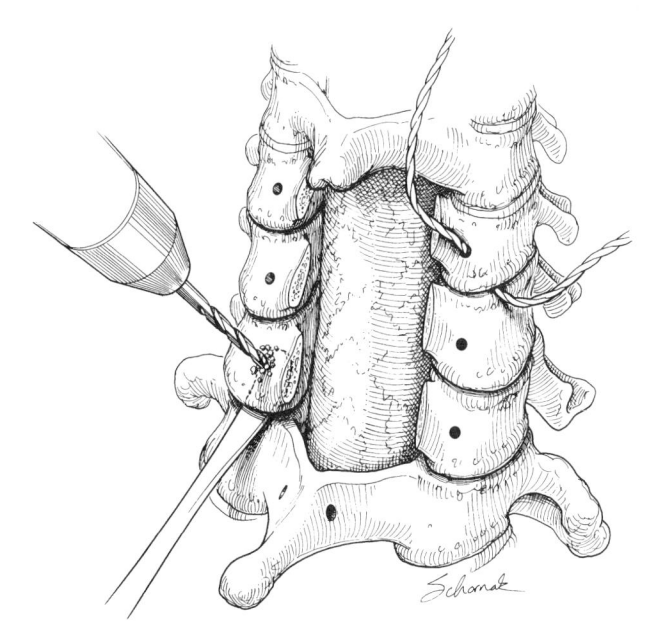

FIG. 5-4. Facet wire passage. Holes are drilled into the inferior facets after opening the joints with a curette. With permission of Barrow Neurological Institute.

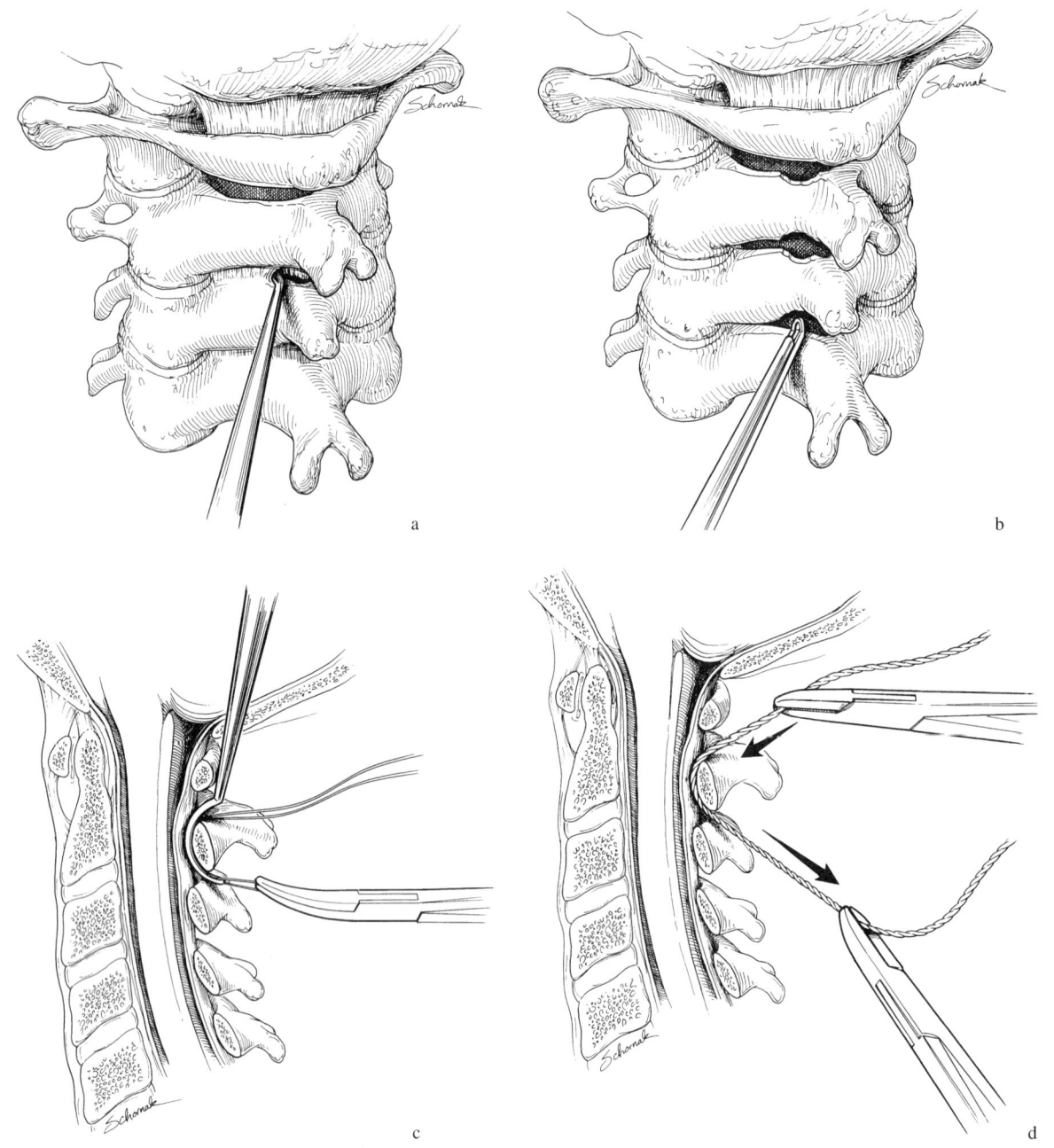

FIG. 5-5. (a and b) Sublaminar wires are passed only while directly visualizing the dura to avoid neural compression. The ligamentum flavum is removed and laminotomies are created. (c) A wire passer can be used to pass the wire beneath the laminae. (d) The wire is simultaneously fed and pulled beneath the bone to avoid displacing the wire against the spinal cord. With permission of Barrow Neurological Institute.

Sublaminar Wiring

Sublaminar wires can be used to fixate adjacent motion segments or to attach bone struts or metal implants to the vertebrae (Abdu & Bohlman, 1992; Boerre & Dove, 1993; Furgeson & Allen, 1992; Geremia et al., 1985; Stauffer, 1988); it is important to remember that using sublaminar wires risks neurologic injury, especially at the middle and lower cervical levels (Geremia et al., 1985). To avoid complications, precise techniques are required. Compressive pathology should be removed and the dura should be visualized directly prior to passing sublaminar wires, because passing sublaminar wires in a stenotic canal could cause neurologic injury (Geremia et al., 1985). The ligamentum flavum is removed from the upper and lower surfaces of the laminae to facilitate wire passage (Fig. 5-5, a). Small laminotomies are made in the medial edges of the laminae (Fig. 5-5, b); however, an extensive laminotomy should be avoided so that the bone is not weakened.

A wire passer or a heavy silk suture is used to position and guide the wire beneath the undersurface of the laminae (Fig. 5-5, c). The wire is first contoured to conform to the shape of the laminae and the end of the wire should be bent into a blunt loop to prevent the sharp wire tip from penetrating the dura. The suture is passed beneath the lamina by grasping the tip of a curved needle with a needle holder and passing the blunt end of the needle with the attached suture beneath the laminae. A hemostat or needle holder is used to grasp the needle on the other side of the laminae. The suture is tied to the end of the wire and is pulled so that the wire is fed in a controlled fashion.

Sublaminar wires should be passed with a two-handed process, simultaneously feeding and pulling the wire in order to avoid displacing the wire or manipulating the unstable vertebrae (Fig. 5-5, d). During sublaminar passage, the wire should hug the undersurface of the bone. After the wires are positioned, they are bent across the bone surface to avoid displacing a loop of wire against the spinal cord. Spanning multiple laminae during sublaminar wire passage should be avoided because the risk of neurologic injury is increased (i.e., it is safer to pass wire beneath one lamina only) (Geremia et al., 1985). Although sublaminar wires are strong and mechanically effective, they have risks that necessitate maximal caution and precision (Boerre & Dove, 1993; Geremia et al., 1985; White & Panjabi, 1978).

ATLANTOAXIAL WIRING TECHNIQUES

Interspinous Fusion

A midline posterior subperiosteal exposure of C1 and C2 is performed (Dickman, Sonntag, Papadopoulos, & Hadley, 1991). To facilitate fusion, the ligamentum flavum and posterior occipitoatlantal membrane are removed from the surfaces of C1 and C2. Bone surfaces that will contact the graft (the superior edges of the C2 spinous process and laminae and the inferior edge of the C1 ring) are decorticated with a high-speed drill or Kerrison rongeur. Also, to facilitate bone healing, the decortication exposes cancellous bone in the fusion bed for apposition with cancellous bone of the graft. To seat the wire, notches are made bilaterally in the inferior surfaces of the C2 laminae where they join the C2 spinous process (Fig. 5-6).

An autologous, curved, tricortical bone graft (4 cm long by 3 cm high) is obtained from the posterior iliac crest (Fig. 5-6, a). The rounded upper cortical edge of the graft is removed with a Leksell rongeur in order to create a bicortical curved strut graft. The strut graft is precisely fitted between C1 and C2 in order to recreate the normal C1-2 height.

The curve of the graft approximates the curve of the ring of C1. The inferior margin of the bone graft is notched in the midline to match the contour of the spinous processes of C2, and the graft is temporarily removed to allow for wire placement.

Twenty-gauge monofilament wire or double-stranded, twisted, 24-gauge wire is halved, looped, and passed beneath the posterior arch of C1 in the midline, directed superiorly (Fig. 5-6, b). The graft is repositioned between the atlas and axis. The loop of wire is passed over the ring of C1, behind the graft, and is secured beneath the base of the C2 spinous process. The free ends of the wire are positioned anteriorly to the graft and are then passed beneath the C2 spinous process (Fig. 5-6, b and c). The wires are then tightened, which compresses the bone graft between the posterior arches of C1 and C2 and entraps the graft between the wires anteriorly and posteriorly (Fig. 5-6, c).

Using a high-speed drill, the surfaces of the posterior arches of C1-2 and the bone graft are segmentally decorticated. Cancellous bone grafts are compressed against the fusion surfaces. To maximize the fusion rate, a rigid or semirigid orthosis is used postoperatively.

Unlike other methods of C1-2 wiring, the interspinous method for atlantoaxial arthrodesis can be used when C1 is dislocated posteriorly. Using this method precludes the risk of sublaminar wire passage at C2, minimizes the risk of neural injury, and in addition, provides excellent translational and rotational stability.

Gallie Fusion

In the 1930s Gallie (1937, 1939) referred to the principle of performing a cervical fusion using wires and bone grafts; however, he did not publish the details of his wiring technique. Because of Gallie's technique, several authors refer to a midline wiring technique for C1-2 fusion as the "Gallie fusion" (Figs. 5-7, a to c) (Abdu & Bohlman, 1992; Fielding, 1988; Grob et al., 1992; Hanley & Harvell, 1992; McGraw & Rusch, 1973; Stauffer, 1988). A unicortical plate of autologous bone (5 to 8 mm thick) is harvested from the iliac crest and a notch is created for the graft to straddle the C2 spinous process. The upper margin of the graft is positioned dorsal to the C1 arch.

Wire is halved, looped, and passed in a sublaminar position at C1, directed superiorly, and the loop is secured beneath the C2 spinous process. The graft is positioned and the free ends of the wire are wrapped dorsally in order to fix the graft into position. A routine wound closure is performed and a supplemental orthosis is used. This technique is simple but cannot be performed when C1 is posteriorly dislocated. Mechanically, this construct weakly resists translation and rotation compared with other wiring techniques for C1-2 fixation (Grob et al., 1992; Hanley & Harvell, 1992; Ulrich et al., 1991; White & Panjabi, 1978). Although this technique is mechanically inferior to other methods of C1-2 fixation, it is presented here because of its historical value.

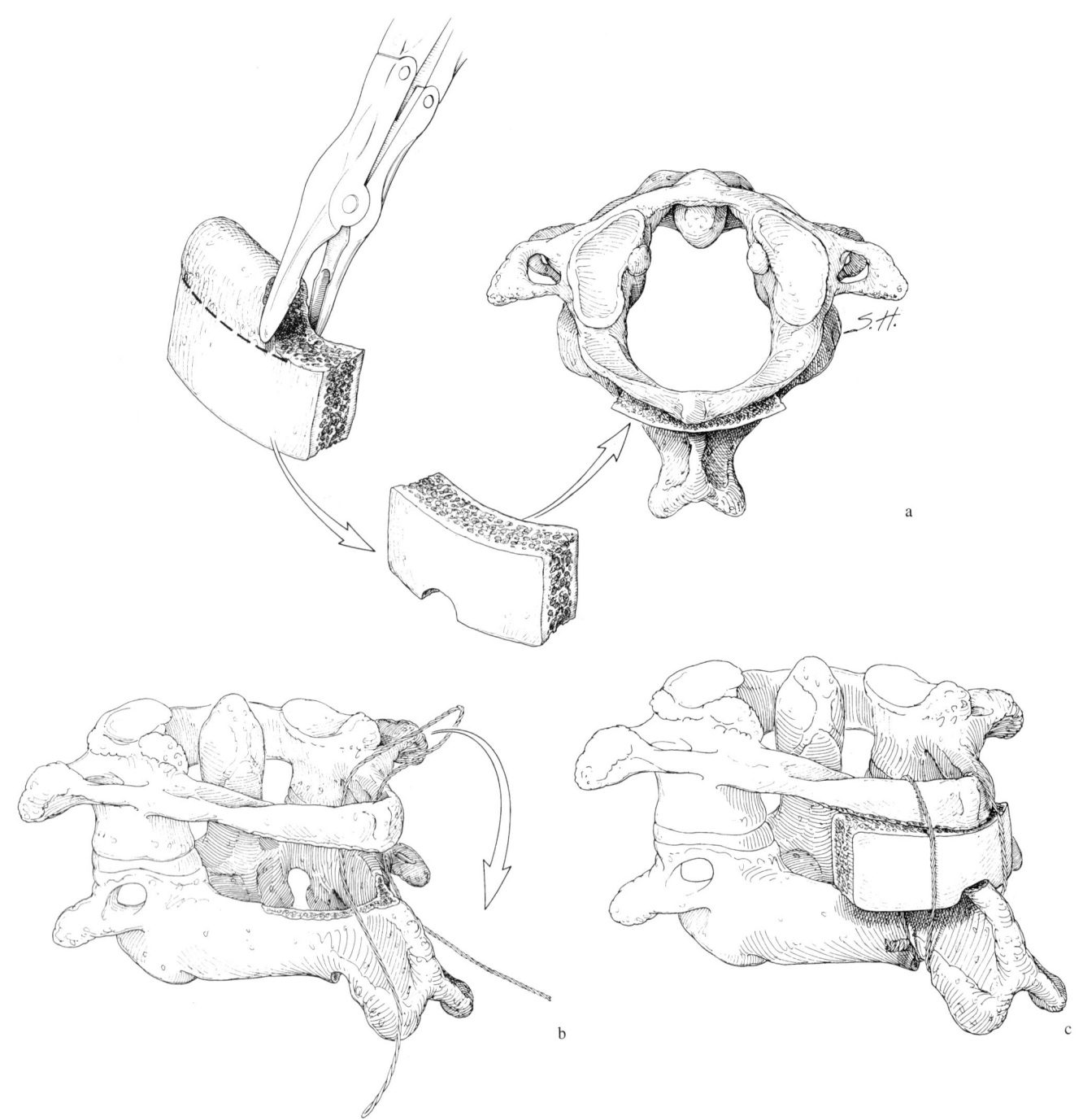

FIG. 5-6. (a) Interspinous fusion. An autologous, curved, bicortical iliac crest strut is fitted between C1 and C2. (b) A wire is halved, looped, passed sublaminar at C1, and secured beneath the C2 spinous process. Notches made at the spinolaminar junction of C2 help to seat the wire. (c) The free ends of the wire are wrapped beneath the C2 spinous process. The graft is entrapped by wire anteriorly and posteriorly, and it is compressed between the bone surfaces of C1 and C2. (*From Dickman CA, Sonntag VKH, Papadopoulos SM, Hadley MN: The interspinous method of posterior atlantoaxial arthrodesis. J Neurosurg 74: 190–198, 1991. Reprinted with permission.*)

Brooks Fusion

In 1978 Brooks and Jenkins described a wedge compression method of C1-2 fixation, which Griswold et al. (1978) subsequently modified (Figs. 5-8, *a* and *b*). Using routine techniques, the atlas and axis are exposed. Bilaterally, two sublaminar wires are sequentially passed beneath C1 and then beneath C2. The dura is visualized to prevent injury during wire passage. Two rectangular corticocancellous wedges of autologous iliac crest bone are harvested and positioned bilaterally between the C1 ring and C2 laminae. The

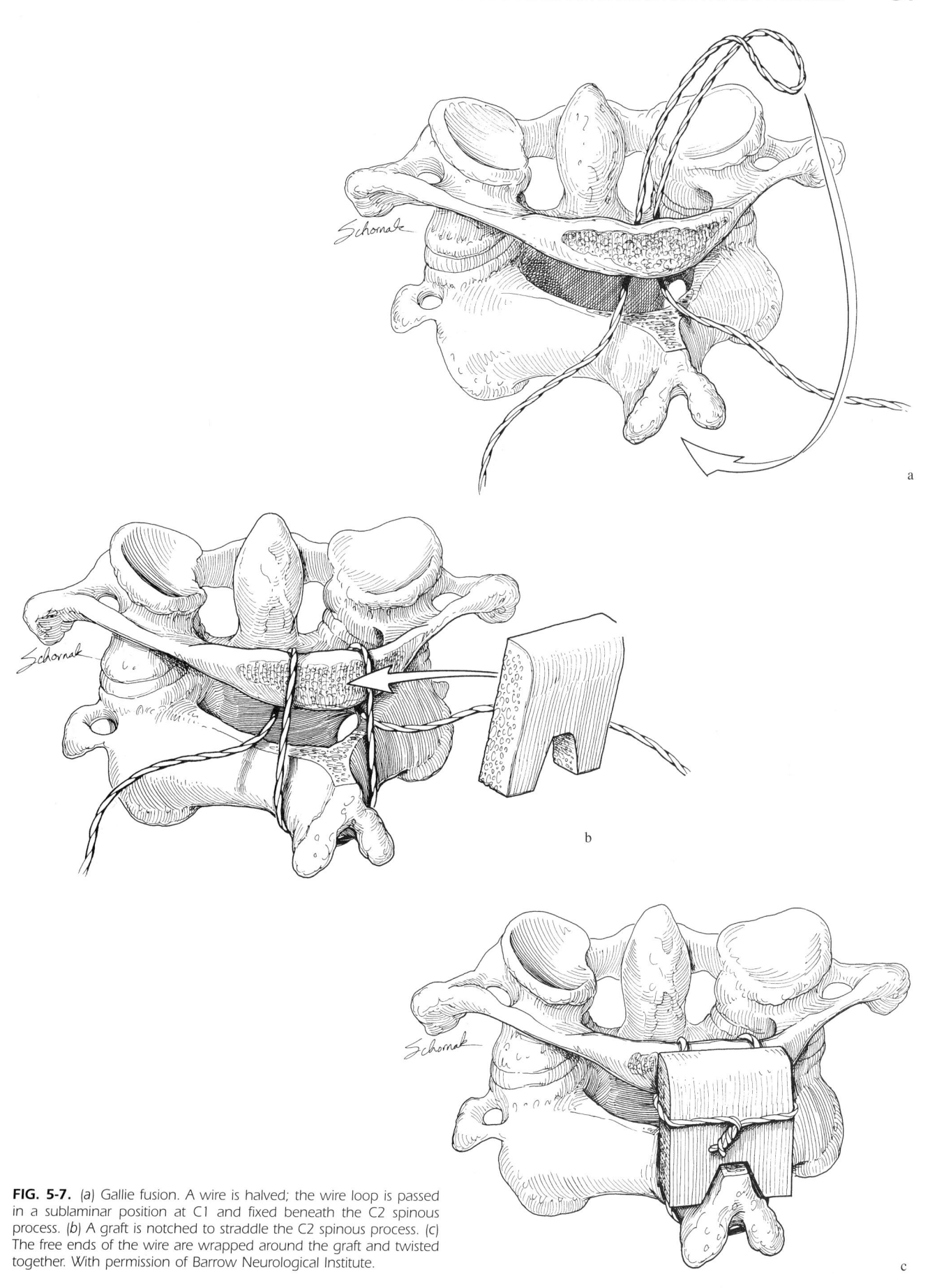

FIG. 5-7. (a) Gallie fusion. A wire is halved; the wire loop is passed in a sublaminar position at C1 and fixed beneath the C2 spinous process. (b) A graft is notched to straddle the C2 spinous process. (c) The free ends of the wire are wrapped around the graft and twisted together. With permission of Barrow Neurological Institute.

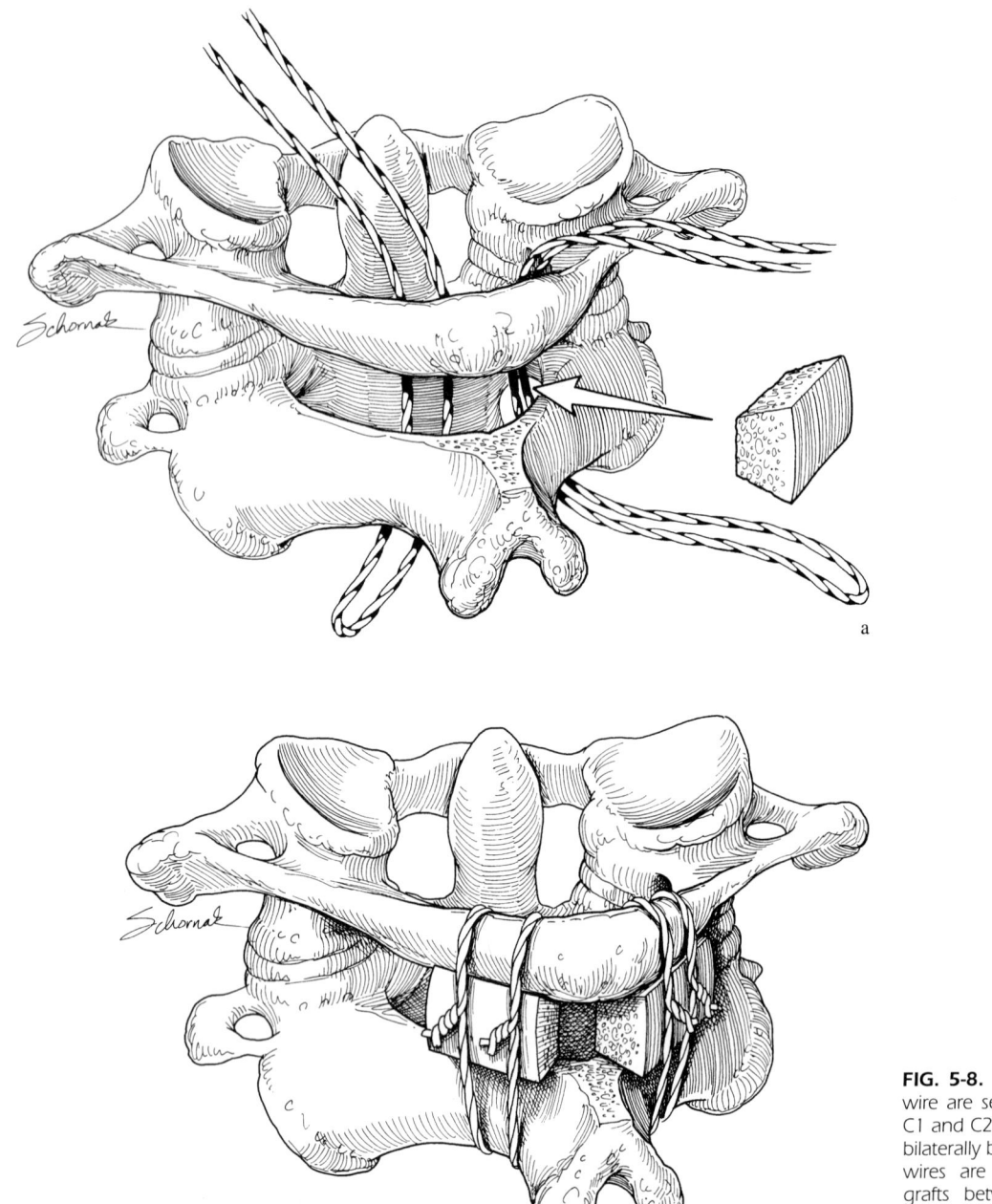

FIG. 5-8. (a) Brooks fusion. Loops of wire are sequentially passed beneath C1 and C2. Wedges of bone are fitted bilaterally between C1 and C2. (b) The wires are twisted to compress the grafts between the bone surfaces. With permission of Barrow Neurological Institute.

bone grafts are wedged into the interlaminar space on each side, and the two wires on each side are tightened behind the grafts, securing the bone wedges into position. The wounds are closed routinely and a postoperative orthosis is used. Mechanically, this technique provides stiffer rotational fixation than the Gallie wiring (Grob et al., 1992; Hanley & Harvell, 1992; Ulrich et al., 1991; White & Panjabi, 1978). The major disadvantage of this technique is that it requires sequential sublaminar wire passage between C1 and C2 and consequently risks neurologic injury.

OCCIPITOCERVICAL WIRING TECHNIQUES

Occipitocervical fixation requires exposure of the occipital squamosa, the rim of the foramen magnum, and the cervical levels to be fused. The occiput should be wired at locations where the bone is thick (near the foramen magnum, at the nuchal line, and along the midline crest). Laterally, the occipital squamosa is thin and wires can easily pull out. To wire the bone adjacent to the foramen magnum, the posterior lip of the foramen magnum is enlarged with a Kerrison rongeur (Fig. 5-9). Two burr holes are placed into the occipital bone, 5 mm superior to the rim of the foramen magnum. In order to prevent intradural wire penetration, the dura is separated from the inner table of the skull and the tip of the wire is bent into a blunt loop. Wire is passed between each burr hole and the foramen magnum.

Midline wiring of the occiput can be performed by positioning burr holes bilaterally, adjacent to the midline crest. The dura is separated, and the thick midline crest is wired. With this procedure care must be taken to avoid injury to the cerebellum and dural venous sinuses. As an alternative, the midline crest can be wired by using holes drilled tangentially to the bone into the crest (Fig. 5-10, *a*).

Stabilization is achieved by wiring bone struts or metal struts to the occiput, spinous processes, cervical laminae, or facets. Metal fixation devices achieve immediate, relatively rigid, spinal fixation; however, in order to ensure fusion they should be used with autogenous bone grafts. Metal contoured loops, rectangular rods, threaded Steinmann pins, or titanium rods can be used (Dickman, Douglas, & Sonntag, 1990; MacKenzie, Uttley, Marsh, et al., 1990; Ransford, Crockard, Pozo, et al., 1986; Sakou, Kawaida, Morizono, et al., 1989). Bone struts (ribs or iliac crest struts) are wired directly against the spine and occiput (Fig. 5-10) (Grantham, Dick, Thompson, et al., 1969; Hamblen, 1967; Wertheim & Bohlman, 1987). The struts provide immobilization and bone tissue to promote fusion. Because bone struts can be weak and fracture, a rigid or semirigid orthosis may be needed postoperatively until fusion occurs.

Another technique for occipitocervical fusion uses a wide (5/32-in. diameter), stainless-steel threaded Steinmann pin (Fig. 5-11, *a*) (Dickman et al., 1990). When postoperative magnetic resonance imaging (MRI) is desired, a titanium grooved rod and titanium wires or titanium braided cables can be used. The threaded rod prevents settling of the construct. The Steinmann pin is bent into a U-shape and secondary bends are placed to match the contour of the occipitocervical region. The curves of the pin need to be smooth because sharp angles create stress risers and encourage pin breakage. The pin is measured and the ends are cut to a length at which the ends of the pin do not extend beyond the fused segments.

The Steinmann pin is wired against the occiput and cervical laminae or facets. In order to achieve optimal fixation, the pin needs to contact the bone surfaces at each level. Gaps between the pin and the bone surfaces will loosely fixate the vertebrae, which will result in excessive motion.

The wide diameter and smooth bends of the Steinmann pin are needed to minimize postoperative pin breakage. A threaded pin is essential because the threads of the pin prevent vertical settling of the construct. The occiput and posterior arches of the cervical levels to be fused are segmentally decorticated with a burr, and autologous cancellous bone grafts are compressed against the levels to be fused. If a suboccipital craniotomy or cervical laminectomy has been performed, a plate of cortical iliac crest bone can be sutured or wired to the central portion of the Steinmann pin (Fig. 5-11, *b*). This bone plate provides a template for the fusion to develop and preserves the dural decompression. A routine multilayered wound closure is performed.

SUMMARY

Various wiring constructs can be used to stabilize the craniovertebral junction and upper cervical spine. To maximize

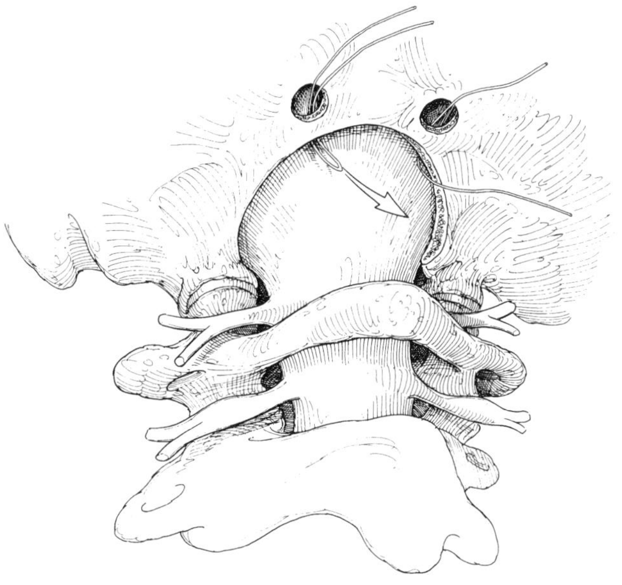

FIG. 5-9. The occiput is wired after enlarging the dorsal rim of the foramen magnum and after placing burr holes 5 mm above the edge of the foramen magnum. With permission of Barrow Neurological Institute.

Table 5-2
Indications and Contraindications for Use of Wiring Techniques for Occipitocervical and Atlantoaxial Pathology

Indications	
Spinous process wiring	fixate single or multiple cervical motion segments with stable anterior columns
Facet wiring	fixate single or multiple cervical motion segments after laminectomy
Sublaminar wiring	fixate single or multiple cervical motion segments
Gallie fusion	C1-C2 instability
Brooks fusion	C1-C2 instability
Contraindications	
Spinous process wiring	three column instability incompetent posterior elements
Facet wiring	osteoporosis incompetent anterior and middle columns
Sublaminar wiring	previous laminectomy incompetent anterior and middle columns
Gallie fusion	posterior dislocation of C1 C1 or C2 laminectomy
Brooks fusion	C1 or C2 laminectomy

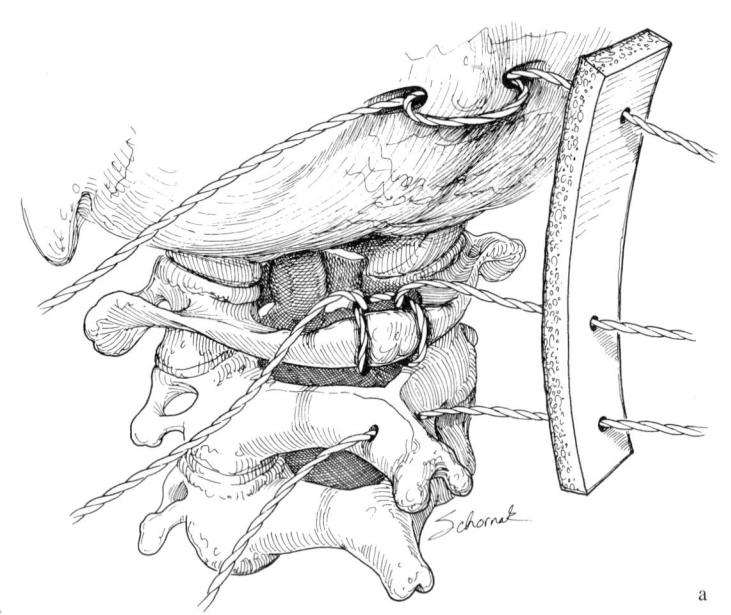

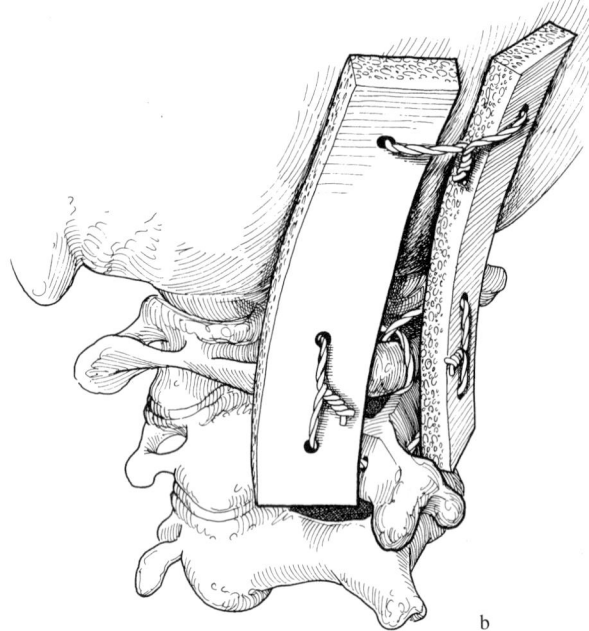

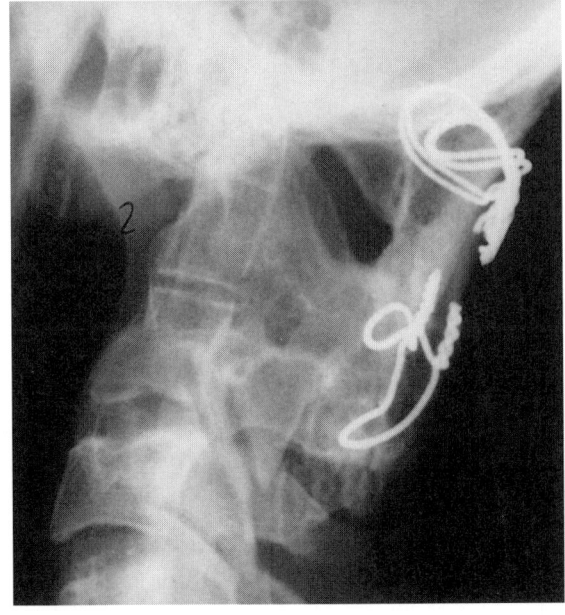

FIG. 5-10. Wertheim-Bohlman technique for occipitocervical fusion (a and b). (a) Midline wires are used in the occiput, C1, and C2 to fixate bone struts to the fusion bed. (b) Final appearance of the wired grafts. (c) This postoperative lateral cervical radiograph reveals a solid bone fusion. With permission of Barrow Neurological Institute.

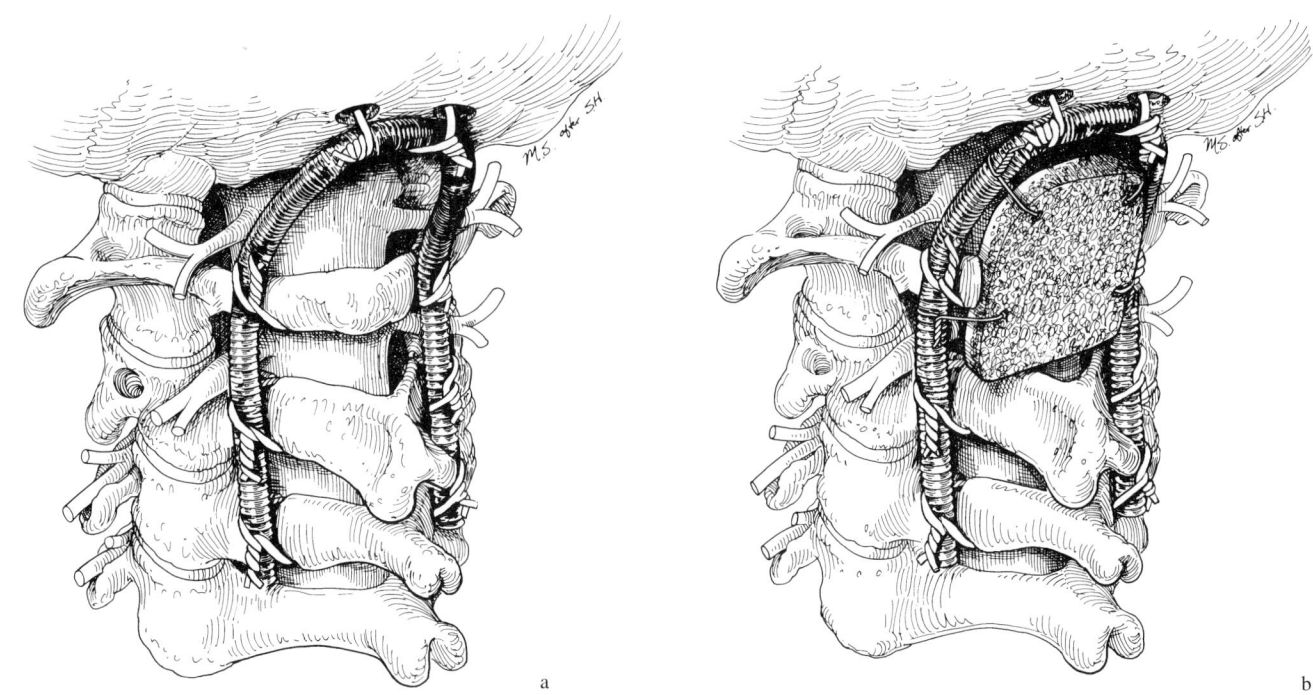

FIG. 5-11. (a) Steinmann pin fusion. A threaded 5/32-in.-diameter Steinmann pin is shaped to match the contour of the craniovertebral junction. The threaded pin is wired to the occiput, C1 ring, and lower cervical laminae or facets. (b) After a suboccipital decompression or cervical laminectomy has been performed, a plate of cortical bone is wired to preserve the decompression and provide a template for fusion. With permission of Barrow Neurological Institute.

success and to avoid complications, wire must be handled carefully and applied correctly. When wired to the spine and skull, bone struts or metal implants provide reasonably good motion control. See Tables 5-2 and 5-3.

A supplemental orthosis is recommended to help control motion and reduce loads on the fixation while solid bone fusion is developing. A Philadelphia collar or a sternal-occipital-mandibular immobilizer (SOMI) brace may be appropriate when the bone quality is good, the fixation is strong, and the deforming forces are minimal. However, a halo brace or Minerva brace may be needed if there is excessive deformity, soft bone, poor fixation, extensive instability, or excessive loading of the vertebrae. The treatment is tailored to appropriate therapy for the individual patient.

Wiring techniques are fundamental skills that need to be incorporated into the surgical armamentarium of every spine surgeon. The merits and limitations of these techniques should be considered when comparing wiring to other methods of fixation.

Table 5-3
Advantages and Disadvantages for Use of Wiring Techniques for Occipitocervical and Atlantoaxial Pathology

Advantages

Spinous process wiring	safe, simple procedure
	avoids sublaminar risks
Facet wiring	can be used after laminectomy
	avoids sublaminar risks
Sublaminar wiring	relatively simple and familiar procedure
Gallie fusion	simple procedure
Brooks fusion	simple procedure
	greater resistance to translation and rotation than Gallie fusion

Disadvantages

Spinous process wiring	poor resistance to extension, lateral bending or rotation
	cannot be used after laminectomy
Facet wiring	frequent pull-out due to thin facets
	need rigid or semi-rigid orthosis to augment wires
	poor resistance to extension
Sublaminar wiring	increased risk of passing sublaminar wires
	poor resistance to extension
Gallie fusion	weakly resists translation and rotation
Brooks fusion	increased risk of passing sublaminar wires

ACKNOWLEDGMENTS

The authors wish to thank Mark Schornak, medical illustrator; Pamela A. Smith, medical photographer; and the editorial staff at the Barrow Neurological Institute for their assistance in the preparation of this manuscript.

REFERENCES

Abdu, W.A., & Bohlman, H.H. (1992). Spinal trauma management update: Techniques of subaxial posterior cervical spine fusion: An overview. *Orthopedics, 15*(3), 287–294.

Boerre, N.R., & Dove, J. (1993). The selection of wires for sublaminar fixation. *Spine, 18*(4), 497–503.

Brooks, A.L., Jenkins, E.B. (1978) Atlanto-axial arthrodesis by the wedge compression method. *Journal of Bone and Joint Surgery, American Volume, 60,* 279–284.

Callahan, R.A., Johnson, R.M., Margolis, R.N., et al. (1977). Cervical facet fusion for control of instability following laminectomy. *Journal of Bone and Joint Surgery, American Volume, 59,* 991–1002.

Dickman, C.A., Douglas, R.A., & Sonntag, V.K.H. (1990). Occipitocervical fusion: Posterior stabilization of the craniovertebral junction and upper cervical spine. *Barrow Neurological Institute Quarterly, 6*(2), 2–14.

Dickman, C.A., Sonntag, V.K.H., Papadopoulos, S.M., Hadley, M.N. (1991). The interspinous method of posterior atlantoaxial arthrodesis. *Journal of Neurosurgery, 74,* 190–198.

Fielding, J.W. (1988). The status of arthrodesis of the cervical spine. *Journal of Bone and Joint Surgery, American Volume, 70,* 1571–1574.

Furgeson, R.L., Allen, B.L., Jr. (1992). Biomechanical principles of spinal correction. In J.M. Cotler & H.B. Cotler (Eds.), *Spinal Fusion.* Berlin: Springer-Verlag.

Gallie, W.E. (1939). Fractures and dislocations of the cervical spine. *American Journal of Surgery, 46,* 495–499.

Gallie, W.E. (1937). Skeletal traction in treatment of fractures and dislocations of cervical spine. *Annals of Surgery, 106,* 770–776.

Garfin, S.R., Moore, M.R., & Marshall, L.F. (1988). A modified technique for cervical facet fusions. *Clinical Orthopaedics and Related Research, 230,* 149–153.

Geisler, F.H., Mirvis, S.E., Zrebeet, H., et al. (1989). Titanium wire internal fixation for stabilization of injury of the cervical spine: Clinical results and postoperative magnetic resonance imaging of the spinal cord. *Neurosurgery, 25,* 356–362.

Geremia, G.K., Kim, K.S., Cerullo, L., et al. (1985). Complications of sublaminar wiring. *Surgical Neurology, 23,* 629–634.

Grantham, S.A., Dick, H.M., Thompson, R.C. Jr., et al. (1969). Occipitocervical arthrodesis: Indications, technic and results. *Clinical Orthopaedics and Related Research, 65,* 118–129.

Griswold, D.M., Albright, J.A., Schiffman, E., et al. (1978). Atlanto-axial fusion for instability. *Journal of Bone and Joint Surgery, American Volume 60,* 285–292.

Grob, D., Crisco, J.J., III, Panjabi, M.M., et al. (1992). Biomechanical evaluation of four different posterior atlantoaxial fixation techniques. *Spine, 17,* 480–490.

Hamblen, D.L. (1967). Occipito-cervical fusion: Indications, technique and results. *Journal of Bone and Joint Surgery, British Volume, 49,* 33–45.

Hanley, E.N. Jr., & Harvell, J.C., Jr. (1992). Immediate postoperative stability of the atlantoaxial articulation: A biomechanical study comparing simple midline wiring, and the Gallie and Brooks procedures. *Journal of Spinal Disorders, 5,* 306–310.

Heywood, A.W., Learmonth, I.D., & Thomas, M. (1988). Internal fixation for occipito-cervical fusion. *Journal of Bone and Joint Surgery, British Volume, 70,* 708–711.

Huhn, S.L., Wolf, A.L., & Ecklund, J. (1991). Posterior spinal osteosynthesis for cervical fracture/dislocation using a flexible multistrand cable system: Technical note. *Neurosurgery, 29,* 943–946.

Kaufmann, H.H., Jones, E. (1989). The principles of bony spinal fusion. *Neurosurgery, 24,* 264–270.

MacKenzie, A.I., Uttley, D., Marsh, H.T., et al. Craniocervical stabilization using Luque/Hartshill rectangles. *Neurosurgery, 36,* 32–36.

McGraw, R.W., & Rusch, R.M. (1973). Atlanto-axial arthrodesis. *Journal of Bone and Joint Surgery, British Volume, 55,* 482–498.

Peek, R.D., Wiltse, L.L. (1992). History of spinal fusion. In J.M. Cotler & H.B. Cotler (Eds.), *Spinal Fusion.* Berlin: Springer-Verlag.

Ransford, A.O., Crockard, H.A., Pozo, J.L., et al. (1986). Craniocervical instability treated by contoured loop fixation. *Journal of Bone and Joint Surgery, British Volume, 68,* 173–177.

Rogers, W.A. (1957). Fractures and dislocation of the cervical spine: An end-result study. *Journal of Bone and Joint Surgery, American Volume 39,* 341–376.

Sakou, T., Kawaida, H., Morizono, Y., et al. (1989). Occipitoatlantoaxial fusion utilizing a rectangular rod. *Clinical Orthopaedics and Related Research, 236,* 136–144.

Scuderi, G.J., Greenberg, S.S., Latta, L.L., et al. (1992) *A biomechanical evaluation of MRI compatible wire for use in cervical spine fixation* (abstract) (pp. 57–58). Cervical Spine Research Society.

Songer, M.N., Spencer, D.L., Meyer, P.R., Jr., et al. (1991). The use of sublaminar cables to replace Luque wires. *Spine, 16*(8 Suppl), S418–S421.

Stauffer, E.S. (1988). Wiring techniques of the posterior cervical spine for the treatment of trauma. *Orthopedics, 11,* 1543–1548.

Taitsman, J.P., Saha, S. (1977) Tensile strength of wire-reinforced bone cement and twisted stainless steel wire. *Journal of Bone and Joint Surgery, American Volume 59*(3), 419–425.

Ulrich, C., Woersdoerfer, O., Kalff, R., et al. (1991). Biomechanics of fixation systems to the cervical spine. *Spine, 16*(3 Suppl), S4–S9.

Wertheim, S.B., & Bohlman, H.H. (1987). Occipitocervical fusion: Indications, technique, and long-term results in thirteen patients. *Journal of Bone and Joint Surgery, British Volume 69,* 833–836.

White, A.A., III, & Panjabi, M.M. (1978). *Clinical Biomechanics of the Spine.* Philadelphia: J.B. Lippincott.

CHAPTER 6

Posterior Cervical Arthrodesis Using the Songer Cable System

Matthew N. Songer

HIGHLIGHTS

The advent of the use of cables for fixation of the spine originated from the frustration incurred with the use of monofilament wire. The Songer cable system was developed to address three main deficiencies inherent in plain wire, as discussed below.

Ease of Use

Plain wire is relatively rigid and must be annealed to soften it and make it more pliable. Despite this processing, wire is stiff and difficult to use, especially in small confined areas. The diameter of the monofilament wire must be of a minimum caliber to obtain adequate strength. This results in a stiff wire that is difficult to manipulate in hard-to-reach areas. Cables designed properly are very flexible, making insertion and removal easy.

Strength

The tensile strength of wire is decreased by the annealing process. A solid wire compared to a cable of an equal diameter made of the same material and heat treated equally, subjected to a straight pull longitudinally is stronger than the cable. However, the mode of failure of monofilament wire is due to stress risers that occur at bends in the wire. The individual wires in a cable are very thin. The force required to bend a wire is proportional to the radius to the fourth power (stiffness = I (moment of inertia) = τ radius^4/4). Hence, the smaller wires are exponentially more flexible and may be made out of hardened steel. The bundle of wires are less subject to stress points, conform to uneven or irregular surfaces, and have a tremendously greater strength (Songer, Jayaraman, & Iwanski, 1993; Songer, Spencer, Meyer, & Jayaraman, 1991) (Figs. 6-1 and 6-2). Cable loops have a far greater static yield and tensile strength than monofilament wire loops (Fig. 6-1). Wire constructs usually fail through fatigue failure rather than by exceeding the maximum tensile strength. Cables have a tremendous advantage over wires in fatigue strength. Fig. 6-2 is a logarithmic curve demonstrating that cables have from 9 to 48 times greater fatigue strength than monofilament wires (Songer et al., 1993).

Safety

The number one reason I began to work on a cable system to replace wires was to develop a safer method of sublaminar passage. The passage of sublaminar wires even in experienced hands has neurologic risks (Johnston, Happel, & Norris, 1986; King, 1984; Thompson, Wilbur, Shaffer, Scoles, et al. 1985; Wilbur, Thompson, Shaffer, & Nash, 1984; Winter & Lonstein, 1989). In the correction of spinal deformities the greater neurologic risk occurs during the manipulation of the wires as the spinal construct is secured with the tightening of the wires. Careful study of the SSEP (somatosensory evoked potential) recordings during the manipulation of wires reveals that there are frequent fluctuations in the amplitude during tightening of the wires (Songer et al., 1991). This fluctuation of the amplitude is notably absent during tightening of the cables. In a fluoroscopic study (Songer & Davenport, 1994) of the passage of sublaminar wires and cables in an animal model, the depth of penetration of the leader portion of the cable and the initial portion of the wire was similar. However, the cable remained in intimate contact with the anterior surface of the lamina, whereas the monofilament wire protruded significantly into the spinal canal even with constant upward pressure. Arthroscopic viewing of the unsecured cable revealed that hydrostatic pressure of the cerebrospinal fluid was enough to prevent indentation of the spinal cord.

Tensile Test of Stainless Steel Cables and Wire in a Loop Configuration
(A typical graph)

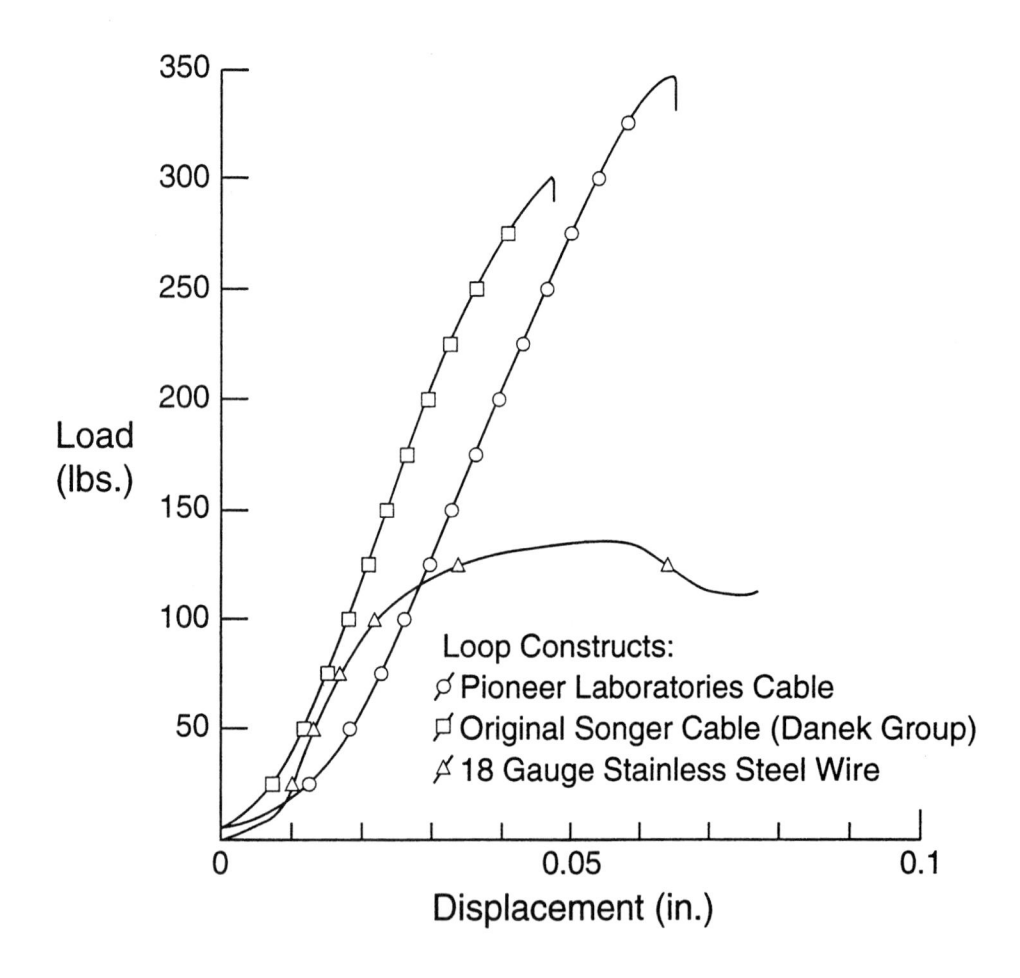

Loop Constructs:
- ○ Pioneer Laboratories Cable
- □ Original Songer Cable (Danek Group)
- △ 18 Gauge Stainless Steel Wire

	Maximum Load
Pioneer Laboratories Cable	$\bar{x}$=346.4 lbs.
Original Songer Cable (Danek Group)	$\bar{x}$=299.9 lbs.
18 Gauge Wire Loop	$\bar{x}$=135.0 lbs.

Test performed: Michigan Technological University, May 1993
Equipment: Instron 8500 Test System with MTS Load Frame & FLAPS Software
Machine Parameters: 10 KN Load Cell
Digital Data Logging 2 hz.
Crosshead Speed 0.05 in./min.

FIG. 6-1. This is a stress-strain curve of the static loading of the cable versus wire. Note, the linear displacement of the cable versus the wire. Hence, the wire stretches before it breaks.

Constant Amplitude Axial Fatigue Test (5 Hz) of Stainless Steel Wire and Cable Loop Constructs

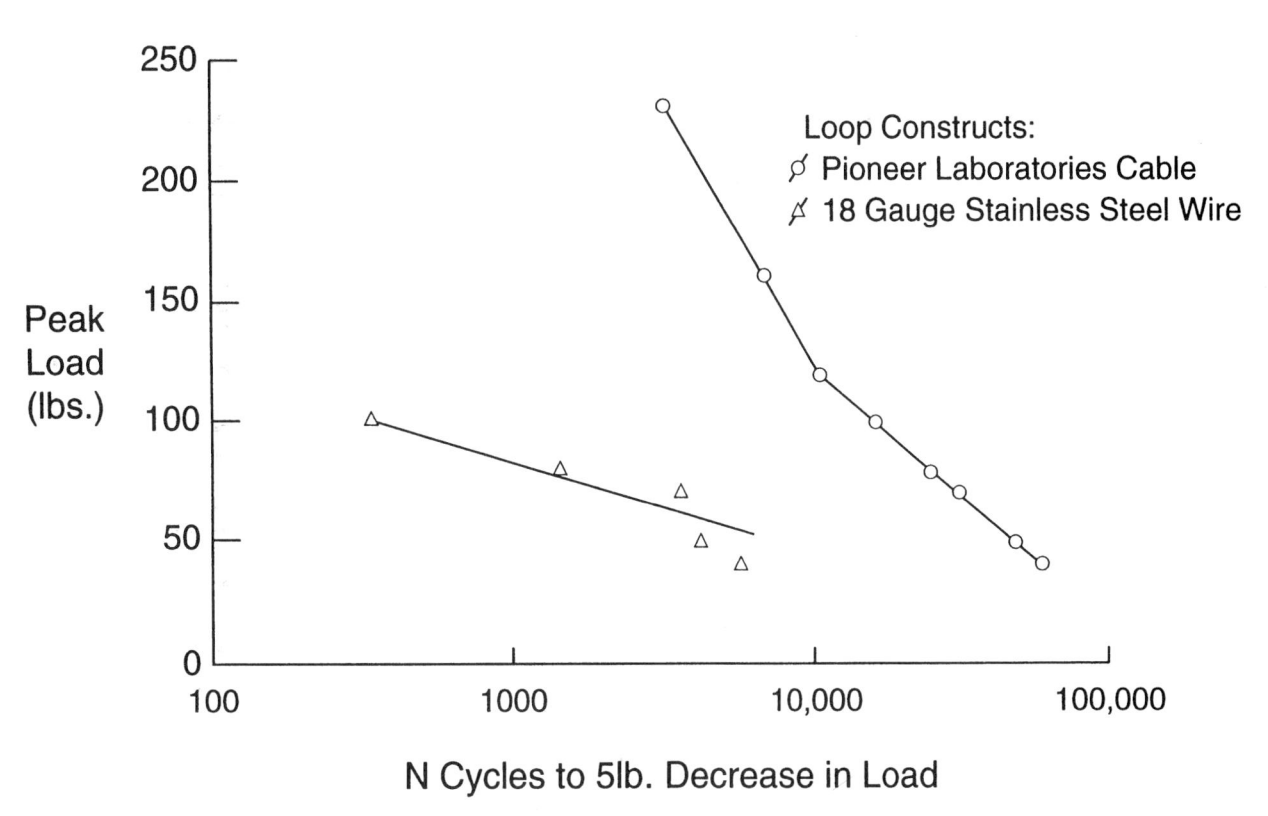

FIG. 6-2. This is a S & N curve of the fatigue strength of the cable versus wire. Since this is a logarithmic curve, it demonstrates that cable has many times the fatigue strength of wire.

BIOMECHANICAL PRINCIPLES OF CABLE FIXATION

Any spinal cable construct should be designed with the least stress risers possible. Sharp bends or kinks in the cable should be avoided. The implanted portion of the cable should not be grasped with any sharp instruments or even a hemostat if possible. When the cable is tensioned and crimped, the loop and crimp should be carefully positioned to avoid stress concentration. A simple loop is the best configuration because a complicated construct is difficult to evenly distribute the load throughout the cable loop. Also, a simple loop is easier to obtain even tension during the tensioning process of the cable. If part of the cable configuration is not evenly tightened, with time the entire cable construct may loosen.

When sequentially tightening cables at multiple levels, care must be taken to ensure that the cables are equally tensioned at each level. This is especially important when a deformity is being corrected. The tension of the cable is easily accomplished by threading two crimps onto the cable and initially crimping the outer crimp. Later, the inner crimp can be grasped by leapfrogging the outer crimp, retensioning the cable, and crimping the inner crimp. This is NOT necessary when performing a fusion in situ.

Cables are primarily used in conjunction with posterior spinal fusions. The cables are applied to create a tension band posteriorly. They may be used alone or applied in conjunction with rods, plates, and/or screws. The goal is to recreate the normal sagittal alignment, by correcting any subluxation or translation, and restoring lordosis in the cervical spine. This can be done simultaneously during the tensioning of the cables.

INDICATIONS FOR USE OF THE SONGER CABLE SYSTEM

The Songer cable system is ideally suited for posterior cervical fusions and occipital-cervical fusions (Table 6-1). The cables may be used with or without other implants such as

Table 6-1
Indications for Use of Songer Cables

Posterior cervical fusion
Cervical instability
   Trauma
   Tumor
   Infection
   Congenital disorders
   Degenerative arthritis
   Destabilizing surgery

rods, plates, and/or screws. The cables are available in stainless steel or titanium. Implants made of different metals should not be used in the same location.

The Songer cable system is indicated for posterior cervical fusion of the upper and lower cervical spine for correction of instability from trauma, tumors, infection (see contraindications below), congenital disorders, degenerative arthritis (both osteoarthritis and rheumatoid arthritis), and from destabilizing procedures such as wide laminectomies (Abdu & Bohlman, 1992; Fielding, 1988; Meyer & Heim, 1989; Stauffer, 1988). White and Panjabi (1984) defined instability as the ability of the spine, under physiologic loads, to prevent initial or additional neurologic damage, severe intractable pain, and gross deformity.

Trauma

Trauma to the upper cervical spine (C1-2) includes odontoid fractures, nonunion of the odontoid, and rupture of the apical ligament of dens.

Examples of trauma to the lower cervical spine (C3-T1) include facet subluxation and/or dislocation, or fracture dislocation involving the facet joint. If the lamina or pedicles are fractured, the fusion must be extended to the vertebra above the level of the subluxation and fractured vertebra. A posterior lateral mass plate may be used in conjunction with the cable to limit the levels of the fusion (Fig. 6-3).

Tumors

A posterior cervical fusion is useful for the correction or the prevention of collapse and kyphosis when the tumor is destroying vertebral body but the posterior elements are preserved. The Songer cable system is ideally suited when there is impending collapse of the vertebral body and the tumor is either not resectable or best treated by radiation and/or chemotherapy. Examples of this are breast cancer and lymphoma.

Congenital and Degenerative Disorders

Os odontoideum is due to the lack of fusion of the odontoid to the body of C2. This may lead to an instability of C1-2, which is best treated with a posterior fusion with cable instrumentation (Fig. 6-4).

Rheumatoid arthritis primarily affects the ligamentous structures, leading to instability. A classic example of this is C1-2 subluxation due to destruction of apical ligaments of the dens. Facet subluxation may occur, leading to subluxation in the lower cervical spine. Bone destruction may lead to basilar invagination, which may require an occipital-cervical fusion to prevent further collapse.

This cable system is also useful for fusion in situ for painful degenerative disease. The quality of bone is an important factor in the stability of the construct. If the quality of bone is poor, which may occur in many rheumatologic diseases or some congenital disorders, then external stabilization may be necessary.

Deformity

The Songer cable system is ideally suited to the application of spinal deformities. The ability to control the tension of the cable allows the correction of deformities by the approximation of the spine to the rod.

There are many different techniques for cervical wiring, and the cable may be adapted to each of them (Abdu & Bohlman, 1992; Brooks & Jenkins, 1978; Fielding, 1988; Gallie, 1939; Garfin, Moore, & Marshall, 1988; Huhn, Wolf, & Ecklund, 1991; Meyer & Heim, 1989; Stauffer, 1988; Weiland & McAfee, 1991; White & Panjabi, 1984). The techniques described below are a few that have passed the test of time. I have a good deal of experience with these and can recommend them. This is by no means an inclusive list of all possible wiring techniques.

CONTRAINDICATIONS FOR USE OF THE SONGER CABLE SYSTEM

The principle contraindication is the lack of posterior elements of good bone quality (Table 6-2). Examples of this are comminuted fracture/dislocations involving the lamina and spinous process, destruction of the posterior elements from a tumor or infectious process, severe osteoporosis, or surgical laminectomy.

An active bacteriologic infection in the posterior surgical spine is another contraindication. It may be safe to proceed during infection from tuberculosis or fungus if the infectious process is being adequately treated. If the anterior column is significantly destroyed from tumor, infection, or trauma, a posterior fusion alone is contraindicated.

POSTERIOR CERVICAL FUSION TECHNIQUES USING THE SONGER CABLE SYSTEM

General Principles of Instrumentation

The newly designed and improved cable system available from AcroMed consists of either a 316L ASTM F-138 stainless steel or titanium 6V-4A ASTM F-136 alloy cable, crimp, and related components (Fig. 6-5). The stainless steel cable is 0.040 in. (~ 1.0 mm) in diameter (18 gauge) and is comprised of 75 strands in a 8x7 + 1x19 configuration. The titanium cable is made up of 75 stands with the identical

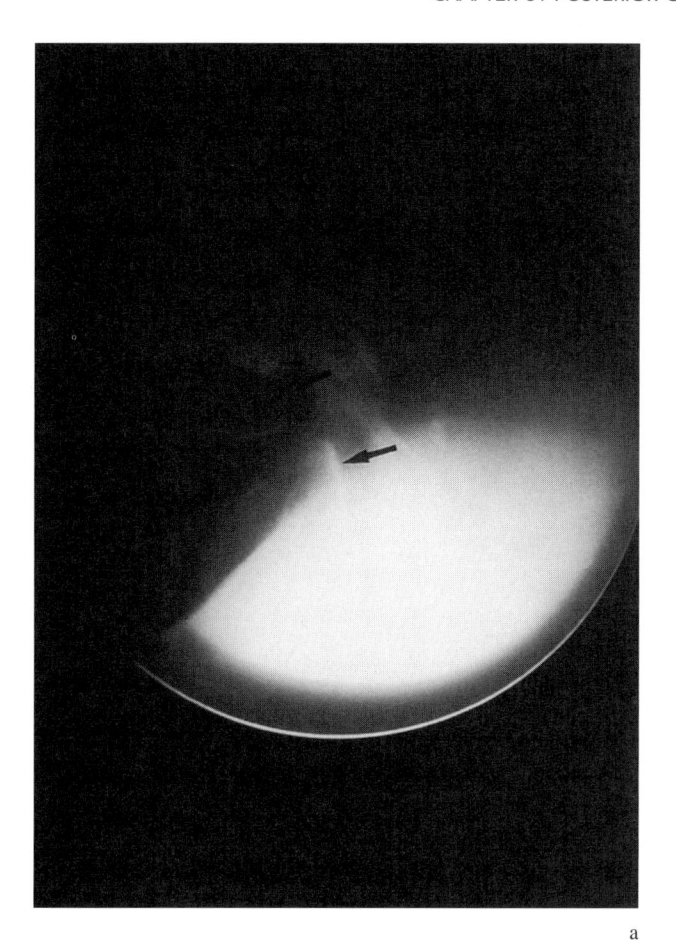

FIG. 6-3. (a) The cervical spine is unstable from a bilateral facet dislocation. (b) Lateral x-ray demonstrating restored alignment and fixation with interspinous cables and two lateral mass plates. (c) AP x-ray demonstrates the interspinous fusion with cables centrally and the lateral mass plates.

weave but is 0.047 in. (1.2 mm) in diameter (17 gauge). The reason for the slightly larger cable with the titanium material is to increase the breaking strength to equal the stainless steel cable's breaking strength. Titanium cable is more flexible and has a greater fatigue life as compared with stainless steel but is weaker in static stress tests. Titanium has less artifact on magnetic resonance imaging than stainless steel and therefore is preferred in the cervical spine (Geisler, Mirvis, Zerbet, & Joslyn, 1989; Mirvis, Geisler, Joslyn, & Zerbet).

There are three types of cables that are available: the double cable, the single cable, and the single Isola cable (Fig. 6-5). The double cable and single Isola cable are similar in that a soft malleable leader is attached to one end and a cable loop or islet is fashioned at the other end. The difference is that the double cable has two cables attached to one leader. The single Isola leader has a small loop at the end of the leader for ease of passage and retrieval during sublaminar passage. The standard single cable has a slightly longer and more rigid leader. The opposite end of the cable has a hat top crimp swagged to the cable. This cable is used with the

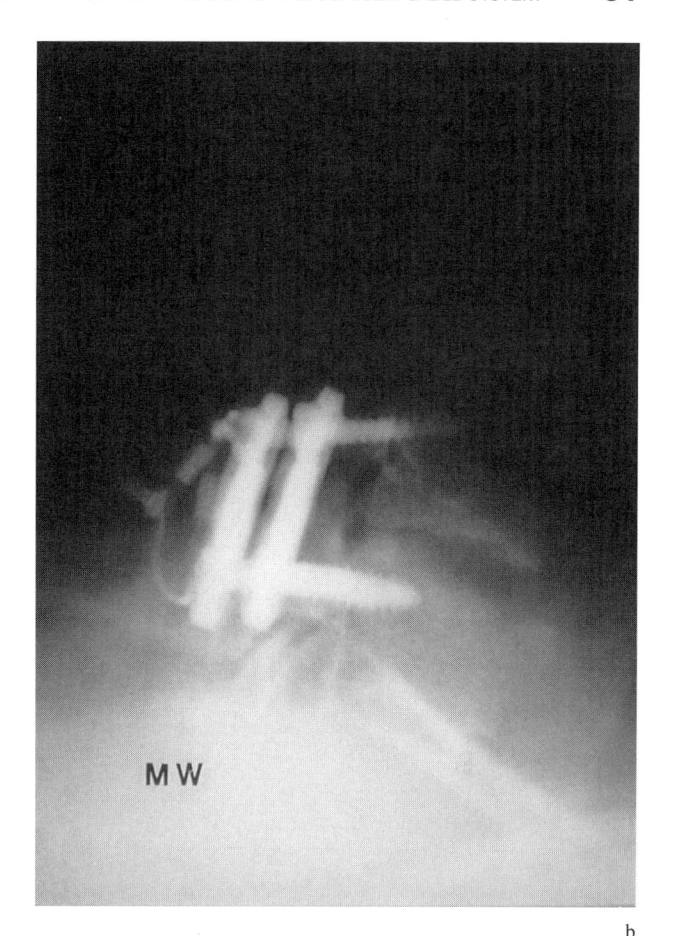

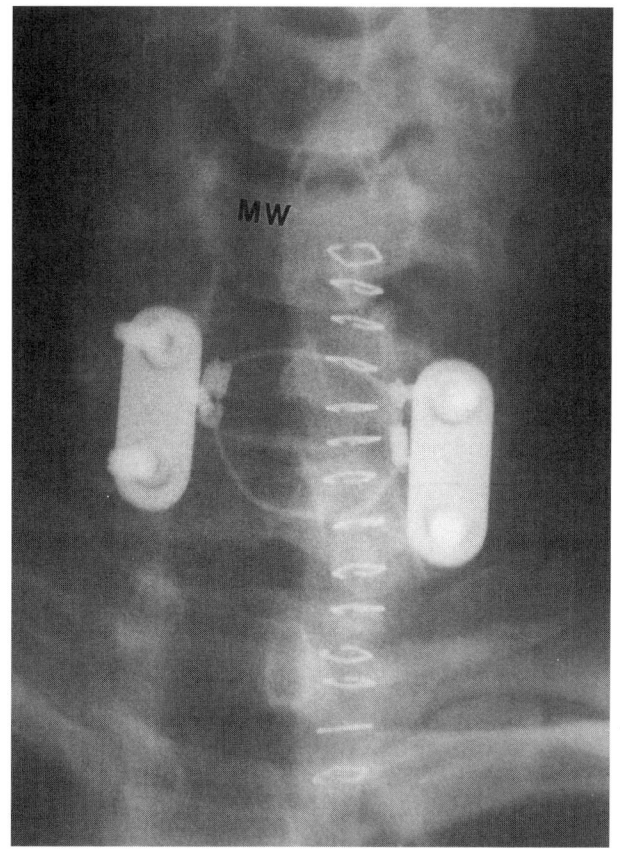

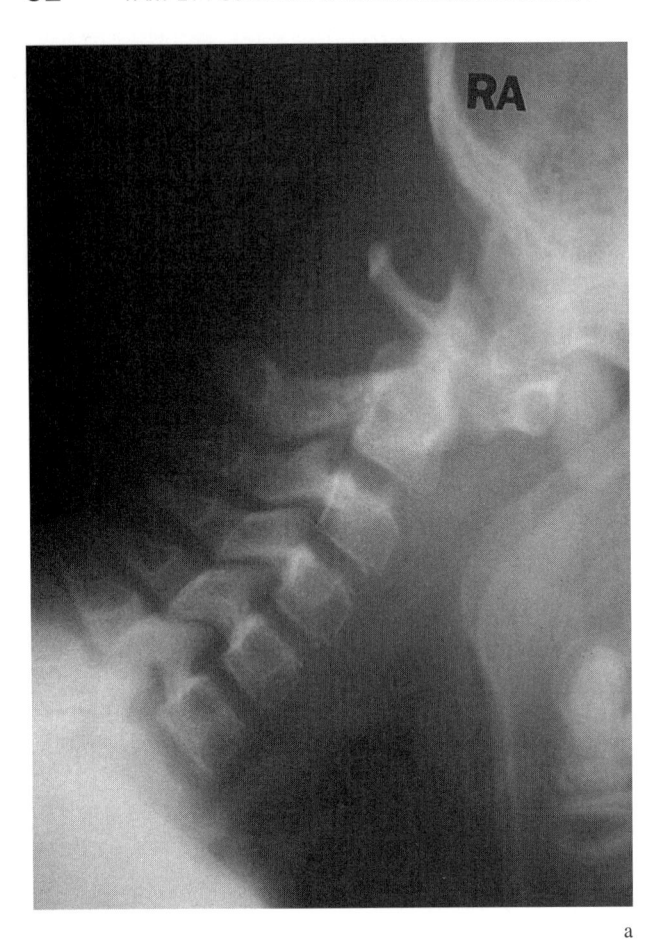

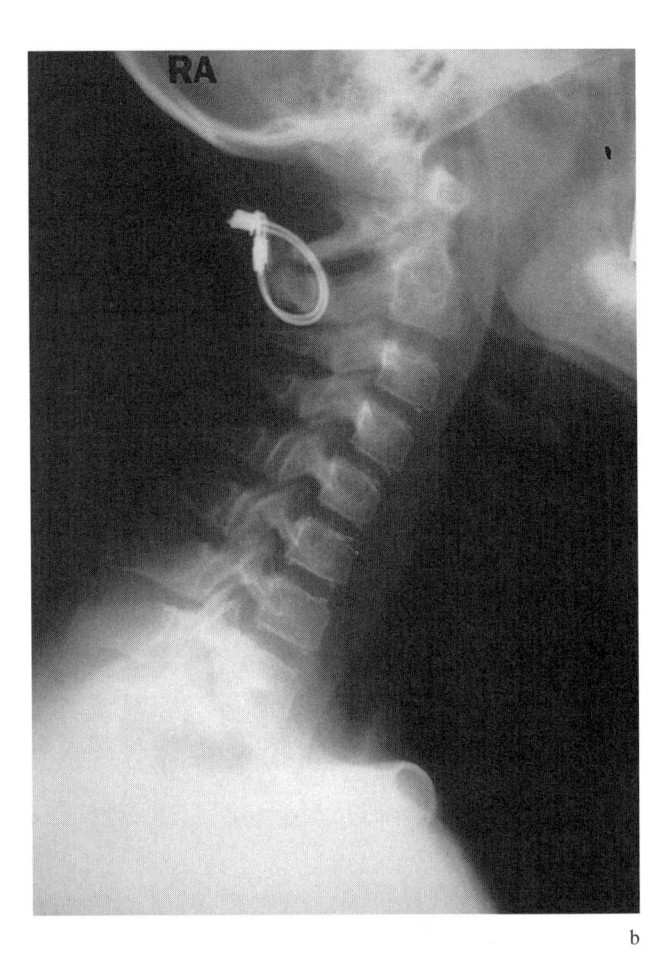

FIG. 6-4. (a) Lateral pre-op x-ray shows C1-2 instability as a result of os odontoideum. (b) Post operative x-ray demonstrates the reduction and stabilization of C1-2 with cables.

flat or round bar. This cable is not designed for the cervical spine and is better suited for the thoracic or lumbar spine (i.e., Drummond technique), or for cerclage applications in the appendicular skeleton.

Technique

The general technique for cable fixation is similar in all cases. First, the cable is wrapped around the objects to be fixed by the cable. With either the double or single Isola cables, the tip of the leader is cut off after the cable is passed (Fig. 6-6, *a* and *b*). Care must be taken to ensure that enough leader is left attached to the cable to allow threading of the crimp onto the cable. Next, the leader is passed through the islet of the cable loop at the end of the cable and pulled

Table 6-2
Contraindications for Use of Songer Cables

Lack of posterior elements of good bone quality
    Comminuted fracture/dislocations
    Tumor-destroying posterior elements
    Severe osteoporosis
    Laminectomy
    Active infection

snugly as one would tighten a noose (Fig. 6-6, *c*). The top hat crimp is grasped with the crimp inserter and set into the jaws of the crimper-tension device. The brim of the top hat crimp must be on the *outside* of the jaws of the crimper (Figs. 6-6, *d*, and 6-7). The crimper-tensioner is ratcheted one click after the jaws make contact with the crimp. The leader of the cable is threaded through the crimp and then through the tensioner component of the crimper-tensioner device (Fig. 6-6, *e*). The slack is pulled out of the cable and the set screw in the tension component is tightened to secure the cable for tightening (Fig. 6-8).

The torque wrench is then adjusted to the desired level depending on the location, the purpose, and most importantly, the quality of bone. In the cervical spine the usual range is 8 to 10 in.-lbs. In rheumatoid arthritis the torque range should be decreased to 6 to 8 in.-lbs. The torque wrench is now keyed into the hex of the tensioner and turned clockwise until the torque wrench slips, which indicates that the desired tension has been achieved (Fig. 6-6, *f*). The reversible worm gear in the tensioner has a 5-to-1 gear ratio. Therefore, the ideal tension generated in the cable is between 40 and 50 lbs. Once the cable has tension, the handles are squeezed until the ratchets release. This indicates that the

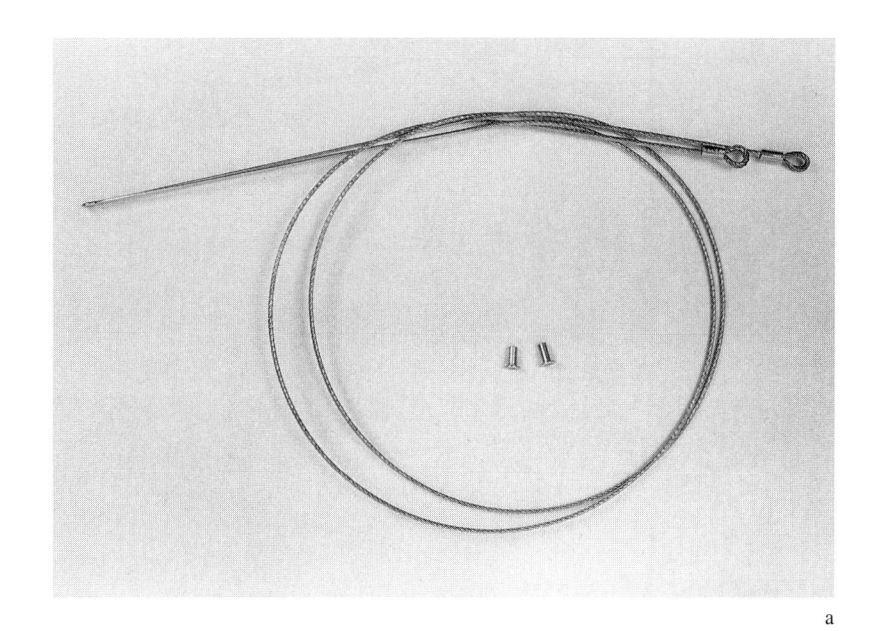

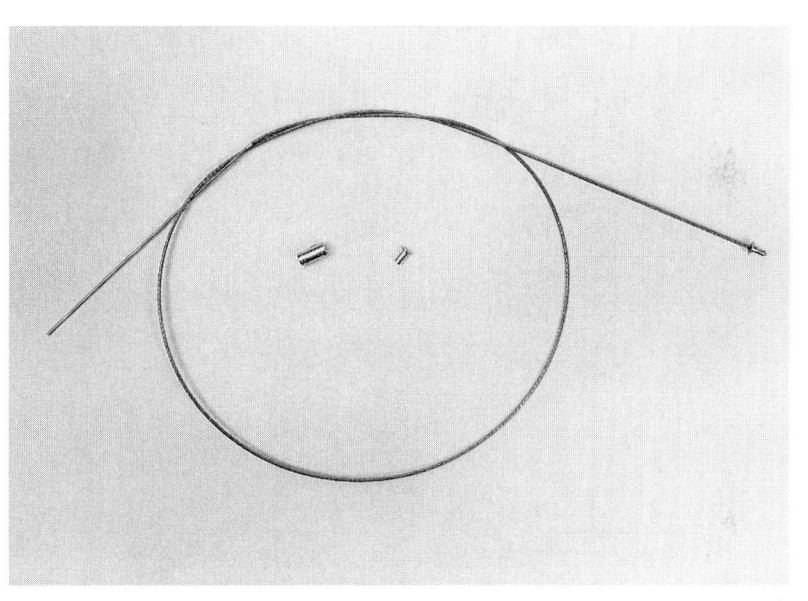

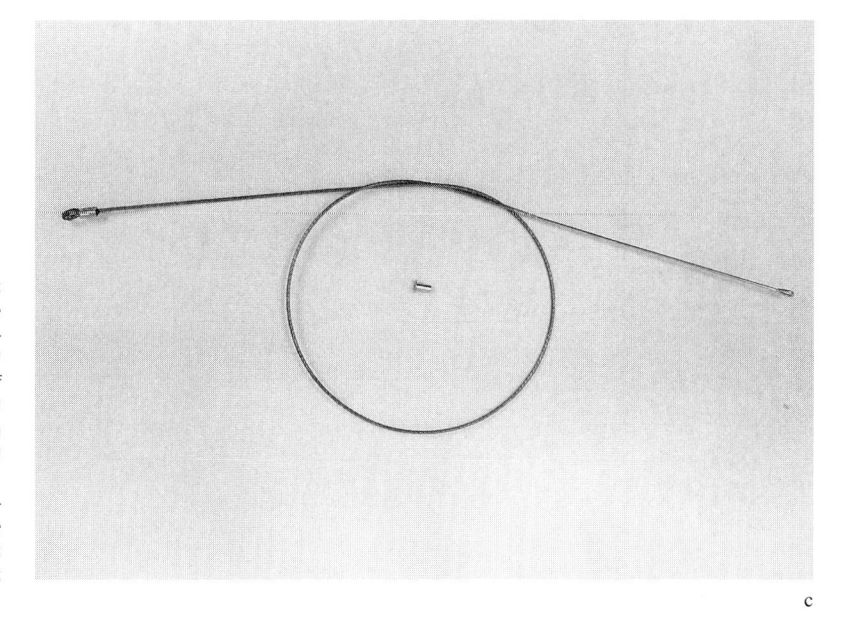

FIG. 6-5. Types of Songer cables: (a) Double cable consists of two cables connected to one soft malleable leader. This cable is ideal for sublaminar passage as two cables are passed at one time. (b) Single cable consists of one longer cable connected to a rigid leader. This cable must be used with a round bar, flex bar, or flat bar. It should not be used for sublaminar passage. (c) Single Isola cable consists of one cable connected to a soft malleable leader with an islet for grasping. This is designed for sublaminar or subpars passage.

64

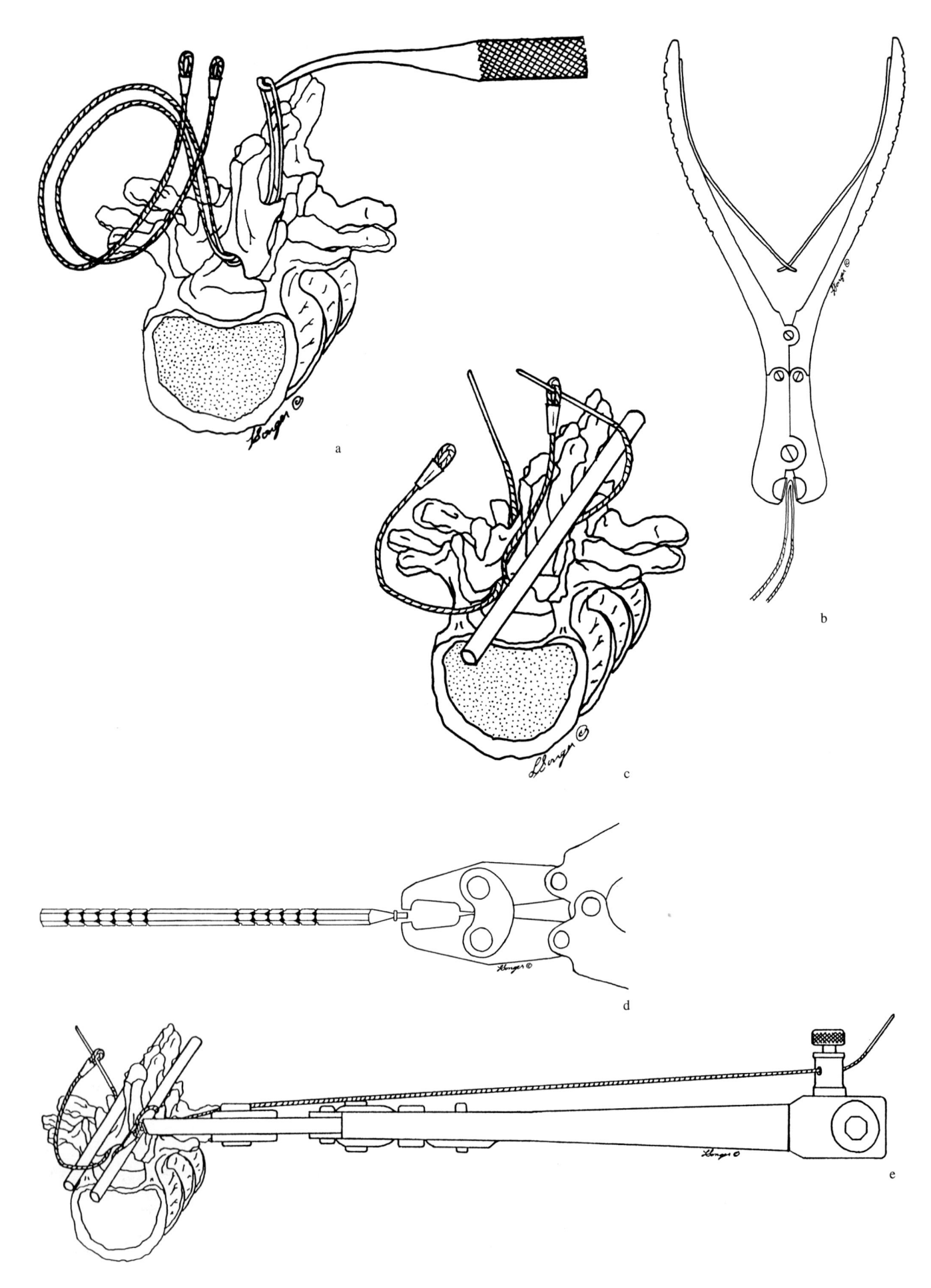

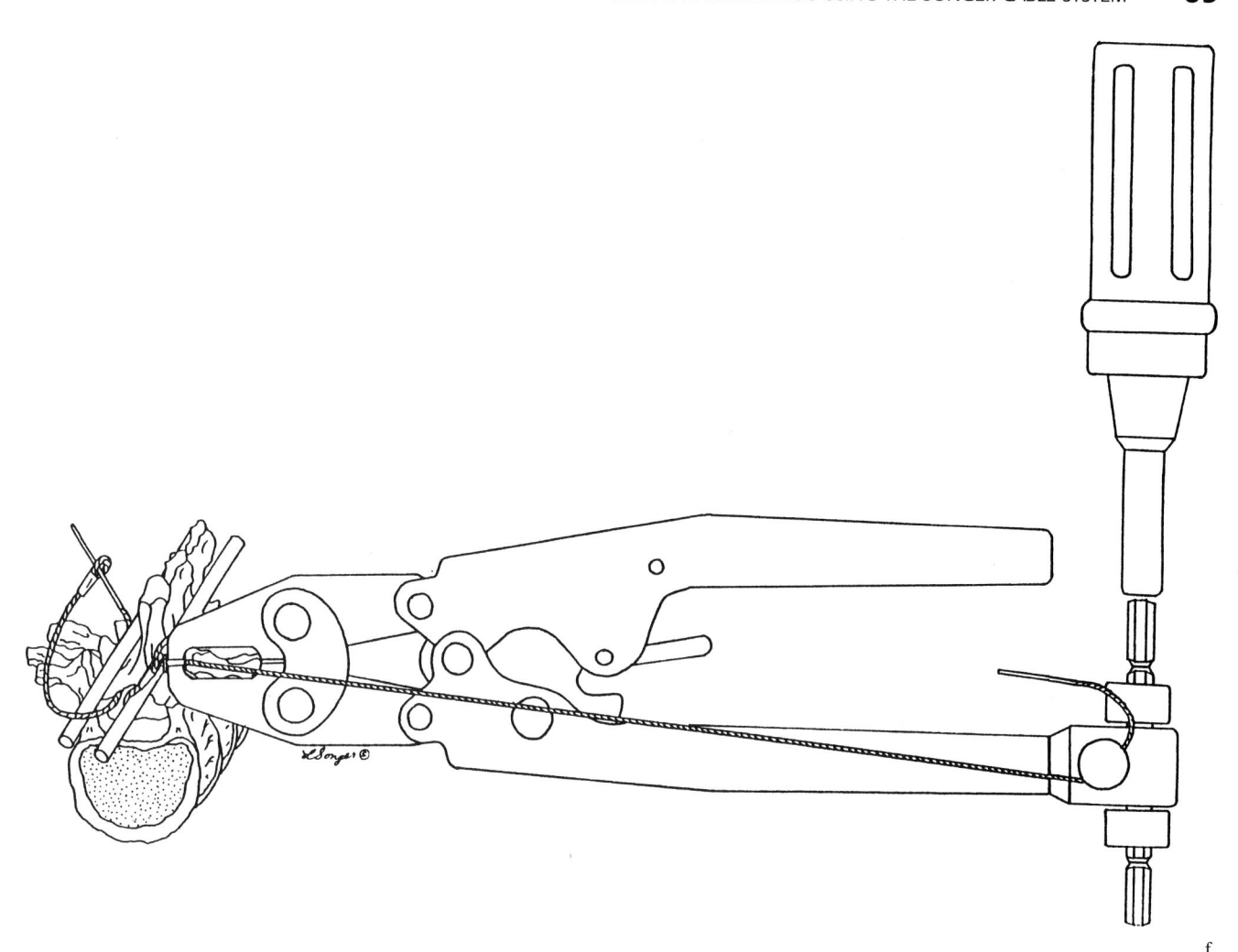

FIG. 6-6. (a) General technique for use of a double cable. The cable is first passed sublaminar. (b) The tip of the leader is cut off to separate the cables. (c) The leader is passed through the loop at the end of the cable. (d) The crimp is loaded into the jaws of the crimper and the jaws are ratcheted one click after contact is made with the crimp. (e) The leader is fed into the spool at the end of the tensioner and the set screw tightened. (f) The torque wrench is keyed into the tensioner and turned until it slips at the desired preset tension.

crimp has been fully crimped. There is a safety release trigger that may be used to release the crimp if crimping is not desired. The excess cable is cut off flush with the crimp. When a flat or round bar is used in conjunction with the cable, the tensioning and crimping process is identical with that described above. The important difference is that the flat or round bar is threaded onto the cable prior to cable insertion, and the leader is passed through the bar instead of the cable islet (Fig. 6-5, b).

Atlantoaxial Cervical Fusion

There are several wiring techniques that have been described for posterior C1-2 fusions. The two most common techniques that will be described are the Brooks (1978) and Gallie (1939) fusion techniques. The cable may be adapted to almost any wiring technique, but these two are the most commonly used. A transarticular atlantoaxial screw may be added in addition to the cable to reinforce the construct if the bone is osteopenic, such as frequently occurs in severe rheumatoid arthritis.

Brooks C1-2 Fusion

The upper cervical spine is exposed and soft tissue cleaned from the posterior elements in the usual manner. The laminae of C1 and C2 are lightly decorticated with a high-speed burr. This is done before the cables are passed to avoid possible damage to the cables from the burr. The ligamentum flavum is removed between the occiput and the atlas, between the atlas and axis, and between the axis and C3.

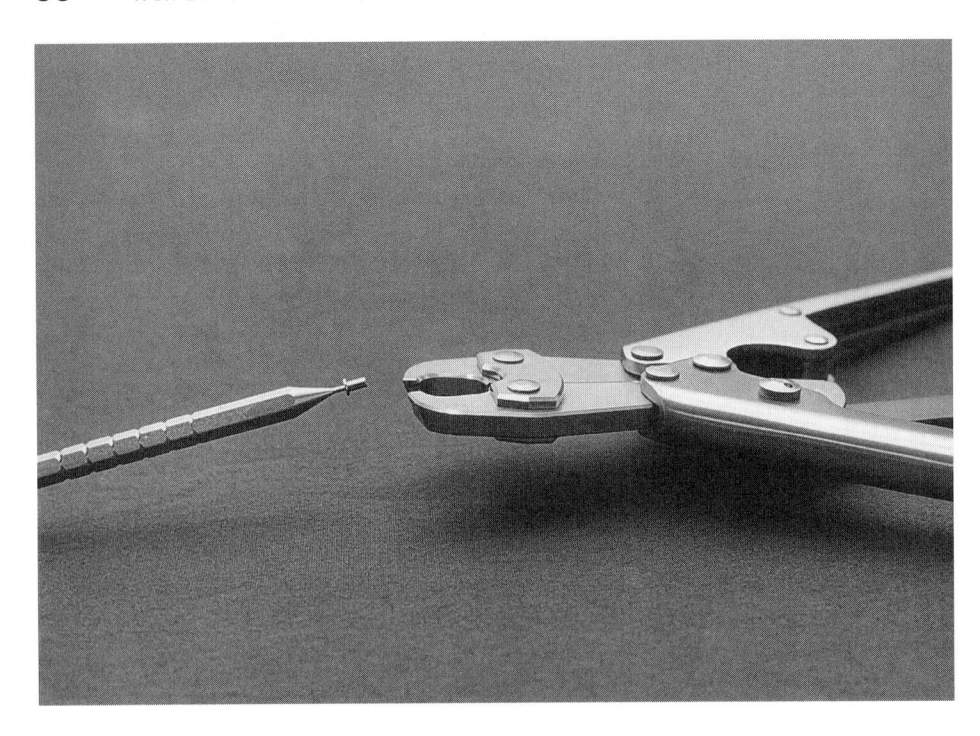

FIG. 6-7. The crimp must be inserted into the crimper with the brim or outer flange facing outward.

The double cable is used for this technique. The leader is fashioned into a gentle C curve. Care must be taken to make only a gentle bend near the tip of the leader and the cable-leader junction to prevent excessive protrusion into the spinal canal during sublaminar passage. The method that I prefer is to pass the cables upward, first under C2 then under C1 (Fig. 6-9, *a* and *b*). The technique of sublaminar passage is very important to prevent protrusion of the leader into the spinal canal. In a fluoroscopic study of sublaminar wire passage in the animal model, we discovered that attempts to pass the wire around the upper corner of the lamina caused the greatest canal protrusion of the wire. The canal protrusion was limited if the wire was passed under the lamina until the tip was visualized, then gently retrieved with a wire retriever or nerve hook. A smooth bend in the leader, especially at the tip and wire cable junction, was important in limiting canal protrusion. Previous work calculated that the ideal radius of curvature of the bend in the leader is 1.5 times the width of the lamina.

Once the leader is pulled out by the wire retriever, it is grasped with a Kocher clamp and steady upward pressure is applied to both ends of the cable. The leader is slowly fed through until it clears the lamina, then the cable can be passed with ease. I prefer to pass the cable under each lamina individually. The curve in the leader is refashioned with a sharper C curve and passed in a similar manner under the lamina of the atlas. During passage of the cables, care should be taken not to cross the cables. After the passage of the cables under the lamina of C1, the slack is gently pulled out of the cable in the C1-2 interspace (Fig. 6-9, *b*). The cables

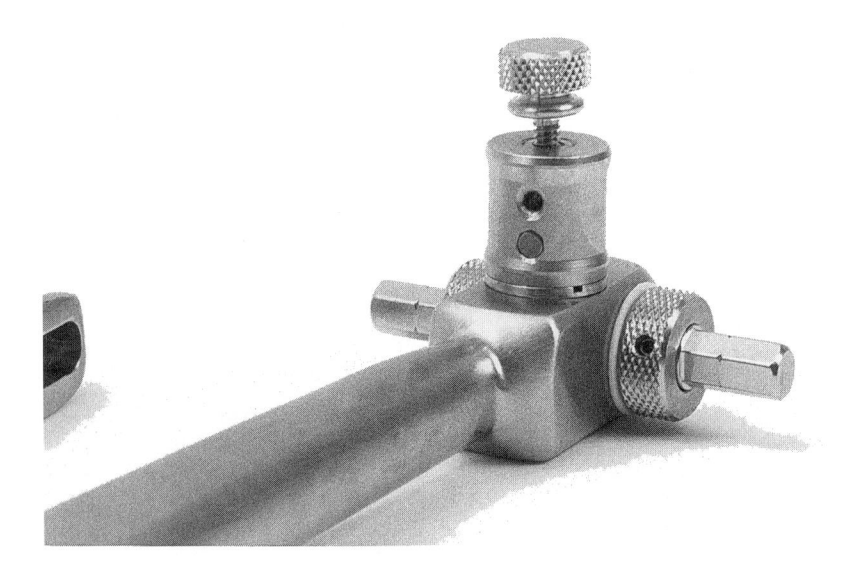

FIG. 6-8. The set screw must be firmly tightened to hold the cable.

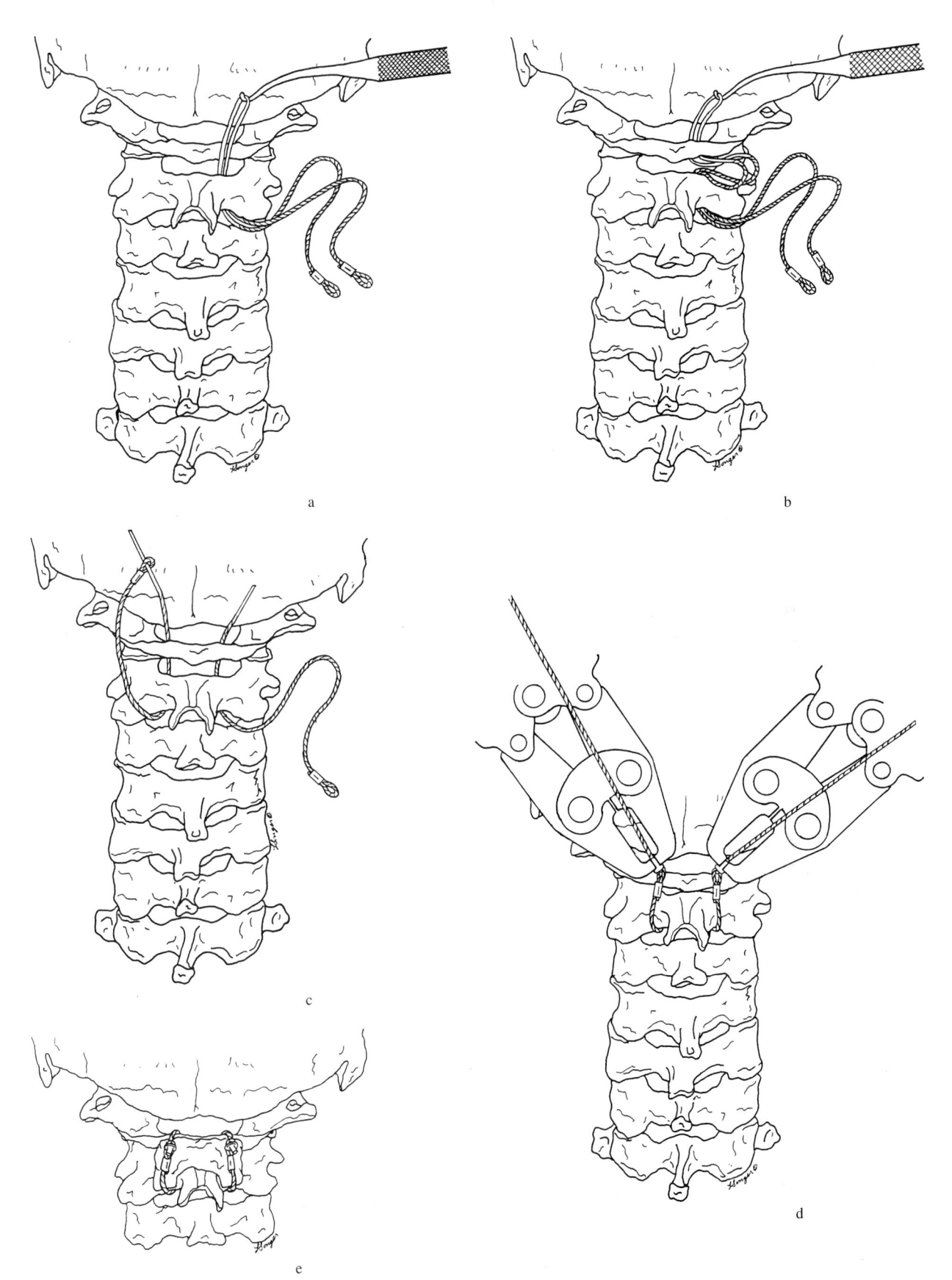

FIG. 6-9. Brooks C1-2 fusion technique: (a) The double Songer cable is inserted between C2 and C3 and passed sublaminarly upward to the C1-2 interspace. (b) The leader is reinserted and passed upward sublaminarly under C1. The leader is pulled out of the C1-occiput interspace. (c) The tip of the leader is cut off, the cables separated to each side, and the leader is passed through the loop at the end of the cable. (d) The cables are simultaneously tensioned and crimped. (e) The excess cable is cut off flush with the crimp. Generally the cables are tensioned over a U-shaped corticocancellous iliac crest bone graft.

are so flexible that this can be done easily and safely. This step was recorded by fluoroscopy in surgery and no canal protrusion occurred when the slack was pulled out of the cable between C1 and C2. Only the tip of the leader is cut off and the cables are separated and draped over each side.

A cortical-cancellous autologous bone graft is laid over the lamina of C1 and C2. A notch is cut out of the graft for the spinous process of C2. The leader is now threaded through the islet of the cable to form a noose (Fig. 6-9, *c*). The cables are then tensioned over the graft and the top hat crimp is crimped as described earlier (Fig. 6-9, *d*). The excess cable is cut off flush with the crimp and removed (Fig. 6-9, *e*). Small cancellous chips may be added laterally to enhance the fusion.

Gallie C1-2 Fusion

A prerequisite for this technique is good quality of bone of the arch of C2. Also, this technique should be used when there is anterior instability of C1 (C1 subluxes anteriorly with respect to C2). The correction force pulls the atlas posteriorly and extends C1 and C2. This technique is contraindicated if the quality of bone is poor or there is posterior instability. If the fixation is less than ideal due to poor bone stock, then a transarticular atlantoaxial screw can be added to enhance the strength of the construct.

The preparation for the fusion is the same as the description for the Brooks fusion technique except that the ligamentum flavum is not removed between C2 and C3. A double cable is passed under the lamina of C1 from caudal to cranial (Fig. 6-10, *a*). The tip of the leader is cut off, the leaders are passed through the islet of each cable, and two loops around C1 are created (Fig. 6-10, *b*). There are two techniques for wrapping the cable around the spinous process of C2. The free ends of each cable are thread in opposite directions through a round bar and are then tensioned with two crimpers simultaneously. Ideally, the bar should be positioned to one side of the spinous process of C2. Both crimps are crimped and the excess cable is cut off.

The new revised technique of completing the Gallie construct is to thread the free ends of each cable through a double-islet cable "bow-tie" (*flex bar*) connector (Fig. 6-10, *c*). In this case the free end of the cable is threaded in the same direction through the double-islet cable connector. Two crimpers are used to put tension on and crimp the cable on each side of the spinous process simultaneously (Fig. 6-10, *d*). Finally, cancellous chips of bone graft are packed posteriorly and laterally over C1 and C2.

Occipital-Cervical Fusion

The Songer cable system is very useful for occipital-cervical fusions (Fig. 6-11). The indications are severe degenerative disease such as that accompanying rheumatoid arthritis, basilar invagination, atlantoaxial instability accompanied by deficiency of the posterior arch of C1, and destruction of the lateral masses of C1 from tumor or infection (Ransford, Crockard, Pozo, Thomas, & Nelson, 1986; Wertheim & Bohlman, 1987). Occipital-cervical fusions are also indicated for cervical stabilization in certain muscle and neurologic disorders such as Duchenne's muscular dystrophy, spinal muscular atrophy, and cerebral palsy.

This procedure is contraindicated in the presence of an active bacteriologic infection posteriorly. Poor bone stock is a relative contraindication, as this system has been used very successfully for occipital-cervical fusions in rheumatoid arthritis.

Technique

The occiput is best positioned and stabilized by a Mayfield frame or similar device. The position of the head and neck is carefully checked by radiography prior to commencing surgery. The posterior cervical spine and occiput is exposed in the usual manner. The posterior elements are cleaned of soft tissue and lightly decorticated with a high-speed burr. The facet joints of the fused levels are decorticated. Laminotomies are completed between the levels to be fused. Two burr holes are placed on each side of the external occipital protuberance of the skull at least 1 cm apart.

Double cables are passed individually under each lamina that is incorporated into the fusion as described above. A double cable is passed between the two burr holes on each side of the occiput (Fig. 6-12, *a*). A double cable is then passed under the lamina of C1 and C2 (Fig. 6-12, *a*). The tip of the leaders are cut off and the cables separated. A solid rectangle rod, or two L-rods connected to form a rectangle, is contoured to fit the occipital-cervical junction and the cervical lordosis. Because of the difficulty in contouring a solid rectangle, I have developed an L-rod that connects to another L-rod, forming a rectangle. Each L-rod can first be contoured then connected to each other prior to implantation.

The contoured rectangle rod is inserted into the neck and the cables fastened as shown in Fig. 6-12, *b*. First, the cables at the lowest cervical level to be incorporated into the fusion are tensioned around the rod and crimped as described above. Second, the inner cables on each side of the occiput are interconnected in a figure-of-eight fashion to form one continuous loop (two cables connected end-to-end). Third, the remaining cables are tensioned around the rod and crimped and the excess cable is cut off (Fig. 6-12, *c*). The cancellous or cortical-cancellous bone graft is primarily packed laterally to the rod on each side.

Lower Cervical Fusion—C3 to T1

The use of cables below the axis is primarily indicated for correction of posterior column instability. This includes facet dislocation or subluxation from ligamentous injury, and certain facet fractures accompanied by subluxation. Other less common indications include impending pathologic fracture or pathologic fracture of the body that is inoperable or the anterior approach is contraindicated. Posterior fusions for degenerative disease are usually indicated only for post-

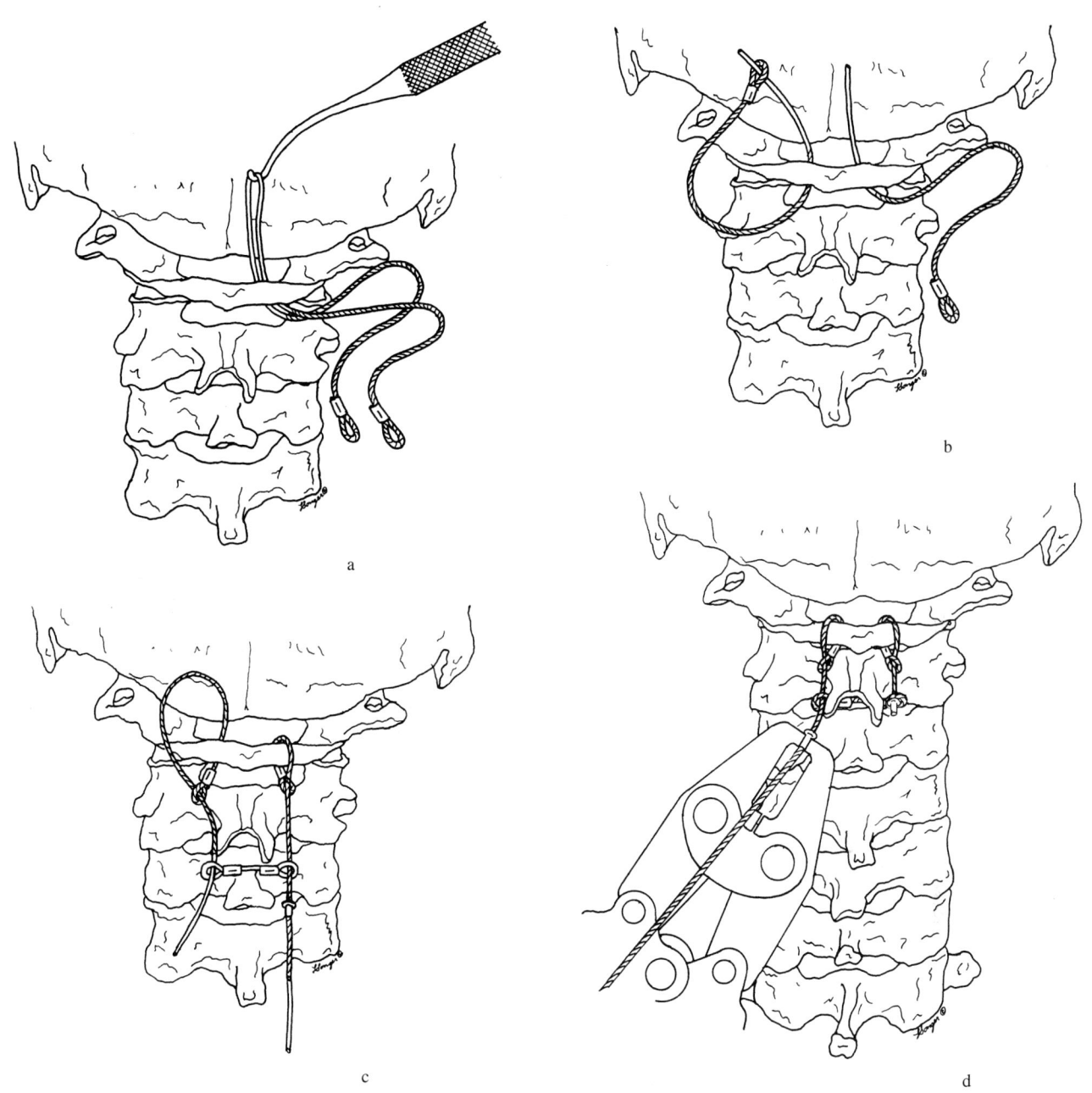

CHAPTER 6 / POSTERIOR CERVICAL ARTHRODESIS USING THE SONGER CABLE SYSTEM   69

FIG. 6-10. Gallie C1-2 fusion technique: (a) The double Songer cable is inserted between C1 and C2 and passed upward sublaminarly. (b) The tip of the leader is cut off, the cables separated to each side, and the leader is passed through the loop at the end of the cable. (c) After the U-shaped graft is inserted, each free end of the cable is passed through a flex (cable) bar, which has been placed through the interspinous C2-3 ligament and below the spinous process of C2. (d) The cables are simultaneously tensioned, then crimped and the excess cable is cut off flush with the crimp.

traumatic degenerative disorders with residual kyphotic deformity. The techniques described below are not applicable to correction of deformities resulting from muscular or neuromuscular disorders.

Techniques

Interspinous Posterior Cervical Fusion. If this technique is carried out properly, the subluxation and kyphosis can be simultaneously corrected with the incorporation of the bone graft (Fig. 6-13). Also, for additional stabilization in a noncompliant patient or a patient with questionable bone quality, a lateral mass plate can be added after the deformity is corrected with the interspinous fusion (Fig. 6-3).

In the case of posterior cervical instability, I prefer to use the Stryker frame with cervical tong traction. The spine is approached in the usual manner, and the posterior elements

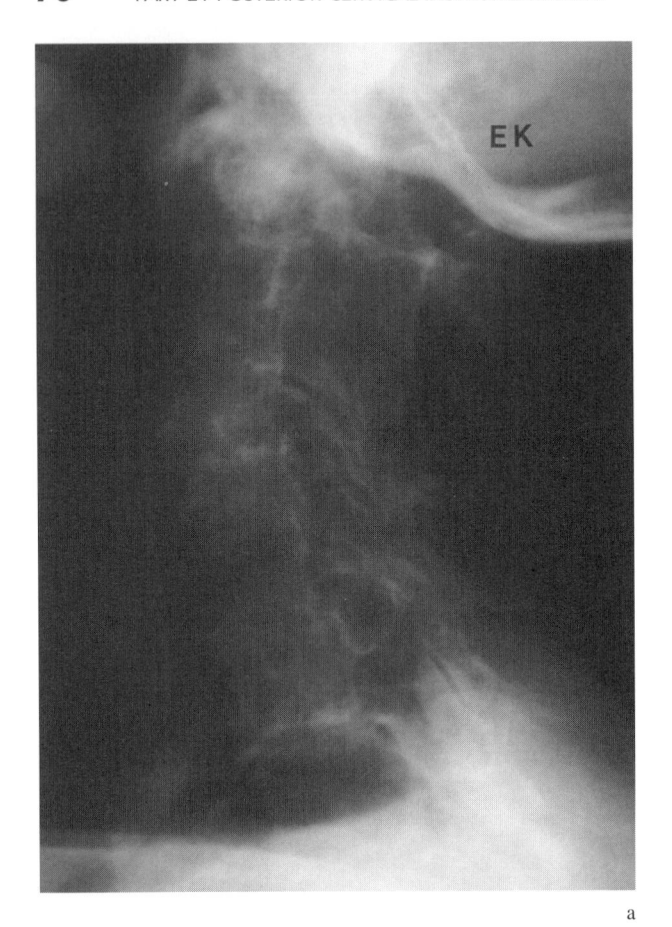

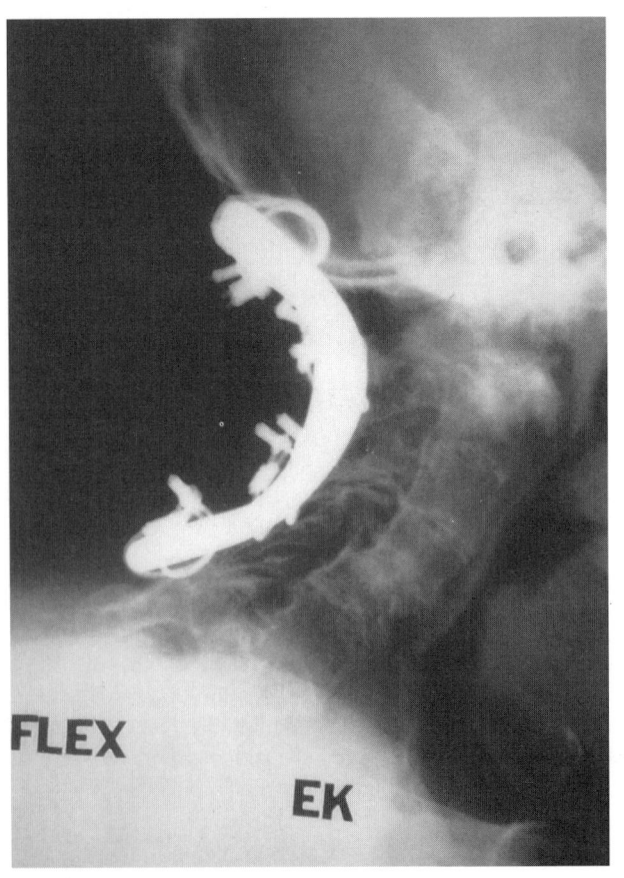

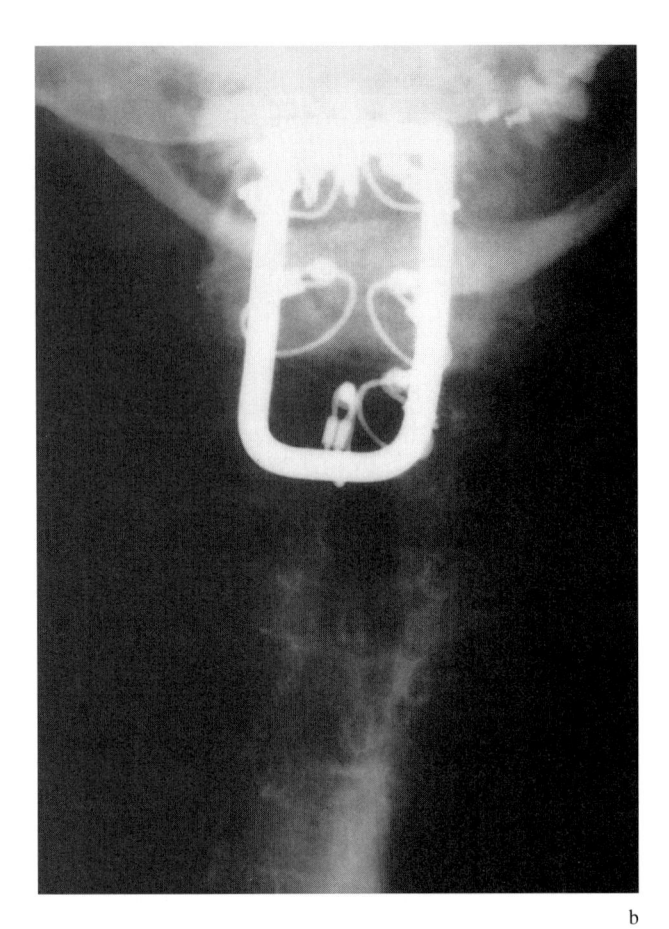

FIG. 6-11. (a) This lateral x-ray of the cervical spine in a patient with rheumatoid arthritis demonstrates basilar invagination. (b) AP x-ray shows the occipital-cervical fusion with the rectangular rod and cable fixation. (c) Lateral x-ray illustrates the use of the sublaminar cables and rectangular rod to perform an occipital-cervical fusion. The occiput is supported by the upper end of the rod.

are lightly decorticated. If a facet is dislocated, this is reduced prior to instrumentation. A small 90-degree-angle dental burr is used to make a small hole at the base of the spinous process. This is done as far cranially as possible in the cranial vertebra to be fused. A hole is created on each side of the spinous process and the holes connected by a towel clip. The holes are made in the middle to caudal side of the base of the spinous process of the caudal vertebra to be fused.

Two cortical-cancellous autologous bone graft strips approximately 1.5 cm by 3.0 cm for a single-level fusion are harvested. The burr is used to create two holes which are angled toward the center of each graft. These holes should be closer together than the holes in the spinous process in order to provide a corrective force during tensioning of the cables. The cortical side faces out and the cancellous side is on the spinous process.

The tip of a double cable is cut off, separating the two cables. Each cable is passed in opposite directions. The leader is first passed through one hole of the bone graft, then through the base of the spinous process, the bone graft

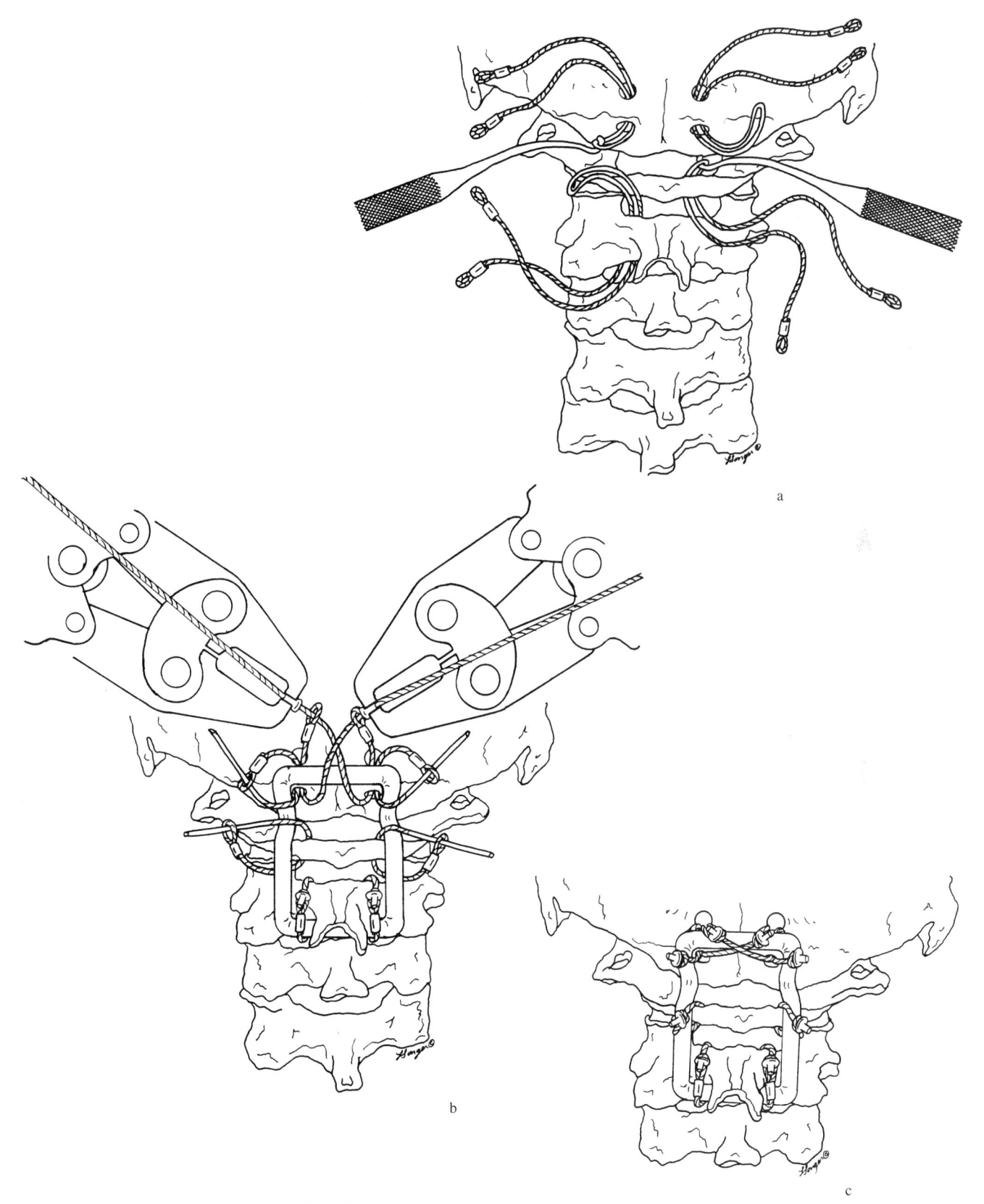

CHAPTER 6 / POSTERIOR CERVICAL ARTHRODESIS USING THE SONGER CABLE SYSTEM   71

FIG. 6-12. Occipital-Cervical fusion technique: (a) A double Songer cable is passed under the lamina of C2 and another double is passed under the lamina of C1. A double cable is passed *downward* under the cranium between the burr holes on each side of the occiput. (b) The rectangular rod is bent to match the occipital-cervical junction. Cable loops around the rod are completed. The two inner cranial cables are locked together in a figure of eight in the midline. (c) The completed construct is shown. Bone graft is placed around the rod.

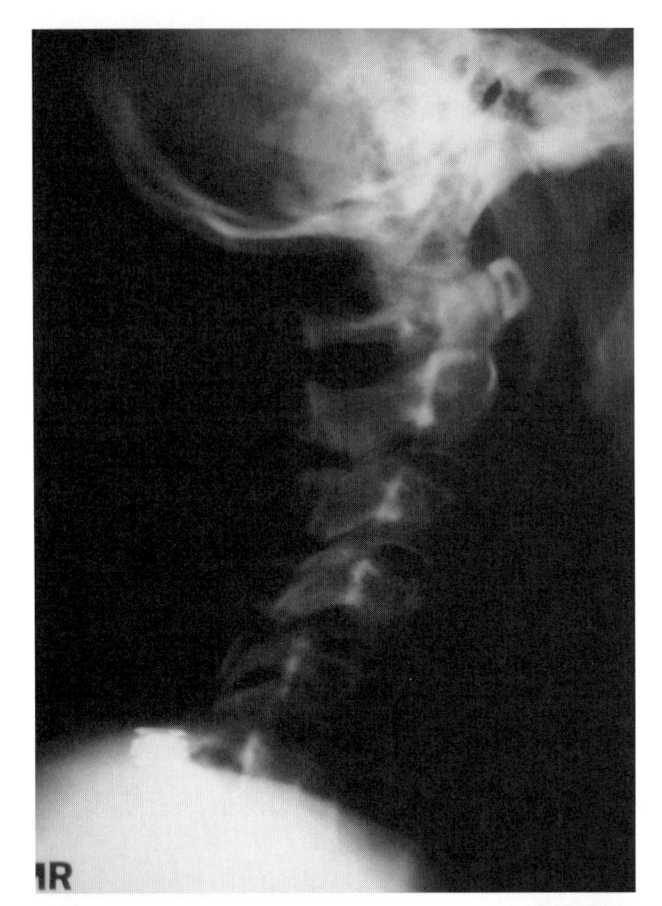

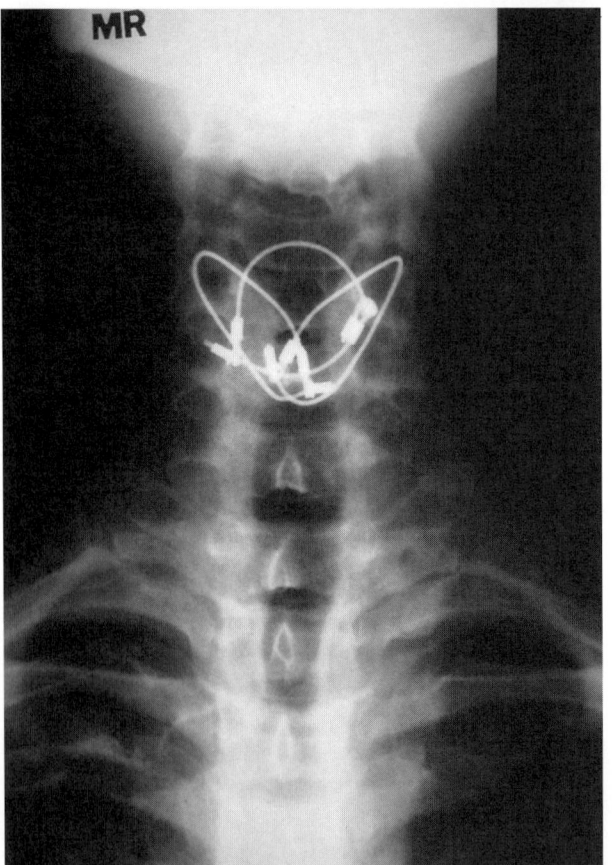

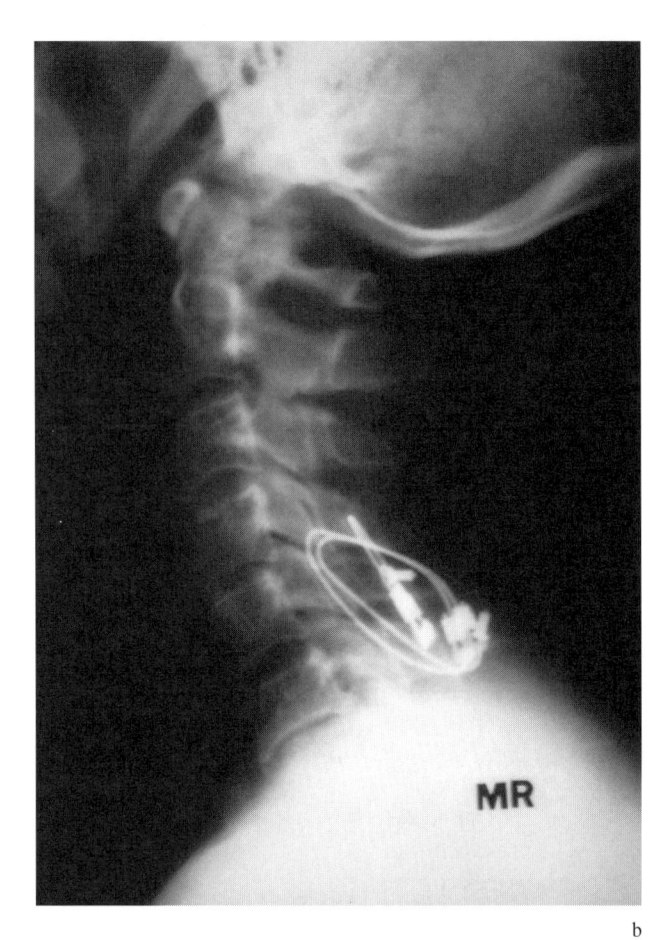

FIG. 6-13. Interspinous posterior cervical fusion: (a) Lateral x-ray demonstrates an example of a bilateral facet dislocation. (b) Lateral post operative x-ray shows the anatomic reduction and the posterior fusion with a combination of facet cables and interspinous cables. (c) AP x-ray demonstrating the posterior facet and interspinous cables.

on the opposite side, and finally through the islet of the other cable (Fig. 6-14, *a*). The second cable is passed in the same way in the opposite direction. A crimp is loaded into two crimpers and fed onto the free end of the cable on each side (Fig. 6-14, *b*). The cables are tensioned simultaneously and the reduction is carefully observed. As the cables are tensioned, the spinous processes should be brought closer together, correcting the kyphosis. If the bone quality is poor or the reduction difficult, a compressor can be used to assist in the reduction (compressor is available from AcroMed and sold with the Isola instruments). The facet cabling technique described next is also a very good adjunct to reducing the subluxation of the facets. Once the reduction is complete and the cables properly tensioned, the crimps are crimped and the excess cable is cut off and removed. Cancellous bone chips may be packed over the lamina and facet joints. A lateral mass plate may be added at this time as noted earlier.

Facet Cabling Technique. The facet joint is good cortical bone and provides an excellent means of fixation and reduction (Garfin et al., 1988). It is very difficult to wire the facet joint because of its rigidity, but using a cable makes this task tremendously easier. The primary indication for facet cabling is facet subluxation or dislocation. It must be a pure ligamentous injury posteriorly, as a fractured facet usually is not amendable to wire fixation. This technique is used as an adjunct to other methods of fixation such as spinous process wiring or sublaminar wiring (Fig. 6-13). The facet cabling technique is also useful for fusions after a laminectomy has been performed.

A facet dislocation must first be reduced. A small drill bit or a fine burr is used to make a hole in the center of the superior facet of the level to undergo instrumentation. Care should be taken to make this hole 5 mm or about a 0.25 in. from the edge of the facet. A Penfield 3 or similar instrument is inserted into the facet joint to protect from penetration into the inferior facet. Once the portal is created, a small hemostat or fine clamp is inserted into the facet joint. The tip of a double cable is cut off and the two cables are separated. Take one of the cables with about 2 in. of leader and pass the leader through the hole in the superior facet. Grab the leader with the clamp and pull the cable through the facet (Fig. 6-15, *a*). The cable is wrapped around the spinous process of the inferior vertebra to be incorporated into the fusion. The leader is passed through the islet of the cable. Usually the interspinous fusion is in place at this time and the cable is laid over or around this construct. I put tension on the facet cables first because this creates the greatest reduction force. As the cable is tensioned, the facet joints should be watched closely because it is possible to overreduce the facet joints (Fig. 6-15, *b*). Also, during the tension process, it is possible to tear the cable out of the facet. The tensioning should be done by feel and observation and not to a specific tension. I usually set the torque wrench between 8 and 10 in.-lb but do continue to add tension until the torque wrench slips if the desired reduction has been achieved or if the cable starts to cut out of the facet. Once the cables are at the proper tension, the crimp is crimped and the excess cable is cut off.

The facet cabling technique is a very good adjunct in the reduction and fixation of the subluxed cervical spine. It is my preference, however, to use a lateral mass plate in combination with the interspinous fusion technique described above. The lateral mass plates are much more expensive, may not be readily available, and may not be approved in certain countries. Under these circumstances, I feel the facet cabling technique is a good alternative.

Sublaminar Cabling Fusion Technique. The lamina has the most cortical bone of the cervical vertebrae and hence is ideally suited for fixation with wire or cables. Sublaminar passage of wires has always carried the risk of neurologic injury. The most significant advantage of cables is the flexibility, which decreases the risk of neurologic injury. In over $7\frac{1}{2}$ years I have never seen a neurologic injury associated with the use of the Songer cables, nor have I heard of a neurologic injury, nor has one been reported that I am aware of.

The indications for this technique are the same as interspinous cabling noted earlier. This technique is particularly useful if the spinous process is fractured or osteoporotic or if the patient is noncompliant with bracing. Laminar fixation with cables provides the strongest fixation against flexion or anterior translation forces. This technique is contraindicated in laminar fractures or destruction of the lamina from tumor or infection.

The sublaminar cabling technique in the lower cervical spine is basically identical to the technique described above for the C1-2 fusion. After the posterior cervical spine is exposed and lightly decorticated and laminotomies created, a double cable is passed under the **lower** cervical vertebrae to be incorporated into the fusion (Fig. 6-9, *a*). The leader is pulled through and then passed under the more cranial lamina (Fig. 6-9, *b*). Care must be taken to make sure that the cables are not crossed and that the loop between the two vertebrae to be fused is gently pulled out. I prefer to guide this with a needle holder as tension is applied to both ends of the cable. An **H**-shaped cortical-cancellous iliac crest graft is fashioned and laid over the lamina. I prefer to create notches on each side of the graft for placement of the cables. The cables are simultaneously tensioned around the lamina and H-shaped graft, crimped, then the excess cut off flush with the crimp (Figs. 6-9, *c* and *d*, and 6-16).

Postoperative Care

The postoperative immobilization for interspinous cabling, facet cabling, and sublaminar cabling is the same. A hard collar such as the Miami collar is worn for three months and the fusion is followed monthly radiographically. If the patient is noncompliant or the bone is poor quality, then a halo is applied for three months.

Experience with the Songer Cable System

After review of my last $7\frac{1}{2}$ years of experience with the Songer cables, I have had one C1-2 nonunion in a large rheumatoid patient who was braced only with a hard collar. He was re-fused with the addition of bilateral C1-2 transarticular screws in conjunction with two titanium cables, and immobilized postoperatively with a halo for three months. One noncompliant young man was in an altercation three weeks postop and fractured a spinous process of an interspinous fusion and was reinstrumented anteriorly and posteriorly. Review of the literature does not indicate that there have been any other problems with the Songer cables in the cervical spine. In my entire experience with Songer cables in the spine, I have had two cases with cable breakages at the cranial end of a Luque-Galveston fusion. Now, I use the Isola system and apply a claw at the cranial end of the construct and have not had any subsequent failures.

To my knowledge there have not been any reported neurologic injuries attributed to the use of Songer cables in any region of the spine. Also, I have not had any infections in the cervical spine to this date.

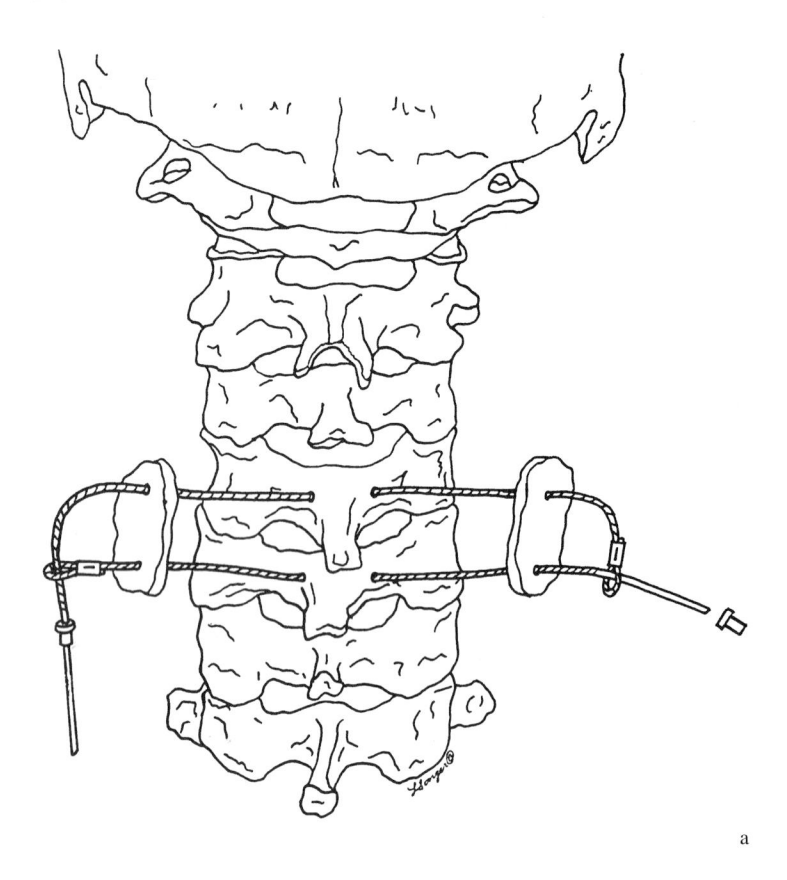

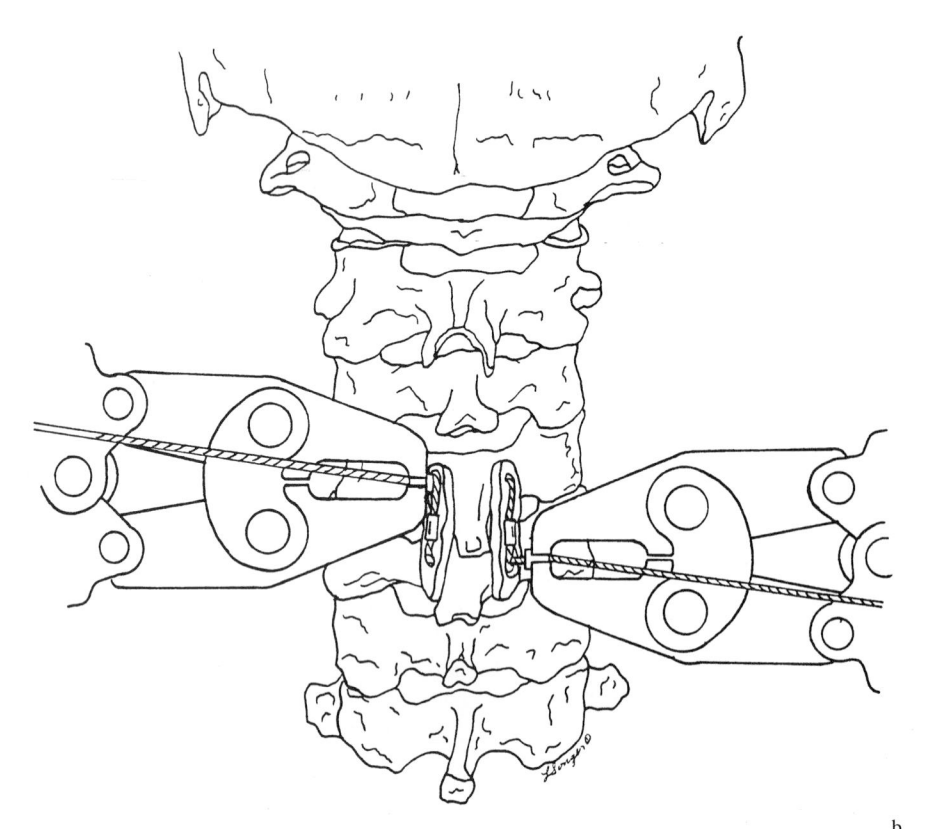

FIG. 6-14. Interspinous fusion technique: (a) After a double cable is cut in two, each cable is passed in opposite directions. First the leader is thread through the bone graft, next through the base of the spinous process, then through the bone graft and loop of the other cable. (b) The cables on each side are simultaneously tensioned and crimped.

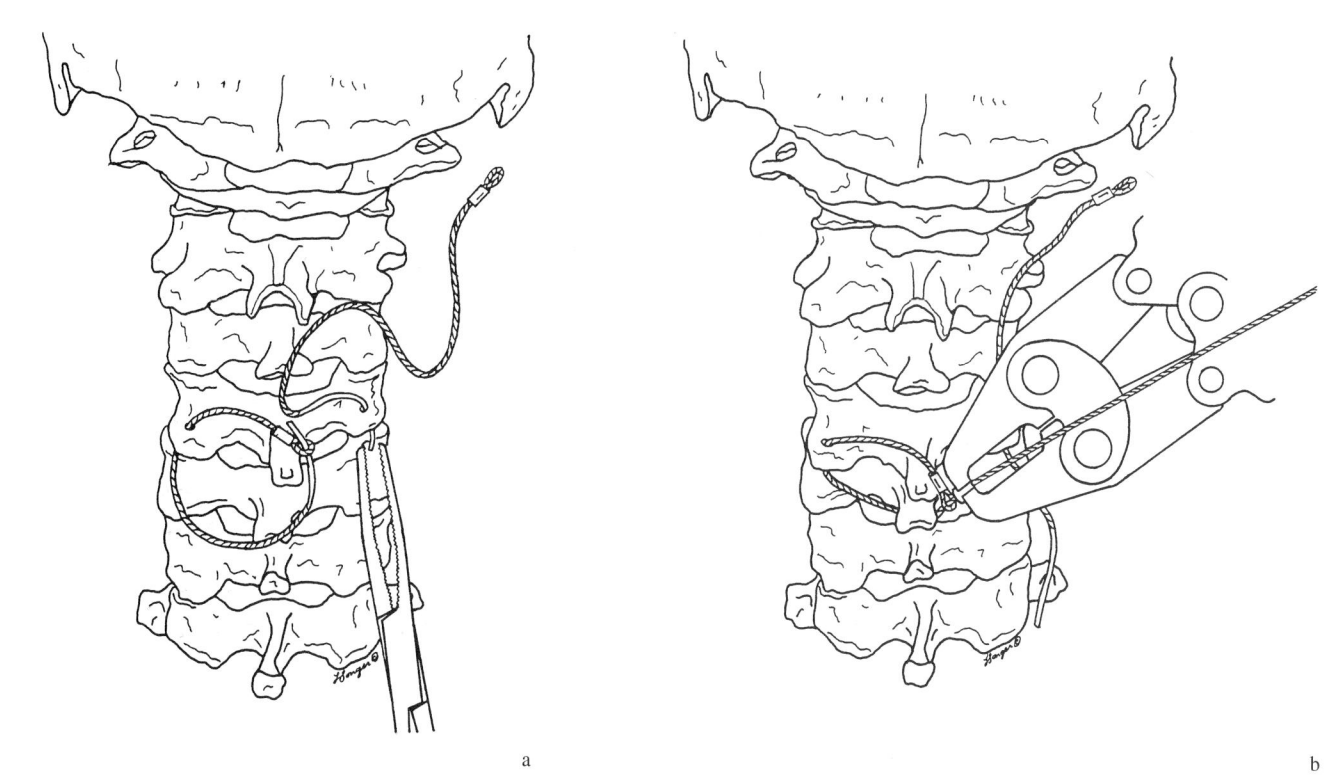

FIG. 6-15. Facet cable fusion technique: (a) A small hole is drilled into the facet. A double cable is cut into two single cables and the leader is passed through the facet. (b) A cable loop is formed around the spinous process below the level of the disruption. As the cable is tensioned, the facet is reduced. The bone graft may be placed under the cables.

The development of the Songer cable system is an evolutionary process. The system is constantly undergoing refinement and improvement (Table 6-3). The original cables were 49 strands and the new improved AcroMed cables are comprised of 75 stands. This was done to increase strength and flexibility (Figs. 6-1 and 6-2). The cables also undergo a special swaging process to smoothen the cable and limit the potential that the cable would cut through soft bone.

Table 6-3
Advantages and Disadvantages of the Songer Cable System

	Songer Cable	Monofilament Wire
Advantages:		
Strength	Far superior	Breaks at twist
Flexibility	Easier to use, safer neurologically	Rigid, difficult to use, neurologic risk
Tension	Known	Unknown
Reproducible	Yes	Variable
Fiddle factor	Less with experience	Always present
Time	Initially longer, less with experience	Constant
Insertion	Easy—especially in deep hole	Difficult
Removal	Easy—no dural tears	Difficult, risk of dural tears
Disadvantages:		
Cost	More expensive	Less expensive
Technique	Sequential tightening requires two crimps	Sequential tighten unlimited

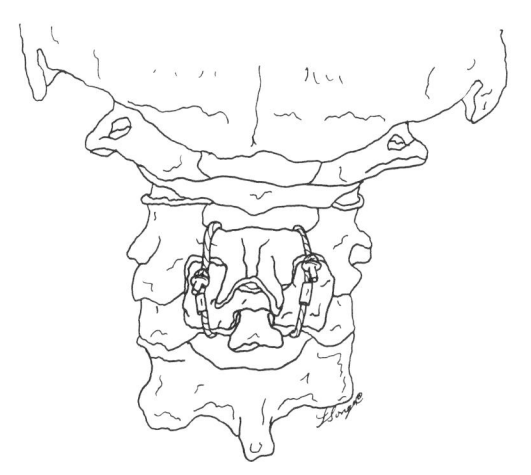

FIG. 6-16. Sublaminar cable fusion: A double Songer cable is passed upward, first under the lower lamina and then repassed sublaminarly under the upper lamina (see Fig. 6-9). The cables are tensioned and crimped over a H-shaped graft.

REFERENCES

Abdu, W.A., & Bohlman, H.H. (1992). Techniques of subaxial posterior cervical spine fusions and overview. *Orthopaedics, 15,* 287–295.

Brooks, A.L., & Jenkins, A.B. (1978). Atlantoaxial arthrodesis by the wedge compression method. *Journal of Bone and Joint Surgery, American Volume, 60,* 279–284, April 1978.

Fielding, J.W. (1988). The status of arthrodesis of the cervical spine. *Journal of Bone and Joint Surgery, American Volume, 70,* 1571–1574.

Gallie, W.E. (1939). Fractures and dislocations of the cervical spine. *American Journal of Surgery, 46,* 495–499.

Garfin, S.R., Moore, M.R., & Marshall, L.F. (1988). A modified technique for cervical facet fusions. *Clinical Orthopaedics and Related Research, 230,* 149–153.

Geisler, F.H., Mirvis, S.E., Zerbet, H., & Joslyn, J.N. (1989). Titanium wire internal fixation for stabilization of injury of the cervical spine: Clinic results and postoperative magnetic resonance imaging of the spinal cord. *Neurosurgery, 25,* 356–362.

Huhn, S.L., Wolf, A.L., & Ecklund, J. (1991). Posterior spinal osteosynthesis for cervical fracture/dislocation using a flexible multistrand cable system: Technical note. *Neurosurgery, 25,* 943–946.

Johnston, C.E., II, Happel, L.T., Norris, R., et al. (1986). Delayed paraplegia complicating sublaminar spinal instrumentation. *Journal of Bone and Joint Surgery, American Volume, 68,* 556–563.

King, A.G. (1984). Complications in segmental spinal instrumentation. In: E.R. Luque (Ed.), *Segmental Spinal Instrumentation* (303–305). Thorofare, NJ: Slack.

Meyer, P.R., & Heim, S. (1989). Surgical stabilization of the cervical spine. In: P.R. Meyer, Jr. (Ed.), *Surgery of Spine Trauma* (397–524). New York: Churchill Livingstone.

Mirvis, S.E., Geisler, F., Josyln, J.N., & Zerbet, H. (1988). Use of titanium wire in cervical spine fixation as a means to reduce MR artifacts. *American Journal of Neuroradiology, 9,* 1229–1231.

Ransford, A.O., Crockard, H.A., Pozo, J.L., Thomas, N.P., & Nelson, I.W. (1986). Cranial cervical instability treated by contoured loop fixation. *Journal of Bone and Joint Surgery, British Volume, 68,* 173–177.

Songer, M.N., & Davenport, K.A. (1994). Fluoroscopic study of depth of wire and cable penetration during sublaminar passage in an animal model. Presented at 6th Annual Ski Snowbird with the Spine Center Meeting; and ISSLS June 21, 1994. Seattle, WA.

Songer, M.N., Jayaraman, G., & Iwanski, G. (May 1993). Comparison of biomechanical properties of stainless steel cable vs stainless wire. Unpublished study, Michigan Technological University.

Songer, M.N., Spencer, D.L., Meyer, P.R., & Jayaraman, G. (1991). The use of sublaminar cables to replace Luque wires. *Spine, 16,* S418–S421.

Stauffer, S.E. (1988). Wiring techniques of the posterior cervical spine for the treatment of trauma. *Orthopaedics, 11,* 1543–1548.

Thompson, G.H., Wilbur, R.G., Shaffer, J.W., Scoles, P.B., et al. (1985). Segmental spinal instrumentation in idiopathic spinal deformities. *Orthopedic Transactions, 9,* 123–124.

Weiland, D.J., & McAfee, P.C. (1991). Posterior cervical fusion with triple-wire strut wrap technique: 100 consecutive patients. *General Spinal Disorders, 4,* 15–21.

Wertheim, S.B., & Bohlman, H.H. (1987). Occipital cervical fusion: Indications, technique, and long-term results in 13 patients. *Journal of Bone and Joint Surgery, American Volume, 69,* 833–836.

White, A.A., & Panjabi, M.M. (1984). Role of stabilization in the treatment of cervical spine injuries. *Spine, 9,* 512–522.

Wilbur, R.G., Thompson, G.H., Shaffer, J.W., & Nash, C.L. (1984). Postoperative neurological deficits in segmental spinal instrumentation: A study using spinal cord monitoring. *Journal of Bone and Joint Surgery, American Volume, 66,* 1178–1187.

Winter, R.B., & Lonstein, J.E. (1989). Adult idiopathic scoliosis treated with Luque or Harrington rods and sublaminar wiring. *Journal of Bone and Joint Surgery, American Volume, 71,* 1308–1313.

CHAPTER 7

Interlaminar Fixation of the Posterior Cervical Spine for Atlantoaxial Instability

Regis W. Haid
Cargill H. Alleyne, Jr.

HIGHLIGHTS

The C1-2 articulation is multiaxial with great mobility and accounts for approximately 47 degrees of cervical rotation (White & Panjabi, 1978). The indications for surgical intervention include instability secondary to trauma with ligamentous damage or odontoid fractures, inflammatory or degenerative arthritis, or rotatory instability. Congenital malformations or skeletal dysplasias presenting with C1-2 instability may also require surgical intervention. A variety of surgical techniques have been advocated for the stabilization of this region. Most of the current techniques use wire or cable internal fixation (with the wire or cable placed around the ring of C1 or encircling both C1 and C2) with autogenous bone grafts. The methods described by Gallie (1939) and Brooks and Jenkins (1978) have been used frequently. The former makes use of onlay bone graft. The Brooks fusion is performed by passing doubled wires deep to the posterior ring of C1 and lamina of C2 and tightened over corticocancellous bone grafts bilaterally. This is a more stable construct than that of the Gallie fusion. Several variations of the above techniques have been described (Fielding, Hawkins, & Ratzan, 1976; Mitsui, 1984; Yashon, 1988). Dickman, Sonntag, Papadopoulos, and Hadley (1991) reported a 97% osseous union rate using a modified interspinous wiring technique. Methods of screw fixation include anterior odontoid screw fixation (Barbour, 1971; Etter, Coscia, Jaberg, & Aebi, 1991; Geisler, Cheng, Poka, & Brumback, 1989; Lesoin, Autricque, Franz, Villette, & Jomin, 1987; Weidner, 1989) as well as anterior or posterior atlantoaxial transfacet screw fixation (Grob, Dvorak, Panjabi, Forehlich, & Hayek, 1990; Hanson, Montesano, Sharkey, Raushning, 1990; Magerl & Seemann, 1985; Weidner, 1989).

There are several risks to "wiring" techniques. The techniques require sublaminar passage of wire or cable at C1 (and at C1 and C2 in the Brooks fusion). Damage to the cord and other neural elements can result. There also exists a potential for the wires/cables to "cheese-cut" through the bone as the wire is tightened, especially in the softer rheumatoid bone. The use of posterior interlaminar clamps may decrease the risks of wire/cable fixation. Immediate stability is also provided by the posterior clamp construct. H.H. Tucker of Halifax, Nova Scotia, first introduced this technique in 1975. Holness, Huestis, Howes, and Langelle (1984) subsequently reported their experience using stainless steel clamps. Since then, various authors have reported high success rates for posterior cervical arthrodesis using interlaminar clamps. Most of these reports have involved C1-2 fusion, but others have included lower cervical levels (Aldrich, Crow, Weber, & Spagnolia, 1991; Aldrich, Weber, & Crow, 1993; Cybulski, Stone, Crowell, Rifai, Gandhi, & Glick, 1988; Moskovich & Crockard, 1992; Seek & Johnston, 1991; Statham, O'Sullivan, & Russell, 1993). In this chapter we will discuss the fixation technique for atlantoaxial instability, and highlight the three systems currently in use.

GENERAL INFORMATION ON SYSTEM

Description

Codman Interlaminar Clamp

The Codman interlaminar clamp is designed for the correction of posterior cervical subluxation with damage of ligamentous structures. It is also indicated for cervical stabilization in patients with rheumatoid arthritis. The construct is made of titanium, and each clamp assembly consists of three components: a screw, an unthreaded clamp, and a threaded clamp. The screw is placed through the unthreaded clamp and screwed into the threaded clamp. Bone grafts are then placed (see "Technique") and each assembly is attached to the laminae bilaterally on either side of the spinous process. The clamps are then tightened with a 90-degree locking wrench. Each screw has a hole distally that facilitates placement of titanium SOF'WIRE (Codman, Inc., Randolph, MA) or a heavy-gauge braided silk suture. This design reduces the degree of screw pullout. The Codman interlaminar clamp is designed to achieve fixation over two to three levels. The contents of the kit include: C1-2 clamps; 7- and 13-mm C3-7 clamps; 10-, 20-, and 30-mm screws; a 90-degree locking wrench; and a storage/sterilizing tray (Fig. 7-1, *a*). The C1-2 clamps have a more contoured design to accommodate the thick inferior lamina of C2 and the rounded anatomy of the posterior arch of C1.

Halifax PLUS Interlaminar Clamp

The Halifax interlaminar clamp (American Medical Electronics, Inc., Richardson, TX) is designed for stabilization of the posterior spine. The system is made of titanium alloy and consists of color-coded clamps (one threaded and the other unthreaded), a screw, and a threaded boss, which retains the screw and reduces the risk of backout.

After the graft is fitted (see "Technique"), the threaded and unthreaded clamps are assembled in the applicator forceps. The screw is then inserted into the clamps and the system is applied to the cervical lamina bilaterally.

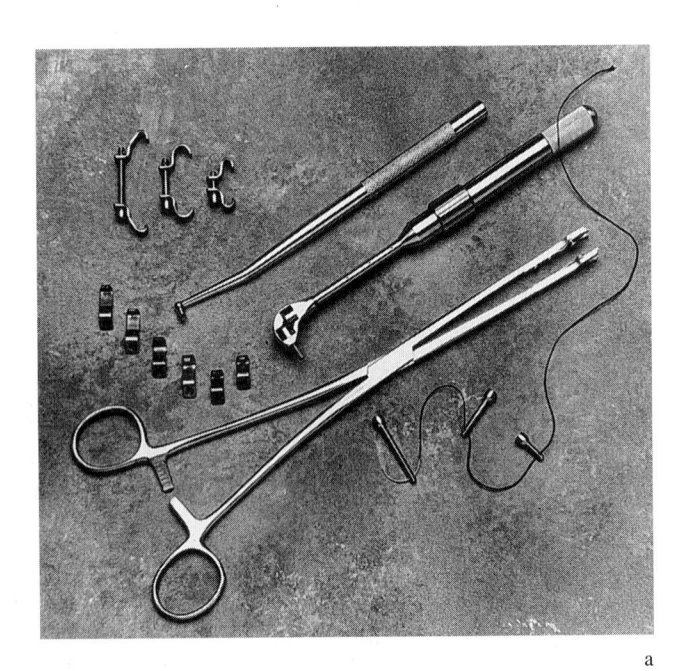

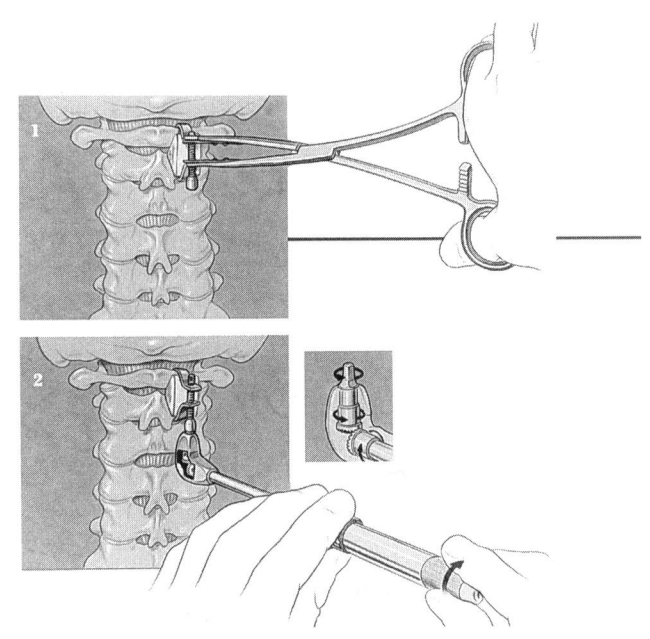

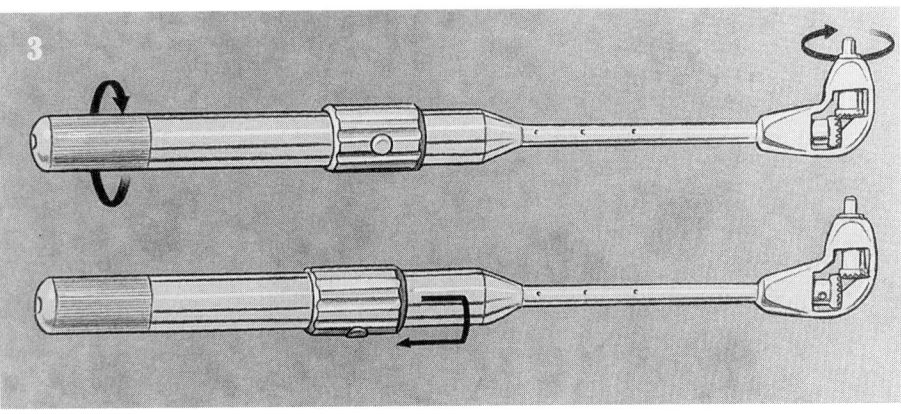

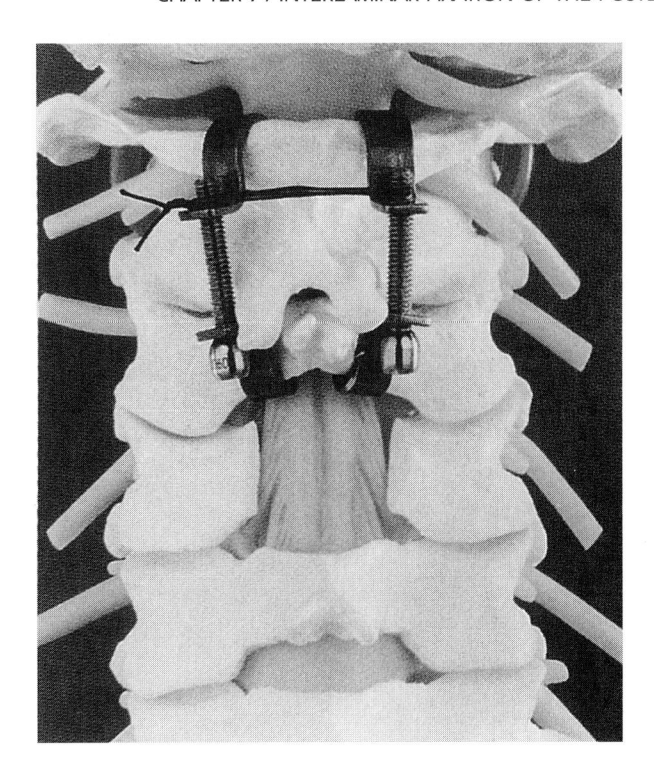

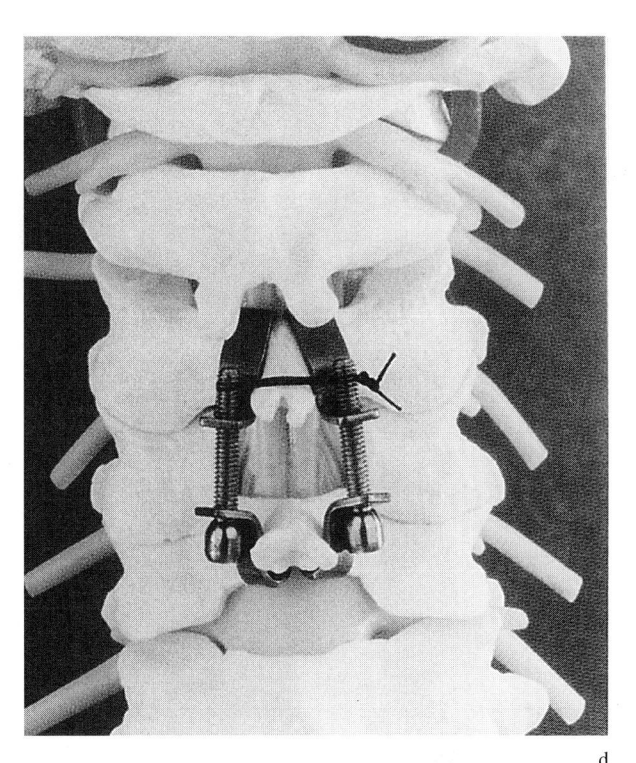

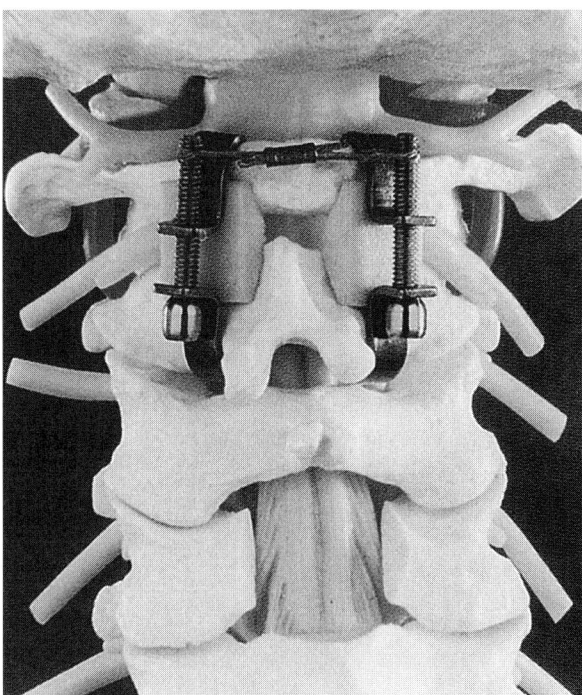

FIG. 7-1. (a) Components of the Codman interlaminar clamp kit. (b) The two halves of the Codman interlaminar clamp and the screw of appropriate length are placed with the forceps. The 90-degree adjustment wrench is used to tighten the screw. (c) A fine adjustment mode is obtained by moving the collet upward and to the right. (d and e) Final placement of the Codman interlaminar clamp using suture and wire, respectively, to decrease the risk of screw backout.

A 90-degree wrench is used to tighten the clamps bilaterally. Included in the set are threaded and unthreaded C1 titanium clamps; 7- and 13-mm titanium clamps; 10-, 20-, and 30-mm titanium screws; a clamp applicator; a sterilization tray; a fine adjustment wrench; and a 90-degree wrench (Fig. 7-2, a and b). Details of the surgical technique can be found in the "Technique" section.

Apofix Fixation Device

The Apofix fixation device (Sofamor-Danek, Inc., Memphis, TN) was designed by Dr. Richard Assaker of Lille, France. The system is used for posterior cervical stabilization using interconnecting laminar hooks that are secured by crimping. The construct is magnetic resonance imaging (MRI)-

80 PART 2 / POSTERIOR CERVICAL INSTRUMENTATION

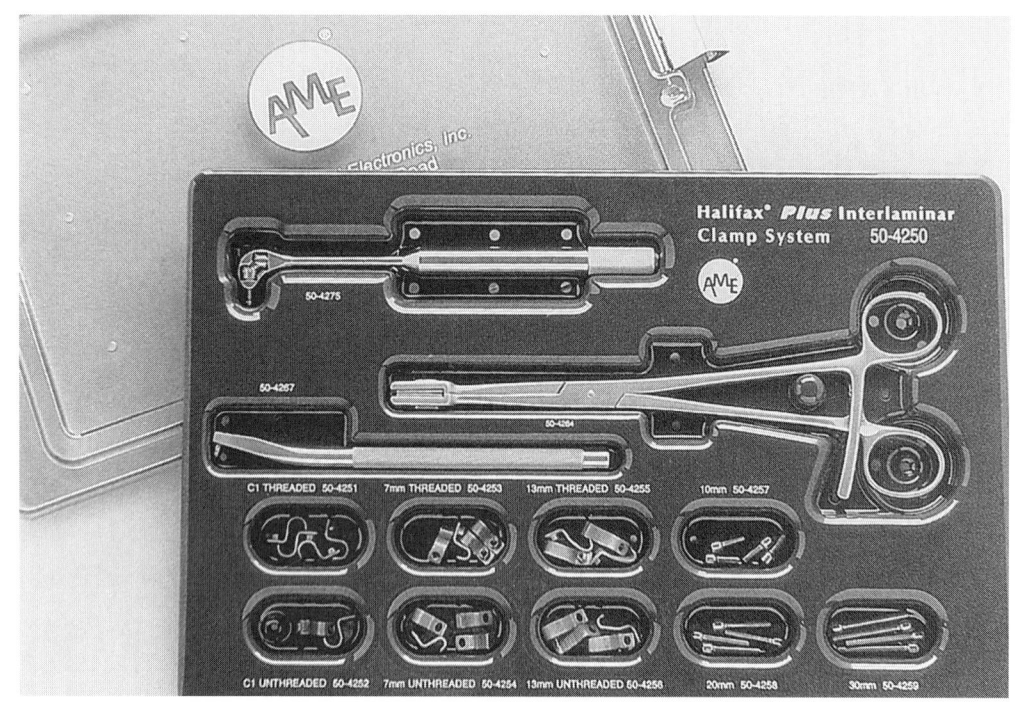

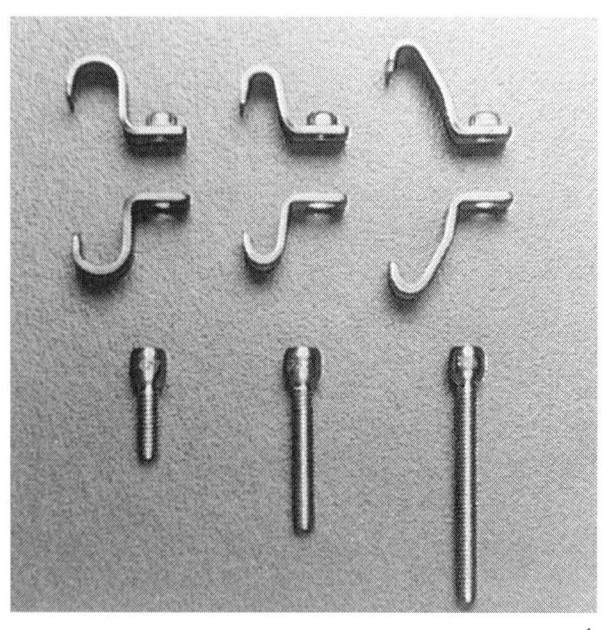

FIG. 7-2. (a and b) Components of the A.M.E. Halifax PLUS interlaminar clamp system. (c) The C1 and C2 clamps of the A.M.E. Halifax system with the screw of appropriate length are placed in the forceps. (d) The screws are tightened with the 90-degree wrench. (e) Final placement of the A.M.E. Halifax PLUS interlaminar clamp system.

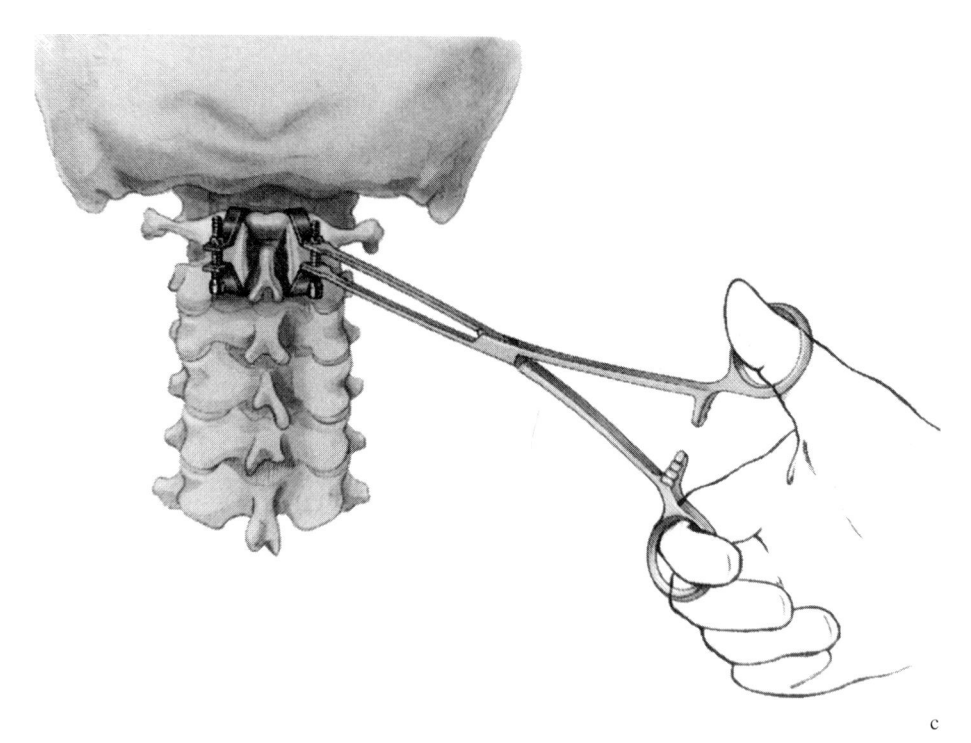

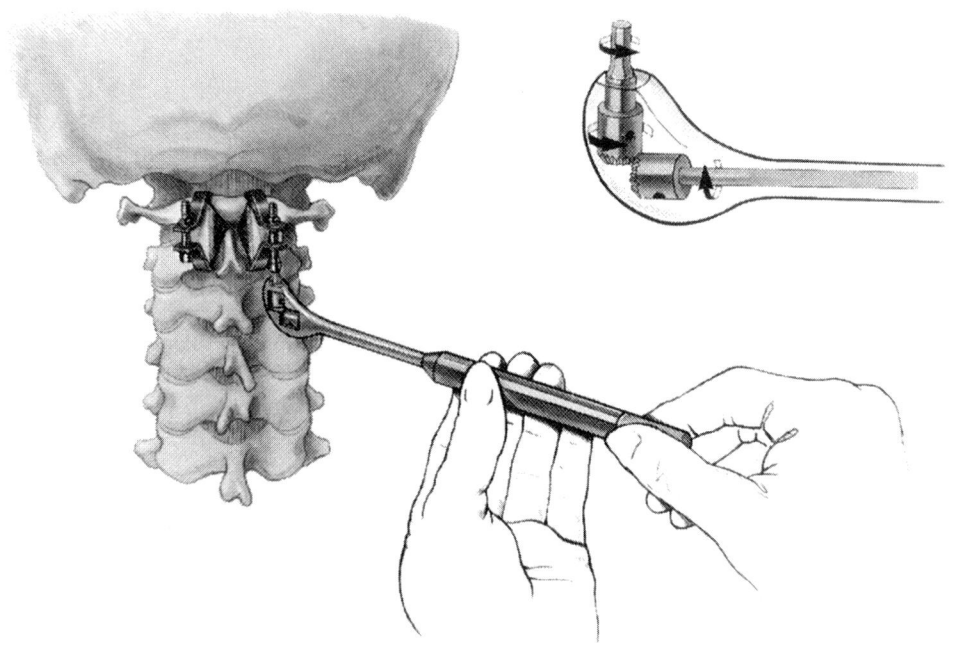

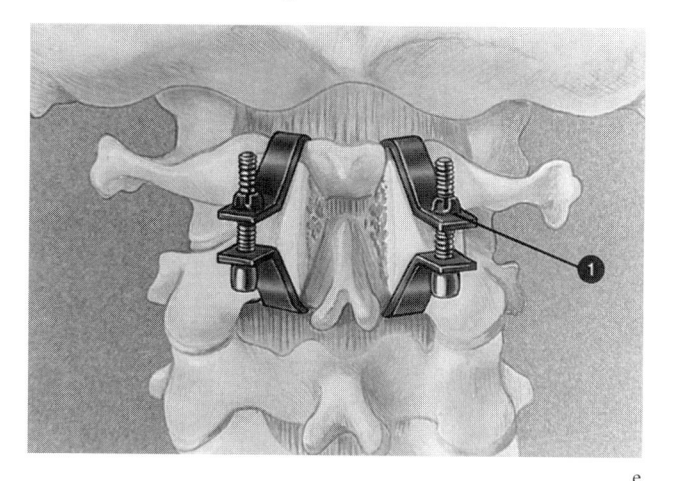

c

d

e

81

compatible and consists of a cranial and a caudal hook (which are hollow along their long axes) and a connecting tube. After the graft is placed, the cranial hook is attached to the connector and applied to the lamina. The caudal hook slides over the connector and the system is compressed with a compressor. The lower hook is then crimped and the excess connector is cut. Included in the basic set are 12 lower and 6 upper hooks, 3 connecting tubes, cutting pliers, an implant holder, 2 compressors, and crimping pliers. Figure 7-3, *a*, shows the upper hooks, lower hooks, and connecting tubes of the Apofix system, and Fig. 7-3, *b*, shows the Apofix instruments.

INDICATIONS, CONTRAINDICATIONS, ADVANTAGES, AND DISADVANTAGES OF THE SYSTEM

The indications for placement of a posterior interlaminar clamp system are posterior stabilization of the cervical spine in patients with instability secondary to ligamentous damage or odontoid fractures, inflammatory or degenerative arthritis, or osseous malformations. The clamp systems can be placed at C1-2 or at lower cervical levels. The advantages of these systems include immediate stabilization and decreased risk of dural penetration and neurologic injury as compared with the wire techniques since the sublaminar passage of wire is eliminated. The risk of "cheese-cut" through the bone is virtually eliminated because of the large surface area of hardware in contact with the bone. The three systems discussed are also MRI-compatible, which facilitates postoperative imaging. An advantage specific to the Halifax PLUS clamp is that a threaded boss on the screw reduces the risk of screw backout. These clamps are also color-coded for ease of use. The Apofix system uses direct crimping to assemble the construct, thus eliminating the need for nuts, screws, or wires and facilitating application. This system also has increased fatigue life, torsional strength, and traction strength as compared with other systems.

Disadvantages of the interlaminar clamp system include an inherent potential for rotational dislocation, and the "fiddle factor." A disadvantage specific to the Codman interlaminar clamp is that wire or suture material must be used with the system to reduce the risk of screw backout. The interlaminar clamp systems are contraindicated in posterior atlantoaxial subluxation or odontoid fractures with posterior subluxation since clamp tightening would tend to pull the ventral elements into the spinal canal. A summary of the preceding points can be found in Table 7-1.

TECHNIQUE

Details

Bone-Graft Harvesting

In preparation for placement of the interlaminar clamp system a standard posterior approach to the cervical spine is first performed. Consideration may be given to using either awake nasotracheal or fiberoptic endotracheal intubation, general anesthesia, and continuous somatosensory evoked potential monitoring. The patient is carefully turned prone onto lateral rolls and the forehead supported on a horseshoe headrest or three-point skull fixation with the arms at the patient's side. Alternatively, a Stryker frame can be used. The head may be stabilized in Gardner-Wells tong traction

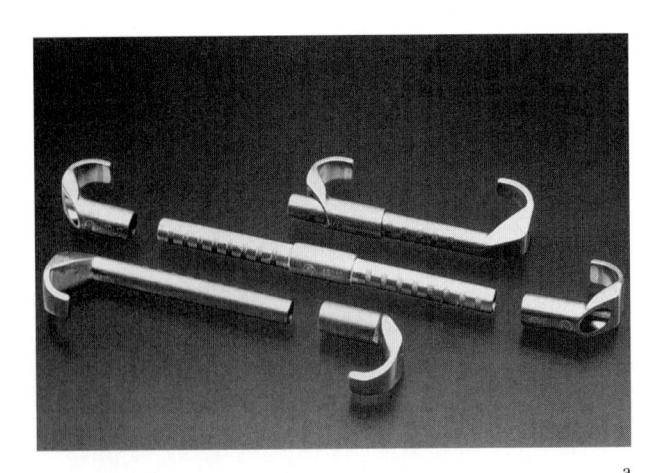

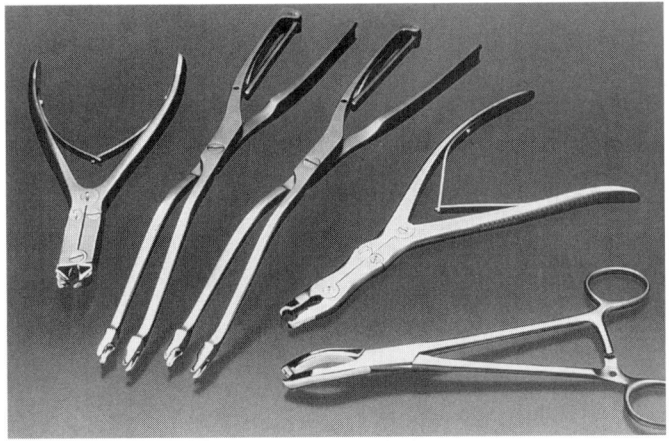

FIG. 7-3. (a) Upper and Lower hooks and connecting tubes of the Apofix system. (b) Apofix instruments.

Table 7-1
Highlights of the Posterior Cervical Interlaminar Clamp Systems

	Codman interlaminar clamp	*A.M.E. Halifax PLUS interlaminar clamp*	*Apofix fixation device*
Basic features of each unit	Screw, unthreaded clamp, threaded clamp	Screw, unthreaded clamp, threaded clamp, threaded boss	Upper hook, lower hook, connecting tube
Indications	Posterior stabilization of the cervical spine in patients with ligamentous instability, in patients with rheumatoid arthritis, and in patients with certain osseous malformations	Posterior stabilization of the cervical spine in patients with ligamentous instability, in patients with rheumatoid arthritis, and in patients with certain osseous malformations	Posterior stabilization of the cervical spine in patients with ligamentous instability, in patients with rheumatoid arthritis, and in patients with certain osseous malformations
Contraindications	Posterior atlantoaxial subluxation or odontoid fractures with posterior subluxation	Posterior atlantoaxial subluxation or odontoid fractures with posterior subluxation	Posterior atlantoaxial subluxation or odontoid fractures with posterior subluxation
Advantages	Decreased risk of dural penetration and neurologic injury as compared with wire techniques Risk of wire cut is eliminated because of the larger surface area in contact with bone MRI-compatible	Decreased risk of dural penetration and neurologic injury as compared with wire techniques Risk of wire cut is eliminated because of the larger surface area in contact with bone MRI-compatible Threaded boss helps prevent screw backout Color-coded clamps for ease of use	Decreased risk of dural penetration and neurologic injury as compared with wire techniques Risk of wire cut is eliminated because of the larger surface area in contact with bone MRI-compatible Construct is joined by direct crimping and does not require any additional devices such as nuts, screws, or wire Ease of application Increased fatigue life, torsional strength, and traction strength
Disadvantages	Fiddle factor Potential for rotational dislocation SOF'WIRE or braided silk must be used	Fiddle factor Potential for rotational dislocation	Fiddle factor Potential for rotational dislocation

using a 4-kg weight. We use either portable C-arm fluoroscopy or portable lateral cervical radiographs to verify cervical spine alignment. The lower occiput and the posterior iliac crest are sterilely prepared and draped. The skin is infiltrated with lidocaine and 1:1,000,000 epinephrine, and a midline incision made from the inion to the upper C4 region. The paraspinal muscles are reflected subperiosteally to expose the posterior rim of C1, the laminae, and the spinous processes of C2 (and C3 if C1-3 arthrodesis is planned). The subperiosteal dissection should be extended superiorly over the ring of C1 and then deep to the ring. This facilitates seating of the C1 clamp. Similarly, the caudal edge and undersurface of the C2 lamina should be prepared to receive the lower clamp. The ligamentum flavum can be removed between laminae to prevent in-buckling when the laminae are compressed with the clamps. Using a Kerrison rongeur or high-speed drill, the graft site is prepared by decorticating the inferior edge of the ring of C1 and the superior portion of the C2 lamina and the spinous process. A tricortical bone graft is then obtained and converted to a bicortical strut by removing the top edge of the graft. Figure 7-4 illustrates the technique for bone-graft harvesting.

The Codman Interlaminar Clamp

Two appropriate clamp halves are selected. The C1-2 clamps are used for atlantoaxial stabilization while either the 7-mm or the 13-mm clamps are selected for subaxial fixation. The two clamp halves are preassembled with an appropriate length screw and then placed in the jaws of the Codman clamp placement forceps. After the bone graft is inserted, the clamps are placed bilaterally over the appropriate cephalad lamina and under the appropriate caudad lamina. The screw head can be oriented either caudad or cephalad. The screw is tightened by placing the tip of the 90-degree adjustment wrench in the hex head of the screw and rotating the knurled end of the handle clockwise. The latter instrument can perform both coarse and fine adjustments of the Codman screw. The collet of the wrench must be in the unlocked position for coarse adjustment, while to lock the gears of the wrench for fine adjustment, the collet is moved in an upward motion and rotated to the right. To loosen the screw, the knurled handle is simply turned counterclockwise. To guard against counterrotation of the screws and subsequent loosening of the clamp, a braided silk suture (2-0 or heav-

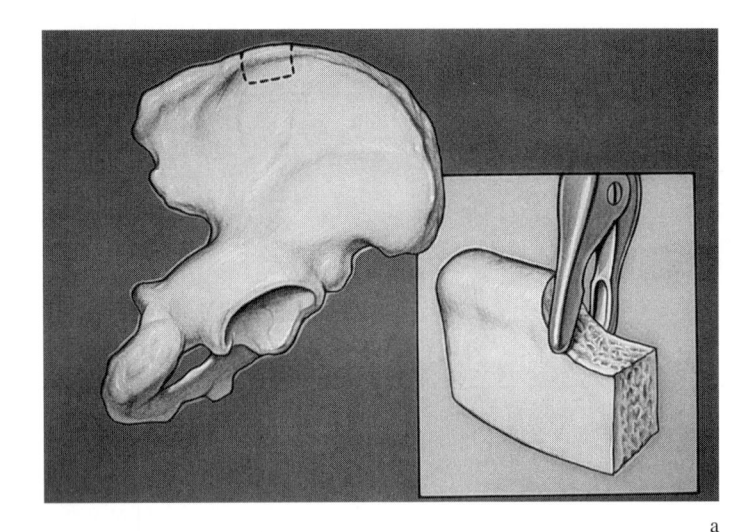

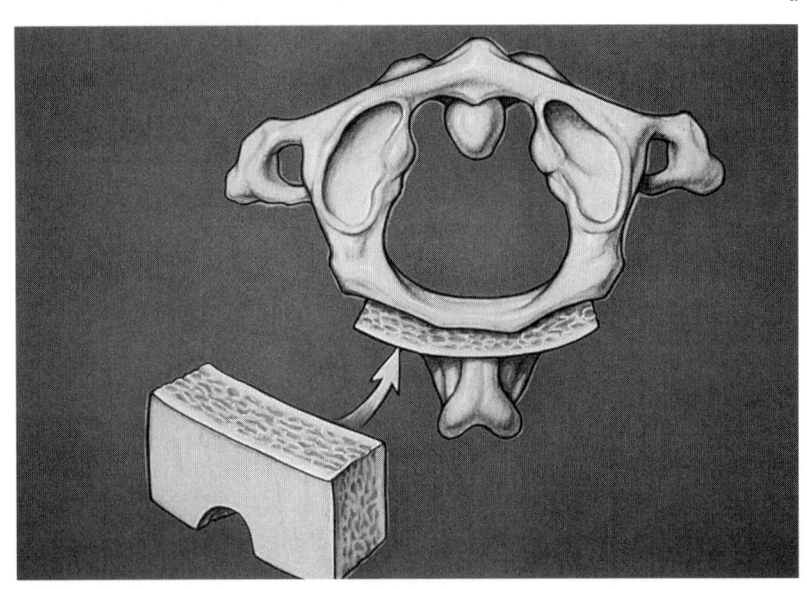

FIG. 7-4. (a) Harvest of the tricortical bone graft. (b) Placement of the bone graft.

ier gauge) on a needle is passed through the cross-holes located at the distal end of the screws. Several passes may be made depending on the suture gauge. The suture should be tied with minimal tension. An alternative method of preventing screw counterrotation is by the use of 22- or 24-gauge titanium surgical wire (SOF'WIRE) and a cinch. Figures 7-1, b to e, show placement of the Codman interlaminar clamp. Figures 7-1, d, and 7-1, e, show the use of suture and wire, respectively, to decrease the risk of screw backout.

The Halifax PLUS Interlaminar Clamp

After the bone graft is inserted, the C1 threaded and the C2 unthreaded clamps are placed in the applicator forceps. The appropriate length screw is inserted into the clamps. Placement of the screw head and unthreaded clamp caudally generally facilitates wrench access. The clamp and interposed bone are gently compressed with the applicator forceps and the clamp partially tightened with the 90-degree wrench. The contralateral clamp is placed and this procedure repeated. The clamps are alternately tightened bilaterally until equal tension is achieved. The fine-adjustment wrench can be used for final tightening. Figures 7-2, c, and 7-2, d, show placement of the Halifax PLUS interlaminar clamp system; Fig. 7-2, e, shows the finished product.

APOFIX Fixation System

C1-2 Level. The cervical spine is prepared for insertion of the graft and implants. The upper hooks are then placed over the cephalad laminae bilaterally using the implant holder. The lower hooks are also placed. The C2-3 interlaminar space is widened to facilitate insertion of the implants by gently pushing the spinous process of C2 cranially. The graft is then positioned between C1 and C2 and the compressors each positioned bilaterally so that the cephalad and caudad hooks are within the jaws. The hooks are compressed symmetrically and maximally. The lower hook is fastened to the upper hook by placing the crimper on the lower hook and crimping. The distal part of the upper hook is cut with the cutting pliers.

Subaxial Levels. For arthrodesis of the lower cervical spine using a long construct, the connecting tube can be used by placing two lower hooks on the cephalad and caudad aspects of the tube. The excess tube can then be cut caudally with the pliers.

Figures 7-5, *a*, *b*, and *c* show the sequential steps in placement of the Apofix system. Figure 7-5, *d*, shows a postoperative lateral radiograph of the Apofix system.

Pearls, Suggestions, Pitfalls

The interlaminar clamps of all three systems are designed to be placed bilaterally. The respective screws should be tightened gradually and alternately to achieve balanced compression of the bony structures.

When using the Apofix system, it may be necessary to use a high-speed drill on the laminae to facilitate placement of the crimper.

The manufacturers of the Codman interlaminar clamp recommend that all instruments be thoroughly lubricated after every cleaning and before sterilization with a water-soluble lubricant. Steam sterilization is recommended.

CLINICAL RESULTS

Personal Experience and Summary of the Literature

The Codman Interlaminar Clamp

Aldrich et al. (1993) reported 50 consecutive patients requiring posterior cervical fusion for various reasons. The etiology of instability included trauma, rheumatoid arthritis, Down's syndrome, os odontoideum, infection, tumor, and degeneration. Presenting signs and symptoms included neck pain, radiculopathy, myelopathy, quadriparesis, quadriplegia, occipital neuralgia, Lhermitte's sign, and Brown-Sequard syndrome. Fusion involved the C1-2 level in 17 cases and lower cervical levels (C2-7) in 32 cases. Follow-up ranged from 6 to 40 months (average, 21). Atlantoaxial arthrodesis was achieved in 14 (82%) of 17 patients. Traumatic C1-2 instabilities fused in all cases, while fusion failed in two of the three patients with Down's syndrome and in the one patient with rheumatoid arthritis.

Moskovich and Crockard (1992) followed 25 patients with atlantoaxial instability treated with posterior C1-2 arthrodesis using the Codman interlaminar clamp. Diagnoses included rheumatoid arthritis, trauma, Down's syndrome, seronegative arthritis, spondyloepiphsyeal dysplasia, C1-2 facet arthrosis, and posterior instability. Atlantoaxial union was achieved within 12 weeks in 20 of 25 patients (80%).

Seek and Johnston (1991) reported on one patient with a C1-3 construct and four with C1-2 Halifax constructs. In two of these patients, hook loosening developed very early postoperatively. They used angular clamps on C1 and not the rounded clamps designed specifically to conform to the rounded anatomy of the posterior rim of C1.

Haid et al. (Haid, McCafferty, & Sypert: unpublished data) described a series of 42 patients who underwent C1-3 Halifax clamp fixation. Eight patients had previously had failed C1-2 fusions (including five with failed C1-2 Halifax clamping). The diagnoses included rheumatoid arthritis, type II odontoid fracture, os odontoideum, transverse ligament rupture, and Down's syndrome. Follow-up ranged from 18 to 57 months, with a mean of 35.6 months. All but one patient (97.6%) achieved stability and osseous union. One patient experienced hardware failure. This patient was one of the earlier patients in this series, and the screws were not crimped during the surgical procedure. They were found to be loose at the 8-week follow-up visit, but flexion-extension films did not demonstrate instability and fibrous union was assumed. The patient reported neck pain but refused further surgical therapy.

Haid et al. believe that although the C1-2 clamp technique is a stable construct, it has a higher potential for failure than a C1-3 construct because of inadequate control of axial rotation and anterioposterior translation and because of relatively poor interspinous bone graft technique at C1-2. Haid et al. believe that in cases of anterior atlantoaxial instability, the Halifax C1-3 construct has superior biomechanical properties because when a "tension band" is placed between C1 and C3, the C2 facet joint and laminae are used as a fulcrum, thus decreasing rotatory and translatory motion.

Halifax Interlaminar Clamp

Statham et al. (1993) reported their experience with the Halifax interlaminar clamp. Forty-four patients underwent atlantoaxial arthrodesis and one underwent C1-3 stabilization. Twenty-six patients underwent stabilization of the lower cervical spine. The diagnoses were trauma, rheumatoid arthritis, seronegative arthritis, spondyloepiphyseal dysplasia, os odontoideum, Down's syndrome, C1-2 facet arthrosis, and postoperative instability. At the C1-2 level, satisfactory fusion was achieved in 36 patients (80%). Complications occurred in 14 cases (31.1%). Twenty-five patients with unstable lower cervical spine injury involving one motion segment underwent arthrodesis without complication.

The initial series of eight patients who underwent C1-2 arthrodesis with the Halifax clamp was reported in 1988 by Cybulski et al. Loosening of the clamp developed in one patient, who required additional operations.

Apofix Fixation Device

Since this system is new to the United States, the largest experience with this system comes from Dr. Richard Assaker of Lille, France. From January 1992 to October 1994 he operated on 37 patients from 8 to 77 years of age (mean, 42.4) using the Apofix system (unpublished data). There were 19 men and 18 women, and the follow-up ranged from 1 to 34 months with a mean of 14 months. There were 29 cases of trauma, 6 cases of rheumatoid arthritis, 1 tumor at C6, and 1 bony malformation at C2. Of the 29 trauma cases, 20 involved the C1-2 level, 4 involved the C6-7 level, 2 each involved the C4-5 and the C5-6 levels and one involved the C7-T1 level. Twenty-six patients presented with cervical pain, 6 with quadriparesis, and 5 with cervical radiculopathy. The average hospital stay (in 31 patients) was 9.7 days. One patient died of a pulmonary embolus on the eighth hospital day. Results in 23 patients with follow-up for more than 6 months were good in 22 (defined as good bony fusion). One patient had recurrence of pseudarthrosis.

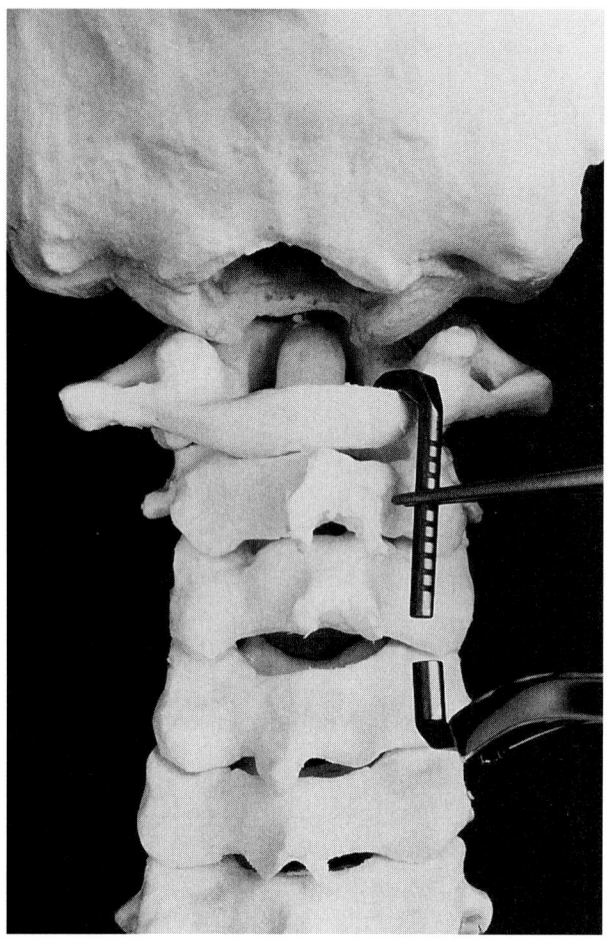

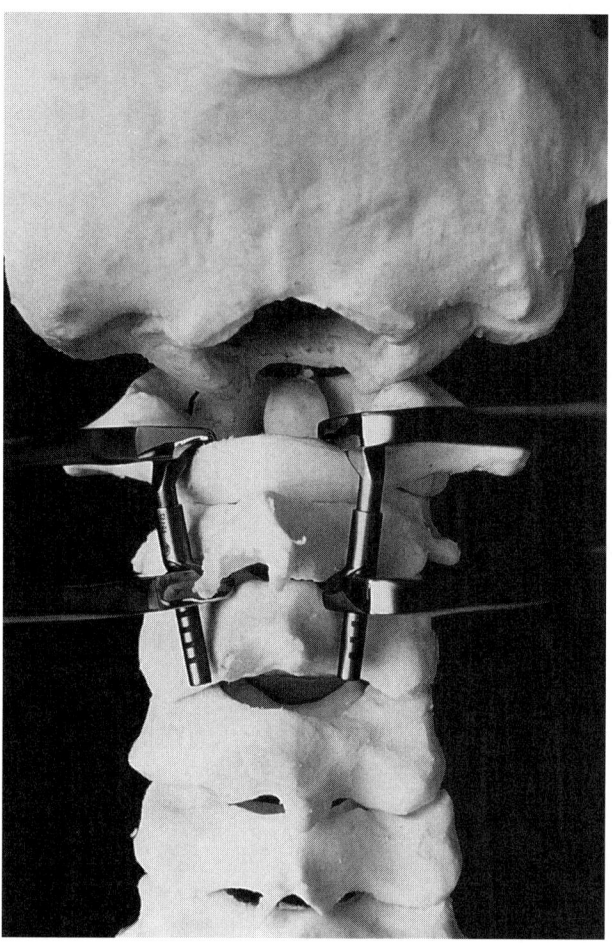

Complications

In the series by Aldrich et al. (1993) in which 50 consecutive patients underwent Codman Halifax interlaminar clamping, surgical failure occurred in 5 patients. These were identified either because the patient became symptomatic or because routine diagnostic studies revealed instability at the operative level. Atlantoaxial fusion failed in 3 of 17 cases. Failure occurred in 2 patients with atlantoaxial instability secondary to Down's syndrome. One patient became myelopathic 5 months after surgery, and radiographic data revealed a C1 arch fracture. In another patient screw loosening was identified. Both patients underwent additional surgery to achieve stability. Asymptomatic screw loosening with instability on flexion-extension films developed in one patient with rheumatoid arthritis. The screws were retightened at reoperation and more bone grafting was performed. Fusion subsequently occurred, and the patient did well. Another patient underwent C1-3 fusion that failed because of screw loosening after 3 weeks. An alternative fusion method was used, and the patient did well. Still another patient had screw loosening with C2-3 instability 4 weeks postoperatively. Reoperation was performed and the patient did well.

Statham et al. (1993) reported complications in 14 of 44 patients (31.8%) who underwent posterior cervical stabilization with the A.M.E. Halifax interlaminar clamp. They all occurred at the C1-2 level. Screw loosening occurred in 10 patients, and clamp disengagement occurred in 4 patients. Complications were symptomatic in 9 cases and discovered radiographically in the others. They occurred at a median of 9 weeks after surgery. Five patients already had solid fusion, while 9 patients required further operation. They found a statistically significant difference in the complication rate between the use of clamps at C1-2 and the use of clamps below C2.

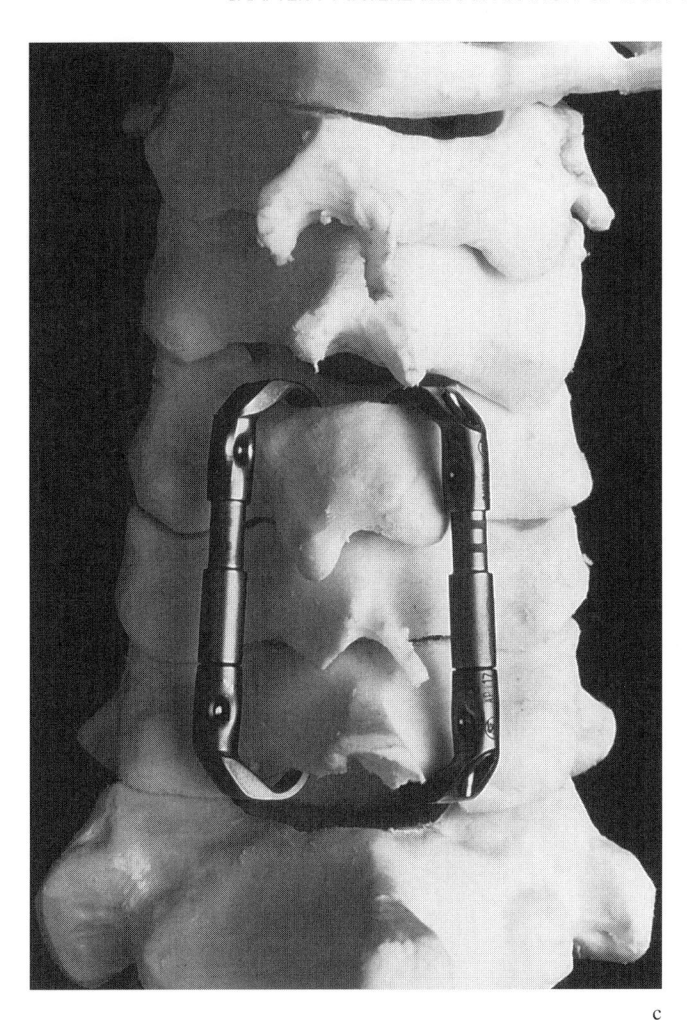

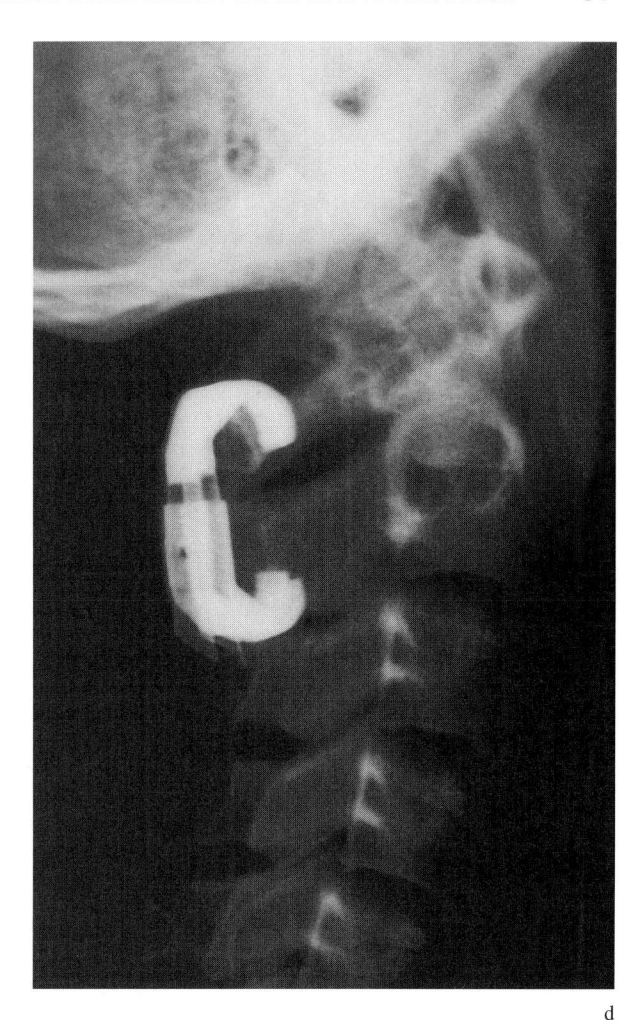

FIG. 7-5. (a and b) Placement of the upper hooks of the Apofix system. (c) Upper and lower hooks in place after crimping. (d) Postoperative lateral radiograph of the Apofix system.

Moskovich and Crockard (1992) had unsuccessful fusions in 5 of 25 patients. Four of these carried a diagnosis of rheumatoid arthritis. Screw loosening occurred in 4 patients. The patient without rheumatoid arthritis subsequently underwent a Brooks fusion, which also failed. The screws were inadequately tightened at surgery in 3 patients because of the limited availability of clamps of the correct length. The clamp fixation was revised in 2 patients with subsequent fusion. Three other patients required repeat surgery for nonunion due to loosening of the clamp. This was usually caused by incomplete tightening of the screws. Moskovich and Crockard pointed out that nonunion is more likely in patients with rheumatoid arthritis and that if nonunion occurs, the pseudarthrosis is usually between the posterior bone graft and the ring of C1.

Haid et al. (unpublished data), documented 2 cases in which overtightening of the clamps produced a contralateral fracture of the C1 arch in 42 patients who underwent C1-2 Halifax clamp fixation. Both patients were treated with bone wedged between the fracture and C2 while a single contralateral clamp was placed. The patients were managed in a halo brace for an average of 14.1 weeks. Somatosensory evoked potential changes developed during the initial tightening in another patient with an os odontoideum. The clamp was repositioned, the changes resolved, and the clamp was tightened with no further change. The patient awoke neurologically intact. Two patients were treated for superficial wound infections. Of the 22 patients treated with a halo brace, 8 (36.4%) had pin-site infections.

SUMMARY

Posterior interlaminar clamp fixation offers a safe, effective, alternative method of cervical stabilization at the atlantoaxial junction (and below) and is indicated in cases of instability of the cervical spine in patients with ligamentous instability, rheumatoid arthritis and certain osseous malformations. The design of the clamps, though not perfect, offers some distinct advantages over standard wiring techniques. The three systems discussed in this chapter, although not differing significantly in basic design, do differ slightly in application and design detail. It is still too early to tell if long-term results will differ with the three systems.

REFERENCES

Aldrich, E.F., Crow, W.N., Weber, P.B., & Spagnolia, T.N. (1991). Use of MR imaging-compatible Halifax interlaminar clamps for posterior cervical fusion. *Journal of Neurosurgery, 74,* 185–189.

Aldrich, E.F., Weber, P.B., & Crow, W.N. (1993). Halifax interlaminar clamp for posterior cervical fusion: A long-term follow-up review. *Journal of Neurosurgery, 78,* 702–708.

Barbour, J.R. (1971). Screw fixation in fracture of the odontoid process. *South Australian Clinics, 5,* 20–24.

Brooks, A.L., & Jenkins, E.B. (1978). Atlanto-axial arthrodesis by the wedge compression method. *Journal of Bone and Joint Surgery, American Volume, 60,* 279–284.

Cybulski, G.R., Stone, J.L., Crowell, R.M., Rifai, M.H., Gandhi, Y., & Glick, R. (1988). Use of Halifax interlaminar clamps for posterior C1-C2 arthrodesis. *Neurosurgery, 222,* 429–431.

Dickman, C.A., Sonntag, V.K.H., Papadopoulos, S.M., & Hadley, M.N. (1991). The interspinous method of posterior atlantoaxial arthrodesis. *Journal of Neurosurgery, 74,* 190–198.

Etter, C., Coscia, M., Jaberg, H., & Aebi, M. (1991). Direct anterior fixation of dens fractures with a cannulated screw system. *Spine, 16,* S25–S31.

Fielding, W.J., Hawkins, R.J., & Ratzan, S.A. (1976). Spine fusion for atlanto-axial instability. *Journal of Bone and Joint Surgery, American Volume, 58,* 400–407.

Gallie, W.E. (1939). Fractures and dislocations of the cervical spine. *American Journal of Surgery, 46,* 495–499.

Geisler, F.H., Cheng, C., Poka, A., & Brumback, R.J. (1989). Anterior screw fixation of posteriorly displaced Type II odontoid fractures. *Neurosurgery, 25,* 30–38.

Grob, D., Dvorak, J., Panjabi, M., Forehlich, M., & Hayek, J. (1990). Posterior occipitocervical fusion: A preliminary report of a new technique. *Spine, 16,* S17–S24.

Hanson, P.B., Montesano, P.X., Sharkey, N.A., & Rauschning, W. (1990). Anatomic and biomechanical assessment of transarticular screw fixation for atlantoaxial instability. *Spine, 15,* 1141–1145.

Holness, R.O., Huestis, W.S., Howes, W.J., & Langelle, R.A. (1984). Posterior stabilization with an interlaminar clamp in cervical injuries: Technical note and review of the long term experience with the method. *Neurosurgery, 14,* 318–322.

Lesoin, F., Autricque, A., Franz, K., Villette, L., & Jomin, M. (1987). Transcervical approach and screw fixation for upper cervical spine pathology. *Surgical Neurology, 27,* 459–465.

Magerl, F., & Seemann, P.S. (1985). Stable posterior fusion of the atlas and axis by transarticular screw fixation. In: P.A. Weidner (Ed.), *Cervical Spine I* (pp. 322–327). New York: Springer-Verlag.

Mitsui, H. (1984). A new operation for atlanto-axial arthrodesis. *Journal of Bone and Joint Surgery, British Volume, 66,* 422–425.

Moskovich, R., & Crockard, H.A. (1992). Atlantoaxial arthrodesis using interlaminar clamps: An improved technique. *Spine, 17,* 261–267.

Seek, K., & Johnston, R.A. (1991). Interlaminar clamp for posterior fusions. *Journal of Neurosurgery, 75,* 495.

Statham, P., O'Sullivan, M., & Russell, T. (1993). The Halifax interlaminar clamp for posterior cervical fusion: Initial experience in the United Kingdom. *Neurosurgery, 32,* 396–399.

Tucker, H.H. (1975). Technical report: Method of fixation of subluxed or dislocated cervical spine below C1-C2. *Canadian Journal of Neurological Sciences, 2,* 381–382.

Weidner, A. (1989). Internal fixation with metal plates and screws. In: Cervical Spine Research Society (Ed.), *The Cervical Spine* (2nd ed.) (pp. 404–421). Philadelphia: J.B. Lippincott.

White, A.A., III, & Panjabi, M.M. (1978). *Clinical Biomechanics of the Spine* (p. 66). Philadelphia: J.B. Lippincott.

Yashon, D. (1988). Surgical management of trauma to the spine. In: H.H. Schmidek & W.H. Sweet (Eds.), *Operative Neurosurgical Techniques: Indications, Methods and Results* (2nd ed) (Vol. 1, pp. 1449–1470). Orlando, FL: Grune & Stratton.

CHAPTER 8

Application of the Luque Rectangle Fixation for Occipital-Cervical and Atlantoaxial Instability

Brian Pikul
Gary L. Rea

Congenital or acquired pathology of the upper cervical spine and craniovertebral junction can lead to bony instability and neural compression. Congenital anomalies include os odontoideum, basilar impression, platybasia, occipitalization (assimilation) of the atlas, Klippel-Feil and Morquio's syndromes. Acquired abnormalities such as posttraumatic instability, rheumatoid arthritis, neoplastic disease, Reiter's syndrome, Down's syndrome, ankylosing spondylitis, osteoarthritis, postpoliomyelitic instabilities, and postlaminectomy instability can also lead to occipital-cervical (OC) problems (Coria, Quintana, Villalba, Rebollo, & Berciano, 1983; Halla, Bliznak, & Hardin, 1988; Menezes, VanGilder, Graf, & McDonnell, 1980; Ransford, Crockard, Pozo, Thomas, & Nelson, 1986; Rea, Mullin, Mervis, & Miller, 1993; Wertheim & Bohlman, 1987).

Patients with neural compression or instability in the OC region may experience a wide range of symptoms and display a multitude of neurologic signs. If the anatomic changes are minor, they can be asymptomatic. Headache, usually occipital, neck pain, vertigo, diplopia, cranial-nerve dysfunction (internuclear ophthalmoplegia, facial diplegia), dysphagia (IX, X, XII involvement), nystagmus, apnea, ataxia, limb paresthesias, cervical myelopathy with progressive quadriparesis/spasticity/hyperreflexia, central cord syndrome, and neurogenic bladder, have all been described with OC pathology.

Full and accurate anatomic evaluation may require several radiographic studies (Menezes et al., 1980; Menezes, VanGilder, Clark, & Khoury, 1985; Rea et al., 1993; Weijun, Zhaoyan, & Shifen, 1981). Plain radiographs of the occiput through T1 reveal subluxation, abnormal dens position, bony destruction, and osteopenia (Fig. 8-1). Computed tomography (CT) with and without myelography can detail the relationship of the neurovascular and bony elements, any bony destruction, and axial rotation (Fig. 8-2). Magnetic resonance imaging (MRI) provides visualization of spinal cord medullary compression, neoplasia, and the appearance of the ligaments, disks, and any pannus formation (Fig. 8-3). With these imaging techniques, an accurate assessment of neural compression, bony offset, bony destruction, and instability can be made (Braunstein, Weissman, Seltzer, Sosman, Wang, & Zamani, 1984; Castor, Miller, Russell, Chiu, Grace, & Hanson, 1983; Menezes et al., 1985; Rea et al., 1993).

The most common indications at our institution for OC fixation are the significant destruction of the atlas-axis interface resulting from cancer, or more likely, inflammatory disease. In this situation, often C1 and C2 cannot be fused as a unit, and the occiput must be included. OC fusions have been used extensively in the past in concomitant C1-2 fractures or in unstable C1-2 situations with an absent C1 arch. These latter indications however, are decreasing with increasing experience with C1-2 anterior or posterior transfacet screw fixation.

The basic tenets of occipitalcervical fusion include neural decompression with restoration of normal anatomic relationships and bony fusion (Menezes et al., 1980). Decompression may be done via cervical traction if the pathology is reducible. However, surgical decompression is often necessary. Posterior decompression can be accomplished through a suboccipital incision of the upper cervical vertebrae, and irreducible symptomatic anterior compression is corrected via a transoral approach before posterior fixation (Menezes & VanGilder, 1988).

A variety of surgical techniques have been introduced to treat occipitocervical instability. Bony fusion and fixation with wires, screws, plates, pins, rods, and methylmethacrylate have all been used to deal with this problem. Cervical collars, halos, sternal-occipital-mandibular (Somi) braces,

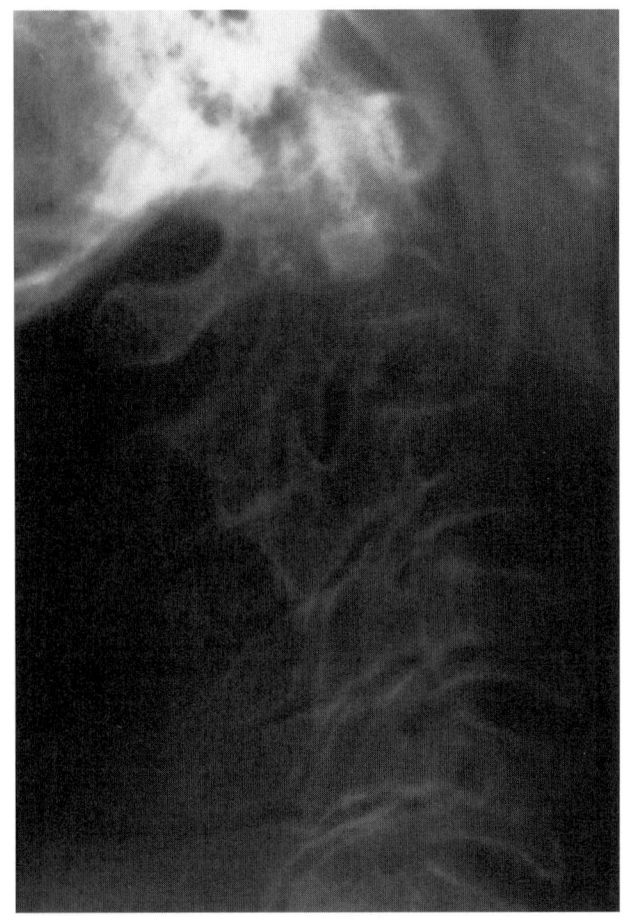

FIG. 8-1. Lateral radiograph in 73-year-old man with severe occipital headache and quadriparesis and no cranial nerve symptoms. X-ray film shows destruction and collapse of C2 body and dens.

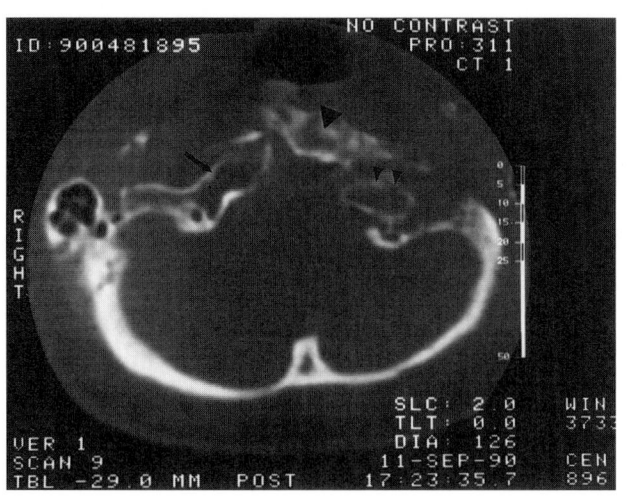

FIG. 8-2. CT scan of 67-year-old woman with rheumatoid arthritis with severe occipital headaches, head tilt, and progressive quadriparesis. In this single CT the occipital condyles (*arrow*), C1 (*double arrowhead*), and the rotated body of C2 (*large arrowhead*) can be seen, showing destruction and instability of the OC complex.

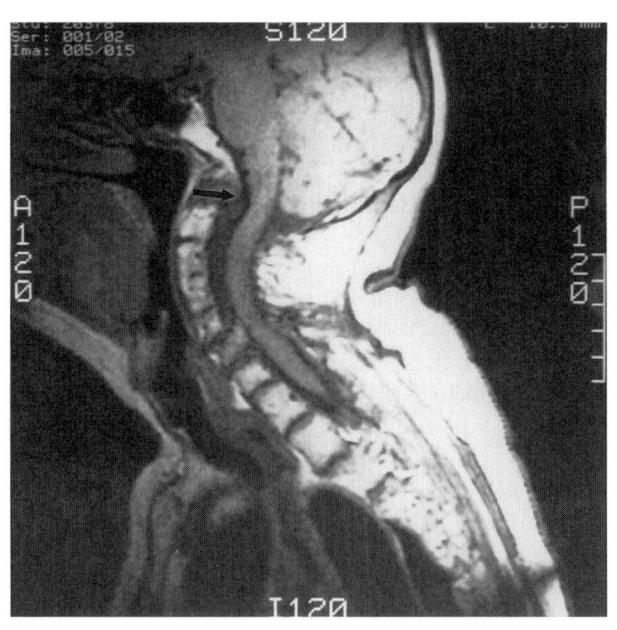

FIG. 8-3. MRI scan of patient in Fig. 8-2. Pannus (*arrows*) at C1-2 are easily seen. She improved after fixation and the pannus was not removed.

and casting have also been proposed to ensure postoperative immobility until adequate bony fusion occurs (Dickman, Sonntag, & Marcotte, 1992).

The technique described here has been used in over 20 patients with OC instability (Table 8-1). It has proven to be simple, direct, successful, and importantly, cost efficient as compared with preformed OC fixation devices (Rea et al., 1993).

The occiput and the upper cervical spine are approached through a posterior midline longitudinal incision. After the occiput, the foramen magnum region and the appropriate cervical vertebrae are exposed, and a stylet template is bent and cut to conform to the OC region. The template is the standard sterilized stylet used with endotracheal tubes. A Luque rectangle of the appropriate length, and the template, are sent to the hospital machine shop for customized bending (Fig. 8-4). Bone is harvested for the fusion while this is being completed. The shaped rectangle is returned, sterilized, and tested for positional accuracy. A high-speed drill removes bone overlying the dura for wire fixation holes on

Table 8-1
Technical Points

1. Bend sterile endotracheal tube stylet into a template for desired fit of the Luque rectangle.
2. Take bone graft while the rectangle is being customized.
3. Wire the rectangle to occiput at the rectangle's cephlad corners and appropriate cervical vertebra to inferior corners to decrease any cephalad-caudad movement.
4. Use wires around foramen magnum and rectangle to improve fixation, especially when cannot wire to C1 lamina.
5. Multiple fixation points via sublaminar or spinous process wiring improves the rigidity of the construct.

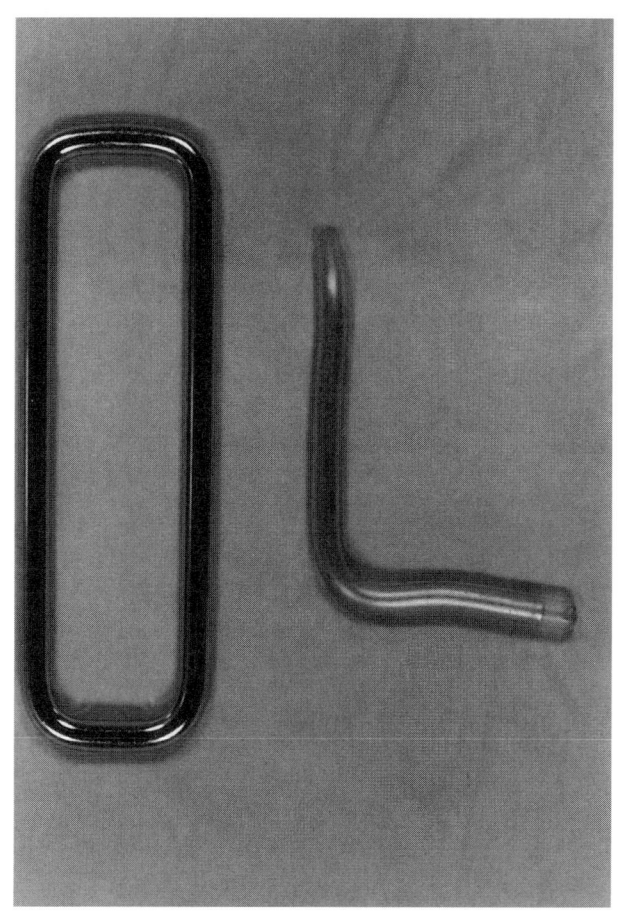

FIG. 8-4. Stylet bent to conform to OC junction and Luque rectangle of appropriate length before customized bending.

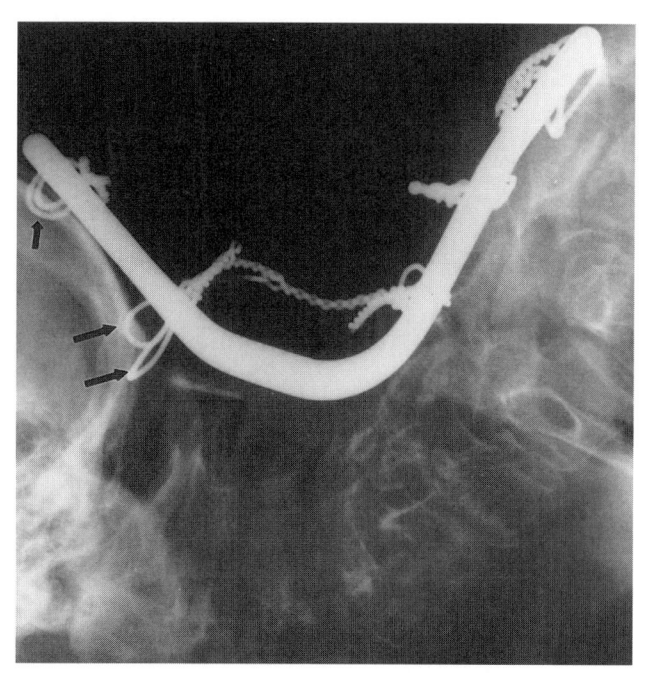

FIG. 8-5. Postfixation placement x-ray film of patient in Fig. 8-2. Note wires at cephlad corners of occipital attachment (*small arrow*), around the foramen magnum (*double arrows*), and at the caudal end of the rectangle.

both sides of the cephalad corners of the Luque rectangle, and single holes on the right and left sides of the foramen magnum, for the attachment to the foramen magnum (Fig. 8-5). The Luque rectangle is then attached to the basiocciput, foramen magnum, and appropriate cervical lamina via sublaminar wiring or spinous process wiring (Fig. 8-6). One must take care to place wires at the corners of the rectangle to avoid cephlad-caudad movement of the device. Although it can be tedious, because of the strength of the cortical bone around the foramen magnum, it is recommended that a wire be placed on each side of the rectangle for fixation. Since C1 is often deficient in these cases, the anchoring at the foramen magnum is very important.

This method provides rigid internal fixation. Cortical and cancellous bone can then be placed over the decorticated occiput and cervical regions. For patients with neoplastic disease, the use of methylmethacrylate may be substituted or added to the bony fusion.

The technique provides a stable construct such that the only postoperative external fixation necessary is a cervical (Philadelphia) collar for 4 to 6 weeks. This type of

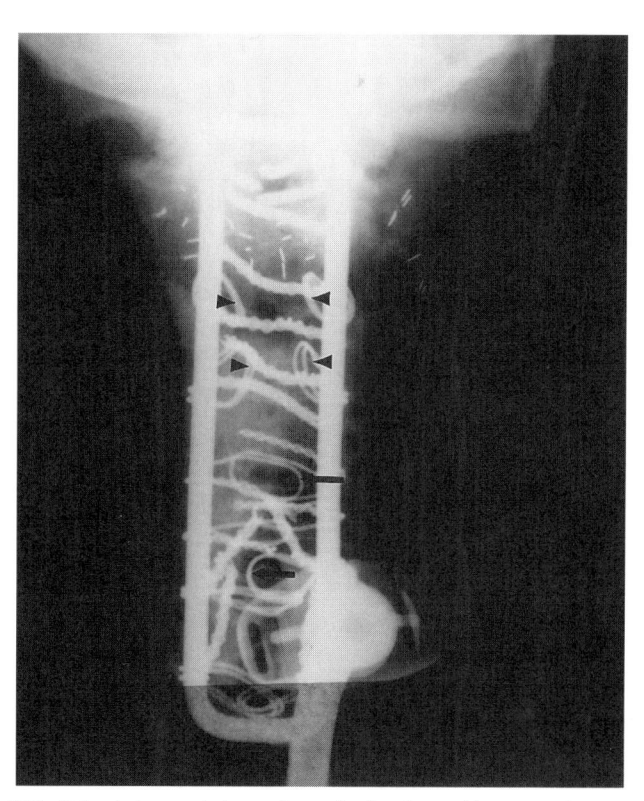

FIG. 8-6. Anteroposterior radiograph of patient with metastatic cancer at the OC region. The construct includes sublaminar wires (*arrowhead*), wires around spinous process (*arrows*), and methylmethacrylate.

Table 8-2
Luque Rectangles* for OC Instability

Indications
   Occipitoatlantial instability
   Atlantoaxial instability with bony destruction preventing fixation of C1-2 alone.
Advantages
   Rigid
   Easily customized in the hospital machine shop during surgery
   No need for postoperative halo
   Low cost
Disadvantages
   Smooth rod requires fixation at corners or at bends
   Difficult to bend by hand
Cost
   Approximately $250

*Zimmer (Warsaw, IN).

rigid internal fixation can allow early patient mobilization, and therefore early rehabilitation (MacKenzie, Uttley, Marsh, & Bell, 1990; Ransford et al., 1986). We have found this technique to be safe, effective, and cost-efficient (Table 8-2).

REFERENCES

Braunstein, E., Weissman, B., Seltzer, S., Sosman, J., Wang, A., & Zamani, A. (1984). Computed tomography and conventional radiographs of the craniocervical region in rheumatoid arthritis—A comparison. *Arthritis and Rheumatism, 27,* 26–31.

Castor, W., Miller, J., Russell, A., Chiu, P., Grace, M., & Hanson, J. (1983). Computed tomography of the craniocervical junction in rheumatoid arthritis. *Journal of Computer Assisted Tomography, 7,* 31–36.

Coria, F., Quintana, F., Villalba, M., Rebollo, M., & Berciano, J. (1983). Craniocervical abnormalities in Down's syndrome. *Developmental Medicine and Child Neurology, 25,* 252–255.

Dickman, C., Sonntag, V., & Marcotte, P. (1992). Techniques of screw fixation of the cervical spine. *Barrow Neurological Institute Quarterly, 8* (2), 9–26.

Halla, J., Bliznak, J., & Hardin, J. (1988). Involvement of the craniocervical junction in Reiter's syndrome. *Journal of Rheumatology, 15,* 1722–1725.

MacKenzie, A., Uttley, D., Marsh, H., & Bell, B. (1990). Craniocervical stabilization using Luque/Hartshill rectangles. *Neurosurgery, 26,* 32–36.

Menezes, A., & VanGilder, J. (1988). Transoral-transpharyngeal approach to the anterior craniocervical junction—Ten-year experience with 72 patients. *Journal of Neurosurgery, 69,* 895–903.

Menezes, A., VanGilder, J., Clark, C., & El-Khoury, G. (1985). Odontoid upward migration in rheumatoid arthritis—An analysis of 45 patients with "cranial settling." *Journal of Neurosurgery, 63,* 500–509.

Menezes, A., VanGilder, J., Graf, C., & McDonnell, D. (1980). Craniocervical abnormalities—A comprehensive surgical approach. *Journal of Neurosurgery, 53,* 444–455.

Ransford, A., Crockard, H., Pozo, J., Thomas, N., & Nelson, I. (1986). Craniocervical instability treated by contoured loop fixation. *Journal of Bone and Joint Surgery, British Volume, 68,* 173–177.

Rea, G., Mullin, B., Mervis, L., & Miller, C. (1993). Occipitocervical fixation in nontraumatic upper cervical spine instability. *Surgical Neurology, 40,* 255-261.

Weijun, W., Zhaoyan, Y., & Shifen, S. (1981). Diagnosis and surgical treatment of congenital anomalies of the atlanto-occipital region. *Chinese Medical Journal, 94,* 449–454.

Wertheim, S., & Bohlman, H. (1987). Occipitocervical fusion. *Journal of Bone and Joint Surgery, American Volume, 69,* 833–836.

CHAPTER 9

Application of the Posterior Interfacet Screw for Atlantoaxial Pathology

Andreas Weidner

HIGHLIGHTS

In atlantoaxial instability, there is a high risk of damage to the spinal cord, and even sudden death resulting from cord compression has been reported (Davis & Markley, 1951; Marks & Sharp, 1981). Knowledge of such complications leads to psychological stress to the patients. A C1-2 fusion prevents this situation. Fusion is performed by inserting bone blocks between laminae of C1 and C2 and fixing these by means of wire or clamps. These techniques are well described by Gallie (1939), Brooks and Jenkins (1978), Holness, Huestis, Howes, and Langille (1984) and Cybulski, Stone, Crowell et al. (1988). A rate of pseudarthrosis between 7 and 10% is the disadvantage of using wires or clamps (Brooks & Jenkins, 1978; Holmes & Hall, 1978). In addition, there is a prerequisite for an intact dorsal arch of C1. Instead of employing wires or clamps for fixation of the laminae, there is a better possibility of rigid coupling using screws placed through the C1-2 joints. This technique of posterior interfacet screws (PIS) was developed by Magerl in 1979, and the first follow-up results were published in 1987 (Magerl & Seemann, 1987).

PRINCIPLES

Screws are inserted bilaterally just above the inferior facet of C2 and 2 to 3 mm laterally of the medial border of C2-3 facet. The screws cross the C1-2 joints from dorsal caudally to ventral cranially. A three-point fixation is achieved by a bone block between laminae of C1 and C2 (Figs. 9-1 and 9-2).

BIOMECHANICS

Hanson, Montesano, Sharkey, and Rauschning (1990) reported, that PIS has biomechanical advantages over the techniques using wires. Grob, Crisco, Panjabi, Wang and Dvorak (1992) determined the immediate three-dimensional stability of four different posterior techniques in vitro: (1) wire with one bone graft (Gallie type), (2) wire with bilateral grafts (Brooks type), (3) two posterior clamps (Halifax), and (4) two interfacet screws with bone graft (Magerl). Specimens were subjected to loads of pure moments of flexion-extension, axial rotation and lateral bending. Each technique decreased motion in all directions, but the PIS was the most stable construction for lateral bending and axial rotation. Not only stiffness (quotient derived from applied forces divided by the resulting motion) but also the irreversible plastic deformation is important to evaluate stabilization techniques. Wilke, Fischer, Kluger, Magerl, Claes, and Woersdoerfer (1992) determined this deformation as the difference between the original position of the atlas with respect to the axis before the first load cycle and the final position after unloading of the third cycle. This plastic deformity is of clinical significance since after only a few head movements new conditions might be established. In vitro experiments show a large standard deviation due to the difficulties encountered in standardizing the wire techniques, but the highest stability was achieved with PIS fixation.

INDICATION

PIS fixation is suitable for all forms of C1-2 instability caused by rheumatoid arthritis, trauma, and malformation (Table 9-1). Painful therapy-resistant degenerative arthrosis at C1-2 is also an indication for fusion.

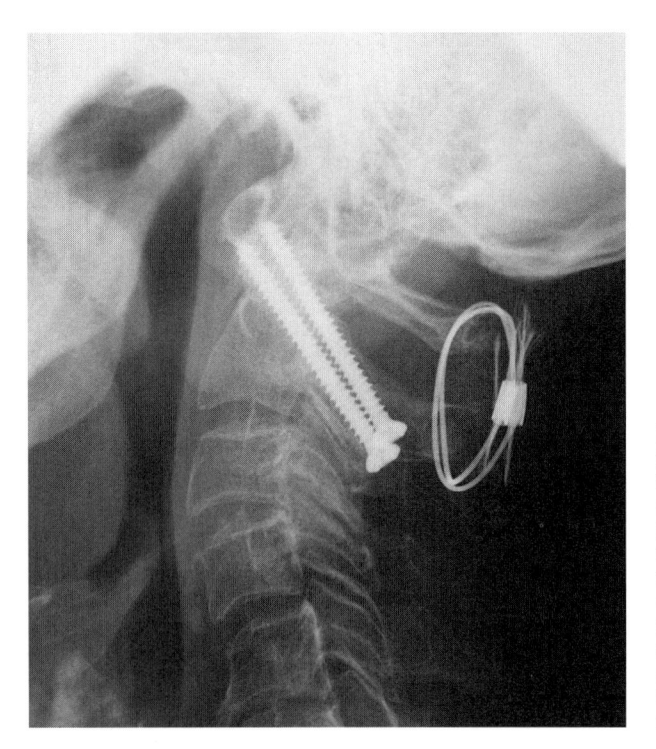

FIG. 9-1. Lateral x-ray view of a 72-year-old woman with rheumatoid arthritis; 3.5-mm cortical screws are used. A bone block from the iliac crest is inserted between the dorsal arch of the atlas and the spinous process of the axis and secured by a cable cerclage. With this technique a three-point fixation is achieved. The target area for the tip of the screw is the middle/upper part of the ventral arch of the atlas, seen on the x-ray screen as an oval.

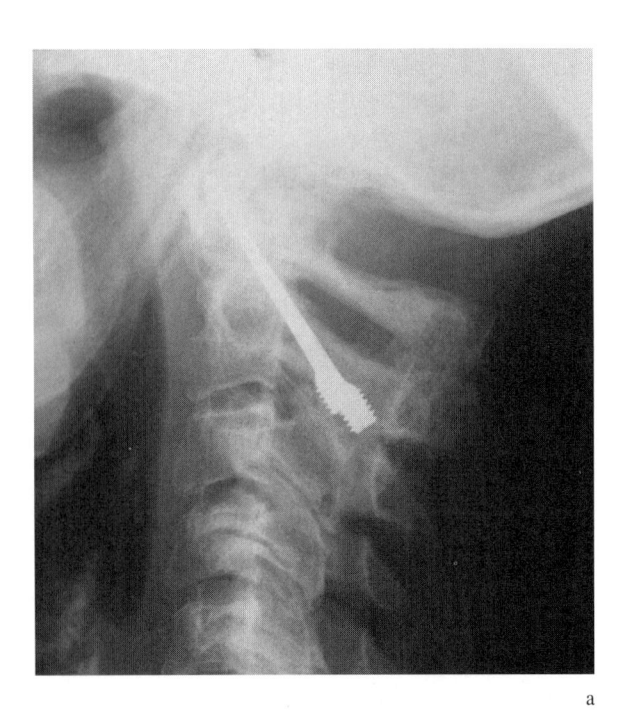

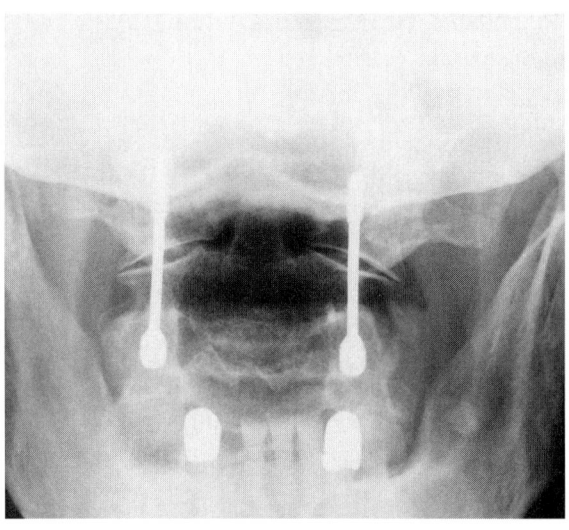

a b

FIG. 9-2. Lateral (a) and anteroposterior (b) x-ray views of a 55-year-old woman with rheumatoid arthritis and a split atlas. After dorsal clamp surgery a pseudarthrosis developed. The clamps were removed and a dorsal fusion by means of interfacet screwing technique with 2.2-mm screws was performed. Fixation of a bone block could not be achieved because of the split atlas. Therefore, bone chips were placed between the remains of the arches of atlas and axis. In addition, bone chips were packed into the joints between atlas and axis. Bony fusion occurred. Screw direction should project into the middle third of the joints as shown in x-ray view b. The 3.5-mm screws are now applied in preference to weaker 2.2-mm screws.

Table 9-1
Indications for Posterior Interfacet Screw Fixation

Instability of C1-2 due to:
   Rheumatoid arthritis
   Trauma
      Dens fracture with ligamentum tranversum rupture
      Pseudarthrosis of dens fracture after ventral spondylodesis
      Jefferson fracture
      Combined Jefferson and dens fracture
      Rotatory subluxation
   Malformation
      Mobile os odontoideum
   Degeneration
      Arthrosis of C1-2

CONTRAINDICATION

Severe osteoporsis is a contraindication to the use of PIS fixation (Table 9-2). There is a risk of screw breakage when solid bony fusion has not been obtained. In very rare cases the route of the vertebral artery at the level of the transverse foramen of the atlas is abnormally medial and therefore prevents the insertion of screws in the lateral mass of the atlas (Tokuda, Myasaka, Abe, et al., 1985). Literature also describes an ectatic vertebral artery not passing through the transverse foramen of the atlas, but instead piercing the dura mater below the posterior arch of the atlas in the atlantoaxial interlaminar space. This occurrence is, likewise, exceptionally rare (Sharma, Parekh, Prabhu, & Gurusinghe, 1993).

Marked cervical lordosis or kyphosis of the upper thoracic spine prevents drilling at the correct angle.

PREOPERATIVE EVALUATIONS

Radiographic Evaluations

Anteroposterior, lateral, and flexion-extension views should be taken. Attention should be given to any possible obstruction of drilling direction (lordotic cervical or kyphotic thoracic spine). Furthermore, a split dorsal arch of the atlas is detectable preoperatively.

Table 9-2
Contraindications for Posterior Interfacet Screw Fixation

Severe osteoporosis
Abnormal course of vertebral artery
Hyperlordosis of lower cervical spine
Kyphosis of upper thoracic spine

Computed Tomography (CT)

To rule out any abnormal routing of the vertebral artery, a CT scan is mandatory (Fig. 9-3).

Magnetic Resonance Imaging (MRI)

It is advisable to observe any displacement of cerebellar tonsils below the foramen magnum level (Chiari malformation Type I). In such cases it is dangerous to enter the spinal canal at the atlas level (Fig. 9-4).

SPECIAL INSTRUMENTS

1. Image intensifier
2. Rigid head fixation (Mayfield clamp)
3. Two drill bits (minimum length, 16 cm), diameter 2.5-mm, calibrated
4. Measurement probe, only when using uncalibrated bits
5. 3.5-mm cortical bone screws of between 38 and 48 mm
6. Flexible multistranded cable to secure the bone block

CONSENT

1. General surgical complications
2. Damage to vertebral artery (see "Complications")
3. Damage to dura (fistula) or spinal cord (see "Complications")
4. Damage to nervus occipitalis major (dysesthesia of back part of the scalp)
5. Overloading adjacent levels (instability)
6. 40 to 50% impairment of cervical rotation (well tolerated in most cases)
7. Fatigue and cramp symptoms during desk work
8. Halo-immobilization as an alternative to C1-C2 fusion

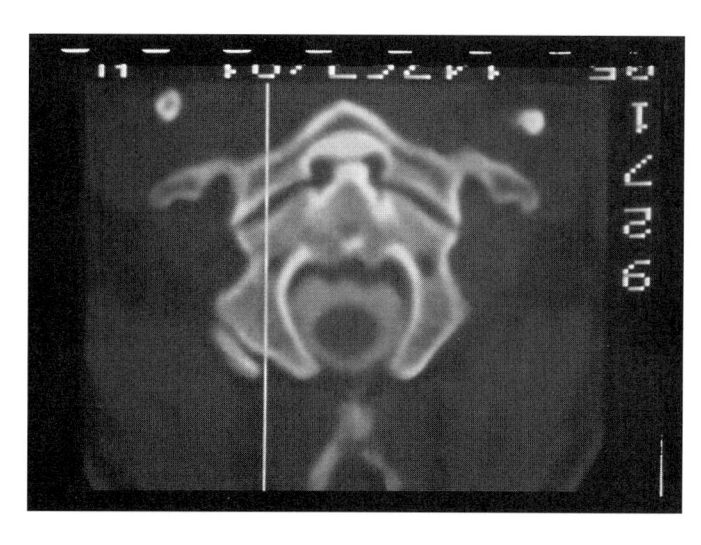

FIG. 9-3. Preoperative CT scan after myelography. The sagittal line represents the direction of the interfacet screw. The screw must always be within the spongiosa of atlas and axis. Any erosion of the cortical bone of the atlas or axis resulting from an abnormal course of the vertebral artery must be excluded by a CT scan. In such rare cases, interfacet screwing is contraindicated.

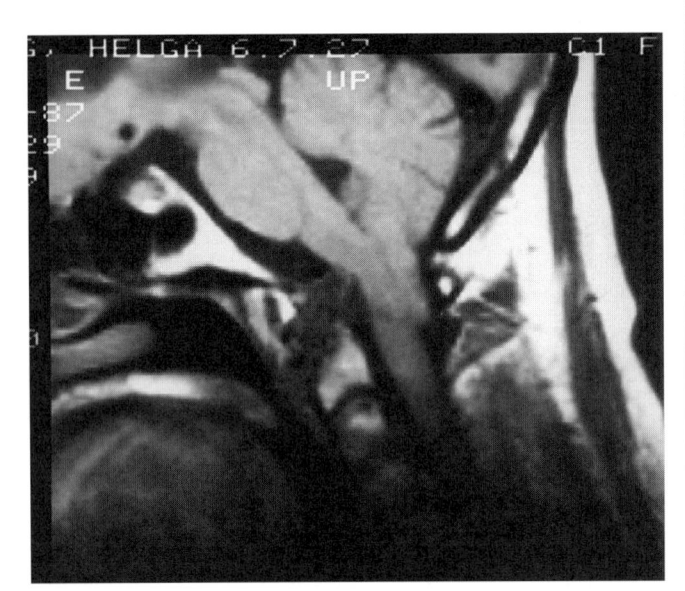

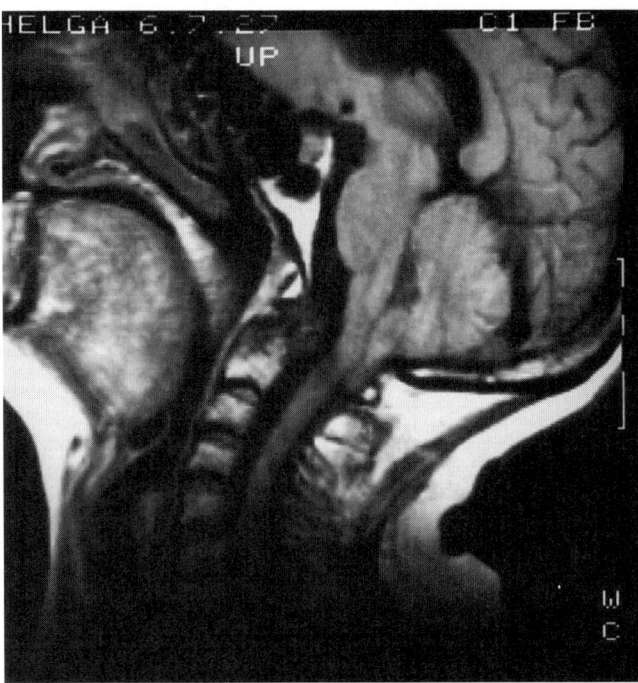

FIG. 9-4. MRI scan in flexion (a) and extension (b) of a 60-year-old woman suffering from a combination of rheumatoid arthritis and a Chiari Type I malformation. The spinal cord is ventrally compressed by the rheumatoid arthritis pannus tissue. The cerebellar tonsils are caudally displaced into the foramen magnum. In extension they compress the spinal cord additionally from the dorsal direction. Application of a wire cerclage around the dorsal arch of the atlas is contraindicated because of possible injury to the cerebellar tonsils. Removal of the dorsal arch and interfacet screws is recommended. Bone chips must be packed into the joints and placed between the remaining arch and lamina of the axis (see Fig. 9-7).

PREOPERATIVE PREPARATIONS

1. Fitting for cervical collar
2. Shaving

POSITIONING

1. Prone position with slightly flexed head.
2. The head is fixed firmly in a Mayfield clamp.
3. The shoulders are pulled down, so the venous vessels in the muscles are compressed to reduce bleeding.
4. X-ray confirmation of drilling direction in order to establish the length of skin incision (Fig. 9-5).
5. Preparation of the iliac crest for removal of bone graft.
6. The surgeon is positioned on the left or right side of the patient; the anesthesiologist is in front of the head.

APPROACH

1. An incision is made in the midline from occiput to vertebra prominens. Fascia nuchae in the midline is prepared. The application of wound retractors of unequal tension prevents exact preparation in the midline.
2. Fascia nuchae incised from occiput to vertebra prominens.
3. Superficial neck muscles are likewise incised in the midline, but only as far as the spinous process of C4-5.
4. Star-shaped insertion of the deep cervical muscles to the spinous process of C2 detached by means of chisel or oscillating saw. Muscles retracted laterally together with a bone fragment attached to their insertion.
5. Subperiosteal preparation of the laminae of C2 and the C2-3 joint.
6. Subperiosteal detachment of musculus rectus capitis minor from dorsal arch of the atlas. Lateral preparation not quite as far as the sulcus for the vertebral artery (10–14 mm).
7. Removal of atlantoaxial membrane. Transition from lamina to isthmus of C2 should be visible. Preparation should be done with a sharp dissector superiosteally. Medial border of isthmus C2 (lateral border of the spinal canal) serves later as important landmark for sagittal drilling direction.
8. Preparation of C1-2 joints as described by Magerl and Seemann (1987) is not absolutely necessary in order to reduce the risk of bleeding of the venous plexus around the joints. Bleeding is controlled by bipolar coagulation or applying hemostatic sponge.
9. Flexible multistranded cable placed around dorsal arch of the atlas, which serves initially as a repositioning aid and later to secure bone block. Screwing should be done after repositioning, which is carried out either with the cable system around the dorsal arch of the atlas pulling dorsally or by ventrally pressing the spinous process C2.

DRILLING DIRECTION

1. Entry point for drilling just above inferior facet of C2 and 2 to 3 mm laterally of the medial border of C2-3 facet (Fig. 9-6).

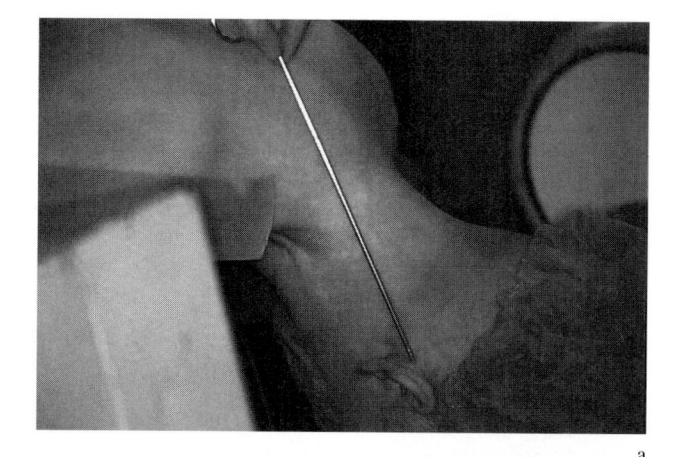

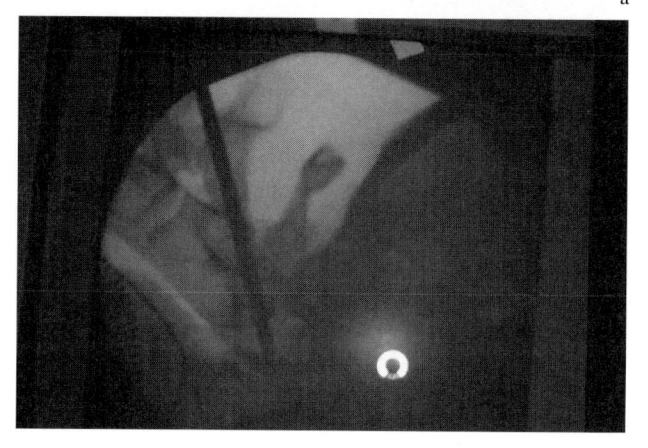

FIG. 9-5. Drilling direction is checked preoperatively (a) by means of an image intensifier (b).

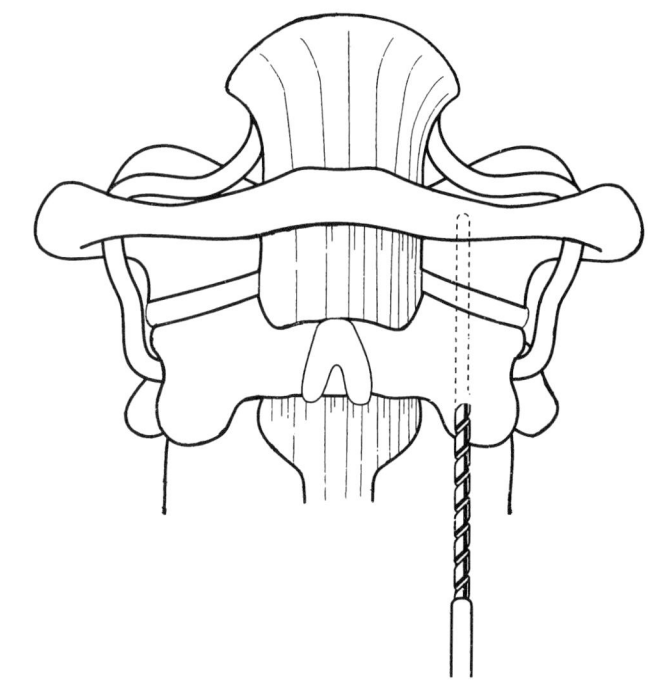

FIG. 9-6. Entry point of the drill bit is the inferior facet of the axis and 2 to 3 mm laterally of the medial border of C2-3 facet. Drilling direction is strictly sagittal.

2. Drilling is strictly sagittal. Guidance of drilling direction is a nerve hook at the inner concavity of the isthmus C2. Any lateral deviation may endanger the vertebral artery.
3. Lateral drilling direction determined by means of image intensifier. Target point is middle/upper part of ventral arch of atlas (see Figs. 9-1 and 9-5, b). If neck cannot be flexed, then percutaneous drilling is performed. A guide to protect paraspinal muscles not necessary when using smooth-shafted drill bit.
4. Perforation of cortex of entry point with an awl.
5. Resistance of joint surfaces noticeable when drilling. Ventral cortex perforation of lateral mass of atlas of 1 to 2 mm is harmless because lateral mass is ventrally covered by muscles.
6. It has proved helpful to leave the drill bit in its present position and to use an identical drill bit for the opposite side. This has the advantage of creating temporary fixation, which not only aids drilling of the second hole but also eases insertion of the first screw. Calibration of the drill allows direct measurements of the screw length, which, as a rule, is between 38 and 48 mm.
7. After drilling second hole, both bits are replaced by 3.5-mm cortical bone screws. Screw length should be chosen so that screw tip does not project into lateral x-ray view beyond the ventral position of the anterior arch of the atlas (see Fig. 9-1).
8. After having inserted both screws, coupling of C1 and C2 must be examined to exclude any possibility of movement. A towel clamp gripping the spinous process of C2 is pressed and pulled to ensure this.
9. Image intensifier turned to anteroposterior position to check screw position, which must be projected into middle third of C1-2 joints (see Fig. 9-2, b). Sometimes it is difficult to recognize the bony structures because of head position and fixation system.

BONE GRAFT

1. Tricortical bone graft (4 cm long and 1 cm wide) removed from posterior iliac crest (Dickman, Sonntag, Papadopoulos, & Hadley, 1991). This graft is reformed into bicortical graft by removing rounded cortical side.
2. Laminae of C1 and C2 decorticated.
3. Flexible, multistranded cable may be used to secure the position of the bone graft. Cable loop passed beneath dorsal arch of atlas in midline from caudally to cranially. A notch must be cut bilaterally in lamina near spinous process of C2 into which the loop is introduced. Graft wedged between arch of atlas and spinous process of C2. The two free ends of the cable are pulled slightly and crimped over the bone block (Fig. 9-1).
4. Remaining decorticated areas covered with bone chips.

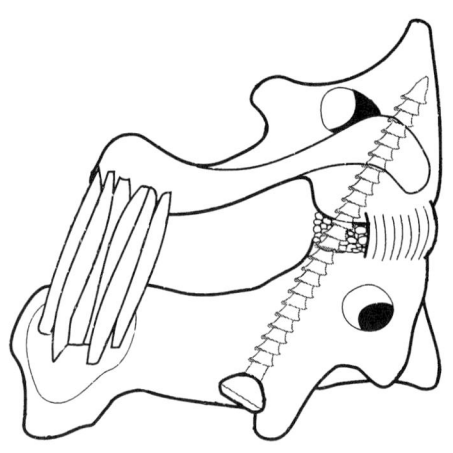

FIG. 9-7. In cases of defective dorsal arch, bone chips must be packed into the cavity between the decorticated joint surfaces and also placed on the remaining dorsal arches.

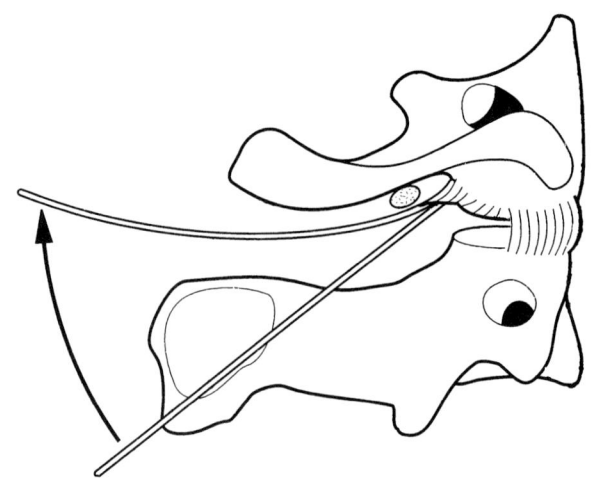

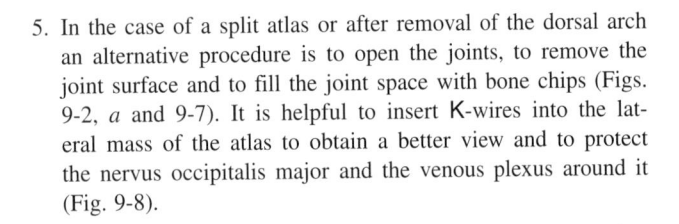

FIG. 9-8. In order to open the joint between atlas and axis it is recommended to insert a K-wire into the massa lateralis and bend the end cranially. This protects the occipital nerve and the surrounding venous plexus.

5. In the case of a split atlas or after removal of the dorsal arch an alternative procedure is to open the joints, to remove the joint surface and to fill the joint space with bone chips (Figs. 9-2, *a* and 9-7). It is helpful to insert K-wires into the lateral mass of the atlas to obtain a better view and to protect the nervus occipitalis major and the venous plexus around it (Fig. 9-8).

CLOSURE

1. Detached bone fragments with insertion of deep cervical muscles fixed to spinous process of C2.
2. Wound closed in multilayer fashion.
3. At end of surgery, anteroposterior and lateral radiographs taken to documentate screw positions.
4. Cervical collar applied.

POSTOPERATIVE TREATMENT

1. Observation for 12 to 24 hours; risk of epidural and retropharyngeal hematoma
2. Cervical (Philadelphia) collar for 6 weeks
3. Radiographs after 6 to 8 weeks; isometric physical therapy started when any screw loosening ruled out

COMPLICATIONS

Vascular, Dura Mater, Spinal Cord, and Nerve Complications

In the published series of Magerl and Seemann (1987) (23 cases), Grob, Jeanneret, Aebi, and Markwalder (1991) (161 cases from 4 spine centers), and Marcotte, Dickman, Sonntag, Karahalios, and Drabier (1993) (17 cases) and in our own 86 cases of transarticular screwing, no injuries to the vertebral artery, dura mater, or spinal cord were observed. Grob et al. (1991) described an injury to 1 of 161 patients, in whom the nervus hypoglossus was damaged by a screw that was too long. The paresis of the hypoglossus nerve resolved after removal of the screw. In another patient, the atlantooccipital joint was irritated by an overly long screw, necessitating its removal.

Pseudarthrosis

In a series of 126 cases with isolated atlantoaxial fusion Grob et al. (1991) found in 1 patient a detectable movement on bending and extension radiographs between C1 and C2 (see Table 9-3). Marcotte et al. (1993) reported fusion in all of their 17 patients. In our own 65 patients, after a follow-up of 6 to 84 months, we did not find any evidence of screw loosening with the above-mentioned technique. We did, however, observe a pseudarthrosis in one patient in whom no bone block was inserted (Fig. 9-9). Absorption of the bone surrounding the screws as a result of movement was the cause of this pseudarthrosis.

Table 9-3
Advantages and Disadvantages of Posterior Interfacet Screw Fixation

Advantages
   Higher fusion rate
   Does not require intact laminae of C1 or C2
   Three-column fixation

Disadvantages
   Requires thorough three-dimensional comprehensions of occiput to C2 anatomy
   Greater risk to vertebral artery
   Occasionally difficult to complete secondary thoracic kyphosis

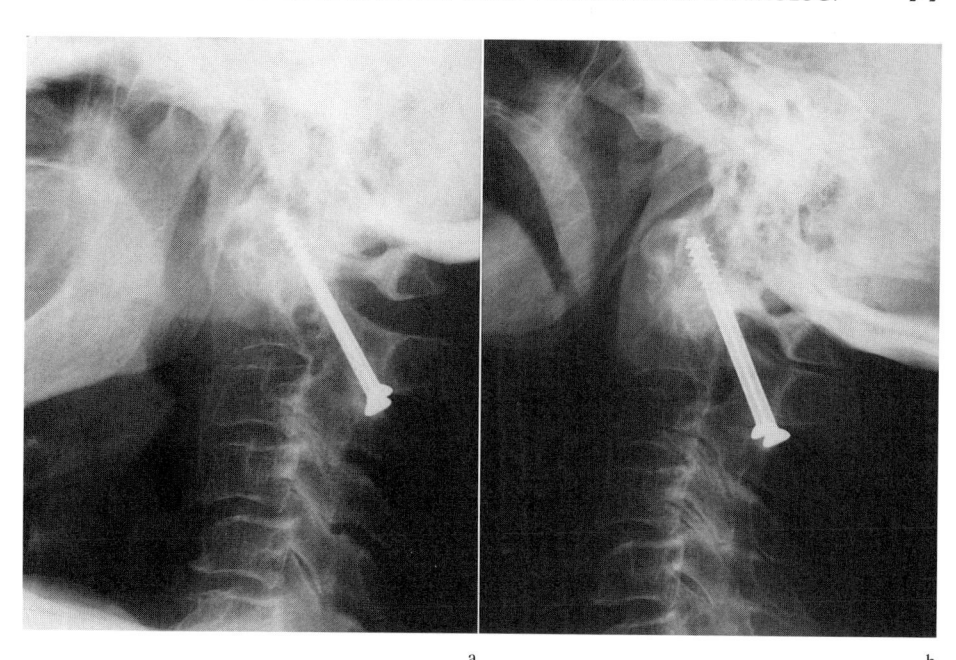

FIG. 9-9. Lateral x-ray view in flexion (a) and extension (b) of a 71-year-old woman with rheumatoid arthritis. A pseudarthrosis developed as a consequence of not placing bone between the arches. Interfacet screwing is inadequate alone.

Instrumentation Failure

No screw loosening or breakage was reported in the 126 patients of Grob et al. (1991) and in the 17 patients of Marcotte et al. (1993). We observed screw breakage in one patient who underwent fusion without a bone graft. There were no clinical consequences. Insertion of a bone graft is therefore mandatory.

REFERENCES

Brooks, A.L., & Jenkins, E.B. (1978). Atlanto-axial arthrodesis by the wedge compression method. *Journal of Bone and Joint Surgery, American Volume, 60,* 279.

Cybulski, G.R., Stone, J.L., Crowell, R.M., et al. (1988). Use of Halifax interlaminar clamp for posterior C1-C2 arthrodesis. *Neurosurgery, 22,* 429–431.

Davis, F.W., & Markley, H.E. (1951). Rheumatoid arthritis with death from medullary compression. *Annals of Internal Medicine, 35,* 451.

Dickman, C.A., Sonntag, V.K.H., Papadopoulos, S.M., & Hadley, M.N. (1991). The intraspinous method of posterior atlantoaxial arthrodesis. *Journal of Neurosurgery, 74,* 190–198.

Gallie, W.E. (1939). Fractures and dislocations of the cervical spine. *Journal of Bone and Joint Surgery, American Volume, 46,* 495–499.

Grob, D., Crisco, J.J., Panjabi, M.M., Wang, P., & Dvorak, J. (1992). Biomechanical evaluation of four different posterior atlantoaxial fixation techniques. *Spine, 17,* 480–490.

Grob, D., Jeanneret, B., Aebi, M., & Markwalder, T.-M. (1991). Atlantoaxial fusion with transarticular screw fixation. *Journal of Bone and Joint Surgery, British Volume, 73,* 972–976.

Hanson, P.B., Montesano, P.X., Sharkey, N.A., & Rauschning, W. (1990). Anatomic and biomechanical assessment of transarticular screw fixation for atlantoaxial instability. *Spine, 16,* 1141–1145.

Holmes, J.C., & Hall, J.E. (1978). Fusion for instability and potential instability of the cervical spine in children and adolescents. *Orthopedic Clinics of North America, 9,* 923–943.

Holness, R.O., Huestis, W.S., Howes, W.J., & Langille, R.A. (1984). Posterior stabilization with an interlaminar clamp in cervical injuries: technical note and review of the long term experience with the method. *Neurosurgery, 14,* 318–322.

Magerl, F., & Seemann, P. (1987). Stable posterior fusion of the atlas and axis by transarticular screw fixation. In: P. Kehr & A. Weidner (Eds.), *Cervical Spine I, Strassbourg 1985* (pp. 322–327). Wien: Springer.

Marcotte, P., Dickman, C.A., Sonntag, V.K.H., Karahalios, D.G., & Drabier, J. (1993). Posterior atlantoaxial facet screw fixation. *Journal of Neurosurgery, 79,* 234–237.

Marks, J.S., & Sharp, J. (1981). Rheumatoid cervical myelopathy. *Quarterly Journal of Medicine, 50,* 307.

Sharma, R.R., Parekh, H.C., Prabhu, S., & Gurusinghe, N.T. (1993). Compression of the C-2 root by a rare anomalous ectatic vertebral artery. *Journal of Neurosurgery, 78,* 669–672.

Tokuda, K., Myasaka, K., Abe, H., et al. (1985). Anomalous atlantoaxial portions of vertebral and posterior inferior cerebellar arteries. *Neuroradiology, 27,* 410–413.

Wilke, H.-J., Fischer, K., Kluger, A., Magerl, F., Claes, L., & Woersdoerfer, O. (1992). In vitro investigations of internal fixation systems of the upper cervical spine. *European Spine Journal, 1,* 191–199.

CHAPTER 10

Application of the Occipitocervical Plate for Occipitocervical and Atlantoaxial Pathology

Dieter Grob

HIGHLIGHTS

Rheumatoid arthritis, tumorous lesions, or infections may require stabilization of the uppermost part of the vertebral column and head. The indication for the occipitocervical fusion is instability of the suboccipital region due to ligamentous or bony destruction. The literature offers several operative techniques. The main concern is the immobilization between head and cervical spine for solid bony fusion. From simple onlay techniques with autologous bone graft to more or less sophisticated internal fixation systems as wires (Brooks & Jenkins, 1978; Gallie, 1939; Wertheim & Bohlman, 1987), plates (Privat, 1988), rods (Bridwell, 1986; Itoh, Tsuji, Katoh, Yonezawa, & Kitagawa, 1988; Ransford, Crockard, Pozo, Thomas, & Nelson, 1986), and clamps (Guyotat, Perrin, Pelissou, Daher, & Bachour, 1987), most of these systems offer enough stability to allow incorporation of the additional bone graft. However, several disadvantages might be detected.

Wiring techniques require intracranial manipulation to fix the cranium and intraspinal handling of the wire loops to fix the laminae. Therefore, there is an inherent potential risk of injury to neurologic structures. The application of forces to reduce dislocations with wires especially in the translational dislocation of C1-2 may be limited. Here, there is a risk of the wire cutting through the soft bone, in such conditions as rheumatoid arthritis with soft and brittle bone. Conditions requiring laminectomy need a long fusion extending into the unaffected cervical spine in order to achieve sufficient stability. Finally, postoperative stability may be jeopardized by difficult wire tightenings or loosening due to repeated loading. An increased incidence of pseudarthrosis may be a consequence.

Techniques with rod systems may carry the risk of a telescoping effect in the lower cervical spine, because of gliding of the wires along the rods. The extent of the fusion is determined by the stability of the wire fixation to the cervical spine and therefore must go at least down to C3 or C4 (Itoh et al., 1988), even in cases in which the pathology is restricted to the suboccipital era, thus including healthy segments in the fusion.

The use of *plates* has been favorized by some authors (Privat, 1988). The drawback of these systems is usually the bilateral weakness of the bone of the occiput, with insufficient purchase of the screws. The atlas remains unfixed by the conventional techniques with plates and screws.

This chapter presents a new technique of posterior occipitocervical fixation with plate and screws with elimination of most of the unfavorable aspects of formerly presented procedures.

INDICATIONS

Any suboccipital instability including the C1-2 complex justifies a posterior fixation of the occipitocervical area (Table 10-1). The main concern is the protection of neurologic structures of the brain stem and medulla. To obtain a completely free spinal canal, it may be necessary to add decompressive maneuvers such as anterior dens resection (Crockard, Calder, & Ransford, 1990) or posterior widening of the occiput and/or laminectomy. Patients with rheumatoid arthritis who have not only isolated atlantoaxial dislocation but also upward migration of the dens with signs of neurogenic compression are candidates for occipitocervical fusion and decompression. Tumorous lesions of the suboccipital area and infectious bony destruction also may require therapeutic or prophylactic stabilization of this anatomic region.

Table 10-1
Indications and Contraindications for Causes and Effects of Occipitocervical Instabilities

Indications: Instability	Causes	Effects
Bony instabilities	Tumors	Compression Bone destruction Pain
	Infection	Bone destruction Joint destruction Pain
	Basilar impression	Pain Compression of the spinal cord or of the brain stem
	Degenerative changes	Joint deformation (osteophytes) Pain
	Fractures	Inveterated joint fractures Malalignment
Ligamentous instabilities	Inflammatory Posttraumatic	Rheumatoid arthritis Rupture of the ligamenta alaria Rupture of the transverse ligament
Iatrogenic instability	Resection of the odontoid Excessive bone resection (tumors)	Insufficiency of the ligamenta alaria
Contraindications:	Reduced general health Short neck in obese patients Anatomical malformation	Poor surgical risk Technically difficult application Increased risk of neurovascular injury

CONTRAINDICATIONS

The contraindications to use of the occipitocervical plate include reduced general health status of the patient. Also, a short neck in obese patients makes access to the occiput and C1-2 impossible, and screw placement difficult. Anatomical malformations such as congenital anomalies of the occipitocervical junction require further preoperative investigations such as computed tomography (CT), magnetic resonance imaging (MRI), and angiography.

SURGICAL PROCEDURE

The principle of this intervention is to fix the occipitocervical region by applying a Y-shaped plate from the occiput down to the desired level of the cervical spine. The plate is fixed with screws in the midline of the occiput and in the posterior elements of the vertebrae. An additional transarticular atlantoaxial screw fixation ensures the stability of the C1-2 segment.

Patient Positioning (Fig. 10-1)

Any intraoperative skull fixation system may be used, provided an extension of the cervical spine and a rotation along a transverse axis through the meatus externus on both sides (flexion in the atlantooccipital joints) is possible. With the patient lying prone on the table, the ideal position of the head is moderate extension of the lower cervical spine and flexion in the atlantooccipital joint. If the rotation is not carefully completed, the drill for the C1-2 fixation may not be lowered enough to guarantee ideal screw placement, especially in obese patients. Ideally, the anesthesist is situated at

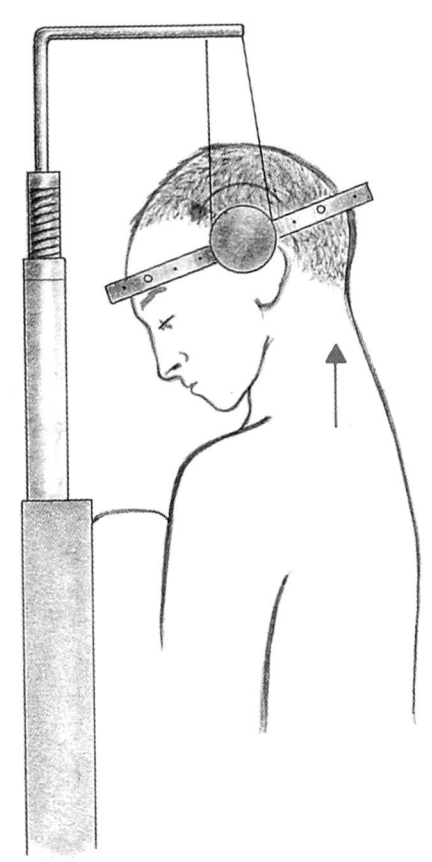

FIG. 10-1. Fixation of the head during the operative procedure may be performed with a halo or any other clamp system that provides enough stability and has its axis of rotation approximately at the level of the atlantooccipital joint. The position for the atlantoaxial screw positioning is slight distraction of the lower cervical spine and flexion in the atlantooccipital joint.

CHAPTER 10 / APPLICATION OF THE OCCIPITOCERVICAL PLATE FOR OCCIPITOCERVICAL AND ATLANTOAXIAL PATHOLOGY

the feet of the patient, in order to give free access for the C-arm of the image intensifier, which is placed laterally during atlantoaxial drilling.

Surgical Approach (Fig. 10-2)

A midline approach from the protuberantia occipitalis down to the midcervical spine is performed. In obese patients it is necessary to have a sufficient-length incision or to insert the drill for the C1-2 screws through separate stab incisions in order to obtain correct positioning of the screws. The fascia nuchae is divided strictly in the midline to avoid excessive hemorrhage. The prominent spinous process of C2 serves as landmark. The muscular insertions are detached here, together with their bony attachment, using a bone saw. A subperiosteal dissection of the lamina of C2 and the posterior arch of the atlas is now possible. The occiput is exposed only in the midline. The laminae of the lower cervical spine should be visualized if the fusion is planned to extend caudally.

Atlantoaxial Screw Fixation (Fig. 10-3)

The atlantoaxial screw fixation is performed with two bilateral screws in the sagittal plane crossing the C1-2 joint. This may be done separately or may be integrated into the Y-plate. In the latter case the screws are placed primarily as described below and secondarily inserted in the corresponding holes of the plate. Additional dissection of the lamina of C2 is

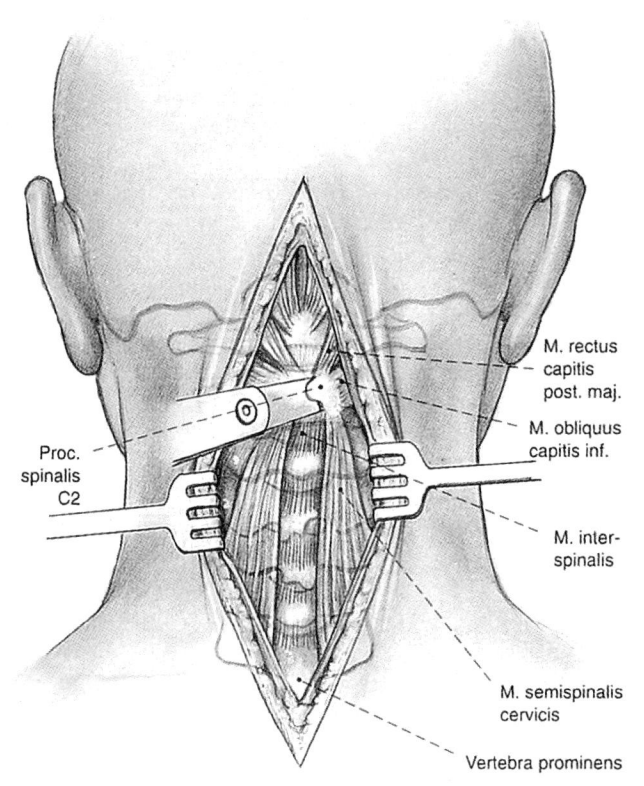

FIG. 10-2. Surgical approach. The prominent spinous process of C2 is the landmark for orientation in the suboccipital era. The muscles are detached by leaving intact their bony attachment at the tip of the spinous process.

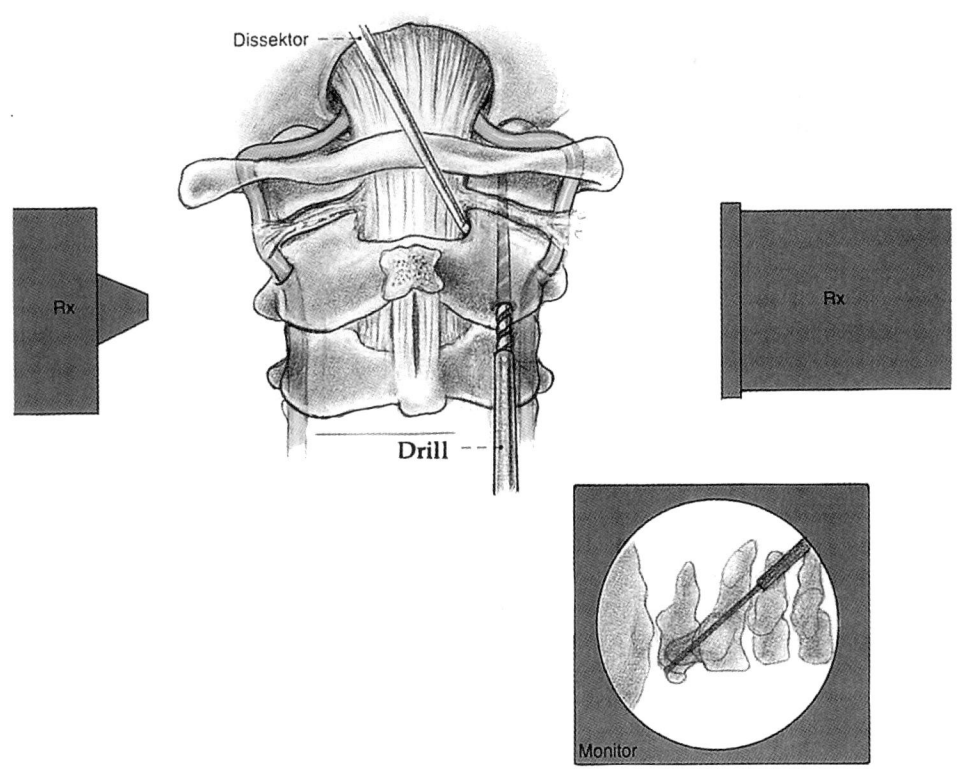

FIG. 10-3. The medial part of the isthmus of C2 has to be well visualized by careful subperiosteal dissection of the area. The lateral part with the transverse foramen and the vertebral artery are not visualized. The soft tissues with the greater suboccipital nerve root are held rostrally by a retractor. The direction of the drill is strictly sagittal in the anteroposterior direction or pointing at the upper part of the projection of the anterior ring of the atlas in the lateral view.

Table 10-2
Guidelines for Correct C1-2 Screw Placement

Patient Position	Neutral C1/C2 Rotation	Lateral C-Arm Control	Sagittal Drilling
Extension of lower cervical spine Flexion of occiput-C1	Verify intraoperatively	Inclination of drill important to cross joint in posterior part	Too lateral, risks injury of the vertebral artery Too medial enters the spinal canal

necessary for correct screw placement. It must be completed in order to show the medial border of the isthmic part of C2 on both sides. For this purpose the atlantooccipitalis membrane extending from C1 to C2 is dissected subperiostally. Reduction of an atlantoaxial dislocation may be held in a reduced position by manipulation of a towel clamp attached to the spinous process of C2 during the drilling and screw insertion. The drilling must be performed in a strictly sagittal direction a few millimeters laterally of the previously exposed medial border of the isthmus of C2. The point of entry of the bore hole lies on the medial border or the posterior aspect of the C2-3 joint. During this procedure, the use of an image intensifier is recommended (Table 10-2). The inclination of the drill can be controlled in the lateral x-ray beam. The tip of the drill must point at the superior half of the lateral oval projection of the anterior ring of the atlas. The ideally positioned screw crosses the atlantoaxial joint in its posterior half and ends in the center of the ventral aspect of the lateral mass of the atlas.

Fixation in the Lower Cervical Spine (Fig. 10-4)

If there is an indication to extend the fusion into the lower cervical spine, the screw fixation of the plate may be performed as follows: The screws are entirely situated in the articular mass of the cervical vertebrae and are inserted according to the technique of Magerl (Grob & Magerl, 1987; Magerl & Grob, 1986). (The screws in the lower cervical spine are not intrapedicular screws.) After tailoring the Y-plate to the desired length, the plate is molded and fit to the posterior parts of the cervical spine, respecting the physiologic lordosis. Drilling is performed through the holes in the plate in a plane parallel to the joint surfaces and diverging ventrally 20 to 25 degrees. Ideally, the point of entry lies between the lamina and the medial border of the articular mass, thus obtaining a length of screw of 18 to 20 mm in adults.

Fixation of the Occiput

The thickness of the bone is more than double in the midline than on the lateral aspects (Grob, 1992); it can be studied with CT or MRI. Therefore the Y-plate is fixed with its single branch in the midline of the occiput. (A safety drill guide with a stop at 10 mm may be used.) Before drilling, the flexion in the head fixation has to be corrected to a neutral position. The midline of the occiput, the posterior part of the atlas and the spinous process of C2 are decorticated. A bone graft is harvested from the posterior iliac crest. Its

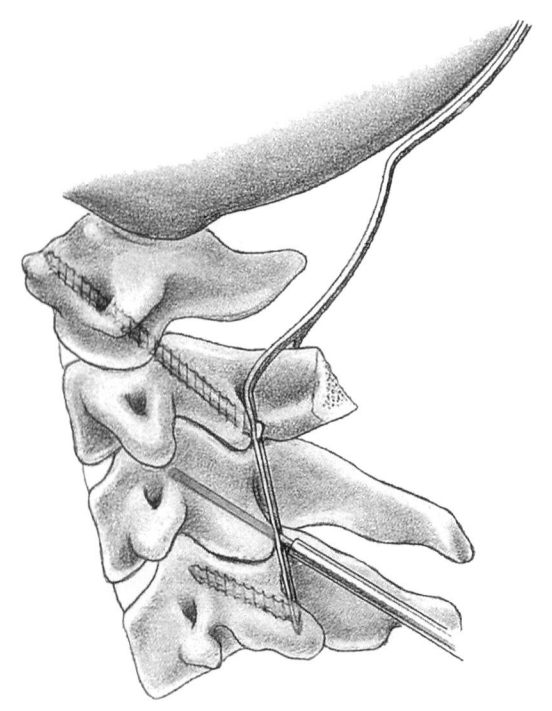

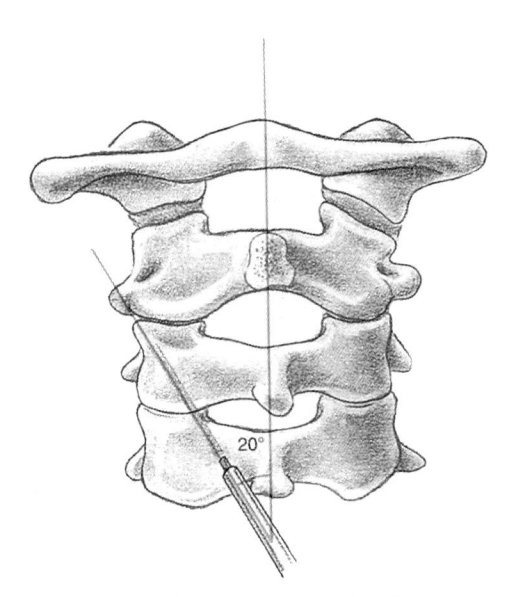

FIG. 10-4. Screw insertion techniques in the lower cervical spine. In the lateral view the direction of the drilling is parallel to the facet joints. In the frontal plane, the drill has to diverge 20 degrees laterally in order to avoid nerve root and vertebral artery on the ventral aspect of the facets.

shape has to be tailored to fit underneath the plate between the occiput and C2. By firmly tightening the screws in the plate, the bone graft is pressed against the underlying bony structures, thus facilitating bony ingrowth. The rest of the bone graft is arranged posteriorly to the plate and the spinous process of the vertebrae to be fused. It is important to make sure that the bone graft between C2 and the occiput is in contact with the bone graft of the subaxial spine (Fig. 10-5)

After adequate hemostasis, the muscle insertions of the spinous process of the axis are reinserted by a transosseous suture and the continuity of the nuchal fascia is reestablished in a separate layer.

Biomechanical Considerations

The Y-plate provides a direct link between the cervical spine and the skull. Flexion of the cervical spine in the fused area is blocked by the tension band mechanism of the plate, while extension is prevented by the rigidity of the plate and the underlying cortical bone graft. The rotation in the upper cervical spine takes place between C1 and C2, while the normal rotation between the occiput and the atlas is small. Because the transarticular screw fixation is an integrated part of the Y-plate construct, it is able to block the rotation effectively (Grob, Crisco, Panjabi, Wang, & Dvorak, 1992). The lateral bending of the upper cervical spine is coupled to the axial rotation of the joints: An attempt to bend the head laterally will result in a combined axial rotation. Thus, the fixation of the Y-plate also prevents lateral bending.

Fixation with the Y-plate provides a multidirectional, immediate postoperative stability. A soft collar, worn out of bed, is therefore sufficient for postoperative immobilization. Six weeks after the surgical procedure an x-ray study is performed and usually confirms the consolidation of the fusion.

PATIENTS

Between 1986 and 1992 33 patients had undergone this surgery. There were 6 men and 27 women whose average age at operation was 60 years (range, 39–81). In all these patients the indication was intractable pain due to instability and/or medullary compression in the cervical spine due to rheumatoid arthritis. Twenty-one patients were determined by the use of Redlund-Johnell technique to have an additional upward migration of the dens. The radiologic classification was done according to the rules of Larsen (1974). According to this classification, 9 patients were Stage V, 13 patients Stage IV, 10 patients Stage III, and 1 patient Stage II. The preoperative atlantodental distance was 7.9 mm and the dens migration according to the Redlund-Johnell method was 11 mm. Of 33 patients, 22 (66%) had clinical neurologic deficit and neurophysiologically verified myelopathy and/or radiculopathy.

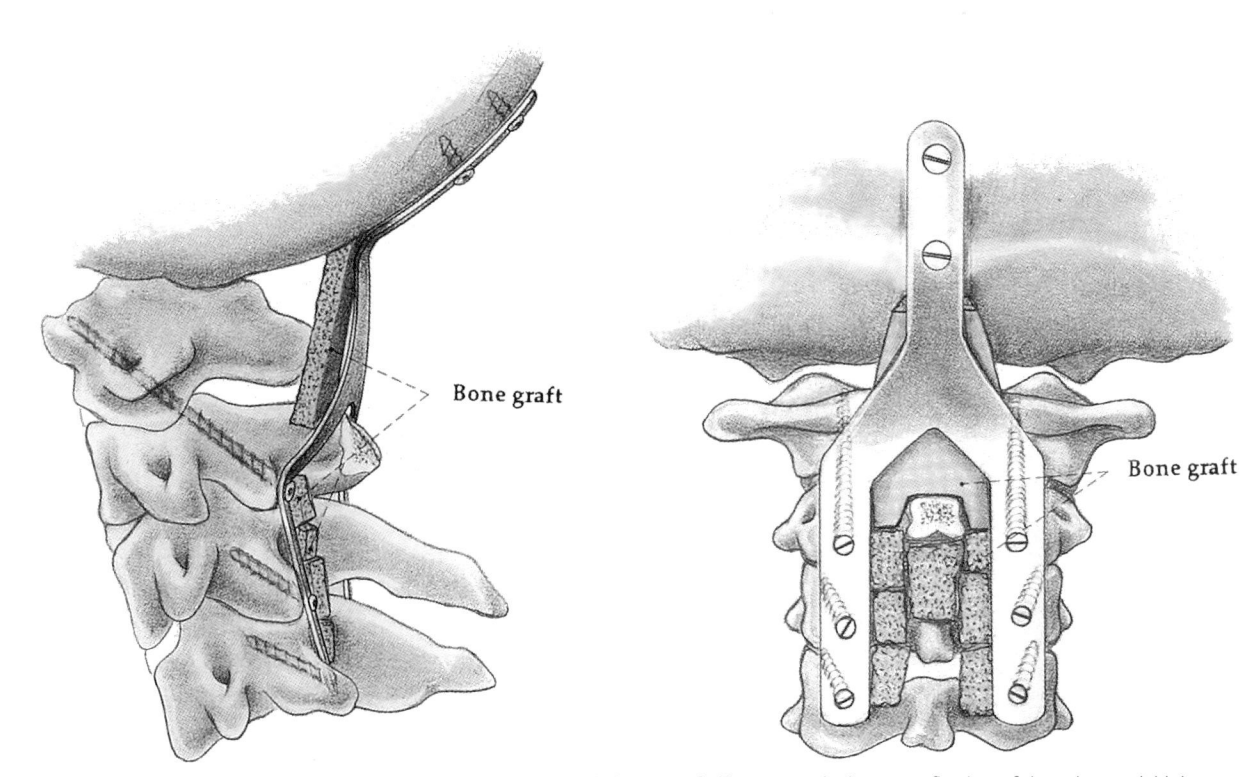

FIG. 10-5. Final construct with bone graft. The transarticular screw fixation of the atlantoaxial joint may be integrated in the plate (as shown) or performed separately, if the fusion extends into the lower cervical spine. Care has to be taken to position the bone graft along the fusion as shown.

RESULTS

The follow-up examination was performed an average of 18 months postoperatively (range, 6–62). The atlantodental distance could be significantly reduced to 1.8 mm postoperatively, while the upward migration of the dens showed no progression. This was also correct for the 10 cases in which a transoral dens resection for decompression was performed. The neurologic deficit could be improved in 19 of 22 patients. However, 3 patients remained unchanged. Two patients died for reasons that were not surgically related. Radiologically, in 29 of 31 patients a solid fusion could be documented by lateral functional x-ray study. The subjective results, according to the criteria of Conaty and Morgans (1981), were 30 satisfactory outcomes and 1 unsatisfactory outcome.

Complications

Screw loosening occurred in 1 patient, with a fusion from occiput to C6 at the lower end of the plate. As the patient was pain-free and no pseudarthrosis was detected in functional radiographs, no additional surgery was needed. Breakage of a Y-plate with pseudarthrosis was seen in a patient with a fusion from the occiput down to T1. The patient had to undergo reoperation after 2 weeks because of unfavorable and uncomfortable head position. Because of flexion due to incomplete correction to neutral position intraoperatively, it was impossible to maintain a horizontal view without excessive lordosis of the lumbar spine. In this case it may be assumed that the blood supply of the bone graft was severely disturbed by this reintervention and pseudarthroses at the level of C2 occurred with the sequelae of implant failure. Additional bone graft and replacement of the plate was performed with a good final outcome. No neurologic damage or vascular disturbances were detected in this series.

DISCUSSION

The titanium Y-plate has proven to be a useful tool for posterior occipitocervical fusion. It offers several advantages over conventional techniques (Table 10-3). Immediate postoperative multidirectional stability is ensured by this procedure. There is a possibility of individually tailored selective fusion with appropriate length of the implant without the need for inclusion of healthy segments into the fusion. There is no need for insertion of hardware or manipulation in the spinal canal, a point especially important in atlantoaxial dislocation in rheumatoid arthritis, in which the posterior ring of the atlas is in firm contact with the medulla. An effective reduction and maintenance of the reduced position is ensured by the described technique of atlantoaxial fusion. The immediate postoperative stability is sufficient to allow easy postoperative treatment with a soft collar. A comparatively high union rate could be demonstrated in clinical experience. MRI and CT scan for follow-up studies are possible because the plate and screws are made of titanium.

Table 10-3
Advantages and Disadvantages of the Use of the Occipitocervical Plate Technique

Advantages
  Decreased risk of neurologic injury
  Decreased risk of "telescoping" compared to rod system
  Requires fixation of fewer motion segments

Disadvantages
  Possible screw pull out
  Not able to fixate atlas

REFERENCES

Bridwell, K.H. (1986). Treatment of markedly displaced hangman's fracture with a Luque rectangle and a posterior fusion in 71 year old men: Case report. *Spine, 11,* 49.

Brooks, A.L., & Jenkins, E.G. (1978). Atlanto-axial arthrodesis by the wedge compression method. *Journal of Bone and Joint Surgery, American Volume, 60,* 279.

Conaty, J.P., & Morgans, E.S. (1981). Cervical fusion in rheumatoid arthritis. *Journal of Bone and Joint Surgery, American Volume, 63,* 1218–1227.

Crockard, H.A., Calder, I., & Ransford, A. (1990). One-stage transoral decompression and posterior fixation in rheumatoid atlanto-axial subluxation. *Journal of Bone and Joint Surgery, British Volume, 72,* 682–685.

Gallie, W.E. (1939). Fractures and dislocations of the cervical spine. *American Journal of Surgery, 46,* 495–499.

Grob, D. (1992). Dorsale Fixation des okzipitozervikalen Uebergangs. *Operative Orthopedic Traumatology, 4,* 151–160.

Grob, D., Crisco, J., Panjabi, M., Wang, P., & Dvorak, J. (1992). Biomechanical evaluation of four different posterior atlantoaxial fixation techniques. *Spine, 17,* 480–490.

Grob, D., Dvorak, J., & Antinnes, J.A. (1993). Surgical management of the subaxial cervical spine (C3-T1). *European Spine Journal, 2,* 60–64.

Grob, D., & Magerl, F. (1987). Dorsale Spondylodese der Halswirbelsäule mit der Hakenplatte. *Orthopäde, 16,* 55–61.

Guyotat, J., Perrin, G., Pelissou, I., Daher, T., & Bachour, E. (1987). Utilization du matériel de Cotrel Dubousset dans les instabilités C1/C2. *Neurochirurgie, 33,* 236–238.

Itoh, T., Tsuji, H., Katoh, Y., Yonezawa, T., & Kitagawa, H. (1988). Occipito-cervical fusion reinforced by Luque's segmental spinal instrumentation for rheumatoid diseases. *Spine, 11,* 1234–1238.

Larsen, A. (1974). *A radiological method for grading the severity of rheumatoid arthritis.* Unpublished master's thesis, University of Helsinki, Helsinki, Finland.

Magerl, F., & Grob, D. (1986). Dorsal fusion of the cervical spine with the hook plate. In: P. Kehr & A. Weidner (Eds.), *Cervical Spine I* (pp. 217–221). Wien: Springer.

Privat, J.M. (1988). Instabilités rhumatismales du rachis sous-occipital. Indications et résultats de la plaque occipito-rachidienne monobloc. In: J. Privat (Ed.), *Osteosynthèse Rachidienne.* (pp. 159–162). Monpellier: Sauramps Médical.

Ransford, A., Crockard, H., Pozo, J., Thomas, N., & Nelson, I. (1986). Craniocervical instability treated by contoured loop fixation. *Journal of Bone and Joint Surgery, British Volume, 68,* 173–177.

Wertheim, S.B., & Bohlman, H.H. (1987). Occipito-cervical fusion. *Journal of Bone and Joint Surgery, American Volume, 69,* 833–836.

Section B
Lower Cervical Spine

CHAPTER 11

Wiring Techniques of the Lower Cervical Spine

Andrew Cappuccino
Paul C. McAfee

HIGHLIGHTS

Traumatic injuries to the cervical spine, a common cause of death and disability, range in severity from simple soft-tissue injuries to fractures with paralysis and/or death resulting. These injuries are often seen in the emergency department and must be carefully evaluated to minimize adverse long-term sequelae. Early diagnosis and restoration of spinal cord function and stabilization are keys to successful management of subaxial cervical spine injuries. The preponderance of cervical spine injuries result from either motor vehicle accidents, falls, or injuries sustained in athletic events or through violent crimes or acts of war. The preponderance of cervical spine injuries occur in young, active individuals during adolescence or early adulthood. The second largest group comprises individuals in their sixth and seventh decades. Preexisting canal stenosis and cervical spondylosis predispose the older age group to severe neurologic injuries when a small amount of force is applied to the cervical spine. The advent of spinal cord injury centers has significantly improved the emergency, medical, and surgical care, as well as the rehabilitation, of the patient who has sustained a spinal cord and bony spine injury. Modern advances in the pathophysiologic basis of spine and spinal cord injuries have allowed improvement in the nonoperative and operative approaches, including both internal fixation and conservative methods of treating the injured spine. Mortality from cervical spine injuries was 80% just 80 years ago (Hartwell, 1917). The current mortality rate with spine injury centers is now 6% (Brachen, Shepard, Collins, et al., 1990). The initial therapeutic goals are to preserve life, maintain neurologic function or restore cord or nerve-root function through appropriate decompression, provide stabilization of the cervical spine, and allow optimal rehabilitation. These goals are attainable if proper care is provided.

PRINCIPLES OF TREATMENT: EMERGENCY RESUSCITATION

Care for a patient with a possible injury to the cervical spine should begin at the scene of the accident. All patients with high-energy trauma and a neurologic deficit or a complaint of neck, shoulder, or arm pain in the absence of gross deformity, must be assumed to have a cervical spine injury. Often, spinal cord injuries, especially cervical spine injuries, will be missed, and the cause for missing these injuries usually relates to the patient's mental status (either intoxication or coma) or to the presence of multiple trauma, with attention being paid to other obviously traumatized parts of the body. The cervical spine should be immobilized at the scene of the injury using a rigid Philadelphia collar and/or sand bags with full spinal precautions, including a spine board. For children, there are special spine boards that accommodate the increased size of the cranium as compared to the body, and proper techniques must be observed in the field. Care should obviously be taken in the field to prevent further injury, which can be caused by inadvertent axial load, flexion, extension, distraction or rotational forces, or even from the application of overzealous traction. On arrival in the emergency department, resuscitation should be performed with the usual priority being airway first, breathing second, and circulation third. In the process of securing an airway, appropriate precautions should be taken to prevent further cervical injury. Once the patient has been fully resuscitated, an initial history must be obtained from either the patient, the paramedics, or witnesses to determine the mechanism of injury. A history of loss of consciousness or paralysis at the scene of an accident is important. Any patient who has a loss of consciousness or a concussion may have no objective findings at the time of the evaluation in the emergency department, thus important neck injuries may be overlooked. In Bohlman's evaluation of 300 cervical spine injuries (1979), 100 of these injuries were initially missed at the time of presentation. Great care must also be taken not to miss concomitant cervical spine injuries. As many as 16% of patients will have noncontiguous spine fractures, with the most common cervical pattern being a fracture of the C1-2 complex and a second remote subaxial fracture (Vaccaro, An, Lin, et al., 1992). Any patient who presents with an obvious cervical spine fracture will require very rigorous screening for associated bodily injuries.

RADIOGRAPHIC EVALUATION

As the initial evaluation proceeds, the radiographic examination of the cervical spine must be planned and executed. A lateral view of the cervical spine, while immobilized in a collar, must include visualization of the entire cervical spine, including the anterior and posterior elements of C3-7. A swimmer's view, tomography, or computed tomographic (CT) scan may be necessary to delineate the C7-T1 relationship if manual distraction of the shoulders is not sufficient. After the lateral view is examined, the anteroposterior and oblique views can be obtained in succession. If substantial osseous injury is found on the anteroposterior (AP) and lateral views, then pillar views should be obtained in the caudal to cranial angle of 30 to 35 degrees so that the facets can be visualized without turning the head. An open-mouth view is necessary to assess the odontoid and the C1-2 lateral mass relationships. Other studies that can subsequently be obtained to provide invaluable information for evaluation of space available for the cord, bony or soft-tissue encroachment on the neural elements, or mechanical alignment of the spine are contrasted CT scan and magnetic resonance imaging (MRI). At present, MRI is gaining in popularity, and there is some evidence that it may even be a better predictor of potential for neurologic recovery as well as to predict risks for neurologic injury with certain fractures and fracture/dislocations (Colter, Kulkarni, & Bondurant, 1993). After the initial views are interpreted, one can assess the clinical stability of the spine using the biomechanical criteria of White and Panjabi (1978) (Table 11-1). Before assessing stability, it is important to determine the fracture pattern. The anterior, posterior, and lateral elements can be involved solely or in combination in many cervical spine injuries. White and Punjabi (1978) have defined clinical instability as the loss of the ability of spinal elements to maintain a relationship between the

Table 11-1
Guidelines for Biomechanical Interpretation of Radiographs

Element	Point Value
Anterior elements destroyed or unable to function	2
Posterior elements destroyed or unable to function	2
Relative sagittal plane translation >3.5 mm	2
Relative sagittal plane rotation >11 degrees	2
Positive stretch test	2
Spinal cord damage	2
Nerve-root damage	1
Abnormal disk narrowing	1
Dangerous loading anticipated	1

Total of 5 or more = unstable

SOURCE: White & Panjabi (1978) reprinted by permission.

vertebral segments under physiologic loads. This loss leads to irritation or damage of the spinal cord and nerve roots, and the structural changes resulting from instability may lead immediately or later to deformity or pain. The anatomy of the spine is critical in the maintenance of stability. The annulus fibrosis is the most important anterior structure. Sharpey's fibers form strong attachments to the vertebral bodies. The well-developed posterior longitudinal ligament also provides considerable strength and stability, but the posterior elements, facet joints, and capsules are the most important sources of tensile and rotational stability. The ligamentum flavum also provides stability in the extremes of motion.

CLASSIFICATION OF CLOSED FRACTURES AND DISLOCATIONS OF THE LOWER CERVICAL SPINE

Over the years, many classifications have been proposed for cervical injuries. In 1982, Allen and colleagues presented a universally accepted classification for lower cervical spine fractures and dislocations. They described a study of 165 cases demonstrating the various spectra of injury, and developed a classification based on the mechanism of injury. In their classification, they described injuries resulting from distraction, from flexion, from compression, and from extension and various permutations, including distractive flexion, or distractive extension, compressive flexion, compressive extension, and the various subcategories of each of these moments. In the literature and in the daily management of cervical spine injuries, it is difficult to remember the various stages of Allen's classification. Further delineation of the Ferguson-Allen classification includes five subtypes of compressive flexion injuries, three subtypes of vertical compression injury, and four subtypes of distractive flexion injuries. There is also noted a five-category subclassification of compressive-extension injury, a two-subcategory classification of distractive-extension injuries as well as two subcategories, Stage 1 and Stage 2 of lateral flexion injury.

TREATMENT OF LOWER CERVICAL SPINAL INJURIES

Spinal alignment can be corrected after the patient is medically stabilized. If there is compression or neurologic tissue, vertebral fractures, or dislocations, they must be reduced to minimize ischemia and edema formation around the cord. Reduction can be accomplished with skull traction and this can be a determinant for long-term outcome. Evidence also suggests improved neurologic outcome if methylprednisone is given within 8 hours of the injury in a bolus of 30 mg/k body weight followed by an infusion of 5.4 mg/k body weight for 23 hours (Brachen et al., 1990). When skeletal traction via tongs is required to obtain alignment of the fracture/dislocation, the tongs should be left in place with the patient in bed with the head of the bed elevated 30 degrees to reduce disorientation and to reduce cervical edema and subsequent airway problems. Cervical dislocations are associated with substantial disruption of anterior and posterior ligamentous structures and clinical instability. Patients who are undergoing realignment and traction must be constantly monitored and examined to prevent iatrogenic injury to neural elements resulting from stretching across the injured segments. Unilateral facet dislocation may be difficult to reduce. We perform an open reduction and posterior fusion if closed reduction fails when more than 40 or 50 lb of traction is applied. There are varying reports in the literature, though, in which the use of tong traction in excess of 120 lb has been used to reduce unilateral and bilateral facet dislocations without any complications. After the tongs are placed in a sterile manner, initially 15 to 20 lb of traction is applied. This is usually preceded by the appropriate sedation, and a lateral radiograph is obtained. Weight is then added in 5-lb increments with a lateral radiograph following each change until the reduction is documented radiographically. Our preference is to use Gardner-Wells tongs initially, because they can easily be applied by one person in an emergency setting. We prefer to apply a halo later under elective surgical circumstances with multiple skilled individuals present after the fracture/dislocation has been reduced and a thorough radiographic evaluation is complete. Some surgeons prefer to apply the halo first because they believe it facilitates closed reduction, and provides better quality radiographs and is also MRI-compatible, although Gardner-Wells tongs may also be MRI-compatible. In patients in whom there is no compression of the neural elements and the stability of the spine has not been jeopardized, a course of bracing in a rigid orthosis for 6 to 12 weeks may be appropriate. Follow-up radiographs must be obtained at regular intervals to assess the healing. Isolated fractures of the posterior and lateral elements may be stable injuries and can be treated in a rigid orthosis. If there is an associated dislocation or neurologic deficit, operative stabilization and fusion is indicated and preferred.

INDICATIONS FOR EARLY OPERATIVE THERAPY

The criteria for urgent early operation in patients who have sustained cervical spinal cord injuries are progression of neurologic signs and complete block of subarachnoid space on myelography (Table 11-2). A cervical root may require decompression to allow the patient increased function and independence. Acute anterior spinal cord injury requires operative intervention. Open fractures and penetrating injuries require irrigation and debridement. Acute cervical teardrop fracture/dislocations and facet fracture/dislocations may cause anterior cord compression and instability. Locked unilateral or bilateral facet dislocations may not reduce with traction and require early surgical intervention.

The absolute indication for urgent operation is myelographic evidence of spinal cord compression by hematoma, bone, or disk elements after alignment has been optimized. Our clinical experience over the past nine years at The Johns Hopkins Hospital and The Maryland Spine Center continues to demonstrate the value of early decompression in optimizing neurologic recovery and stabilization.

POSTERIOR WIRING TECHNIQUES

The purpose of this chapter is to describe posterior wiring techniques of the subaxial cervical spine. Aside from wiring techniques, there are other methods of fusing the lower cervical spine, which will be described elsewhere in this

Table 11-2
Indications and Contraindications for the Use of Wiring Techniques of the Lower Cervical Spine

Indications	
Rodgers technique	fractures and fracture dislocations of cervical spine
Sublaminar wiring	fracture and fracture dislocations of cervical spine
Bohlman's triple wire technique	fracture and fracture dislocations of cervical spine
	revision of failed anterior surgery
	cervical tumors
Dewar fusion	fracture and fracture dislocations of cervical spine

Contraindications	
Rodgers technique	compromised posterior elements
	three column instability
	incompetent anterior and middle column
Sublaminar wiring	previous laminectomy
	cervical stenosis
	incompetent anterior and middle columns
Bohlman's triple wire technique	incompetence of posterior elements
	previous laminectomy
Dewar fusion	incompetence of posterior elements
	previous laminectomy
	incompetent anterior and middle columns

textbook. The mainstay of operative treatment of the posterior cervical spine is to obtain rigid fixation and bony fusion. After the patient has been resuscitated, placed in tong traction, and been fully stabilized, operative intervention is carefully planned. All procedures for posterior cervical wiring are performed through a midline posterior approach. The patient is placed under adequate anesthesia, and this may be either general or local while in bed or preferably on a Stryker frame. Usually, for general anesthesia, these patients will require a fiberoptic intubation to allow for as little trauma to the cervical spine as possible. Once the patient is fully anesthetized, on either the Stryker frame or carefully positioned, he or she is placed in the prone position on the operating room table. If no Stryker frame is available, the five-man roll technique should be performed using two attendants on either side of the patient and the primary operating surgeon controlling the head during the turn with the assistance of the anesthetist to maintain both cervical spinal integrity as well as airway patency. Once in the prone position, the patient is fully positioned and all bony prominences are padded and carefully secured to avoid any iatrogenic complications of the surgery. Longitudinal traction of the shoulders is pulled toward the end of the bed and held with adhesive tape. The posterior aspect of the neck is prepped with povidone-iodine. The neck and iliac crest are prepped with antiseptic solution and the field is draped with surgical towels and an antibiotic-impregnated sterile drape. Cervical spinous processes should be palpated in the midline. A posterior midline incision is made and cautery is used freely to minimize blood loss. Other options are the use of a cell saver, but usually this is not required for posterior cervical spine surgery. A midline subperiosteal dissection is performed, and Cobb elevators are used more for retraction, rather than dissection. If there is any question about which spinal level to operate on, intraoperative radiography may be performed. For the reduction of a unilateral or bilateral facet dislocation, a high-speed bur is used to remove a small portion of the superior articular process, which blocks the reduction. It is helpful to use motor or somatosensory evoked potentials throughout the course of the reduction. Once the spine has been adequately reduced and its reduced position has been confirmed by lateral radiography, internal fixation in preparation for fusion is undertaken. There are many techniques of posterior cervical wiring. Among these are the Rodgers wiring technique, Bohlman triple wire technique, Southwick wiring, the Dewar posterior fusion, sublaminar wiring, and for the very rare occasion of unilateral laminar fracture with rotational instability, an oblique facet to spinous process wire can be performed. This chapter will concentrate on describing in detail the Rodgers technique, sublaminar wiring, the Bohlman technique, and the Dewar technique. It will also describe the biomechanics of the above-mentioned processes. Relative advantages and disadvantages of each technique are listed in Table 11-3.

Table 11-3
Advantages and Disadvantages of Wiring Techniques of the Lower Cervical Spine

Advantages

Rodgers technique	minimal risk to neurologic structures
	segmental control
Sublaminar wiring	simple, familiar procedure
	segmental control
Bohlman's triple wire technique	easily performed
	high fusion rate
	minimal risk to neurologic structures
	superior biomechanical strength than other posterior wiring techniques
Dewar fusion	simple technique
	stiffer than Rodgers technique

Disadvantages

Rodgers technique	bone graft not rigidly attached
	poor resistance to extension and rotation
	requires intact posterior elements
Sublaminar wiring	risk of neurologic injury with sublaminar wire pass
	poor resistance to extension
Bohlman's triple wire technique	poor resistance to extension
Dewar fusion	poor resistance to extension

Rodgers Technique

The Rodgers technique for posterior cervical wiring is used for all disrupted fractures and dislocations of the lower cervical spine. It will be described here for historical purposes. It was first described in 1942 by Dr. Rodgers in the *Journal of Bone and Joint Surgery.* This process is begun by placing a transverse hole at the junction of the spinous process and the lamina, usually by using either a high-speed bur or a towel clip or an awl from a Bankart shoulder reconstruction kit. The start hole is made on either side of the laminar base and completed using either the towel clip or tenaculum. Great care must be taken not to place the hole too far anteriorly so that no injury to the spinal cord or dural sac will be created. Once the holes are completed at the bases of the spinous processes at the levels to be used, an 18-gauge wire is passed. The wire is then looped around the superior border of the cephalad spinous process and the ends are passed through the drill holes of that process in opposite directions. In a similar manner, the wires are then passed distally in a caudad direction parallel to the interspace to the next inferior spinous process. The wire ends are then passed in opposite directions through the drill holes in the caudad spinous process. They are then twisted after looping them around the inferior border of the caudad process. Usually, it is customary to leave some slack on both the right and left lateral parallel wires so that tightening loops can be tethered on either side of the spinous process to ensure equal compression across the posterior elements bilaterally. Corticocancellous graft is then placed on either side of the construct. Cancellous graft can then be carefully placed in the decorticated facets or any defects left in the posterior elements. Limitations to this technique can be the fact that the bone graft is not rigidly fixed in place and also you are bound by the strength of the posterior elements themselves.

Sublaminar Wiring

The technique for passing sublaminar wires in the human spine has been described in several papers. Ideally, the fixation attained by passing wires around a lamina on a segment-by-segment basis would be desirable. The potential pitfalls and risk for neurologic injury have been delineated (Coe, Warden, Sutterlin, & McAfee, 1989; Gaines, Munson, Satterlee, Lising, & Betten, 1983). The technique for passing sublaminar wires involves careful subperiosteal dissection of the cervical spine, isolation of the levels to be fused, and dissection of the ligamentum flavum from the underside of the lamina using a 3-0 angled curette to be sure that all soft tissues have been swept free from the underside of the lamina. A 20-gauge stainless steel wire is contoured into a semilunar position after being folded in half (so as to have a blunted tip for a leader) and can be passed underneath the lamina from a cephalad to caudad direction. In this manner, excellent purchase on the lamina above and below the injured level can be performed. This procedure should be performed bilaterally and the wires synchronously tightened to obtain adequate bilateral compression posteriorly. In a similar manner, corticocancellous bone graft from the iliac crest can be packed along the decorticated posterior elements in and around the wires to obtain a bony fusion at this level.

Bohlman's Triple-Wire Technique

In 1985, McAfee, Bohlman, and Wilson described a triple-wire fixation technique for stabilization of acute fractures and dislocations of the cervical spine. This technique can be applied to revision of failed anterior surgery (Weiland & McAfee, 1991) and to tumors or any other pathology requiring posterior cervical stabilization and fusion. Once again, after confirming the level of fusion and obtaining reduction, a 20-gauge wire is placed through a hole at the base of the spinous process and at the junction of the spinous process and lamina. The use of wires through and around the base of the spinous process prevents a cheese-cutter effect on the bone. One midline tethering wire of 20-gauge stainless steel is passed through and around the involved spinous processes. At this point, a 20-gauge wire is then passed through and around the superiormost and inferiormost involved spinous processes. Full thickness corticocancellous bone struts taken from the posterior iliac crest, after having drill holes made in them, are then wired in placed across the site of the injury after decorticating the bone of the posterior elements of the spine. The cancellous surface of the strut is placed against the bony posterior elements in order to allow for maximum fusion potential. The grafts are oriented to maximize bone-to-bone contact and then the wires are tightened, thus compressing the cancellous bone of the graft against the cancellous bone of the lamina. In some written reports, this fusion technique has as high as a 100% fusion rate for injuries to the lower cervical spine and as high as a 98% fusion rate for injuries to the upper cervical spine. In general, it is an easily performed and highly reliable technique for fusion methods in the subaxial spine. Compared to all other posterior cervical wiring techniques biomechanically, this technique proves to be superior. A full description of biomechanics will follow in subsequent sections.

Dewar Fusion

Frederick P. Dewar, of the University of Toronto, described a posterior cervical stabilization and fusion technique that is less well known but has been proven to be biomechanically sound (Bernstein, Simmons, Capicotto, Simmons, & Delahunt, 1992). Steinmann pins are passed percutaneously through corticocancellous strut grafts, which have been contoured to the posterior elements, through the spinous process, and then cut short. Over these Steinmann pins, which have fixed the corticocancellous grafts to the posterior elements, is placed a figure-of-eight 20-gauge stainless steel wire in order to provide even greater compression. Simmons, Burke, Haley, & Medige (1992) describe the biomechanics and the results of testing of this technique in comparison with Rodgers wiring. They found the Dewar technique to be significantly stiffer immediately following fixation than the Rodgers wiring technique in both flexion and in torsion. In general, the technique was described as being easily applicable and extremely effective (Fig. 11-1).

BIOMECHANICS OF POSTERIOR CERVICAL STABILIZATION DEVICES

In our laboratory, both a bovine and cadaveric model was developed for biomechanical evaluation of surgical procedures for stabilizing traumatic cervical injuries, disrupting the anterior and posterior spinal column (Coe et al., 1989; Sutterlin, McAfee, Warden, Rey, & Farey, 1988). As flexion distraction injuries are the most common cervical spinal injuries, bilateral facet fracture/dislocations were created in bovine species at the C4-5 level and in human cadaveric cervical spines at the C5-6 level. Cyclic testing was performed to compare the following stabilization methods: (a) the intact cervical spine; (b) the Rodgers posterior wiring method; (c) the Bohlman triple-wire technique, which used a midline tethering wire and bilateral 22-gauge wires to fix an iliac strut against the posterior aspect of the facet joints; and (d) sublaminar wiring. Other methods tested were anterior Caspar plating and the Magerl posterior hook plate, which will not be considered in this chapter. The results of the biomechanical studies showed that anterior cervical plate instrumentation alone provided inadequate fixation and was the least rigid with axial and flexural loading with a p value less than 0.05. There was no significant difference among

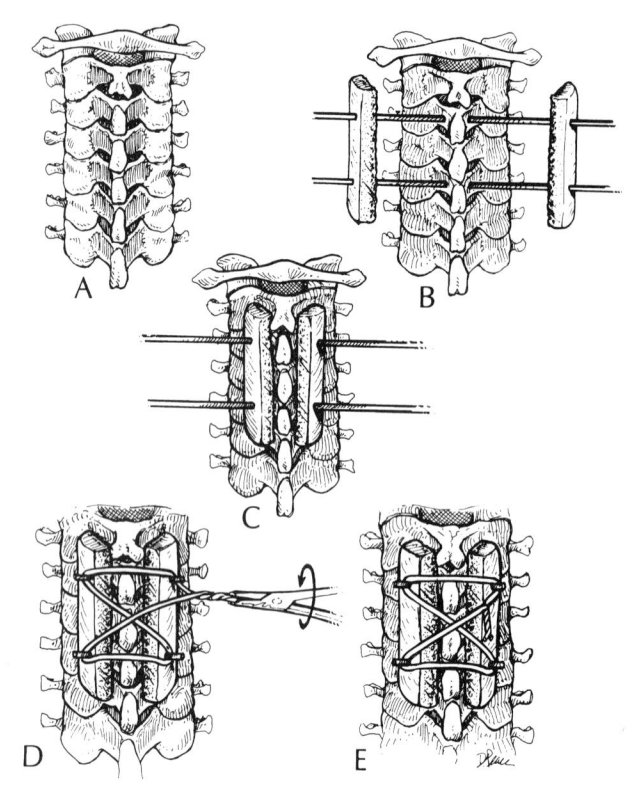

FIG. 11-1. Dewar fusion. (a) Decorticated cervical spine. (b) Percutaneous Steinmann pins passed through corticocancellous strut-spinous process-corticocancellous strut. (c) Pins firmly fixing strut grafts to cervical spine. (d) Cut pins with 20-gauge figure-of-eight wire around pins. (e) Final fusion/stabilization construct by Dewar technique.

the three posterior wiring methods and all generally restored stability to the uninjured intact cervical spine. Cyclical in vitro testing was the most sensitive method in highlighting mechanical differences among instrumentation systems, particularly with online continuous measurement of anterior and posterior strains. Anterior cervical plate stabilization did not appear to confer enough stability in cervical facet injuries to obviate the need for posterior cervical stabilization procedures (Ulrich, Uorsdorer, Claes, & Magerl, 1987). In 1989, Coe and colleagues confirmed previous studies by using the human cadaveric cervical spine and created distractive flexion injuries at the C5-6 level. Flexural torsional testing once again was performed and the stability of eight cervical stabilization constructs were tested cyclically and nondestructively. The Roy-Camille posterior plate fixation technique, the AO posterior hook plate fixation technique, and the anterior Caspar plate fixation techniques were compared with the traditional wiring methods. Biomechanical testing demonstrated no significant differences in any of the posterior stabilization methods tested. There was little biomechanical justification after all the testing was carefully evaluated for the use of potentially dangerous sublaminar wire fixation and posterior plating methods in these biomechanical studies since equally efficacious results were obtained with simple relatively safe posterior wiring techniques. In conclusion, posterior cervical wiring of the subaxial spine has proven over time to be an efficacious and biomechanically sound method for restoring alignment and stability to the unstable or injured cervical spine after adequate resuscitation and support.

REFERENCES

Allen, B.L., Ferguson, R.L., Lehmann, T.R., & O'Brien, R.P. (1982). A mechanistic classification of closed, indirect fractures and dislocations of the lower cervical spine. *Spine, 7,* 1–27.

Bernstein, A.J., Simmons, G.H., Capicotto, W.N., Simmons, E.D., & Delahunt, S.P. (1992). The Dewar posterior cervical fusion: description and comparative results. Orthopaedic Transactions, 16, 151.

Bohlman, H.H. (1979). Acute fractures and dislocation of the cervical spine: An analysis of 300 hospitalized patients and review of literature. *Journal of Bone and Joint Surgery, American Volume, 61,* 1119–1142.

Brachen, M.B., Shepard, M.H., Collins, W.F., et al. (1990). A randomized controlled trial of methylprednisolone or naloxone in the treatment of acute spinal cord injuries. *New England Journal of Medicine, 322,* 1405–1411.

Coe, J.D., Warden, K.E., Sutterlin III, C.E., & McAfee, P.C. (1989). Biomechanical evaluation of cervical spinal stabilization methods in human cadaveric model. *Spine, 14,* 1122–1131.

Colter, H.B., Kulkarni, M.V., & Bondurant F.J. (1993). MRI of acute cord trauma: A preliminary report. *Journal of Orthopaedic Trauma, 2,* 1–4.

Gaines, R.W., Munson, G., Satterlee, C., Lising, A., & Betten, R. (1983). Harrington rods supplemented with sublaminar wires for thoracolumbar fracture dislocation: Experimental and clinical investigation. *Orthopaedic Transactions, 7,* 15.

Hartwell, J.B. (1917). Analysis of 133 fractures of the spine treated at Massachusetts General Hospital. *Boston Medical and Surgical Journal, 177,* 31–41.

McAfee, P.C., Bohlman, H.H., & Wilson, W.L. (1985). Triple wire fixation technique for stabilization of acute fracture, dislocations of the cervical spine: A biomechanical analysis. *Orthopaedic Transactions, 9,* 142.

Rodgers, W.A. (1942). Treatment of fractures and dislocations of the cervical spine. *Journal of Bone and Joint Surgery, American Volume, 24,* 245–258.

Simmons, E.D., Burke, T.G., Haley, T., & Medige, J. (1992). Biomechanical comparison of the Dewar and Rodgers cervical spine fixation techniques. Presented at the SSAF Meeting, December 1992, New York.

Sutterlin C.E., III, McAfee, P.C., Warden, K.E., Rey, R.N., & Farey, I.D. (1988). A biomechanical evaluation of cervical stabilization methods in a bovine model—Static and cyclic loading. *Spine, 13,* 795–802.

Ulrich, C., Uorsdorer, O., Claes, L., & Magerl, D. (1987). Comparative study of the stability of anterior and posterior cervical spine fixation procedures. *Archives of Orthopaedic and Trauma Surgery, 106,* 226–231.

Vaccaro, A.R., An, H.S., Lin, S.S., et al. (1992). Non-contiguous injuries of the spine. *Journal of Spinal Disorders, 5,* 320–329.

Weiland, D.J., & McAfee, P.C. (1991). Posterior cervical fusion with triple-wire strut graft technique: One hundred consecutive patients. *Journal of Spinal Disorders, 4,* 15–21.

White, A.A., & Panjabi, M.M. (1978). Clinical biomechanics of the spine. Philadelphia: J.B. Lippincott, p. 223.

CHAPTER 12

Application of the Codman Sof'wire System for Stabilization of the Lower Cervical Spine

Michael MacMillan

HIGHLIGHTS

Wiring of the posterior cervical spine is the oldest documented method of spinal stabilization and remains the most widely applied cervical fixation technique today. It was first advocated by Hadra in 1891, but its specific application to cervical spine fractures was described by Rogers in 1942. From a purely biomechanical standpoint, however, wires have several inherent limitations. For example, Oh, Sander, and Treharan demonstrated in 1985 that even an extremely small notch (1%) in a wire can reduce its fatigue strength by 63%. They also showed that wire breakage usually occurred within 2 mm from where the wire was twisted. In order to maintain the technical versatility of cervical wiring, but improve the biomechanical performance, cables have been developed for use in the cervical spine.

The Codman Corporation (Randolph, MA) has introduced new multistranded cable available for use in the cervical spine. The cable consists of approximately 103 fine strands intertwined to a diameter of 0.034 in. (20-gauge wire is 0.032 in.). The end of the cable becomes confluent and forms a malleable wire leader on one end and a burnished tip on the other. The cable is manufactured out of both titanium and stainless steel. The cable is attached together by means of a cinch—a small cylinder through which both cable ends are passed. The cinch is then compressed around the cables, thus, linking them together (Fig. 12-1).

The central instrument for placement of these cables is the tensioner. This is a high-density plastic, disposable instrument. It has a long forked extension and the cinch is clipped between the two tines of the fork (Fig. 12-2). The cable ends are passed through the cinch in opposite directions. In order to develop tension in the cable, the ends are then passed up the sides of the fork. The handle of the tensioner has two capabilities. First, it has a tunnel through the stem of the handle, which has a plastic thumb screw in it. Secondly, the handle can be turned. Thus, the cable going up the side of the tensioner can be secured within the tunnel and the handle turned. As this is turned, the cable is pulled up and wrapped around the handle and tension is gradually applied. To obtain maximal tension, a metal extension can be placed on the tensioner handle to increase the torque that can be generated.

Once the construct is appropriately tightened, the ratcheting mechanism in the handle will maintain the tension. The cinch around the cables can now be secured. The cinch pliers are placed around the cinch and compressed until the handles touch. Finally, the cable is cut—first, where it runs up the side of the tensioner in order to release and remove it; then down near the cinch.

This system has FDA 510(k) approval for both distribution and sale. This approval is for small bone fixation. In the cervical spine, Sof'wire is approved for interspinous, interfacet, and sublaminar fixation. Using these approved applications, we will discuss the indications for primary use of Sof'wire in the lower cervical spine.

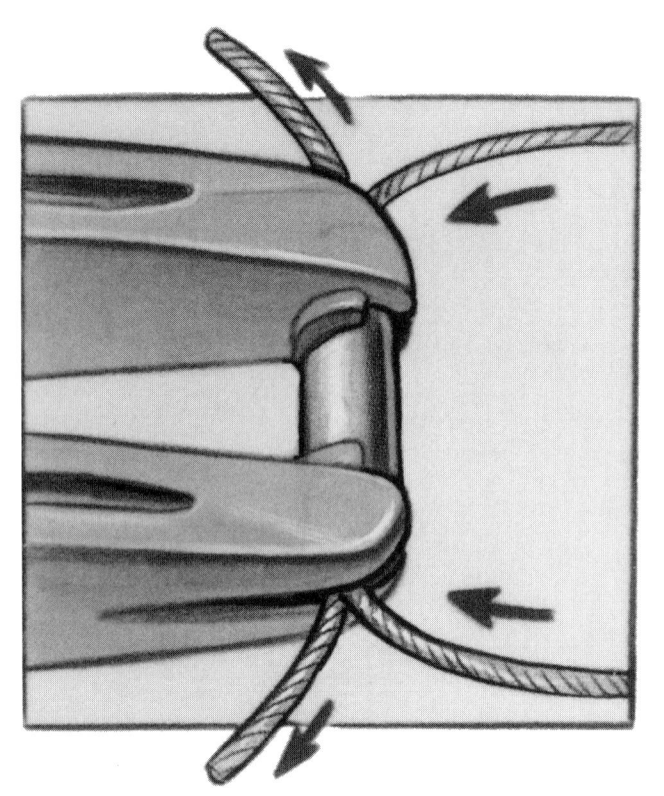

FIG. 12-1. The cinch is held in the tensioner and the cable ends are passed through in opposite directions.

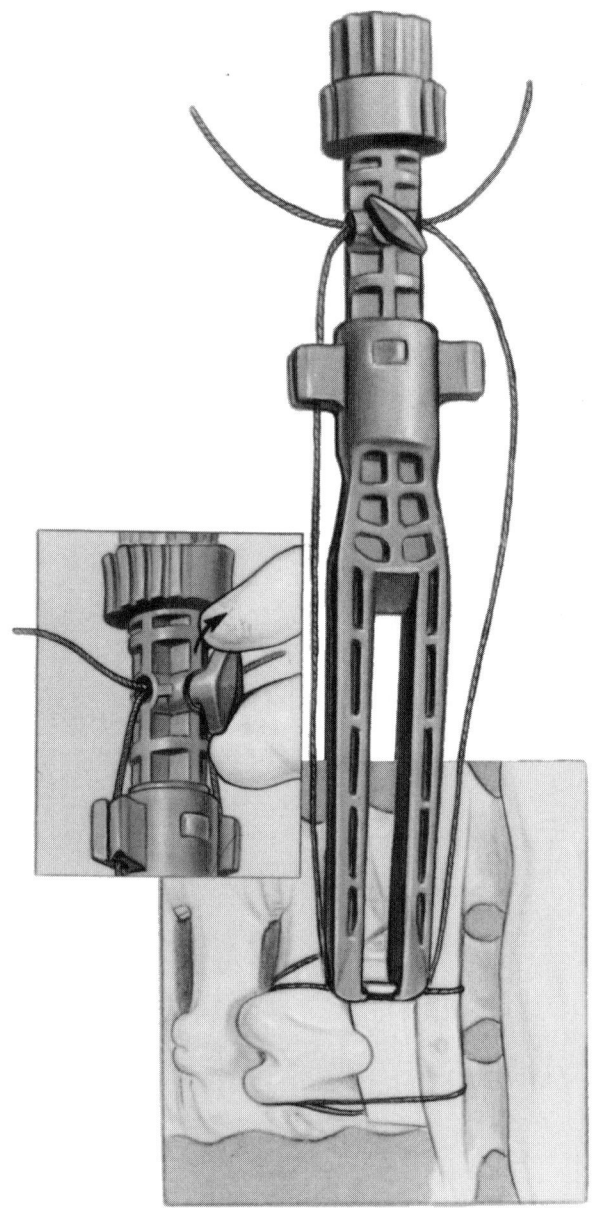

FIG. 12-2. The tensioner.

INDICATIONS

Whether the site of application is interspinous, interfacet or sublaminar, the cable will function as a tension band (Table 12-1).

Interspinous fixation is indicated when there is pure flexion instability in sagittal plane. (Table 12-2) The midline position of the cable does not adequately control rotation. There are two indications for this technique. The first is a flexion/distraction injury, which is in fact, a pure flexion instability pattern. This injury implies disruption of the supraspinous, interspinous, and facet capsular ligaments. A single midline tension band is usually sufficient for this problem because the facet joints are typically not fractured (Fig. 12-3). When the facets are reduced, they prevent rotational displacement.

Interspinous fixation can also be used for simple unilateral facet dislocations. In this rotational injury, the inferior facet of the suprajacent vertebra is dislocated over the superior facet of the subjacent vertebra. After reduction, the intact facet complex can prevent rotational displacement. Therefore, midline interspinous fixation is suitable for this injury.

Another possible application of posterior tension band fixation is facet fixation. In this use the cable runs from the spinous process out laterally to the inferior facet of the suprajacent vertebra (Fig. 12-4). The most common indication for this is the unilateral facet dislocation with fracture of the superior facet. The incompetent facet complex allows rotational redisplacement. Therefore, fixation from the midline out laterally to the facet prevents this.

The final approved fixation site of the Sof'wire cable is in the sublaminar position. The major advantage of this fixation style is its strength. The sublaminar position has the highest pullout strength (Brooks & Jenkins, 1978). However, sublaminar placement also has had the highest possibility of neurologic injury. In the vast majority of cervical spine injuries associated with spinal cord trauma, sublaminar placement should not be used because of possible spinal cord swelling. However, in cervical spine fractures without neurologic deficit, or in cervical reconstruction, this fixation site can be very helpful. One potential use is a flexion-distraction injury in a patient with osteoporosis. Also, this tension band can be used when a higher assuredness of fix-

CHAPTER 12 / APPLICATION OF THE CODMAN SOF'WIRE SYSTEM FOR STABILIZATION OF THE LOWER CERVICAL SPINE

Table 12-1
Indications and Contraindications for Primary Fixation Techniques

Interspinous	
Indications	Contraindications
Flexion/distraction injuries	Three-column instability
Facet dislocation without fracture	Posterior element fractures
Simple degenerative instability	Previous laminectomy
	Osteoporosis

Facet	
Indications	Contraindications
Facet dislocations without fracture	Facet fractures
Fractured spinous processes	Anterior column or three-column instability

Sublaminar	
Indications	Contraindications
Postlaminectomy instability	Swollen spinal cord
Eliminate external immobilization	Stenosis
Poor bone quality	Previous laminectomy

Multisegmental	
Indications	Contraindications
Degenerative instability	
Fractures in the degenerated spine	
Rheumatoid instability	

Table 12-2
Advantages and Disadvantages for Interspinous Fixation

Advantages	Disadvantages
Very malleable	Expensive
Allows simultaneous tightening of multiple levels	Using multiple tensioners simultaneously can be clumsy
Greater strength and fatigue life than 18- or 20-gauge wire	Usually not adequate for stabilization of three-column instability

ation is required. The increased strength comes from the ability to use two cables and the placement around fully cortical surfaces. This application may be helpful in patients who cannot tolerate external immobilization.

In addition to the primary use of Sof'wire cable, this system can also be used as supplemental fixation in conjunction with other implants. One important supplemental use of Sof'wire cable is in cervical burst fractures. In this situation, anterior cervical plating is routinely used after decompression. However, a large number of cervical burst fractures have associated posterior ligamentous disruption. Sutterlin, McAfee, Warden, Rey, & Farey (1988) have shown that anterior fixation alone is not sufficient to prevent flexion resistance. Therefore, posterior disruption associated with a cervical burst fracture is an indication for a supplement posterior tension band (Fig. 12-5).

Supplemental tension bands may sometimes be indicated in conjunction with multiple-level corpectomies. When three or more cervical vertebral bodies are removed, very high forces are generated on the anterior fixation construct. In noncompliant patients or those with poor bone quality, a posterior tension band can enhance the stability of the construct.

Finally, supplemental tension bands should also be considered in conjunction with lateral mass plates. Plates on the lateral mass are more inherently rigid than other forms of cervical fixation. However, in the sagittal plane, they lie close to the posterior wall of the vertebral body. This position gives them little mechanical advantage in preventing

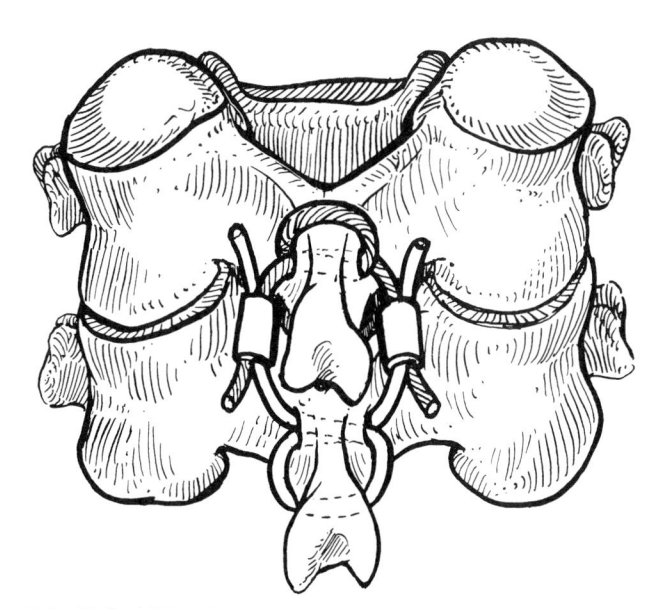

FIG. 12-3. Midline interspinous placement of Sof'wire cable. Note that the cable is passed twice through each spinous process. Using two cables permits symmetrical tightening.

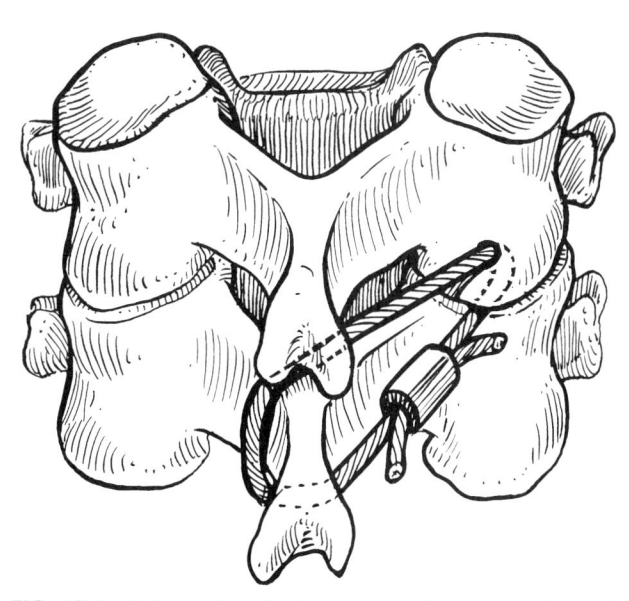

FIG. 12-4. Unilateral facet fixation is achieved by passing the cable through the inferior facet of the suprajacent vertebra.

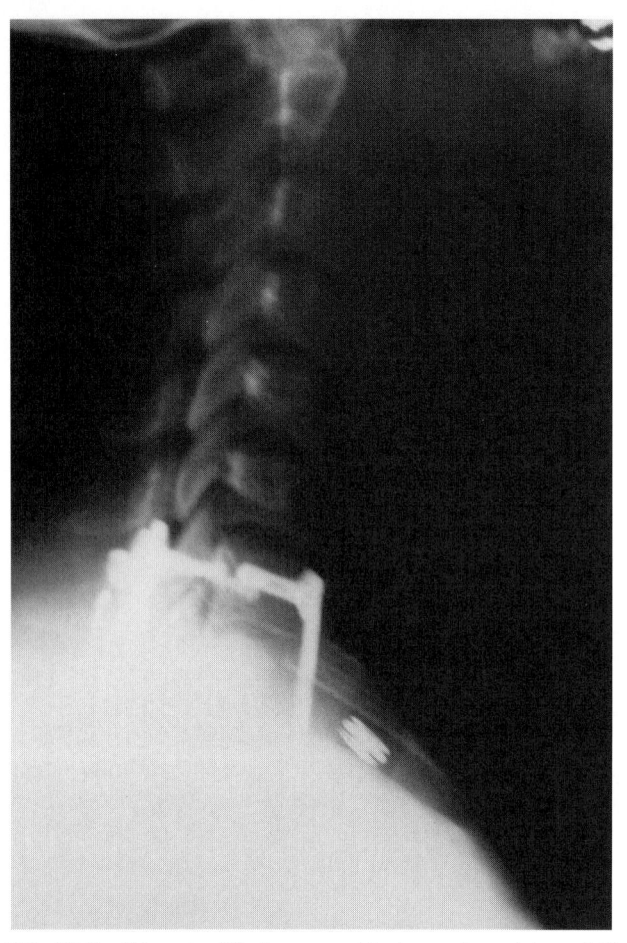

FIG. 12-5. Although difficult to see, this three-column injury of T1 used a Sof'wire cable posteriorly to supplement other fixation methods.

flexion. A supplemental tension band spanning the length of the construct can enhance the flexion stability (Fig. 12-6).

A final application of Sof'wire cable is its use in combination with other implants. The most common of this technique is sublaminar cables attached to rods. This is one of the most versatile implant combinations in the spine. Also called Luque rods or L-rods, this technique can be applied to the cervical, thoracic, or lumbar spine. However, because the cables are not rigidly attached to the rod, there is little resistance to subsidence under axial loading (Fig. 12-7).

Rigidity in all planes can be achieved by combining cables with other instrumentation systems that use hooks and rods. Although additional cable may be attached anywhere along a rod system, we have found sublaminar cables to be most helpful for thoracic rods that extend across the cervicothoracic junction. By fixing C7 or C6 to a thoracic construct with sublaminar cable, not only is secure fixation obtained, but also the bulkiness of hook attachment can be avoided (Fig. 12-8).

In some special situations, we have found that using sublaminar cable in conjunction with multiholed plates to be helpful. When used in conjunction with plates, the cable is placed sublaminarly, then each end is placed through an adjacent hole in the plate. This technique allows segmental fixation with stability against axial loading (Fig. 12-9).

In deciding which implant is best for the needs of your patient, several factors need to be considered. These include biomechanical performance, local anatomy, pathology of injury, technical difficulty, canal intrusion, and cost.

In deciding between the use of surgical wire or Sof'wire cable, it is clear that wire is less expensive. However, if the implant is to be placed in the sublaminar position, the property of soft deflection makes Sof'wire the superior selection. Biomechanically, cable has significantly higher ultimate strength and fatigue life than either 20- or 18-gauge wire (Fig. 12-10). Also, Sof'wire cable has significantly less elongation prior to failure. Since anatomic applications are similar for both cables and wires, the only other significant difference is the technical ease of application. Proper wire tightening requires that the two free ends approach each other at a 45-degree angle and equal tension be applied while they are rotated around one another. Failure to accomplish this can result in either "wrapping" of the wire (one end wraps around the other) or asymmetric stress creating microscopic fatigue cracks in the first twist. Often in the deep recess of a posterior cervical spine wound, twisting the wire can be difficult. However, wire may be useful in patients with more stable pathology and whose surgeons are experienced with proper wire handling techniques.

In choosing cabling techniques over lateral mass fixation, the local anatomy and biomechanical properties of the implant become more important. One relative indication for lateral mass fixation is absence of the posterior elements. In the presence of posterior elements, the nature of instability problems becomes a major factor. Lateral mass plates have two biomechanical advantages over tension band fixation. The first is that the plating construct imparts rigidity in all planes and is superior to posterior tension bands (Gill, Paschal, Corin, Ashman, & Bucholz, 1988). Therefore, plates are superior for three-column fractures or anterior-posterior degenerative instability. Also, since lateral mass plates are located at a distance from the central axis, they have biomechanical superiority in controlling rotation as well. Rotational control is significant when there is failure of the bony surfaces of the facet complexes. Cusick, Yoganandan, Pintar, Myklebust, and Jussain (1988) noted that loss of facet joint opposition causes significant loss of strength as compared with the intact spine. Therefore, lateral mass plates have two possible advantages over Sof'wire fixation and other posterior tension band techniques. The first is that in the presence of three-column disease, the enhanced rigidity of lateral mass plates makes them the preferred construct. A relative indication is in the presence of facet fracture. Wiring or cabling of a facet to the inferior spinous process can restore rotational stability (Cusick et al., 1988). However, if the facet cannot be attached to midline then lateral mass plates should be used to restore stability.

Sof'wire also has similar biomechanical properties to interlaminar clamps. Gill et al. (1988) found interlaminar

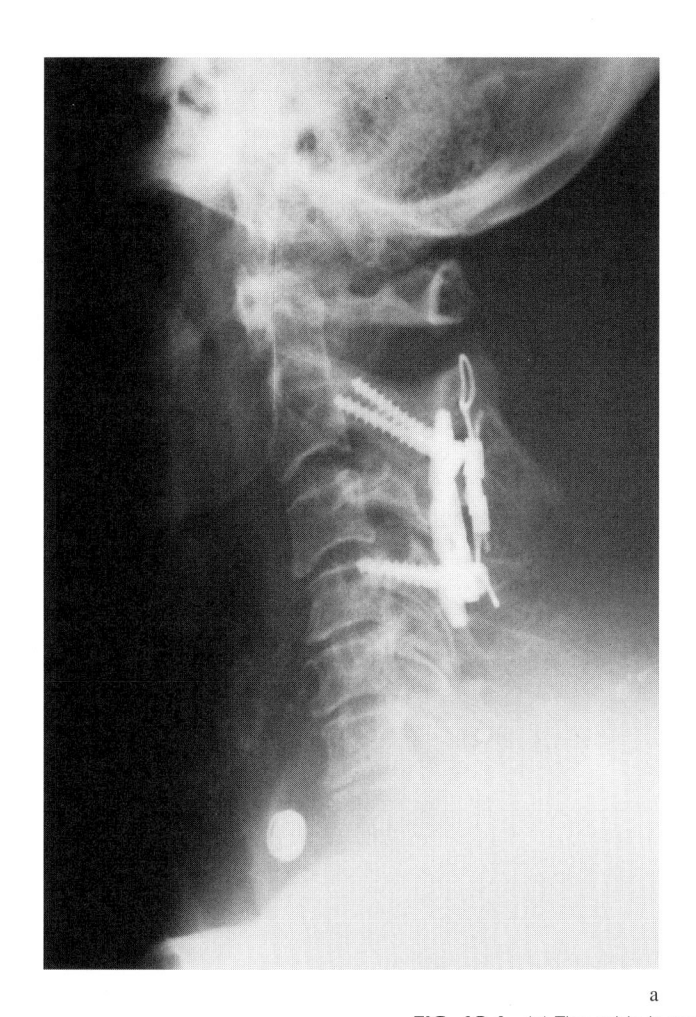

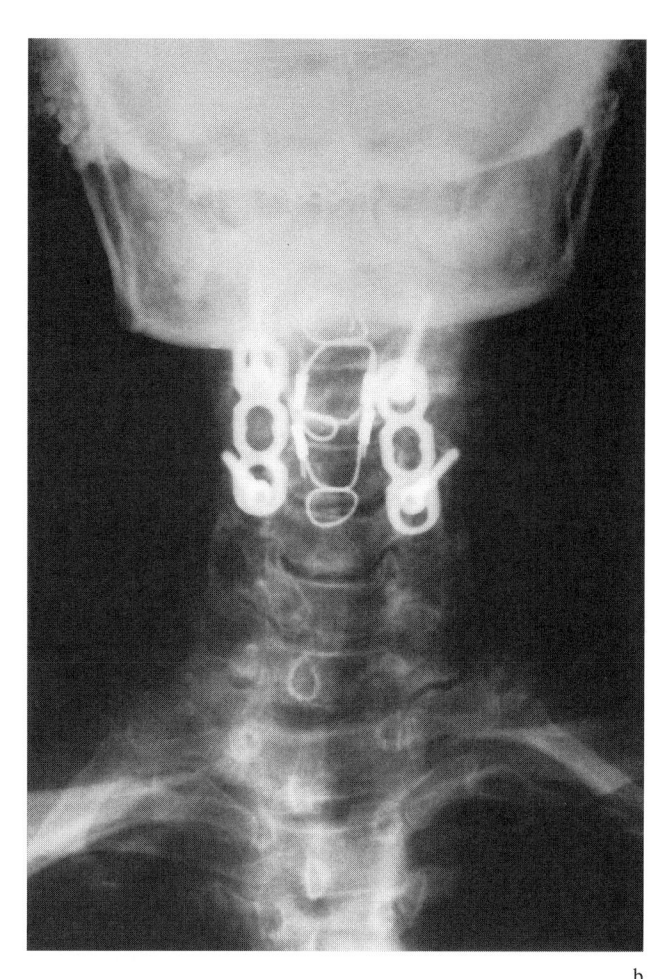

FIG. 12-6. (a) The cable is seen on this lateral view supplementing lateral mass plates. The patient suffered a C3-4 flexion injury. (b) The anteroposterior view demonstrates how three cables can be used to wire three successive spinous processes.

FIG. 12-7. Cables used on smooth rods offer little resistance by themselves to axial loads.

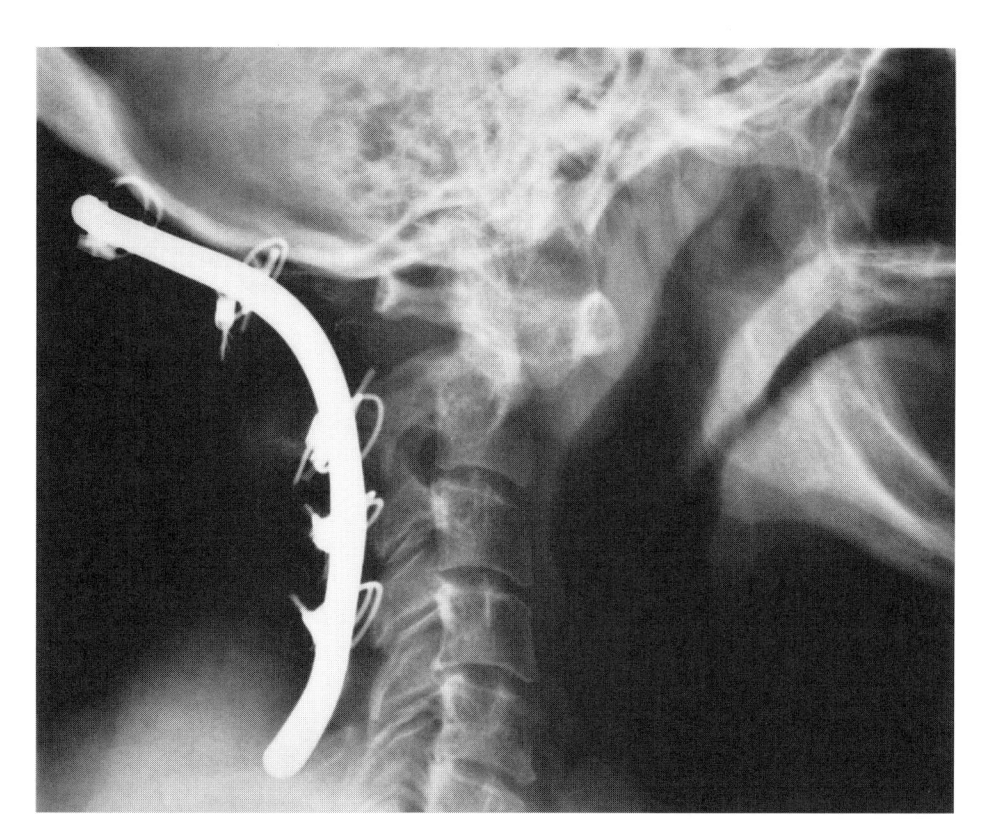

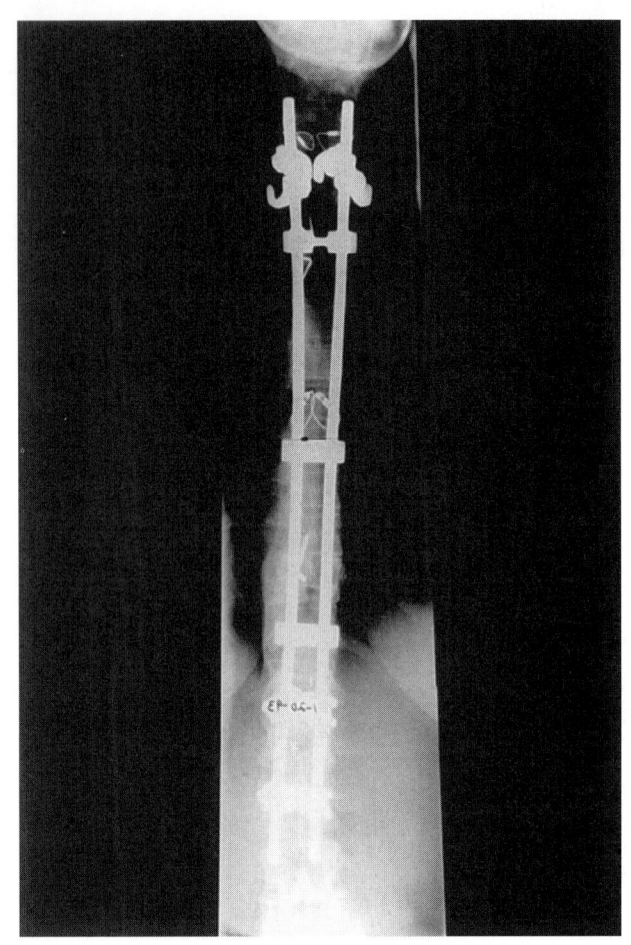

FIG. 12-8. This anteroposterior view shows cables being used to gain additional purchase at the cervicothoracic junction.

clamps to have no increased fixation strength over interspinous wiring techniques. Therefore, in comparing clamps to cables, the technical ease of application should be addressed. The longitudinally oriented screw of the clamp can be difficult to place and requires multiple turns to tighten fully. Also, clamp failure from screw loosening has been reported (Holness, Huestis, Howes, & Langille, 1984). One of the main considerations of choosing interlaminar clamps over interspinous fixation is the issue of canal intrusion. Clamps must extend into the spinal canal to some extent. In the presence of neurologic injury, avoidance of cord manipulation is necessary and extracanal fixation should be employed.

Finally, Sof'wire should be compared with other cables available for spinal fixation. Once again, there is little difference in the ability of these implants to establish an effective posterior tension band and provide stability to the injured spine. In lower cervical spine injuries, the material difference of these implants becomes important. The primary difference between Sof'wire and other cables is pliability. Low resistance to bending has two advantages. The first is that Sof'wire is easier to manipulate in the relatively small confines of the cervical wound. However, the primary advantage of decreased stiffness is in the sublaminar passage, since Sof'wire is 60 times more flexible than 20-gauge wires

(Report on Biomechanics Performance of Sof'wire, February 1993) during passage. In our experience, Sof'wire can be safely advanced on the surface of the dura underneath the lamina with no tendency toward cord impingement. Larger, stiffer cables have more of a tendency to bow downward toward the dura during passing.

Another biomechanical difference is the method of securing the cables. Previously, we have shown that when wires are fatigued, they tend to fracture near the first bend in the twist (Oh et al., 1985). The Sof'wire cables are "cinched" together in a parallel fashion without a terminal 90-degree bend. The Songer (Danek Corporation) cable, however, has a terminal crimp, which requires that the cable makes a 90-degree bend. This bend can predispose to fatigue failure (Fig. 12-11).

TECHNIQUE

We have just discussed the relative advantages of Sof'wire cable in the lower cervical spine. We will now discuss the technique of Sof'wire application.

There are three sites where Sof'wire can be applied in the lower cervical spine: interspinous, facet, and sublaminar.

Interspinous fixation can be done with either a single cable or with double cables. With a single cable, a simple loop is created between two adjacent spinous processes. This fixation method has some potential disadvantages. The major problem is the minimal bone available for fixation. A single pass through a spinous process means that the cable only has a half-width of the spinous process preventing pullout. In addition, a simple loop can allow micromovement of the cable back and forth through the hole in the interspinous process. For these reasons, we recommend a "double pass/double cable" method (see Fig. 12-3). This technique enhances the cable's bone fixation.

As stated earlier, a cable extending from a spinous process out laterally to facet joint is effective in controlling rotational instability. The inferior facet of the suprajacent vertebra must be intact in order to place a facet wire. A hole for passage of the cable is drilled through the dorsal surface of the inferior facet into the facet joint. The cable is placed through the hole then retrieved from the facet joint. Since facet fixation usually accompanies interspinous fixation, the cable attached to the facet may not be able to be passed through a spinous process. In this case, we loop the end of the cable under the spinous process (see Fig. 12-4).

The final position for cable placement is sublaminar. Because of the many reported problems with sublaminar wire passage, there is an understandable hesitance to perform this technique in the cervical spine (Nicastro, 1986). The existence of Sof'wire as a highly pliable cable, however, now allows two different methods of cable passage to be performed.

The first method is the standard wire passing method. This is possible with Sof'wire cable because there is a wire

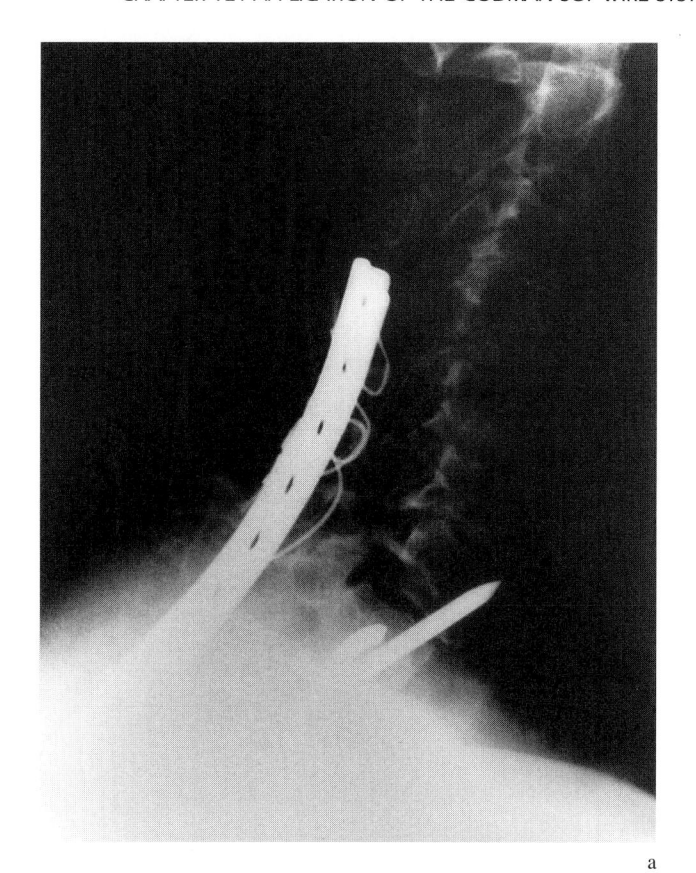

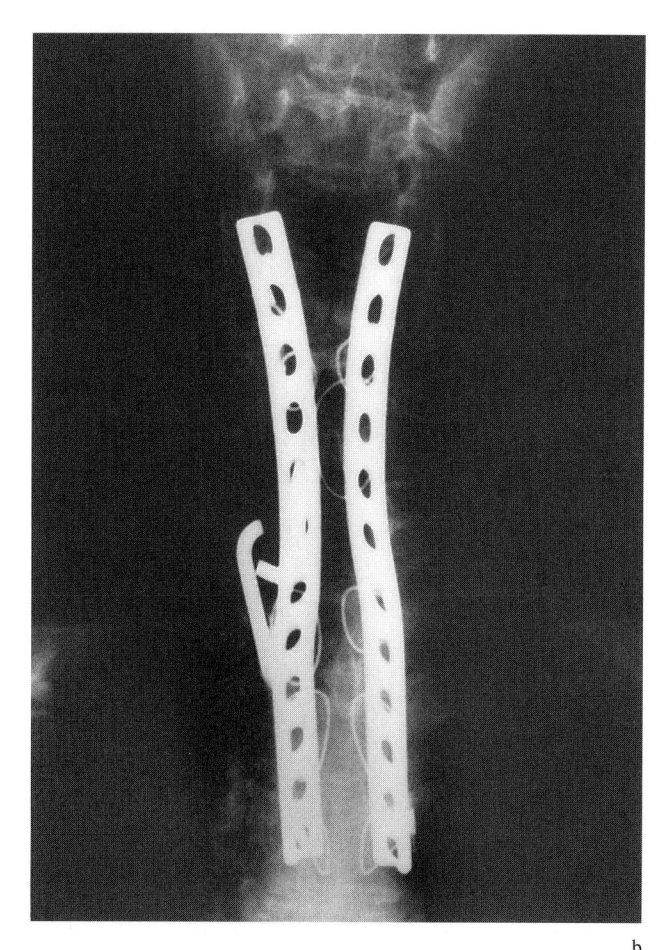

FIG. 12-9. (a) This lateral view shows Sof'wire cables placed through dynamic compression plates. This was used to reconstruct a T1 metastatic melanoma. (b) Anteroposterior view of cables attaching plates to cervicothoracic junction.

leader on one end that can be bent to the appropriate shape. In nonneurologically involved spines and adequate canal diameters, standard wire leader passage can carefully be performed in the cervical spine. However, in most circumstances, we try to utilize the pliability characteristics of Sof'wire cable to improve the safety of sublaminar passage. The technique we prefer is the same used for the placement of epidural catheters. This "catheter method" requires a small laminotomy in the interspaces above and below the lamina. One end of the Sof'wire is a simple burnished tip. This tip is simply advanced cephalad under the lamina until it appears in the interspace above. Because the cable is very supple, it can be retrieved with simple forceps. Because of high conformation of the cable, simple tension at either end of the cable will cause it to pull up against the lamina, again preventing any canal stenosis.

FIG. 12-10. Ultimate strength of Sof'wire as compared with monofilament wire.

Wire/Cable Tensile Strength (Kg.)

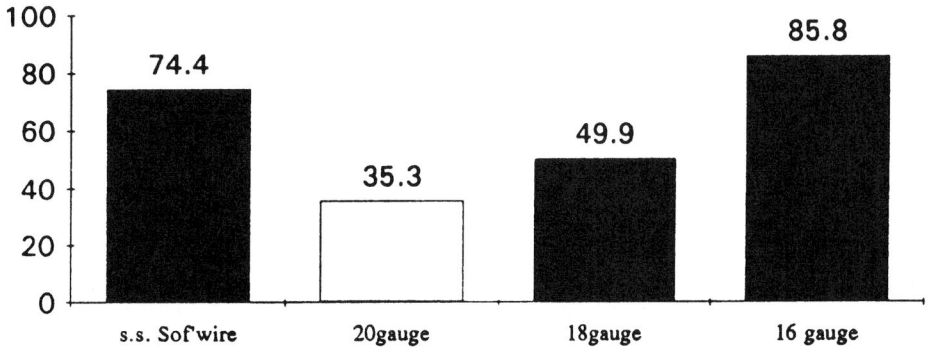

s.s. Sof'wire	20 gauge	18 gauge	16 gauge
74.4	35.3	49.9	85.8

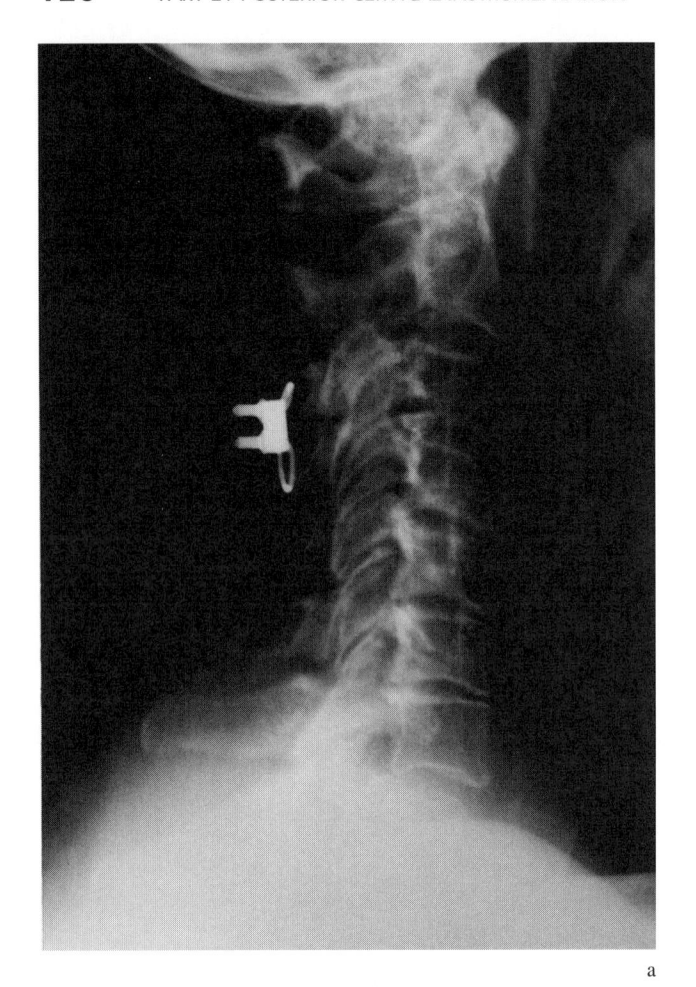

There is one special method that allows more than two spinous processes to be secured together. This is done by first performing the "double wire/double pass" technique over one interspace, but not cutting the loose cable ends. A third cable is then doubly passed through the spinous process inferior with these cable ends directed superiorly. Then the loose cable ends from the interspace above are placed in the same cinch as the cables from the additional spinous process below. By applying tension to the inferior and superior cables together, the additional segment becomes incorporated into the construct (Fig. 12-12). This can be repeated simply by leaving the loose cable ends uncut.

Therefore, although many factors enter into the decision as to which implant to use in the lower cervical spine, the existence of a soft, pliable cable allows many more alternatives for the surgeon to choose from. In addition, the cable can function in concert with other fixation methods to solve difficult problems.

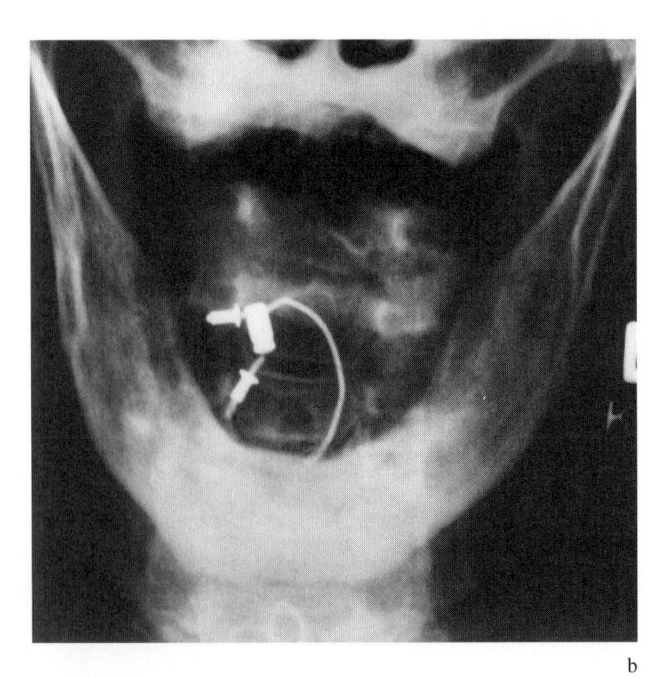

FIG. 12-11. (a) Cable turning at 90 degrees prior to crimping. (b) Anteroposterior view showing cable failure at 90-degree bend.

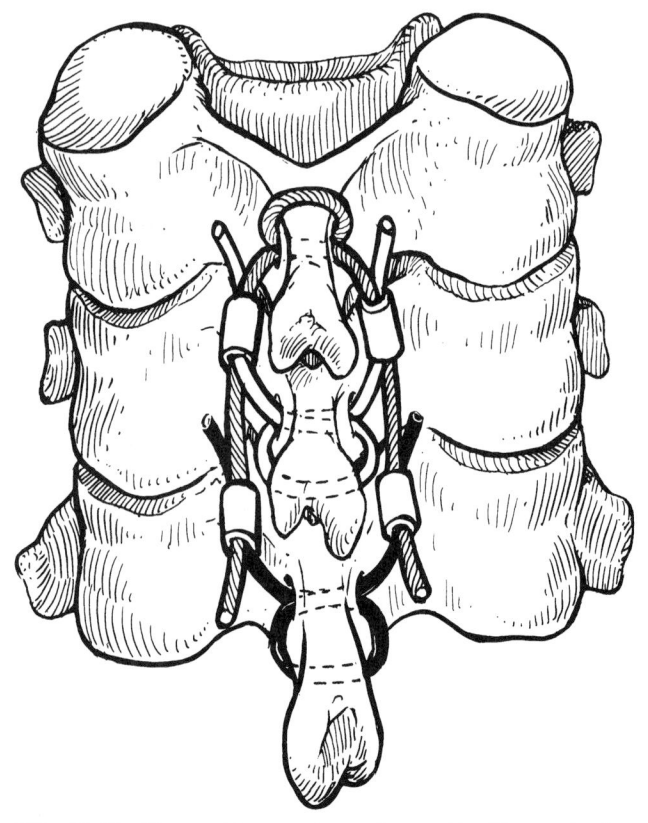

FIG. 12-12. Three cables are shown here with different shading marks. Note how successive levels can be included in a fixation construct.

REFERENCES

Brooks, A.L., & Jenkins, E.B. (1978). Atlanto-axial arthrodesis by the wedge compression method. *Journal of Bone and Joint Surgery, American Volume, 60,* 279–284.

Cusick, J.F., Yoganandan, N., Pintar, F., Myklebust, J., & Jussain, H. (1988). Biomechanics of cervical spine facetectomy and fixation techniques. *Spine, 13,* 809–812.

Gill, K., Paschal, S., Corin, J., Ashman, R., & Bucholz, R.W. (1988). Posterior plating of the cervical spine: a biomechanical comparison of different posterior fusion techniques. *Spine, 13,* 813–816.

Hadra, B.E. (1891). Wiring of the vertebra as a means of immobilization in fracture and Pott's disease. New York and Philadelphia: *The Times and Register, 22* (21), 423.

Holness, R.O., Huestis, W.S., Howes, W.J., & Langille, R.A. (1984). Posterior stabilization with an interlaminar clamp in cervical injuries: technical notes and review of the long term experience with the method. *Neurosurgery, 14,* 318–322.

Nicastro, J.F., et al. (1986). Intraspinal pathways taken by sublaminar wires during removal: An experimental study. *Journal of Bone and Joint Surgery, American Volume, 68,* 1206–1209

Oh, I., Sander, T.W., & Treharen R.W. (1985). The fatigue resistance of orthopaedic wire. *Clinical Orthopaedics and Related Research,* 192, 228–235.

Report on Biomechanics Performance of Sof'wire Cable. (February 1993). Randolph, MA: Codman.

Rogers, W.A. (1942). Treatment of fracture-dislocation of the cervical spine. *Journal of Bone and Joint Surgery, American Volume, 24,* 245.

Sutterlin, C.E., McAfee, P.C., Warden, K.E., Rey, R.M., & Farey, J.D. (1988). A biomechanical evaluation of cervical spinal stabilization methods in a bovine model; static and cyclical loading. *Spine, 13*(7), 795–802.

CHAPTER 13

Application of the Halifax Clamp for Pathology of the Lower Cervical Spine

Michael G. O'Sullivan
Patrick Statham
Thomas Russell

HIGHLIGHTS

In 1975 Tucker reported the use of interlaminar clamps in conjunction with facet joint fusion to provide internal fixation of the unstable cervical spine below C1-2. The clamps, contoured to hook around adjacent laminae were placed separately and linked with a screw, avoiding the need for sublaminar wiring and its potential complications (Geremia, Kim, Cerullo, et al., 1985) (Fig. 13-1). A further report by Holness, Huestis, Howes, et al. (1984) from Halifax, Nova Scotia, confirmed its usefulness, and since then the term *Halifax clamp* has been used. Other authors have reported satisfactory results with this technique in the lower cervical spine (Aldrich, Crow, Weber, et al., 1991; Aldrich, Weber, & Crow, 1993; Statham, O'Sullivan, & Russell, 1993). A titanium alloy clamp offers the advantage of magnetic resonance imaging (MRI) compatibility (Aldrich et al., 1991) (Table 13-1). Cybulski, Stone, Crowell, (1988) and colleagues were the first to report its use for atlantoaxial arthrodesis but later reports questioned its reliability at this level (Statham et al., 1993).

INSTRUMENTATION

The Halifax Interlaminar Clamp System (AME, Richardson, TX) consists of clamps, screws, clamp holding forceps, a right-angled wrench, and a fine wrench. A similar kit is available from Codman & Shurtleff, Randolph, MA.

Clamps

Anatomical differences between the atlantoaxial articulation and subaxial articulations necessitate different-shaped clamps for use at C1-2 and in the lower cervical spine (Fig. 13-2). Color-coded clamps for use at C1-2 and at C2-7 simplify selection. The clamps must be carefully selected to fit the appropriate laminae. They vary in length from 7 to 13 mm, and each pair of clamps contains one unthreaded and one threaded clamp into which the screw is threaded. A modification incorporating four and one half turns in the boss of the threaded clamp prevents screw loosening.

Screws

Screws are of uniform diameter and vary in length from 10 to 30 mm. Screw heads are hexagonal, which necessitates special wrenches for tightening. Three additional instruments are also necessary: placement forceps for handling and positioning the clamps, a 90-degree locking adjustment wrench for tightening the screws, and a fine adjustment wrench for final tightening of the screws (Fig. 13-3).

BIOMECHANICS

Grob, Crisco, Panjabi (1992) and colleagues compared the biomechanical properties of Halifax clamps, Gallie fusion, Brooks fusion, and transarticular screw fixation for atlantoaxial arthrodesis in human cadaveric specimens and found no significant difference between the Halifax clamps and the other systems. To our knowledge similar testing has not been performed in the lower cervical spine.

INDICATIONS

Halifax clamps are indicated when posterior column instability is present in one motion segment and the posterior elements are intact (Table 13-2). It is usually necessary to perform an associated anterior fusion in cases of three-column instability (Cybulski, Douglas, Meyer, et al., 1992). Pre-

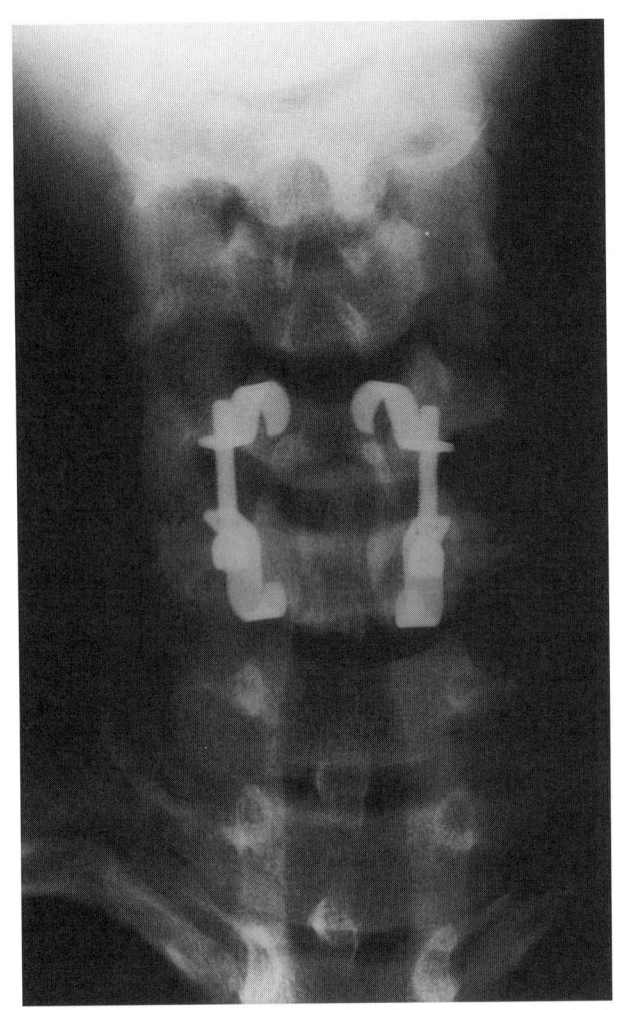

FIG. 13-1. Anteroposterior (AP) radiograph of Halifax clamps in situ in the lower cervical spine. Note bilateral clamps stabilizing one motion segment.

Table 13-1
Advantages and Disadvantages of the Halifax Clamp

Advantages	Disadvantages
Simple	Stabilizes only one motion segment
Avoids sublaminar wires	Requires intact posterior elements
MRI-compatible	Screw loosening
	Clamp disengagement

operative evaluation with flexion/extension radiographs, computed tomographic (CT) scanning, and MRI is necessary. Particular attention is paid to the posterior elements to ensure their continuity.

SURGICAL TECHNIQUE

General anesthesia with due care during intubation is used in all cases. An appropriate prophylactic antibiotic is administered at induction of anesthesia. We routinely record somatosensory evoked potentials during positioning and surgery which is performed with the patient in the prone position.

Normal spinal alignment must be attained before proceeding with internal fixation. This may be achieved by cervical traction or open reduction and must be confirmed by cross-table radiography or perioperative screening prior to internal fixation. Decompression of nerve roots must also be performed prior to internal fixation.

When necessary we perform anterior stabilization before proceeding to posterior stabilization. If open reduction is required the reverse applies.

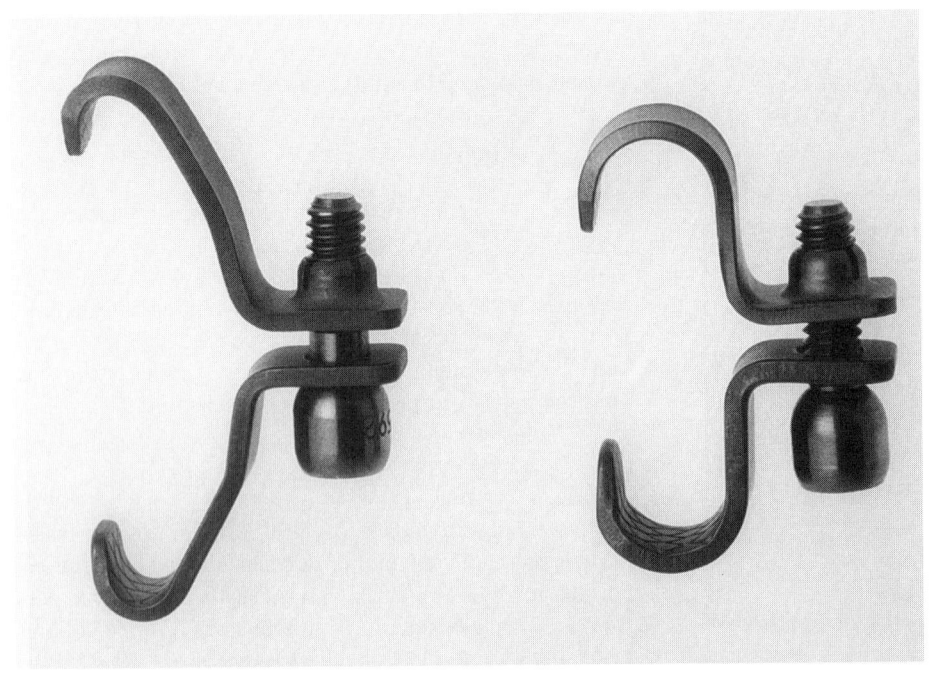

FIG. 13-2. Photograph demonstrating the different shape of the C1-2 Halifax clamp (right) and the clamp for use in the subaxial cervical spine (left).

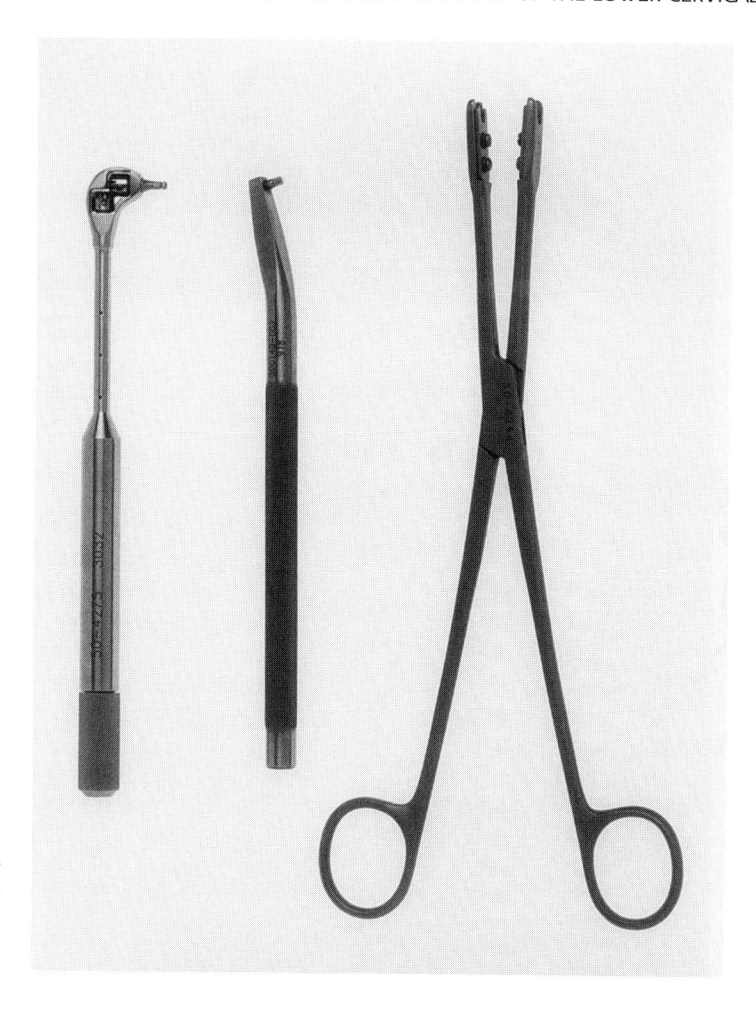

FIG. 13-3. Instrumentation necessary for clamp placement: right-angled locking adjustment wrench (*left*), fine adjustment wrench (*center*), and clamp-holding forceps (*right*).

Exposure

A posterior midline cervical incision and subperiosteal dissection exposes the spinous processes, laminae, and facet joints comprising the unstable motion segment and the adjacent laminae. The exposure must be adequate to enable correct placement and tightening of the clamps. Open reduction and nerve-root decompression is performed if necessary.

Preparation for Clamping

The superior border of the superior laminae and the inferior border of the inferior laminae are dissected to enable the clamps to be placed as close as possible to the midline. It is usually necessary to divide the ligamentum flavum to enable correct positioning of the clamp.

Preparation for Grafting

The exposed cortex of the laminae, lateral masses, and spinous processes of the unstable segment is roughened with a high-speed drill until it bleeds freely. Cancellous bone chips are harvested from the preferred site. Alternatively, the articular surfaces of the facet joints may be curetted to promote fusion.

Clamp Placement

Clamps for use in the lower cervical spine are selected such that the shortest possible screw is used (Table 13-3). One threaded (superior) and one unthreaded (inferior) clamp are employed on each side. The clamps are then held in position and a screw inserted from the unthreaded to the threaded clamp and partially tightened (Fig. 13-4). This maneuver is repeated on the contralateral side, and the clamps are alternately tightened until equal tension is achieved. Final tightening is performed with the fine adjustment instrument. The bone chips are positioned under the clamps and over the prepared sites. Adequate fixation in flexion, extension, and rotation is assessed by stressing the construct.

Table 13-2
Indications and Contraindications for the Use of the Halifax Clamp

Indications
    Posterior instability at one motion segment
    Posterior elements intact
    Anterior stabilization may be necessary in a three-column injury
Contraindications
    Previous laminectomy
    Multilevel stabilization
    Incompetent posterior elements

Table 13-3
Surgical Technique

Appropriate clamps (lower cervical spine)
One threaded and one unthreaded clamp per side
Use clamps such that shortest screw is required
Tighten sides alternately
Bone graft required
Be prepared to use alternative method

Closure

The wound is closed with absorbable sutures over a closed suction drain.

POSTOPERATIVE CARE

The need for a Philadelphia collar is determined by the adequacy of three-column fixation. Cervical radiography is performed immediately postoperatively to ensure correct placement of the clamps and at 6-weekly intervals until radiologic bone fusion occurs.

COMPLICATIONS

Neural injury is rare if adequate reduction is obtained prior to surgery. Infection and hematoma occur in less than 1% of cases. Two specific complications are loosening of the screws and clamp displacement. A modification to the threaded clamp mitigates against loosening of the screws, and proper selection of clamps together with adequate preparation of the laminae makes clamp displacement an unusual complication in the lower cervical spine.

DISCUSSION

Several unresolved issues persist regarding the use of the Halifax clamp.

Bone Graft

The aim of stabilization is solid bone fusion, which usually requires a bone graft. Fixation maintains stability until bone fusion occurs but cannot be relied on for long-term stability. We agree with Aldrich and colleagues (1991, 1993) that bone grafting or facet joint fusion is necessary when the Halifax clamps are used. Nevertheless Holness (1991) reported satisfactory results without the use of bone grafts in the lower cervical spine.

Unilateral or Bilateral Clamps

In the original description by Tucker (1975), clamps were used on one side only. Holness and colleagues (1991) reported few problems in 175 patients who had unilateral

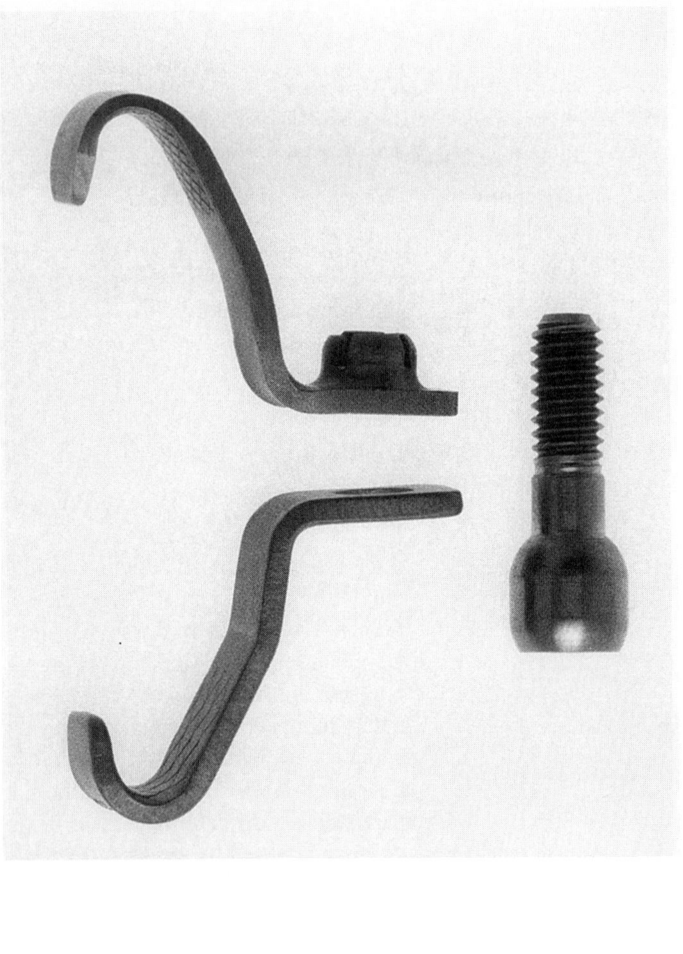

FIG. 13-4. Direction of screw placement from unthreaded to threaded Halifax clamp.

placement of the clamp (although fixation was supplemented with interspinous wires in an unknown number of patients). Other authors (Aldrich et al., 1991, 1993; Statham et al., 1993) routinely employ bilateral clamps. The application of bilateral clamps adds little to the operating time or morbidity and results in a more stable construct.

Multiple-Level Clamping. Authors (Aldrich et al., 1991, 1993; Holness, 1991; Statham et al., 1993) are agreed that for optimal performance only one motion segment should be stabilized. If clamps are applied over more than one motion segment the intermediate level can remain mobile. In cases in which more than one motion segment require stabilization, bilateral alternate clamps have been employed (e.g., C4-5 on one side and C5-6 on the other). However, the number of cases is too small for a definitive statement on reliability.

CONCLUSION

Halifax interlaminar clamps have proven to be safe and reliable for stabilization of the posterior elements in the lower cervical spine. Correct placement is essential for successful stabilization. If there is doubt about the stability of the construct, an alternative method should be employed (Fielding, 1988).

REFERENCES

Aldrich, E.F., Crow, W.N., Weber, P.B., et al. (1991). Use of MR imaging-compatible Halifax clamps for posterior cervical fusion. *Journal of Neurosurgery, 74,* 185–189.

Aldrich, E.F., Weber, P.B., & Crow, W.N. (1993). Halifax interlaminar clamp for posterior cervical fusion: a long-term follow-up review. *Journal of Neurosurgery, 78,* 702–708.

Cybulski, G.R., Douglas, R.A., Meyer, P.R., et al. (1992). Complications in three-column cervical spine injuries requiring anterior-posterior stabilization. *Spine, 17,* 253–256.

Cybulski, G.R., Stone, J.L., Crowell, R.M., et al. (1988). Use of Halifax interlaminar clamps for posterior C1-2 arthrodesis. *Neurosurgery, 22,* 429–431.

Fielding, J.W. (1988). Current concepts review: The status of arthrodesis of the cervical spine. *Journal of Bone and Joint Surgery, American Volume, 70,* 1571–1574.

Geremia, G.K., Kim, K.S., Cerullo, L., et al. (1985). Complications of sublaminar wiring. *Surgical Neurology, 23,* 629–634.

Grob, D., Crisco, J., Panjabi, M., et al. (1992). Biomechanical evaluation of four different posterior atlantoaxial fixation techniques. *Spine, 17,* 480–490.

Holness, R.O. (1991). Halifax clamps for posterior cervical fusion. *Journal of Neurosurgery, 75,* 836–838.

Holness, R.O., Huestis, W.S., Howes, W.J., et al. (1984). Posterior stabilization with an interlaminar clamp in cervical injuries: technical note and review of the longterm experience with the method. *Neurosurgery, 14,* 318–322.

Statham, P., O'Sullivan, M.G., & Russell, T. (1993). The Halifax interlaminar clamp for posterior cervical fusion: Initial experience in the United Kingdom. *Neurosurgery, 32,* 396–399.

Tucker, H.H. (1975). Technical report: Method of fixation of subluxed or dislocated cervical spine below C1-C2. *Canadian Journal of Neurological Sciences, 2,* 381–382.

CHAPTER 14

Use of Lateral Mass Plates for Stabilization of the Lower Cervical Spine

Paul R. Cooper

HIGHLIGHTS

The use of posterior plates and screws for the internal fixation of the cervical spine represents an important advance in the treatment of patients with cervical instability. Although posterior instrumentation using plates and screws has been used most frequently for patients with cervical instability resulting from trauma, this technique is also appropriate for instability caused by degenerative, infectious, and neoplastic disorders or instability resulting from prior surgery.

Application of plates and screws similar to those originally described and popularized by Roy-Camille is technically simple, easily learned, and associated with a low incidence of complications. Moreover, instrumentation produces immediate and long-term stability without the need for complex orthoses such as the halo-vest, and is not dependent on the integrity of the laminae or spinous processes (Cooper, Cohen, Rosiello, et al., 1988; Roy-Camille, Saillant, Berteaux, et al., 1979; Roy-Camille, Saillant, Judet, et al., 1983). Because instrumentation does not intrude on the spinal canal, as is the case with hooks or wires, there is little risk of neurological injury. The advantages of lateral mass plating are summarized in Table 14-1.

INITIAL ASSESSMENT AND MANAGEMENT

Although posterior plates and screws may be used for the management of instability caused by nontraumatic conditions as noted above, for the purpose of this discussion we will assume that the patient has instability resulting from trauma.

After cervical alignment and the anatomy of the fracture are assessed with plain films the patient is placed in cervical traction using Gardner-Wells tongs. If the cervical spine is unstable but the alignment is satisfactory, 5 kg of weight is used to maintain alignment. If a subluxation is present, 5 to 10 kg of weight is initially applied and is increased in 2-kg increments until the subluxation is reduced, or a maximum of 20 kg is used. The effectiveness of this management in restoring alignment is followed with lateral cervical spine films taken just before additional weight is applied. If the subluxation is not reduced with this amount of weight, open reduction is performed at the time of posterior stabilization.

Although some authors believe that a better neurologic outcome is obtained in patients who have reduction of their subluxations in the first 6 hours after injury as compared with those who have reduction after this time, there is no agreement on the effect of early reduction on neurologic outcome in the literature (Aebi, Mohler, Zach, et al., 1986; Roy-Camille et al., 1983).

IMAGING

After initial evaluation with plain films, patients who are neurologically intact and those with residual neurologic function below the level of the injury should undergo magnetic resonance imaging (MRI) scanning to determine the presence of dural compression by a herniated disk, hematoma, or bone. If MRI scanning is not available or is otherwise precluded by clinical circumstances a myelogram and postmyelogram computed tomographic (CT) scan should be performed.

In patients with complete neurologic deficit below the level of the injury, evaluation of the bony anatomy with CT is sufficient. This author believes that operative decompression in such patients does not improve neurologic function and therefore does not assess the presence of continued compression by bone or soft-tissue with CT/myelography or MRI.

Table 14-1
Advantages and Disadvantages of Lateral Mass Plating

Advantages
    Technically simple
    Bone grafting generally unnecessary
    Superior rotational stability
    Intact laminae and spinous processes unnecessary
    No instrumentation within spinal canal
    High success rate

Disadvantages
    Increased risk of screw pullout in osteoporotic bone
    Minimal ability to "reduce" fractures or kyphotic deformities

Table 14-2
Indications for Posterior Cervical Plating

Traumatic facet dislocation
Absent or fractured posterior elements
Subaxial cervical instability unless severe vertebral-body injury
Instability from degenerative, infectious, or neoplastic processes

Regardless of whether MRI scanning or myelography is performed, it is essential that the bony anatomy of the fracture be fully defined at some point by a CT scan with bone windows to determine the correct level of plate placement and size of the plate. Particular scrutiny should be directed to the lateral masses and facet joints. If there is a fracture of the lateral mass, the level should be carefully noted. There is no point in placing a screw in a lateral mass that is disconnected from the vertebral body because of a fracture of the lateral mass or pedicle. In this instance operative strategy must be altered in a manner that will be detailed in a subsequent section. However, fracture of a facet has little significance because screws are placed in the lateral mass and not the facet.

INDICATIONS AND CONTRAINDICATIONS FOR POSTERIOR CERVICAL PLATING

Indications

Posterior cervical plating is an effective means of producing immediate stability of the cervical spine whether the injury involves the vertebral body or the facet joints and their ligamentous attachments. This technique is ideal for facet dislocations caused by fractures or ligamentous injuries. It is particularly suitable for patients with laminar and spinous process fractures when these structures cannot be wired. Because the plates are placed bilaterally at the site of movement they provide greater rotational stability than can be achieved with wiring of posterior midline structures.

In theory, stabilization using anterior cervical plates is a superior means of fixation for injuries of the vertebral bodies. In practice, however, posterior plates are an extremely effective means of stabilizing injuries of the vertebral bodies unless there is severe vertebral body collapse. Moreover, their application is simpler than is the use of cervical corpectomy, grafting, and anterior plating. The indications for lateral mass plating are summarized in Table 14-2.

Contraindications

There are few contraindications to posterior plating. However, the technique should not be used in patients with osteoporosis, metabolic bone disease, or conditions, such as ankylosing spondylitis, in which the bone is soft; in these situations screw pullout and loss of reduction is likely. Posterior plating is also contraindicated in patients with residual neurologic function and persistent anterior compression of the spinal cord by bone, disk, or soft tissue. In this situation anterior decompression, bone grafting, and anterior plating is the most appropriate means of achieving the combined goals of neural decompression and stabilization. If there is also a facet dislocation that cannot be reduced, the facet dislocation can be reduced and lateral mass plates and screws applied through a posterior approach after anterior decompression is achieved.

Posterior plates and screws are frequently ineffective in the treatment of fixed or progressive kyphotic deformities. If the deformity is fixed it is unlikely that it can be reduced with posterior instrumentation. If the deformity is chronic and progressive but reducible, posterior plates and screws will frequently not be sufficient to hold the patient in lordosis, and screw pullout may occur. Patients with such disorders are generally better treated by an anterior approach with reduction of the kyphos using the Caspar distraction apparatus, bone grafting, and anterior plating. However, these patients may need supplemental posterior plates and screws. Contraindications to lateral mass plating are summarized in Table 14-3.

OPERATIVE MANAGEMENT

Timing of Operation

Residual subluxations and locked facets are usually easiest to reduce in the first 3 or 4 days after injury. The same dislocations are frequently irreducible when operation is performed several weeks after trauma. Therefore, every attempt should be made to operate as soon as possible after injury.

In patients with incomplete neurologic deficit, early operation with reduction and stabilization also has the theoretical advantage of improving neurologic function (Ducker, Bellegarrigue, Saleman, et al., 1984). Early stabilization also reduces the risk of secondary neurologic injury as a result of movement at unstable spinal segments. In patients with complete deficit, early operation allows mobilization and will minimize pulmonary complications. Delaying surgery for as little as 2 or 3 days frequently allows septic complications to be manifest and sometimes precludes operation for many weeks.

Perioperative Management

Patients are brought to the operating room in cervical traction. In patients with normal neurologic function or residual function below the level of their injury, electrodes for evoked potential monitoring are placed.

Table 14-3
Contraindications for Cervical Plating

Osteoporotic bone
Residual anterior spinal cord compression
Fixed kyphotic deformity
Anterior injury with severe vertebral-body collapse

Extension is usually the position of safety for patients with fractures of the mid and lower cervical spine; because oral endotracheal intubation usually entails extension of the neck, intubation by this method is unlikely to produce spinal cord injury. Fiberoptic intubation while the patient is awake is indicated when extension is likely to result in an increase in subluxation. If somatosensory evoked potentials are to be monitored, a low concentration of halogenated inhalation agents should be used; ideally, patients should be maintained on muscle relaxants, narcotics, and nitrous oxide.

After intubation a cervical collar is placed and the patient is turned to the prone position. The head may be placed on a horseshoe head rest or fixed in a three-pin head holder. The latter method provides more reliable fixation and precludes the occurrence of pressure necrosis of the face. A radiopaque marker is placed on the neck to establish the optimal site for placement of the incision and an x-ray film is taken to confirm that alignment has been maintained. Intraoperative fluoroscopy is unnecessary and is not used.

Operative Technique

A midline incision is made and the posterior elements of the levels to be plated are exposed. The muscles must be dissected off the bone far laterally to expose the entire lateral mass of the vertebrae to be plated. If there is any doubt as to the level of the fracture or subluxation when the posterior elements are exposed, a lateral x-ray film is taken.

Several plating systems for achieving fixation of the lateral masses of the cervical spine are commercially available in the United States. None of these is currently approved by the Food and Drug Administration for fixation of the lateral masses of the cervical spine. The original Roy-Camille plates specifically designed for lateral mass fixation and manufactured by the Howmedica Company are available everywhere except the United States.

Haid Universal Bone Plates

This author has had the most experience with the Haid Universal Bone Plates manufactured by American Medical Electronics (AME; Dallas, TX). The plates are made of titanium and contain two, three, four, or five holes for stabilizing one, two, three, or four motion segments respectively. The plates cannot be bent or otherwise shaped but are curved slightly to recreate the normal lordotic curve of the cervical spine when they are screwed in place. The distance from the center of one hole to the center of the adjacent hole is either 13 or 15.5 mm. Two-hole plates with the shorter interhole distance are almost always adequate for stabilizing one motion segment. Occasionally, a three-hole plate with a 15.5-mm interhole distance is necessary to stabilize two motion segments; usually plates with the shorter interhole distance are satisfactory (Fig. 14-1).

If four- or five-hole plates are needed to stabilize three or four motion segments it is essential that plates with a 15.5-mm interhole distance be used. The plates are held in place by 3.5-mm-diameter self-tapping titanium screws. Although screws are now available from AME in a variety of lengths, this author has used exclusively the 16-mm screws.

Small Notched Titanium Reconstruction Plates

Small notched titanium reconstruction plates are available from Synthes (Paoli, PA). These plates have holes either 8 or 12 mm apart. The plates with 8-mm hole spacing come

FIG. 14-1. Two- and three-hole Roy-Camille lateral mass plates and 16-mm screw 3.5 mm in diameter. The Haid plates manufactured by American Medical Electronics are almost identical in appearance. Plates shown have holes 13 mm apart. Haid plates have holes 13 or 15.5 mm apart.

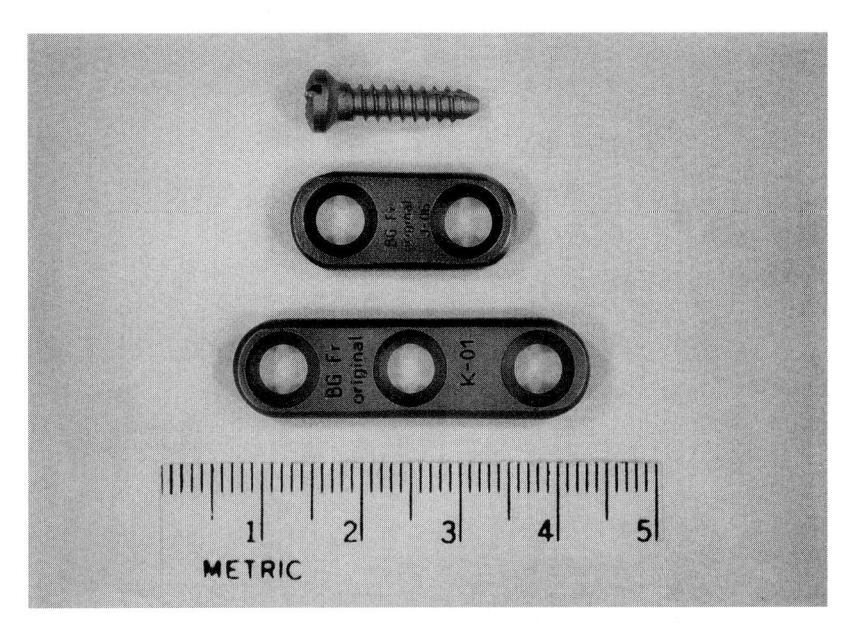

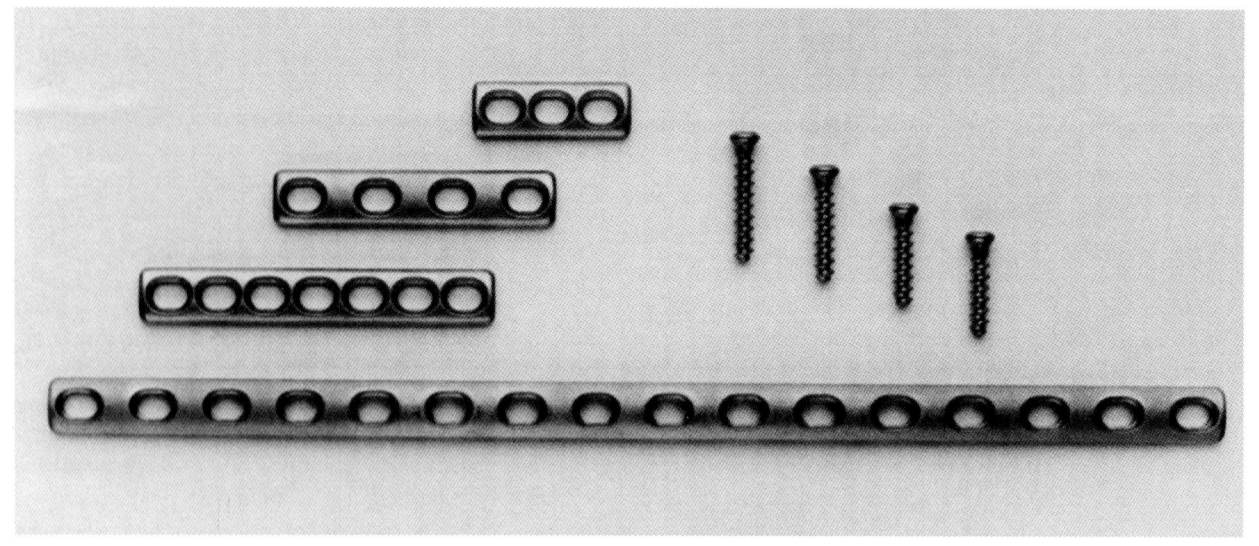

FIG. 14-2. Small notched titanium reconstruction plate marketed by Synthes. The plates come in the lengths shown as well as additional sizes (see text). Plates shown have an interhole distance of either 8 or 12 mm. The cancellous screws shown are 3.5 mm in diameter.

with 3, 5, 7, or 24 holes. The plates with 12-mm hole spacing come in 2-, 3-, 4-, 5-, and 6-hole models A plate with 16-mm spacing is now available. The plates can be bent with appropriate plate benders or cut to the desired length. Holes are drilled with a 2.0-mm bit for fully threaded titanium cancellous bone screws 3.5 mm in diameter, which are available in 2-mm increments from 12 to 24 mm. However, I have used exclusively the 16-mm screws (Fig. 14-2).

Two-hole plates with a 12-mm interhole distance should be used when stabilizing one motion segment. When utilizing plates with three, four, five, or six holes for stabilizing two or more motion segments, plates with an interhole distance of 8 mm should be used. By using every other hole for a screw, the holes will line up at the center of each lateral mass, which are approximately 16 mm apart.

Choice of Plating System

The Haid Universal Bone Plate or the Synthes small notched reconstruction plate set may both be used successfully to achieve lateral mass fixation. The Haid Universal Bone Plate (in spite of its name) has been designed specifically for cervical lateral mass plating and is preferred by this author. The longest plates contain five holes and may be used for stabilizing up to four motion segments. If five or more motion segments must be stabilized, the six-hole plates marketed by Synthes must be used. Although the Synthes plates offer the advantage of being malleable and able to be bent to fit the contour of the cervical spine, in practice the Haid plates fit the contour of the cervical spine in virtually all patients very nicely.

Both AME and Synthes market their plates and screws separately or in sets with a tray with multiple screws and plates of varying sizes. Depending on the company, drill guides, drill bits, screwdrivers, bending templates, plate holders, awls, and so forth are also included in the set. In practice none of these adjuncts to implantation is absolutely necessary. Drill bits, awls, and screwdrivers are standard in most operating rooms and money may be saved by using readily available equipment.

Screw and Plate Placement

The screws are placed in the center of the lateral masses adjacent to the motion segment to be stabilized. Thus, if the C4-5 motion segment is to be stabilized, screws are inserted into the lateral masses of C4 and C5. The plates and screws must be placed symmetrically. If a two-hole plate is used to secure the lateral masses of C4 and C5 on the left, a two-hole plate must be used at the same levels on the right.

The center of the lateral mass in a rostral-caudal direction is midway between the upper and lower facet joints; in a medial-lateral direction the center is midway between the valley that marks the lateral margin of the lamina and the edge of the lateral mass laterally (Fig. 14-3). An awl is used to make a shallow hole in the center of the lateral mass or 1 mm lateral to the center. AME supplies a 2.7-mm-diameter drill bit that has a stop at 1 cm, preventing more than 1 cm of bone penetration. If the Synthes system is used, a 2.2 mm drill bit is used.

Utilizing the technique described by Roy-Camille, and co-workers (Roy-Camille, Saillant, Berteaux, et al., 1979; Roy-Camille, Saillant, Judet, et al., 1983) the drill is directed straight anteriorly and 10 degrees laterally. However, I prefer to direct the drill 20 to 30 degrees laterally, which provides more assurance that the screw tip will lie lateral to the foramen transversarium and the vertebral artery (Fig. 14-4). Magerl, Grob, & Seemann (1987) have described screw placement with a point of entry just above and medial to the exact center of the lateral mass. The screw is directed 25 degrees laterally and rostrally in the same plane as the facet joint. The Roy-Camille technique carries less risk of nerve-

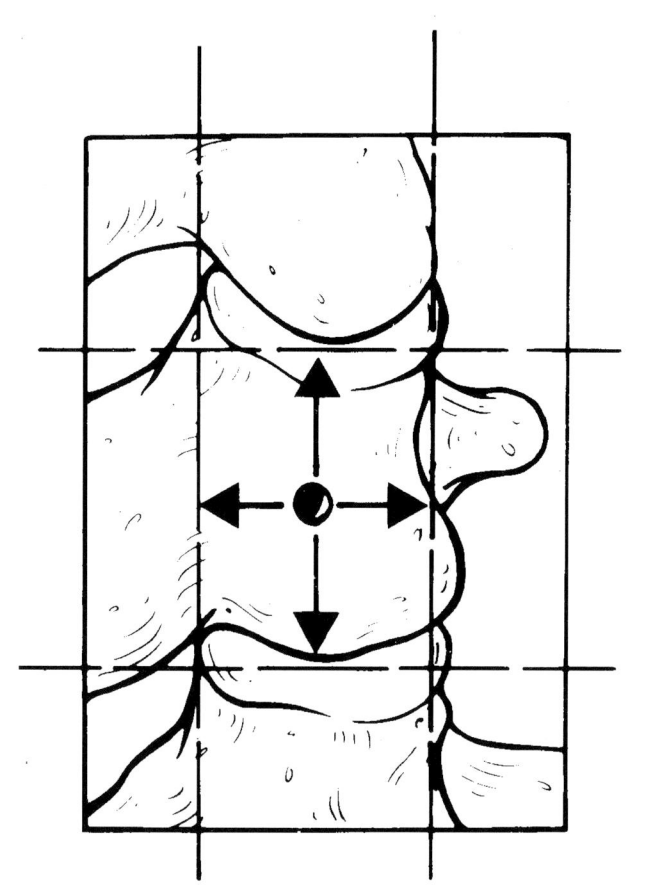

FIG. 14-3. The borders of the lateral mass are defined superiorly and inferiorly by the facet joints, laterally by the bone edge, and medially by the valley where the lateral mass ends and the lamina begins. A hole is then drilled in the center of the lateral mass for screw placement and angled directly anterior and 20 to 30 degrees laterally. (Reproduced courtesy of American Medical Electronics, Dallas, TX.)

root injury but a greater chance of facet-joint violation and inadvertent incorporation of an additional motion segment by the lower screw (Heller, Carlson, Abitbol, et al., 1991). Biomechanical studies indicate that the upward trajectory preferred by Magerl gives stronger screw purchase. In clinical practice screw pullout is unusual and results in loss of fixation very infrequently (Errico, Uhl, Cooper, et al., 1992).

When two-hole plates are used, the holes are first drilled on the side of the jumped facet or greatest subluxation. Any residual subluxation is first reduced, drilling off the facet, if necessary. Because the screws are placed in the lateral mass, the presence of a fractured facet (in reality an appendage of the lateral mass) does not preclude the placement of lateral mass plates.

After the subluxation is reduced, an assistant maintains reduction by grasping the posterior elements with a Kocher clamp or other appropriate instrument. This will have the effect of bringing the lateral masses closer together and enabling a plate that at first might seem too short to fit nicely. The plate is secured in place by screwing the self-tapping screws into the holes that have been drilled to two-finger tightness. The screws are tightened sequentially until the plate is secured. The same procedure is then followed on the opposite side. If three- or four-hole plates are to be used, the most rostral and caudal holes are drilled and the plate secured using screws inserted in these holes (Fig. 14-5). The one or two intervening holes are drilled last, after the plate has been secured. Should a screw be stripped it should be removed and replaced with a larger-diameter rescue screw. AME markets a 4.5-mm-diameter "recovery screw" for this purpose.

Lateral mass plating of the cervical spine is most appropriate for the management of fractures and subluxations from C3 to C7. The anatomy of T1 is different from the cervical vertebrae. This author has preferred not to use lateral mass plates and screws for the unusual case of C7-T1 instability. However, screws may be directed more medially at T1 and placed in the T1 pedicle if necessary.

Posttraumatic instability at C2-3 is uncommon and usually occurs in the presence of a hangman's fracture, which is usually best managed with a halo vest. When C2-3 instability necessitates internal fixation, lateral mass plates and screws may be used. However, the technique of screw placement in C2 differs from the techniques used in the subaxial cervical spine. Unlike the remainder of the cervical spine, C2 has a large pedicle, which may be used for engaging the screw.

The point of entry for the screw is at the inferior medial aspect of the lateral mass. The screw is directed rostrally at an angle of approximately 60 degrees. The superior-medial aspect of the pedicle of C2 is felt using a nerve hook. The drill hole and screw are directed into the C2 pedicle just lateral to its medial border to avoid the spinal canal. The screw must not be directed too laterally lest the vertebral artery be injured. The technique is identical to that described by Magerl and Seemann (1987) for C1-2 transarticular screw fixation. However, the screw must not pass into the C1-2 articulation. Once the hole is drilled, a 20-mm-long screw is used to secure the plate to C2. Screw placement in the lateral mass of C3 is identical to that described in the preceding paragraphs.

Bone Grafting

The necessity for bone grafting with the use of posterior cervical plates is controversial. Posterior plates stabilize the facet joint so effectively that spontaneous fusion occurs here or at sites of bony injury. Therefore, in patients who have sustained trauma within several weeks of operation this author does not use bone grafts. Although I have had patients who have lost reduction this has always occurred in the first weeks after operation as a result of faulty screw placement or placement of the plates at inappropriate levels.

In patients who are stabilized long after their trauma and those with nontraumatic conditions, bone grafting is usually indicated; the synovial cartilage of the facet joint is curetted and small chips of bone, which may be taken from the spinous processes of the exposed vertebrae, are inserted into the joint. If there is a bilaminar fracture the lamina can be removed and cut into small pieces and used to pack the facet joint.

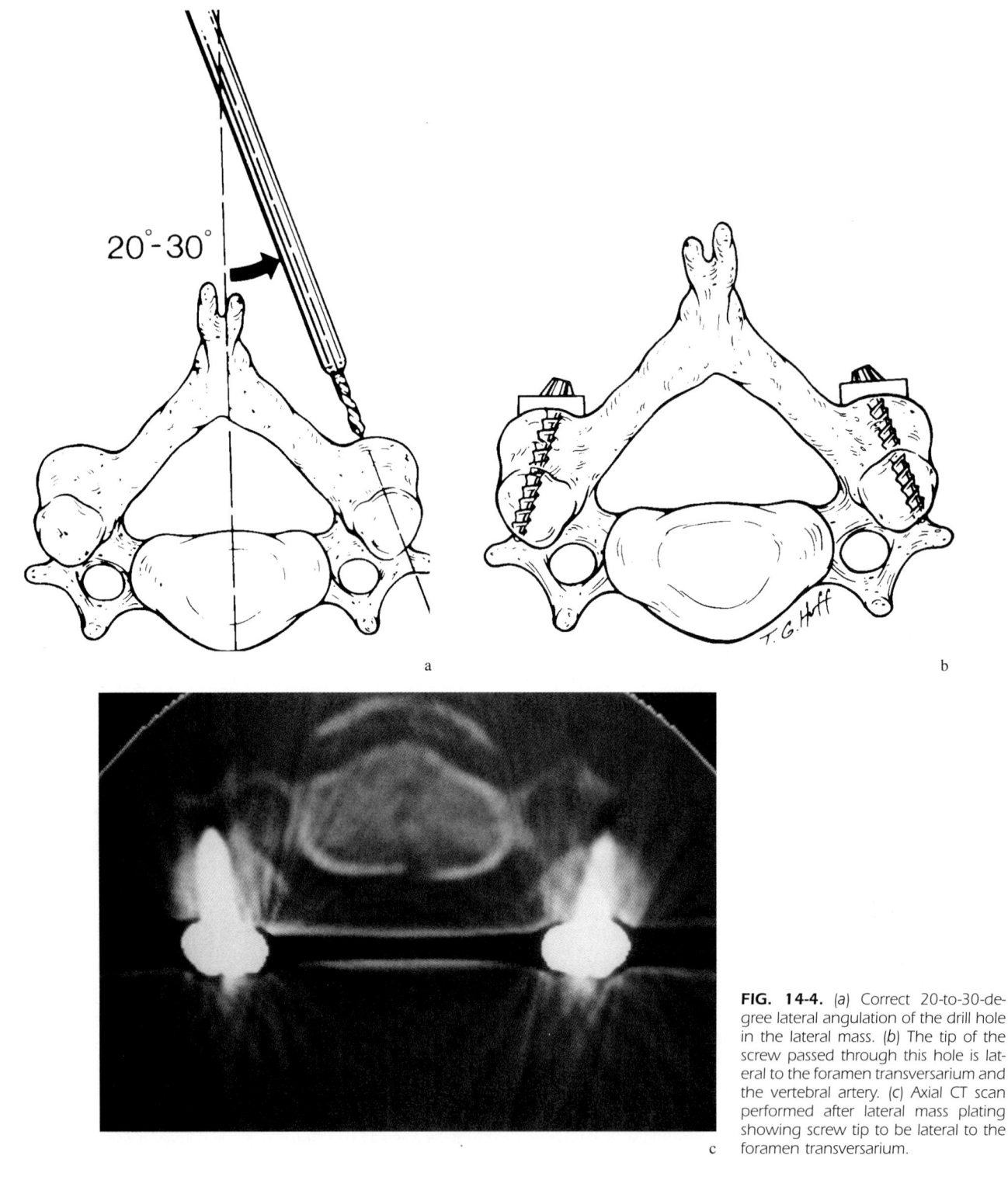

FIG. 14-4. (a) Correct 20-to-30-degree lateral angulation of the drill hole in the lateral mass. (b) The tip of the screw passed through this hole is lateral to the foramen transversarium and the vertebral artery. (c) Axial CT scan performed after lateral mass plating showing screw tip to be lateral to the foramen transversarium.

Operative Decision Making: Plate Length and Site of Placement

The technical details of operative placement of posterior cervical plates and screws are relatively straightforward. However, decision making regarding the location of plates and the number of motion segments requiring stabilization is frequently more complex; conceptual mistakes in the location of plate placement probably account for more cases of plate failure than technical errors in insertion.

Two-hole plates are ideal for patients with single-level subluxations or facet dislocations (Fig. 14-6). At the time of operation it is essential that exposure be obtained of adjacent motion segments. If there is instability at the level above or below the facet subluxation this motion segment must be stabilized by using a three-hole plate.

Three-hole plates are also used when there is injury to the vertebral body and adjacent disk spaces, even though there may only be a subluxation at one level. Thus, when

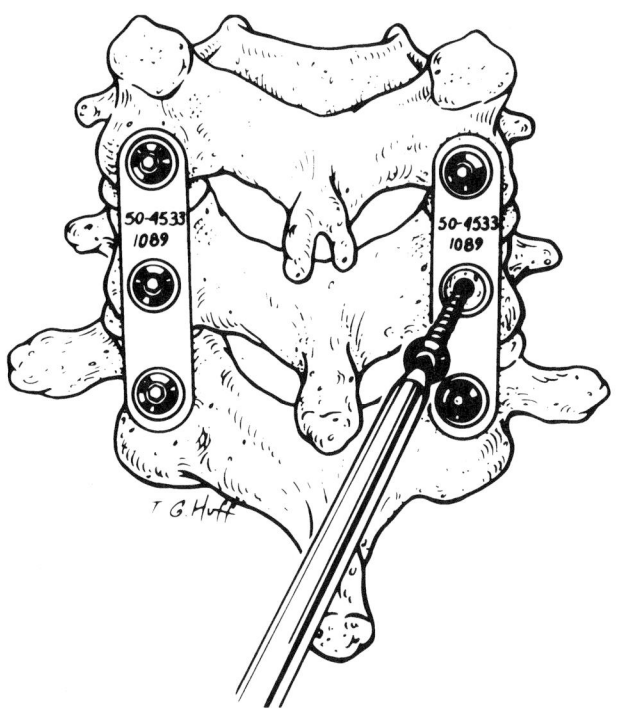

FIG. 14-5. Three-hole plate in correct position with the center screw being placed last.

there is a subluxation at C5-6 with injury to the C5 vertebral body stabilization of the C5-6 motion segment alone may result in late instability at the C4 level. Plating from C4-6 will avoid this complication.

When there is a fracture of the lateral mass or pedicle, plating of that lateral mass will do nothing to restore stability because it has lost its connection with the vertebral body. In this situation an additional adjacent motion segment must be stabilized using a three-hole plate. Thus, if there is a subluxation at C4-5 with an associated fracture of the lateral mass of C4, placing two-hole plates between C4 and C5 will immobilize this motion segment unilaterally only on the side of the intact lateral mass. Rotational stability will not be achieved, and screw pullout and loss of alignment may occur. Application of three-hole plates from C3 to C5 will be necessary in this situation (Fig. 14-7).

The use of three-hole plates is also appropriate when there is instability of two motion segments. The need to stabilize three or four motion segments using four- or five-hole plates is infrequent, but if necessary these longer plates provide excellent posterior fixation. They may be particularly

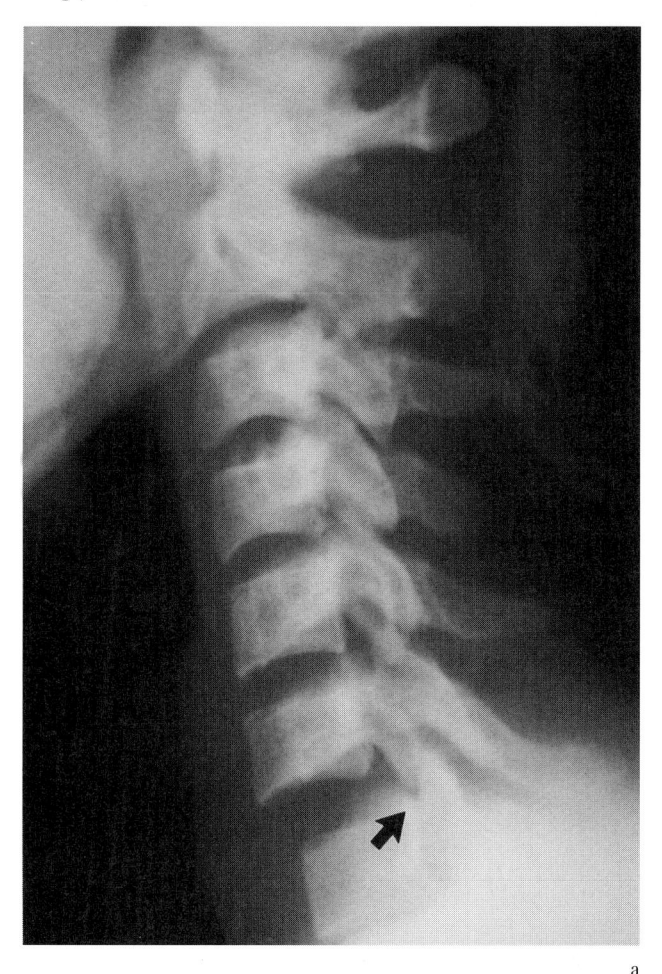

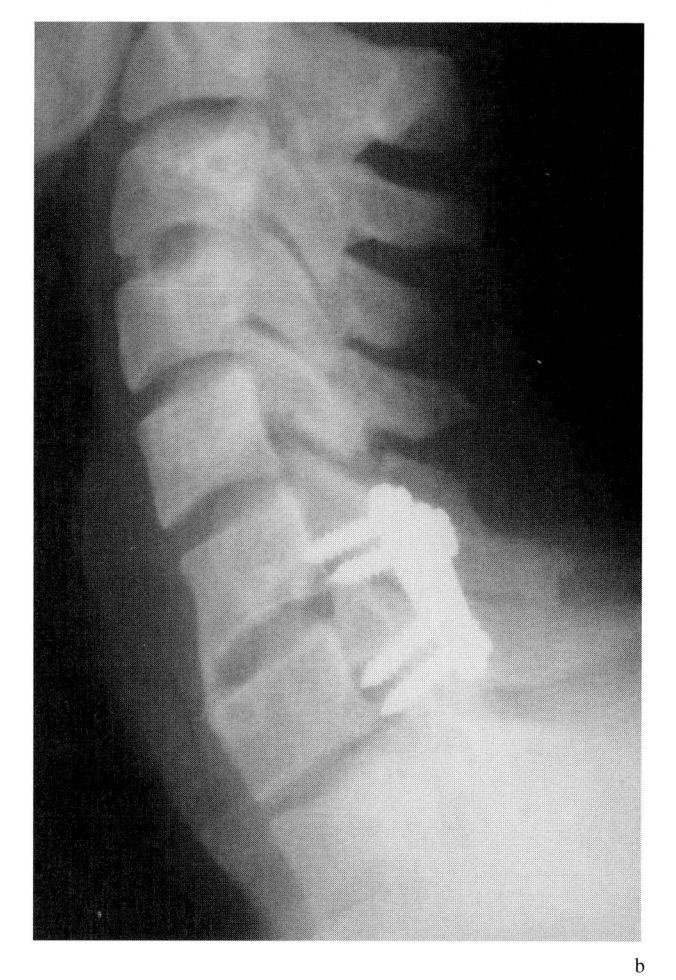

FIG. 14-6. (a) Lateral x-ray film taken on admission of a patient with a C6-7 jumped facet (*arrow*). (b) Lateral x-ray film taken 1 year after reduction of jumped facet and stabilization using two-hole plates. Note bone bridging at the anterior aspect of the C6-7 vertebral bodies.

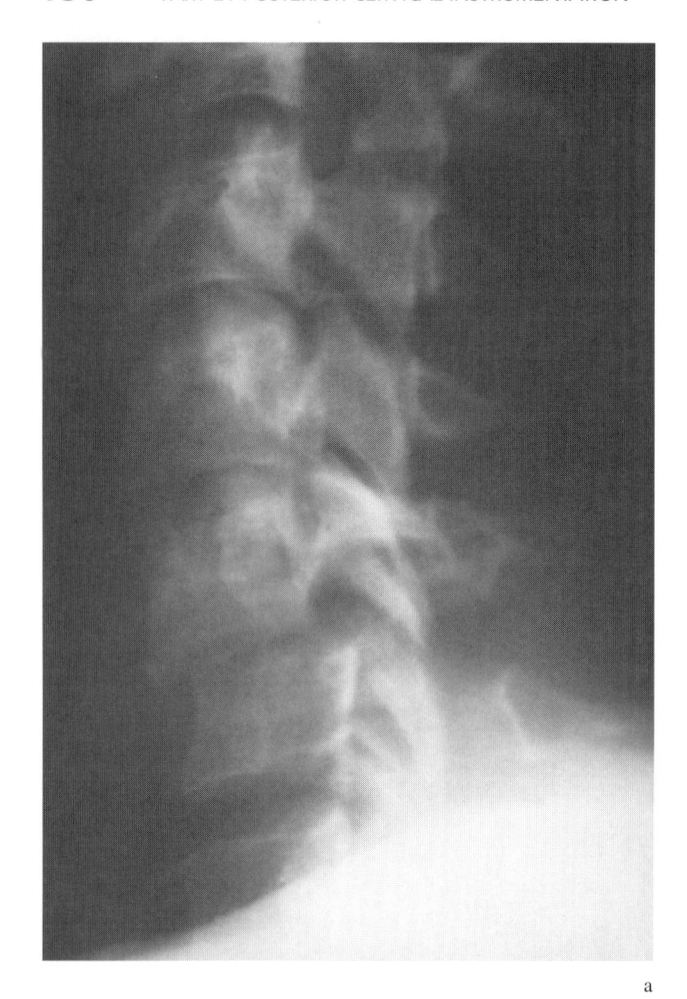

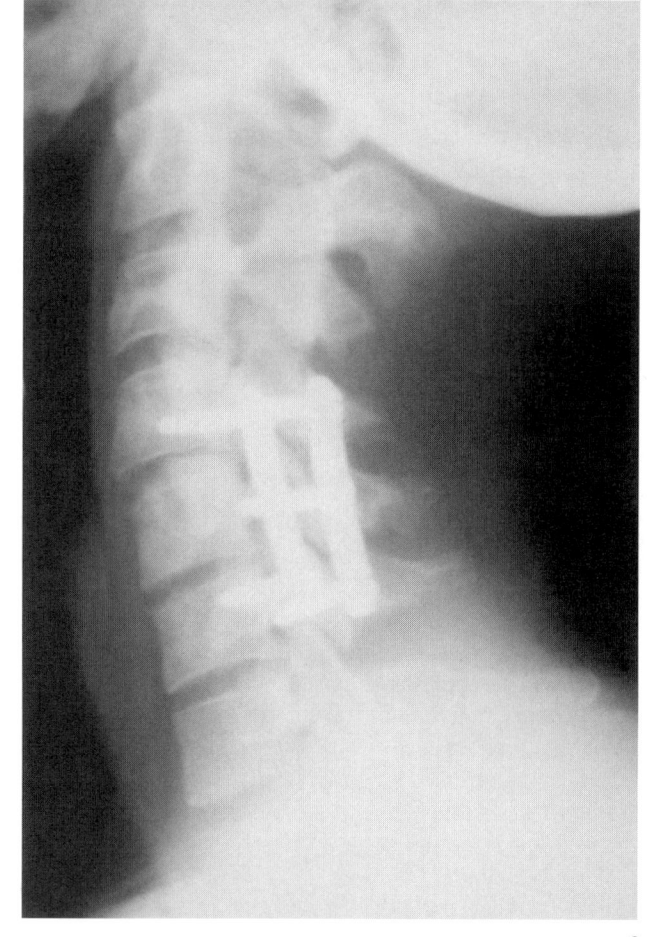

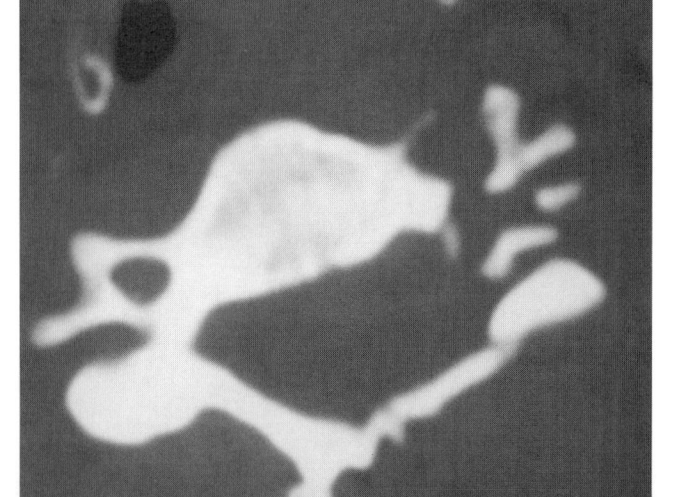

FIG. 14-7. (a) Plain lateral x-ray film of the cervical spine showing a C5-6 subluxation. (b) CT scan of the same patient reveals a fracture separation of the left lateral mass and pedicle of C5. (c) Three-hole plates were placed from C4 to C6 bilaterally. Fracture of the C5 lateral mass necessitated instrumentation to C4 to achieve C4-6 stability. Note that there is only one screw in the lateral mass of C5. No screw has been placed in the fractured C5 left lateral mass.

useful when applied prophylactically after laminectomy in patients in whom a kyphotic deformity might be expected to develop.

POSTOPERATIVE MANAGEMENT

Patients are allowed out of bed the day after surgery. The neck is immobilized for 3 months using a Philadelphia collar. Lateral cervical spine films are taken once or twice in the first week after operation and monthly until the collar is removed. An increase in neck pain or worsening of the patient's neurologic deficit is an indication for a lateral x-ray study of the cervical spine. At the end of 3 months the collar is removed and flexion and extension films of the cervical spine are taken.

COMPLICATIONS

Loss of alignment is infrequent and almost always occurs in the first days or weeks after application of plates. Screw pullout almost always accounts for loss of alignment at the plated level and may occur if the screw is placed too laterally in the lateral mass and there is too little bone lateral to the screw to hold it in place. If the screw has been tightened excessively it may be stripped, in which case pullout is almost inevitable. If the bone is soft as a result of osteoporosis or metabolic bone disease, screw pullout is likely, and other means of stabilizing the spine such as wiring should be used.

Loss of alignment at levels adjacent to the plated level may occur if ligamentous injury is not recognized. Flexion and extension films are quite appropriately not obtained in patients with obvious subluxations or instability at one level. Therefore, a second level of ligamentous injury may not be suspected if the patient's alignment is satisfactory at the time of evaluation with lateral cervical spine radiography. In all patients, careful inspection of the facet joints adjacent to the level of plating should be carried out. This may reveal ligamentous injury (presumptive evidence of instability) that had not been appreciated prior to operation. The joints may be stressed by grasping and distracting the spinous processes with clamps. If there is abnormal movement, this additional motion segment should be stabilized using a three-hole plate.

Injury to the vertebral artery during drilling is not possible using a drill bit with a stop at 1 cm. Vertebral artery penetration during screw placement is theoretically possible but will not occur if the screw is angled 20 to 30 degrees laterally and the screw penetrates the center of the lateral mass. Moreover, in many patients screws 16 mm in length will be too short to reach the vertebral artery even if the angle of the screw is incorrect.

Root injury caused by screw penetration has not been seen by this author and should not occur if the screws are pointed directly anteriorly or slightly rostrally. Should a patient awaken after operation with severe radicular pain or motor deficit, a CT scan should be obtained to determine whether a screw has penetrated the neural foramen.

An increase in neurologic deficit is unusual but may result from injury to the spinal cord during turning of the patient or overvigorous manipulation of the spine during intraoperative reduction of subluxations or plate placement. Disk herniations may occur or be exacerbated when the spine is moved into a kyphotic position as the screws are tightened. Preexisting disk herniations will usually be apparent on a preoperative MRI scan and are a contraindication to posterior cervical plating. A summary of complications encountered in 44 patients followed for a mean of almost 4 years is seen in Table 14-4.

Table 14-4
Complications of Cervical Plating*

Complication	No.
Perioperative death (<3 mo postoperatively)	0/44
Neurologic deterioration	0/44
Vascular	0/44
Revision required	3/44
Loose screw	8/202
Increased kyphosis	2/38
Superficial infection	2/44
Deep venous thrombosis	2/44
Sacral decubitus	2/44
Renal sepsis	1/44
Neck pain	2/38
Occipital decubitus	1/44

*Perioperative complications are listed for all 44 patients; long-term complications are limited to the 38 followed for >24 months.

SOURCE: Reproduced with permission from Fehlings, Cooper, & Errico (1994).

OUTCOME

Lateral mass fixation is now the procedure of choice for posterior instability of the cervical spine. Initial encouraging results reported in 20 patients followed for less than 1 year were reported in 1988 by Cooper, Cohen, Rosiello, et al. (1988). In a review of long-term outcome in a larger series with a mean follow-up of nearly 4 years in 41 patients we reported an overall fusion rate of 92.7% (Fehlings, Cooper, & Errico, 1994). Of 210 screws implanted only 8 (3.8%) loosened. The mean preoperative kyphosis was 24.4 degrees, which had decreased to 5.5 degrees postoperatively. A more detailed analysis of this patient series is seen in Table 14-5. Roy-Camille (1979) reported results in 221 patients who had lateral mass plating, none of whom received a bone graft. Over 85% had no loss of correction and only 3% had an increase of 10 degrees or more of angulation in the sagittal plane. Other authors have reported similar gratifying results (Domenella, Berlanda, & Bassi, 1989; Ebraheim, An, Jackson, et al., 1989) using the techniques and instrumentation similar to that popularized by Roy-Camille.

Anderson, Hanley, Grady, et al. (1991) reported their results in a series of 30 patients treated with lateral mass fixation utilizing Synthes reconstruction plates. Bone graft-

Table 14-5
Outcome Analysis in 41 Patients*

Factor	Finding
Fusion	
Overall fusion rate	38/41 (92.7%)
Patients without bone grafting	31/34
Patients with bone grafting	7/7†
Correction of sagittal plane kyphosis	
Mean preoperative kyphosis	24.4 ± 3.2 degrees
Mean preoperative kyphosis	5.0 ± 6.4 degrees
Mean correction	19.4 ± 5.5 degrees‡
Incidence of loose screws	8/210 (3.8%)
Extension of fusion beyond instrument segments	1 (Case 1)
Incidence of chronic significant neck pain§	2/38 (5.2%)

*Patients with less than 6 months of follow-up monitoring were excluded; 38 of the remaining 41 were followed for more than 2 years.

† Difference not significant ($\chi^2 = 0.67$; df = 1; $p = 0.41$).

‡ Degree of postoperative correction of sagittal plane kyphosis significant (t = 3.53; df = 37; $p < 0.01$).

§ Pain requiring analgesics or interfering with activities of daily living.

SOURCE: Reproduced with permission from Fehlings, Cooper, & Errico (1994).

ing was used in all patients, and supplemental wiring was used in many. Results were comparable to that reported by others using the instrumentation and techniques of Roy-Camille.

Biomechanical studies provide an explanation for the excellent clinical results. Flexion stiffness is increased by 92% with posterior plating but only 33% with wiring (Roy-Camille, 1979). Montesano, Juach, Anderson, et al. (1991) and others (Gill, Paschal, Corin, et al., 1988) have confirmed the superiority of lateral mass plates compared to all other means of posterior fixation.

SUMMARY AND CONCLUSIONS

Posterior cervical fixation using lateral mass plates and screws is now the procedure of choice for stabilization of the subaxial cervical spine. Careful definition of the nature of the bony injury and location of the subluxation using plain films and CT with bone windows is crucial for correct operative planning and satisfactory outcome. MRI is essential to identify the presence of neural compression that might preclude the safe placement of lateral mass plates. Implantation of plates and screws is straightforward and safe and easily learned. Bone grafting is usually not necessary, and long-term fixation can be achieved in over 90% of patients.

REFERENCES

Anderson, P.A., Hanley, M.R., Grady, M.S., et al. (1991). Posterior cervical arthrodesis with AO reconstruction plates and bone graft. *Spine, 16* (Suppl 3), S72–S79.

Aebi, M., Mohler, J., Zach, G.A., et al. (1986). Indication, surgical technique, and results of 100 surgically-treated fractures and fracture-dislocations of the cervical spine. *Clinical Orthopaedics and Related Research, 203,* 244–257.

Cooper, P.R., Cohen, A., Rosiello, A., et al. (1988). Posterior stabilization of cervical spine fractures and subluxations using plates and screws. *Neurosurgery, 23,* 300–306.

Domenella, G., Berlanda, P., & Bassi, G. (1989). Posterior-approach osteosynthesis of the lower cervical spine by the R. Roy-Camille technique. *Italian Journal of Orthopaedics and Traumatology, 3,* 23–28.

Ducker, T.B., Bellegarrigue, R., Salcman, M., et al. (1984). Timing of operative care in cervical spinal cord injury. *Spine, 9,* 525–531.

Ebraheim, N.A., An, H.S., Jackson, W.T., et al. (1989). Internal fixation of the unstable cervical spine using posterior Roy-Camille plates: Preliminary report. *Journal of Orthopaedic Trauma, 3,* 23–28.

Errico, T., Uhl, R., Cooper, P., et al. (1992). Pullout strength comparison of two methods of orienting screw insertion in the lateral masses of the bovine cervical spine. *Journal of Spinal Disorders, 5,* 459–463.

Fehlings, M.G., Cooper, P.R., & Errico, T.J. (1994). Posterior plates in the management of cervical spinal in instability: long-term results in 44 patients. *Journal of Neurosurgery, 81,* 341–349.

Gill, K., Paschal, S., Corin, J., et al. (1988). Posterior plating of the cervical spine: A biomechanical comparison of different posterior fusion techniques. *Spine, 13,* 813–816.

Heller, J.G., Carlson, G.D., Abitbol, J.-J., et al. (1991). Anatomic comparison of the Roy-Camille and Magerl techniques for screw placement in the lower cervical spine. *Spine, 16,* S552–S557.

Magerl, F., Grob, D., & Seemann, D. Stable dorsal fusion of the cervical spine (C2-Th 1) using hook plates. In: P. Kehr & A. Weidner (Eds.), *Cervical Spine I* (pp. 217–221). New York: Springer-Verlag.

Magerl, F., & Seemann, D. (1987). Stable posterior fusion of the atlas and axis by transarticular screw fixation. In: P. Kehr & A. Weidner (Eds.), *Cervical Spine I* (pp. 322–327). New York: Springer-Verlag.

Montesano, P.X., Juach, E.C., Anderson, P.A., et al. (1991). Biomechanics of cervical spine internal fixation. *Spine, 16* (Suppl 3), S10–S16.

Roy-Camille, R., Saillant, G., Berteaux, D., et al. (1979). Early management of spinal injuries. In: B. McKibbon (Ed.), *Recent Advances in Orthopedics* (pp. 57–87). New York: Churchill Livingstone.

Roy-Camille, R., Saillant, G., Judet, T., et al. (1983). Traumatismes recents des cinq dernières vertèbres cervicales chez l'adulte (avec et sans complication neurologique). *Seminars d'Hôpital, Paris, 59,* 1479–1488.

Roy-Camille, R., Saillant, G., & Mazel, C. (1989). Internal fixations of the unstable cervical spine by a posterior osteosynthesis with plates and screws. In: H.H. Sherk, E.J. Dunn, F.J. Eismont, et al. (Eds.), *The Cervical Spine* (2nd ed.) (pp. 390–403). Philadelphia: J.B. Lippincott.

CHAPTER 15

AXIS Fixation System Surgical Technique

Chester E. Sutterlin, III
David E. Jenkins

HIGHLIGHTS

The AXIS fixation system (Sofamor Danek Group, Memphis, TN) is labeled by the manufacturer and approved by the U.S. Food and Drug Administration (FDA) as a device for internal fixation of long bones and pelvis. The device is valuable for internal fixation of the posterior cervical spine utilizing the lateral mass fixation techniques described by Roy-Camille, Magerl, and An (Roy-Camille, Mazel, and Saillant, 1987; Magerl, Grob, and Seemann, 1987; An, Gordin, and Renner, 1991). This is considered an off-label use of the device and all patients should be so informed. The obvious advantages of lateral mass plate and screw fixation are usually apparent to all who have taken the time to review available information (surgeons, patients, family members, and on occasion attorneys and U.S. government officials). Along with obvious advantages of lateral mass plate and screw fixation, there are inherent risks that are unique in comparison with more traditional methods of cervical fixation. These benefits, risks, and potential complications should be clearly outlined for patients and their families, along with the approximate chances of success/failure in terms that the patient and family can understand, and ample time should be allowed to answer all of their questions.

These general measures, along with proper surgeon training and meticulous execution of technique will maximize beneficial and minimize adverse outcome.

TECHNIQUE OUTLINE

1. Preoperative plan
2. Position
3. Exposure
4. Step-by-step technique
   a. Curette facets
   b. Choose template
   c. Mark entry point
   d. Awl
   e. Drill
   f. Depth gauge
   g. Tap
   h. Contour plate
   i. Insert screws
   j. Bone graft
   k. Tighten screws

Preoperative Plan

Posterior segmental lateral mass fixation may be indicated in a variety of spinal disorders, including:

- degenerative,
- traumatic,
- rheumatologic,
- neoplastic,
- iatrogenic,
- and others.

It should be considered as a surgical option whenever outcome can be improved or enhanced by use of a fixation device. This is most often the case when the patient demonstrates cervical:

- instability,
- deformity, or the
- potential for pseudarthrosis (or failure of fusion).

Prior to lateral mass fixation of the cervical spine, computed tomographic (CT) scans are highly recommended in order to assess any anatomical variations that may affect the plating technique or surgical outcome.

Position

Proper patient positioning will facilitate and enhance the application of segmental lateral mass fixation. The patient is placed in the prone position and padded accordingly to ensure that no pressure is applied to the ocular orbits. Traction is applied to the patient's head via Gardner-Wells tongs, a head halter, or a similar device. Care should be taken to ensure that the cervical spine is in optimal sagittal contour (lordosis, if possible). The shoulders and arms should be gently retracted caudally. A radiographic examination of the cervical spine is indicated to confirm position and visualization of the involved vertebral levels.

Exposure

For adequate surgical exposure, it may be necessary to shave and cleanse a portion of the occipital region of the skull. A standard midline incision and dissection should be performed. The operative level must be verified. Soft tissue and muscle are dissected and elevated from the lamina and lateral masses. Care should be taken to avoid disturbing the facet joints above and below the involved levels as this may result in spontaneous fusion or instability. The articular cartilage of the involved facet joints should be removed and the joints packed with bone graft. The dorsal and lateral surfaces of the lateral masses are lightly decorticated prior to plate placement.

Surgical Technique

Step One—Determine Proper Plate Size and Screw Entry Point with Template

The entry point for the screw is at or near the center of the lateral mass. The center is defined by the medial, lateral, cephalad, and caudal borders of the lateral mass. The screw entry point should be visualized through the proper template. The AXIS templates correspond to the plate sizes and are color coded: blue, 11 mm; green, 13 mm; and gold, 15 mm. Once you have chosen the proper template, bend it to match the curvature of the spine. You may use this as a guide when bending the plate into the appropriate configuration. Holding the template in the desired position next to the lateral mass, mark the screw entry point at each level with a sterile marking pen, or in some other reliable manner. In virtually all cases, the multiple options for screw placement allow for a screw to be inserted into each and every lateral mass because of the AXIS system's variable plate sizes and "figure-eight" screw holes (Fig. 15-1).

Step Two—Use Awl to Place Starter Holes in Lateral Masses

The retractable awl is useful to place a pilot hole in the bone of the lateral mass exactly where you wish the screw entry point to be. This lessens the risk of drill-bit wandering,

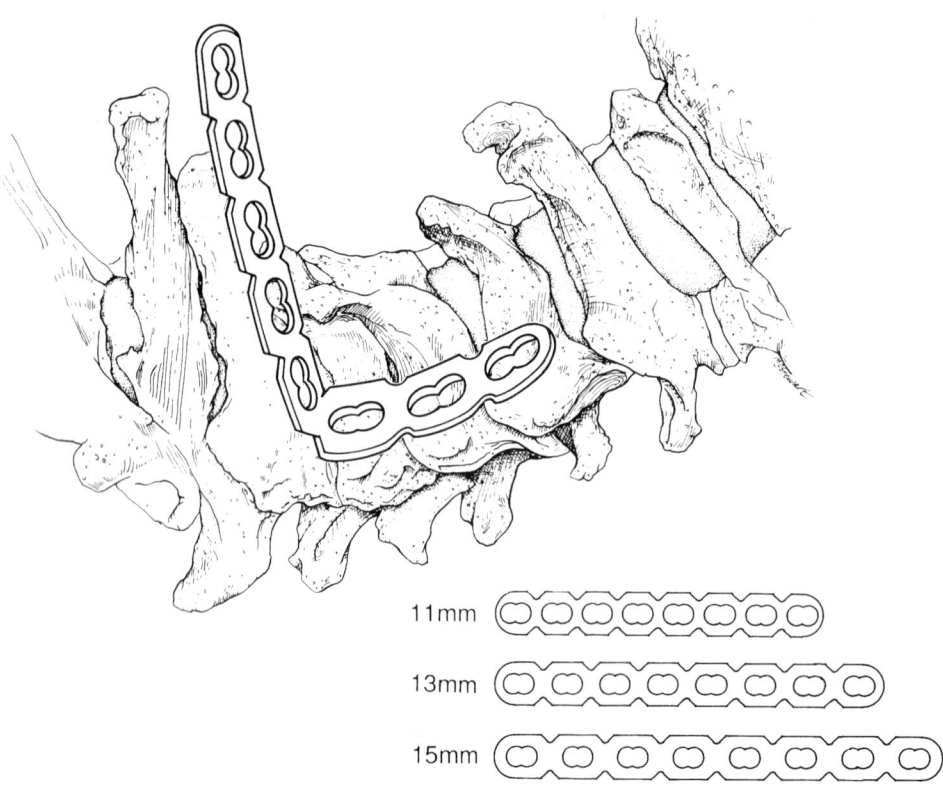

FIG. 15-1. The AXIS templates are color coded and are utilized to determine plate size and contour for optimal screw placement.

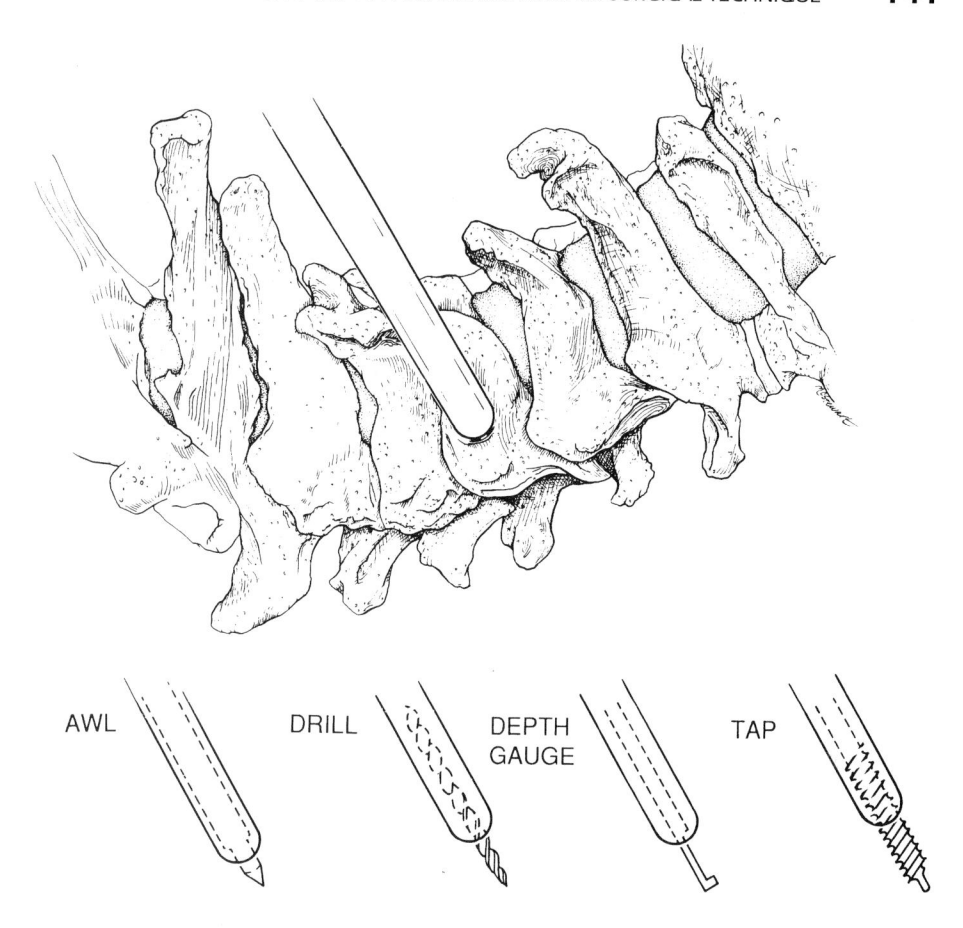

FIG. 15-2. To prepare each screw hole in the lateral mass, the technique requires sequential use of the awl, drill, depth gauge, and tap.

which could result in neurovascular injury. Create a starter hole in every involved lateral mass. The retractable sleeve of the awl protects the patient, surgeon, and others from injury. The awl point is very sharp and caution should be exercised during its use (Fig. 15-2).

Step Three—Drill Screw Holes with Desired Angulation and Depth of Purchase with Adjustable Drill Bit, Drill Stop, and Drill Guide

Slide the adjustable drill stop onto the cancellous drill bit and lock the stop in the groove that corresponds to your chosen hole length. The notches on the upper end of the drill bit correspond to the length of the cutting portion exposed when put through the drill guide. To achieve bicortical purchase, the average length is between 14 and 16 mm by the Magerl method (Magerl, Grob, and Seemann, 1987). If you wish unicortical purchase only, set the drill guide at 14 mm, or use the preset 14-mm drill bit. The drill guide and bit should be angled 20 to 30 degrees laterally. If the Roy-Camille technique is to be used, then no cranial angulation is necessary (Roy-Camille, Mazel, and Saillant, 1987). If you choose a technique that allows for a longer screw with more screw threads interfacing with the patient's bone, then the Magerl technique with enough cranial angulation to parallel the facet joint should be employed.

A K-wire, Penfield elevator, or other instrument placed within the facet joint can assist in determining the proper cephalad angulation. Drill every involved lateral mass (see Fig. 15-2).

Step Four—Use Depth Gauge to Verify Depth of Drill Hole

The reading on the depth gauge corresponds directly to the length of the screw within bone. If the depth gauge reads 16-mm, choose a 16-mm screw. It is also useful to measure the lateral border of the drill hole and the medial border of the drill hole because a difference of several millimeters may occur between the two. Measure all the drill holes. It is useful for an assistant to record the varying screw lengths at different levels (see Fig. 15-2).

Step Five—Tap Drill Holes with Appropriate Tap

For lateral mass fixation, 3.5-mm cancellous screws are satisfactory. Choose the 3.5-mm cancellous tap. It is not necessary to tap as far as the deepest cortex; however, you should tap through the posterior cortex. The tap is graduated to display depth of thread penetration; 4.0 cancellous screws and tap are available for use as salvage screws. This step is not necessary if self-tapping screws are used. Tap every drill hole of the involved lateral masses (see Fig. 15-2).

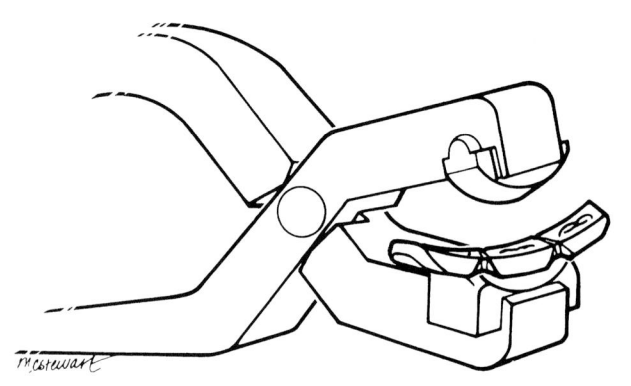

FIG. 15-3. The AXIS plates should be contoured with the plate bender included in the AXIS instrument set and no other because excessive contouring may weaken the plate. A new double action plate bender is available.

Step Six—Contour Plate with Plate Bender and Bending Irons

In its proper position the concave side of the AXIS plate faces the bone and the flat surface faces the surgeon. Line up each notch in the plate with the center of the plate bender; the plates are designed to bend at the scored sections and not through the screw holes. Use only the AXIS plate bender to contour the plate. AXIS plates are made of titanium alloy. They cannot withstand contouring that exceeds the radius of curvature of the plate bender. AXIS plates cannot withstand back bending to a lesser contour once they are bent too much. Both situations reduce the plate's strength as occurs with any titanium implant. Bending irons may be used to add medial-lateral or torsional bends as desired. Using the template as a guide for plate contouring is helpful (Fig. 15-3).

Step Seven—Use Plate Holder and Screw Drivers to Secure Plate and Insert Screws

The plate holder will connect to the plate at any of the screw holes. Place the plate on the lateral mass in the desired position and insert screws. Inserting the most cranial and caudal screws first and second will aid in easy screw placement. Screws should be provisionally tightened to allow for a space beneath the plate for placement of bone graft. If the threads in bone are inadvertently stripped during insertion of a 3.5-mm cancellous screw, a 4.0-mm cancellous salvage screw should be inserted (Fig. 15-4).

Step Eight—Place Bone Graft under Plate and Tighten Screws

The concavity of the bone side of the AXIS plate is designed to allow for the placement of bone graft under the plate. After the desired amount of bone graft is placed, tighten all of the screws to two-finger tightness (Fig. 15-5).

The wound should be irrigated, drains should be placed if necessary, and the wound should then be closed in layers.

SUPPLEMENTAL FIXATION TECHNIQUES

Placement of an Interspinous Titanium Cable

Use of Atlas Cable System to Enhance Biomechanical Strength of Lateral Mass Fixation

The application of a tension band from the uppermost involved spinous process to the lowermost involved spinous process may supplement the overall strength of the AXIS fixation system when used as a lateral mass plate. The cable assists against possible screw failure in flexion by acting as a load-sharing tension-band component. Application

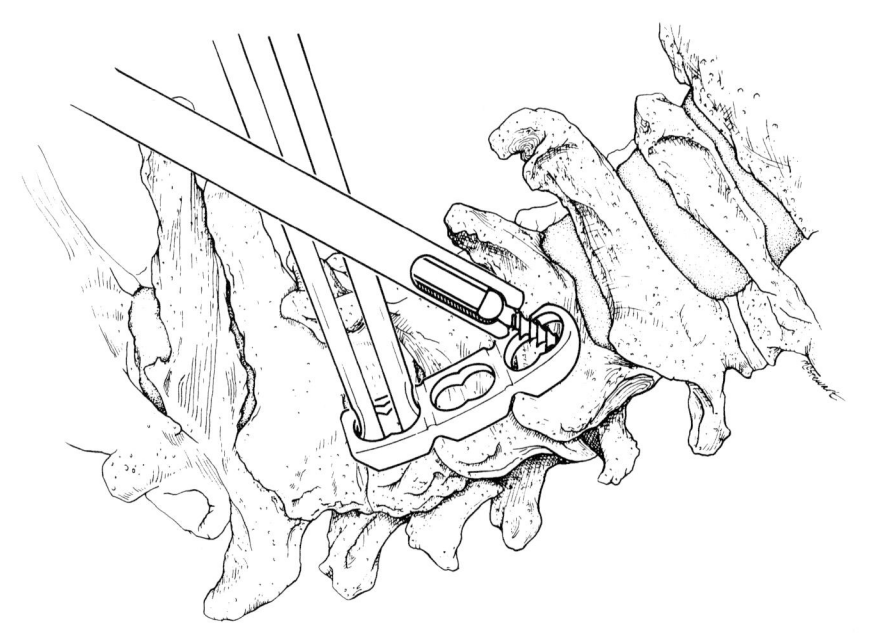

FIG. 15-4. The AXIS plate is secured with the pronged plate holder during screw insertion.

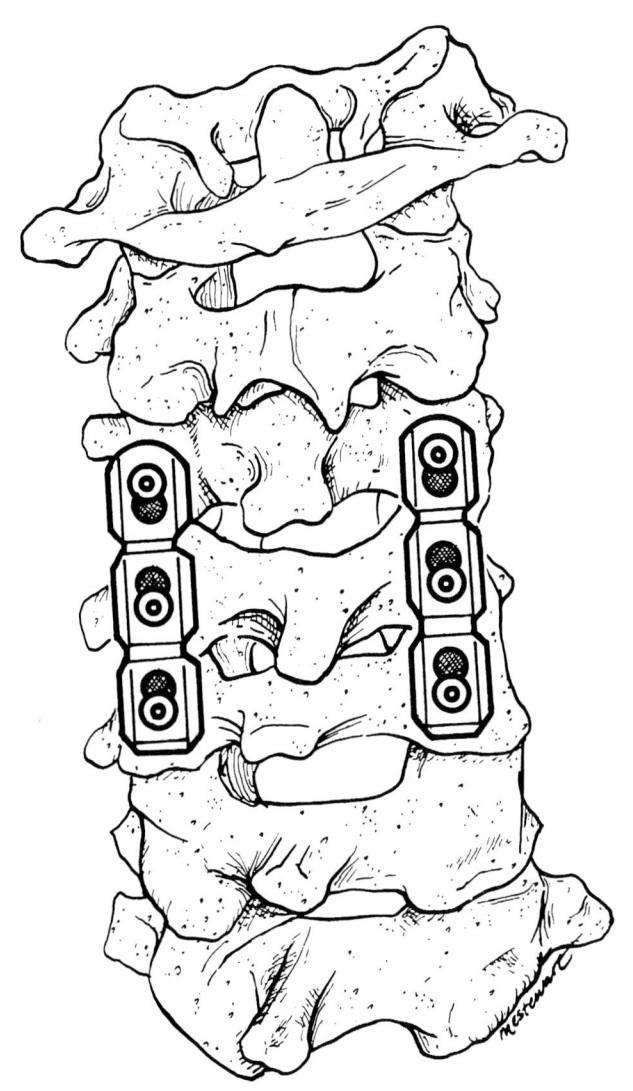

FIG. 15-5. The AXIS fixation system achieves optimal versatility in screw placement by providing various plate sizes and figure-of-eight slots in each segment of the plate.

of the cable prior to plate fixation can also improve the lordotic contour of the cervical spine. The cable should be placed after the facets are prepared for bone grafting and before the template is used to determine plate size and contour. Tension greater than 20 lb is rarely needed.

Indications and Placement of 4.0-mm Cortical Screws in Lateral Masses of the Atlas (C1) via Pedicles of Axis Vertebra (C2)

Use of AXIS Fixation System Screws for Atlantoaxial Stabilization and Promotion of Fusion

The screws of the AXIS fixation system can be used for stabilization of the atlantoaxial complex by the technique originally described by Magerl (Magerl and Seemann, 1985). This technique does not require utilization of AXIS plates, although they can be incorporated into multilevel occipitocervical, cervical, and cervicothoracic constructs along with the Magerl atlantoaxial fixation technique. In most cases, supplemental C1-2 posterior wiring should also be incorporated into the atlantoaxial Magerl screw construct. The AXIS fixation system also has instrumentation that allows for the percutaneous insertion of screws by the Magerl technique with fluoroscopic guidance. This minimally invasive technique minimizes soft-tissue trauma and maximizes early postoperative recovery.

Stabilization of the atlantoaxial complex is most often indicated for traumatic or rheumatoid instabilities. The Magerl technique itself is clearly outlined elsewhere in this book and use of AXIS screws in this application employs similar methods of insertion. Cortical screws of 4.0 mm are recommended.

Indications and Placement of 4.0-mm Cortical Screws in Vertebral Pedicles of Cervicothoracic Spine

Placement of Screws in Lower Cervical and Upper Thoracic Spine in Long Posterior Constructs

The insertion of 4.0-mm cortical AXIS screws into the pedicles of the cervicothoracic spine can increase the biomechanical strength of posterior cervical plate fixation. The lateral masses of C7 and T1 are often insufficient for screw placement and provide tenuous bony purchase at the caudal end of long constructs with significant flexural lever arms. This can result in implant failure due to screw pullout on cervical constructs that extend to the upper cervical spine or cross the cervicothoracic junction. In these situations AXIS 4.0-mm cortical screws can be placed into the pedicles of C7 and/or T1.

Screw Insertion Technique

Prior to consideration or placement of screws into the pedicles at the cervicothoracic junction, a CT scan is needed to assess any anatomical anomalies that may be present, such as congenital absence of a pedicle, pedicles that are too small and narrow to receive a screw, or vascular anomalies and abnormalities. The pedicle insertion sites should be determined prior to Step 1 of the AXIS lateral mass technique. This will allow for good screw alignment with the future cephalad screw sites. To assess the pedicular isthmus, it may be necessary to perform a laminotomy at C7 and/or T1. This window will allow for direct pedicle palpation with a narrow nerve hook or similar instrument. The medial and cranial borders of the pedicle can be defined, and the screw entry point thus marked. The approximate location of the T1 pedicle can be found at the intersection of a vertical line along the lamina-transverse process junction ("the valley") near the midpoint of the facet and a horizontal line along the middle of the transverse process. The intersection of these two lines is usually 1 to 2 mm caudal to the C7–T1 facet joint.

Step 1—Create Pilot Hole in Dorsal Cortex at Screw Entry Point. Decorticate the dorsal cortex with a burr until cancellous bone is seen. It may be necessary to drill through the caudal edge of the C6 facet for the C7 pedicle or C7 facet for the T1 pedicle.

Step 2—Establish Entry into Pedicle with Small Straight Curette. Using a 3-0 curette, create a funnel into the pedicle. Cancellous bone should be visualized in the center of the pedicle and cortical bone visualized on all sides of the pedicle. A straight-beaded tip probe (Holt) can be used to palpate the inner walls of the pedicle. The beaded probe can also be used to create a channel through the pedicle into the vertebral body by gently pushing the probe manually or tapping the probe with a mallet.

Step 3—Drill Pedicle with 4.0-mm Cortical Drill. Lock the drill stop at the desired depth, usually 28 to 30 mm for C7 and T1. Angle the drill 25 to 30 degrees medially. If there is a laminotomy, directly palpate the medial wall of the pedicle while drilling. Caution should be exercised if purchase on the ventral cortex is attempted; however, ventral cortical purchase is usually not necessary.

Step 4—Use Depth Gauge to Determine Exact Depth. The length on the depth gauge corresponds with the screw length. The depth gauge can also be used to confirm drill-hole placement by palpating the inside walls of the pedicle.

Step 5—Tap Drill Hole with 4.0-mm Cortical Tap. It is not necessary to tap the deepest cortex, but the posterior cortex and the pedicular isthmus should be tapped. The tap is graduated to display the depth of instrument penetration.

Step 6—Continue with Lateral Mass Fixation. The screw holes in the pedicles should be used as a guide for lining up the other more cephalad lateral mass entry points.

POSTOPERATIVE PLAN

The AXIS fixation system can provide secure vertebral stabilization when used as a lateral mass fixation system. Postoperatively, most patients need minimal orthotic support for comfort only, such as a soft cervical collar. A more rigid orthotic device may be needed at times, and a supplemental halo-vest orthotic device may be necessary on rare occasions. Regular postoperative examinations and radiographs are recommended.

INDICATIONS AND CONTRAINDICATIONS

Indications for application of the AXIS fixation system to the posterior cervical spine may be deduced from a clear understanding of the expected function of the implant (Table 15-1). Therefore, the surgeon may find the AXIS system useful, and at times essential, in treating patients with an extensive variety of spinal disorders (Table 15-2). Indications for use of the implant may be found in any disease process that renders the spine unstable, malaligned, unreduced, or painful provided that the nature of the condition is improved by decreasing spinal motion with a rigid implant system.

Other spinal disorders may be included when the clinical situation warrants. Of course, successful outcome relies heavily on the surgeon's understanding of the basic disease process, its role in production of the patient's symptoms and signs, the natural history of the disease process both without and with surgical intervention, the mechanical nature of the spinal disorder, and how the AXIS implant is expected to function to improve the clinical situation. Always keep in mind the basic functional capabilities of the AXIS system discussed previously.

Table 15-1
Functions of the AXIS System When Applied to Posterior Cervical Spine

1. Effect reduction and restore alignment
2. Maintain reduction and alignment
3. Restore stability
4. Promote fusion
5. Relieve mechanical pain
6. Protect neurovascular and other vital structures by attaining goals 1 through 4
7. Improve outcome of, increase safety factor of, and/or salvage or supplement anterior procedures

Table 15-2
Indications for Posterior Fixation with the AXIS System

1. Degeneration of the spine
   Spondylosis
   Degenerative disk disease
   Degenerative facet arthrosis

2. Inflammation and/or rheumatologic
   Rheumatoid arthritis
   Ankylosing spondylitis

3. Trauma to the spine
   Fractures
   Dislocations
   Subluxations

4. Neoplasia
   Benign
   Malignant

5. Congenital/developmental disorders
   Os odontoideum
   Aplastic dens

6. Iatrogenic instability
   Postlaminectomy
   Postfacetectomy
   Failed fusion

7. Deformity of the spine

Table 15-3
Contraindications to Posterior Lateral Mass Stabilization with the AXIS System

Active local or systemic infection
Significant risk of infection (immunocompromise)
Shortened life expectancy (malignant neoplasia)
Debility
Mental incompetence
Poor bone quality (osteoporosis, osteomalacia, osteodystrophy, etc.)
Anatomic constraints (congenital anomaly, infancy and early childhood, etc.)
Metal allergy
Inadequate hospital facilities and/or support personnel
Inadequate surgeon training and/or preparation

Relative contraindications to use of the AXIS implant exist and should be assessed adequately prior to its use. Contraindications are listed in Table 15-3. This list, although not exhaustive or complete, may serve as a guide to assist the surgeon in analyzing the factors that may adversely affect eventual outcome.

Finally, a comparison of AXIS fixation system to other methods of posterior cervical fixation is made in Table 15-4.

CASE REPORT

H.H. was a 54-year-old electrician with chief complaints of pain, paresthesiae, weakness, and incoordination of the upper extremities when first evaluated in 1993. MRI revealed severe stenosis C3-C7. Same day anterior/posterior cervical decompression and reconstruction was performed. Laminectomy C4-C6 with keyhole foraminotomies, bone grafting with freeze dried allograft cancellous chips, and posterior segmental plate and screw fixation of the lateral masses

Table 15-4
AXIS Fixation System Comparison Chart

		Wire/Bone	Wire/Rod	AO Reconstruction Plate (Anderson)	Haid Plate	AXIS
1.	Requires intact lamina and spinous processes	Yes	Yes	No	No	No
2.	Mechanical stability in all planes of motion	Poor	Fair	Better	Good*	Best†
3.	Occipitocervical and cervicothoracic fixation	Yes	Yes	Yes	No	Yes‡
4.	Versatility for screw location and angulation in lateral mass	NA	NA	Minimal	Minimal	Maximal
5.	Screw diameter, length, and thread types	NA	NA	Many options	Few options	Many options
6.	Static and fatigue strength of plates	NA	NA	Good§	NT	Best§
7.	Difficult reconstructive problems: deformity, instability, multilevel constructs, osteoporosis	Poor	Fair	Fair	Poor	Best
8.	Cost of device	Cheapest	Moderate	More expensive	More expensive	More expensive
9.	FDA issues: Off-label use of device, requires specific patient consent	NA	Unknown	Yes	Yes	Yes
10.	Overall versatility	Poor	Fair	Good	Poor	Best

*Mechanical stability compromised compared to other two plating systems due to poor pullout strength of screw design.

†When compared with AO reconstruction plate (Anderson): (a) stronger plate (static and fatigue); (b) more fixation points in long multilevel constructs (maximal versatility of screw placement points); (c) much stronger occipital fixation with maximal bony purchase of custom device.

‡AXIS custom device allows seven screws in occiput with three screws (10–14 mm) in thick midline bone. AO reconstruction plate allows 2–3 screws only (4 mm) in each thin lateral occipital bone. European Y plate (Allopro, Switzerland) allows only 2 screws in midline.

§Four point bending test to simulate flexion in static loading and fatigue. NA = not applicable; NT = not tested. *Source:* Sutterlin, C.E. (1994). AXIS fixation system for posterior cervical reconstruction. In: P.W. Hitchon, S. Reganachary, & V. Traynclis (Eds.) (1994) *Techniques in Spinal Fusion and Stabilization* (pp. 159–169). New York: Thieme.

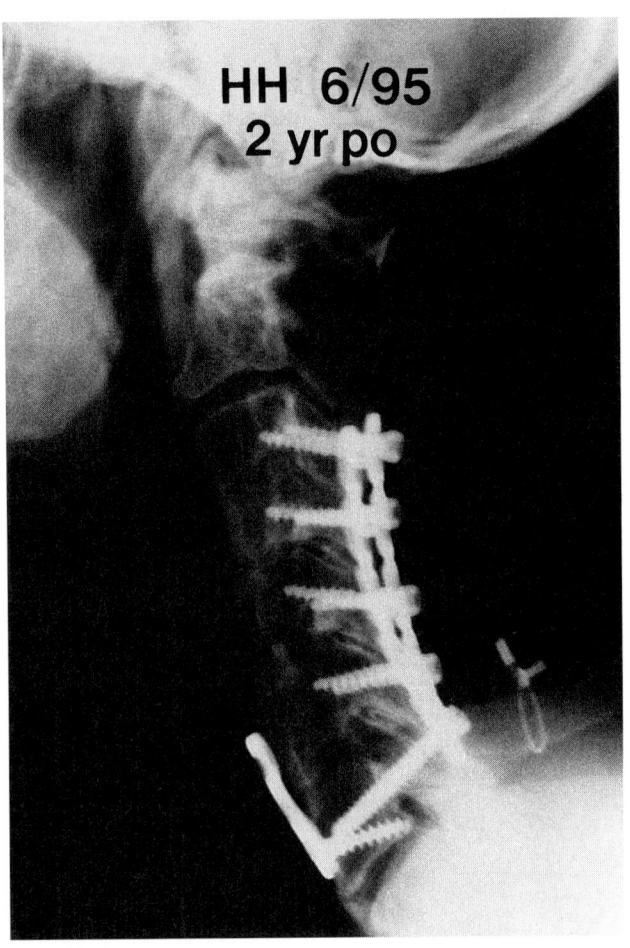

FIG. 15-6. C3-C7 anterior and posterior fusion and fixation using AXIS plates and anterior buttress plate fixation.

tress plate fixation. On the two year postoperative lateral radiograph (Fig. 15-6) note:

1. Excellent cervical lordosis.
2. Anterior and posterior bone grafting optimize fusion rate even when utilizing allograft.
3. Anterior buttress plate minimizes potential for strut graft dislodgment at caudal end, but does not stress shield strut graft and is easier to insert than plate extending from C2-C7.
4. Posterior plate and screw fixation of the lateral masses with supplemental tension band cable C2-C7 optimize ability to create cervical lordosis while minimizing mechanical failure due to segmental fixation obtained. The construct is not entirely rigid, however, which is less likely to result in stress shielding of bone grafts.
5. Pedicle screws in C7 minimize possibility of mechanical failure at caudal end of long constructs caused by pullout of screws during flexion. The lateral masses of C7 are less thick than other cervical levels accepting only shorter screws. Pedicle screws can also be inserted at upper thoracic levels.

The patient returned to full employment 11 weeks after surgery with minimal symptoms and remains so at the time of this report 2.5 years after surgery.

C3-C7 with supplemental tension band cable was followed by corpectomy C4, C5, and C6, bone grafting with freeze dried allograft tricortical iliac strut C3-C7, and anterior but-

REFERENCES

An H.S., Gordin R., & Renner K. (1991). Anatomic considerations for plate-screw fixation of the cervical spine. *Spine, 16,* No. 10-S, S549-S553.

Roy-Camille R., Mazel C.H., & Saillant G. (1987). Treatment of cervical spine injuries by a posterior osteosynthesis with plates and screws. In: P. Kehr, & A. Weidner (Eds.), *Cervical Spine I* (p. 163). New York, Springer-Verlag.

Magerl F., Grob D., & Seemann P. (1987). Stable dorsal fusion of the cervical spine (C2-T1) using hook plates. In: P. Kehr, & A. Weidner (Eds.), *Cervical Spine I* (p. 217). New York: Springer-Verlag.

Magerl F., & Seemann P.S. (1985). Stable posterior fusion of the atlas and axis by transarticular screw fixation. In P. Kehr, & A. Weidner (Eds.) *Cervical Spine I* (p. 332–327). New York: Springer-Verlag.

CHAPTER 16

Application of the Roy-Camille Posterior Screw Plate Fixation System for Stabilization of the Cervical Spine

R. Roy-Camille
Claude Laville

HIGHLIGHTS

Most of the lesions of the cervical spine can be treated posteriorly by screw plate fixation. In an emergency, the posterior approach is safe, quick, and simple, and the screw plate fixation will give a safe and strong osteosynthesis. We have used posterior fixation for 25 years on all traumatic lesions of the cervical spine, except for body fractures, which are treated with an anterior procedure.

THE PLATES AND SCREWS

The plates and screws are made of stainless steel or titanium (Fig. 16-1).

Lower Cervical Spine

The Plates

At the level of C2 to T1, the osteosynthesis is performed with premolded plates to restore cervical lordosis. These plates are 2 mm thick and 1 cm wide. The holes are positioned every 13 mm, which corresponds to the average distance between two articular masses. Four types of plates are available, to bridge two to five vertebrae.

Special tile plates have been designed to treat fracture dislocation of the articular masses or separation fracture of the mass. These tile plates are made either to replace an upper facet or to support a lower one while healing. These plates are made up of two parts. One vertical part with two holes is available in two different sizes in order to bridge one or two articular masses. The second part of the plate is oblique, with a 60-degree angulation on the first part, and corresponds to the angle of the facets on the mass.

The Screw

The screw diameter is 3.5 mm. Length varies from 15 to 18 mm. The screws are self-tapping.

Upper Cervical Spine

To stabilize the occipitocervical junction, we use a special premolded plate. Its shape is designed to restore the normal curve of the occipitocervical junction with a 105-degree angulation.

These plates are thickened in their middle at the top of the curve. The occipital part of the plates has been flattened in order to prevent skin compression and scarring. On the cervical part the holes are circularly reinforced.

Two types of plates are available to bridge the occiput to C4 or the occiput to C5. The fixation on the occiput is lateral and is achieved with 9- to 13-mm-long screws, diameter 3.5 mm. The screws in the masses are the same as those used in the normal procedure (16 to 18 mm long).

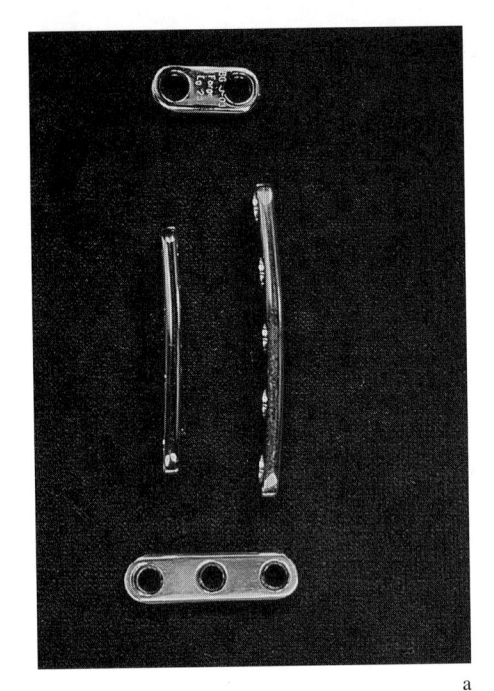

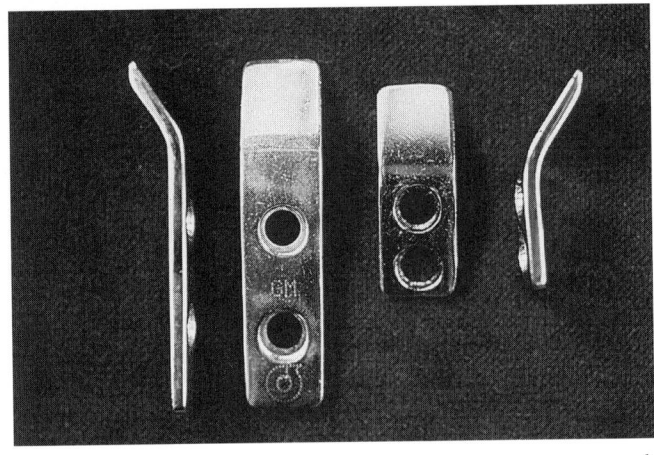

148 PART 2 / POSTERIOR CERVICAL INSTRUMENTATION

FIG. 16-1. (a) Roy-Camille cervical plates, 2 to 5 holes. (b) Roy-Camille tile plates to replace a broken facet.

SURGICAL TECHNIQUE

Approach

The procedure is performed through a midposterior approach (Fig. 16-2). The patient is placed in a prone position and the head is firmly fixed in a head holder that enables flexion-extension. Local lidocaine and adrenaline infiltration helps the approach—dividing the muscles on the midline—and diminishes the bleeding.

The posterior approach is achieved primarily with electrocautery. One must go down to the lateral side of the articular masses in order to locate exactly the reference marks to implant the screws.

Lower Cervical Spine

Fixation of the cervical spine is performed in the articular masses. The screws are not implanted into the pedicle of the vertebra at the cervical level, as we do at the thoracic or lumbar level, because the pedicle is too thin to admit a screw at this level, and it is too close to the vertebral artery.

To implant a screw in an articular mass, one must know the exact anatomy of the cervical spine in order to avoid the

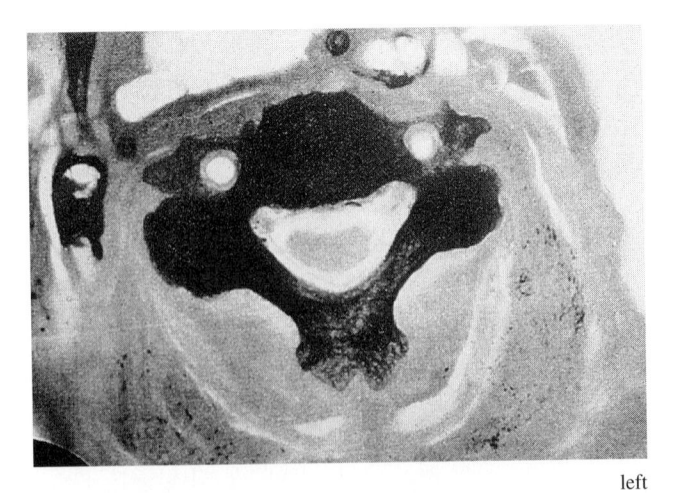

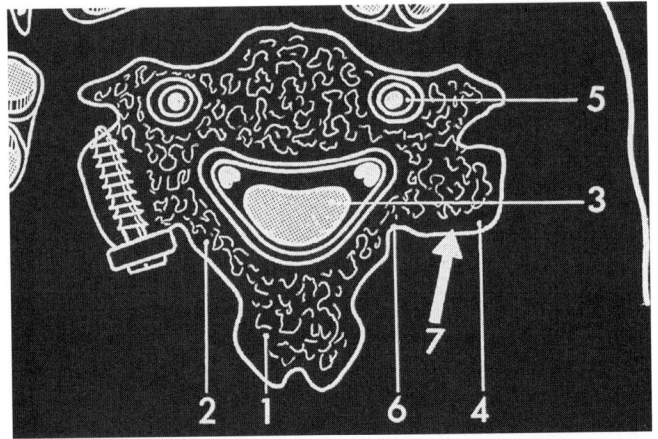

FIG. 16-2. (Left and Right) Slice through C4 showing the correct point of penetration of the cervical screw: (1) spinous process, (2) lamina, (3) cord, (4) articular mass, (5) vertebral artery, (6) valley, and (7) point of penetration and direction of the screw.

three main elements: the cord, the vertebral artery, and the roots. In fact, through the posterior approach one can see only the posterior aspect of the vertebra. From this posterior aspect, the landmarks must be precisely known in order to avoid the previous elements.

Through the posterior approach, the spinous processes are on the midline, the laminae and the articular masses more laterally. In front of the laminae is the cord. Between the articular mass and the laminae is a depression that can be compared with a valley. The articular mass can in this way be compared to a hill. This helps to remind one that in front of the depression (valley) flows the vertebral artery, as it can be demonstrated on a slice through C4. The valley must be avoided during the procedure. On a lateral view of the articular mass, one can see that the roots are in the gutter of the superior aspect of the pedicles distant from the center of the articular masses.

According to these different anatomical features, the best point of penetration of the screw will be exactly in the middle and at the top of the hill that can be seen through the posterior approach. Therefore, this point has to be exactly in the center of the articular mass (Fig. 16-3).

From this point of penetration, drilling should be oblique, 10 degrees lateral, to be sure to avoid the vertebral artery. The first cortex of the mass will be stopped with an awl, and a 2.8-mm drill bit with a stop at 18 mm will be used. This will go through the two cortices. Some surgeons prefer to stop the drill bit before the second cortex and to go through this one only with the self-taping screw.

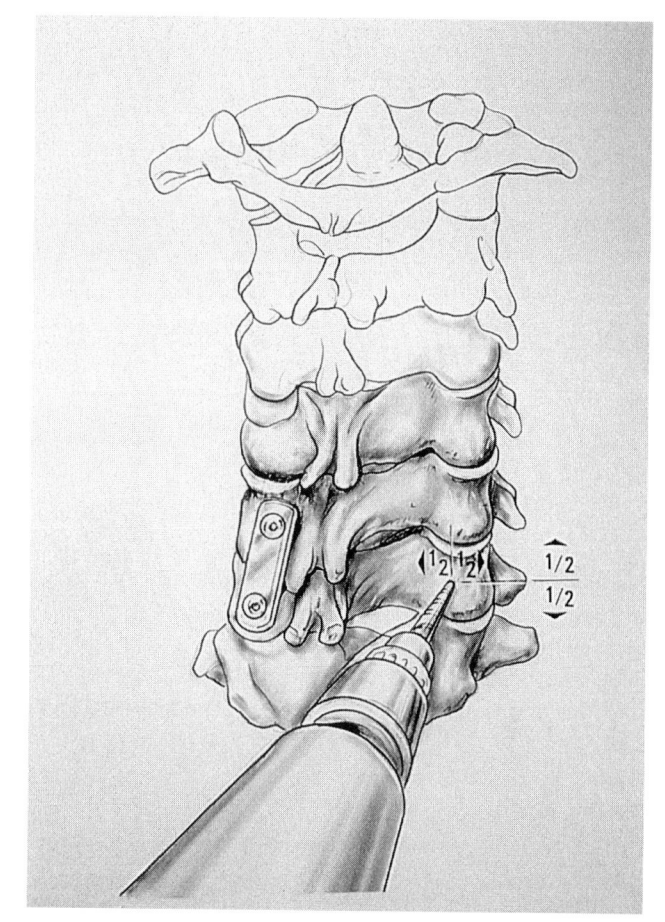

FIG. 16-3. Correct position of the drilling. Note the position of the drill bit on the articular mass and the direction.

UPPER CERVICAL SPINE

The lower screws of the plates from C2 to C4 or C5 are implanted in the articular mass as previously described. The fixation of the occiput is lateral in order to avoid the median venous sinus. Fixation is achieved with 9- to 13-mm-long screws and the drilling is performed straightforwardly with a depth gauge drill of 12 mm. The screw penetrates into the skull through the deep cortex without any neurologic damage because of the protection of the cerebrospinal fluid.

The table head holder allows one to bring the occipito-cervical junction to the premolded plates, and therefore, to restore the normal position of the head. This is important for horizontal vision postoperatively. Implantation of the screws is usually started from the occiput because some flexion of the head can help to drive the lower occipital screws.

INDICATIONS

Lower Cervical Spine

In our 25-year experience, and in a continuous series of 221 cases, all lesions of the lower cervical spine except body fractures can be treated posteriorly (this includes 90% of the cervical traumas). This posterior approach is safe and simple, and the stability provided by plating shortens the time of hospitalization. The patient is able to walk the day after surgery if there is no neurologic involvement, and will be discharged from the hospital on the fourth or fifth postoperative day (Table 16-1).

Traumatic lesions of the cervical spine can be divided in three types: (1) posterior lesions (67% of the series), includes: dislocations that can be unilateral or bilateral, fracture-dislocations, and articular mass separation fracture (AMSF); (2) midvertebral segment lesions (22%), include: severe sprains and teardrop fractures; and (3) anterior vertebral segment lesions (11%), or body fractures.

Dislocation (21%)

Unilateral Dislocation (13%). In these cases reduction is achieved operatively with a spatula introduced between the laminae at the dislocated level. The first spatula is introduced near the midline close to the spinous process and starts the reduction with a lever maneuver. While the first spatula is kept in place, a second one is introduced laterally and improves the reduction (Figs. 16-4, 16-5 and 16-6).

150 PART 2 / POSTERIOR CERVICAL INSTRUMENTATION

Table 16-1
Indications for Roy-Camille Posterior Screw Plate Fixation of the Lower Cervical Spine

Vertebral segment	Approach	Type of lesion	Fixation
Posterior	Posterior	Unilateral or bilateral dislocation	Operative reduction—2 two-hole plates
	Posterior	Fracture dislocation	Reduction—Removal of the fragment Tile plate: short *porte-manteau*—1 disk level
	Posterior	Articular mass separation fracture	Reduction of the mass Tile plate: long *porte-manteau* + opposite 3-hole plate levels
Middle	Post	Severe sprains Teardrop fractures	Fixation with 2 two-hole plates
Anterior	Anterior	Body fracture	Corporectomy + iliac graft + staple

The first spatula is then placed further on, between the dislocated articular facets, and the lever maneuver achieves the reduction by moving the upper articular facet backward over the lower one. Reduction is then stabilized by the table head holder positioned in extension and with the special "sea urchin" reduction forceps applied on the spinous processes or on the laminae.

A first posterior two-hole plate is implanted on the dislocated side and the fixation is completed with a second plate on the opposite side. Drilling the screws is normally

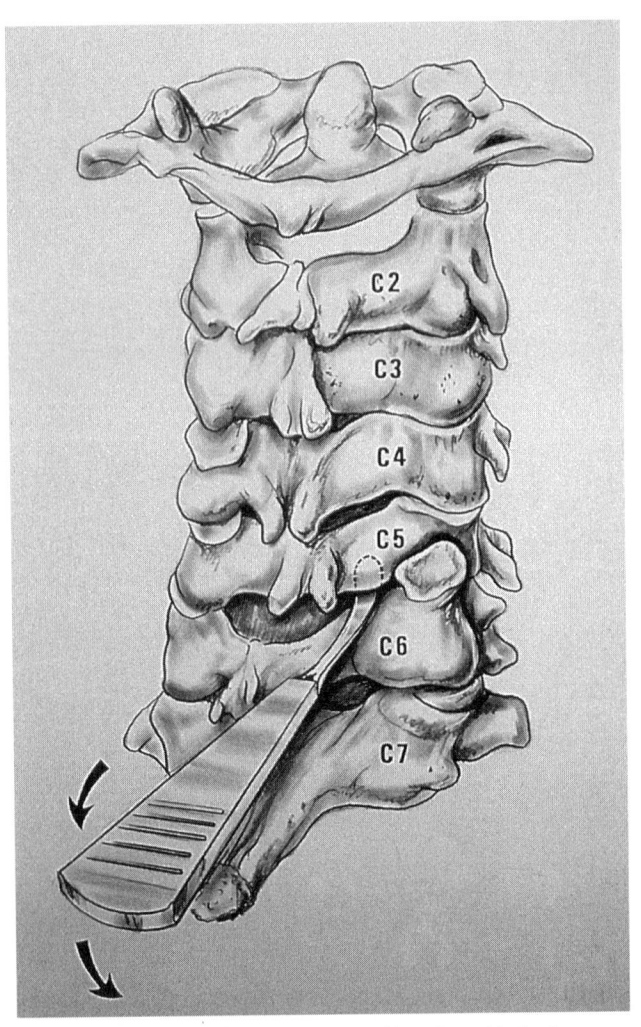

FIG. 16-4. Reduction of a C5-6 unilateral luxation with the lever maneuver.

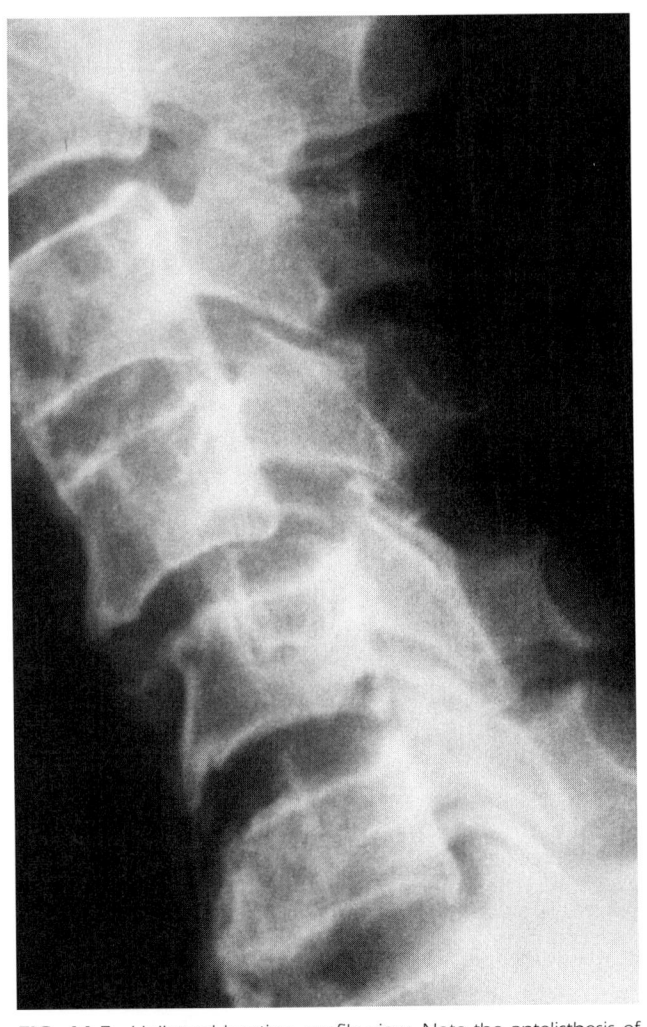

FIG. 16-5. Unilateral luxation, profile view. Note the antelisthesis of the vertebral body and the rotation of the articular mass.

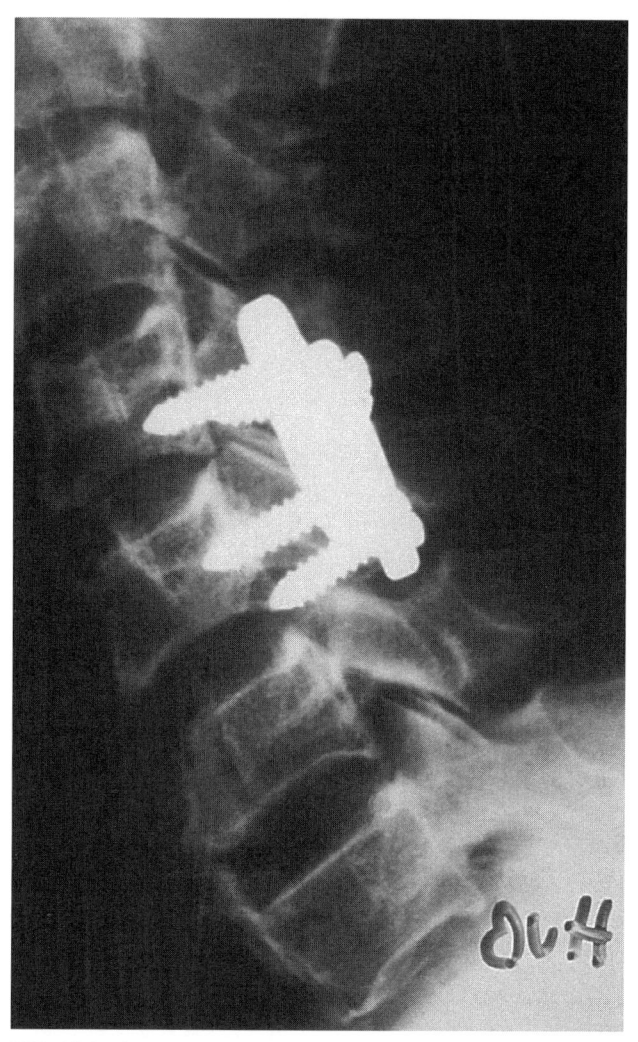

FIG. 16-6. Same patient as in Fig. 16-5, postoperatively, profile view reduction and fixation with 2 two-hole plates.

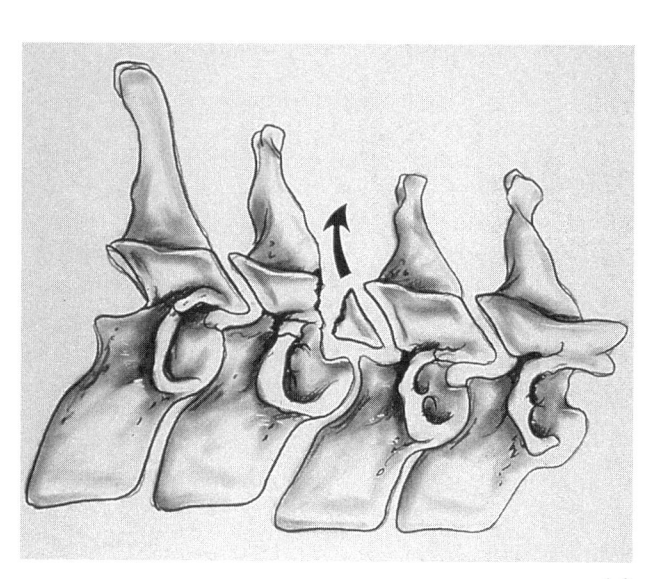

performed on the top of the articular mass. Because reduction is usually not complete, the holes are more than 13 mm distant. One screw is normally implanted but not tightened; then the second one is driven obliquely to the second hole, and during its implantation it will achieve the perfect reduction. The two screws are finally firmly tightened.

Bilateral Dislocation (8%). The same maneuver with the spatula is performed on both sides symetrically. Once again the stabilization is achieved with two posterior two-hole plates. The fixation of one-level dislocation with the two-hole plate is strong enough to prevent any secondary displacement.

This procedure is very simple and quick and it provides very good stability of the damaged level.

Facet-Joint Fractures and Dislocations (37%)

A facet-joint fracture will induce a dislocation that is much more unstable than a simple dislocation (Fig. 16-7). This is usually a fracture of the upper articular facet. The support of the vertebra above disappears unilaterally and a rotational displacement occurs. The broken fragment is pushed into the foramen and can compress the ipsilateral cervical nerve root.

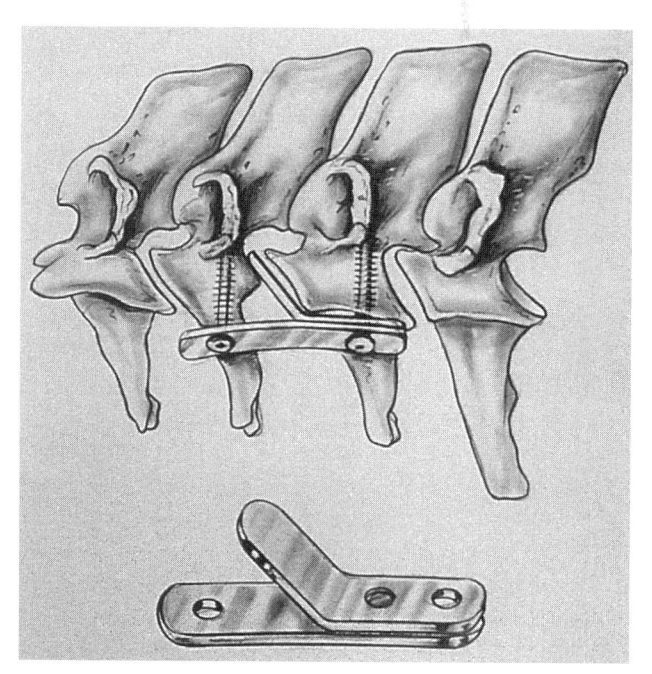

left   right

FIG. 16-7. (*Left* and *Right*) Fracture of the upper facet. Note the antelisthesis. Treatment: *porte-manteau* procedure with the tile plate after removal of the broken facet.

The displaced compressive fragment must be removed from the foramen before achieving fixation. This can be performed only with a posterior approach through the facet joint.

After the removal of the broken fragment, reduction and fixation are then achieved with reconstruction of the broken articular facet using a tile-shaped plate. This is a true joint replacement. The upper oblique part of the plate is slipped beneath the facet of the upper rotated vertebra. The lower part of the plate is pushed forward, reducing the rotation, and then is fixed in the articular mass with screws. We combine a tile plate with a standard two-hole plate. The normal plate is placed over the tile plate like a *porte-manteau.* Fixation is achieved with a lower screw driven through the lower holes of the two plates and an upper screw is implanted into the articular mass of the vertebra above through the two-hole plate. A simple two-hole plate is also implanted on the opposite side.

In some cases there is a sprain of the level below. It is then recommended to use a long tile plate with a long *porte-manteau* fixation bridging three vertebrae.

Separation-Fracture of Articular Mass (9%)

This fracture is difficult to stabilize (Figs. 16-8 and 16-9). Two fracture lines separate the articular mass from the rest of the vertebra. The first one is on the pedicle, the second one is on the lamina on the same side. Thus, the articular mass is completely liberated from the vertebra and will rotate with the upper or the lower adjacent vertebra. On lateral x-ray films it appears horizontal and no longer parallel to the adjacent facets; this is pathognomonic.

The fracture lines can be demonstrated on the lamina (anteroposterior view), or on the pedicle (oblique view). The correct reduction and fixation of such fractures is achieved with a long *porte-manteau* on the side of the articular mass fracture. In our experience to obtain a stable construct a simple three-hole plate is mandatory on the opposite side, symmetrical in length.

Severe sprains (14%)

These need to be well understood because they are often misdiagnosed. The whole mobile vertebral segment is involved by the trauma but without any bony lesion. Induced by the continuous movement of the neck, displacement occurs a few weeks or months later and is characterized by the following: interspinous widening, facet joint subluxation, posterior disk opening, and anterior slipping of the upper vertebra. In such cases dynamic lateral radiographs, performed 2 weeks after the injury when the muscle spasm has disappeared are very important to avoid missing the diagnosis. Fixation with two-hole posterior plates and screws is a simple and perfect technique for stabilization of these lesions. A Hibbs fusion is helpful in such cases.

Teardrop Fracture (8%)

The teardrop fracture is more like a severe sprain than a fracture. The lesions are indeed mainly on the disk and the ligaments, and the small broken bony fragment of the vertebral body is not important. Instability comes from the severe sprain. When the injury is primarily posterior with demonstrable interspinous widening and posterior facet joint opening, the surgical treatment can be performed posteriorly with posterior plates to reduce and to bridge just the involved level with two-hole plates. Anterior grafting would have to bridge two levels to have good support on the normal adjacent vertebral plateaux.

Failure of Anterior Stabilization

Posterior fixation with plates and screws is a very simple and elegant method to achieve a fusion after a failed anterior procedure. Posterior stable fixation induces the anterior fusion. A Hibbs fusion is usually done on the laminae.

Complementary Procedures

The posterior approach and the use of posterior plates and screws implanted into the articular masses enables different associated procedures. A laminectomy is easily performed when necessary because the plates are lateral to the laminae on the articular masses.

It was pointed out that grafting is not necessary for patients with pure dislocation. But for those with associated fractures a Hibbs fusion on the laminae is always possible, if desired.

The only contraindication to this plating method is a severe degree of osteoporosis.

Postoperative Care and Results

Simple injuries such as unilateral dislocations are immobilized by a simple collar for 5 weeks. More unstable lesions with associated fractures are immobilized for 2 to 3 months by a light plastic or leather Minerva jacket. In case of cord injury with tetraplegia, the stable fixation induced by the plates facilitates the nursing care.

The mechanical stability of this fixation is demonstrated by the study of a series of 221 patients with lower cervical spine injuries treated by this technique. There has been no secondary displacement in 85.2% of the patients and displacement of less than 5 degrees in 8.8%, of 5 to 10 degrees in 3%, and over 10 degrees in 3%. No breakage of plates or screws has been observed.

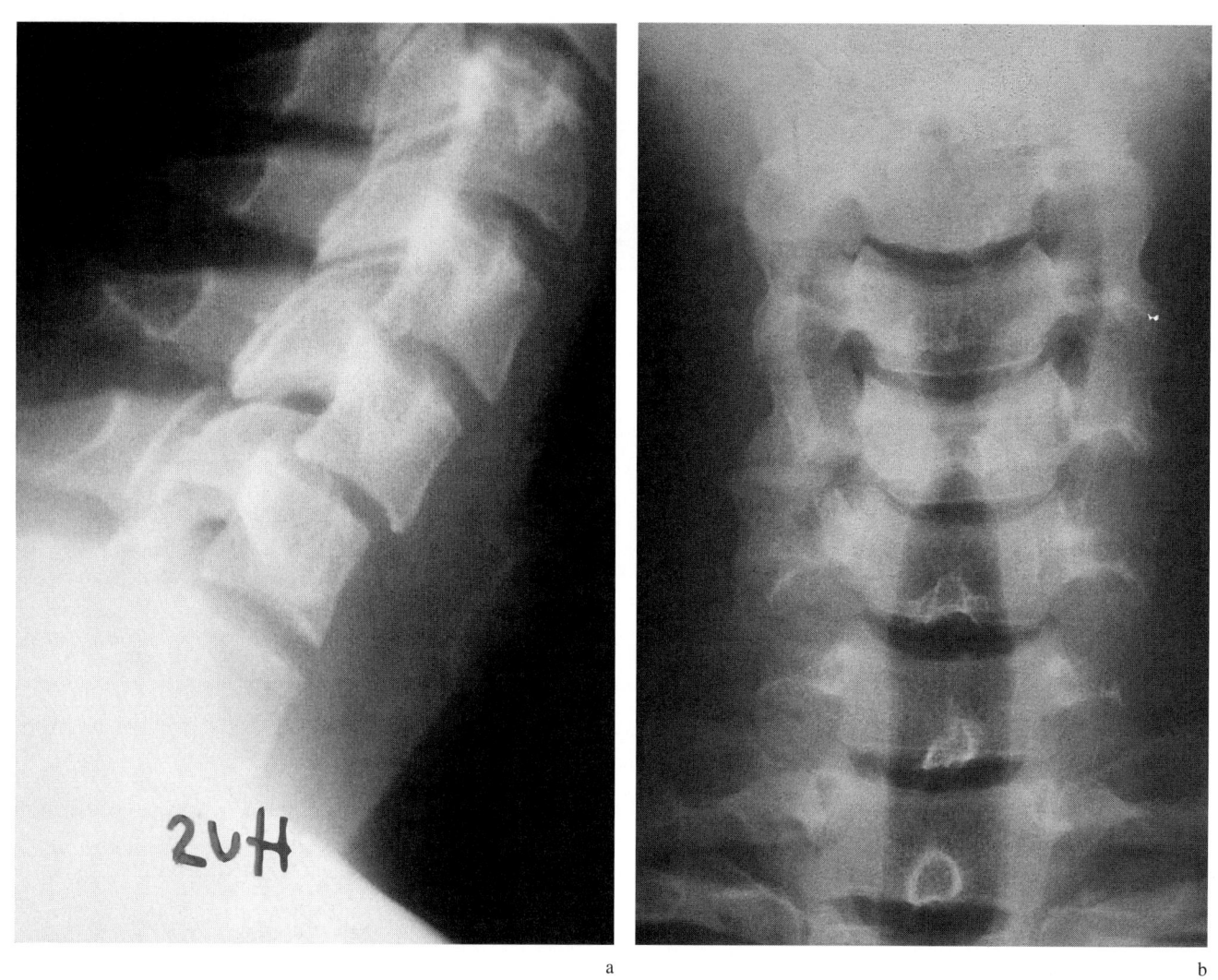

FIG. 16-8. (a and b) Articular mass separation fracture. Note the position of the mass on the profile view.

Upper Cervical Spine

Upper cervical spine lesions can be treated with a screw plate fixation through a posterior approach (Table 16-2).

Hangman's Fracture

When the fracture is stable and displacement minimal, without important damage to the disk and ligaments, healing will occur with conservative treatment. But when there is severe damage of the C2-3 mobile segment (anterior displacement plus posterior opening of the disk), and in the presence of an associated C2-3 facet dislocation, surgical treatment is necessary to reduce and stabilize the lesion. In the latter case, reduction of the facet joints is impossible with traction alone and must be achieved through a posterior surgical approach. Fixation will be performed with 2 two-hole plates, which stabilize C2-3. The upper screws must be driven into the C2 pedicles, achieving the direct fixation of the fracture lines.

This technique is difficult and demands very precise anatomic landmarks to prevent vertebral artery injury.

The superior border of the C2 lamina has to be cleared. Then a slightly curved spatula is introduced into the large vertebral canal along the medial aspect of the pedicle. The posterior aspect of the articular mass of C2 can be divided in four quarters. The optimal point of screw penetration is in the upper and medial quadrant. Once this point of penetration has been determined and prepared with the awl, drilling can be performed with control of the spatula in the vertebral canal. This drilling is directed obliquely upward and inward 10 to 15 degrees. The drill bit must be as close as possible to the medial and the upper cortices of the

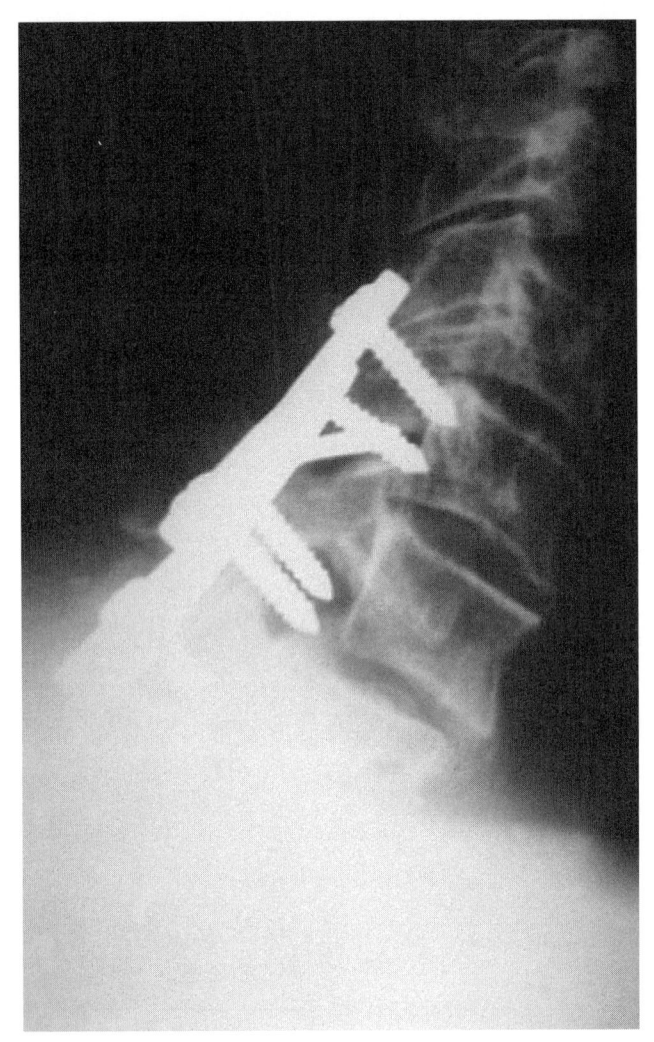

FIG. 16-9. Articular mass separation fracture. Treatment: long *portemanteau* procedure.

pedicle. Depth should be 35 mm deep. The vertebral artery, therefore, remains lateral and inferior to the drill bit. A 35-mm-long screw can be inserted up to the anterior cortex of the C2 vertebral body.

Once the C2 pedicle has been drilled, the C3 articular mass has to be drilled in the middle of the mass going 10 degrees laterally. Then a two-hole plate is inserted with a 15-mm-long screw in C3 and a 35-mm-long screw in the pedicle of C2.

Occipitocervical Fusion

This indication is more frequent in degenerative lesions. However two indications of trauma lesions exist, as discussed below.

Occipitocervical Dislocation. This type of dislocation is usually immediately fatal. We have observed two patients who survived. One patient needed a simple fusion with two molded plates and graft and the other needed reduction with light traction followed by a two-plate fixation for the fresh one. It is important to recognize the difficulty of this diagnosis and the importance of the anterior occipitocervical line, which is normally continuous and regular.

Surgery is performed through the posterior approach. The plates are implanted normally in the articular masses from C2 to C4 or C5 and in the occiput. The occiput and the spinous processes are decorticated and a corticocancellous graft is placed on the spinous processes and screwed on to the occiput.

Teardrop Fracture of C2. If there is significant instability, these fractures have to be fixed by an occipitocervical fusion. In cases of lesser instability, a simple C2-3 stabilization is sufficient. This fixation is then performed with two posterior two-hole plates with the screws implanted into C2 pedicles and C3 articular masses.

CONCLUSION

Posterior screw plate fixation is safe, strong, and simple and may be indicated in over 90% of lower cervical traumas. This fixation is effective, as demonstrated by the mechanical results in our patients: 85.2% have perfect stability and 8.8% have secondary displacement of less than 5 degrees.

At the upper cervical spine, the use of special occipitocervical plates increases confidence in the immediate postoperative stability when an occipitocervical fusion is necessary.

Table 16-2
Indications for Roy-Camille Posterior Screw Plate Fixation of the Upper Cervical Spine

Hangman's fracture	Stable	Conservative treatment	
	Displaced with C2-3 sprain	C2-3 plating with C2 pedicle screws	
Occipitocervical dislocation	New	Reduction—Occipitocervical fusion	2 Occipitocervical plates Corticocancellous graft
	Old	In-place fixation	
C2 teardrop fracture	Stable	C2-3 plating	
	Unstable	Occipitocervical fusion with occipitocervical plates + corticocancellous graft	

BIBLIOGRAPHY

Roy-Camille, R. (1988). Rachis cervical inferieur. In: R. Roy-Camille (Ed.), *Sixième Journée d'Orthopédie de la PITIE*. Paris: Masson.

Roy-Camille R., Mazel, C., & Saillant G. (1990). Rationale and techniques of internal fixation in trauma of the cervical spine. In: *Treatment of Surgical Spine Disease* (163–191). New York: Springer-Verlag.

Roy-Camille, R., Saillant, G., & Lazennec, J.Y. (1987). Chirurgie par abord posterieur du rachis cervical. In: Techniques Chirurgicales (Orthopédie). *Encyclopédie Médico-Chirurgicale*. Paris.

Roy-Camille, R., Saillant, G., & Mazel, C. (1989). Internal fixation of the unstable cervical spine by a posterior osteosynthesis with plates. In: M.M. Sherk (Ed.), *The Cervical Spine* (390–421). Philadelphia: J.B. Lippincott.

Roy-Camille, R., Saillant, G., & Mazel, C. (1979). Rachis cervical traumatique non neurologique. In: R. Roy-Camille (Ed.), *Première Journées d'Orthopédie de la PITIE*. Paris: Masson.

Roy-Camille, R., Saillant, G., & Sagnet P. (1985). Luxation fracture du rachis. In: P.H. Detrie (Ed.), *Chirurgie d'Urgence*. Paris: Masson.

PART 3

Anterior Thoracolumbar Instrumentation

CHAPTER 17

Application of the Kaneda Anterior Spinal Stabilization System

Terry J. Coyne
Michael G. Fehlings

HIGHLIGHTS

Kaneda anterior spinal instrumentation was developed by Kiyoshi Kaneda of the Hokkaido University School of Medicine in an effort to improve the management of thoracolumbar burst fractures. This type of injury had been characterized in 1970 (Holdsworth, 1970), with the standard treatment options traditionally being bed rest, cast, and brace (Reid, Hu, Davis, & Saboe, 1988); posterior fusion (classically extending from three levels above to two levels below the fracture) with Harrington instrumentation (Dickson, Harrington, & Erwin, 1978); and anterior decompression with strut grafting, followed by posterior stabilization to prevent graft collapse and kyphosis (Whitesides & Shar, 1976). The early 1980s saw the introduction of treatment of these injuries with one-stage anterior decompression, strut grafting, and internal fixation. Anterior instrumentation devices such as the Dwyer (Dwyer, Newton, & Sherwood, 1969) and Zielke (Kaneda, Hashimoto, & Albumi, 1986) systems had been developed for scoliosis correction, and these led to the development of devices for the treatment of thoracolumbar fractures, such as the Kostuik-Harrington system (a modified anterior Harrington instrumentation system) (Kostuik, 1983), and the Dunn (1986) device, which although biomechanically sound was associated with a number of catastrophic late vascular erosions (Jendrisak, 1986). Using concepts similar to those of Kostuik and Dunn, Kaneda developed an anterior device utilizing vertebral plates, screws, and threaded rods with nuts. The results of the use of this device in thoracolumbar burst fractures were initially presented in 1982, and subsequently published in 1984. Since then, the Kaneda device has been used for a wide range of spinal disorders, with later modifications enabling multisegmental fixation to be performed. With the development of flexible rods, this multisegmental device has been adapted for use in the correction of scoliosis.

In essence, the Kaneda anterior device was designed to allow one-stage anterior decompression, realignment of kyphotic angulation, and stabilization with fixation at a single level above and below the site of decompression.

Kaneda anterior spinal instrumentation is manufactured and supplied in North America by AcroMed (Cleveland, OH).

INDICATIONS

In general terms, anterior instrumentation in the thoracolumbar spine is appropriate to provide stabilization following loss of integrity of the anterior and middle columns, either as the result of a pathologic process or when corpectomy has been required to decompress the thecal sac (Tables 17-1 and 17-2).

Thoracolumbar Fractures

Although some aspects of management remain controversial, we believe an anterior procedure is indicated for thoracolumbar burst fractures (anterior and middle column disruption) with neurologic deficit with any degree of canal compromise, ≥50% canal compromise without neurologic deficit, ≥50% loss of vertebral-body height, or ≥20 degrees kyphosis.

Table 17-1
Indications and Contraindications for Use of the Kaneda Anterior Spinal Device

Indications
  Thoracolumbar instability due to loss of anterior and middle column integrity, as the result of disease or in the process of anterior decompression of the thecal sac.
  Burst fracture with:
    Neurologic deficit with any canal compromise
    ≥ 50% canal compromise with no neurologic deficit
    ≥ 50% loss of vertebral-body height
    ≥ 20 degrees of kyphosis
  Late posttraumatic kyphosis with:
    Progressive deformity
    Progressive neurologic deficit
    Pain
  After anterior decompression for neoplasm or infection
  Scoliosis repair

Contraindications
  Posterior column disruption (associated anterior compression may require anterior decompression, but if so this needs to be accompanied by posterior stabilization)
  Difficult to apply Kaneda device above T10 or below L4

Table 17-2
Advantages and Disadvantages of the Anterior Approach with Instrumentation for Anterior Lesions

Advantages
  Assured decompression of thecal sac
  Decompression plus stabilization possible by one approach at one procedure
  Shorter length of instrumentation required than with posterior procedure for same lesion

Disadvantages
  Does not provide sufficient stability by itself when posterior column disruption is present
  Potential morbidity with transthoracic and retroperitoneal approaches; Kaneda device in particular requires dissection posterior to the great vessels

Rarely, an anterior wedge compression fracture (anterior column disruption) may produce significant kyphosis (≥20 degrees) or loss of vertebral-body height (≥50%), in which case an anterior stabilization procedure is indicated to prevent progression of kyphosis.

While the timing of surgery has been one of the areas of controversy, we reserve emergency surgery for patients who show progressive neurologic deterioration with canal compromise and who are not able to undergo postural reduction. Otherwise, surgery is preferably performed electively within 7 to 10 days following injury, when the patient's general medical condition has stabilized and all appropriate imaging has been obtained.

Posttraumatic Kyphosis

Anterior decompression and stabilization is the treatment of choice for kyphosis after a thoracolumbar fracture that is progressive, causing pain, or causing neurologic deficit (Errico & Bauer, 1990; McAfee, Bohlman, & Yuan, 1985; Roberson & Whitesides, 1985). Following decompression, a rod system such as the Kaneda device allows a distraction force to be applied, reducing the kyphosis. With plate systems, manual reduction is required.

Neoplasms and Infections

When surgery for spinal tumor is indicated, an anterior approach should be performed when the tumor is primarily located anterior to the thecal sac, which is the most commonly encountered situation (Cooper, Errico, Martin, Crawford, & DiBartolo, 1993; Sundaresan, Galicich, Bains, Martini, & Beattie, 1984). Following resection of tumor and involved vertebral body, stabilization may be achieved by the use of bone graft (or methylmethacrylate when appropriate), and application of the Kaneda device.

When surgical intervention is required for thoracolumbar vertebral osteomyelitis, an anterior approach is usually indicated to provide adequate access to the involved tissue and thus enable adequate debridement (Eismont, Bohlman, Soni, Goldberg, & Freehafer, 1983; Kemp, Jackson, Jeremiah, & Cook, 1973). Subsequent stabilization is achieved with bone graft, with the addition of anterior (Kaneda) instrumentation if there are any doubts about continuing instability. Our experience and that of others (Dickman, Fessler, MacMillan, & Haid, 1992) has been that placement of graft and instrumentation at the site of the debrided infection does not lead to perpetuation of infection. Granulomatous infections such as tuberculosis, in which the disease is again primarily anteriorly situated, are approached in a similar manner when surgery is indicated.

Thoracolumbar Degenerative Disease and Scoliosis

Spinal canal compromise and neurologic deficit resulting from osteoporotic compression fracture is uncommon, but when they occur they may be amenable to anterior decompression and stabilization. Kaneda has reported a satisfactory outcome in a series of 22 patients utilizing his device (Kaneda, Asano, Hashimoto, Satoh, & Fujiya, 1992). This series included the use of a bioactive ceramic vertebral prosthesis instead of iliac crest graft, the use of which had led to a high incidence of late kyphosis after graft sinkage into adjacent osteoporotic vertebral bodies.

A multisegmental modification of the Kaneda system has been used for instrumentation in correction of thoracic and thoracolumbar scoliosis (Kaneda, 1992). The device has been shown to be biomechanically sound in this setting (Shono, Kaneda, & Yamamoto, 1991), but long-term outcome is not yet known.

CONTRAINDICATIONS

Anterior procedures alone are contraindicated when there is posterior column disruption, such as after fracture-dislocations of the thoracolumbar spine. These injuries require posterior reduction and stabilization.

Relative contraindications are lesions cephalad to T10 and caudad to L4. Above T10, the small size of the vertebral bodies makes screw placement difficult, and below L4, the iliac veins and inferior vena cava origin tend to impede safe placement of the Kaneda system.

BIOMECHANICS

Sheno et al. (1991) and Krag (1991) have described the biomechanics of thoracolumbar anterior fixation devices when loss of anterior and middle column integrity is present. The two rod and screw groupings of the Kaneda device give rigid stabilization against forces of axial compression, flexion, extension, and rotation. The quadrangular construct created by two independent rods linked by the two cross-linking bars provides greater resistance to flexion-extension and rotation than a single-rod system, such as the Zielke system. The insertion of the vertebral-body screws in nonparallel (triangular) alignment controls anterior and downward displacement. In the anteriorly destabilized spin, the Kaneda construct provides superior fixation as compared with posterior instrumentation (such as laminar hook or pedicle screw systems), particularly in flexion and axial compression. If posterior element disruption is present, anterior instrumentation alone will be insufficient to provide stability.

Regardless of the rigidity of the instrumentation, it will ultimately fail unless solid bony fusion occurs. One of the key concepts of anterior fusion is that the bone graft is placed under compression, which enhances graft stability and fusion (Kaneda, 1992).

APPLICATION OF THE KANEDA ANTERIOR DEVICE

Components

The components of the Kaneda anterior device (Fig. 17-1) are a four-spiked vertebral plate that is fitted into the cortex of the lateral vertebral body, tapered self-tapping vertebral-body screws (6 mm diameter at neck), 5.5-mm-diameter paravertebral rods, screw nuts (fixed onto the rod on each side of the screw head), transverse fixators for coupling the rods, and one-hole vertebral plates, for use with multisegmental fixation.

Preoperative Imaging

We have found it helpful to obtain a thorough radiologic assessment of the thoracolumbar spine and associated pathology prior to surgery. Plain radiographs and computed tomographic (CT) scans define bony anatomy and alignment, three-column integrity, and compromise of the spinal canal diameter. Magnetic resonance imaging (MRI) assesses integrity of the vertebral bodies, intervertebral disks, and spinal ligaments, demonstrates the presence and extent of tumor and infection, defines compromise of the thecal sac, and images the spinal cord. With the use of these procedures, myelography is unnecessary.

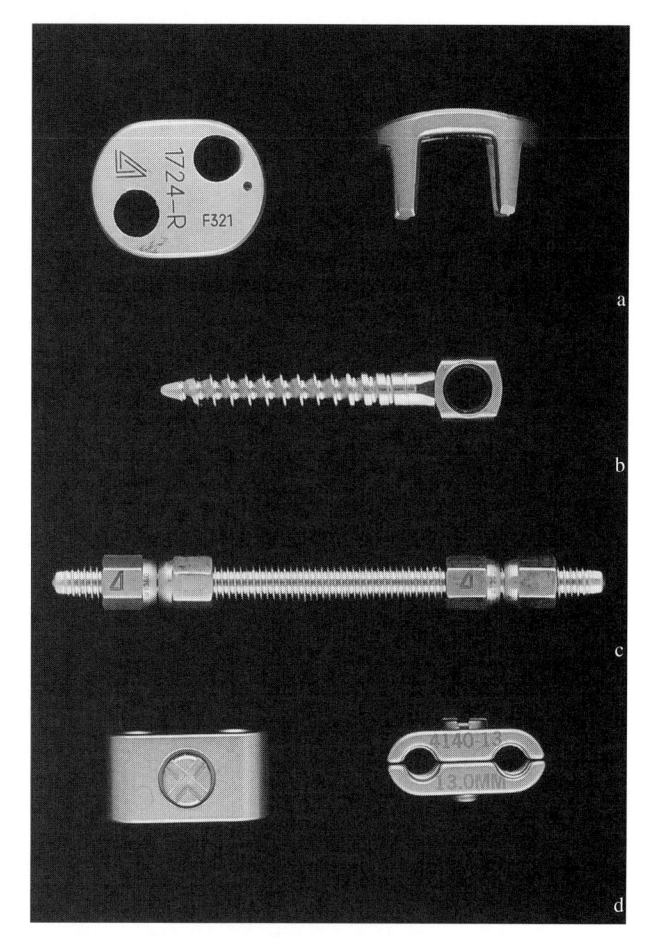

FIG. 17-1. Components of Kaneda anterior device: (a) vertebral-body plate, (b) vertebral-body screw, (c) paraspinal rod with nuts, (d) transverse fixator.

Surgical Approach

When exposure of T12 or L1 is required, we use a transthoracic retroperitoneal approach, with resection of the 10th rib. For exposure of L2 and lower, our approach is retroperitoneal via the 11th rib. A standard thoracotomy approach is chosen for exposure of T10-11 and above.

Positioning

Following the induction of general anaesthesia, leads for monitoring of somatosensory evoked potentials (SSEPs) are placed, and positioning is carried out under SSEP control. Conventional ventilation is used, as it is not necessary to collapse the lung for these approaches.

The patient is placed in the lateral decubitus position. A left-sided approach is generally chosen, as the aorta is easier to manage than the vena cava, and the spleen is less intrusive than the liver (Fig. 17-2).

The position should be made secure with operating table supports and strapping, with care taken to protect peripheral nerves and potential pressure points. An axillary roll protects the neurovascular structures of the contralateral axilla.

Exposure of the Spine

With the 10th rib transthoracic retroperitoneal approach, a curved incision is made from the lateral border of the paraspinal musculature over the 10th rib, along the 10th rib to its tip, and is carried down to the edge of the lateral rectus. The periosteum of the 10th rib is incised and stripped. The rib is cut posteriorly at the angle of the rib and anteriorly at the junction of the rib and costal cartilage and is removed. The pleural space is entered, the lung retracted and packed away, and the rib bed fully opened. The costal cartilage is then split and retracted, and the three layers of the abdominal musculature are opened. The retroperitoneal fat pad and peritoneum are identified, and the peritoneum is swept forward from the undersurface of the diaphragm and posterior abdominal wall. The spine is now displayed, with the diaphragm remaining in the wound. It is divided circumferentially, leaving a cuff of 2 cm of attachment to the chest wall to allow reapproximation. The spine is further exposed by opening the parietal pleura (for the thoracic spine), cutting the crus of the diaphragm and elevating it from the spine (for T12-L1), and removing the attachments of the psoas, arcuate ligaments, and crus (for the lumbar spine). The intervertebral disks and vertebral bodies are identified. The fascia over the spine is divided longitudinally in the midsection of the vertebral bodies, and the segmental vessels are identified. Those along the length of the spine to be instrumented are ligated and divided at the midsection of the vertebral body, and remaining soft tissue dissected off the spine. Good exposure of the lateral and anterior aspects of the vertebral bodies must be obtained.

When the 11th-rib retroperitoneal approach is employed, a curved incision is made over the length of the rib. The periosteum is divided and stripped from the rib and the rib resected from the angle to its junction with the costal cartilage. The cartilage is divided, and the underlying retroperitoneal space is identified and bluntly dissected a short distance. The peritoneum is identified. The incision is extended medially a further 8 cm from the tip of rib, and the abdominal muscle layers are divided. Having identified the peritoneum, the parietal pleura is identified, bluntly dissected cephalad from the rib bed, and protected with a laparotomy sponge. The rib bed may then be incised, and the approach continues under the diaphragm, dissecting the peritoneum forward. In the retroperitoneal space, the psoas muscle is identified, over the transverse processes and bodies of T12 and L1. The left crus of the diaphragm is cut and elevated from the L1 and L2 vertebral bodies, and the medial and lateral arcuate ligaments are detached from the transverse process of L1. The vertebral fascia is opened, and the segmental vessels spanning the length of spine to be instrumented are ligated and divided. Remaining soft tissue may then be dissected to expose the spine. Again, good lateral and anterior exposure is required for application of the Kaneda system.

Preparation for Grafting and Instrumentation

The correct spinal level is often apparent, as the pathologic process that is the indication for surgery is usually visualized. If there is any doubt, the heads of the 11th and 12th ribs may be used as a guide to the equivalent vertebral bodies, or a cross table x-ray film may be taken.

A subperiosteal exposure to the disk spaces above and below the levels to be instrumented is obtained. The disk spaces above and below the lesion are excised. It is important for future graft fusion to remove the end plates of the vertebral bodies above and below the lesion. We prefer to then identify the spinal canal and thecal sac. The landmarks used are the head of the rib and its underlying pedicle. The head of the rib may be drilled down to identify the posterior part of the pedicle. The exiting nerve root is visualized, which is followed back to the thecal sac. The corpectomy

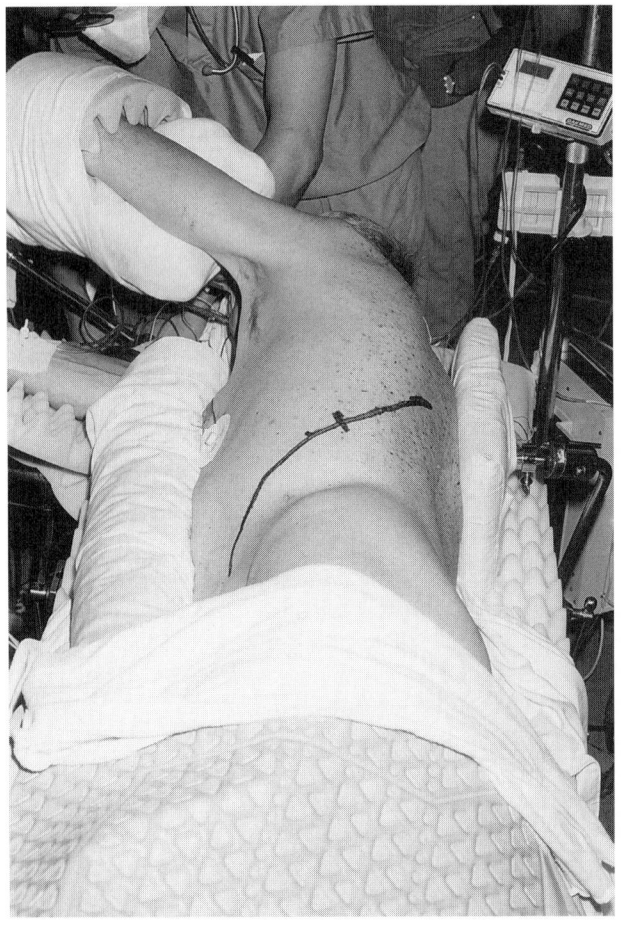

FIG. 17-2. Position and skin incision for thoracoabdominal approach to T12 vertebral body.

and decompression is then performed. This may be done with rongeurs, punches, osteotomes, a high-speed drill, or a combination of these, depending on the consistency of the bone and disease process. The canal is carefully cleared of bone and pathologic tissue. We prefer to remove the posterior longitudinal ligament and to visualize directly the complete decompression of the thecal sac. If there are tightly impacted retropulsed bone fragments, we have sometimes found that inserting the vertebral screws and applying distraction with the Kaneda distractor as an initial step can make it easier to disimpact the fragments.

Application of the Kaneda Device and Graft Placement

Following the decompression, appropriately sized vertebral plates, one each for the top and bottom vertebral bodies spanning the corpectomy are selected. These are held in the plate holder, and tapped into place (Fig. 17-3). The Kaneda device is designed to be a trapezoidal construct, with the anterior rod longer than the posterior one, so the plates are placed with the screw holes oriented to permit this.

The vertebral-body screws are then selected. The transverse diameter of the vertebral body as measured on the preoperative CT scan is a useful guide to screw length. The vertebral gauge may be used to confirm the required length. The Kaneda system's accompanying gouge is used to start the screw holes (Fig. 17-4), and the screws are driven through the screw holes in the vertebral plate into the vertebral body (Fig. 17-5). The screw heads must be firmly seated against the vertebral plate and should penetrate the opposite cortex by 2 to 3 mm; by fixing the opposite cortex, the holding strength of the screws is doubled (Kostuik, 1983). In order for this to be done safely, the contralateral psoas muscle and associated soft tissue must be dissected away from the contralateral side of the vertebral body, so that the penetration of the screws can be palpated. In doing this great care must be taken not to injure the great vessels or the contralateral segmental vessels. If this dissection is difficult, such as in the presence of a large tumor mass, we accept the screw lengths as calculated from the CT scan. The anterior screw is placed transversely across the vertebral body, while the posterior screw is placed at an angle of 10 to 15 degrees anteriorly away from the spinal canal, giving a triangular fixation.

With the screws in place, the distractor is placed between the anterior screw heads, and any kyphotic deformity is corrected (Fig. 17-6). In patients with fixed kyphotic deformity resulting from previous trauma, division of the anterior longitudinal ligament may enable reduction.

The corpectomy defect is measured with calipers, and an appropriate length of graft is chosen and inserted under distraction. There is debate as to the most appropriate graft material. Kaneda (1992) favors the use of tricortical iliac crest autograft, along with the resected rib and bone chips from the resected vertebral body. We use allograft bone, finding a strut of humerus to be of ideal size and strength. This type of allograft strut has greater biomechanical strength than iliac crest, with fusion rates similar to that of autologous bone, although the high cortical bone content means that it may take up to a year for the graft to incorporate (Bernard & Whitecloud, 1987). The use of allograft also avoids donor site morbidity. With metastatic disease, we generally bridge

FIG. 17-3. Application of vertebral-body plates.

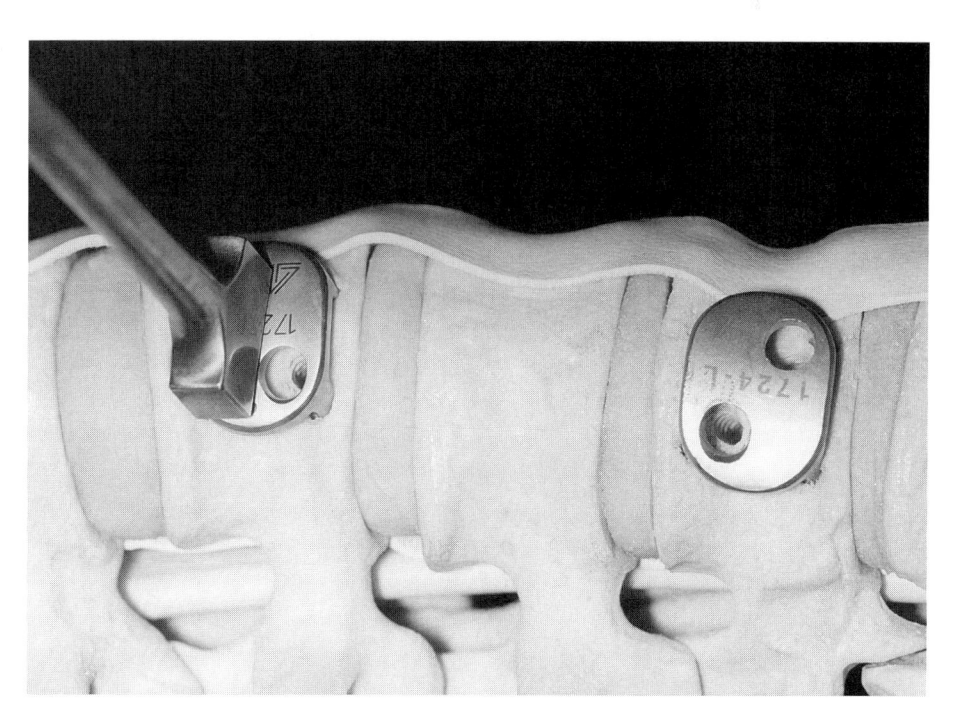

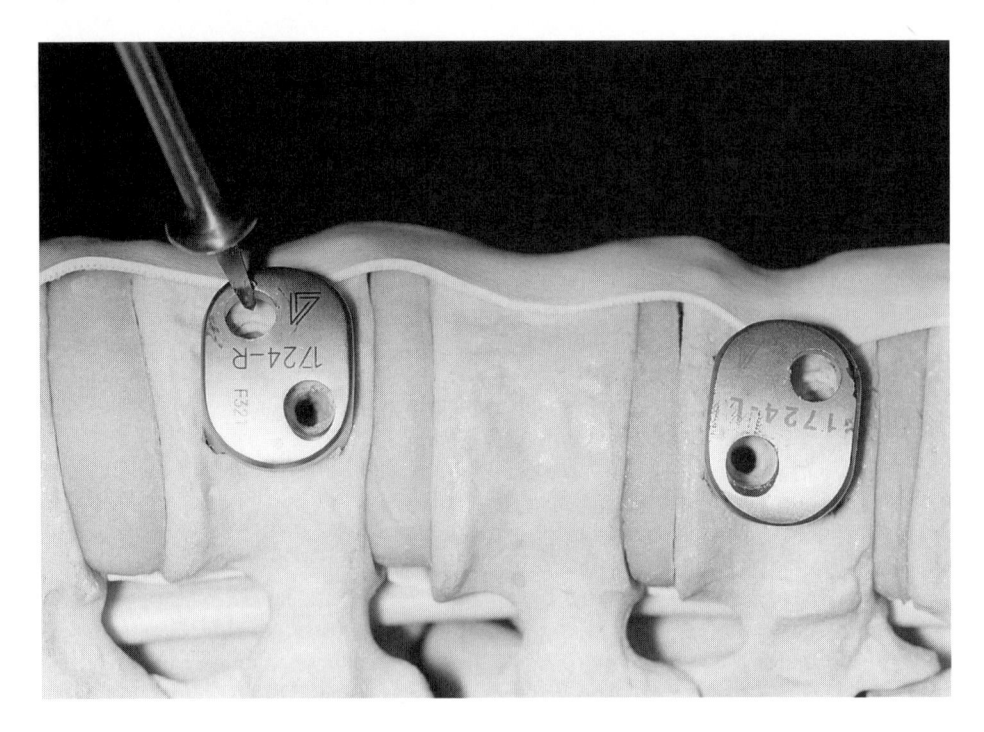

FIG. 17-4. Beginning of each screw hole is made with Kaneda gouge.

the gap created by the corpectomy with methylmethacrylate-filled Silastic tubing, as described by Cooper et al. (1993), prior to application of the Kaneda instrumentation.

Appropriate-length paraspinal rods are then selected. There are two nuts for each screw. The inner nuts are placed in correct orientation on the rods, which are then inserted through the screw heads (Fig. 17-7). The distal nuts are then placed onto the rod, and by tightening the nuts at each end of the rods, a compressive force is applied to the graft (Fig. 17-8). If the posterior rod is inserted first, it may be used as a fulcrum to maintain kyphosis correction.

The transverse fixators are then applied, creating the quadrangular construct (Fig. 17-9). Following completion of the instrumentation, an anteroposterior x-ray film is obtained to confirm a satisfactory position and spinal alignment (Figs. 17-10 and 17-11).

Multisegmental Fixation

If kyphotic deformity and instability over several levels is being treated, such as occurs with thoracolumbar spondylosis, the newer Kaneda multisegmental fixation device may be used. Anterior decompression is achieved by multiple

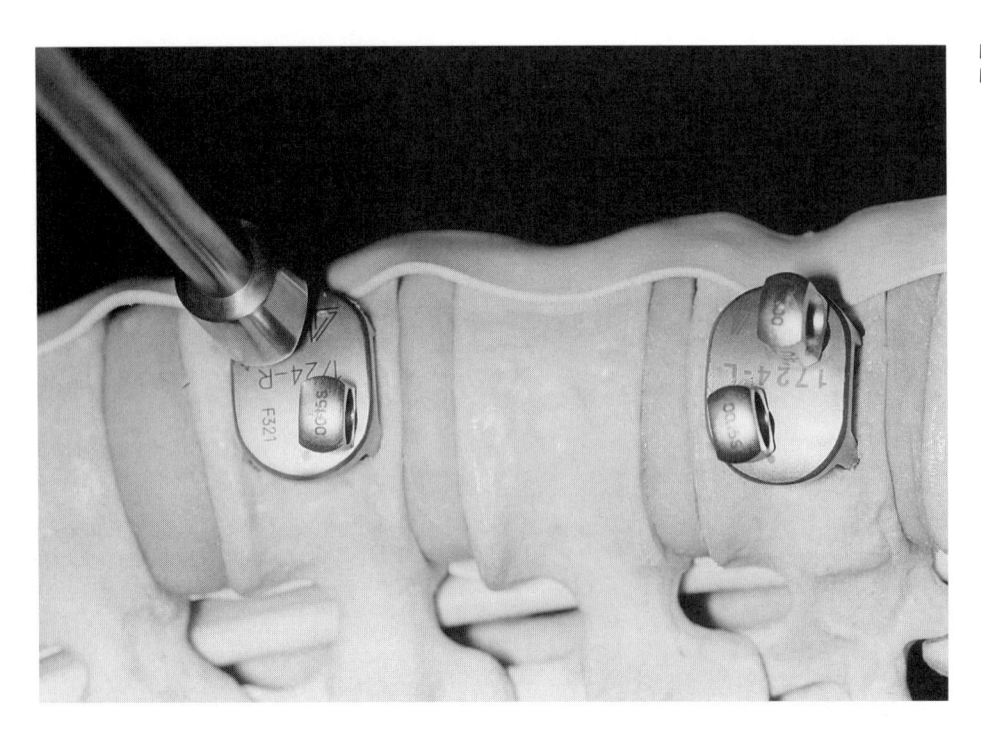

FIG. 17-5. Placement of vertebral-body screws.

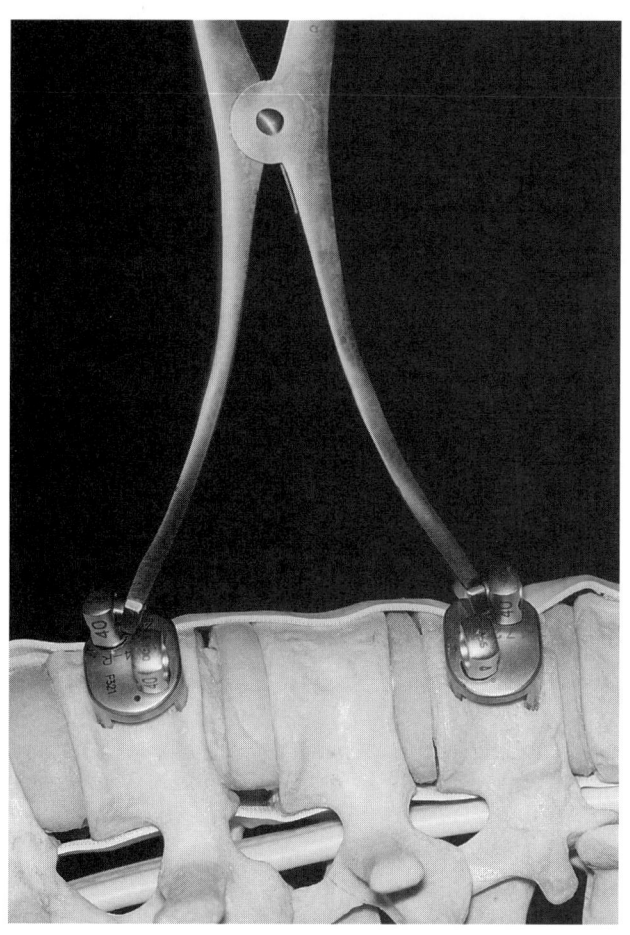

FIG. 17-6. Correction of kyphosis with distractor.

diskectomies and removal of osteophytes. In these cases, long-term stability is obtained by packing the disk spaces with bone chips. When placing the instrumentation, the usual vertebral plates and screws are placed in the cephalad and caudad vertebral bodies as described previously. The one-hole plates (one for each intervening vertebral body), with nuts on either side of each plate, are threaded onto the paravertebral rods, which are then placed through the screw heads fixing the cephalad and caudad plates. The posterior rod is applied and the screws tightened before anterior rod application. The one-hole plates are then fixed with screws to the intervening vertebrae, and their respective nuts are tightened. Three-dimensional correction of deformity is obtained by placement of bone graft in the disk spaces and sequential tightening of the screw nuts.

When using Kaneda multisegmental instrumentation for correction of scoliosis, a similar procedure is followed, although if the scoliotic curve is quite rigid, 4-mm-diameter flexible paravertebral rods are available. The screw nuts are tightened while force is applied at the apex of the curve to correct the deformity. This may be achieved by an assistant's palm pushing on the deformity, as suggested by Kaneda (1992) or by the use of Zielke derotation instruments.

Closure

Following completion of instrumentation via the transthoracic retroperitoneal approach, the diaphragm is carefully reapproximated. The 10th costal cartilage is also reapproximated. We insert two chest drains, placing one anterosuperiorally, and the other posterobasally. Each layer of the abdominal wall is closed separately, and the chest is closed in the standard thoracotomy fashion.

FIG. 17-7. Placement of anterior paraspinal rod through vertebral-body screw heads.

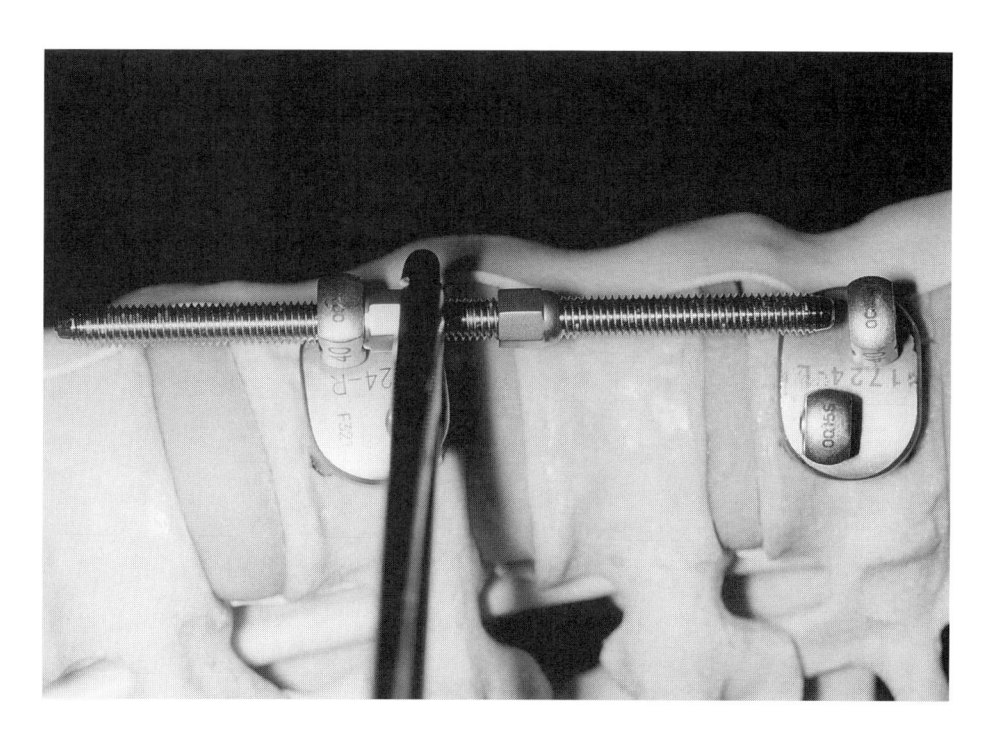

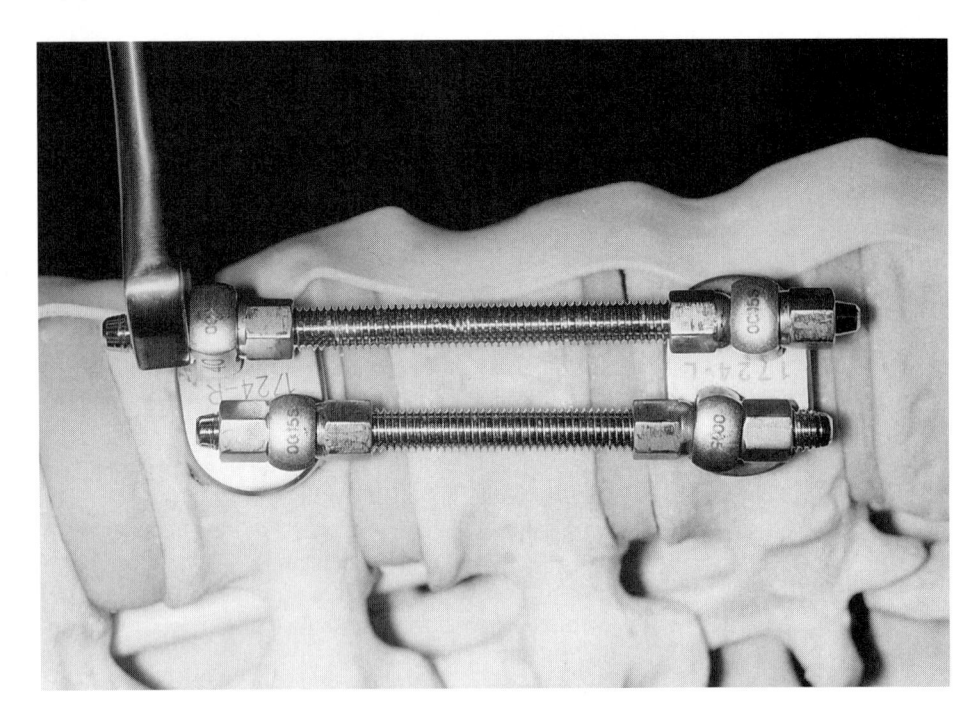

FIG. 17-8. Tightening of nuts on paraspinal rods.

When the approach has been an 11th-rib retroperitoneal one, the sites of diaphragm detachment are reapproximated. The 11th costal cartilage is reapproximated and the remainder of the wound closed in separate layers. We have not found it necessary to drain the retroperitoneal space.

Postoperative Care

For postoperative analgesia, we use narcotic agents administered via a patient-controlled analgesia system. Chest drains are kept in until drainage is ≤ 100 ml per 12-hour shift (this usually takes 48–72 hours). Patients begin walking on the second postoperative day (or whenever the chest drains are removed) in a thoracolumbosacral orthosis (TLSO), which is worn for 6 months. An orthosis is not employed if methylmethacrylate has been used.

RESULTS

The most extensive experience with Kaneda instrumentation has been accumulated by Kaneda himself (1992). His first 100 patients treated for thoracolumbar burst fracture with neurologic deficit were reviewed at a time when the mean

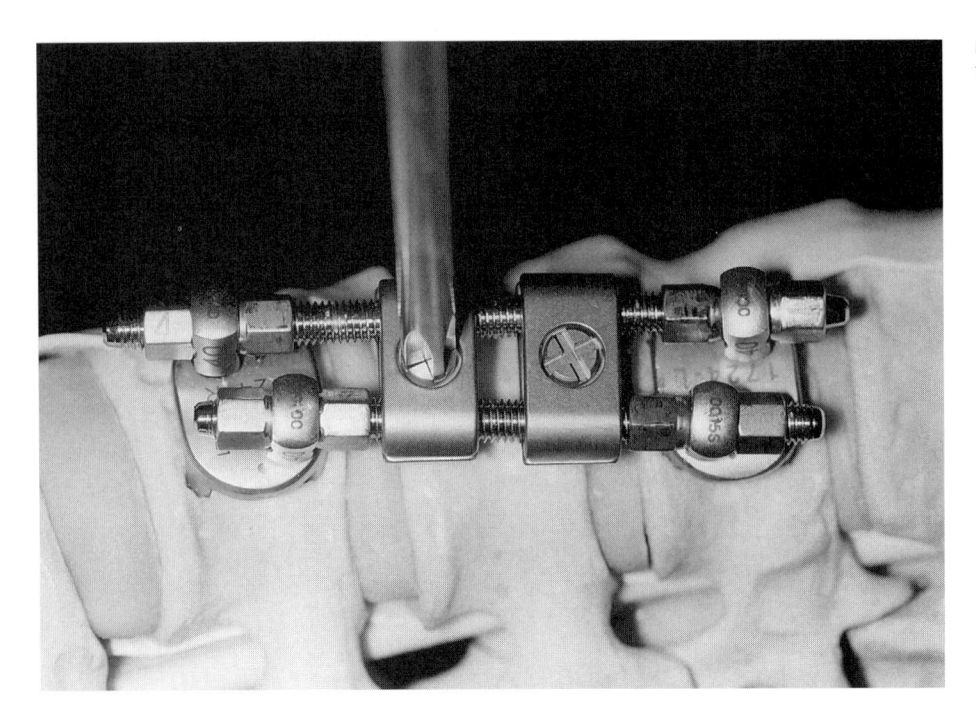

FIG. 17-9. Application of transverse fixators.

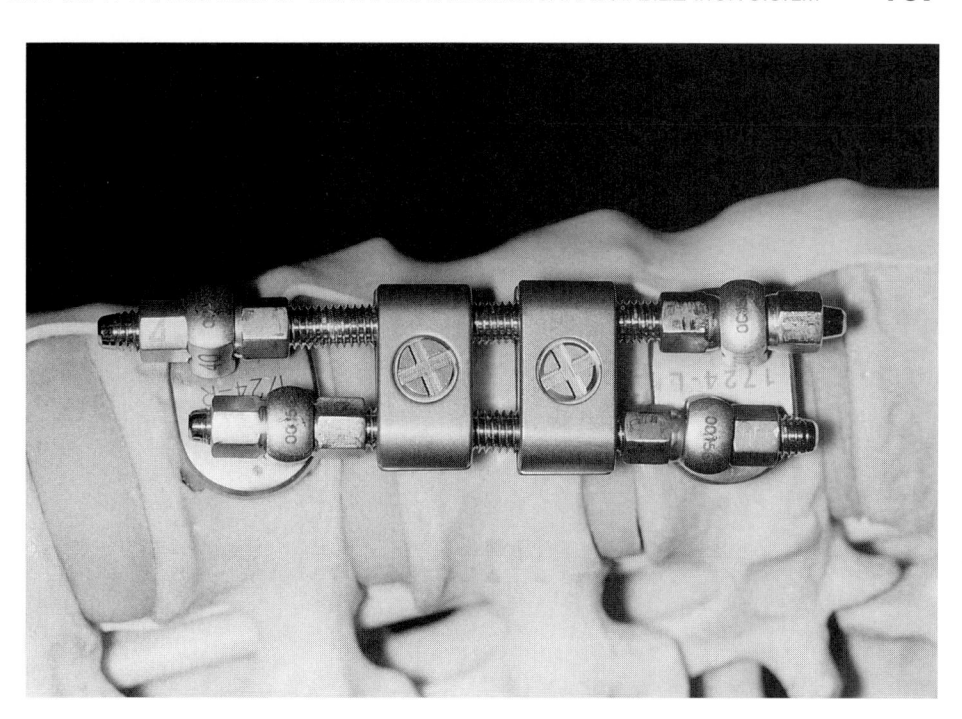

FIG. 17-10. Completed Kaneda construct.

follow-up period was 4 years, 5 months. Excluding 10 patients with pure conus medullaris lesions, Frankel grade (Frankel, 1969) improved from preoperatively: A—2 patients; B—5; C—4; and D—79; to postoperatively: A—2 patients; B—0; C—1; D—8; and E—79. There were no instances of worse neutrologic function postoperatively. Solid bony fusion was achieved in 48 of 54 (88.9%) when transverse fixators were not used, and in 44/46 (95.7%) when transverse fixators were applied. Average kyphosis was 20.2 degrees at the time of surgery, and 9.8 degrees at follow-up.

Kaneda has reported the use of Kaneda anterior instrumentation in association with a bioactive ceramic vertebral spacer in 21 patients with metastatic spinal tumor (Kaneda, 1992). In all instances, spinal stabilization was obtained. Eleven patients had died at the most recent follow-up, all from metastases to other organs. Mean survival time for these patients was 11 months (range, 3–29).

COMPLICATIONS

Complications may be classified into those of the approach and those relating to the instrumentation. A thoracoabdominal approach to the thoracolumbar spine is a significant undertaking. The thoracotomy carries pulmonary risks such as atelectasis and pneumonia. The retroperitoneal exposure may injure the spleen, kidney, or ureter, and a prolonged postoperative ileus may occur. Any unrepaired defect in the abdominal wall or diaphragm may be a site of a later visceral herniation. As mentioned, Kaneda recommends that placement of the vertebral body screws be performed with manual confirmation of bicortical penetration. This requires significant dissection of the contralateral aspect of the vertebral body, placing the aorta, inferior vena cava, and iliolumbar vessels at risk if this is not done carefully. Injury to the lumbar sympathetic chain may result in warm lower extremities, although this is not usually a clinically significant problem. Of course, there is also potential for neurologic injury when decompressing the thecal sac in any of these procedures.

The only reported complications directly related to the Kaneda device have been those of instrument failure (screw or rod breakage) and pseudarthrosis. Kaneda reports a pseudarthrosis rate of 4% for thoracolumbar burst fractures treated with the Kaneda device when the transverse fixators have been incorporated (Kaneda, 1992). Pseudarthrosis is treated by posterior fusion and instrumentation. No vascular, neurologic, or other system injuries related to the Kaneda device have been described.

SUMMARY

Anterior instrumentation is appropriate for thoracolumbar instability resulting from loss of anterior and middle column integrity, which may occur with trauma (burst fracture), tumor, infection, or degenerative disease. The Kaneda device allows decompression, correction of kyphosis, and stabilization to be performed as a one-stage procedure. The biomechanical principles of anterior instrumentation and the rigid fixation provided by the Kaneda device allows stability with fixation one level above and one level below the site of instability. Postoperatively, excellent fusion rates are obtained, and complications directly attributable to the instrumentation appear to be minimal.

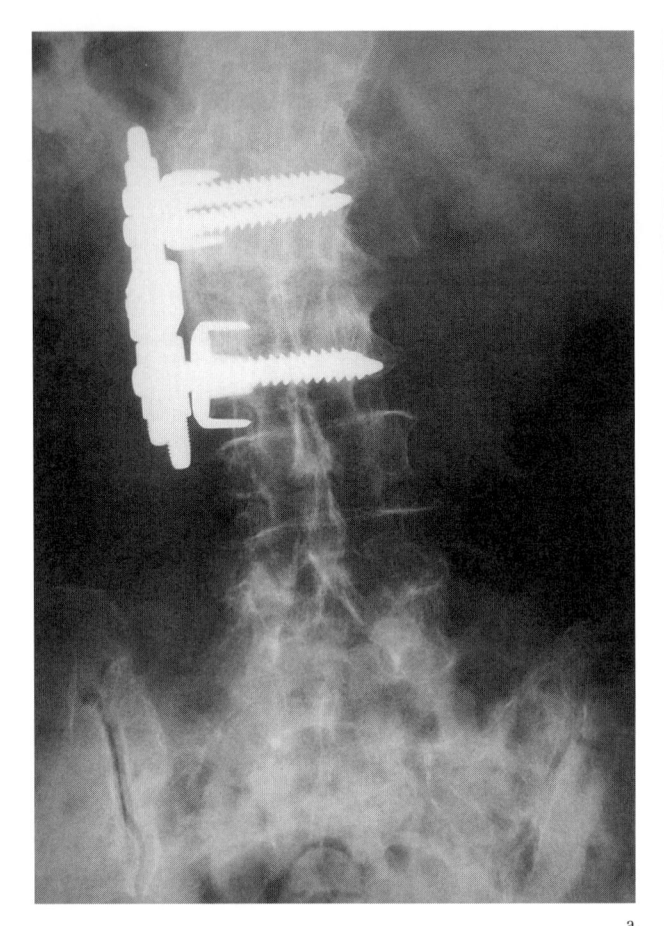

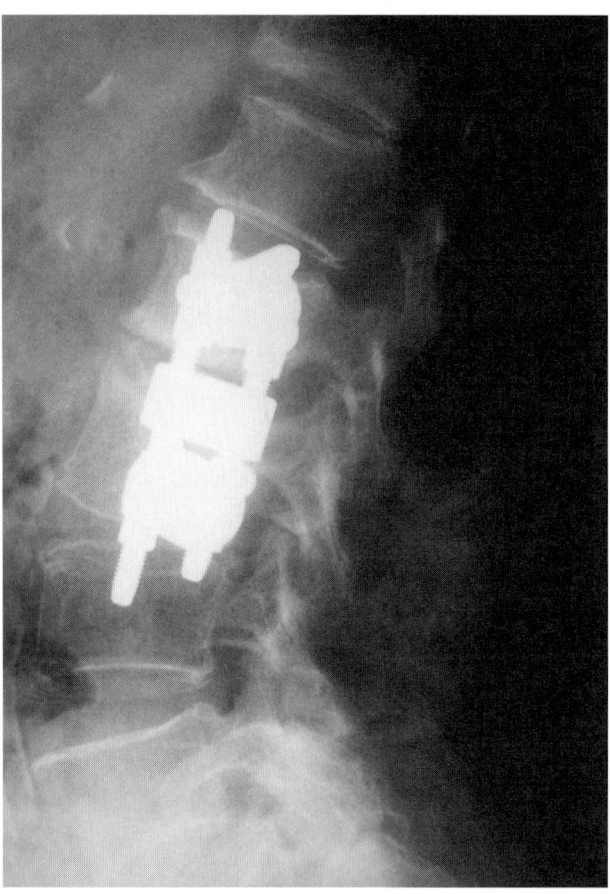

FIG. 17-11. (a) Anteroposterior and (b) lateral radiographs showing Kaneda device spanning segment where bony fusion has occurred. In this case, there was only sufficient space to apply a single transverse fixator.

REFERENCES

Bernard, T.N., & Whitecloud, T.S., III. (1987). Cervical spondylotic myelopathy and myeloradiculopathy—anterior decompression and stabilization with autogenous fibula strut graft. *Clinical Orthopaedics and Related Research, 221,* 149–160.

Cooper, P.R., Errico, T.J., Martin, R., Crawford, B., & DiBartolo, T. (1993). A systematic approach to spinal reconstruction after anterior decompression for neoplastic disease of the thoracic and lumbar spine. *Neurosurgery, 32,* 1–8.

Dickman, C.A., Fessler, R.G., MacMillan, M., & Haid, R.W. (1992). Transpedicular screw-rod fixation of the lumbar spine: operative technique and outcome in 104 cases. *Journal of Neurosurgery, 77,* 860–870.

Dickson, J.H., Harrington, P.R., & Erwin, W.D. (1978). Results of reduction and stabilization of the severely fractured thoracic and lumbar spine. *Journal of Bone and Joint Surgery, American Volume, 60,* 799–805.

Dunn, H.K. (1986). Anterior stabilization and decompression for thoracolumbar injuries. *Orthopedic Clinics of North America, 17,* 113–120.

Dwyer, A.F., Newton, N.C., & Sherwood, A.A. (1969). An anterior approach to scoliosis-preliminary report. *Clinical Orthopaedics and Related Research, 62,* 192–202.

Eismont, F.J., Bohlman, H.H., Soni, P.L., Goldberg, V.M., & Freehafer, A.A. Pyogenic and fungal vertebral osteomyelitis with paralysis. *Journal of Bone and Joint Surgery, American Volume, 65,* 19–29.

Errico, T.J., & Bauer, R.D. (1990). Thoracolumbar spine injuries. In: P.R. Cooper (Ed.). *Management of Posttraumatic Spinal Instability* (pp. 135–162). Park Ridge, IL: American Association of Neurological Surgeons.

Frankel, H.L. (1969). The value of postural reduction in the initial management of closed injuries of the spine. *Paraplegia, 7,* 179–192.

Holdsworth, F. (1970). Fractures, dislocations, and fracture dislocations of the spine. *Journal of Bone and Joint Surgery, American Volume, 52,* 1534–1551.

Jendrisak, M.D. (1986). Spontaneous abdominal aortic rupture from erosion by a lumbar spine fixation device: A case report. *Surgery, 99,* 631.

Kaneda, K. (1992). Kaneda anterior spinal instrumentation for the thoracic and lumbar spine. In: H.S. An & J.M. Cotler (Eds.), *Spinal Instrumentation* (pp. 413–433). Baltimore: Williams & Wilkins.

Kaneda, K., Abumi, K., & Fujiya, M. (1984). Burst fractures with neurologic deficits of the thoracolumbar spine: Results of anterior decompression and stabilization with anterior instrumentation. *Spine, 8,* 788–795.

Kaneda, K., Asano, S., Hashimoto, T., Satoh, S., & Fujiya, M. (1992). The treatment of osteoporotic-posttraumatic vertebral collapse using the Kaneda device and a bioactive ceramic vertebral prosthesis. *Spine, 17,* S295–S303.

Kaneda, K., Hashimoto, T., & Abumi, K. (1986). Results with Zielke instrumentation for idiopathic thoracolumbar and lumbar scoliosis. *Clinical Orthopaedics and Related Research, 205,* 195–203.

Kemp, H.B.S., Jackson, J.W., Jeremiah, J.D., & Cook, J. (1973). Anterior fusion of the spine for infective lesions in adults. *Journal of Bone and Joint Surgery, British Volume, 55,* 715–734.

Kostuik, J.P. (1983). Anterior spinal cord compression for lesions of the thoracic and lumbar spine: Techniques, new methods of internal fixation, results. *Spine, 8,* 512–531.

Krag, M.H. (1991). Biomechanics of thoracolumbar spinal fixation: A review. *Spine, 16* (3 Suppl), S84–S99.

McAfee, P.C., Bohlman, H.H., & Yuan, H.A. (1985). Anterior decompression of traumatic thoracolumbar fractures with incomplete neurological deficit using a retroperitoneal approach. *Journal of Bone and Joint Surgery, American Volume, 67,* 89–104.

Shono, Y., Kaneda, K., & Yamamoto, I. (1991). A biomechanical analysis of Zielke, Kaneda, and Cotrel-Dubousset instrumentations in thoracolumbar scoliosis: A calf spine model. *Spine, 16,* 1305–1311.

Reid, D.C., Hu, R., Davis, L.A., & Saboe, L.A. (1988). The non-operative treatment of burst fractures of the thoracolumbar junction. *Journal of Trauma, 28,* 1188–1194.

Roberson, J.R., & Whitesides, T.E. (1985). Surgical reconstruction of late posttraumatic thoracolumbar kyphosis. *Spine, 10,* 307–312.

Sundaresan, N., Galicich, J.H., Bains, M.S., Martini, N., & Beattie, E.J., Jr. (1984). Vertebral body resection in the treatment of cancer involving the spine. *Cancer, 53,* 1393–1396.

Whitesides, T.E., Jr., & Shar, S.G.A. (1976). On the management of unstable fractures of the thoracolumbar spine: Rationale for use of anterior decompression and fusion and posterior stabilization. *Spine* 1, 99–107.

CHAPTER 18

Anterior Kostuik-Harrington Distraction Systems for the Treatment of Acute and Chronic Kyphotic Deformities

John P. Kostuik

HIGHLIGHTS

Based on the biomechanical principles of anterior distractive forces combined with instrumentation to decrease sagittal bending moments, an anterior system using a modification of Harrington instrumentation has been developed for the correction of kyphotic deformities, including the treatment of acute burst fractures in 125 patients, flat-back syndrome in 80, posttraumatic kyphosis in 60, postlaminectomy in 50, Scheuermann's kyphosis in 40, kyphosis secondary to tumor in 12, kyphosis secondary to osteoporosis with fracture in 7, acute rigid kyphosis (congenital) in 6, and rigid round backs in 4. A total of 384 patients have been treated with anterior instrumentation. Complications include breakage of 40 screws and 5 rods. There have been no early or late vascular or neurologic sequelae related to instrumentation. The biomechanical basis for the treatment of kyphotic deformities includes an anterior distractive force to resist compressive loads and where possible segmental fixation to decrease sagittal bending moments combined with bone grafts far from the neutral axis. This system provides these benefits with minimal risk and morbidity.

HISTORY

The first surgical procedure for a spinal cord injury was performed by Paul of Aegina (625 to 690). Since that time, the treatment of injuries of the spine with or without neurologic deficit and in particular those involving the thoracic and lumbar spine has moved from bed rest, to postural reduction, to laminectomy with or without posterior fusion. The fusion, when done, has sometimes been in conjunction with varying forms of internal fixation used posteriorly, such as wires, plates, and springs.

Because of the high failure rate of posterior fixation devices such as wires and plates, the conservative postural reduction approach of Sir Ludwig Guttman, Frankel, and Bedbrook (Bedbrook, 1979; Freebody, Bendal, & Taylor, 1979; Guttmann, 1969, 1954) for fractures of the spine column was adopted in many spinal centers throughout the world. However, the results of reduction by this method were not universally obtained (Nicholl, 1949; Roberts & Curtis, 1970; Malcolm, Bradford, Winter, & Chou, 1981).

The report of Harrington in 1962 and that of Dickson, Harrington and Erwin in 1978 led to considerable efforts to achieve stabilization of fracture-dislocations of the thoracic and lumbar spine. The improved fixation using the Harrington distraction rods to provide three-point fixation, which results in a more anatomical reduction of the vertebral column, particularly the anterior column, has obviated the need for laminectomy, which not infrequently increases the neurologic deficit and may result in an increasing kyphosis (Morgan, Wharton, & Austin, 1971; Whitesides & Jun, 1977; Malcolm et al., 1981).

In most centers in North America, Harrington instrumentation has become the preferred mode of treatment for injuries of the thoracic and lumbar spine for stabilization. This form of fixation has enhanced the speed with which rehabilitation of patients with spinal injury may commence.

Although accepted by many as a panacea, Harrington instrumentation has not proven to be so with particular reference to burst injuries of the thoracic and lumbar spine. Initial reports on the use of Harrington distraction rods using three-point fixation, failed to differentiate between different fracture patterns (Bradford, Akbarnia, Winter, & Seljescog, 1977; Dickson, Harrington, & Erwin, 1978; Yosipovitch, Robin, & Makin, 1977).

It was thought that applying a distractive force would result in a realignment of bony fragments and disimpact the neural canal, on the theory that the fragments would remain attached to the posterior and/or anterior longitudinal ligament.

Numerous reports have now appeared to show that this is not the case, particularly with reference to burst injuries of the spine (Bohlman, Freeajfel, & Dejak, 1975; Breig, 1972; Dewald, Fister, & Savino, 1982; Kaneda, Abumi, & Fujiya, 1982; Kostuik, 1990, 1988a, 1988b, 1983; Moon et al., 1981; Paul, Michael, Dunn, & Williams, 1975; Riska, 1977; White, Punjabi, and Thomas, 1977; Whitesides, Jun, & Shah, 1976).

As a result of such reports and similar cases in the author's experience, together with cases of late onset of neurologic deficit after old burst injuries that subsequently required anterior cord decompression and fusion with beneficial results, it has become the author's policy to perform anterior surgery together with anterior fixation for some burst injuries of the spine.

Royle (1928) was the first to describe anterior spinal cord decompression. The technique, however, remained unpopular until Hodgson and Stock in 1956 reported on anterior decompression for tuberculous lesions of the spine that had resulted in paraplegia.

Since then there has been an increasing number of reports of anterior decompression for related problems, such as tuberculosis, pyogenic osteomyelitis, rigid kyphotic deformities, and more recently tumor (both primary and metastatic) and burst fractures. Most reports have consisted of anterior debridement and resection and fusion without the use of internal fixation.

Wenger in 1953 (Milgram, 1984) was the first to describe the use of an anterior distractive device. Unfortunately, this failed. The use of anterior devices still remains unpopular largely because of their lack of ready availability and fear of complications.

In 1969 Dwyer was the first in the modern era to illustrate the use of an anterior corrective device in the treatment of certain spinal deformities, namely scoliosis in the thoracolumbar spine. Hall and Micheli in 1977 reported on the use of modified Dwyer instrumentation and anterior stabilization of the spine. Dunn (1984) reported on the use of an anterior distractive stabilizing device for the treatment of burst injuries.

Anterior distractive devices or fixation devices generally fall into the categories of plates or external devices, that is, the rods lie outside the vertebral bodies. Distractive devices include the Kostuik-Harrington (Kostuik, 1990, 1988b), Dunn (1984), Slot (1981), Zielke (1982), Kaneda (1982), and more recently devices such as Moss Miami, Universal Spine Systems, Texas Scottish Rite, amongst others, and plates such as the AO plate, the Armstrong (CASP) plate and the I beam plate of Yuan (1987) and recently Z-plates, Anterior Locking Plate System (ALPS), etc. Interbody devices, such as the Rezaian (Rezaian, Dombrowski, & Ghista, 1983) device or temporary devices such as the Pinto distracter and more recently carbon, titanium, or ceramic interbody devices.

Plates provide fixation only, whereas most distractive devices are corrective as well. Reports of anterior interbody fusion in the lumbar spine indicate varying rates of union, varying from 100% to 18%. In most series the average has been 10 to 20% nonunion. As a result there has been a somewhat general reluctance to perform anterior surgery in the lumbar spine. In the author's experience the incidence of nonunion has been 5% with the use of Kostuik-Harrington (Kostuik, 1990, 1988b) devices for kyphotic deformities, either acute such as in burst injuries or late such as for long fusions for Scheuermann's kyphosis corrected anteriorly with anterior distraction. Morscher (1984) and Malcolm et al. (1981) have reported on the use of interbody grafts. Malcolm et al. (1981), in the case of posttraumatic kyphosis, have reported on the use of interbody grafts and found a 50% incidence of nonunion and loss of correction with the use of interbody grafts alone without fixation or without second-stage posterior surgery. Morscher (1984) stated that interbody grafts were unable to withstand the loads without fixation, White et al. (1977) have stated that iliac crest interbody grafts cannot withstand the loads in the erect position although they may in the recumbent position. Fibular cortical strut grafts may withstand these loads; however, revascularization does not take place until approximately 6 months after surgery. While testing in a cyclical and dynamic fashion in the laboratory, using calf spines, the author has noted that a single anterior fixation rod device used alone does not provide good control over rotation and lateral bending. As a result, when rod systems are to be used, supplementary fixation with a second rod as a neutralization rod is recommended, preferably coupling the two rods. Laboratory testing indicates that these devices, although not as rigid as segmental wiring or posterior Harrington instrumentation, do provide sufficient stability to allow for early rehabilitation and ambulation, generally with the use of an external orthosis rather than a body cast. The use of anterior fixation devices precludes the necessity of posterior fusion or instrumentation in the majority of cases provided that the posterior elements are intact (i.e., not comminuted in the burst fracture or not resected in the other cases). The use of these devices shortens hospitalization and the necessity of a second procedure and its possible morbidity. However, if the posterior elements are absent, comminuted, or if more than one vertebral body has been resected, a second-stage posterior stabilization and fusion, in addition to the anterior fixation, is necessary.

BIOMECHANICS OF KYPHOTIC DEFORMITIES

Definition

In the thoracic spine, angulation in the saggital plane greater than 40 degrees is considered as abnormal. In the cervical and lumbar spine, 5 degrees or more of fixed posterior angulation is defined as a kyphotic deformity.

Anatomical Considerations

The spinal column is essentially divided into two, consisting of the anterior elements and the posterior elements. Everything anterior to the posterior longitudinal ligament is considered to be an anterior element.

From a viewpoint of burst fractures of the spine and computed tomographic (CT) scanning, the three-column concept is used. The anterior column consists of the anterior longitudinal ligament and the anterior two thirds of the body, a middle column consisting of the posterior third and cortex of the body and posterior longitudinal ligament, then the remaining posterior column. Muscles that apply loads to the spine can temporarily alter the spatial arrangement of the vertebra. The resting positions of the spine are dictated by the osseous and ligamentous components. The physiologic thoracic kyphosis is determined primarily by osseous structures, and the lordotic curves of the cervical and lumbar are determined more by ligamentous structure.

The posterior elements are under tension and the anterior elements are under compression. Kyphosis may occur when either of these two components is disrupted. Posteriorly, the laminae and yellow ligaments are major structures resisting tension. Osteoporotic fractures are the most common cause for loss of anterior support.

Unphysiologic loads, both in magnitude and direction (Fig. 18-1) may also result in a kyphotic deformity. An increase in the moment arm (Fig. 18-1) that is the amount of angulation present also plays an important role in the production of kyphosis. The more angulation there is, the greater the chance for additional angulation under a given load.

As a result of an increasing angulation, one gets an increase in the moment arm that results in an increase in eccentric loading and can result in increasing wedging and a subsequent increase in angulation. This may play a role in both adults and children. Wedging accentuates angulation and effectively increases the moment arm, which in turn increases eccentric loading, and a vicious cycle ensues.

BIOMECHANICAL CONSIDERATIONS INVOLVED WITH TREATMENT

The treatment of severe kyphosis involves one or more steps, including, if necessary, adequate decompression of the spinal cord and the application of forces to correct defor-

FIG. 18-1. Biomechanics of kyphosis. *Left,* Kyphotic deformity showing a Cobb angle of 58 degrees. Vertically directed physiologic forces shown by the large arrow work at a moment arm at length (A). *Right,* Deformity depicted schematically, showing that posterior elements (P) resist tensile loading. Anterior elements (A) resist compressive loading. Factors lending to contribute to kyphosis include increase in physiologic load (*white arrow*), increase in moment arm (A), weakening of posterior elements, and weakening of anterior elements.

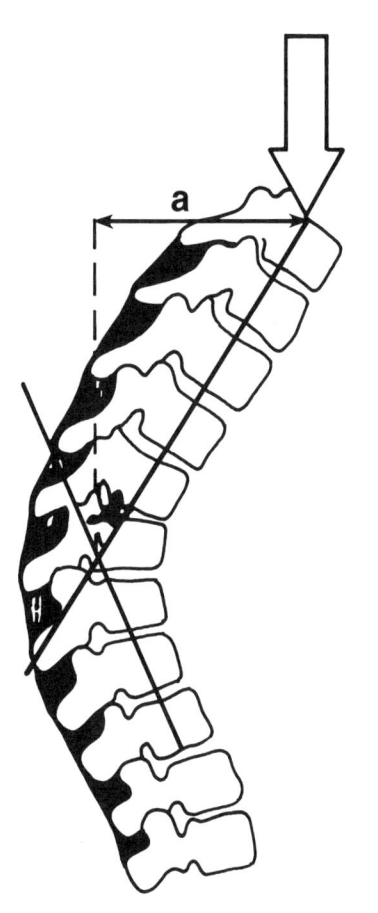

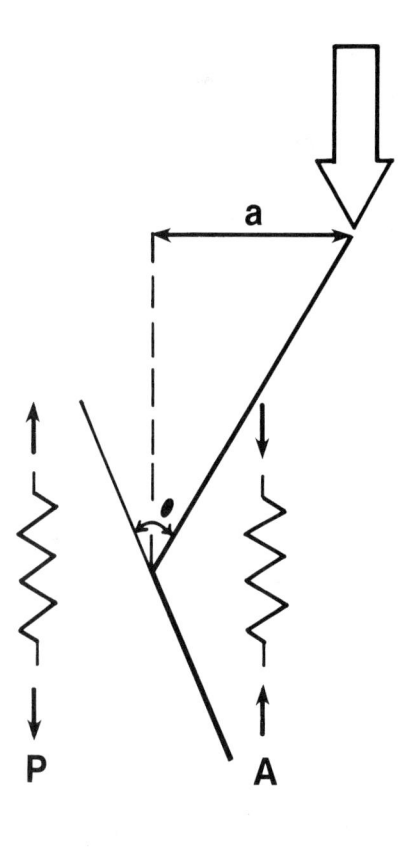

mity. The corrective forces consist of axial traction and sagittal plane bending moments (transverse loading). These correctional forces reverse the role of the anterior and posterior structures. The biomechanical concepts of creep and relaxation play a role in the treatment of spinal deformities. Creep plays a particular role where axial correction is used in the reclining position. Relaxation of tissues plays a role in axial correction with the patient erect. This is due to the viscoelastic properties of bone and ligaments.

PATHOMECHANICS OF FUSION (GRAFTS)

Posterior fusions in a kyphotic deformity are generally under tension and are usually thin and susceptible to stress fractures and indeed may bend. A posterior fusion is usually considered as being more stable the greater its length. Despite this, pseudarthrosis rates and failure to maintain correction are as high as 40% in the treatment of Scheuermann's disease in adults (Kostuik, 1990, 1988b). Conversely, anterior fusions are under compression and therefore ideal.

If one considers a kyphotic deformity as a bent column and the middle of the column the neutral axis, the more one moves away from this neutral axis toward the concavity, the more the moment arms are reduced and the more effective the support. Ideally, bone grafts for fusion kyphosis should be placed as far as feasible from the neutral axis on the compressive side and include all vertebrae that are in the deformity.

INSTRUMENTATION

Kostuik-Harrington instrumentation provides adequate rigidity and stability provided that it is used in a rectangular or parallelogram fashion, (Figs. 18-2 and 18-3).

The assets of the system are its versatility, ease of application, cost, and adaptability (Table 18-1). The system allows for ease of correction of deformity through distraction and/or compression and early ambulation. Long segments (multiple levels) may be instrumented, and the instrumentation is easily applied, in contrast to the Kaneda instrumentation, which although more rigid, cannot be used over long segments and is less adaptable. Instrumentation is simple, and a standard Harrington distraction instrumentation is all that is required together with a crimper to crimp the screw heads where heavy compression rods are used in conjunction with distraction. Crimping the collar-ended heads over the heavy compression rod is faster and as effective as using nuts. Equipment consists of a collar-ended screw and a distraction (ratchet) screw. The heads of either screw are compatible with the standard round end of the Harrington rods. The screw heads are attached to cancellous threads, which come in three lengths. Ideally, the maximum length is used and the excess cut after measuring the depth of insertion required with a depth gauge and adding 2 to 3 mm to ensure penetration of the contralateral cortex of the vertebral body. Cross-linkage is desirable between two rods either by wire or a cross-link.

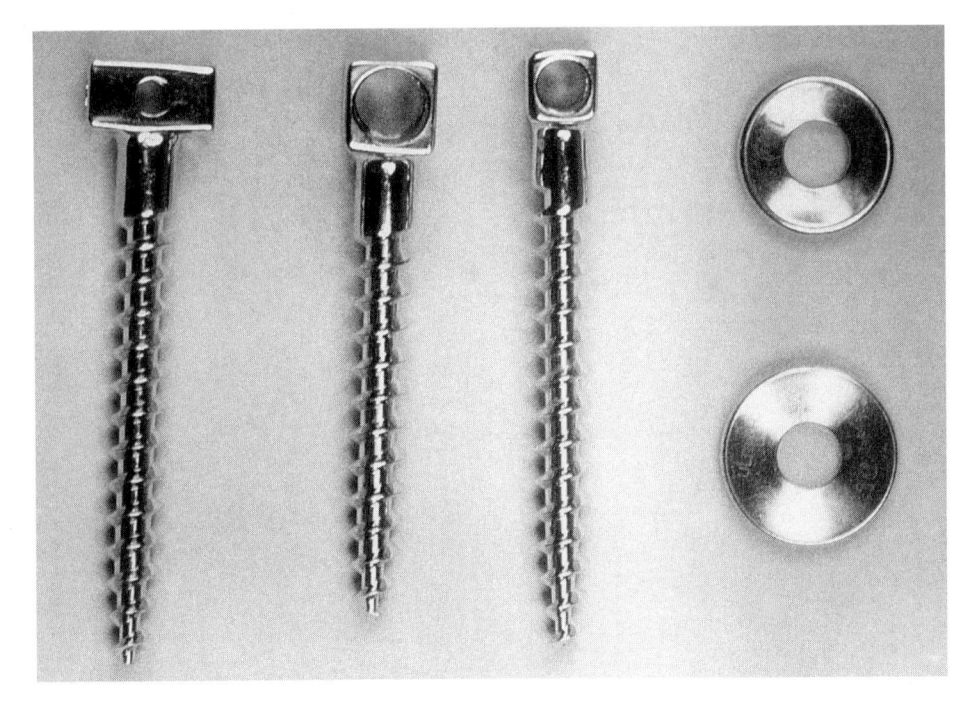

FIG. 18-2. Kostuik screws (*Left to Right*). Distraction screw (ratchet end). Collar-ended screw (for compression rods and end of distraction rod).

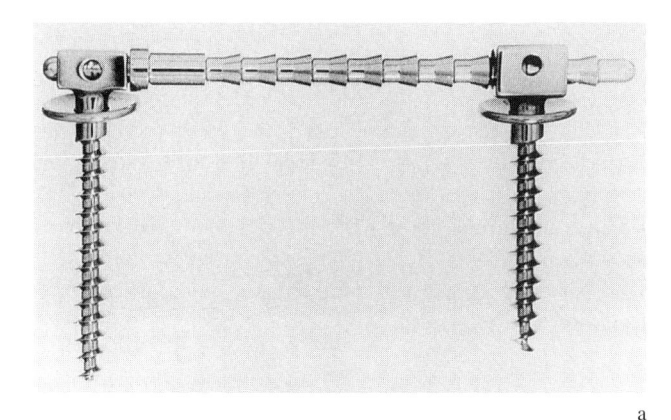

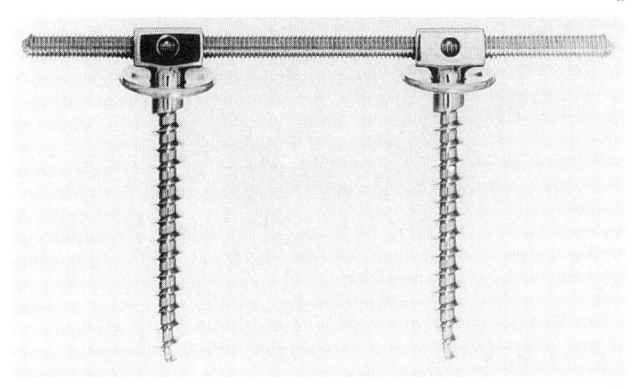

FIG. 18-3. (a) Kostuik-Harrington system. Round-ended Harrington rod, distraction screw (ratchet end), collar-ended screw, and washers. (b) Heavy-compression Harrington rod.

INDICATIONS

The anterior Kostuik-Harrington system is used for all forms of kyphotic deformities, both acute and chronic, for the following indications: burst injuries of the spine, posttraumatic kyphosis, Scheuermann's disease, rigid round back, postlaminectomy kyphosis and instability, iatrogenic lumbar kyphosis (flat-back syndrome), kyphosis secondary to tumor, and kyphosis secondary to osteoporosis with fracture (Table 18-2).

CLINICAL STUDIES

Between 1981 and April 1992, the author (1990, 1988b) has employed the Kostuik-Harrington system in the following

Table 18-1
Advantages and Disadvantages of Kostuik-Harrington System*

Advantages	Disadvantages
Cost (much less)	Less rigid in rotation than other systems
Ease of use	Higher profile than plates
Adaptable	
Relatively low profile (lower than Kaneda device)	
No special equipment	

* Available from Zimmer Corp., Warsaw, Indiana.

Table 18-2
Indications and Contraindications for Anterior Kostuik-Harrington Instrumentation

Indications	Contraindications (Relative)
Diagnosis	Lumbosacral level
Kyphosis (any)	Above T2
Posttraumatic	Lordotic spine (other devices are preferred; i.e., plates)
Burst injuries	
Scheuermann's kyphosis	
Acute rigid kyphosis	
Postlaminectomy kyphosis	
Flat-back syndrome	
Tumor	
Levels	
T2 to L5	

situations: acute burst injuries (125 cases), iatrogenic lumbar kyphosis (flat-back syndrome) (80), posttraumatic kyphsis (60), postlaminectomy kyphosis (50), Scheuermann's disease (40), kyphosis secondary to tumor (12), kyphosis secondary to osteoporosis with fracture (7), acute rigid kyphosis (6), and rigid round back (4), for a total of 384 cases. The screws have also been used posteriorly for pedicle fixation for a variety of reasons (pseudoarthrosis, multiple-level degenerative disease, tumor) in 50 cases.

COMPLICATIONS RELATED TO INSTRUMENTATION AND FUSION

To date, the instrumentation has been used in 384 cases anteriorly and 50 cases of pedicle fixation posteriorly. There have been minimal complications. Screw breakage occurred in 40 cases, the majority (24) were with the older, thin shank, untapered screw. Twenty-five of these occurred with burst fractures and 6 in Scheuermann's kyphosis, 4 in posttraumatic kyphosis, 4 in pedicles and 4 miscellaneous cases. There was no loss of correction despite the fractured screws, except in 4 cases.

Three distraction rods fractured at the junction of the racket rod area, a well-recognized point of stress concentration. There were no abnormal sequelae to this problem. Two heavy compression rods also fractured.

Vertebral-body fracture occurred in 10 cases. All occurred intraoperatively, in osteoporotic bone. Three occurred in the same patient. All cases were salvaged by the insertion of methylmethacrylate bone cement and the application of screws within the fractured body. The use of bone cement in osteoporotic vertebral bodies is recommended and appears to provide excellent holding power. The body is drilled with a standard drill and measured for depth. The drill hole is then enlarged with the aid of a curette and cement is packed in. The screw is then inserted over a washer. The screw can be turned after the cement hardens. There have been no vascular or neurologic injuries.

GENERAL TECHNICAL POINTS

1. Use an awl to start the screw holes.
2. Ideally, place the screws for distraction at midbody (slightly anterior in fractures, slightly posterior in other kyphoses).
3. Pierce the far cortex.
4. Use staples when possible (screw length should be measured with a depth gauge, and add 2 to 4 mm). Staples improve coupling forces.
5. Ideally, placement of the distraction screw(s) should be where the spine proximally or distally is level in order to allow for ease of rod insertion.
6. During distraction, apply manual pressure posteriorly to help correct the kyphotic deformity and lessen forces on the screws.
7. Distract as with posterior Harrington instrumentation.
8. In Scheuermann's disease place both rods first and distract both concurrently.
9. In burst fractures, distract to a predetermined length (normal body plus two disk heights as measured from a lateral x-ray film). Place the bone graft, preferably iliac crest bicortical or tricortical grafts slightly longer than the gap. Rib graft can be added. Add a second heavy Harrington compression rod and crimp the screw heads lightly. (Nuts may be used instead of crimping the screw heads.)
10. Cut any excess rod length.
11. In burst injuries and other short kyphosis such as posttraumatic kyphosis, the compression rod may be used as a neutralization rod or a compression rod.

SURGICAL APPROACHES

For anterior decompression the author prefers the left side. Damage to arterial vascular structures can easily be repaired, damage to venous structures, which frequently results in greater blood loss, is more difficult. For this reason the left side is employed since the aorta tends to protect the venous system.

The only indication for an anterior approach in trauma is for burst injuries associated with neurologic damage as a result of canal intrusion by bone fragments or late posttraumatic kyphosis.

With injuries to L5 and occasionally to L4, posterior decompression can be done by removing the posterior elements preferably "en bloc" and pushing the bony fragments anteriorly and removing any disk fragments or by employed distraction and lordosis by means of an internal fixator. Generally, in fractures proximal to L5, an anterior approach is preferred by the author. A left flank approach is satisfactory for lesions of L3-4 and L5; the iliolumbar and segmental vessels must be ligated and the psoas resected at the lateral aspect of the vertebral bodies. Frequently, the approach for L2 and L3 is through the 12th rib, which is often subdiaphragmatic or at most requires that a small part of the diaphragm be released. For approaches to T11 and L1 an thoracoabdominal approach must be used.

For approaches more proximal in the thoracic spine generally an incision is made two ribs above the desired vertebral level—that is, a fracture of T9 is approached through the bed of the seventh rib. If the ribs are horizonal one can go one rib proximal to the affected vertebral body.

Ligation of the segmental vessels two levels proximal and distal to the affected site at any level allows for satisfactory mobilization of the major vascular structures and prevents their abutment against any foreign materials that might be used. Care must be taken to avoid the abutment of any screw heads or prominent metal components against the aorta or the common iliac artery.

INDICATIONS FOR KOSTUIK-HARRINGTON INSTRUMENTATION

Acute Fractures

Current indications for anterior fixation of spinal fractures with or without decompression of the spinal cord are (1) Acute burst injuries with neurologic injury involving the anterior and middle column with retropulsion of bone fragments into the canal. (2) Late burst injuries, that is 5 to 7 days or more after injury, with or without neurologic injury. The analogy is to a Colles' fracture, which is cancellous bone and is difficult to reduce by standard means 10 days after injury. This has also been the experience with posterior attempts at reduction of late burst injuries using Harrington distraction, or more recently posterior pedicle fixation devices such as the AO internal fixator. (3) Burst injuries without neurologic injury, which on CT scan shows significant retropulsion of material into the spinal canal. (At present, this is greater than 50% but is dependent on bony level of injury.)

The region of the cauda equina will tolerate much greater bone intrusion into the canal than the more proximal cord level. As much as 85% canal occlusion has been noted in the area of the cauda equina without neurologic sequelae, whereas as little as 20% has resulted in severe paraparesis in the area of the cord.

There is no available data on the long-term sequelae, especially spinal stenosis, of significant canal bone intrusion, although this author (1989), Bohlman et al. (1975) and Malcolm et al. (1981) have reported on the late development of spinal stenosis following such injuries.

Current approaches in which surgery is indicated are burst fracture with neurologic injury, anterior decompression, and stabilization with Kostuik-Harrington instrumentation; and burst injuries with no neurologic injury and less than 7 days old with the AO internal fixator. If the injury is older than 7 days, posterior methods are frequently insufficient to restore vertebral-body height and reduce the traumatic kyphosis. Thus, in cases older than 7 days, the anterior approach is used as previously described. A postoperative CT scan is done in all cases in which posterior instrumentation is done and in which there was significant (greater than 20%) canal occlusion by bone fragments.

Technique

A lateral decubitus left-sided approach is preferred. The incision is usually two levels above the fracture (i.e., 10th rib for fracture at T12). The anterior quarter of the body (Figs. 18-4 and 18-5) is left. The dura is fully decompressed (Fig. 18-5). The Kostuik screws are inserted (Figs. 18-5b, and 18-6). Distraction is then done. C-clamps are applied to the ratchet end of the distraction rod after distraction is completed. The bone graft is then inserted (Fig. 17-6). A rib strut is added, if available. A heavy compression rod is inserted into the collar-ended Kostuik screws, which are angled forward from the near posterior part of the body to the contra-anterolateral cortex of the body (Fig. 18-7). Slight compression is applied, and the screw heads are lightly crimped. More recently, cross-linkage has been added to create a more stable quadralateral frame.

Figures 18-8 to 18-13 illustrate a case. A 20 year old male fell 12 m, sustaining a burst injury of L2. His neurologic status was a Frankel grade B. Decompression, correction of deformity, grafting and stabilization were carried out within 24 hours. At 2 years of follow-up, he was functional, and Frankel-graded as D.

Postoperative immobilization has usually been with a plastic molded orthosis. In less accommodating patients a body cast is utilized.

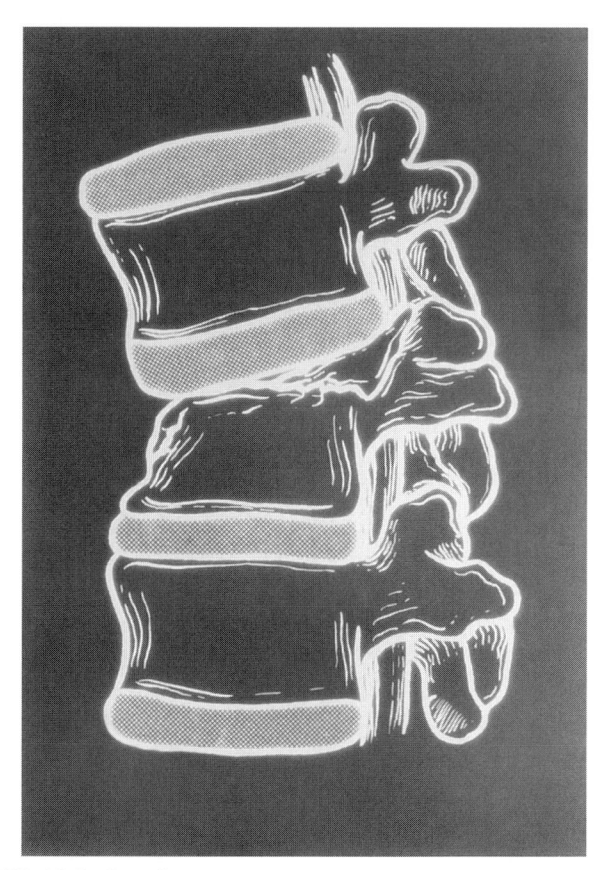

FIG. 18-4. Burst fracture.

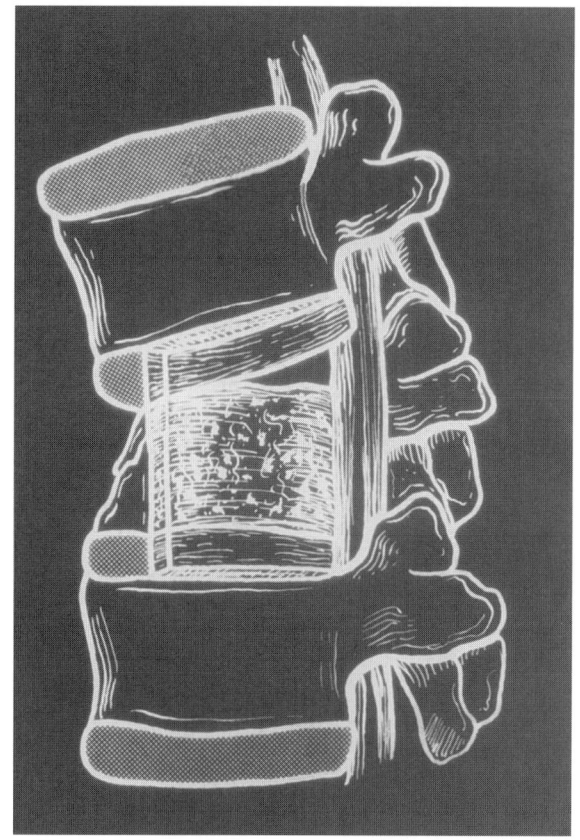

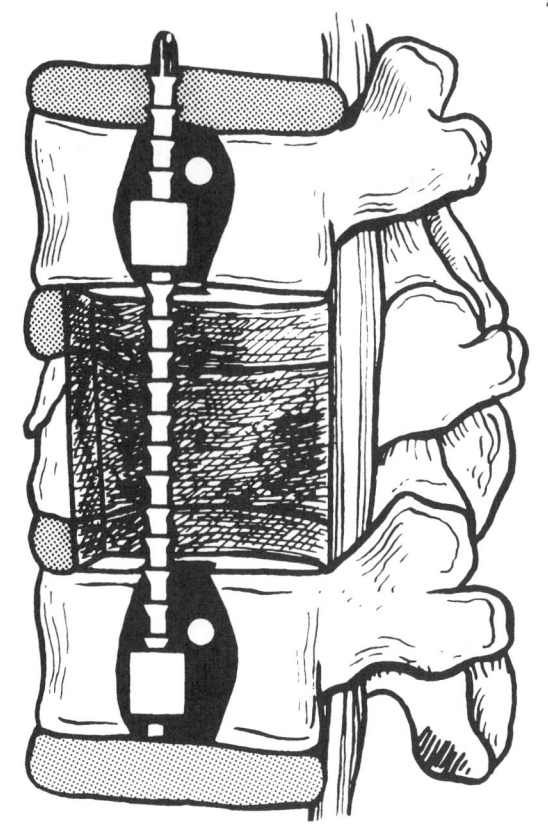

FIG. 18-5. (a) Dura-decompressed anterior quarter of body is left as graft. (b) Kyphosis is reduced with Kostuik-Harrington distraction device.

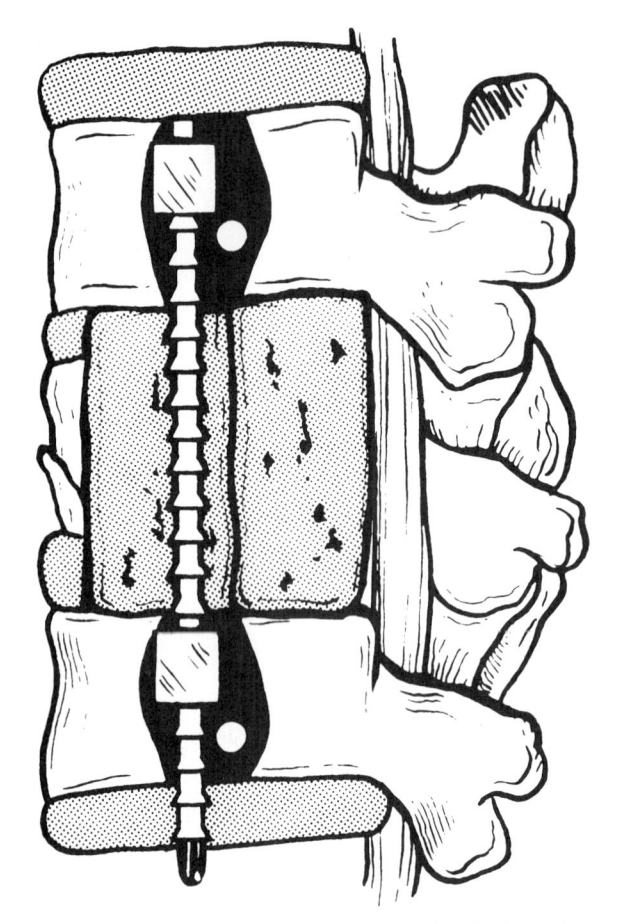

FIG. 18-6. Anterior lateral rod is inserted to reduce kyphosis; bone graft (iliac crest) is added.

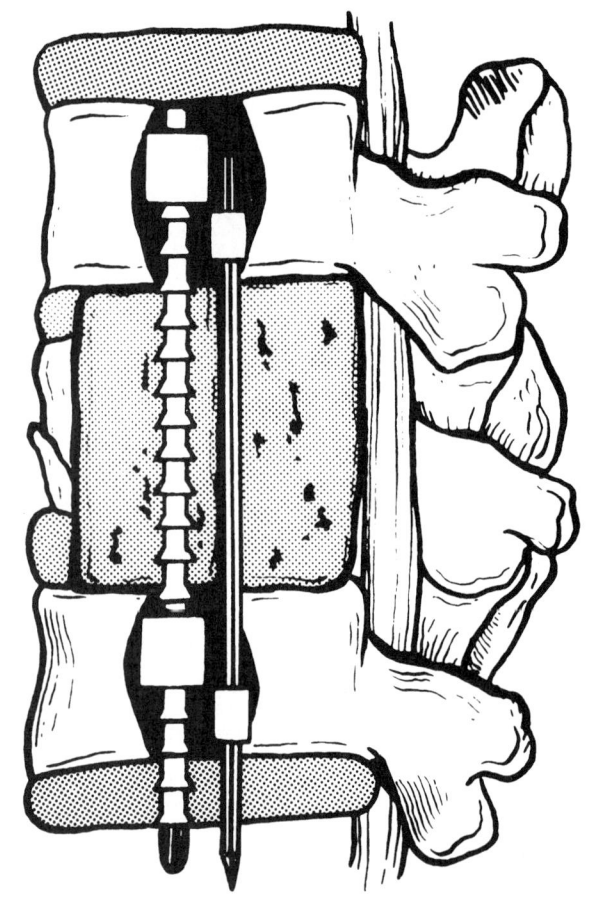

FIG. 18-7. Second heavy Harrington compression rod is added to increase stability. Slight compression is applied. Collar-ended screw heads are crimped.

Ambulation is dependent on the degree of neurologic damage. Early transfers and walking are permitted.

The advent of distractive devices that include building in of lordosis such as the AO internal fixator may decrease the need for anterior surgery for acute burst injuries. A randomized prospective study by Esses, Kostuik, and Botsford (1989) comparing the use of the AO internal fixator with Kostuik-Harrington instrumentation showed no statistical differences for correction of kyphotic angulation, instrumentation, failure fusion rate, or neurologic recovery. The Kostuik-Harrington instrumentation was significantly better at achieving canal clearance by virtue of the anterior decompression.

Results

Up to April 1992, a total of 125 cases were treated with the anterior technique described above (Kostuik, 1988a). There were five nonunions, including three cases early in the series where in retrospect second-stage posterior fusion and instrumentation, because of severe posterior column comminution, should have been added. Screw fracture occurred in 25 screws. The majority in the earlier model of untapered screws. Two rods fractured.

Average neurologic improvement was 1.6 Frankel grades in the partial paraplegics, with a range from 2.0 to 1.0. Greater improvement was seen the earlier the procedure was performed.

There were no early or late neurovascular problems.

If there is severe posterior element comminution or severe posterior instability delayed second-stage posterior instrumentation and fusion is recommended.

Posttraumatic Kyphosis

The indications for surgery included pain and deformity, which were present in all patients. Sixty such patients underwent surgery.

Preoperative assessment included CT scanning, metrizamide myelography, diskography (done above and below the fracture; 4 levels), and facet blocks (if no previous posterior fusion). Diskography and facet blocks are done to make sure all painful levels are incorporated in the subsequent surgery.

The technique is as with burst fractures. If CT scanning shows no or little canal intrusion the dura does not need to be decompressed. Previous posterior fusions do not need an osteotomy (Figs. 18-14 to 18-16).

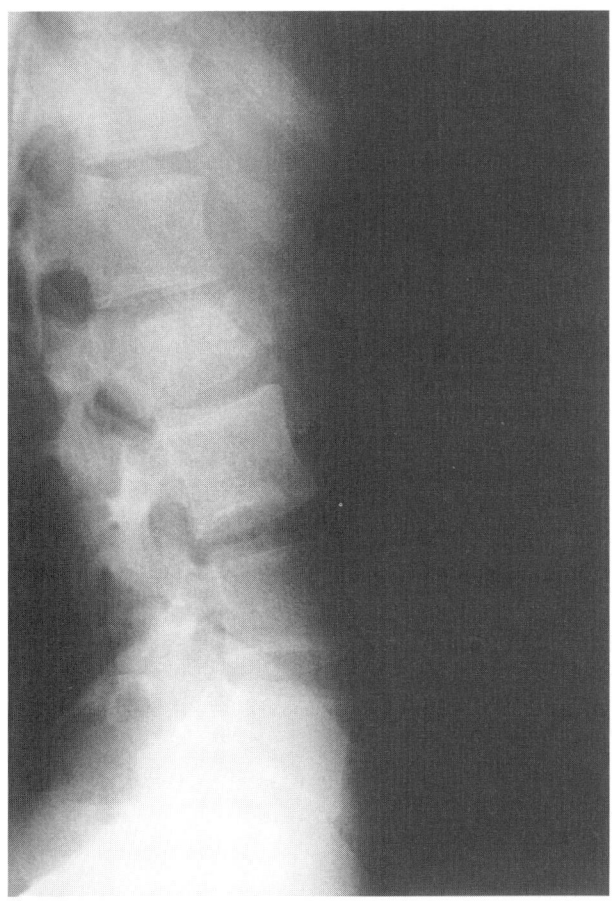

CHAPTER 18 / ANTERIOR KOSTUIK-HARRINGTON DISTRACTION SYSTEMS   **179**

FIG. 18-8. Lateral views of a burst fracture. Neurologic assessment Frankel grade B.

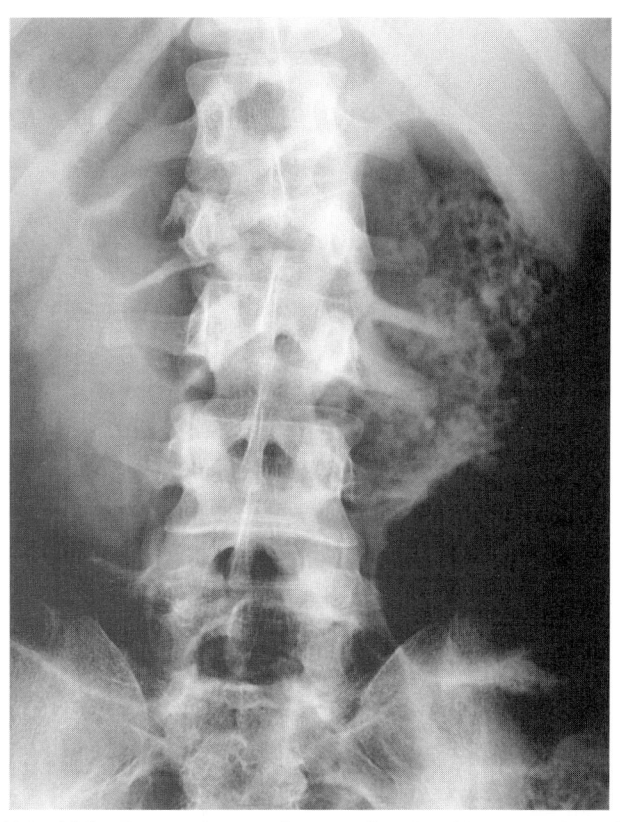

FIG. 18-9. Preoperative anterior posterior view. Note widening of pedicles of L2.

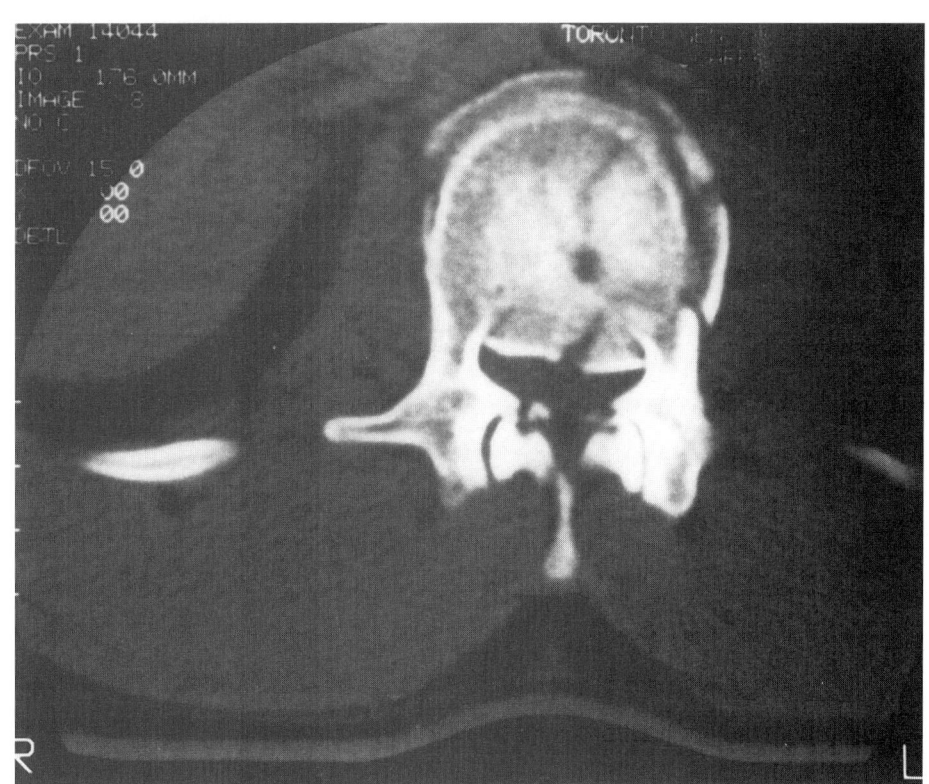

FIG. 18-10. CT scan with saggital reconstruction demonstrates significant canal occlusion.

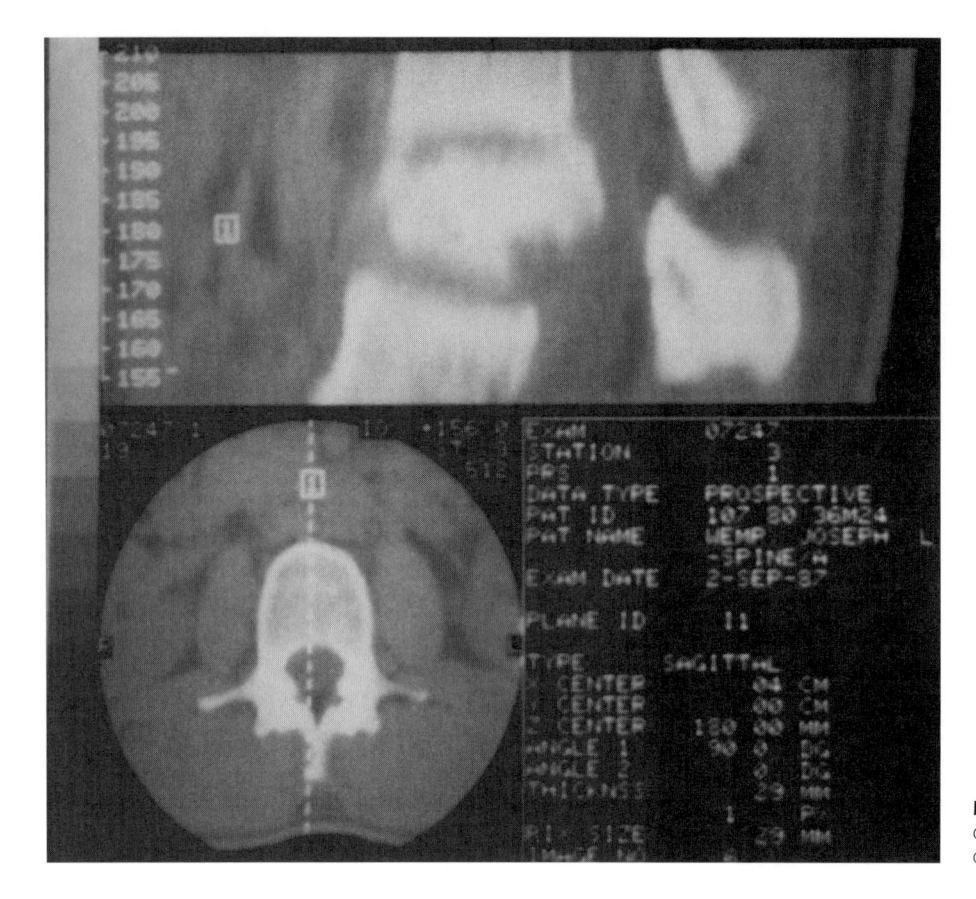

FIG. 18-11. CT scan with saggital reconstruction demonstrates significant canal occlusion.

Results

Screw breakage occurred in four patients. Kostuik and Matsuzaki reported their initial results in 45 patients in 1989. Pain relief was good to excellent in 37 of the 45 patients. Neurologic improvement can be seen 20 years after the initial fracture. Twenty-two of 45 patients had neurologic lesions, including 10 with residual paraparesis from the original injury and 12 in whom late signs and symptoms of spinal stenosis developed.

Of the 10 patients with residual paraparesis, 4 improved more than one grade on the Frankel scale after decompression. All 12 cases of spinal stenosis improved after anterior decompression.

Scheuermann's Kyphosis

Studies of the surgical treatment of Scheuermann's kyphosis by posterior instrumentation indicate a progressive loss at long-term follow-up (Kostuik, 1990, 1988b). Loss of correction is due to fusion on the tensile side of the spine, high pseudarthrosis rates (up to 40%), and late stress fractures due to repetitive cyclic loading on the tensile side of the spine. Anterior interbody fusion alone does not provide adequate correction of the deformity.

The relatively unsuccessful techniques of posterior instrumentation and fusions with high pseudarthrosis rates, complications, and subsequent surgical procedures due to loss of correction from the above causes, led to the development of techniques of anterior instrumentation and interbody fusion.

The general aim is to stabilize and correct the kyphotic deformity by a mechanically sound procedure, with minimal immobilization, with minimal complications, that will not deteriorate within or out of the fusion mass.

The biomechanical aims are to stabilize and correct the kyphotic deformity by providing axial distraction and reducing bending moments and producing a fusion mass which is 1) under compression 2) long 3) far from neutral axis and 4) interbody.

Surgical Technique

For thoracic deformities a thoracotomy via the fifth or sixth rib is performed. The scapula is mobilized. If there is an associated right thoracic scoliosis, a left-sided approach is preferred. The segmental vessels are clipped and the spine is exposed from T2 to T12 (or where appropriate). All disks and end plates back to the posterior annulus are removed. Ratchet and collar-ended screws are inserted. The screws must pierce both cortices of the body and are placed as far posteriorly as possible. The rods are inserted and may be contoured. Distraction of both rods is carried out concurrent with application of pressure manually posteriorly. C-clamps are used to secure the rods. Bicortical iliac crest grafts are inserted under compression (Figs. 18-17 and 18-18). The

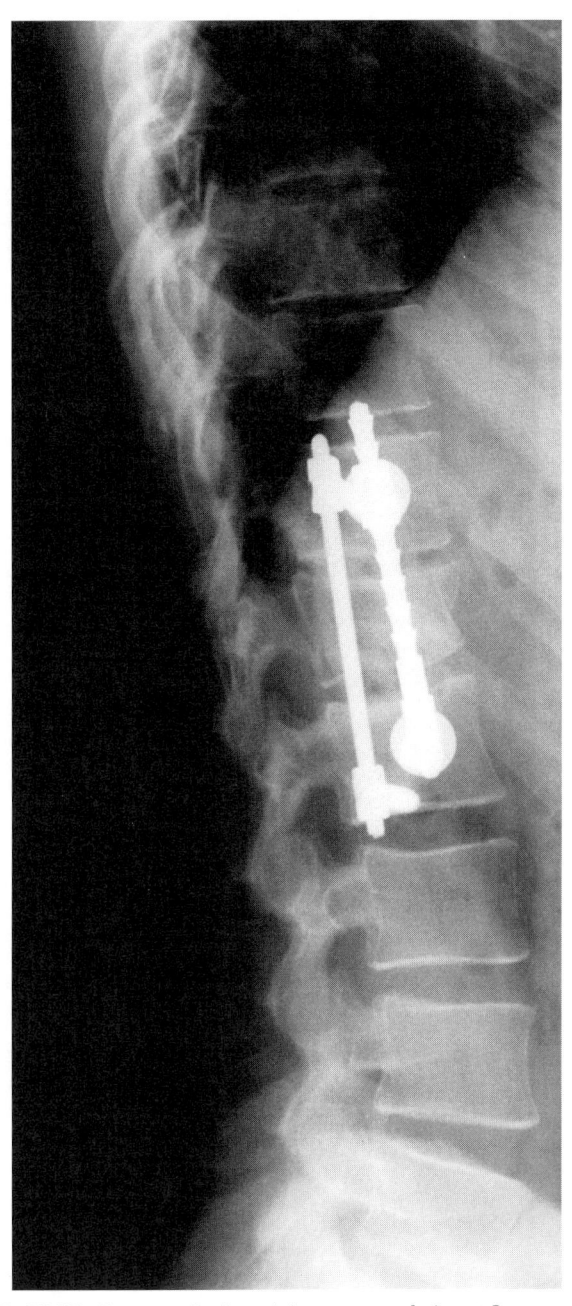

FIG. 18-12. Postoperative lateral demonstrates fusion at 2 years with good correction of deformity after anterior decompression, grafting, and stabilization.

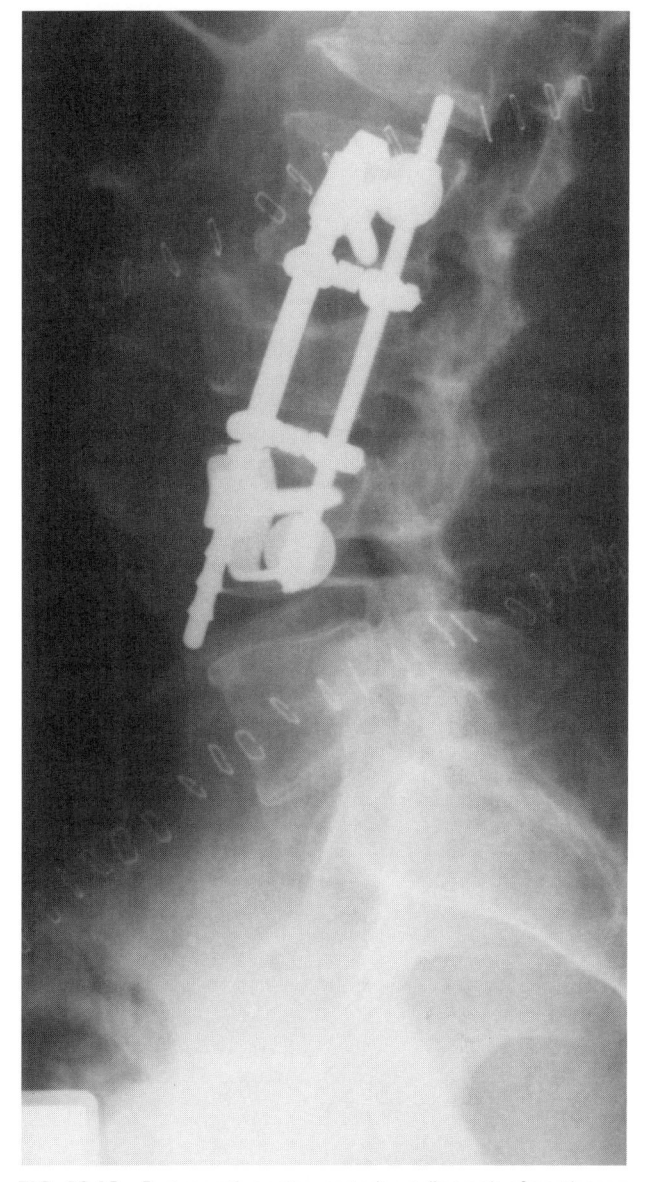

FIG. 18-13. Postoperative anteroposterior radiograph of another patient demonstrating cross-linkage producing a quadrilateral frame and enhancing rotational control.

grafts should be slightly larger than the interspace. Supplementary rib is also used. In osteoporotic bodies, cement may be used to hold the screws in place.

Surgical Indications

Surgical indications include in the skeletally mature pain (apical or low back), deformity (75 degrees or greater), spinal cord compression (rare), and progression of kyphosis; and in the skeletally immature failure of bracing techniques and rigid deformity (65 degrees or greater).

Early Results

The early results (Kostuik, 1990, 1988b) of anterior interbody fusion and modified Kostuik-Harrington anterior instrumentation from 1982 to the present include 40 patients with an average age of 27.5 years (range, 21–62). The preoperative curve was 75.5 degrees. Postoperatively, the curve was reduced to 56 degrees with instrumentation. After follow-up, the average curve was 60 degrees (Figs. 18-19 and 18-20), and six patients had progression of their curves within their fusions. One patient underwent subsequent

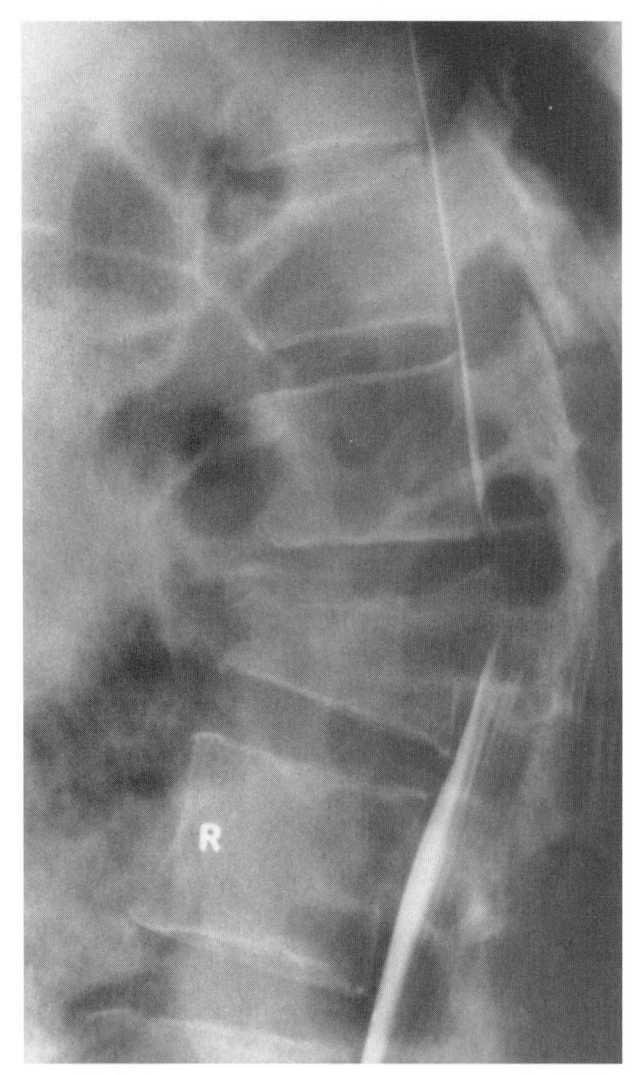

FIG. 18-14. 34-Year-old man with posttraumatic kyphosis resulting from acute burst fracture with neurologic deficit.

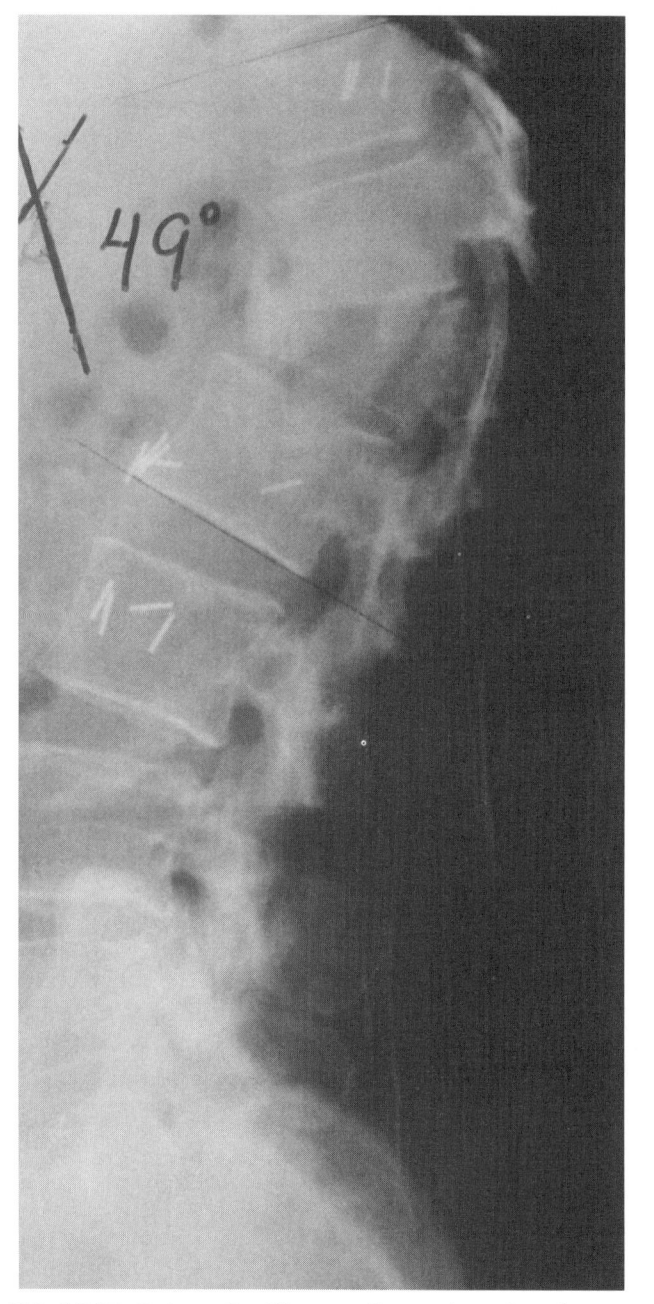

FIG. 18-15. Postoperative CT scan at 2 years shows loss of correction with graft collapse and a recurrence of her neurologic deficit.

surgery, and two patients had a pseudoarthrosis. The complications were minimal, with 6 fractures of 160 screws used.

Postoperatively, patients were immobilized in a plastic orthosis for 6 months. The average hospital stay was 12 days.

Conclusions

The preliminary results of anterior distraction and interbody fusion indicate minimal loss of correction, minimal complications with minimal morbidity, and short hospital stay. This is attributed to the fusion mass being under compression. Anterior instrumentation prevents collapse of interbody grafts. Preliminary results indicate that anterior instrumentation and fusion appear to yield satisfactory results.

Acute Rigid Kyphosis

Moe, Winter and Bradford (1978) have clearly outlined indications and treatment protocol for the treatment of acute angular kyphosis of either a congenital, developmental, or infective nature. General principles in the treatment of acute angular kyphosis consist of (1) decompression of the neural canal, (2) traction for correction of deformity, if indicated,

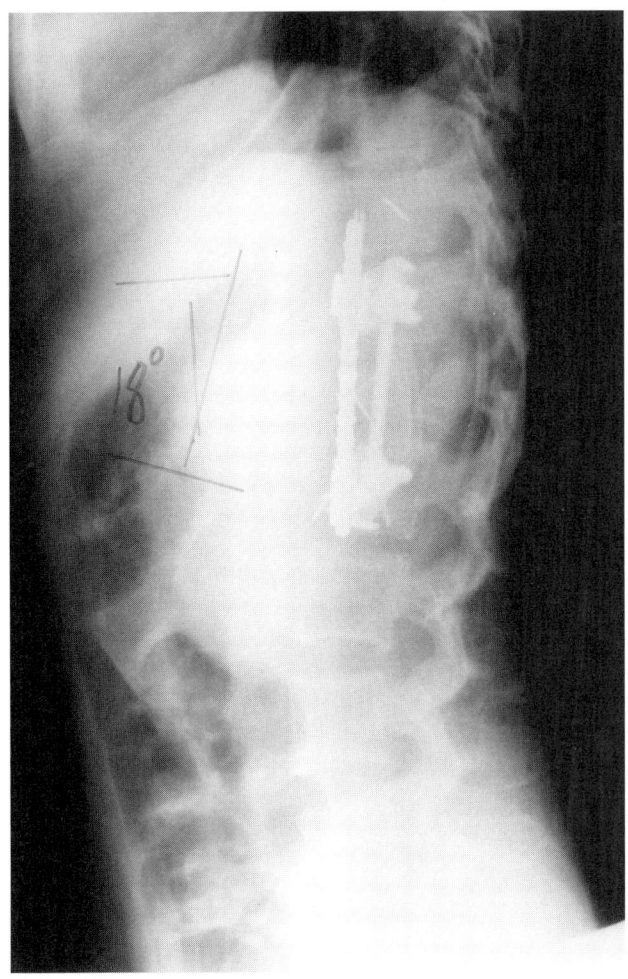

FIG. 18-16. Diskographys revealed a painful degenerative disk at the level below. Correction was obtained, pain relieved, and the neurologic deficit alleviated.

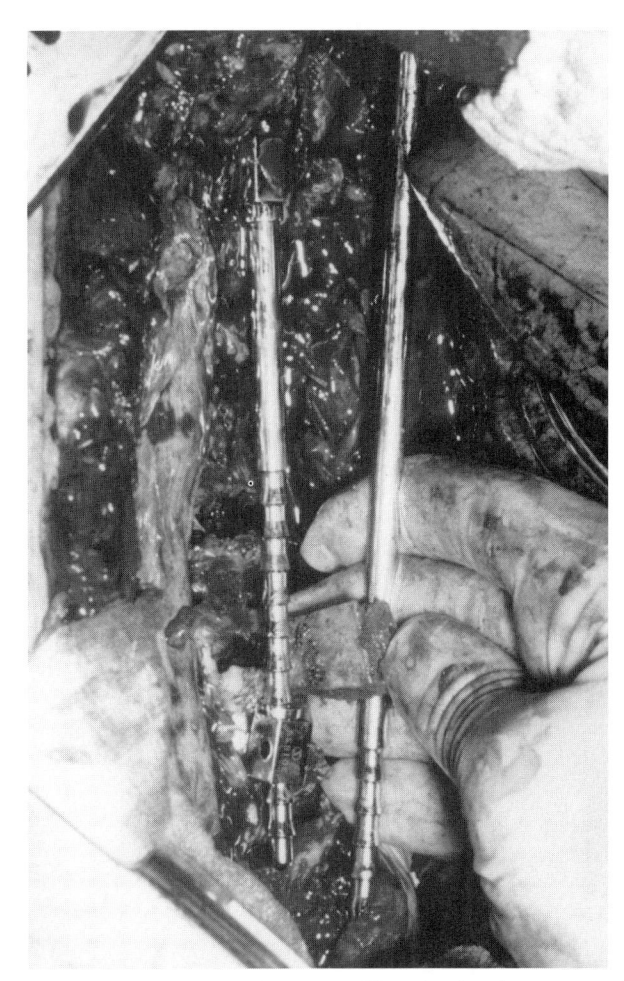

FIG. 18-17. Scheuermann's kyphosis. The spine has been exposed from T2 to L2. The Kostuik-Harrington rods have been inserted to correct the deformity. A bicortical graft is inserted at each disk space together with small bone chips.

FIG. 18-18. Grafting completed.

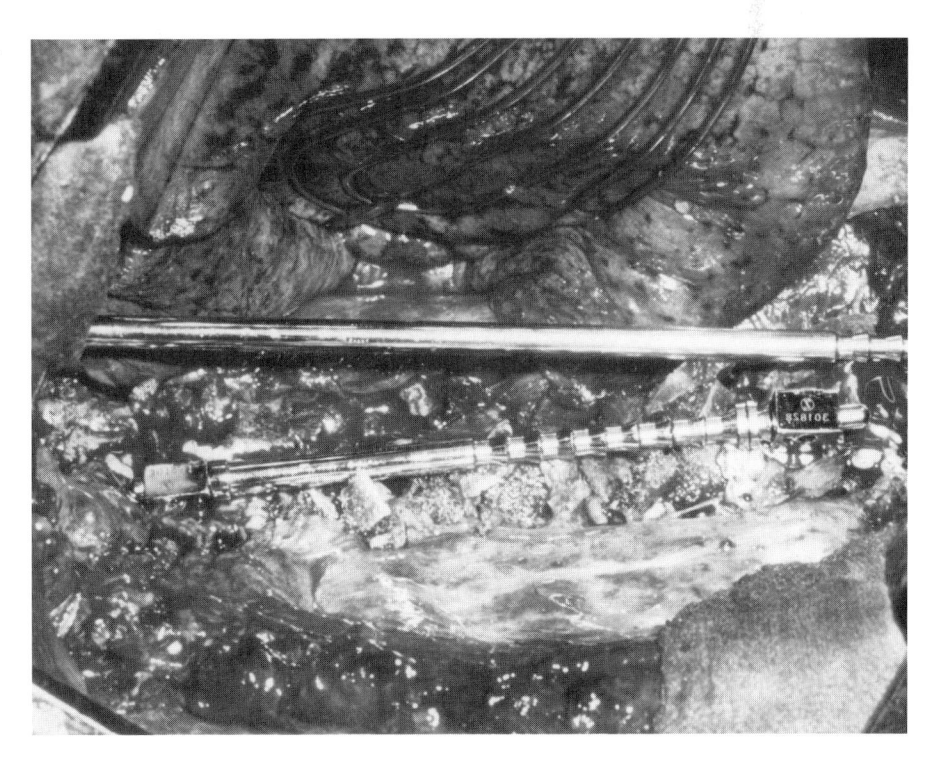

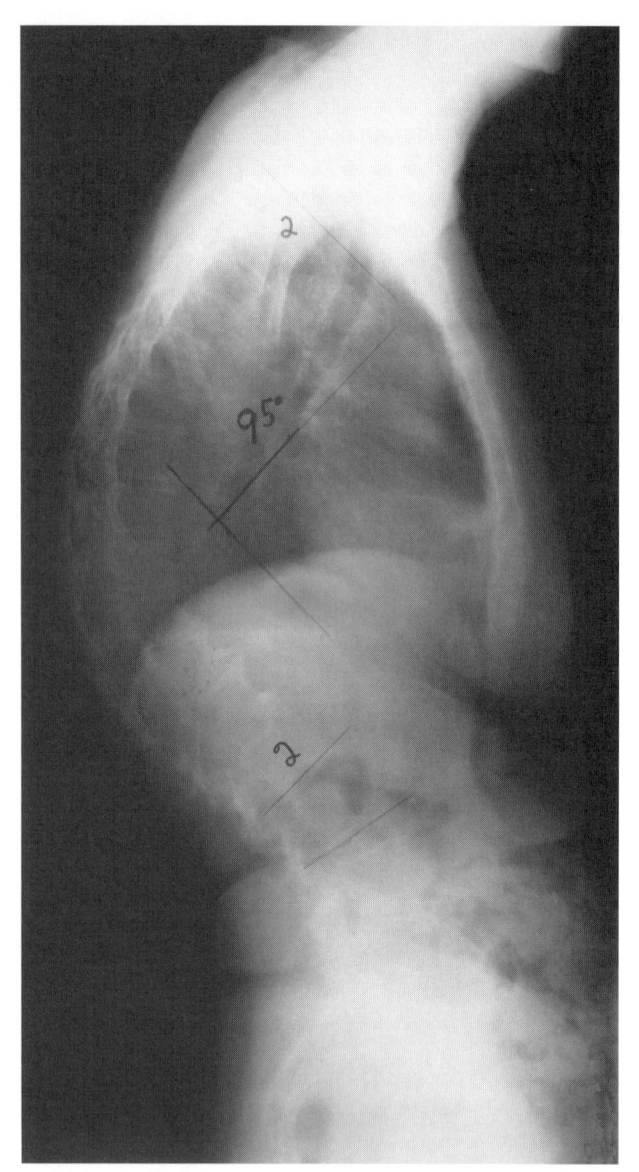

FIG. 18-19. In this 49-year-old woman the deformity increased to 95 degrees from T2 to L2, with associated pain.

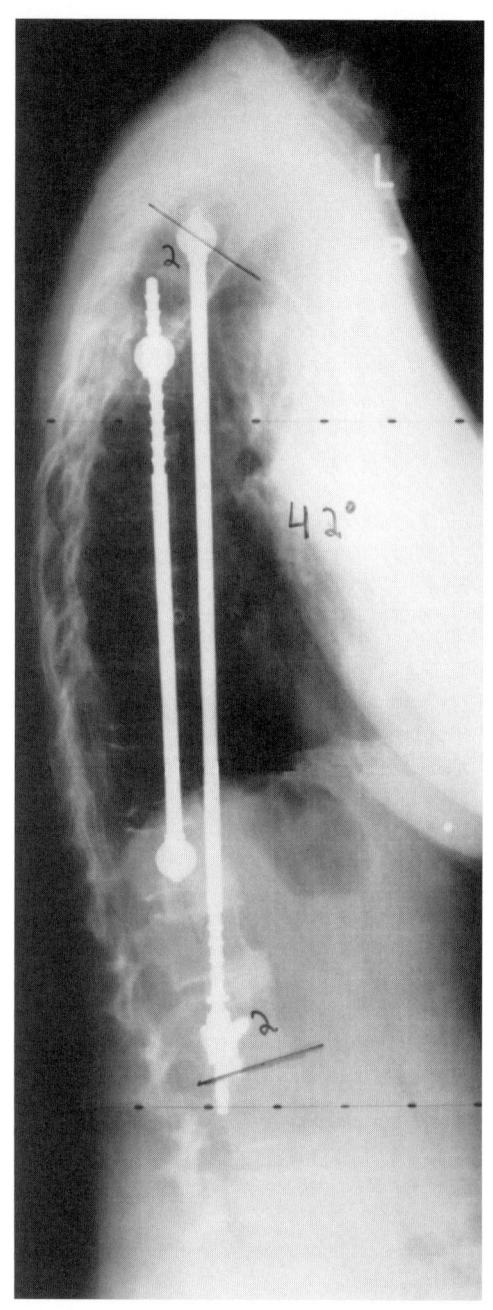

FIG. 18-20. Postoperative lateral radiography demonstrated the deformity reduced to 42 degrees; pain was relieved.

(3) strut grafting anteriorly, and (4) supplementary posterior fusion with instrumentation.

The use of anterior instrumentation has decreased the need for posterior instrumentation and fusion in the treatment of this problem (Figs. 18-21 to 18-25).

The principles of decompression and strut grafting, plus or minus traction where indicated, remain the same. We prefer to use iliac crest strut grafts rather than fibular grafts. The iliac crest grafts were substantiated with rib grafts.

Fibular grafts take up to 2 years to revascularize and are quite weak, particularly at their ends, at 6 months following implantation. Iliac crest grafts revascularize quickly. Bicortical grafts are generally used in the treatment of all forms of kyphosis, but tricortical grafts may be used in the presence of osteoporosis.

Surgical Loss of Lumbar Lordosis

Posterior instrumentation (Harrington) to L5 and S1 may result in excessive loss of lordosis. Pseudarthrosis rates for fusion to the sacrum in adults with Harrington rods are as high as 50% and may lead to loss of lordosis. Pseudoarthrosis rates in adolescents with fusions to L5 or S1 are 12% with

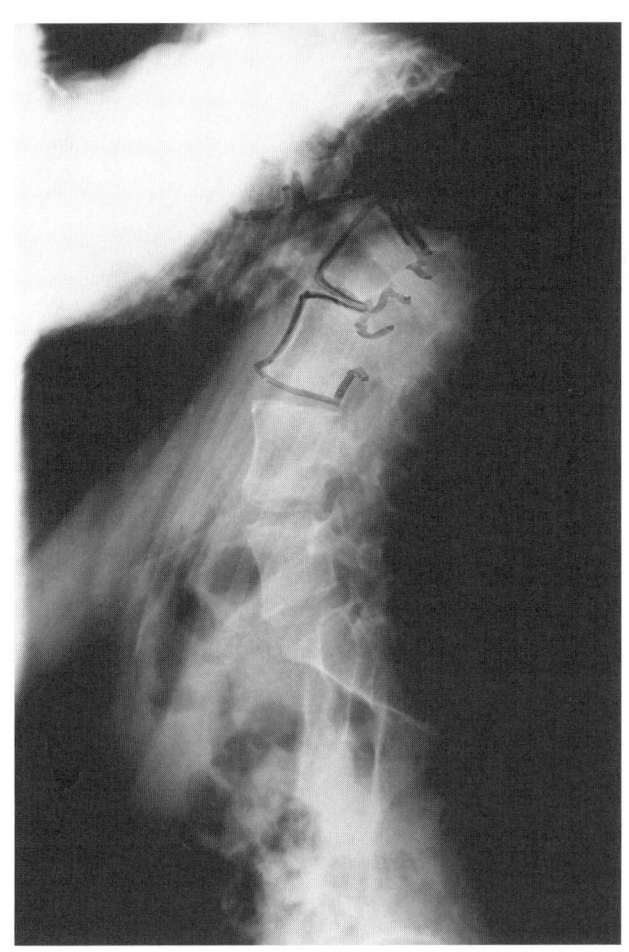

FIG. 18-21. Acute rigid kyphosis in a 23-year-old woman with congenital deformity of approximately 160 degrees with spastic paraparesis.

Harrington rods and may lead to loss of lordosis (Kostuik, 1988c; Kostuik, Richardson, Maurais, & Okajima, 1988). Loss of lordosis (flat back) occurred in 50% of posterior fusions to the sacrum in adults and was significant in half of these. Children with flat backs develop problems as adults, as they no longer can compensate for the loss of lordosis after age 35. Frequently, the development of degenerative changes below a previous fusion ending at L3-4 or L5, as shown by Cochran, Irstam, and Nachemson (1983) may lead to loss of anterior disk height, loss of lordosis, and a flat back.

The prevention of iatrogenic lumbar kyphosis or flat-back syndrome can be achieved with strict attention to detail if fusion to the sacrum is necessary. Preservation or an increase of lordosis is essential. Any distraction in the lumbar spine will lead to loss of lordosis.

The advent of segmental wiring with Luque contoured rods into lordosis (Kostuik, 1988c) has helped and has decreased the pseudarthrosis rates to 20% over Harrington instrumentation, in which fusion to the sacrum is necessary. However, the incidence of pseudoarthrosis is still, we feel, somewhat too high.

In mobile curves, with preservation of lordosis anterior Zielke (1982) instrumentation followed by a second-stage posterior pedicle fixation from L3 to the sacrum will ensure correction, fusion, and preservation of lordosis. In rigid curves, especially kyphoscoliosis the procedures of choice are multiple-level anterior diskotomies filling the disk spaces with morsalized bone graft followed by a second-stage posterior Cotrel-Dubousset instrumentation and fusion in order to derotate the spine and restore lordosis, performed 7 to 10 days after the first stage (Kostuik, 1988c).

Materials

Kostuik et al. in 1988 reported on a retrospective review of 56 scoliotic patients who underwent corrective surgery for loss of lordosis, four of whom were men and 52 women. The average age was 40, with a range of 15 to 60. Of the 56 patients, 45 had idiopathic scoliosis. The number of patients who had previous operative procedures was 27. Previous posterior instrumentation extended to L4 in 4 cases, to L5 in 5 cases, and to S2 in 47 cases.

Surgical Technique

A combined single-stage posterior and anterior approach is used, incorporating two incisions, flank and posterior. Incisions are joined if a quadrilateral wedge removal is required. An anterior osteotomy in the presence of a previous fusion is done. Alternatively, the disk and end plates at the selected level are removed (usually L3-4 or at the same level as a preexisting pseudoarthrosis). The anterior instrumentation is inserted (Figs. 18-26 to 18-31). The posterior osteotomy is done (1–1.5 cm. of bone is removed). Posterior instrumentation consisting of Dwyer screws and cables of more recently placed Cotrel-Dubousset rods in the fusion mass lateral to the dura are used. The anterior osteotomy is opened with the anterior Kostuik-Harrington system simultaneously as the posterior osteotomy is closed. A bone graft (iliac crest) is applied anteriorly in the open wedge. A contoured neutralization plate is applied centrally posteriorly for rotational control together with a posterior bone graft.

Results

The preoperative lordosis prior to initial posterior distraction with Harrington rod surgery measured from L1 to S1 was 49 degrees of lordosis; after the first operative distraction, the average was 21.5 degrees. At minimum of 2 years of follow-up after osteotomy, the average lordosis was again 49 degrees, with a range from five to 78 degrees. Bone union occurred in all cases. Pain relief was obtained in 48 to 56 patients. Three patients lost partial correction due to partial anterior graft collapse. There were three intraoperative major left common iliac vein tears. All three had had previous anterior surgery. There were two neurologic complications, one with persistent loss of bowel and bladder function.

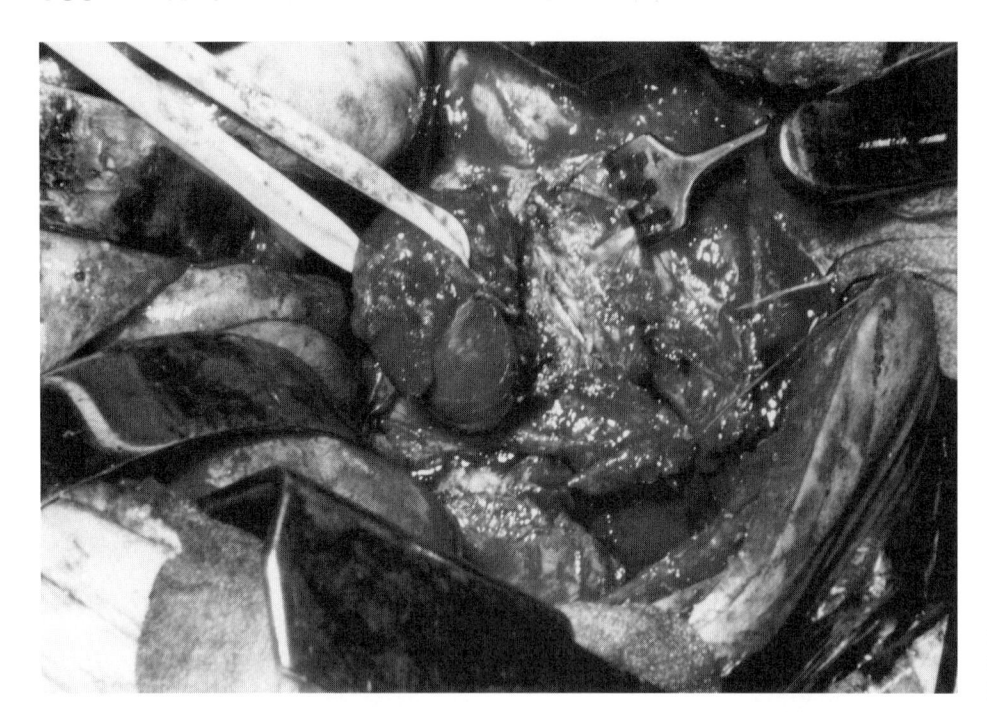

FIG. 18-22. Intraoperative view of anterior spinal elements prior to decompression and reconstruction.

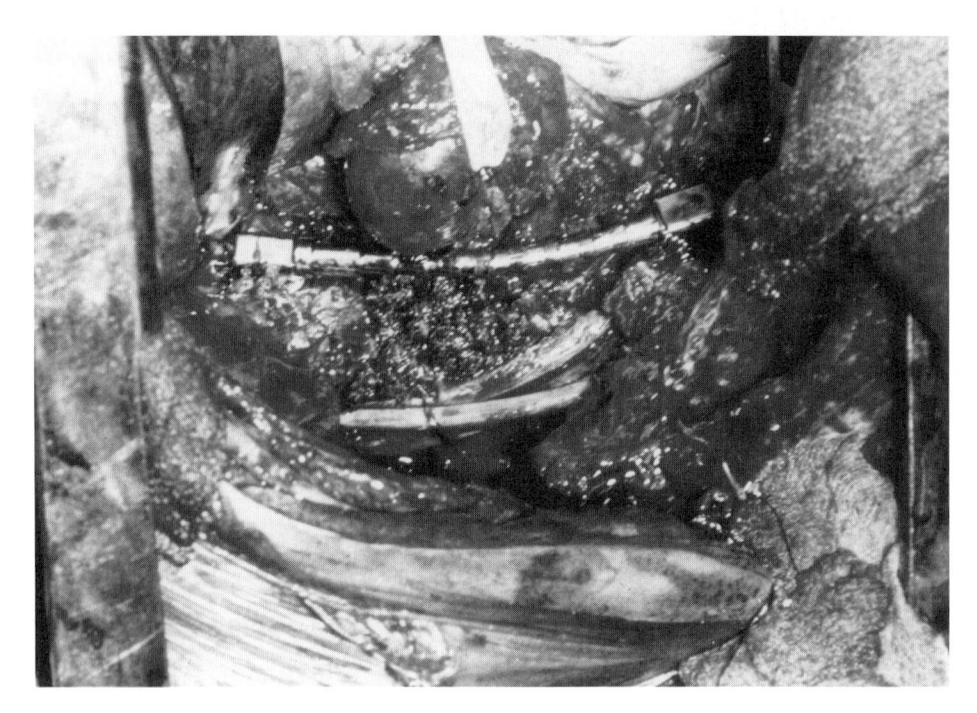

FIG. 18-23. Intraoperative view of anterior spinal elements following decompression and reconstruction. This procedure was preceded by a posterior release and multiple posterior osteotomies. Note decompression posterior to the rib struts. The aorta lies anterior to the rod.

DISCUSSION

The first device described for anterior fixation of the spine and in particular for the correction of kyphosis, was described by Wenger (Milgram, 1984) in New York City in 1953. Unfortunately, this was not successful.

Subsequent reports on anterior lumbar interbody fusion, indicate varying rates of nonunion from 0 to 82% (Bedbrook, 1979; Bohlman et al., 1981; Bradford et al., 1977; Flynn, Anwarul, & Hogue, 1979; Freebody et al., 1971; Goldner, McCollum, & Urbaniak, 1969; Harmon, 1960; Royle, 1928; Sacks, 1966; Stauffer & Coventry, 1972). In most series, the average has been between 10 and 20%. As a result, there has been a somewhat general reluctance to perform anterior surgery in the lumbar spine. In this series of acute fractures, the incidence of nonunion was 4%. Generally, in cases of posttraumatic kyphosis as described by Malcolm et al. (1981) or in cases of trauma in which anterior surgery has been performed, the surgery has been followed by a second-stage posterior fusion and instrumentation. This was done

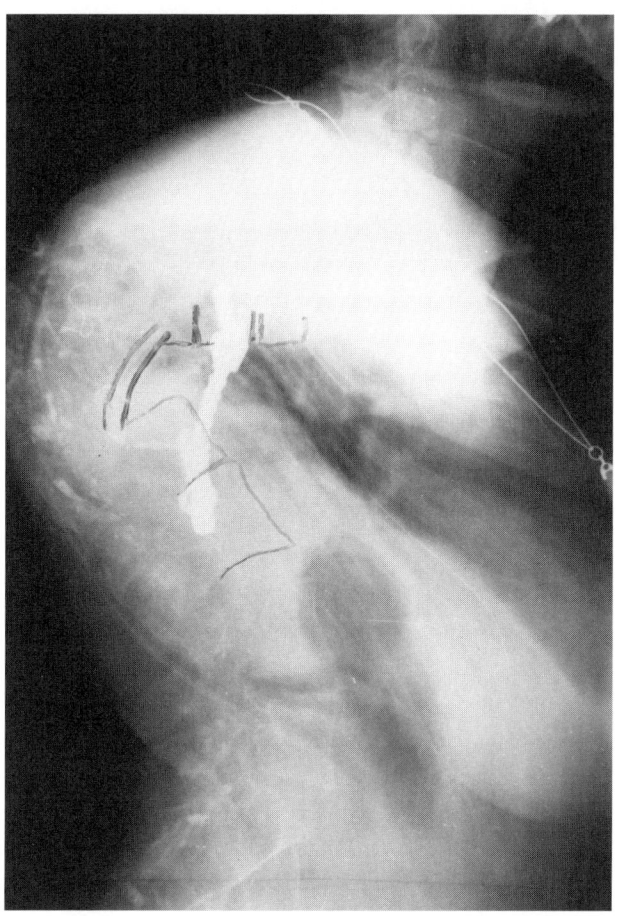

FIG. 18-24. Postoperative lateral x-ray of patient in Figures 18-22 and 18-23.

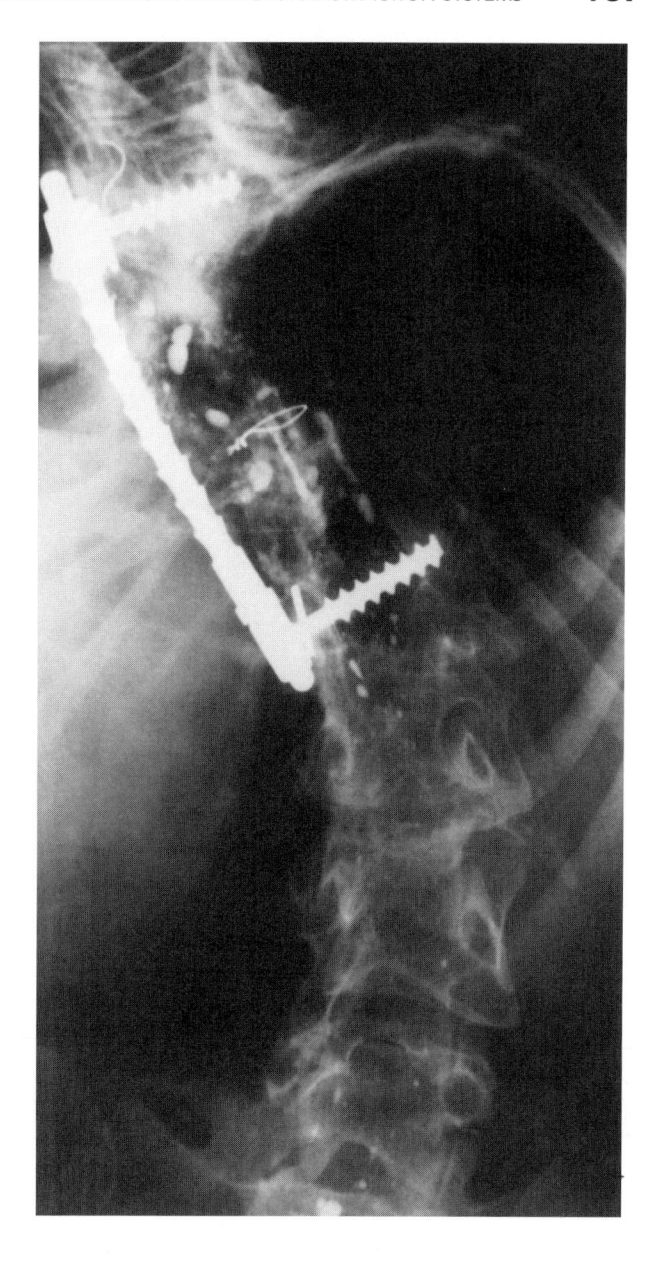

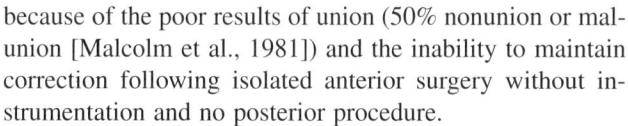

FIG. 18-25. Postoperative anteroposterior view of patient in Figures 18-22 and 18-23. Curve has been reduced to 105 degrees.

because of the poor results of union (50% nonunion or malunion [Malcolm et al., 1981]) and the inability to maintain correction following isolated anterior surgery without instrumentation and no posterior procedure.

In cases of late posttraumatic kyphosis, Malcolm et al. (1981) have recommended the use of supplementary posterior fixation and fusion, as they felt that anterior fusion alone was insufficient. We feel that with the advent of anterior fixation devices, particularly the anterior distraction devices described here, that this is no longer necessary since the device serves to correct the kyphosis and the bone graft is under compressive load. The anterior lumbar spine supports three to four times body weight. Iliac crest grafts, either bicortical or tricortical cannot support these loads in the erect position. Hence, the need for anterior fixation devices.

The anterior Harrington system as described by the author (Kostuik, 1990, 1988b) has been in clinical use for 20 years for a variety of reasons, including the correction of acute kyphosis in burst injuries, late posttraumatic kyphosis, Scheuermann's kyphosis, acute angular kyphosis, and anterior fixation for a variety of other reasons. There have been a total of 40 screw fractures, 25 in acute fractures, 4 in late posttraumatic kyphosis, 6 used anteriorly for correction of Scheuermann's kyphosis, and 5 others in a variety of other cases. There have been five rods break, three in acute burst injuries. A total of 1536 screws and 768 rods have been used to date.

In the treatment of acute burst injuries or late posttraumatic kyphosis, the devices serve to correct the kyphosis readily and to provide stability and allow for early rehabilitation and ambulation. The ease of application allows for

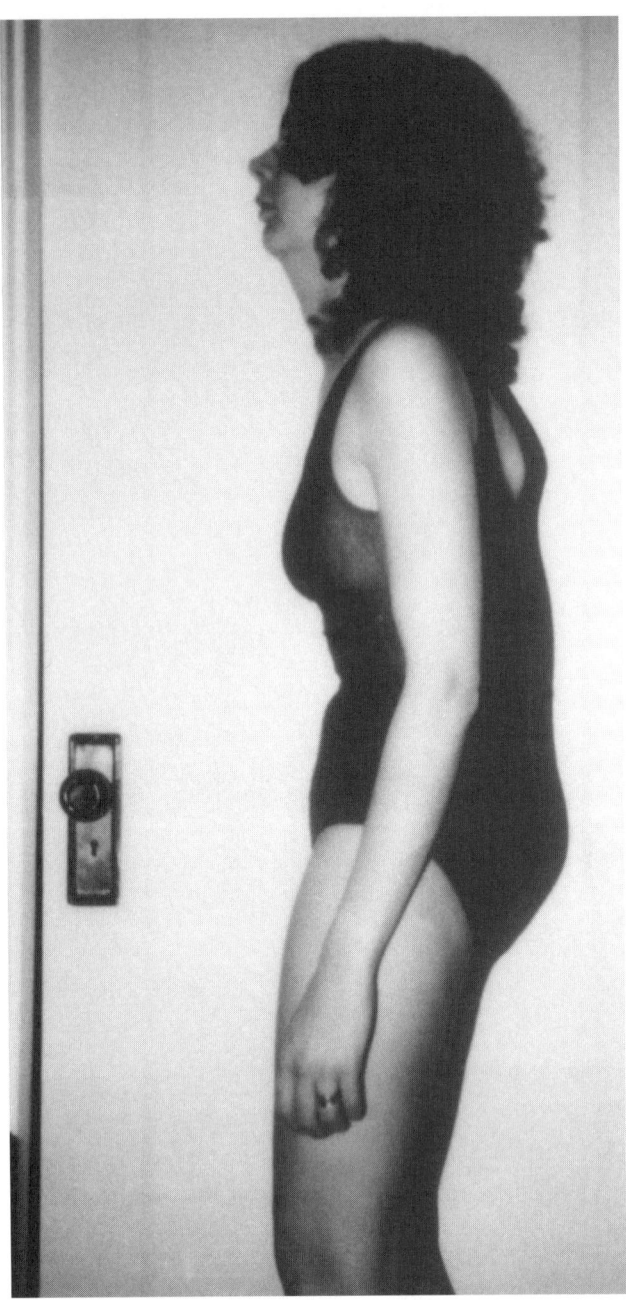

FIG. 18-26. Precorrection painful lumbar kyphosis in a 36-year-old woman that was iatrogenic to lumbar distraction. Distraction rod has been removed.

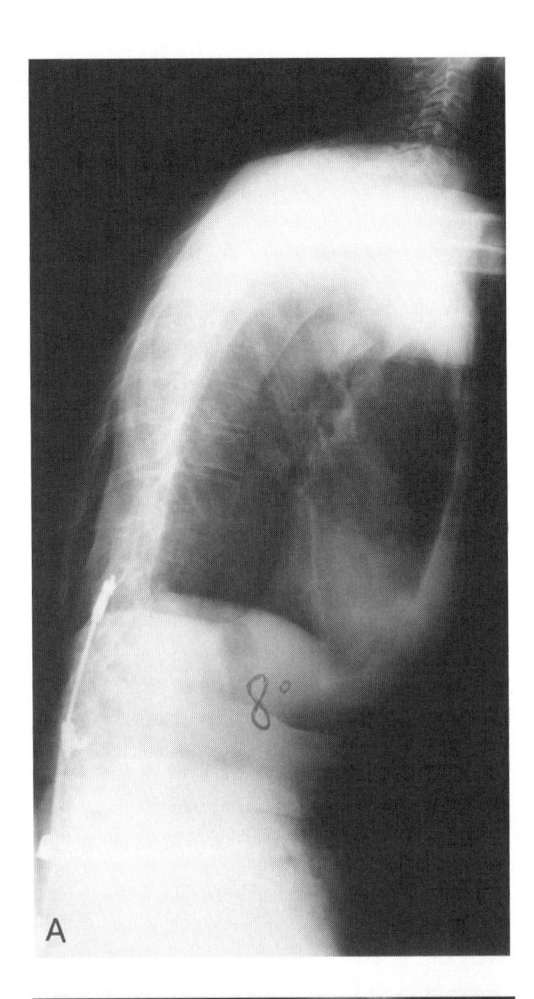

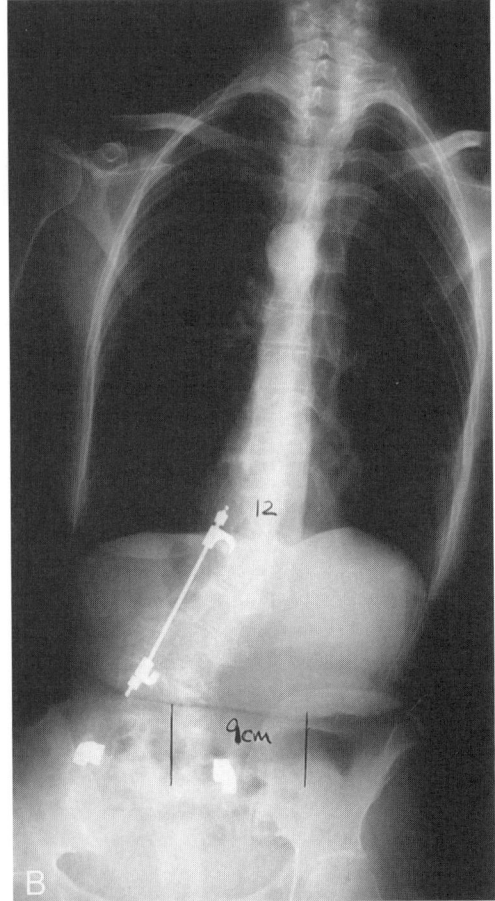

FIG. 18-27. (a) Precorrection lateral and (b) AP x-ray of patient in Figure 18-26.

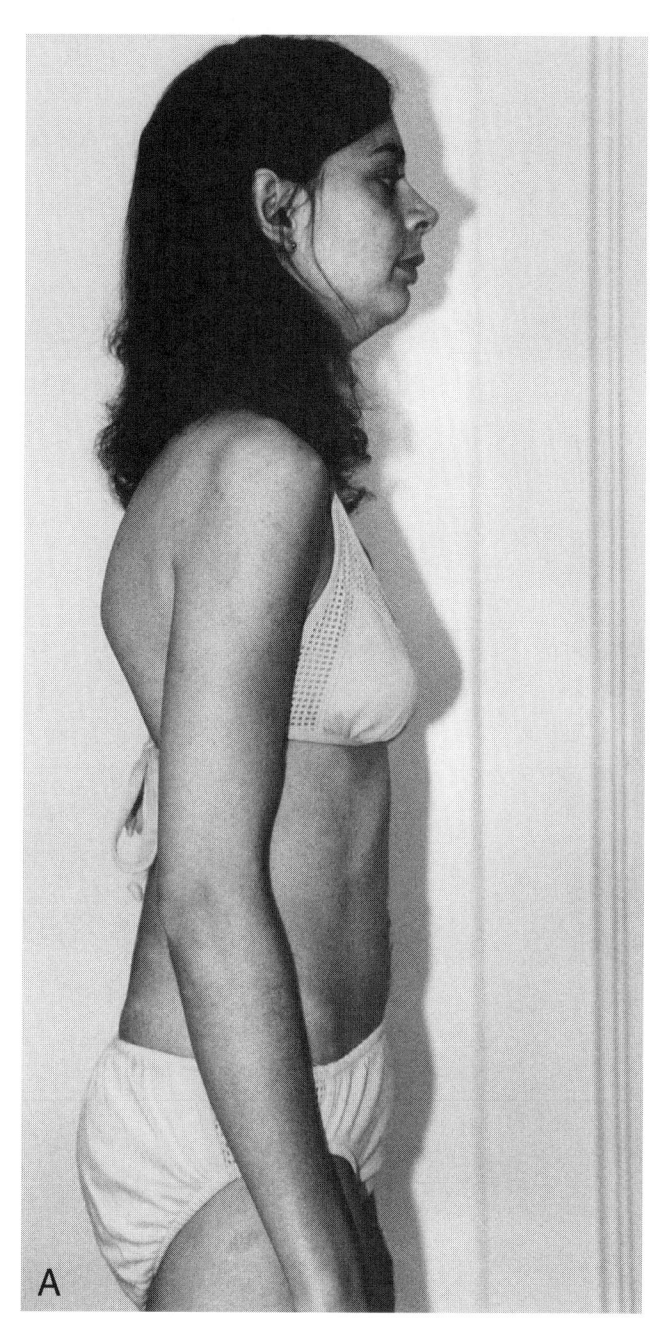

FIG. 18-28. (a) Postosteotomy restoration of lordosis in patient in Figures 18-26 and 18-27. (b) AP x-ray following anterior and posterior reconstruction. (c) Lateral x-ray following anterior and posterior reconstruction.

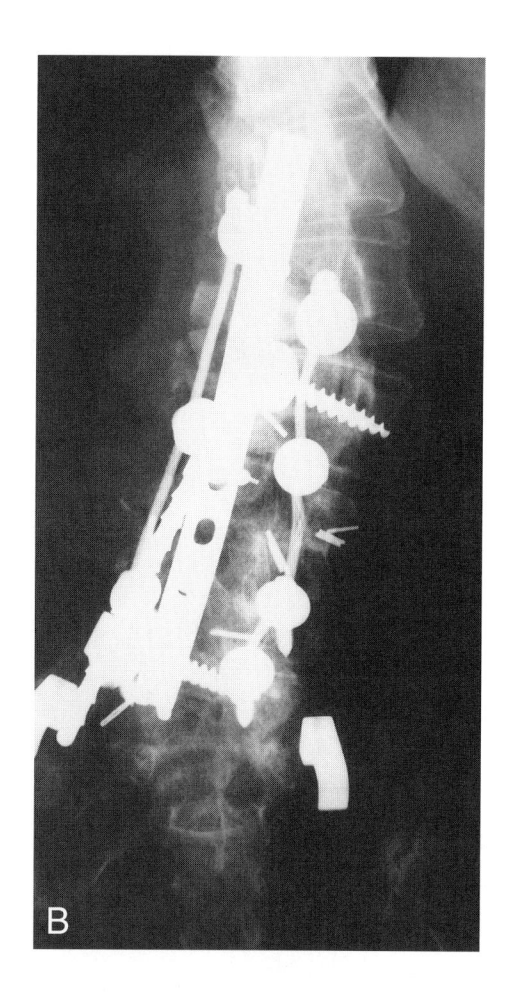

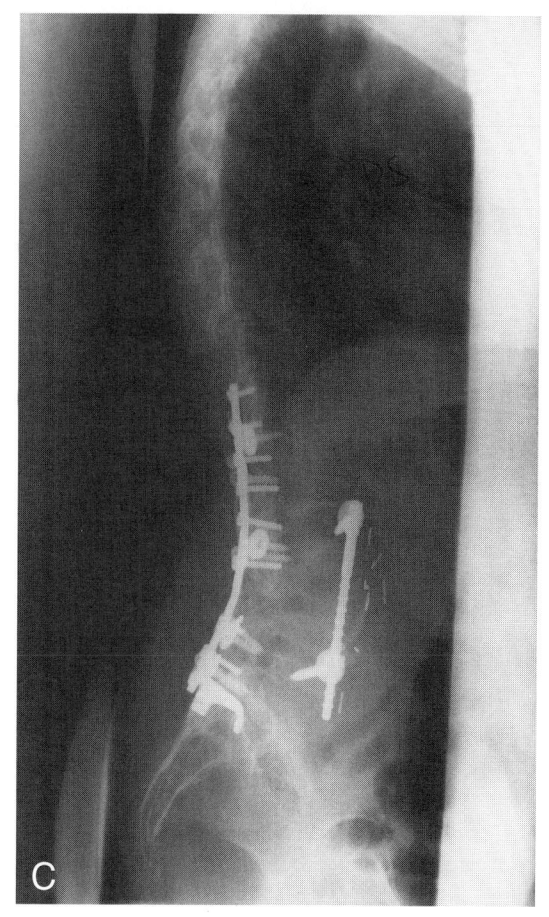

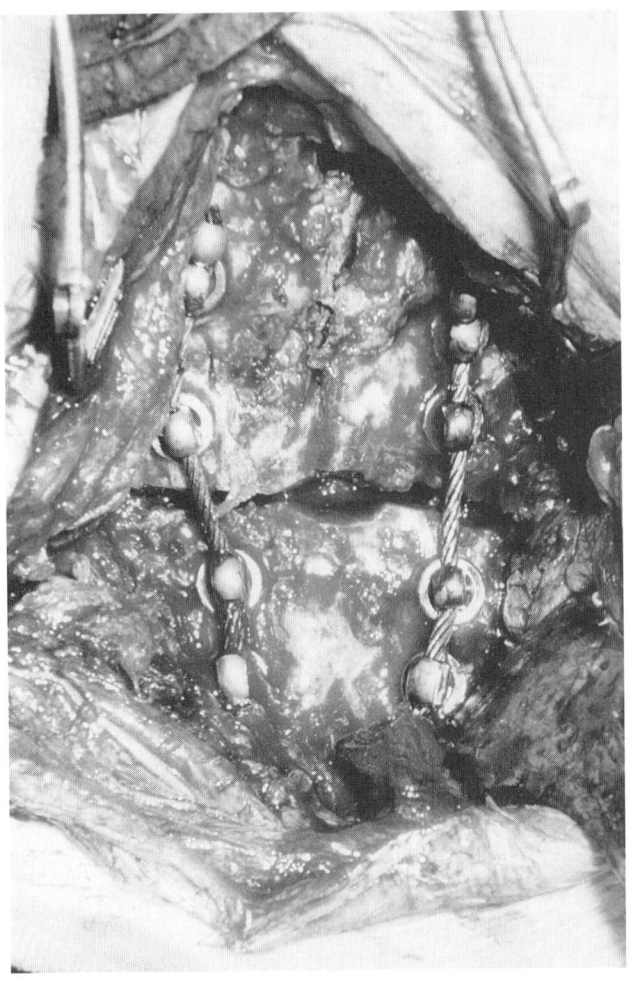

FIG. 18-29. Osteotomy closed posteriorly with Dwyer cables simultaneously as anterior wedge opens with anterior Kostuik-Harrington distraction device. Bone graft has been added.

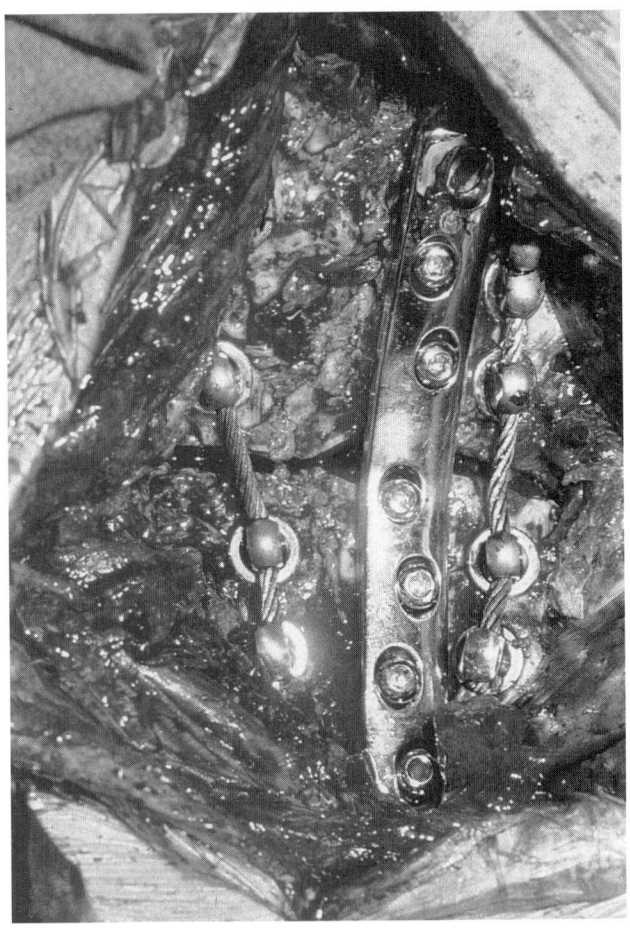

FIG. 18-30. A second compression rod is added and fixed with Kostuik-Harrington screws.

its variable use in many areas of the spine. The uppermost level of vertebral-body insertion has been T2 and the lowest level L5. Although the screws are available in three lengths, they can be readily shortened by cutting the tips. The use of washers or staples serves to prevent toggling of the screw within the cancellous vertebral body. In cases of severe osteopenia, methylmethacrylate bone cement can be used to enhance screw fixation.

Tested cyclically in a dynamic fashion in a laboratory, using calf spines, a single anterior fixation rod device used alone, does not provide good control of rotation and lateral bending. As a result, the use of supplementary fixation with a second rod as a neutralization rod is recommended. Laboratory testing indicates that these devices, although not as rigid as segmental wiring or posterior Harrington instrumentation do provide sufficient stability to allow for early rehabilitation and ambulation with the use of an external orthosis rather than a body cast.

The use of these anterior fixation devices precludes the necessity for any posterior fusion or instrumentation in the majority of cases and shortens hospitalization and the necessity for a second procedure and its possible morbidity. The exception is acute burst injuries that on CT scanning indicate significant posterior element comminution or in which there has been a previous posterior decompression and ambulation is to be allowed.

One early case of a severe T12 burst injury, Frankel grade A, with significant posterior element comminution failed when the patient started transfers in the early postoperative rehabilitation period. Since then we recommend additional second-stage posterior pedicle fixation in cases of severe posterior comminution.

The prime purpose of this chapter has been to describe the uses for anterior fixation in the treatment of acute and chronic kyphosis of the thoracic and lumbar spine. The role

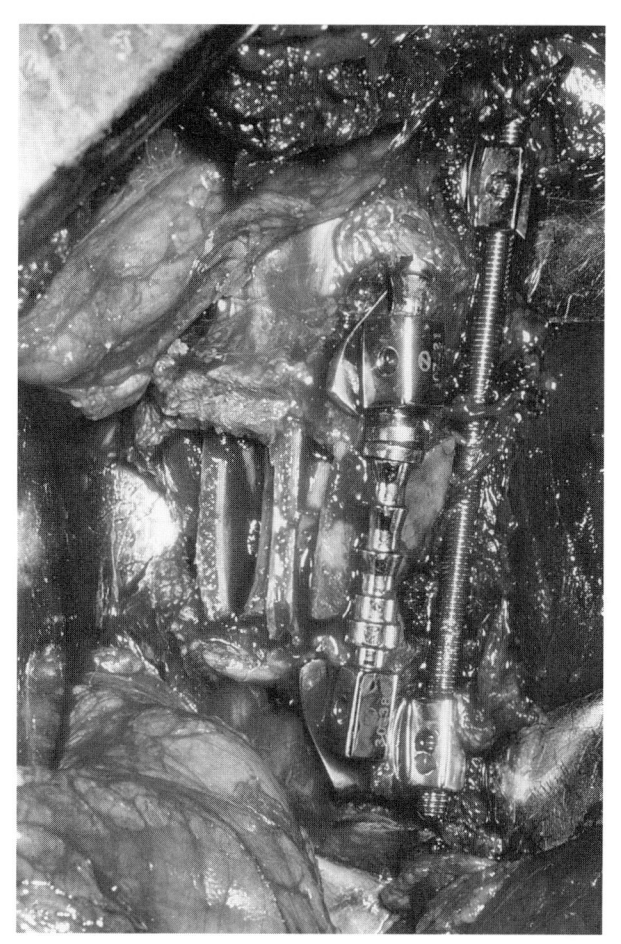

FIG. 18-31. Posteriorly, an AO plate controls rotational Cotrel-Dubousset rods; screws and hooks are alternatives.

of decompression in neurologic injury remains controversial. The results of neurologic improvement were extremely gratifying, with an average improvement of 1.6 grades using the Frankel classification in all cases of incomplete paraplegia resulting from burst fractures.

REFERENCES

Batchelor, J.S. (1963). Anterior interbody spinal fusion. *Guy's Hospital Report, 112,* 61.
Bedbrook, G.M. (1979). Spinal injuries with tetraplegia and paraplegia. *Journal of Bone and Joint Surgery, British Volume, 61,* 267.
Bohlman, H.H., Freeajfel, A., & Dejak, J. (1975). Spinal cord injuries and late anterior decompression of spinal cord injuries. *Journal of Bone and Joint Surgery, American Volume, 57A,* 1025.
Bohlman, H.H., et. al. (1981). Surgical techniques of anterior decompression and fusion for spinal cord injuries. *Clinical Orthopaedics and Related Research, 154,* 57.
Bradford, D.S., Akbarnia, B.A., Winter, R.D., & Seljescog, E.L. (1977). Surgical stabilization of fracture and fracture dislocation of the thoracic spine. *Spine, 2,* 185.
Breig, A. (1972). The therapeutic possibilities of surgical bio-engineering in incomplete spinal cord lesions. *Paraplegia, 9,* 173.
Chou, D., Armstrong, G., O'Neal, J., Gardiner, J., & Black, R. (September 1989). The contoured anterior spinal plate (C.A.S.P.). Presented to the Scoliosis Research Society, Amsterdam, Holland.
Cochran, T., Irstam, L., & Nachemson, A. (1983). Longterm anatomic and functional changes in patients with adolescent idiopathic scoliosis treated by Harrington rod fusion. *Spine, 8(6),* 576–584.
Dewald, R.L., Fister, J.S., & Savino, A.W. (September 1982). The management of unstable burst fractures of the thoracolumbar spine. Presented to the Scoliosis Research Society, Denver, CO.
Dickson, J.H., Harrington, P.R., & Erwin, W.D. (1978). Results of reduction and stabilization of the severely fractured thoracic and lumbar spine. *Journal of Bone and Joint Surgery, American Volume, 60,* 799.
Dunn, H.K. (1984). Anteriorstabilization of thoracolumbar injuries. *Clinical Orthopedics, 189,* 116–184.
Dwyer, A.F. (1973). Experience of anterior correction of scoliosis. *Clinical Orthopaedics and Related Research, 93,* 191.
Esses, S.I., Kostuik, J.P., & Botsford, D. (July 1989). A prospective randomized comparison of the use of the AO internal fixator and Kostuik-Harrington instrumentation for the treatment of burst fractures. Presented to the North American Spine Society, Quebec City.
Flynn, J.C., Anwarul, & Hogue, M.P. (1979). Anterior fusion of the lumbar spine. *Journal of Bone and Joint Surgery, American Volume, 61,* 1143.
Freebody, B., Bendal, R., & Taylor, R.D. (1971). Anterior transperitoneal lumbar fusion. *Journal of Bone and Joint Surgery, British Volume, 53,* 617.
Frankel, B.L., Hancock, D.O., Hyslop, G., Melzak, J., Michaelis, L.S., Ungar, G.H., Vernon, J.D.S., & Walsh, J.J. (1969). The value of postural reduction in the initial management of closed injuries of the spine with paraplegia and tetraplegia. *Paraplegia, 7,* 179.
Goldner, J.L., McCollum, D.E., & Urbaniak, J.R. (1969). Anterior disc excision and interbody spine fusion for chronic low back pain. In: *American Academy of Orthopaedic Surgeons, Symposium of the Spine* (p. 111). St. Louis: C.V. Mosby.
Guttmann, L. (1969). Spinal deformities in traumatic paraplegics and tetraplegics following surgical procedures. *Paraplegia, 7,* 38.
Guttmann, L. (1954). Initial treatment of traumatic paraplegia. *Proceedings of the Royal Society of Medicine, 47,* 1103.
Hall, J.E., & Micheli, L.J. (October 1977, September 1981). The use of modified Dwyer instrumentation in anterior stabilization of the spine. Presented to the Scoliosis Research Society, Hong Kong, Montreal.
Harmon, P.H. (1960). Anterior extra peritoneal disc excision and vertebral body fusion. *Clinical Orthopaedics and Related Research, 18,* 169.
Hodgson, A.R. & Stock, F.E. (1956). Anterior spinal fusion: A preliminary communication on radical treatment of Pott's disease and Pott's paraplegia. *British Journal of Surgery, 44,* 266–275.
Harrington, P.R. (1962). Treatment of scoliosis. *Journal of Bone and Joint Surgery, American Volume, 44,* 591.
Kaneda, K., Abumi, K., & Fujiya, M. (September 1982). Burst fractures of the thoracolumbar and lumbar spine with neurological involvement: Anterior decompression and fusion with instrumentation. Presented to the Scoliosis Research Society, Denver, CO.
Kostuik, J.P. (1990). Anterior Kostuik-Harrington distraction systems for the treatment of kyphotic deformities. *Spine, 15,* 169–180.
Kostuik, J.P. (1988a). Anterior fixation for burst fractures of the thoracic and lumbar spine with or without neurological involvement. *Spine, 13,* 286–293.
Kostuik, J.P. (1988b). Anterior Kostuik-Harrington distraction systems for the treatment of kyphotic deformities. *Iowa Orthopedic Journal, 8,* 68–77.
Kostuik, J.P. (1988c). Treatment of scoliosis in the adult thoracolumbar spine with special reference to fusion to the sacrum. *Orthopaedics Clinics of North America, 2,* 371–381.
Kostuik, J.P. (1983). Anterior spinal cord decompression for lesions of the thoracic and lumbar spine, techniques, new methods of internal fixation, results. *Spine, 8,* 512–531.
Kostuik, J.P., & Matsuzaki, H. (1989). Anterior stabilization, instrumentation, and decompression for post-traumatic kyphosis. *Spine, 14,* 379–386.

Kostuik, J.P., Richardson, W., Maurais, G., & Okajima, Y. (1988). Combined single stage anterior and posterior osteotomy for correction of iatrogenic lumbar kyphosis. *Spine, 13*, 257–266.

Malcolm, B.W., Bradford, D.S., Winter, R.B., & Chou, S.N. (1981). Posttraumatic kyphosis. *Journal of Bone and Joint Surgery, American Volume, 63*, 891.

Milgram, J. (1984). Hospital for Joint Diseases. New York. Personal communication.

Moe, J.H., Winter, R.B., Bradford, D.S., & Lonstein, J.E. (1978). Scoliosis and other spinal deformities. Philadelphia: W.B. Saunders.

Moon, M.S., et. al. (1981). Anterior interbody fusion in fractures and fracture dislocations of the spine. *International Orthopaedics, 5*(2), 143.

Morgan, T.H., Wharton, G.W., & Austin, G.N. (1971). The results of laminectomy in patients with incomplete spinal cord injuries. *Paraplegia, 9*, 14.

Morscher, E., Gerber, B., & Fasel, J. (1984). Surgical treatment of spondylolisthesis by bone grafting and direct stabilization of spondylolysis by means of a hook screw. *Archives of Orthopaedic Trauma Surgery, 103*, 175–178.

Nicholl, E.A. (1949). Fractures of the dorso-lumbar spine. *Journal of Bone and Joint Surgery, British Volume, 31*, 376.

Paul, R.L., Michael, R.H., Dunn, J.E., & Williams, J.P. (1975). Anterior transthoracic surgical decompression of acute spinal cord injuries. *Journal of Neurosurgery, 43*, 299.

Rezaian, S.M., Dombrowski, E.T., & Ghista, D.N. (1983). Spinal fixator for the management of spinal injury (the mechanical rationale). *Engineering in Medicine, 12*, 95.

Riska, E.B. (1977). Antero-lateral decompression as a treatment of paraplegia following a vertebral fracture in the thoraco-lumbar spine. *International Orthopaedics, 1*, 22.

Roberts, J.B., & Curtis, P.H., Jr. (1970). Stability of the thoracic and lumbar spine in traumatic paraplegia following fracture or fracture dislocation. *Journal of Bone and Joint Surgery, American Volume, 52*, 1115.

Royle, N.D. (1928). The operative removal of an accessary vertebra. *Australian Medical Journal, 1*, 467.

Sacks, S. (1965). Anterior interbody fusion of the lumbar spine. *Journal of Bone and Joint Surgery, British Volume, 47*, 211.

Sacks, S. (1966). Anterior interbody fusion of the lumbar spine: indications and results in two-hundred cases. *Clinical Orthopaedics and Related Research, 44*, 163.

Slot, G.H. (September 1981). A new distraction system for the correction of kyphosis using the anterior approach. Presented to the Scoliosis Research Society, Montreal, Quebec.

Stauffer, R.N., & Coventry, M.B. (1972). Anterior interbody lumbar spine fusion: Analysis of Mayo Clinic series. *Journal of Bone and Joint Surgery, American Volume, 54*, 756.

White, A.A., III, Punjabi, M., & Thomas, C.L. (1977). The clinical biomechanics of kyphotic deformities. *Clinical Orthopaedics and Related Research, 128*, 8–17.

Whitesides, T.E., Jun, & Shah, S.G.A. (1976). The management of unstable fractures of the thoracolumbar spine. *Spine, 1*, 99.

Whitesides, T.E., & Jun. (1977). Traumatic kyphosis of the thoracolumbar spine. *Clinical Orthopaedics and Related Research, 128*, 78.

Yosipovitch, Z., Robin, G.C., & Makin, M. (1977). Open reduction of unstable thoracolumbar spinal injuries and fixation with Harrington Rods. *Journal of Bone and Joint Surgery, American Volume, 59*, 1003.

Yuan, H. (1987). Personnal communication.

Zielke, K. (1982). Ventral Derotation Spondylodese: Behandlungsergebnisse bein Idiopathischen Lumbarskoliosen. *Orthopedics, 120*, 320–329.

CHAPTER 19

Application of Rezaian Anterior Fixation System for the Management of Fractures of Thoracolumbar Spine

S.M. Rezaian

HIGHLIGHTS

Aebie, Ettercher, and Thalgott (1988) have stated that "an ideal treatment of spinal fractures would be anterior instrumentation that would provide enough stability and fixation to prevent deformity even in osteoporotic bone, that is not yet available." In 1986, Ferguson and Allen from the University of Texas, Galveston, also gave an algorithm for the treatment of unstable thoracolumbar fractures. After extensive biomechanical testing using the currently available instruments for spinal fixation, they concluded that no one instrument is perfect to handle all thoracolumbar fractures. The experience of others is the same (Emans, 1990; Kaneda, 1984; Kostuik & Matsusaki, 1989; Louis, 1985; Schultz, Belytschko, Andriacchi, & Galante, 1973). In this chapter, I present a new spinal fixator used through the anterolateral approach for anterior instrumentation that will provide enough stability and fixation, and prevent deformity, even in a person with osteoporosis. It is used with bone graft for fusion for long-term results. It is suitable for all types of fractures of the thoracolumbar spine. No external supports (e.g., plastic jacket or cast) are required. Hospitalization is short, just 5 to 10 days. Long-term results have proven that this fixator has stood the test of time, at least for the past 12 years.

PROBLEM

In a serious fracture of the thoracolumbar spine with neurologic deficit, commonly the middle column fails, and fragments of bone and ruptured disk invade into the spinal canal. The vector of gravity that falls anterior to the vertebral body shifts more forward and produces further compromise of the spinal canal. In this scenario, safe decompression of the anterior aspect of the neural tube from the posterior approach is difficult and stabilization of flexion moment by the posterior metallic splintage is mechanically unsound. Consequently, it fails (Francis, 1984; Dunn, 1984; Ghista, 1986; Kaneda, 1984; Kostuik & Matsusaki, 1989; Louis, 1985; Rezaian, 1991, 1982).

SOLUTION

The Rezaian Spinal Fixator has been designed to resolve the problem of burst and compression fractures. It is, essentially, a turnbuckle-like instrument. There is a flat plate on each end, each with four sharp spikes.

When used, this fixator simply replaces the middle column of the damaged vertebral body. The flat plate rests on the intact end plates above and below. By turning the turnbuckle, the sharp spikes penetrate into the end plate and the kyphotic deformity is corrected. There is a locking screw by which one may fix the apparatus in position (Figs. 19-1, 19-2). The Rezaian spinal fixator commercially is available in four sizes. (Spinal and Orthopedic, Inc., Van Nuys, CA.)

BIOMECHANICAL CONSIDERATIONS

The line of gravity of the upper trunk falls ventrally to the transverse axis of motion, at all levels of the spine (Frankel & Nordin, 1980) and the major weight of trunk is based on body of vertebrae in all the time and the vector of gravity is anterior to body at lumbar spine (White & Panjabi, 1990).

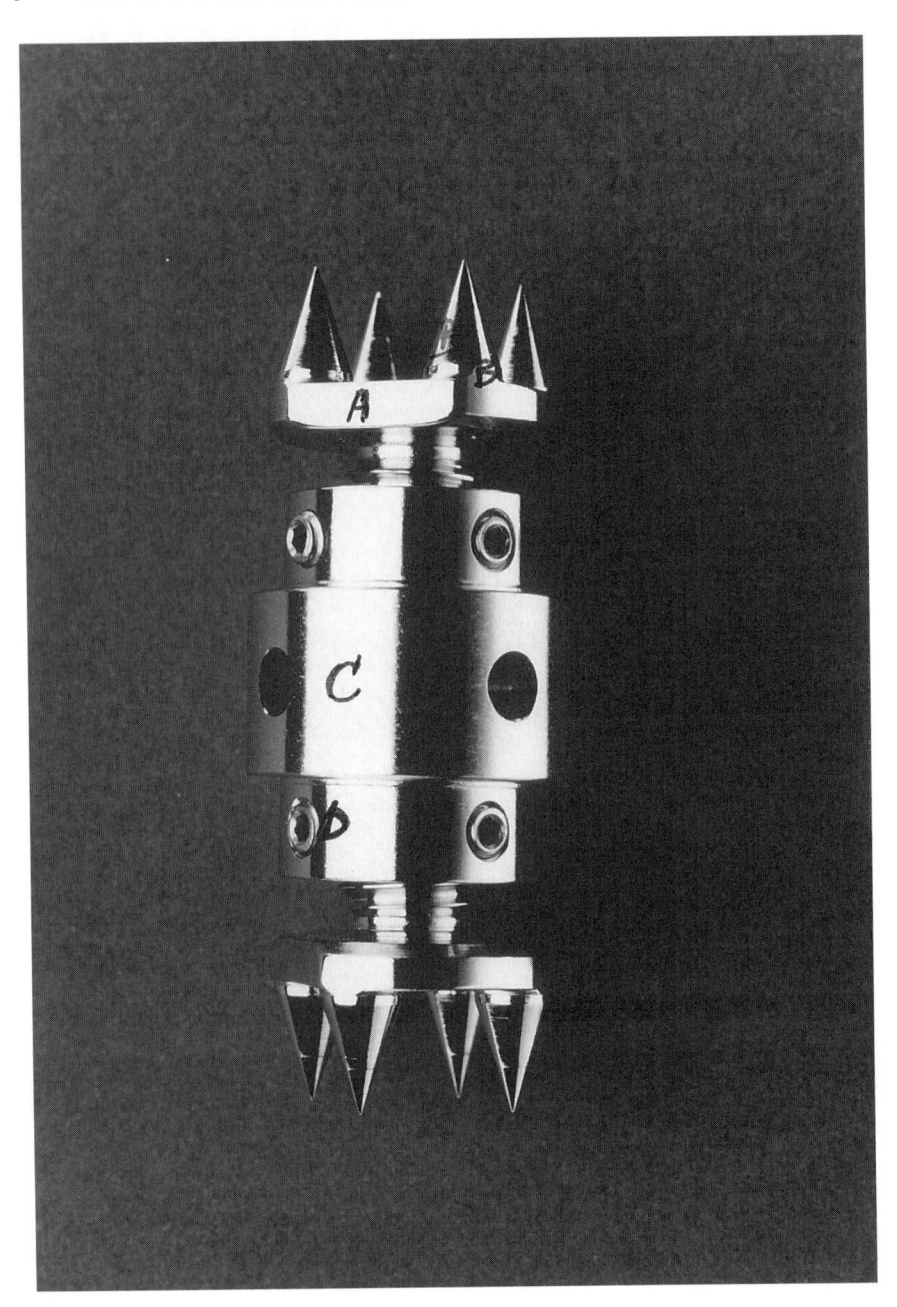

FIG. 19-1. The Rezaian spinal fixator (RSF) consists of flat plate (A), sharp spikes (B), turnbuckle (C), and a locking screw (D).

Any amount of collapsed vertebral body due to fracture shifts the axes of gravity further anteriorly and therefore produces a tension on the posterior elements and compresses the anterior aspect of the spinal canal. The ruptured disks and fragments of bone compress into the spinal canal.

In this situation, the spinal canal will be compromised, and neurologic deterioration will ensue or be aggravated. For this reason, posterior splinting of burst fractures by posterior metallic splinting is not safe, and it may eventually fail (Ghista, 1986).

However, in such a situation, the Rezaian spinal fixator restores the height of the collapsed vertebrae and constructs a pillar between the adjacent intact vertebrae along the line of normal gravity. At the same time, the surgeon will decompress the anterior aspect of the spinal canal. In practice, the spinal fixator is embedded in bone graft for long-term good results.

Independent experimental work on human cadaver spine at two different centers in two different countries has proven that the Rezaian spinal fixator is very stable under flexion moment. The fixed spine with the Rezaian spinal fixation system is more stable than an intact spine (Ghista, 1986).

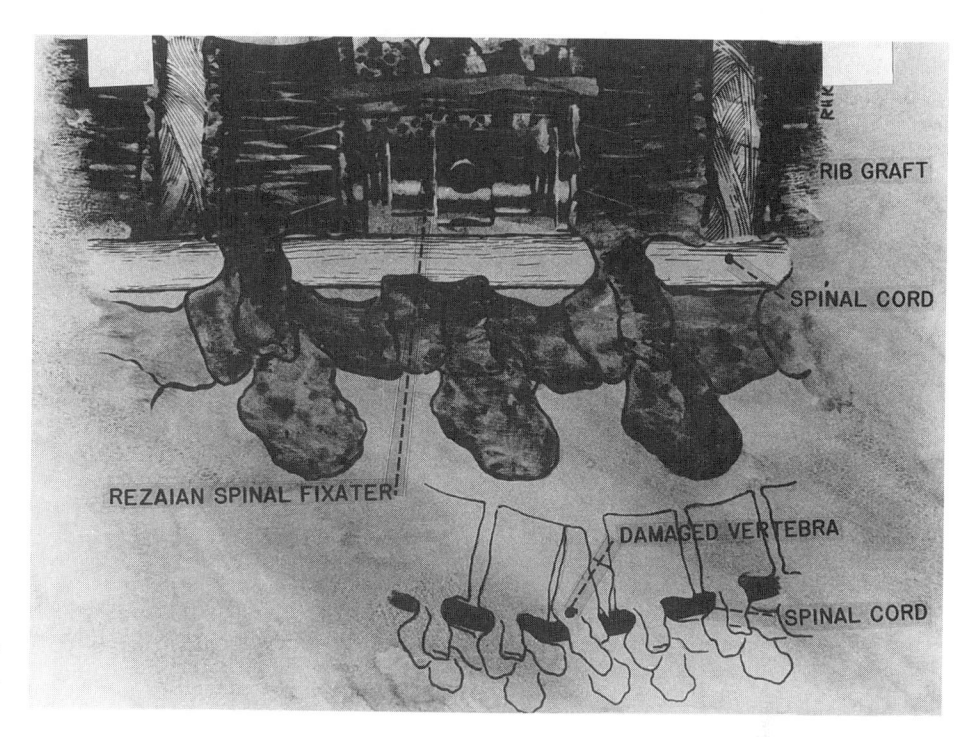

FIG. 19-2. Drawing of Technique. Note on the right side the fracture of the spine and on the left the reconstruction by RSF.

INDICATIONS FOR USE

The Rezaian spinal fixator is indicated in any of the following conditions:

- To replace a diseased or injured vertebral body in tumor patients.
- To restore the height of a collapsed vertebral body due to burst fractures.
- To achieve anterior decompression of the spinal cord and neural tissues.
- To provide stabilization following severe disk degeneration.

Generally, there is a combination of the above-mentioned conditions that present as indications (Table 19–1). The Rezaian spinal fixator is always used with a combination of bone graft for fusion and long-term good results.

CONTRAINDICATIONS

The Rezaian spinal fixator should not be used in cases in which there is:

- No neurologic deficit present.
- Less than 10% compression of the vertebrae.
- Active infection of the involved vertebral bodies.
- Widely disseminated metastatic tumors of the involved vertebrae, affecting more than three vertebrae.
- Severe osteoporosis.
- Sensitivity to implant materials.

PREREQUISITES

- A comprehensive radiologic study of the damaged and adjacent vertebrae must be available. CT and MRI studies are very helpful in preoperative planning.
- A myelogram is still an excellent method of determining whether there is compression of the spinal cord and neural tissues.
- The cell saver should be available during the operation, or at least four units of blood must be available.

Table 19-1
Indications and Contraindications for Use of the Rezaian Spinal Fixator

Indications
  Traumatic burst fractures.
  Traumatic compressed fractures with clinical symptoms not responding to usual nonsurgical treatment.
  Pathologic fracture involving one to three body vertebra. Bridge the gap with the use of bone graft or methylmethacrylate.
  Quiescent infection, after complete debridement, bridging the adjacent vertebrae combination with bone graft.
  Anterior arthrodesis with bone graft after failed-back syndrome.

Contraindications
  Metal sensitivity to stainless steel (e.g., patient cannot use metal watch).
  Complete fracture and dislocation of the spine. (When posterior elements are inside the canal, one must first reduce the posterior element, then proceed with the use of the anterior Rezaian spinal fixator.)

ANAESTHESIA

General anaesthesia is recommended, with endotracheal intubation.

PATIENT POSITIONING

I recommend the left anterolateral approach. The patient should be placed on the operating table on his or her right side, in such a way that the left side of the body is elevated at 45 degrees from the operating table. The right lower limb is flexed and the left is straight. The left arm is suspended. In this situation, the kidney support is elevated in such a way that about 20 to 30 degrees of lateral flexion with convexity to the left side will be produced. The left side, from the midline of the spine to the midline of the anterior body, is prepared and draped in the standard fashion.

SURGICAL TECHNIQUE

For the thoracic and thoracolumbar region, I generally go through the bed of the rib, above the lesion (Fig. 19-3). For example, in order to remove or replace the vertebral body of T12, the suitable approach would be through the bed of the 11th rib. Once through the bed of the 11th rib, one may expose from T10 to L3. Nevertheless, one or two ribs above or one rib below may be selected as the entry site. For the last two lumbar regions, we recommend the kidney approach, which is well documented in orthopedic and urologic textbooks.

We recommend that the subcutaneous tissues along the 11th rib be infiltrated with normal saline mixed with epinephrine (1:1,000,000). This will provide a bloodless field. The skin incision is made along the length of the 11th rib, starting from the costochondral junction anteriorly and continuing to the costovertebral junction posteriorly. The skin is well retracted with a pair of self-retaining retractors, then the periosteum of the 11th rib is cut with a scalpel, sharply along its shaft. Its outer, upper, and lower edges are reflected with the aid of a periosteal elevator.

Now, the rib is cut at its anterior end at the junction of the costochondral area in such a way that about 1 or 2 cm of cartilage, even in an adult, always remain with the soft tissues. Then, gradually working from anterior to posterior, the rib is freed from the soft tissue and is disarticulated at the junction of the costovertebral joints. At this stage, the intercostal neurovascular segments are easily distinguished in the wound.

The intercostal nerve will lead to the intervertebral foramen and is the best guide for later surgery. But first, attention is paid to the anterior part of the incision.

Following removal of the rib, the remnant of its cartilage is just in the anterior part of the incision. This cartilage is vertically split by using a strong pair of scissors or knife. By splitting this cartilage, the diaphragm is actually split.

Through this slit, a hole is made in the undersurface of the diaphragm. Then, by enlarging this hole, one finger (normally the index), may be passed through it, beneath the diaphragm and into the retroperitoneal cavity. Working from anterior to posterior, on the distal part of the wound, one can easily dissect the diaphragm from the chest wall and push toward the proximal section of the wound. Approximately 1 cm of the diaphragm remains attached to the chest wall to facilitate its later repair.

At this point in the procedure, the surgeon requests the anesthetist to inflate the lungs repeatedly so that the boundary of the lung and pleura will be well visualized. The aim is to dissect the diaphragm from the wall of the chest without damaging the parietal pleura. In this way, the whole diaphragm, together with parietal pleura, will be separated from the wall of the chest and gradually will be pushed up toward the head of the patient.

On advancing to the posterior part of the wound, one may feel the pulsation of the aorta, which normally slips from the midline to the right side of the patient.

Careful dissection of the parietal pleura will be continued until the crus of diaphragm (semi-tendinomuscular structure) is visible. The crus must be tied between two nonabsorbable sutures and will be cut off in such a way that a part of it will remain in the chest wall over the body of L2, and another end will be freed over the diaphragm.

Deep retractors are inserted and the chest and abdominal cavity are opened widely. With gentle dissection and with the aid of a wet sponge, the peritoneal cavity is pushed down and the pleural cavity is pushed up. The sympathetic chain of nerves and intervertebral artery and vein may be visible at this point.

The vertebral body from T10 to L3 can easily be palpated. The fracture site or damaged body can be distinguished. In this stage, the sympathetic chain will be dissected and pushed downward carefully, after which, the boundary of damaged bony vertebra is traced.

One or two intervertebral arteries and veins must be ligated and cut off. I strongly recommend that the artery and vein be cut at the midline, or as near as possible to the midline, of the spine.

In this way, through the intercommunications on the lateral side of the spine, the ischemic damage to the nueral tissues will be minimized.

By covering the abdominal and pleural cavity with two large wet sponges, the damaged area will be available for reconstructive surgery. I prefer to use the intercostal nerve as a guide to enter into the lateral side of the vertebral bodies and just in front of the intervertebral foramen, and remove the damaged piece of vertebral body up and forward until the spinal canal and epidural space are fully exposed.

At this time, the anterior part of the cord is exposed. If, however, the radiologic studies have shown that there was compression on the spinal cord, the cord and dura over it will expand and be visualized in the form of a "sausage." The damaged vertebral body (one or more) and the adjacent disks are removed.

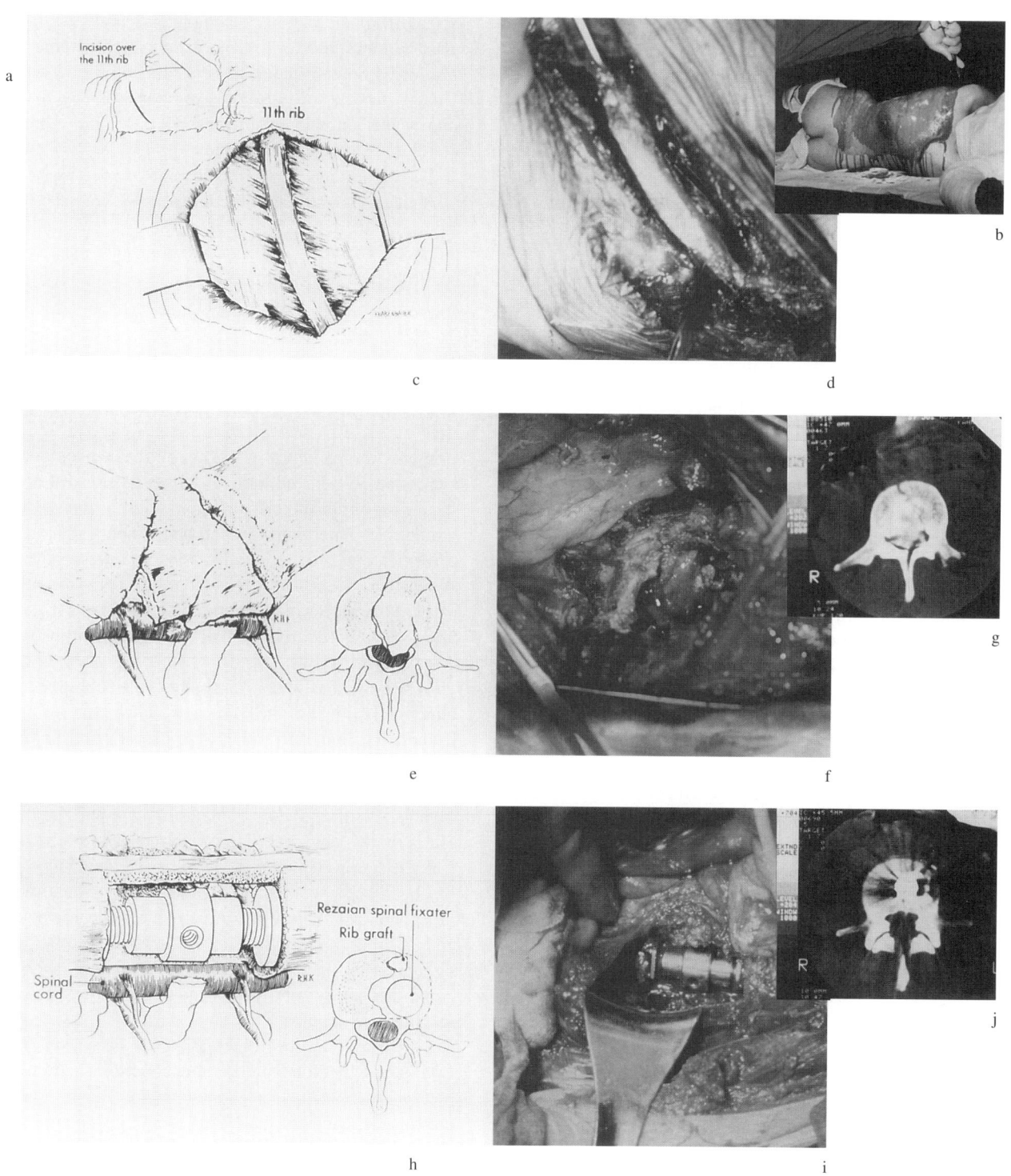

CHAPTER 19 / APPLICATION OF REZAIAN ANTERIOR FIXATION SYSTEM 197

FIG. 19-3. (a) Drawing of position. (b) Patient in operating room. (c) Drawing of incision. (d) Actual operating field, with ribs exposed. (e) Drawing of fracture of spine; transverse and axial section. (f) Operative field. (g) CT scan. (h) Drawing of reconstruction of fracture of spine with Rezaian spinal fixator. (Note the rib graft in front of RSF.) (i) Operative field. (j) CT scan 14 months after surgery. (Note that spinal fixator is embedded with bone graft.)

Normally, I recommend that the anterior part of the canal be completely decompressed. In addition, a space should be made inside the vertebra for placement of the spinal fixator. I generally replace the middle column of the vertebra (the part that makes the anterior aspect of the spinal canal) with the spinal fixator.

After completing this stage, the distance between the adjacent intact vertebrae is measured and one of the sizes of the Rezaian spinal fixator is chosen for insertion. Any displacement at this stage may be completely corrected under direct vision, without damage to neural tissues.

The spinal fixator will be inserted with a special instrument called an "introducer." It will distract the spine until the height of the damaged vertebra is restored.

A small slit about 1 cm in length is then made on the anterolateral edge of the intact vertebrae above and below the area where the damaged vertebra and disk were removed. Suitably sized pieces of the 11th rib, which was removed during the approach, are inserted in these slits in such a way that the adjacent vertebrae are biologically connected and the anterior column of the vertebra is restored. The rest of the spongy bone is inserted between the rib grafts and the remainder of the vertebral body and spinal fixator.

Anteroposterior and lateral x-ray films are taken to confirm satisfactory position of the spinal fixator and alignment of the vertebrae. After documenting the correct position of the spinal fixator on x-ray films, the final step is to lock the fixator by tightening the small locking hexagonal screw. The hexagonal tip at the end of the introducer should be used for this purpose.

We generally recommend that two medium size drains be placed, one in the retropleural cavity and another in the retroperitoneal cavity. The diaphragm should then be replaced. Repair will start with nonabsorbable sutures, first to put the crus of the diaphragm together; then the peripheral part of the diaphragm must be reattached to the remnant of the diaphragm in the thoracic wall in the normal site. In this way, the two halves of the cartilage of the anterior end of the rib will come together exactly.

Next, a second row of nonabsorbable sutures will be placed inside the chest through the diaphragm to the wall of the chest. Subsequently, an approximator is applied to the 12th and 10th ribs and the wall of the chest will be closed in three layers, in the usual manner. A light dressing is then applied to the wound.

All other precautions and measures for major operations and internal implants, including prophylactic, broad-spectrum antibiotics must be taken into account. Electrolytes, blood replacement and blood balance are the most important factors.

POSTOPERATIVE MANAGEMENT

The patient may be allowed to sit up 1 to 3 days after the operation. Hemovac drains are removed 48 hours after the operation. If the patient is completely paralyzed, he or she must be measured for braces. If the patient is able to walk with or without crutches, he or she is allowed to do so 5 to 7 days after the operation. Respiratory therapy for expansion of the lungs is most necessary, particularly during the first 3 days after the operation.

The patient may leave the hospital as soon as the wound has healed. No particular complications have occurred after the wound has completely healed. My experience shows that the spinal fixator is embedded in bone and, therefore, bone healing takes place around it, and it is generally tolerated well by the body. Consequently, it is not necessary to remove this appliance.

A SHORT REVIEW OF THE MEDICAL LITERATURE

Compression of neural elements by retropulsed bone fragments can be relieved indirectly by posterior distraction instrumentation or directly by exploration of the spinal canal through an anterolateral approach. There is no universal agreement as to the indication for these alternatives (Weinstein, 1993). Multiple pieces of bone fragment and particularly pieces of disk retropulsed into the canal may not be completely reduced by distraction posterior instrumentation (Francis, 1984).

When there is a burst fracture with neurologic deficit, blind realignment of the spine with Harrington rods in many patients may not decompress the neural canal. In addition, when using posterior instrumentation, the application of a body cast is recommended; it should be worn for 3 to 6 months (Francis, 1984). Sublaminar wire and the Luque L-rod is more stable, but will not hold distraction for anatomical correction of fractures. Also, passing sublaminar wires has been accompanied by as much as 25% neurologic injury. The risks of pedicle screw fixation include neurologic and vascular injury (McAfee, 1992, 1987). Furthermore, although many plate and screw internal fixation systems are being evaluated, none have been approved by the FDA for use in spine (Emans, 1990).

Anterior spinal instrumentation has been used. In 1973, Dwyer designed the anterior spinal instrumentation for correction of scoliosis. His technique has been modified for the use of management of fractures of the spine by others (Kaneda, 1984; Kostuik & Matsusaki, 1989; Dunn, 1984).

The Dunn apparatus was removed from the market because of serious complications. In the Kaneda and Kostuik techniques, the rods are attached to the side of the vertebrae above and below by means of screws. Therefore, the weight of the trunk is diverged to the lateral side over the instrumentation and loaded on the screws. The author has recommended that the patient should wear external support postoperatively—for example, a body cast plastic jacket. For this reason, the technique seems not to be producing sufficient stability. Practically, both techniques are complicated

(Dunn, 1984; Kaneda, 1984; Kostuik & Matsusaki, 1989; McAfee, 1992, 1987).

In theory, one must choose a technique that will minimize the patient's exposure to the risks of surgery, and avoid the iatrogenic neurovascular injury reported in the literature. In addition one must have confidence that one can achieve the goals of surgery. The goals must include decompression of the neural canal for better recovery and restoration of height of the vertebra for immediate weight-bearing. Finally, one must be able to secure stabilization without the need for external support (e.g., body cast) for early rehabilitation.

The Rezaian spinal fixator has been designed to fulfill these criteria (Table 19–2). The technique has proven to be effective and reliable. It has shown that it will stand the test of time without instrumentation failure (Rezaian, 1991).

Table 19-2
Advantages and Disadvantages of the Rezaian Spinal Fixator

Advantages*
  Approved by FDA since 1984.
  Stabilizes the normal weight-bearing axes.
  Provides a secure stability without need for external support (e.g., plastic jacket)
  Much safer for the patient.
  Easier for the surgeon.
  Simple apparatus with no need for extra instrumentation.
  No instrument failure has been reported (1984–1994).

Disadvantages
  Not adequate as sole stabilization for three-column instability.
  Does not provide stabilization in extension.

*Based on 106 uses by the author and experience with over 1200 sold by the company. (Spinal and Orthopaedic Devices, Inc., Van Nuys, CA).

REFERENCES

Aebie, M., Ettercher, R., & Thalgott K. (1988). The internal skeletal fixation. *Clinical Orthopaedics and Related Research, 227,* 30.

Francis, D. (1984) *Thoracolumbar Spine in Orthopedic Knowledge Update 1 (OKUI)* (p. 231). Rosemont, Illinois: American Academy Orthopaedic Surgeons.

Dombrowski, E.T., & Rezaian, S.M.: Rezaian fixator in the anterior stabilization of unstable spine. *Orthopedic Review, 15,* 30/65.

Dunn, H.K. (1984) Anterior stabilization of thoracolumbar injury. *Clinical Orthopaedics and Related Research, 189,* 116.

Dwyer, A.F. (1973). Experiences of anterior correction of scoliosis. *Clinical Orthopaedics and Related Research, 93,* 191.

Emans, J.B. (1990). *Thoracolumbar Spine in Orthopedic Knowledge Update 3.* (p. 438). Rosemont, Illinois: American Academy Orthopaedic Surgeons.

Ferguson, R.L., & Allen, B.L. (1986). An algorithm for treatment of unstable thoracolumbar spine. *Orthopedic Clinics of North America, 17,* 105.

Frankel, V.M. & Nordin, M.D. (1980). Eds: Biomechanics of the skeletal system. (pp. 255–285). Lea & Febiger, Philadelphia.

Ghista, D.N. (1986). *Spinal Cord Injury.* Springfield, IL: Charles C Thomas.

Kaneda, K. (1984). Burst fracture with neurological deficit of thoracolumbar spine. *Spine, 9,* 788.

Kostuik, J.P., & Matsusaki, M. (1989). Anterior stabilization and decompression for post traumatic kyphosis. *Spine, 14;* 379.

Lamy, C., Bazergui, A., Kraus, H., & Farfan, H.F. (1975). The strength of the neural arc and the etiology of spondylosis. *Orthopedic Clinics of North America, 6,* 215.

Louis, R. (1985). Spinal stability as defined by the three-column spine concept. *Anatomia Clinica, 7,* 33.

McAfee, P.C. (1992). Spinal instrumentation for spinal fractures. In: *The Spine.* (p. 1161) R.H. Rothman & F.A. Simeone (Eds.), Philadelphia: W.B. Saunders.

McAfee, P.C. (1987). *Thoracolumbar Spine in Orthopedic Knowledge Update 2* (p. 297). Rosemont, Illinois: American Academy Orthopaedic Surgeons.

Moore, A.J., & Uttley, D. (1989). Anterior decompression and stabilization of the spine in malignant disease. *Neurosurgery, 24,* 713–717.

Rezaian, S.M. (1991). Rezaian spinal fixator for management of fractures of the thoracolumbar spine. *Neuro Orthopaedic Surgery Journal, 12,* 307.

Rezaian, S.M. (1982). A biomechanical approach to the management of the spinal injury. *Orthopedic Transactions, 6,* 9.

Rezaian, S.M., Dombrowski, E.T., & Ghista, D.N. (1983). Spinal fixator for management of spinal injury (the mechanical rational). *Med Ltd, 12* (2), 95–96.

Schultz, A.B., Belytschko. T.P., Andriacchi, T.P., & Galante, J. (1973). Analog studies of forces in the human spine: Mechanical properties of motion segment behavior. *Journal of Biomechanics, 6,* 373.

Weinstein, J.N. (1993). *Thoracolumbar Spine in Orthopedic Knowledge Update 4* (p. 470). Rosemont, Illinois: American Academy Orthopaedic Surgeons.

White, A.A., Panjabi, M.M. (1990). *Practical biomechanics of Spine Trauma.* In: *Clinical Biomechanics of the Spine* (p. 169). Philadelphia: J.B. Lippincott.

CHAPTER 20

Use of the Syracuse I-Plate and Anterior Locking Plate System (ALPS) for Anterior Spinal Fixation

John D. Schlegel
Rand L. Schleusener
Hansen Yuan

HIGHLIGHTS

Techniques and instrumentation systems associated with spinal fixation have escalated in number and popularity over the past few years. Although posterior fusion and instrumentation remains a mainstay procedure in spinal surgery, anterior approaches for certain conditions are extremely valuable. The authors feel that certain pathologic conditions, especially neoplastic and traumatic disorders, may be better handled by the use of anterior surgery.

Supplemental internal fixation is an accepted procedure for many orthopedic conditions. It has, until recently, maintained a less popular acceptance in spinal fusion. When vertebrectomy is performed, internal fixation anteriorly is an integral portion of the procedure. The chapter will discuss the indications, techniques, and biomechanical background associated with anterior spinal fusion and internal fixation.

HISTORY

Posterior spinal fusion dates back to the early 1900s. Hibbs and Albee described surgical techniques for fusion in 1911 (Albee, 1911; Bick, 1964). Posterior fixation devices including wire techniques were described by Hadra in 1891 and Lang in 1909 (Bick, 1964). Posterior surgery was the procedure of choice until the mid-1930s. During this period, anterior surgery became a viable alternative to address the problems of Pott's disease, degenerative disorders, and spondylolisthesis (Burns, 1933; Capener, 1932; Fang, Ong, & Hodgson, 1964; Harmon, 1963; Hodgson, 1966; Jenkins, 1936; Mercer, 1936; Southwick & Robinson, 1957; Speed, 1938).

Internal fixation for anterior procedures has been much slower to gain acceptance. Humphries, Hawk, and Berndt developed a slotted contoured plate that was used for anterior fixation in 1961. Their clinical results, reported in 27 patients, were moderately successful. Werlinich (1974) reported good results in 127 patients treated with anterior fusion and fixation with an associated staple. Beginning in 1964, Dwyer used a cable system for anterior spinal instrumentation (Dwyer, 1970; Dwyer, Newton, & Sherwood, 1969; Dwyer, O'Brien, Seal, et al., 1977; Hall, 1981; Simmons, Sue-A-Quan, O'Leary, & Garside, 1977). Subsequent to this, Zielke, Dunn, Yuan, Black, Kostuik, Kaneda, and others had developed fixation devices for anterior procedures (Black, Gardner, Armstrong, Oneil, & St. George, 1988; Chan, 1983; Dunn, 1986, 1984, 1983; Kaneda, Abumi, & Fujiya, 1984; Kaneda, Fujiya, & Satoh, 1986; Kostuik, 1988a, 1988b, 1983; Kostuik, Errico, & Gleason, 1986; Kostuik, Maurais, Richardson, & Okajima, 1988; Moe, Purcell, & Bradford, 1973; Ryan, Taylor, & Sherwood, 1986). These are used for patients with instability, for patients who have undergone vertebrectomy, or in situations to correct significant deformity.

The available systems can be divided into three types: cable systems, rod systems, and plate systems (Schlegel, Yuan, & Fredrickson, 1991). Cable systems were initially developed by Dwyer. They are easy to use and have adequate stability. Unfortunately, they have a tendency to place the thoracolumbar spine in kyphosis (Hall, 1981). Multiple rods systems are in use. They show excellent stability on biomechanical testing and provide adequate fixation. Unfortunately, many are bulky and have been associated with complications.

Plate systems make up the final category of devices. Though deformity has to be corrected posturally, they are low profile and technically are quite easy to use (Haas, Blauth, & Tscherne, 1991). This chapter will describe the techniques and indications for utilization of the Syracuse I-plate and the anterior locking plate system (ALPS).

INDICATIONS

The indications for anterior lumbar surgery are fairly well known (Table 20-1). Degenerative disk disease has been treated with anterior diskectomy for some time with varying results (Calandruccio & Benton, 1964; Freebody, Bendall, & Taylor, 1971; Stauffer & Coventry, 1972); usually most authors do not feel that supplemental anterior fixation is necessary for these conditions.

The potential goals of supplemental anterior fixation for anterior fusion are to correct deformity and reduce the risk of neurologic impairment, maintain rigidity and anatomic alignment, decrease pseudarthrosis rate, and enhance postoperative patient mobilization and rehabilitation.

Indications for utilization of anterior fusion and internal fixation are obviously beyond the scope of this text book. Some of these include thoracolumbar burst fracture with or without neurologic deficit, iatrogenic lumbar kyphosis (flat-back syndrome), one- or two-level neoplastic disorder with or without neurologic deficit, repair of failed posterior fusion, instability, possibly secondary to wide laminectomy and posterior decompression, high-grade spondylolisthesis or spondyloptosis, and spinal osteotomy (Schlegel et al., 1991).

Many authors have favored a posterior approach to many traumatic and neoplastic conditions (Starr & Hanley, 1992). Though decompression of the spinal canal can be accomplished indirectly via distraction (Fredrickson et al., 1992), and directly via the posterolateral approach, we feel strongly that in conditions in which the pathology is largely anterior (i.e., burst fracture or metastatic neoplasm), anterior surgery is the safest and most effective way to decompress the canal completely. In traumatic situations in which posterior distraction is utilized, the canal certainly is decompressed but usually not to a maximum effect. This has been supported by the work of Gertzbein and others (Essess, Botsford, & Kostuik, 1990; Freebody et al., 1971; Gertzbein, Crowe, Fazi, Schwartz, & Rowed, 1992; Willen, Lindahl, Irstam, & Nordwell, 1984). Especially in the patient with neurologic impairment, this is not optimal. Therefore, there exists a strong rationale for the anterior approach (Chohisy et al., 1992; Denis, 1983; Essess et al., 1990; McAfee, Bohlman, & Yuan, 1985).

When more than one vertebral body has to be removed, supplemental anterior internal fixation in addition to fusion is a very important adjunct to the procedure. The force placed on the thoracolumbar spine above the level of the waist can approach 2.5 to 3 times body weight. When simple bone grafting without fixation is performed, collapse and reproduction of deformity can occur. Bone graft material may require 6 months to 1 year to incorporate fully. The use of supplemental fixation maintains anatomic alignment during this healing process and can be done safely with very low risk.

TECHNIQUE

The anterior approach to the spinal column is not difficult (Watkins, 1983). For illustrative purposes, the approach described will be for an injury of the L1 vertebral body. Various surgeons use either a right or left approach. We prefer a left approach, since mobilization of the liver on the right side makes that approach somewhat more technically demanding. The patient should be placed in a right lateral decubitus position. Spinal cord monitoring is utilized. All bony prominences are protected. The table is broken at the level of the lower rib cage and angulated about 20 degrees. The appropriate ribs are palpated, and the 10th rib is selected as the entrance point for the surgical dissection. An incision is made over the 10th rib from the posterior margin of the erector spinae muscles to the costochondral junction. The incision is then extended distally in line with and parallel to the lateral border of the rectus abdominal muscle. The external

Table 20-1
Use of the Syracuse I-Plate and Anterior Locking Plate Systems

Indications	Contraindications	Advantages	Disadvantages
Thoracolumbar burst fracture	Multiple-level anterior involvement	Ease of insertion	Difficult to correct deformity
Iatrogenic kyphosis (flat back)	Severe osteoporosis	Attacks pathology directly	Morbidity associated with anterior approach
One- or two-level neoplastic involvement	Multiple previous anterior procedures	Place fusion mass in weight-bearing center	
Failed posterior fusion		Decrease pseudarthrosis rate	
Instability		Enhances postoperative rehabilitation	
High-grade spondylolisthesis			
Osteotomy			

thoracic muscles are divided with electrocautery over the 10th rib to expose the periosteum of the rib. The rib is dissected free of periosteum and removed. The rib is excised at the costal-cartilage junction, which is the key to exposing the diaphragm.

The costal cartilage is then split longitudinally with a knife. Stay sutures are placed to aid in retraction and subsequent closure. The chest cavity is then entered and rib spreaders are placed. Using the gateway created by splitting the cartilage tip of T10, blunt finger dissection is used to dissect the abdominal contents away from the diaphragm in the retroperitoneal space. It is difficult to complete the entire dissection without dividing the anterior portion of the diaphragm. The diaphragm is visualized both inferiorly and superiorly prior to division 1 to 1.5 cm from the costal insertion. Innervation is from the phrenic nerve centrally, allowing for little denervation and loss of function. Sutures are placed on both sides of the divided diaphragm to aid in accurate reapproximation of the diaphragm during closure. Only that portion of the crus necessary for exposure is removed from the spine.

Once the chest cavity is entered, the level is confirmed by palpating the ribs on the interior of the chest cavity, which is much more reliable than external palpation. The vertebral bodies and disks are easily palpable under the pleura. The vertebral bodies are recognizable by their concavity (valleys), and the disks by their convexity (hills). An 18-gauge spinal needle bent at double right angles is then inserted in the desired disk and an anteroposterior (AP) x-ray film is obtained to confirm the correct level.

Once the level has been confirmed by x-ray study, rib spreader retractors are placed over the moist lap sponges on the skin to avoid damage to the segmental vessels. The lung is packed off with a moist lap and may be held in place with a malleable retractor clamped to the rib spreader. The malleable retractor must not be allowed to lie on the pulsating aorta, as this is a potential source of vascular erosion.

The pleura is incised longitudinally over the lateral aspect of the vertebral column. Sharp dissection is used to open the pleura directly over a disk. The dissection is extended as far as needed, taking care to avoid damage to the segmental vessels, which are located directly over the midportion of the vertebral body. The segmental vessels are then ligated and transsected with 2-0 silk and at the midportion of the body. The segmental vessels must not be ligated too close to the aorta, risking avulsion of the artery, nor too close to the spinal column, and risking damage to the collateral circulation of the spinal cord. Once the segmental vessels are ligated, the pleura and soft tissue can be dissected off the spine with a Cobb elevator. The pleura can then be retracted using a stay suture to expose the spine.

Vertebrectomy at this time is then performed. Anatomic landmarks are identified. The pedicle of L1 is an excellent anatomic landmark, and can be removed with a Kerrison rongeur, exposing the posterior aspect of the body more visibly. A no. 15 blade is used to resect the disk between T12-L1 and L1-2. This is done and pituitary rongeurs are used to evacuate the disk totally. A bur or osteotomes are then used to remove the middle portion of the vertebral body of L1. We prefer to try to preserve the very anterior aspect of the body as well as the anterior longitudinal ligament to help provide stability. Certain points need to be emphasized: if the patient has an old fracture, if there is significant canal stenosis, or if there is kyphosis >20 degrees, then it is very important to remove a significant aspect of the mid and anterior vertebral bodies prior to canal debridement. We prefer to take an anterior and middle trough resected down to the opposing cortex of the body. If the dural sheath is exposed on the side of surgical entry or if a wide trough is not cut, then the dura can buttonhole through this entry point, migrate anteriorly, and make surgical decompression of the remainder of the canal essentially impossible. This point cannot be overemphasized. We prefer to cut a deep trough while doing a vertebrectomy and to approach the dural tube, either at its mid or opposite aspect. After that, we bur back to the posterior cortical margin and use a curette or small Kerrison rongeur to try to remove the posterior wafer of the vertebral cortex. Again, if the dura is exposed on the side of surgical entry (in this case, left), it will buttonhole, making decompressions of the far side of the canal difficult. Then an L1 vertebrectomy with associated diskectomy is carried out.

After the spinal decompression is complete, fixation of the spine may be necessary. Anterior strut fusion has a basic biomechanical advantage over posterior fusion as the bone graft is under compression. Posterior fusions, especially in kyphotic situations, are more likely to absorb or progress to pseudarthrosis, as the graft is under tension. Even with the biomechanical advantage of compression, strut grafting alone in certain pathologic conditions is insufficient without supplemental internal fixation. At the thoracolumbar junction, stresses on the vertebral body can approach three times body weight. Bone graft material is a nonphysiologic entity that has to revascularize and heal. This is excessive force to be placed on graft material, and augmentation with instrumentation is necessary. Laboratory data support this philosophy (Mann, Found, Yuan, Fredrickson, & Lubicky, 1987; McGowan, Mann, Yuan, Fredrickson, & Albanese, 1987).

The technique for bone grafting is simple yet important. A slot is fashioned in the vertebral bodies above and below. A slot would be cut on the undersurface of the T12 vertebral body, as well as the superior surface of the L2 vertebral body. This slot should be cut directly left to right with no migration, either toward the spinal canal or anteriorly toward the vascular structures. We actually prefer to start the slot slightly posterior to the midportion of the body of the associated vertebrae and to carry it slightly anteriorly as we go across the body. This helps prevent graft migration or dislodgment. A slot cut beginning at the area of danger and working away from it is the safest and best situation. After the graft is impacted, the table is leveled and the graft is checked for stability. If the graft can be mobilized with a clamp, we redo the entire procedure. The graft should be stable, it should not be allowed to move, and it should be in anatomic position. AP and lateral radiography is performed at this time.

Anterior instrumentation has suffered some controversy over the years. It was used in the 1930s and 1940s as a technique to augment a fusion for spondylolisthesis (Burns, 1933; Capener, 1932). It was gaining favor until certain rare and untoward consequences occurred (Jendrisak, 1986; McMaster & Sibert, 1975). It is our opinion that technical factors, rather than the hardware itself, are responsible for many of these failures. Realize that there is an important specified margin of safety that allows for placement of this hardware.

From a technical standpoint, instrumentation associated with bony fusion is not a new concept. It is routinely used almost without exception in injuries to upper and lower extremities. We have had a much slower acceptance of that in reference to spinal problems. Obviously, potential complications play a role in that. But acceptance of intervertebral fixation for cervical procedures as well as more recently, again, for thoracolumbar procedures appears to be gaining popularity.

Various instrumentation systems exist for anterior thoracolumbar surgery (Dwyer, 1970). They fall into two categories: plating systems (I-plate, DCP plate, ALPS plate, Armstrong plate) and rod systems (Dunn device, Kaneda device, TSRH system, CD system, Zielke system). Whichever system is chosen, it is important to recognize that placement of the device is crucial. If bulkier devices are used (i.e., Dunn device, Kaneda device, TSRH system), then the right-sided approach is safer, as it lessens the chance of vascular complications.

The technique for anterior instrumentation is quite simple. A subperiosteal exposure of the entire vertebral body above and below is necessary. Most anterior systems require some type of screw placement into the vertebral body above and below the injured levels. Some require fixation of the opposing cortex, though this needs to be done carefully. It is important for wide exposure to be obtained, and this necessitates the entire body of T12 and L2 to be exposed in this particular situation. It is important to try to reduce the kyphosis and restore the spinal column to as normal an anatomic alignment as possible. In summary, after this is done, the device is secured to the T12 and L2 bodies and anatomic reduction is restored (Fig. 20-1).

X-ray films are obtained at the time closure has begun. The posterior parietal pleura is closed over the fixation device with absorbable suture. The hemidiaphragm is repaired, utilizing O-silk in an interrupted figure-of-eight fashion, and oversown with a running stitch. A chest tube is placed and the parietal pleura is closed anteriorly. Muscular layers are closed utilizing O-Vicryl or another absorbable stitch. The skin is closed with skin staples. The patient is usually able to be extubated and returned to the intensive care unit, where he or she will be monitored overnight. Careful observation of the patient's neurologic status is carried out. A CT scan is usually obtained on postoperative day 1 to assess the decompression and efficiency of the surgical procedure.

I-PLATE/ANTERIOR LOCKING PLATE SYSTEM

The Syracuse I-plate was developed in the late 1980s (Bayley, Yuan, & Fredrickson, 1991; Yuan, Mann, Found, Halbig, Fredrickson, Lubicky, Albanese, Winfield, & Hodge, 1988). It is a 3.5-mm stainless steel plate in the shape of an I-beam (Fig. 20-2, *a*). It is attached to the vertebral body with four 6.5-mm cancellous screws (Fig. 20-2, *b*). The plates come in a variety of sizes, and essentially can span either one or two vertebrectomy segments. After the patient has been appropriately positioned, the plate is placed directly on the lateral aspect of the vertebral body. Exact lateral placement is important and has been discussed. Once the plate is localized over the vertebral body, the two more anterior screws are placed. Each screw hole anteriorly in the vertebral body above and below is

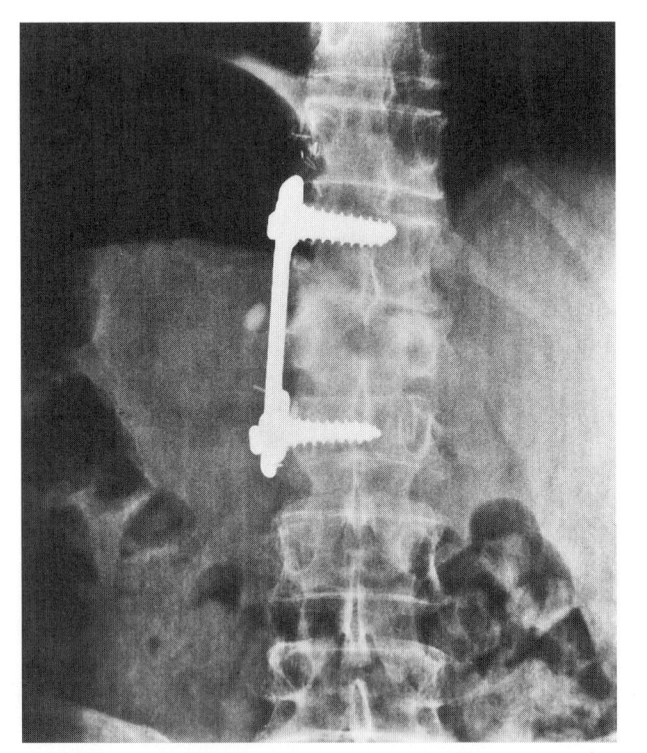

FIG. 20-1. AP x-ray of appropriately positioned I-plate, spanning T12 to L2.

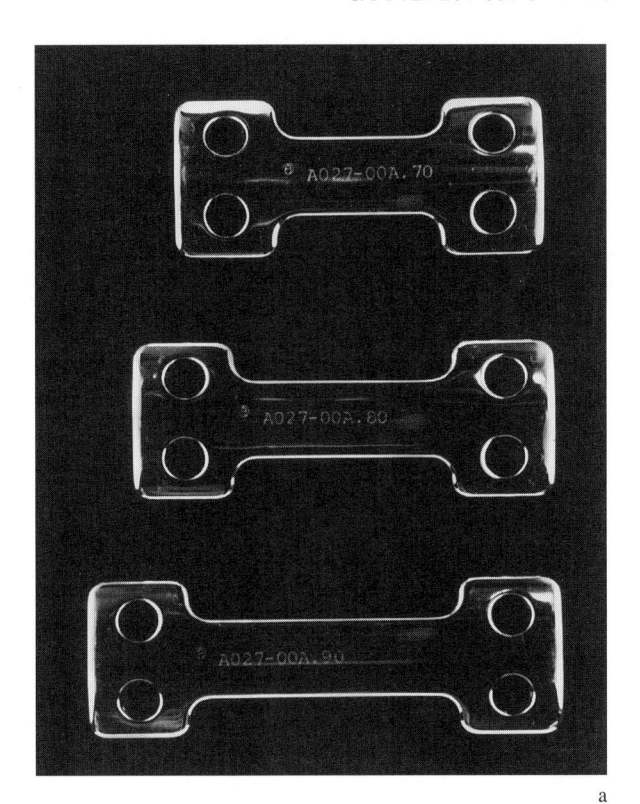

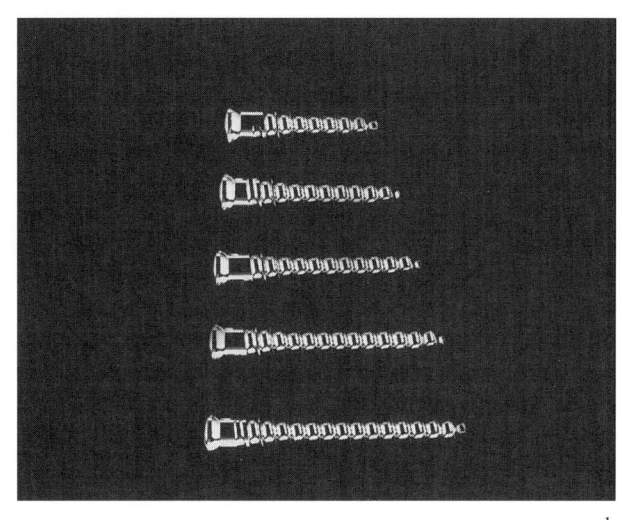

FIG. 20-2. (a) Three sizes of Syracuse I-plates. (b) 6.5 mm cancellous screws for I-plates.

drilled with a 3.2-mm drill. The cortex is tapped with a 6.5-mm cancellous tap, the depth is measured and the appropriate 6.5-mm cancellous screw is put in place. In osteopenic individuals, added strength may be gained by engaging the opposing cortex. If this is done, the authors prefer a subperiosteal dissection around the circumference of the vertebral body to prevent vascular or neurologic compromise as the screw exits the opposing cortex. Many authors favor use of methylmethacrylate in osteopenic individuals, though this needs to be done with great care and judgment. Once the anterior screw holes have been engaged, the posterior 6.5-mm screws are then placed in a similar fashion. After all four screws have been appropriately secured, x-ray evaluation is obtained, documenting optimal placement of the device. Closure is carried out in a standard fashion. Posterior parietal pleura, or the posterior fascia, can usually be reapproximated over the device. Usually a soaked Gelfoam sponge is placed directly over the fixation and closure of the posterior pleura is carried out with O-Vicryl in a running, simple fashion. The diaphragm is then closed with O-silk in an interrupted figure-of-eight fashion and later reinforced with a running, simple stitch. If the chest cavity is entered, a chest tube is placed. The muscle layers are then closed, using O-Vicryl, and the skin is reapproximated in the standard fashion. A supplemental orthosis is usually placed until the fusion is solid. The major difficulty with most plate systems is screw backout. With the I-plate, the proximal part of the screw (adjacent to the head) completely fills the plate screw-hole producing a "press weld" fit. This decreases the incidence of screw backout noted with other 6.5-mm cancellous screws.

Similar to the I-plate, the ALPS is used in thoracolumbar and lumbar conditions in which internal fixation and stability are required. In summary, it can be used safely and effectively from T10 down through L5.

The ALPS is made of 316 LVM stainless steel. It consists of a combination of straight and contoured rectangular vertebral plates, vertebral double-locking screws, and self-locking screws. The plates are 3 mm thick and 25 mm wide. There are two columns of holes in each plate; one column is elliptical and the other is round. The elliptical holes are designed to receive the double-locking screws, and the four round holes are designed for the self-locking screws. A center hole is present in all plates and is used for the plate holder; the straight vertebral locking plates are available in seven lengths ranging from 50 to 110 mm. The contoured plates are used for situations in which the vertebral bodies are malaligned up to 5 degrees; they are available in six lengths ranging from 60 to 110 mm.

After vertebrectomy and debridement are done, the trial plates should be placed over the lateral portion of the vertebral body. A plate holder is placed in the central hole to optimize positioning of the trial plate. The elliptical holes

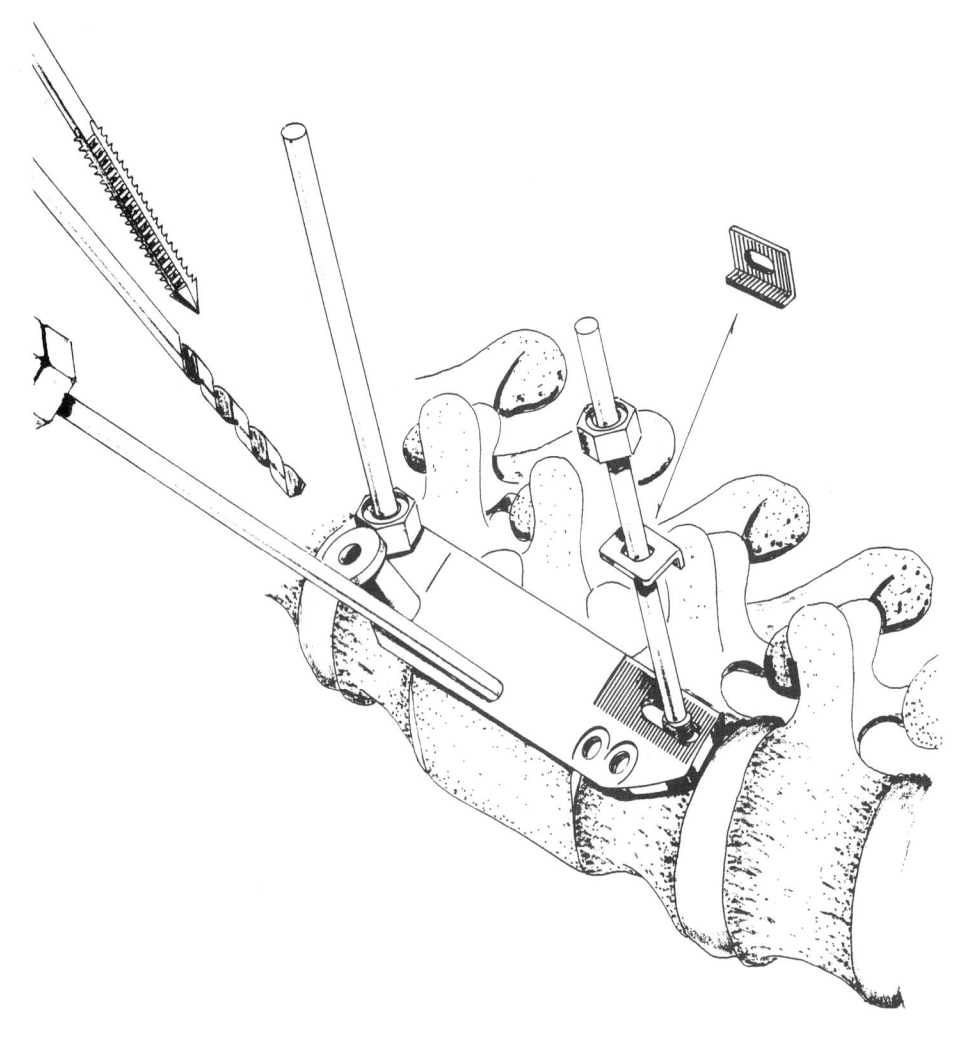

FIG. 20-3. Anterior Locking Plate System (ALPS) held in correct position with plate holder. Note position of screws, washers, and nuts.

are placed posteriorly and the round holes are placed more anteriorly.

Once the trial plate is put into position, a 4-mm drill bit through a drill sleeve is used to drill first the 4-mm superior elliptical hole. The appropriate depth is measured. The opposite cortex is not usually engaged. In a similar fashion, the inferior hole is appropriately drilled and measured. The trial plate is then removed and a seating reamer is used to expand the diameter of the proximal aspect of the screw holes. This allows for flush placement of the plate against the vertebral body. A threaded driver is then used to implant the double-locking screws. After the screws are implanted, the threaded driver is turned in a clockwise motion while the handle of the driver is held into place. This disengages the screw from the driver.

Using the plate holder, the ALPS plate is then placed over the heads of the implanted double-locking screws (Fig. 20-3). The larger, slotted hole is placed over the screw in the inferior vertebral body. The screws should be checked and maintained at a proper height above the plate to facilitate placement of the locking nut. A locking nut is then placed over each screw, using a nut socket wrench to secure it. A hexagonal screwdriver turns the screw in a counterclockwise direction, securing it.

At this time, drill guides are used to facilitate placement of the more anterior screws. The anterior screws are secured via drilling and tapping in the usual fashion. They are introduced with a hexagonal screwdriver (see Fig. 20-4). As with the I-plate, x-ray evaluation is obtained to document placement of the device and overall alignment of the spine. Closure is then carried out as described previously.

BIOMECHANICAL DATA

Limited biomechanical data is available in reference to anterior devices. The underlying biomechanical concept surrounding anterior fusion is that compression is placed directly on the graft material where a fusion is effected. Posterior fusion, especially in a kyphotic deformity, is under tension and is therefore subject to potential failure (Whitesides, 1977). The loads on the thoracolumbar spine are significant. They can approach two to three times body weight at the thoracolumbar junction. The authors feel this

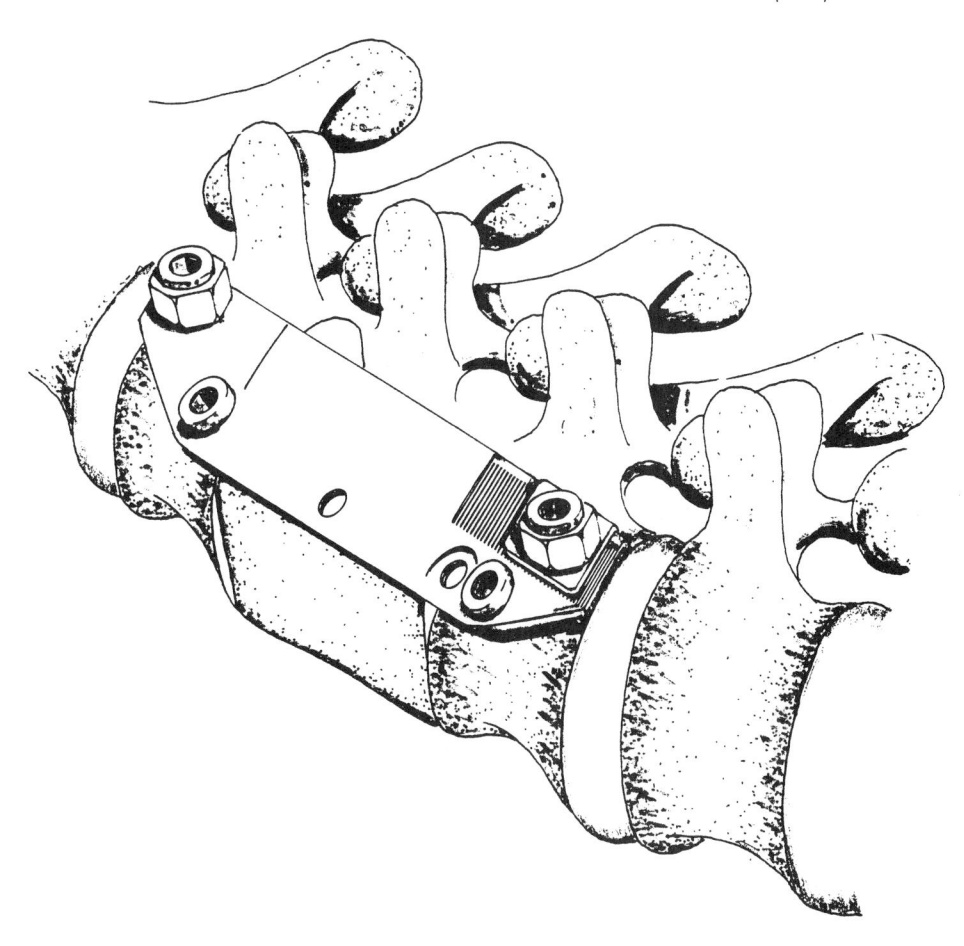

FIG. 20-4. Anterior Locking Plate System with anterior/posterior locking nuts and crossing screws.

is an excessive load to be placed on graft material alone, and that internal fixation is necessary not only to enhance stability but to maintain anatomic alignment.

Biomechanical data is somewhat sparse in reference to anterior fixation devices. Mann et al. (1987) evaluated certain anterior fixation devices. In cadaveric specimens, anterior vertebrectomy was carried out in nine test subjects. The grafted specimen without fixation was evaluated in comparison with the Kostuik device, the Kaneda device and the anterior I-plate system. The results are shown in Table 20-2. It shows that bone graft without instrumentation does not provide adequate support to the spine, and is at risk. All of the devices tested returned stability to at least that of the impact spine. The Kaneda device and I-plate system appear to provide the greatest increase in stability. Laboratory data surrounding the anterior locking plate system are also available.

CLINICAL RESULTS

Early clinical results of I-plate fixation were published in 1988 by Yuan et al. Sixteen cases were reported with minimal complications. Spinal cord compression was improved in all patients. The age range was 14 to 72, with a mean of age 30.

Table 20-2
Bending Moments of the Average Percent Increase in Stiffness of Each Device over the Normal Spine in Each of the Tested Modes*

	Flexion (14 N-m)	Extension (12 N-m)	RL Bend (10 N-m)	LL Bend (10 N-m)
Graft	−6.8% (NS)	−10.0% (NS)	−48.6% ($p<0.0025$)	−12.2% ($p<0.1$)
Kostuik	−24.2% ($p<0.1$)	5.3% (NS)	7.5% (NS)	20.1% ($p<0.05$)
Kaneda	9.6% (NS)	3.3% (NS)	16.1% ($p<0.02$)	37.2% ($p<0.01$)
I-Plate	12.4% ($p<0.15$)	8.6% (NS)	6.8% (NS)	25.5% ($p<0.01$)
Revised I-plate	16.3% ($p<0.1$)	8.7% (NS)	16.9% ($p<0.01$)	29.0% ($p<0.01$)

RL = right lateral; LL = left lateral; NS = not significant; N-m = Newton meters.

*Results for the grafted spine alone, without instrumentation, are included. A negative number indicates a percent decrease in stiffness when compared to the intact spine. Statistical significance levels when compared to the normal spine are listed in parentheses.

Complications were few. One patient had screw breakage, although the patient remained asymptomatic. One graft dislodgment occurred without untoward effect.

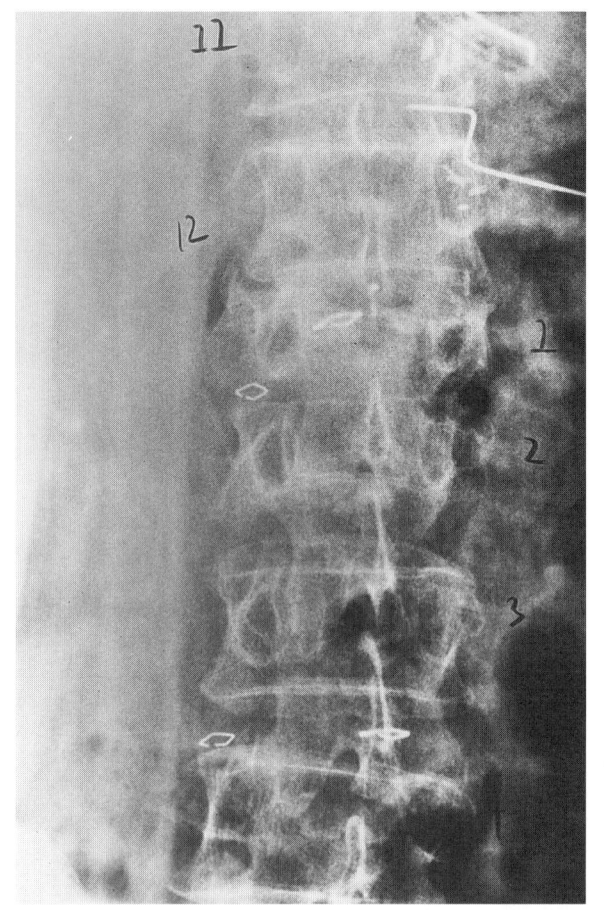

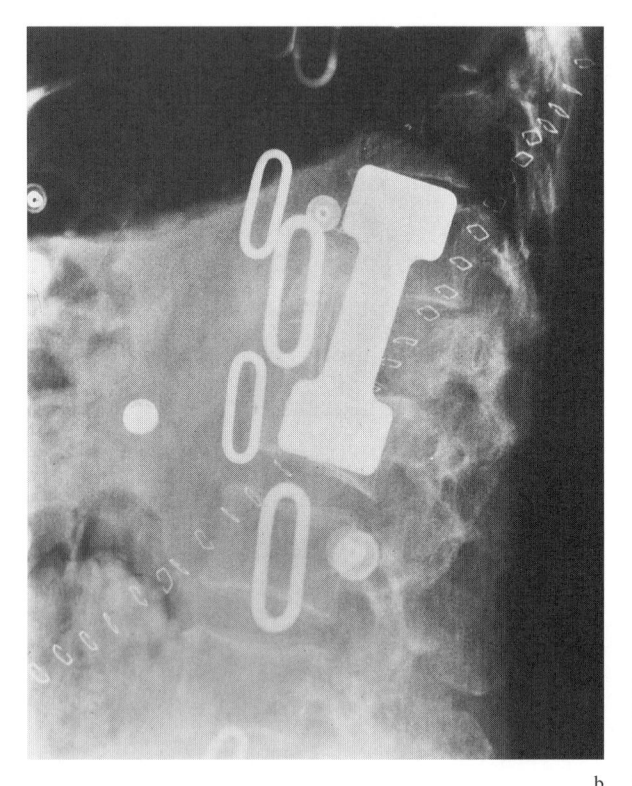

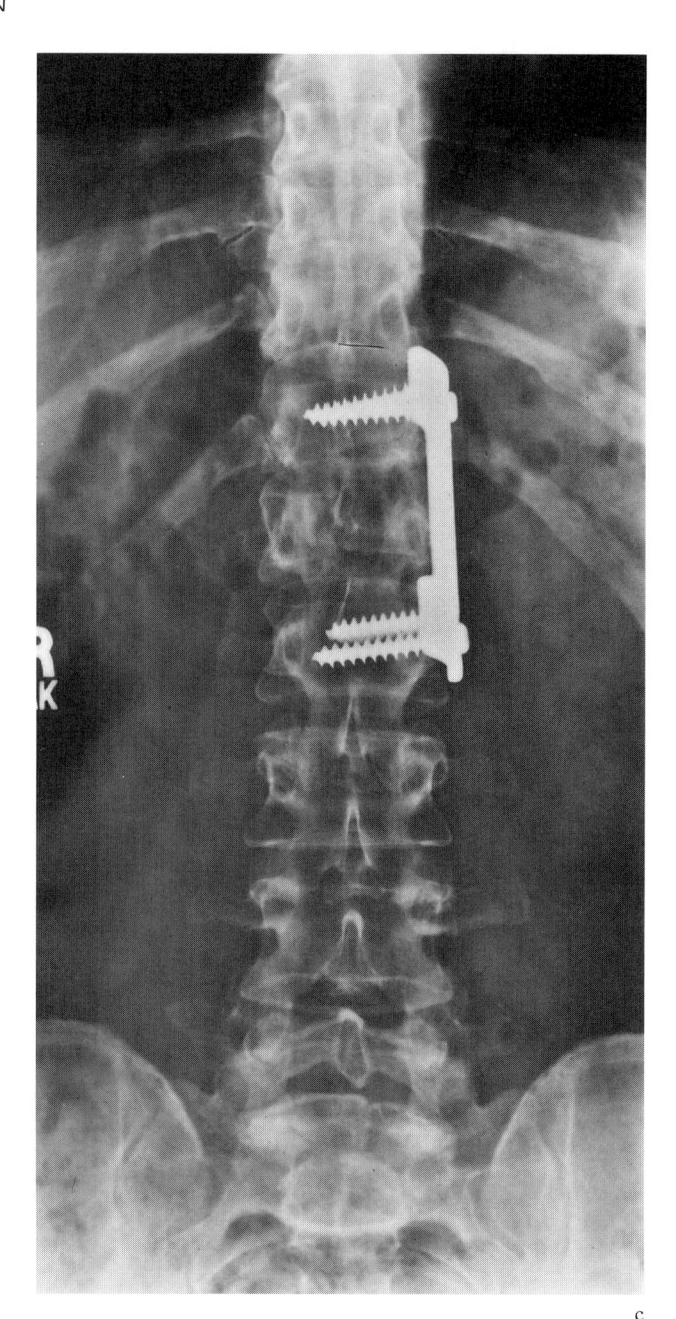

FIG. 20-5. (a) AP x-ray of a 29-year-old male who suffered an L1 burst fracture and partial neurologic deficit. He underwent anterior vertabrectomy, instrumentation and fusion utilizing the Syracuse I-Plate. (b) Lateral x-ray following reconstruction using the I-plate. (c) AP x-ray following reconstruction using the I-plate.

Many patients subsequently have been treated with the I-plate and ALPS with good results. Though limitations exist, both devices are an effective, simple choice for thoracolumbar burst fractures and neoplasms. They are not optimal for multiple-level problems or for patients with significant deformity.

An illustrative case is presented in Fig. 20-5. A 29-year-old man suffered a traumatic injury to the L1 vertebral body. A burst fracture was present with loss of vertebral body height and canal impingement. Fixation with the I-plate was carried out after vertebrectomy and grafting. The patient's initial neurologic deficit resolved and fusion was obtained without problems. The exact placement of the device should be appreciated.

COMPLICATIONS

The popularity of anterior fixation devices has waxed and waned. Exact placement of the device is crucial. There is a very small margin of error with this. If the device is placed too far anteriorly, significant vascular complications can be encountered. Posterior placement obviously can lead to complications, including neurologic compromise. Potential complications are listed in Table 20-3.

The most devastating complications are vascular and neurologic. Kostuik (1988) reported two iliac vein lacerations in 79 patients treated with anterior decompression (2.5%). Urologic complications have been documented after Dwyer instrumentation, although the one case presented involved obstruction of the left ureter, possibly by scar tissue rather than the device itself (McMaster & Sibert, 1975). Significant vascular complications led to the removal of the Dunn device from widespread commercial use (Jendrisak, 1986). Nevertheless, the senior author has done more than 80 cases using the Dunn device, without complications.

Prevention of complications is essential. Most complications can be prevented by adequate, meticulous placement of the device. Mobilization of the great vessels is important, and ligation and appropriate reflection of the segmental vessels is crucial. These vessels need to be ligated at their midportion. Ligation too far anteriorly can lead to avulsion from the aorta. Ligation too far posteriorly can cause neurologic compromise. Spinal cord monitoring or wake-up test should be routinely used in these procedures. The more bulky devices need to be placed on the right side. As mentioned, we feel that the plate systems can be placed adequately and safely on the left side; technically this is somewhat easier since the liver does not have to be mobilized. Careful preoperative planning and attention to detail are crucial in this patient population.

CONCLUSIONS

Internal fixation is widely accepted in the orthopedic community for disorders of the upper and lower extremity. It provides rigidity, maintains anatomy, appears to improve fusion rates, reduces postoperative morbidity and rehabilitation time, and potentially corrects deformity. Anterior spinal surgery augmented with internal fixation is gaining popularity. When indicated, this is an invaluable tool in certain pathologic conditions. It can be performed safely and effectively and can improve patient care. Further scientific investigation with biomechanical testing and implant improvement obviously will improve our knowledge and understanding of these procedures.

REFERENCES

Albee, F.H. (1911). Transplantation of a portion of the tibia into the spine for Pott's disease. *Journal of the American Medical Association, 57*, 885–886.

Bayley, J.C., Yuan, H., & Fredrickson B. (1991). The Syracuse I plate. *Spine, 16*(3), 120–124.

Bick, E.M. (1964). An Essay on the history of spine fusion operations. *Clinical Orthopaedics and Related Research, 35*, 9–15.

Black, R.C. Gardner, V.O., Armstrong, G.W.D., Oneil, J., & St. George, M. (1988). A contoured anterior spinal fixation plate. *Clinical Orthopaedics and Related Research, 227*, 135–142.

Burns, B.H. (1933). Operation of spondylolisthesis. *Lancet, 1*, 1233.

Calandruccio, R.A., & Benton, B.F. (1964). Anterior lumbar fusion. *Clinical Orthopaedics and Related Research, 35*, 63–68.

Capener, N. (1932). Spondylolisthesis. *British Journal of Surgery, 19*, 374–386.

Chan, D.P. Zielke instrumentation. (1983). *AAOS Instructional Course Lectures, 32*, 208–209.

Clohisy, J.C., et al. (1992). Neurologic recovery associated with anterior decompression of spinal fractures at the thoracolumbar junction (T12-L1). *Spine, 17*, 325–330.

Denis, F. (1983). The three column space and its significance in the classification of acute thoracolumbar spinal injuries. *Spine, 8*, 817–831.

Dunn, H.K. (1986). Anterior spine stabilization and decompression for thoracolumbar injuries. *Orthopaedic Clinics of North America, 17*, 113–119.

Dunn, H.K. (1984). Anterior stabilization of thoracolumbar injuries. *Clinical Orthopaedics and Related Research, 189*, 116–124.

Dunn, H.K. (1983). Spinal instrumentation. I. Principles of anterior and posterior instrumentation. *AAOS Instructional Course Lectures, 32*, 192–202.

Dwyer, A.F. (1970). Anterior instrumentation in scoliosis. *Journal of Bone and Joint Surgery, British Volume, 52*, 782–783.

Dwyer, A.F., Newton, N.C., & Sherwood, A.A. (1969). An anterior approach to scoliosis. *Clinical Orthopaedics and Related Research, 62*, 192–202.

Table 20-3
Complications of Anterior Fixation Devices

Retroperitoneal fibrosis
Urologid dysfunction
Major vascular injury/aneurysm
Neurologic impairment
Implant failure
Sympathetic-nerve injury
Infection
Graft migration
Pseudarthrosis
Deep venous thrombosis/embolism

Dwyer, A.P., O'Brien, J.P., Seal, P.P., et al. (1977). The late complications after the Dwyer anterior spinal instrumentation for scoliosis. *Journal of Bone and Joint Surgery, British Volume, 59,* 117.

Essess, S.I., Botsford, D.J., & Kostuik, J.P. (1990). Evaluation of surgical treatment for burst fractures. *Spine, 15*(7), 667–673.

Fang, H.S., Ong., G.B., & Hodgson, A.R. (1964). Anterior spinal fusion: The operative approaches. *Clinical Orthopaedics and Related Research, 35,* 16–33.

Fredrickson, B.E., et al. (1992). Vertebral burst fractures: An experimental, morphologic, and radiographic study. *Spine, 17*(9), 1012–1021.

Freebody, D., Bendall, R., & Taylor, R.D. (1971). Anterior transperitoneal lumbar fusion. *Journal of Bone and Joint Surgery, British Volume, 53,* 617–627.

Gertzbein, S.D., Crowe, P.J., Fazi, M., Schwartz, M., & Rowed, D. (1992). Canal clearance in burst fractures using the AO internal fixation. *Spine, 17*(5), 558–560.

Haas, N., Blauth, M., & Tscherne, H. (1991). Anterior plating in the thoracolumbar spine injuries. *Spine, 16*(3):100–111, 1991.

Hall, J.E. (1981). Dwyer instrumentation in anterior fusion of the spine. *Journal of Bone and Joint Surgery, American Volume, 63,* 1188–1190.

Harmon, P.H. (1963). Anterior excision and vertebral body fusion operation for intervertebral disk syndromes of the lower lumbar spine. *Clinical Orthopaedics and Related Research, 26,* 107–127.

Hodgson, A.R. (1966). Results of anterior fusion. *Journal of Bone and Joint Surgery, British Volume, 48,* 595.

Hodgson, A.R., & Stock, F.E. (1956). Anterior spinal fusion: A preliminary communication on radical treatment of Pott's disease and Pott's paraplegia. *British Journal of Surgery, 44,* 266–275.

Humphries, A.W., Hawk, W.A., & Berndt, A.L. (1961). Anterior interbody fusion of lumbar vertebrae: A surgical technique. *Surgical Clinics of North America, 41,* 1685–1700.

Jendrisak, M.D. (1986). Spontaneous abdominal aortic rupture from erosion of a lumbar spine fixation device: A case report. *Surgery, 99,* 631–633.

Jenkins, J.A. (1936). Spondylolisthesis. *British Journal of Surgery, 24,* 80–85.

Kaneda, K., Abumi, K., & Fujiya, M. (1984). Burst fractures with neurologic deficits of the thoracolumbar-lumbar spine. *Spine, 9,* 788–795.

Kaneda, K., Fujiya, N., & Satoh, S. (1986). Results with Zielke instrumentation for idiopathic thoracolumbar and lumbar scoliosis. *Clinical Orthopaedics and Related Research, 205,* 195–203.

Kostuik, J.P. (1988a). Anterior Kostuik-Harrington distraction systems for the treatment of kyphotic deformities. *Iowa Orthopedic Journal, 8,* 68–77.

Kostuik, J.P. (1988b). Anterior fixation for burst fractures of the thoracic and lumbar spine with or without neurological involvement. *Spine, 13,* 286–293.

Kostuik, J.P. (1983). Anterior spinal cord decompression for lesions of the thoracic and lumbar spine, techniques, new methods of internal fixation results. *Spine, 8,* 512–531.

Kostuik, J.P., Errico, T.J., & Gleason, T.F. (1986). Techniques of internal fixation for degenerative conditions of the lumbar spine. *Clinical Orthopaedics and Related Research, 203,* 219–231.

Kostuik, J.P., Maurais, G.R., Richardson, W.J., & Okajima, Y. (1988). Combined single stage anterior and posterior osteotomy for correction of iatrogenic lumbar kyphosis. *Spine, 13,* 257–266.

Kostuik, J.P., & Matsusaki, H. (1989). Anterior stabilization, instrumentation, and decompression for posttraumatic kyphosis. *Spine, 14,* 379–386.

Mann, K.A., Found, E.M., Yuan, H.A., Fredrickson, B.E., & Lubicky, J. (1987). Biomechanical evaluation of the effectiveness of anterior spinal fixation systems. Presented at the Orthopaedic Research Society 33rd Annual Meeting, San Francisco.

McAfee, P.C., Bohlman, H.H., & Yuan, H.A. (1985). Anterior decompression of traumatic thoracolumbar fractures with incomplete neurological deficit using a retroperitoneal approach. *Journal of Bone and Joint Surgery, American Volume, 67,* 89–104.

McGowan, D.P., Mann, K.A., Yuan, H.A., Fredrickson, B.E., & Albanese, S.A. (1987). A biomechanical study of anterior spinal fixation for thoracolumbar burst fractures with varying degrees of posterior disruption. Presented to the International Society for the Study of the Lumbar Spine.

McMaster, W.C., & Silbert, I. (1975). A urological complication of Dwyer instrumentation. *Journal of Bone and Joint Surgery, American Volume, 57,* 710–711.

Mercer, W. (1936). Spondylolisthesis. *Edinburgh Medical Journal, 43,* 545–572.

Moe, J.H., Purcell, G.A., & Bradford, D.S. (1973). Ziekle instrumentation (VDS) for the correction of spinal curvature: Analysis of results in 66 patients. *Clinical Orthopaedics and Related Research, 93,* 207.

Ryan, M.D., Taylor, T.K.F., & Sherwood, A.A. (1986). Bolt-plate fixation for anterior spinal fusion. *Clinical Orthopaedics and Related Research, 203,* 196–202.

Schlegel, J., Yuan, H., & Fredrickson, B. (1991). Anterior interbody fixation devices. In: Frymoyer, J.W. (Ed.), *The Adult Spine* (pp. 1947–1959). New York: Raven Press.

Simmons, E.H., Sue-A-Quan, E.A., O'Leary, P.F., & Garside, H.J. (1977). An analysis of Dwyer instrumentation of the spine with assessment of its place in spinal surgery. *Journal of Bone and Joint Surgery, British Volume, 59,* 117.

Southwick, W.O., & Robinson, R.A. (1957). Surgical approaches to the vertebral bodies in the cervical and lumbar regions. *Journal of Bone and Joint Surgery, American Volume, 39,* 631–644.

Speed, K. (1938). Spondylolisthesis. *Archives of Surgery, 37,* 175–189.

Starr, J.K., & Hanley, E.N. (1992). Junctional burst fractures. *Spine, 17*(5), 551–557.

Stauffer, R.N., & Coventry, M.B. (1972). Anterior interbody lumbar spine fusion. *Journal of Bone and Joint Surgery, American Volume, 54,* 756–768.

Watkins, R.G. (1983). *Surgical Approaches to the Spine.* New York: Springer-Verlag.

Werlinich, M. (1974). Anterior interbody fusion and stabilization with metal fixation. *International Surgery, 59,* 269–273.

Whitesides, T.E., Jr. (1977). Traumatic kyphosis of the thoracolumbar spine. *Clinical Orthopaedics and Related Research, 128,* 78–92.

Willen, J., Lindahl, S., Irstam, L., & Nordwell, A. (1984). Unstable thoracolumbar fractures. *Spine, 9*(2), 214–219.

Yuan, H.A., Mann, K.A., Found, E.M., Helbig, T.E., Fredrickson, B., Lubicky, J.P., Albanese, S.A., Winfield, J.A., & Hodge, C.J. (1988). Early clinical experience with the Syracuse I-plate: An anterior spinal fixation device. *Spine, 13,* 278–285.

CHAPTER 21

Z-Plate Anterior Thoracolumbar Instrumentation

Thomas A. Zdeblick

HIGHLIGHTS

The treatment of thoracolumbar burst fractures is evolving rapidly. Although fractures of the spine have been recognized for centuries, treatment of burst fractures is a relatively modern development. Historically, burst fractures with paralysis were treated with neglect and/or prolonged bed rest, which led to a 90% mortality rate (Bedbrook, 1975). Lorenz Boehler was the first physician to advocate postural reduction of the kyphotic spine using hyperextension and a body cast. He then encouraged early ambulation and trunk strengthening exercises to ensure patient rehabilitation (Holdsworth, 1970). This treatment was echoed by Holdsworth in 1970 when he first classified spinal injuries and formally described the burst fracture. His recommended treatment was postural reduction followed by bed rest and, eventually, a molded plaster body cast.

The adaptation of the Harrington distraction rods for the treatment of displaced burst fractures was a great step forward (Cotler, Vernace, & Michalski, 1986; Dewald, 1984; Dickson, Harrington, & Erwin, 1978; Flesch, Leider, Erickson, Chou, & Bradford, 1977; Jacobs, Nordwall, & Nachemson, 1982; Keene, Wackwitz, Drummond, & Breed, 1986). Distraction allowed some restoration of the height of the injured vertebrae, and fixation led to a higher percentage of fusions and to earlier patient mobilization. With modifications such as rod contouring and the use of sleeves, some reduction of the kyphosis and spinal canal clearance was possible. However, posterior distraction instrumentation has some drawbacks, such as the need for fixation two levels caudad and three levels cephalad to the fracture. Also, only semirigid fixation is achieved, and supplemental external support is often necessary. Most importantly, posterior distraction utilizing ligamentotaxis may not lead to adequate clearance of the spinal canal and lead to residual neurologic compression (Gertzbein, MacMichael, & Tile, 1982). Direct spinal canal decompression could be achieved only through an anterior or anterolateral decompression.

The anterolateral approach to the thoracolumbar spine was first described by Hodgson and Stock (1956). This approach was a retroperitoneal muscle-splitting approach. Their procedures were developed primarily for the drainage of tuberculous abscesses. In the 1950s, the anterior approach had begun to be used for the anterior fusion of scoliosis. Capener (1954) advocated anterior disk space fusion of the scoliotic curve. In 1953, Wenger (1982) described an anterior distraction device to help reduce scoliotic deformity. Dwyer (1969), Hall (1972), and Zielke (1982) all developed anterior instrumentation devices for the correction of scoliosis. In general, these fixation devices included a single vertebral-body screw placed laterally, connected by a flexible cable or threaded rod, which could then be compressed to help reduce the convexity of the scoliotic curve. This fixation was not rigid, but was primarily a device used for reduction.

The retroperitoneal approach to the thoracolumbar spine for the decompression of late, malunited burst fracture was developed by Bohlman (Bohlman, 1985; Bohlman, Freehafer, DeJak, 1975). These fractures were primarily treated late, after healing with a kyphotic malunion. McAfee, Bohlman, and Yuan (1985) noted substantial neurologic recovery with late anterior decompression. Anterior strut grafting alone, however, cannot stabilize an acutely fractured spine that has disruption of the posterior column. The nonunion rate when anterior fusion is performed without instrumentation ranges from 18 to 100%, but averages 10 to 20% (Benzel & Larson, 1986; Dunn, 1984; Dunn, Goble, McBride, & Daniels, 1981; Flynn & Hoque, 1979; Freebody, Bendall, & Taylor, 1971; Riska, Myllynen, & Bostman, 1987). Because of this, several surgeons began recommending a two-stage operative procedure (Bradford & McBride, 1987; Dall & Stauffer, 1988; Denis, Armstrong, Searls, & Matta, 1984; Eismont, Green, Berkowitz, Montalvo, Quencer, & Brown, 1984; Garfin, Mowery, Guerra, & Marshall, 1985). Typically, this entailed posterior instrumentation with distraction followed by the performance of intraoperative studies such as myelography or ultrasonography to assess canal clearance (Eismont et al., 1984; Garfin et al., 1985). If compression of the canal persisted, an anterior or posterolateral decompression would then be carried out.

To reduce the morbidity of a two-stage operation, anterior instrumentation after anterior decompression has been advocated as a single-stage procedure (Dickson, Harrington, & Erwin, 1978; Dunn, 1984; Kaneda, Abumi, & Fujiya, 1984; Kostuik, 1984, 1983; Krag, Beynnon, Pope, Frymoyer, Haugh, & Weaver, 1986). An anterior fixation device designed by Dunn had initial excellent results in both the reduction and fixation of thoracolumbar burst fractures (Dickson et al., 1978; Dunn, 1984). This device was applied in the anterior/anterolateral spine with a screw and staple used for fixation. Although this device was eventually withdrawn because of late vascular injuries, other surgeons were more successful with the use of anterior thoracolumbar devices. Kostuik (1984, 1983) reported on 80 sequential patients treated with single-stage anterior decompression, bone grafting, and stabilization using the Kostuik-Harrington device. He noted excellent neurologic recovery in patients with incomplete neurologic deficit. He also found a nonunion rate of only 4%, although 16% had some type of hardware failure. Bradford and McBride (1987) compared 20 patients treated by anterior decompression and stabilization with 39 patients treated by posterior decompression and stabilization. The neurologic recovery rate was greater for those with anterior surgery (88% vs. 64%) and inferior results correlated with residual bony canal stenosis identified on postoperative computed tomographic (CT) scans.

Kaneda and coworkers (1984) have developed an anterior fixation device that employs vertebral body staples and screws connected by two threaded longitudinal rods that are cross-linked. In the first 100 cases in the United States, 96% of patients have had some neurologic recovery, and the nonunion rate is 6%. More importantly, no vascular or neurologic complications have occurred with this device. Static devices, such as the Armstrong plate or the Yuan I-plate have also been effective in performing anterolateral fixation following decompression for fracture and/or tumor resection (Yuan, Mann, Found, Helbig, Fredrickson, Lubicky, Albanese, Winfield, & Hodge, 1988). Most recently, Heller, Zdeblick, Kunz, McCabe, and Cooke (1991) and Lowery (1991) have reported their early results using the Texas Scottish Rite Hospital (TSRH) screw and rod system as an anterior fixation device following corpectomy. Both studies have shown low rates of hardware failure, high fusion rates, and excellent neurologic recovery.

Few animal studies have been performed on the efficacy of anterior fixation followed by corpectomy. Zdeblick, Shirado, McAfee, deGroot, & Warden (1991) created a model of burst fracture treated by anterior corpectomy in the dog. They performed anterior corpectomy and spacer application in seven dogs, anterior corpectomy followed by anterior arthrodesis with an ulnar strut in seven dogs, and an ulnar strut plus an anterior Kaneda-type instrumentation in seven dogs. They analyzed their results in terms of the rate of fusion, biomechanical rigidity, neuropathologic findings, and histomorphometric data. They found that the rate of fusion was significantly higher in the group using anterior instrumentation. In addition, the spines were stiffer in torsion than those that were uninstrumented. Minimal device-related osteopenia occurred in the spines treated with the anterior fixation device. Their conclusion was that, in the unstable spine, anterior bone grafting alone led to a high rate of nonunion and less mechanical rigidity than anterior grafting plus instrumentation.

Bench-top testing of anterior thoracolumbar fixation devices has led to a determination of the initial stability provided by these devices (Gurr, McAfee, & Shih, 1988; Gurr, McAfee, Warden, & Shih, 1989; Jacobs et al., 1982; Johnston, 1989; McAfee, 1985; McAfee, Regan, Farey, Gutt, & Warden, 1988; McAfee, Farey Sutterlin, Gutt, Warden, & Cunningham, 1989; Zdeblick, Warden, Zou, McAfee, & Abitbol, 1993). Jacobs et al. (1982) tested the biomechanical stiffness of spinal constructs with simulated spine injuries. Although he tested anterior vertebral body plates, he failed to report on their effectiveness. Gurr et al. (1989, 1988) compared the mechanical stiffness of the Kaneda device construct with traditional posterior spinal constructs in a calf spine model. They found that posterior pedicle screw systems spanning five levels were equivalent to the Kaneda device spanning three levels. Ashman, Bechtold, and Edwards (1989) and Ashman, Birch, and Bone (1988) tested four anterior fixation systems: the Zielke-Slot, the Kostuik-Harrington device, the ASIF T-plate, and a broad compression plate. They found that the broad dynamic compression plate was stiffer in axial load and torsion than the other systems tested, in particular, they found the Kostuik-Harrington system to be less stiff in torsion.

Abumi, Panjabi, and Duranceau (1989) compared an anterior Kaneda-type device with posterior Harrington compression rods and a transpedicular external fixator. They found that the external fixator was superior in returning spinal stability in flexion-extension and rotation. They felt that the Kaneda device, although performing well in flexion and extension, was not as stable in rotation. However, this device did not include cross-link bars. Zdeblick et al. (1982) in a calf spine model, compared the biomechanical stiffness of the Kaneda device, the Kostuik-Harrington device, the TSRH vertebral-body screw construct, and the Armstrong CASP plate. Their tests were performed under torsion, flexion-extension, and axial compression. They found that in torsion the Kostuik-Harrington device was unstable, while the Kaneda device was most rigid. In axial loading and flexion, the Kaneda device and the TSRH construct proved to be the most stiff. They concluded that the TSRH anterior vertebral-body screw construct or the Kaneda device were most effective in restoring the acute stability to the lumbar spine after corpectomy.

CLINICAL INDICATIONS

From the above discussion, it appears clear that anterior decompression and stabilization does play a significant role in the treatment of thoracolumbar burst fractures. For fractures without neurologic deficit and with mild deformity, postural reduction followed by bed rest and casting is still indicated (Reid, Hu, Davis, & Saboe, 1988; Schmidek, Gomes, Seligson, & McSherry, 1980; Weinstein, Collalto, & Lehmann, 1988). In general, patients with less than 20 degrees of local kyphosis and less than 50% canal compromise can be adequately treated in this manner. With greater degrees of deformity but without neurologic deficit, posterior reduction and stabilization with fusion is the treatment of choice. In fractures in the proximal thoracolumbar spine, this is best treated with either rod-hook devices or pedicle screw-rod devices (Aebi, Etter, Kehl, & Thalgott, 1987; Cotrel, Dubousset, & Guillamat, 1988; Dick, 1987; Jelsma, Kirsch, Jelsma, Ramsey, & Rice, 1982; Krag et al., 1986; Levine & Edwards, 1988; Magerl, 1984). In the mid to lower lumbar spine, pedicle screw fixation of one level above and below the fracture is indicated (Krag et al., 1986; Levine & Edwards, 1988).

In patients with neurologic deficit from a thoracolumbar burst fracture, I prefer to perform both anterior decompression and stabilization. This is based on the higher degree of neurologic recovery following anterior decompression, the restoration of the height of the anterior and middle columns possible with the anterior approach, and the lower incidence of late collapse and settling with restoration of the anterior and middle columns.

If one is to treat with a single-stage anterior decompression and stabilization, the most rigid system should be chosen. However, there are numerous perceived difficulties of the current anterolateral fixation devices. Although the Kaneda device and the anterior TSRH system were rigid under biomechanical testing, both are high-profile systems with difficult insertion of the rods and cross-link. In addition, both devices are stainless steel, which makes postoperative imaging difficult. In cases of fracture, imaging for postoperative syringomyelia is best achieved with a magnetic resonance imaging (MRI) scan, which is precluded by the use of a stainless steel fixation device. For patients with tumor decompressions, following the tumor with either CT scan or MRI scan is difficult with these stainless steel devices. Although plate devices such as the CASP or the Yuan plate are low-profile and easier to insert, they have shortcomings as well. With either plate device, one is not able to use the device in reduction of the kyphotic deformity (i.e., distraction). In addition, once the device is placed, placing compression across the bone graft further increases the stability that can be achieved. Neither of these plate devices allow bone graft compression.

Z-PLATE DESIGN CRITERIA

The impetus for the design of a new anterior thoracolumbar fixation system was to remedy some of the difficulties with existing systems (Table 21-1). The results of animal studies have shown that the increased rigidity of a fixation system will lead to an increased fusion rate and more rigid fusion mass. Therefore, we felt that the system should be as rigid as possible in the connections of the screws to the longitudinal member. In addition, it should have high pulloff strength (i.e., the construct should not fail by pulling off of the vertebral body). This system should be low-profile to prevent late vascular complications and to allow easy repair of the diaphragm. In addition, we felt that a

Table 21-1
Indications and Contraindications for Z-Plate Instrumentation

Indications	Contraindications
Burst fracture with neural deficit	Active infection
Burst fracture with severe comminution	Severe osteoporosis
Tumor requiring corpectomy	Scoliosis
Anterior thoracolumbar fusion with instability	Kyphosis >50 degrees (requires posterior instrumentation as well)
Burst fracture with malunion; kyphosis <50 degrees	

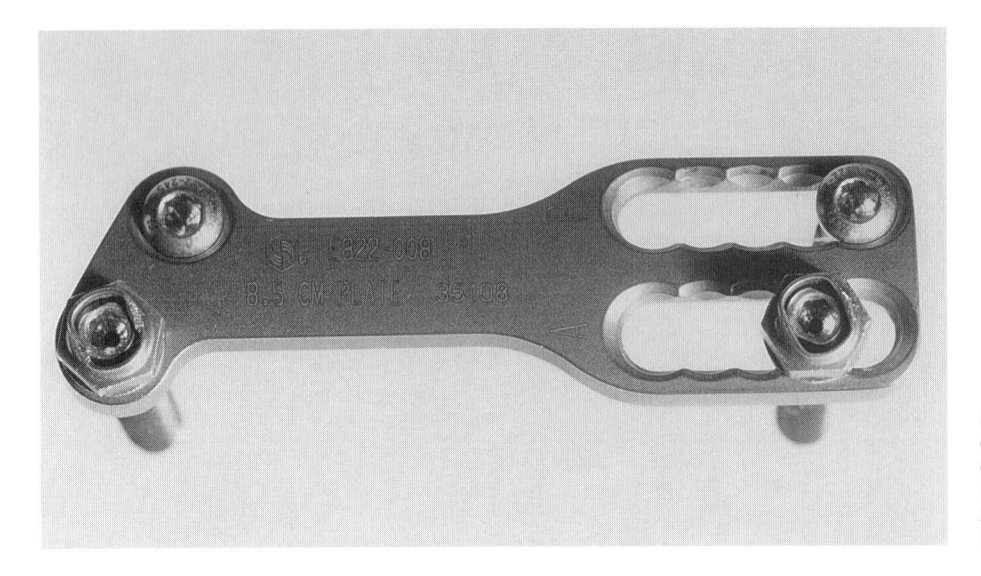

FIG. 21-1. The Z-plate (Danek Medical, Memphis, TN) is a titanium plate designed for use in the anterior thoracolumbar spine. It consists of two slots and two holes through which bolts and screws are placed.

system that was top-loading versus using threaded rods or closed screws would be much easier for a surgeon to insert, with a low "fiddle factor." Due to the success using the Kaneda device as a dynamic device, we felt that the ability to distract, to help in the reduction of kyphosis, as well as the ability to compress after bone grafting were useful criteria. Finally, the materials that were used should be both MRI- and CT-compatible to allow postoperative imaging of the fracture and/or tumor site.

Implant design should incorporate a design for failure and removal. It was felt that this system should fail by loosening rather than screw or plate fracture. This would help reduce the incidence of loose implants in an inaccessible body cavity. It was felt that in-line loosening, that is, loosening of the bolt-plate interface without the loss of alignment, would be the preferred failure mode. We feel that we have met all of these criteria in the design of the Z-plate anterior thoracolumbar system.

The plate is a titanium system with titanium bolts and screws. There are slots at the superior end and fixed holes at the inferior end of the plate (Fig. 21-1). The plate has a radius of curvature so that it is more closely applied to the curvature of the vertebral body (Fig. 21-2). The longer plates and the thoracic plates also have a curvature over their length to adapt to the normal kyphosis of the thoracic spine. There is both a thoracolumbar size and a thoracic size. It is recommended that the thoracic plates be used from T3 to T9, and that the thoracolumbar plates be used from T9 to L4.

The system is used by placing a bolt into the vertebral body above and below, as well as a screw into the vertebral

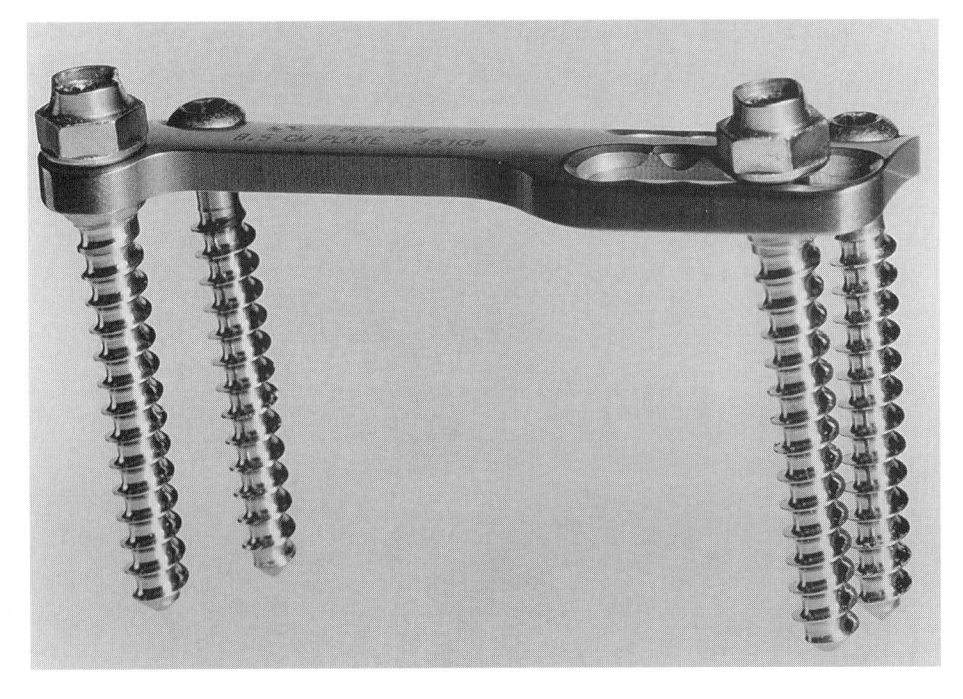

FIG. 21-2. Rigid bolts are placed posteriorly and have a titanium nut that is crimped at the end of the procedure. The bolts are 7 mm in diameter. Titanium 6.5-mm screws are placed in the anterior hole and slot and also engage the opposite cortex.

body above and below. The bolt-plate interface is rigid and the screw-plate interface is semirigid. However, this combination of a bolt and screw in each vertebra allows the system to be top-loading, as well as to allow convergence of the bolt and screw for greater pulloff strength. The bolts, once placed, can be used to provide distraction to help reduce a kyphotic deformity. The plate is then applied and the bolts partially tightened. The slot then allows compression to be placed across the bolts, compressing the bone graft before final tightening. The screws are then placed convergent with the bolts to provide fixation into the vertebrae above and below. Finally, the nuts on the bolts are then crimped, which provides additional stability. Should the nuts ever loosen, the crimp will prevent them from disengaging from the bolt and becoming free in the thoracic or retroperitoneal space.

SURGICAL TECHNIQUE

The Z-plate anterior thoracolumbar system (Danek Medical, Memphis, TN) is indicated for anterior spine stabilization following corpectomy for fracture, tumor, or following diskectomy and anterior bone grafting. The thoracolumbar Z-plate can be used form T8 to L4, and occasionally to L5 if the vascular anatomy permits. The thoracic Z-plate is indicated from T3 to T9. When treating thoracolumbar fractures or tumors with anterior decompression and instrumentation, the approach is usually from the patient's left side. In the thoracolumbar spine, this is because it is easier to deal with the arterial anatomy than the venous, and the patient's liver does not become an obstruction. However, if the tumor or fracture fragments are located primarily on the right side, the approach can be from that side. It is important to ensure that the patient is positioned in a true lateral position, and that this position is held secure throughout the procedure.

The thoracolumbar junction is generally approached through the bed of the 10th or 11th rib, and may require partial division of the diaphragm. After exposure of the spinal segments to be instrumented, the disks above and below the area of abnormal anatomy are excised. At this time, the corpectomy is performed and canal decompression completed. Once the corpectomy is complete, the coronal diameter of the vertebral body is measured using the anterior depth gauge (Fig. 21-3). This will allow determination of the length of

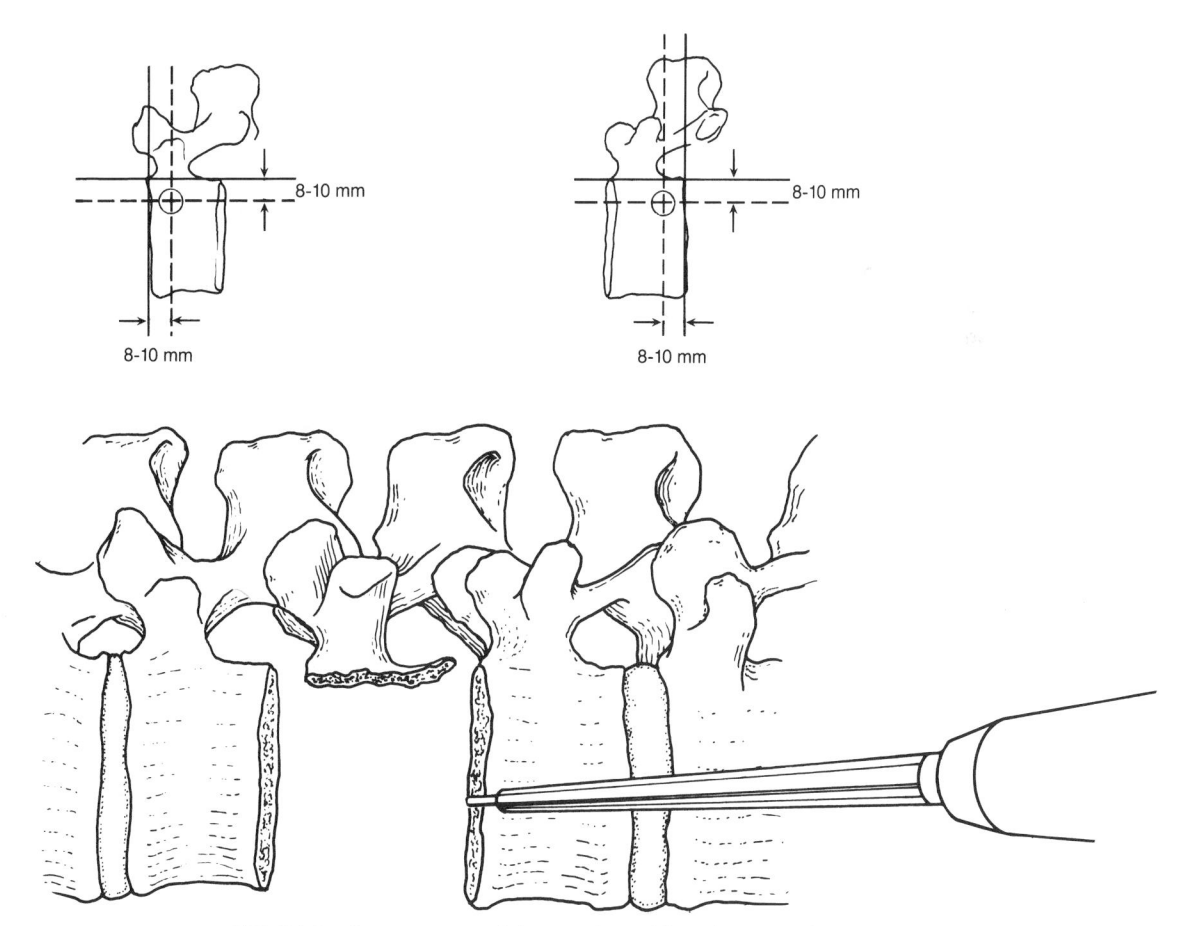

FIG. 21-3. Once exposure of the anterior and lateral aspects of the thoracolumbar spine are achieved and the corpectomy is performed, one can measure across the corpectomy defect to obtain the length of the bolts and screws to be used. The bolt starting points are determined as shown. The superior bolt is placed in the superior posterior corner of the vertebral body and the inferior bolt in the inferior posterior corner of the vertebral body. These starting points are approximately 8 to 10 mm from the vertebral end plate and from the posterior margin of the vertebral body.

the bolts and screws to be used. Measurements from preoperative CT scans and/or x-ray films can also be used to help determine appropriate bolt and screw length. It is recommended that the screws and bolts engage the opposite cortex of the vertebral body for the most secure fixation.

Because the bolts are slightly higher profile than the screws, it is recommended that the bolts be placed posteriorly. In addition, since one is distracting against these bolts, it is recommended that they be placed farther apart than the screws—that is, the inferior bolt should be placed near the inferior end plate of the vertebral body below the fracture and the superior bolt be placed near the superior end plate of the vertebral body above the fractured vertebra.

If no reduction is required, the appropriate plate template can be used to help determine the position of the starting points for the bolts. However, if reduction is required, the bolts should be placed using the hand-held guide only (Fig. 21-4). This guide will allow the bolt to be placed at an angle of 10 degrees away from the spinal canal. The bolt should be placed parallel to the vertebral-body end plate (Fig. 21-5). An awl is first used to perforate the proximal cortex and the bolt is then driven across using the bolt screwdriver. Tapping is generally not necessary in vertebral-body bone. The second, or superior, bolt is then placed in a similar fashion using the hand-held starting guide and angling 10 degrees away from the spinal canal. Both bolts should be sunk into the vertebral body until the shoulder of the bolt is just touching the proximal cortex.

With fracture and kyphosis, reduction should be performed at this time. The reduction maneuver recommended is first to apply manual pressure over the dorsal spine at the apex of the kyphosis. A wide lamina spreader can then be placed between the vertebral end plates within the corpectomy defect to help assist in the reduction. The majority of

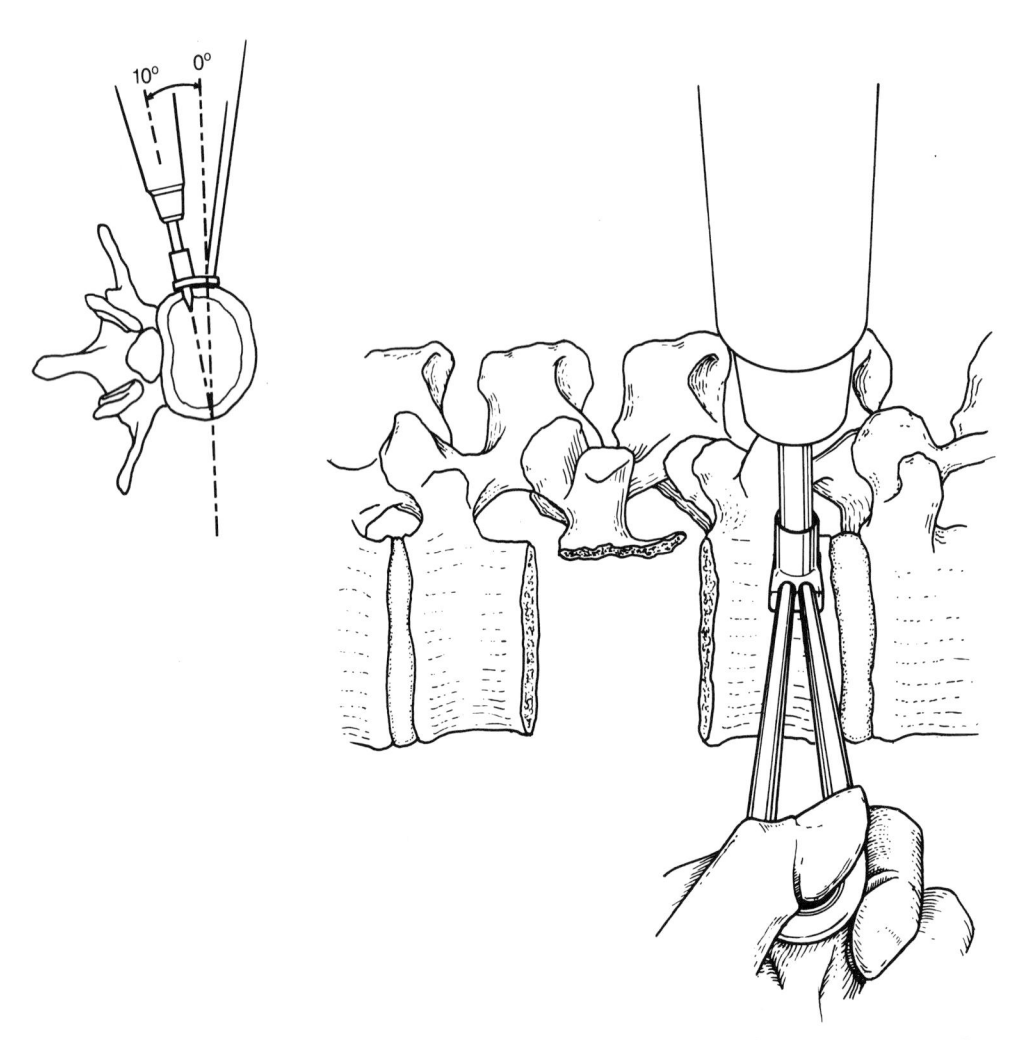

FIG. 21-4. Starting hole is made using an awl angling 10 degrees away from the spinal canal. Only the proximal cortex is perforated.

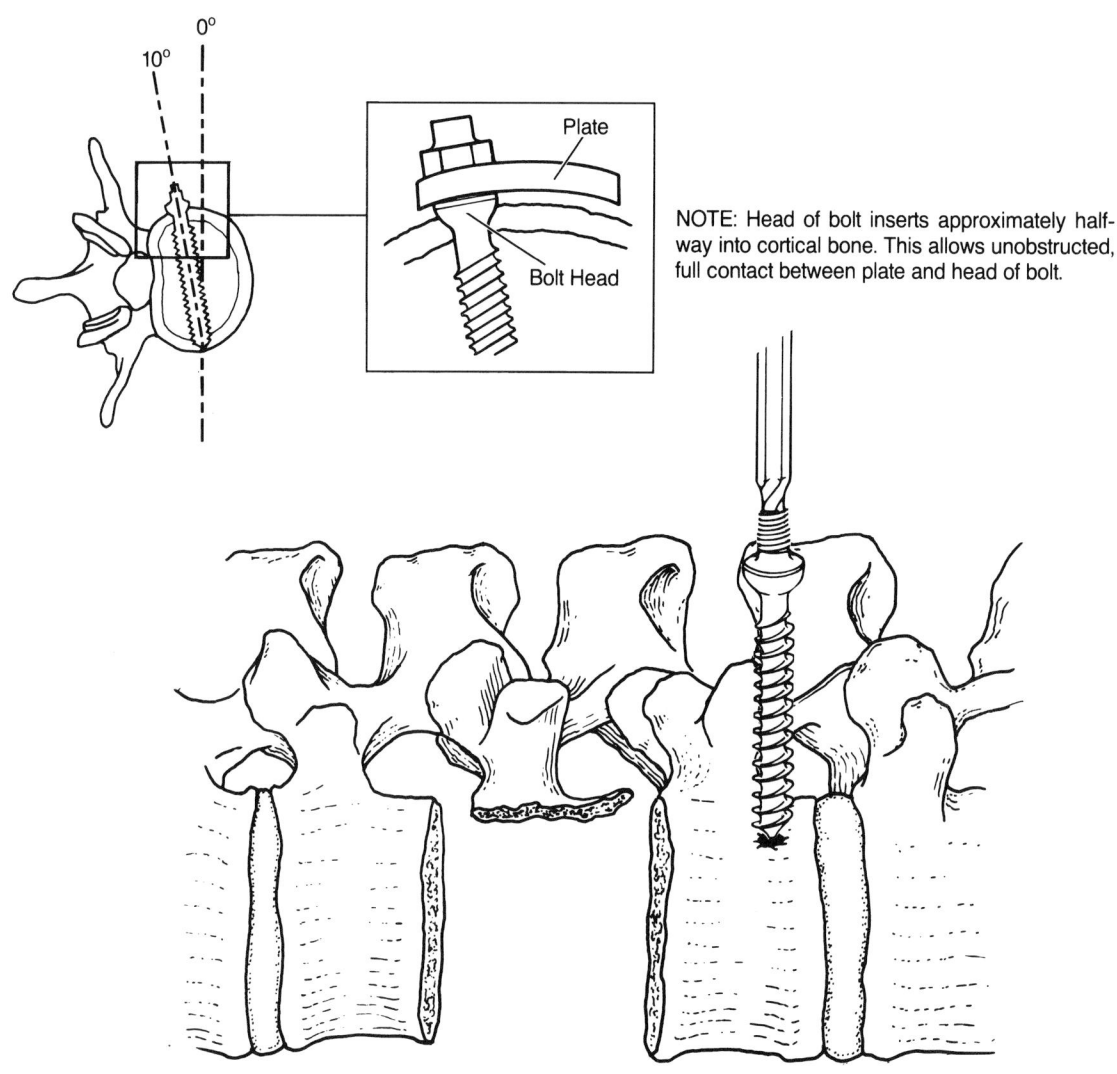

FIG. 21-5. The 7.0-mm bolt is inserted using the screwdriver. Tapping is not necessary. Care should be taken to remain parallel to the vertebral end plate and to angle slightly away from the spinal canal.

NOTE: Head of bolt inserts approximately halfway into cortical bone. This allows unobstructed, full contact between plate and head of bolt.

reduction should be obtained with these two maneuvers. The Z-plate distractor can then be used to help hold the reduction (Fig. 21-6). This distractor is placed against the exposed threads of the vertebral-body bolts. Additional distraction can be obtained using this. Once the reduction is complete, the laminar spreader is removed from the corpectomy defect and the reduction is held with the Z-plate distractor. One can now measure for the length of the bone graft using the anterior caliper. The bone graft can then be harvested and tamped into place, securing the reduced position (Fig. 21-7).

One should then choose the appropriate size Z-plate. The slots should be positioned superiorly. To minimize impingement of the superior disk space and to allow for maximum compression, select the shortest length plate possible.

Prior to placing the plate over the bolts, care should be taken in preparing a flat surface along the lateral aspect of the vertebral bodies. This can be done by removing the lateral prominence of the vertebral end plates using a high-speed bur or rongeur.

Once the plate is in place and fully seated over the bolts, the spiral lock nut is implanted onto the Z-plate nut starter shaft. The collar of the nut is directed toward the handle. The hex end of one of the Z-plate nut starter shafts is inserted into the recessed hex of the inferior bolt. This allows one to hold countertorque on the handle of the shaft, preventing the bolt from being inserted further during tightening of the nut. The nut starter is then turned until the nut drops down onto the bolt; the spiral lock nut is partially tightened at this time (Fig. 21-8). The second Z-plate nut starter

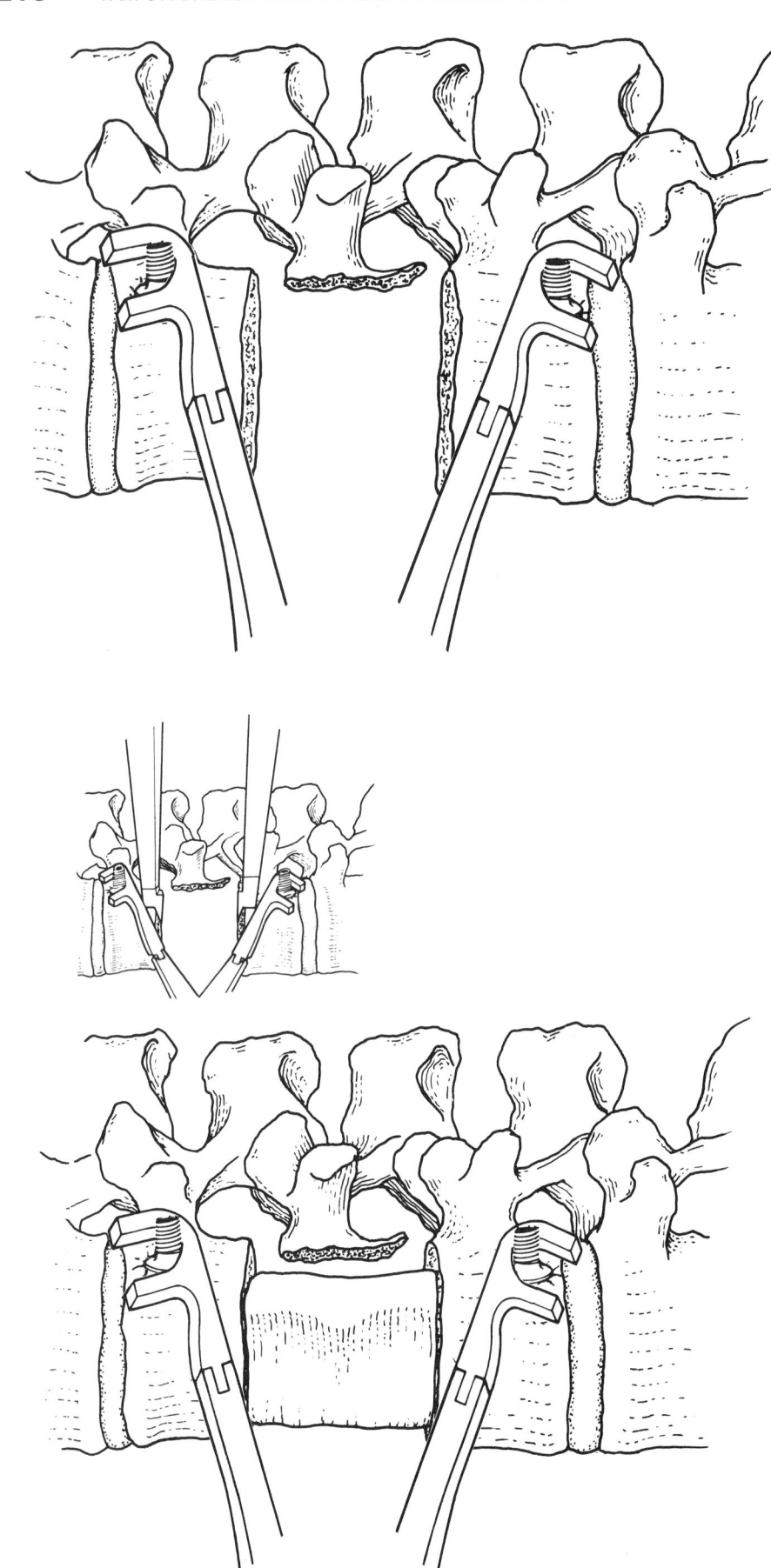

FIG. 21-6. Once both bolts are placed, if fracture reduction is required, reduction maneuvers can be performed at this point. This includes manual pressure on the patient's back, distraction using a laminar spreader within the corpectomy defect, and distraction against the bolts using the Z-plate distractor.

FIG. 21-7. Once distraction is complete, the length of bone graft is measured and an appropriate sized bone graft inserted. This maintains the reduced position of the spine.

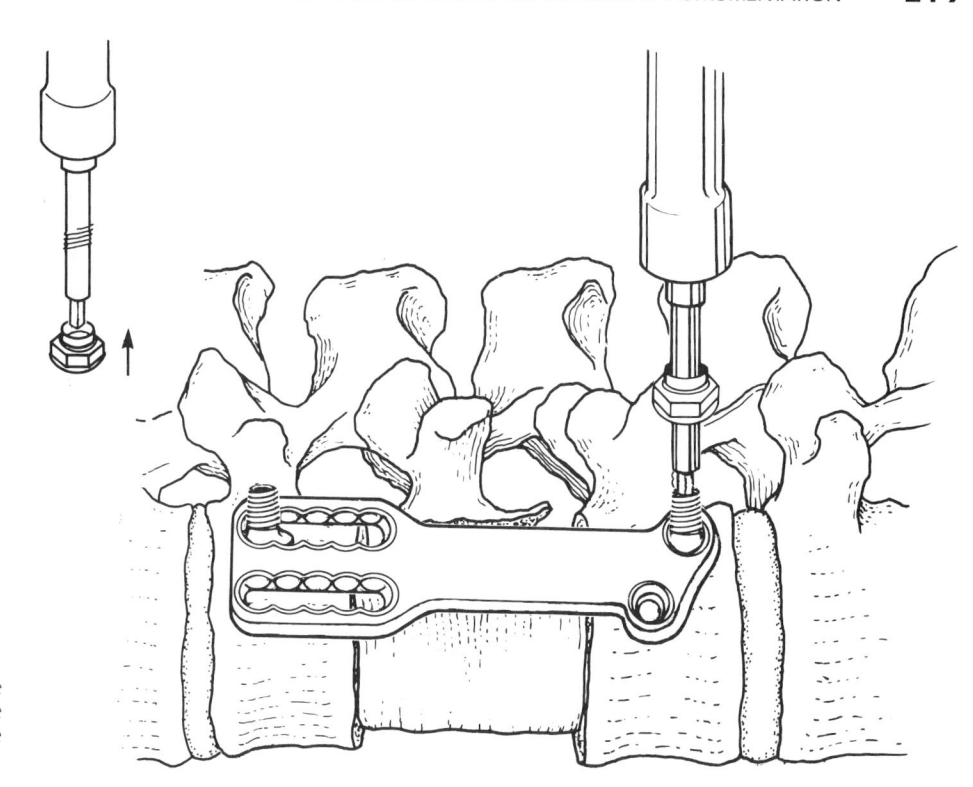

CHAPTER 21 / Z-PLATE ANTERIOR THORACOLUMBAR INSTRUMENTATION   219

FIG. 21-8. Appropriate sized Z-plate is inserted over the bolts. Nuts are started using the nut starter shafts, the inferior nut first.

FIG. 21-9. Starter shaft is left on the inferior nut as the superior nut is seated. Prior to final tightening, compression across the bone graft can be obtained.

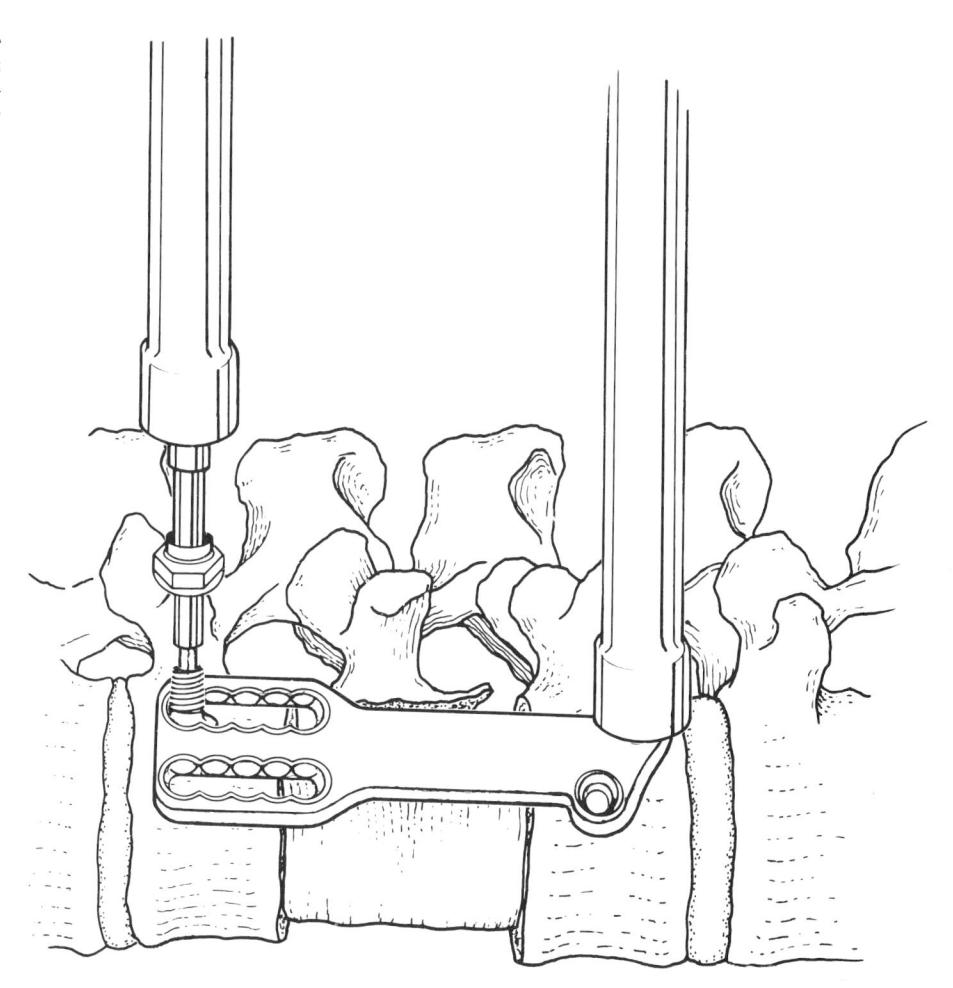

shaft is then inserted onto the superior bolt and this nut threaded as well. The Z-plate nut starter shafts are left in place at this time (Fig. 21-9).

The Z-plate compressor is then used to compress the bone graft prior to final nut tightening (Fig. 21-10). The surgical assistant holds the nut starter shafts in a parallel fashion while the surgeon applies the Z-plate compressor to the base of the nut starter shaft sockets. Compression is then applied and the nuts are fully tightened, while maintaining the parallel plane of the nut starter shafts.

Using the nut starter wrench, the inferior spiral lock nut is tightened while holding countertorque on the shaft handle (Fig. 21-11). Once the inferior nut has been tightened, the superior nut can then also be tightened, again maintaining countertorque on the shaft handle. Compression should be maintained using the compressor during the final tightening of both nuts. The compressor can now be removed. Final tightening of the spiral lock nuts is done using the crow's foot torque wrench. Final tightening should be to a minimum of 80 in.-lb.

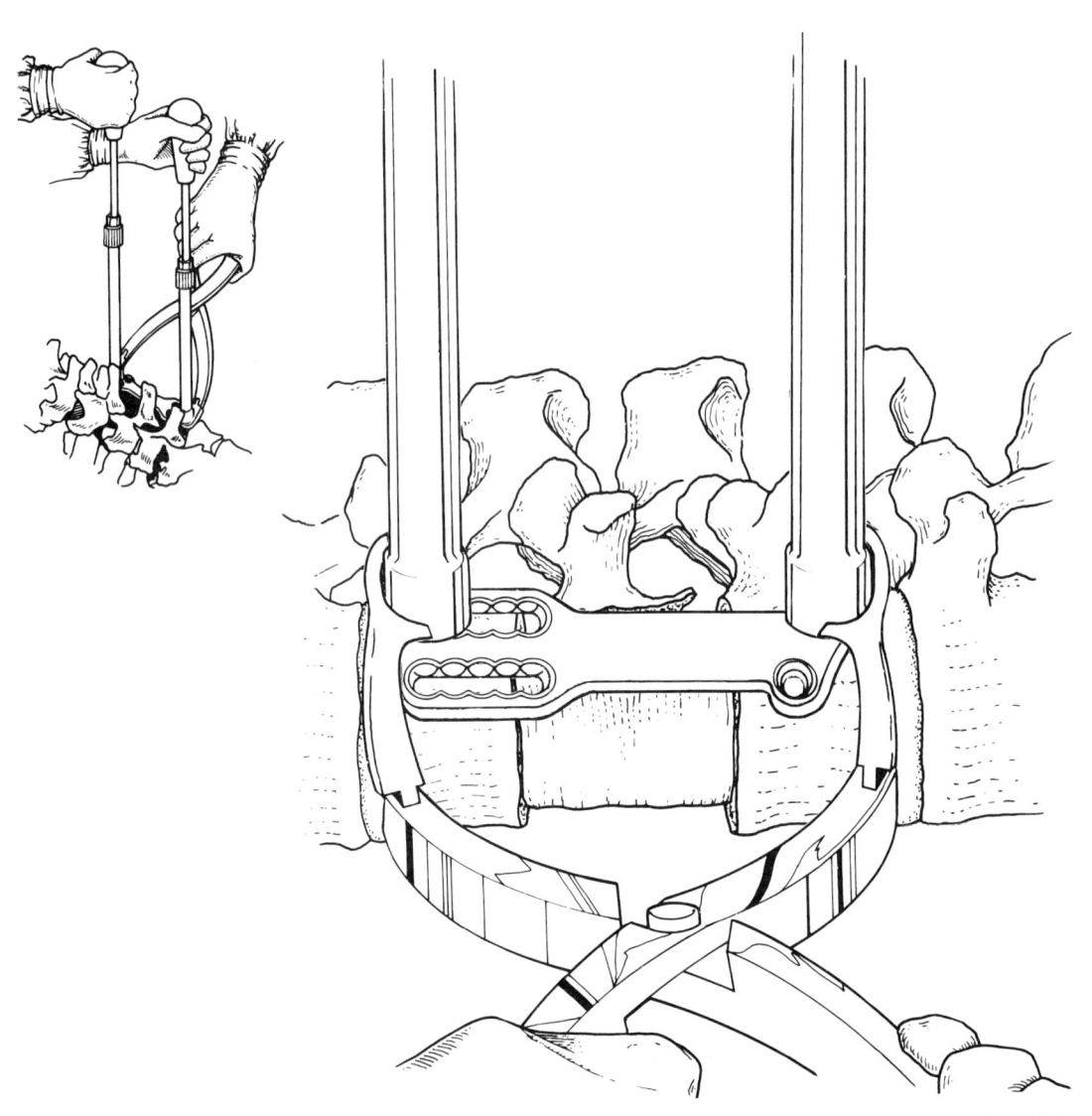

FIG. 21-10. While compression is being applied using the Z-plate compressor, final tightening of the nuts is completed. Care should be taken to maintain the starter shafts in a parallel fashion while compression is being applied.

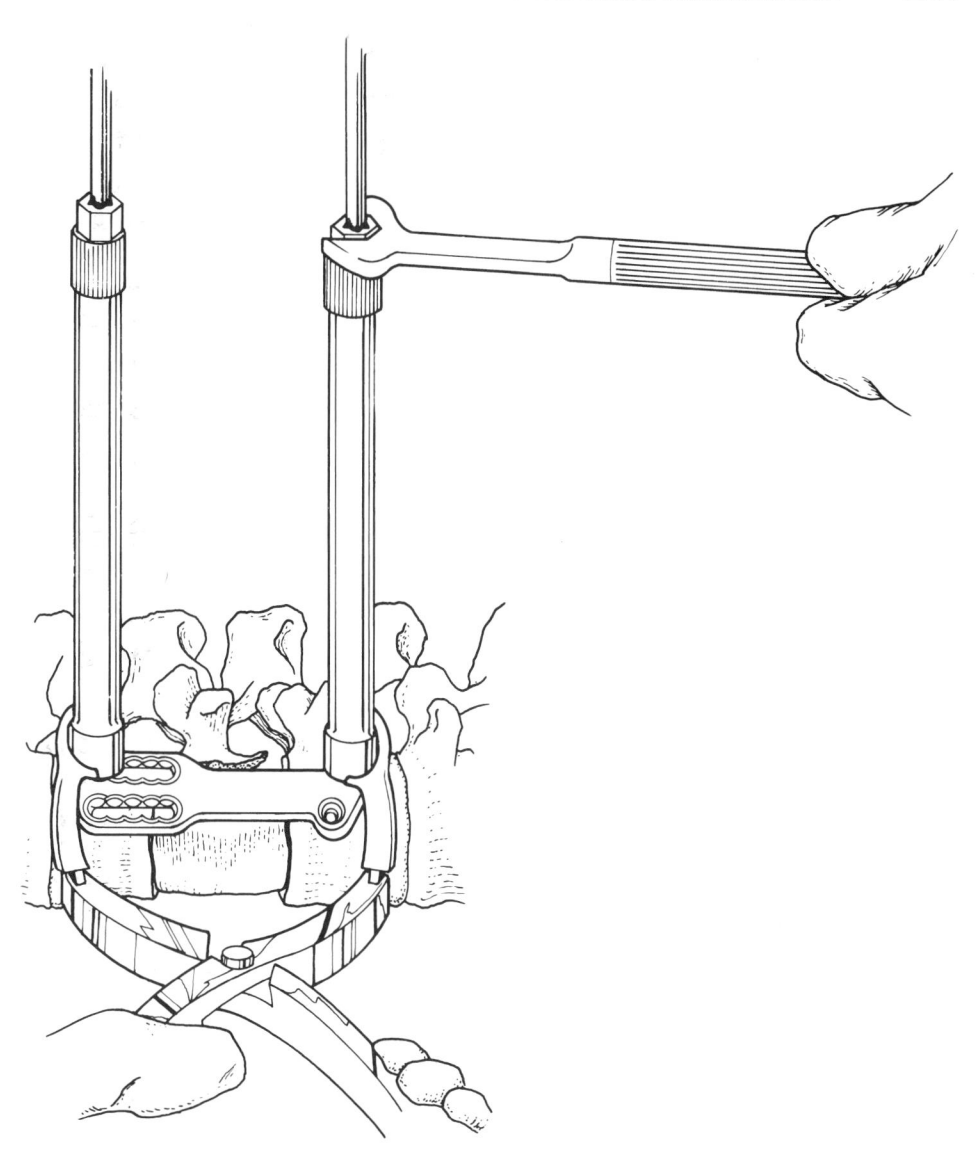

FIG. 21-11. Final tightening is performed using the speed wrench and torque wrench while holding countertorque on the screwdriver shaft.

The two anterior screws are now implanted (Fig. 21-12). Screw placement sites are prepared using the awl. The anterior screws should be placed directly across the vertebral body perpendicular to the proximal cortex. Again, tapping is not necessary, and the screws should engage the opposite cortex. In general, they will need to be 5 mm longer than the bolt implanted in the same vertebral body. When placing the screw in the slot, one should make sure that the starting guide is used with the awl to ensure that the screw head settles firmly into the base of one of the slots. An x-ray film can then be obtained to ensure adequate placement of all spinal hardware. The Z-plate crimper is used to crimp the nut collars onto the flat portion of the bolt. This will prevent postoperative disengagement of the nut from the bolt (Fig. 21-13).

Standard postoperative care should be followed. Typically, a TLSO molded brace is applied on the third postoperative day and ambulation allowed. Bracing is continued for 10 to 12 weeks or until solid fusion is noted on x-ray films.

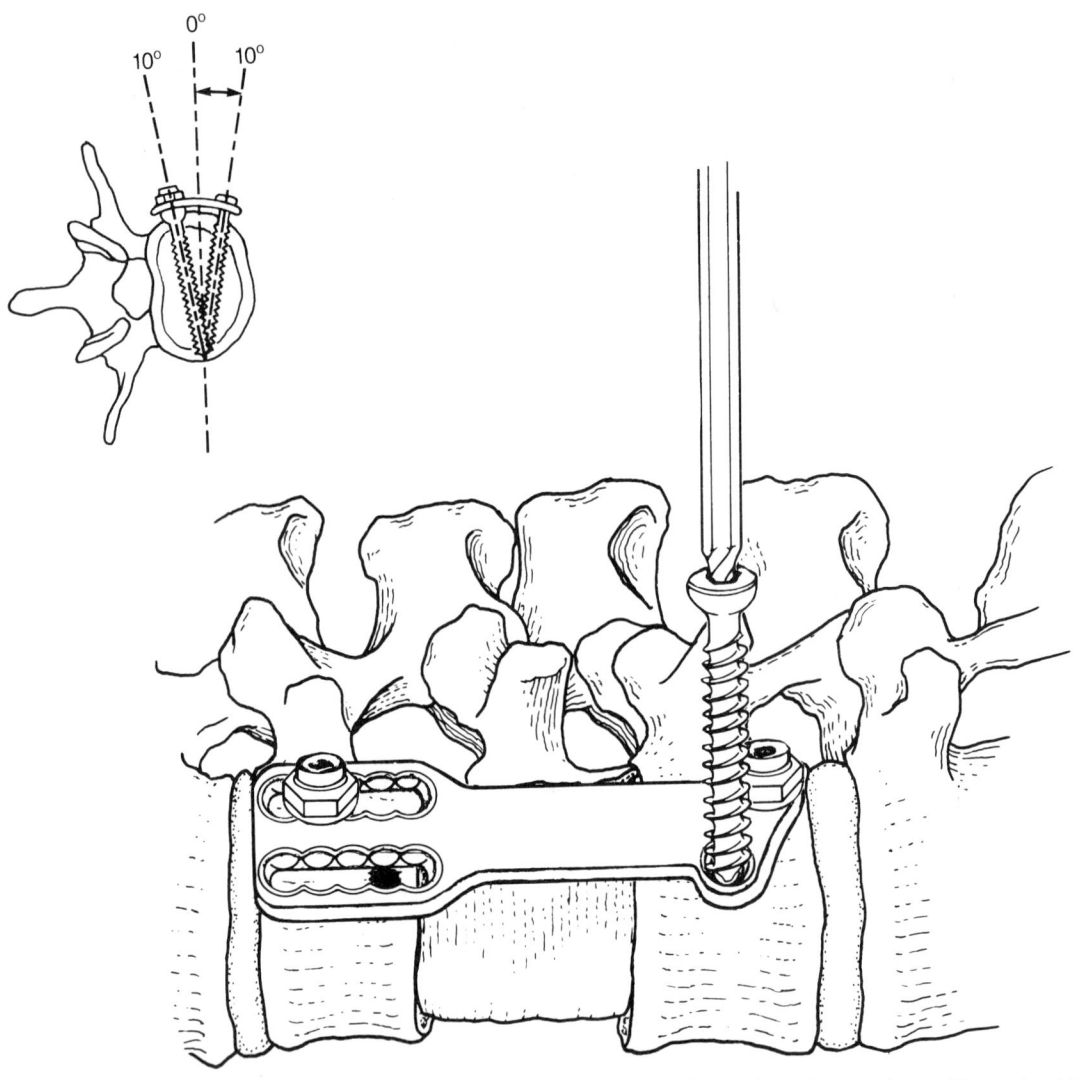

FIG. 21-12. The two anterior 6.5-mm screws are inserted in starting points as shown. These should engage the opposite cortex and angle slightly toward the spinal canal.

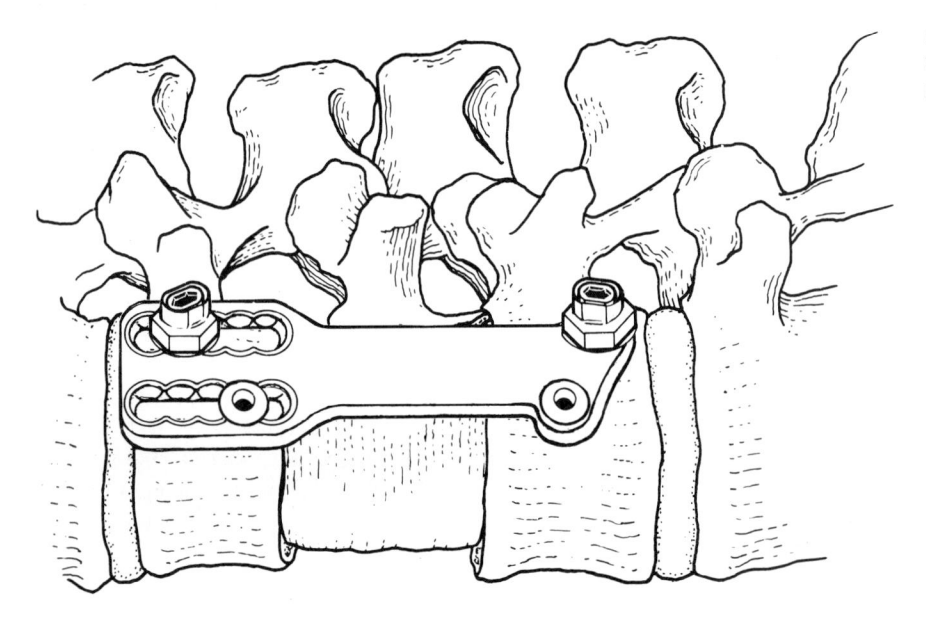

FIG. 21-13. The final step is to crimp the nut collars using the crimp device prior to wound closure.

CONCLUSION

Early clinical results using the Z-plate anterior thoracolumbar system have been quite promising (Table 21-2). The system's low profile and ease of insertion has facilitated anterior instrumentation greatly. Sufficient rigidity is present to provide an excellent biomechanical environment for early anterior fusion. Postoperative maintenance of reduction has been excellent. In addition, the use of the postoperative MRI scan has allowed us to visualize the neurologic elements to assess the presence of syringomyelia, tumor recurrence, and adequacy of decompression postoperatively.

Table 21-2
Advantages and Disadvantages of Z-Plate Instrumentation

Advantages	Disadvantages
Rigid	Not segmental over numerous levels
Low profile	
Allows distraction for reduction, compression of graft	Noncontourable
MRI/CT-compatible	
Simple to insert	
Easy instrumentation	
Multiple sizes	

REFERENCES

Abumi, K., Panjabi, M.M., & Duranceau, J. (1989). Biomechanical evaluation of spinal fixation devices. Part III: Stability provided by six spinal fixation devices and interbody bone graft. *Spine, 14,* 1249–1255.

Aebi, M., Etter, C., Kehl, T., & Thalgott, J. (1987). Stabilization of the lower thoracic and lumbar spine with the internal spinal skeletal fixation system: Indications, techniques, and first results of treatment. *Spine, 12,* 544–551.

Ashman, R.B., Bechtold, J.E., & Edwards, W.T. (1989). In-vitro spinal arthrodesis implant mechanical testing protocols. *Journal of Spinal Disorders, 2*(4), 274–481.

Ashman, R.B., Birch, J.G., & Bone, L.B. (1988). Mechanical testing of spinal instrumentation. *Clinical Orthopaedics and Related Research, 227,* 113–125.

Bedbrook, G.M. (1975). Treatment of thoracolumbar dislocation and fractures with paraplegia. *Clinical Orthopaedics and Related Research, 112,* 127.

Benzel, E.C., & Larson, S.J. (1986). Functional recovery after decompressive operation for thoracic and lumbar spine fractures. *Neurosurgery, 19,* 772–778.

Bohlman, H.H. (1985). Current concepts review: Treatment of fractures and dislocations of the thoracic and lumbar spine. *Journal of Bone and Joint Surgery, American Volume, 67,* 165–169.

Bohlman, H.H., Freehafer, A., & DeJak, J. (1975). Free anterior decompression of spinal cord injuries. *Journal of Bone and Joint Surgery, American Volume, 57,* 1025.

Bradford, D.S., & McBride, G.G. (1987). Surgical management of thoracolumbar spine fractures with incomplete neurologic deficits. *Clinical Orthopaedics and Related Research, 218,* 201–216.

Capener, N. (1954). The evolution of lateral rachitomy. *Journal of Bone and Joint Surgery, British Volume, 36,* 173.

Cotler, J.M., Vernace, J.V., & Michalski, J.A. (1986). The use of Harrington rods in thoracolumbar fractures. *Orthopaedic Clinics of North America, 17,* 87–103.

Cotrel, Y., Dubousset, J., & Guillamat, M. (1988). New universal instrumentation in spinal surgery. *Clinical Orthopaedics and Related Research, 227,* 10–23.

Dall, B.E., & Stauffer, E.S. (1988). Neurologic injury and recovery patterns in burst fractures at the T12 or L1 motion segment. *Clinical Orthopaedics and Related Research, 233,* 171–176.

Denis, F., Armstrong, G.W.D., Searls, K., & Matta, L. (1984). Acute thoracolumbar burst fractures in the absence of neurologic deficit: A comparison between operative and nonoperative treatment. *Clinical Orthopaedics and Related Research, 189,* 142–149.

Dewald, R.L. (1984). Burst fractures of the thoracic and lumbar spine. *Clinical Orthopaedics and Related Research, 189,* 150–161.

Dick, W. (1987). "The fixateur interne" as a versatile implant for spine surgery. *Spine, 12,* 882–900.

Dickson, J.H., Harrington, P.R., & Erwin, W.D. (1978). Results of reduction and stabilization of the severely fractured thoracic and lumbar spine. *Journal of Bone and Joint Surgery, American Volume, 60,* 799–805.

Dunn, H.K. (1984). Anterior stabilization of thoracolumbar injuries. *Clinical Orthopaedics and Related Research, 189,* 116–124.

Dunn, H.K., Goble, E.M., McBride, G.G., & Daniels, A.U. (1981). An implant system for anterior spine stabilization. *Orthopedic Transactions, 5,* 433–434.

Dwyer, A.F., Newton, N.C., & Sherwood, A.A. (1969). An anterior approach to scoliosis. *Clinical Orthopaedics and Related Research, 62,* 192–202.

Eismont, F.J., Green, B.A., Berkowitz, B.M., Montalvo, B.M., Quencer, R.M., & Brown, M.J. (1984). The role of intraoperative ultrasonography in the treatment of thoracic and lumbar spine fractures. *Spine, 9,* 782–787.

Flesch, J.R., Leider, L.L., Erickson, D.L., Chou, S.N., & Bradford, D.S. (1977). Harrington instrumentation and spine fusion for unstable fractures and fracture-dislocations of the thoracic and lumbar spine. *Journal of Bone and Joint Surgery, American Volume, 59,* 143–153.

Flynn, J.C., & Hoque, M.A. (1979). Anterior fusion of the lumbar spine. End-result study with long-term follow-up. *Journal of Bone and Joint Surgery, American Volume, 61,* 1143–1150.

Freebody, D., Bendall, R., & Taylor, R.D. (1971). Anterior transperitoneal lumbar fusion. *Journal of Bone and Joint Surgery, British Volume, 53,* 617–627.

Garfin, S.R., Mowery, C.A., Guerra, J. Jr., & Marshall, L.F. (1985). Confirmation of the posterolateral technique to decompress and fuse thoracolumbar spine burst fractures. *Spine, 10,* 218–223.

Gertzbein, S.D., MacMichael, D., & Tile, M. (1982). Harrington instrumentation as a method of fixation in fractures of the spine: A critical analysis of deficiencies. *Journal of Bone and Joint Surgery, British Volume, 64,* 526–529.

Gurr, K.R., McAfee, P.C., & Shih, C.M. (1988). Biomechanical analysis of anterior and posterior instrumentation systems after corpectomy: A calf spine model. *Journal of Bone and Joint Surgery, American Volume, 70,* 1182–1191.

Gurr, K.R., McAfee, P.C., Warden, K.E., & Shih, C.M. (1989). Roentgenographic and biomechanical analysis of lumbar fusions: A canine model. *Journal of Orthopaedic Research, 7,* 838–848.

Hall, J.E. (1972). The anterior approach to spinal deformation. *Orthopaedic Clinics of North America, 3,* 81–98.

Heller, J.H., Zdeblick, T.A., Kunz, D.N., McCabe, R.P., & Cooke, M.E. (August 1991). Stability of spinal constructs for metastatic disease. Presented at the North American Spine Society Annual Meeting, Keystone CO.

Hodgson, A.R., & Stock, F.E. (1956). Anterior spinal fusion. A preliminary communication on radical treatment of Pott's disease and Pott's paraplegia. *British Journal of Surgery, 44,* 266–275.

Holdsworth, F. (1970). Fractures, dislocations, and fracture-dislocations of the spine. *Journal of Bone and Joint Surgery, American Volume, 52,* 1534–1551.

Jacobs, R.R., Nordwall, A., & Nachemson, A. (1982). Reduction, stability, and strength provided by internal fixation systems for thoracolumbar spinal injuries. *Clinical Orthopaedics and Related Research, 171,* 300–308.

Jelsma, R.K., Kirsch, P.T., Jelsma, L.F., Ramsey, W.C., & Rice, J.F. (1982). Surgical treatment of thoracolumbar fractures. *Surgical Neurology, 18,* 156–166.

Johnson, C. (September 1989). Spinal rigidity following instrumentation. Presented at the combined meeting of the Scoliosis Research Society and the European Spinal Deformities Society, Amsterdam, The Netherlands.

Kaneda, K., Abumi, K., & Fujiya, M. (1984). Burst fractures with neurologic deficits of the thoracolumbar spine: Results of anterior decompression and stabilization with anterior instrumentation. *Spine, 9,* 788–795.

Keene, J.S., Wackwitz, D.L., Drummond, D.S., & Breed, A.L. (1986). Compression-distraction instrumentation of unstable thoracolumbar fractures: Anatomic results obtained with each type of injury and method of instrumentation. *Spine, 11,* 895–902.

Kostuik, J.P. (1984). Anterior fixation for fractures of the thoracic and lumbar spine with or without neurologic involvement. *Clinical Orthopaedics and Related Research, 189,* 103–115.

Kostuik, J.P. (1983). Anterior spinal cord decompression for lesions of the thoracic and lumbar spine, techniques, new methods of internal fixation results. *Spine, 8,* 512–531.

Krag, M.H., Beynnon, B.D., Pope, M.H., Frymoyer, J.W., Haugh, L.D., & Weaver, D.L. (1986). An internal fixator for posterior application to short segments of the thoracic, lumbar, or lumbosacral spine: Design and testing. *Clinical Orthopaedics and Related Research, 203,* 75–98.

Levine, A.M., & Edwards, C.C. (1988). Low lumbar burst fractures: Reduction and stabilization using the modular spine fixation system. *Orthopedics, 11,* 1427.

Lowery, G. (1995). Personal communication.

McAfee, P.C. (1985). Biomechanical approach to instrumentation of the thoracolumbar spine: A review article. *Advances in Orthopaedic Surgery, 8,* 313–327.

McAfee, P.C., Bohlman, H.H., & Yuan, H.A. (1985). Anterior decompression of traumatic thoracolumbar fractures with incomplete neurological deficit using a retroperitoneal approach. *Journal of Bone and Joint Surgery, American Volume, 67,* 89–104.

McAfee, P.C., Regan, J.J., Farey, I.D., Gurr, K.R., & Warden, K.E. (1988). The biomechanical and histomorphometric properties of anterior lumbar fusions: A canine model. *Journal of Spinal Disorders, 1,* 101–110,

McAfee, P.C., Farey, I.D., Sutterlin, C.E., Gurr, K.R., Warden, K.E., & Cunningham, B.W. (1989). Device-related osteoporosis with spinal instrumentation. *Spine, 14,* 919–926.

Magerl, F.P. (1984). Stabilization of the lower thoracic and lumbar spine with external skeletal fixation. *Clinical Orthopaedics and Related Research, 189,* 125–141.

Reid, D.C., Hu, R., Davis, L.A., & Saboe, L.A. (1988). The nonoperative treatment of burst fractures of the thoracolumbar junction. *Journal of Trauma, 28,* 1188–1194.

Riska, E.B., Myllynen, P., & Bostman, O. (1987). Anterolateral decompression for neural involvement in thoracolumbar fractures: A review of 78 cases. *Journal of Bone and Joint Surgery, British Volume, 69,* 704–708.

Schmidek, H.H., Gomes, F.B., Seligson, D., & McSherry, J.W. (1980). Management of acute unstable thoracolumbar (T11-L1) fractures with and without neurological deficit. *Neurosurgery, 7,* 30–35.

Weinstein, J.N., Collalto, P., & Lehmann, T.R. (1988). Thoracolumbar burst fractures treated conservatively: A long-term follow-up. *Spine, 13,* 33–38.

Wenger, D.R., Carollo, J.J., & Wilkerson, J.A. (1982). Laboratory testing of segmental spinal instrumentation versus traditional Harrington instrumentation for scoliosis. *Spine, 7,* 265–269.

Yuan, H.A., Mann, K.A., Found, E.M., Helbig, T.E., Frederickson, B.E., Lubicky, J.P., Albanese, S.A., Winfield, J.A., & Hodge, C.J. (1988). Early clinical experience with the Syracuse I-plate: An anterior spinal fixation device. *Spine, 13,* 278–285.

Zdeblick, T.A., Shirado, O., McAfee, P.C., deGroot, H., & Warden, K.E. (1991). Anterior spinal fixation after corpectomy: A study in dogs. *Journal of Bone and Joint Surgery, American Volume, 73,* 527–534.

Zdeblick, T.A., Warden, K.E., Zou, D., McAfee, P.C., & Abitbol, J.J. (1993). Anterior spinal fixators: A biomechanical in-vitro study. *Spine, 18,* 513–517.

Zielke, K. (1982). Ventral derotation spondylodese: Behandlungsergebnisse bei idiopathischen lumbarskoliosen. *Orthopade, 120,* 320–329.

CHAPTER 22

Application of the AO Titanium Anterior Thoracolumbar Locking Plate System

John S. Thalgott
Mark B. Kabins
Marcus Timlin
Kay Fritts
James M. Giuffre

HIGHLIGHTS

Posterior internal fixation for fractures of the thoracic and lumbar spine has been in practice for decades. The major problem with this procedure is that the devices did not reliably reduce the anterior column and neural canal. The classical Harrington instrumentation did not provide the surgeon with the ability to decompress neural structures completely in patients with an incomplete neurologic injury (Gertzbein, Macmichael, & Tile, 1982). Biomechanically, Harrington rods lacked rotational stability (Aebi, Etter, Kehl, & Thalgott, 1987; Aebi, Mohler, Zach & Morscher, 1986; Gertzbein et al., 1982; Phillips, Brick, & Spenger, 1988). This inadequacy of posterior instrumentation to solve all spinal instability problems necessitated the development of anterior fixation systems.

The anterior column of the spine is primarily loaded with compression forces and the posterior column with distraction forces. Eighty percent of the weight of the forces on the spinal column is supported by the anterior column. Therefore, anterior instability causes a crucial loss of mechanical support of the spine. Direct anterior decompression was first popularized by Bohlman (Aebi et al., 1987; Bohlman, Freeajfel, & Dejak, 1975; Bohlman & Esimont, 1981). Others followed suit, showing the advantages of direct anterior decompression for anterior neural compression in burst fractures (Been, 1991; Haas, Blauth, & Tscherne, 1991; Humphries, Hawk, & Berndt, 1959; Kaneda, Abumi, & Fujiya, 1984; McAfee, Bohlman, & Yuan, 1985; McAfee, Yuan, & Lasda, 1982; Yuan, Mann, Found, et al., 1988). However, early decompression with bone graft still required secondary posterior instrumentation. The first generation of single-stage anterior fixation devices were of two types. The first were static devices such as a plate. The second were variable fixation devices. The basic tenets of AO, rigid fixation and rapid mobilization (Muller, Allgower, Schneider, & Willenegger, 1979), were served by both types of devices, which allowed immediate single-stage fixation and stabilization.

The earliest use of anterior fixation of the spine as reported in the 1950s was by Humphries et al. (1959). The device was a simple plate attached anteriorly to the vertebral body directly beneath the vessels. There was only one reported use of this plate. The next generation of anterior fixation devices were of both the static and variable modes. The static devices were the early plates such as the AO DCP plate (Muller et al., 1979), and the contoured anterior spinal plate (Black, Gardner, Armstrong, O'Neil, & St. George, 1988). These systems had no reduction capabilities and relied mainly on the graft spanning the corpectomy site. Because there was no rigid plate/screw fixation, the adjacent segments often fell into kyphos. One of the earliest variable anterior fixation devices was developed by Kostuik (1983). Although this device has been successful clinically, it does not provide rigid fixation.

The next of the variable devices was developed by Dunn (1984). This device was the most rigid anterior fixation device developed up to that time. However, the Dunn device had severe design problems, which were reported to have caused death by aortic erosion (Jendrisak, 1986). In Japan, Kaneda developed a device similar to Dunn's during the same period. This device was not as rigid as the Dunn device and was technically much more complicated to implant in the anterior column

(Kaneda et al., 1984). A problem with all of the previously named devices is that they were manufactured in 316 stainless steel. Stainless steel is not magnetic resonance imaging (MRI)- or computed tomography (CT)-compatible, making postoperative imaging difficult. Stainless steel also has a high concentration of nickel. Many patients are allergic to nickel and therefore unable to be treated with stainless steel devices.

The AO titanium anterior thoracolumbar locking plate (ATLP) system was created to provide compression and rigid fixation across a bone graft in the anterior thoracolumbar spine. It can be used between T10 and L5, and is inherently low-profile, with a smooth, rounded contour. While the ATLP provides rigid fixation, it does not provide reduction capabilities. Reduction must be attained with supplementary instrumentation and grafting prior to placing the device. The ATLP system includes a titanium plate in various sizes (Fig. 22-1) depending on anatomical differences, and titanium screws (Fig. 22-2). Four screws are permanently seated in the chosen vertebral bodies at the conclusion of implantation. There are also two temporary screws used to hold the plate in place for drilling and seating of the permanent screws, to provide direct compression across the graft, and to secure the plate to the spine. Biomechanically, the system has been tested to dynamic failure at 10,000,000 cycles of a load at approximately 900 nm. The average amount of torque necessary to loosen the screws is 6 nm. A specific set of instruments (AO/ASIF Spinal Instruments for Anterior Surgery) are used to facilitate implantation of this system. The ATLP system and Spinal Instruments for Anterior Surgery are manufactured and marketed by Synthes Spine (Paoli, PA).

INDICATIONS

The major indication for using the ATLP system is instability of the thoracolumbar spine between T10 and L5 (Table 22-1). The classical indication for anterior decompression and fixation is the burst fracture with mechanical and partial neurologic compromise by a retropulsed posterior vertebral-body fracture. It may offer a less traumatic way to decompress the spinal canal as compared with posterior methods. The ATLP system may also be used for reconstruction after resection of primary or metastatic tumors, degenerative diseases of the anterior column in the lumbar spine, and after resection for vertebral body osteomyelitis, both bacterial or fungal. The ATLP may also be used for anterior column support after osteotomies for kyphos deformity.

CONTRAINDICATIONS

Contraindications to using the ATLP system are the presence of severe osteopenia and a fixed scoliosis deformity. It is obvious that the patient with osteopenia will not withstand the loads required for screw placement and the fixation will

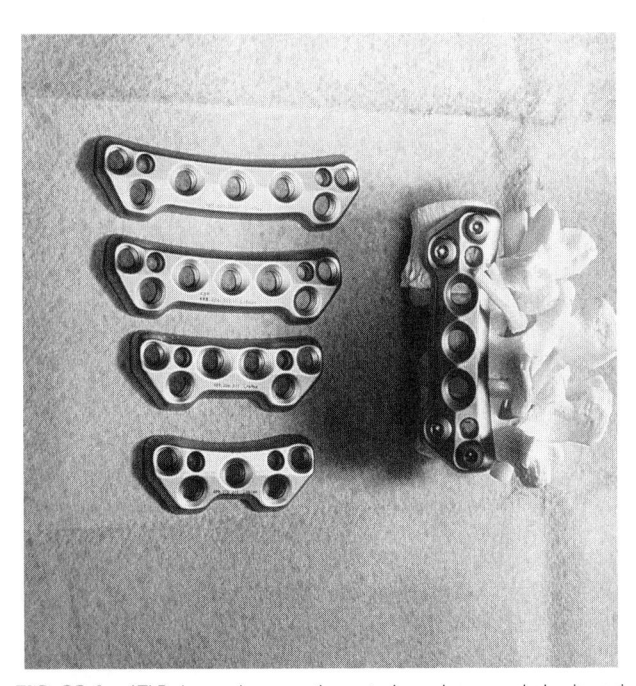

FIG. 22-1. ATLP shown here on the anterior column and also in variable lengths.

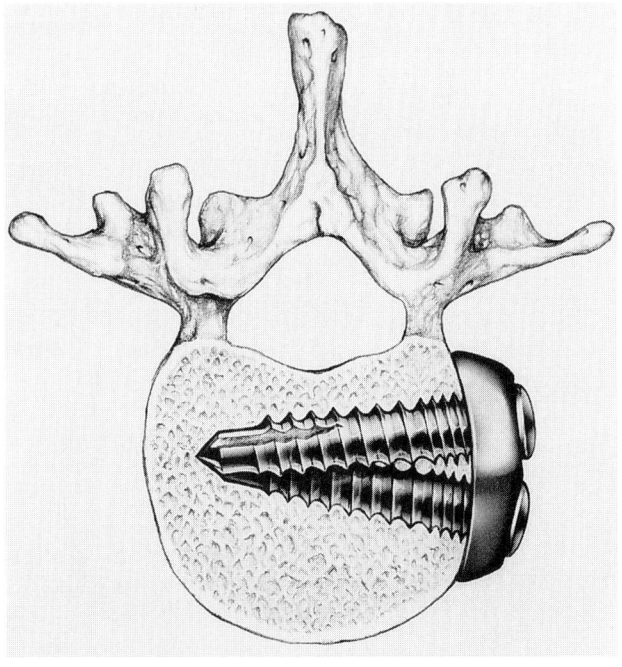

FIG. 22-2. Triangulate-tipped screws shown implanted through the plate into the vertebral body.

Table 22-1
Indications and Contraindications for Use of the AO Titanium Anterior Thoracolumbar Locking Plate System

Indications	Contraindications
T10 to L5	Patients with poor bone
Fractures	quality (osteoporosis)
Metastatic and primary tumor management	Vertebral bodies too small to hold construct
Degenerative diseases	Unreduced fracture dislocations
Anterior column support after osteotomies for kyphos deformity	

Table 22-2
Advantages and Disadvantages of the AO Titanium Anterior Thoracolumbar Locking Plate System

Advantages	Disadvantages
MRI-compatible	Fixed interval sizing
Tissue-compatible	Difficult to use above T10
Wide variety of plate sizes	Limited intrinsic reduction capability
Triangulated screw tips	
Screws countersunk into plate	
Machine thread section locks screw to plate	

fail on loading. Also, in patients with a fixed scoliosis deformity, a straight plate could not be contoured to the annular deformity. There are some spatial constraints with the ATLP. In patients with very small vertebral bodies, such as Asians and children; the vertebral bodies may be too small to accommodate the fixation screws. Also, the ATLP may not be used in the mid or upper thoracic spine because of these same spatial constraints.

DISCUSSION

The ATLP has distinct advantages over other anterior fixation systems (Table 22-2). The system is commercially pure titanium and is more MRI- and CT-compatible than other systems in stainless steel. The design of this plate with its locking fixed angle screws makes it the most rigid anterior system available. The system is highly adaptable to a variety of pathologies and is technically quite straightforward. The screws are triangulated into the plate for greater pullout strength. The screw/plate design is of fixed angle and the screws are self-locking to prevent angular deformity and screw backout. The operator may use nonlocked 6.5-mm full thread cancellous screws to allow more angular freedom. The ATLP system allows direct compression across the cage or graft by the use of dynamic compression holes in the plate.

An entire spectrum of anterior instruments for disk removal, osseous removal, fine osseous removal, and decompression as well as reconstruction have been designed for use with the ATLP. The use of these anterior instruments allow the operator to have mechanically efficient instruments that are long enough to allow the surgeon to operate outside of the chest or abdomen. This anterior instrumentation set includes a set of large reduction forceps that are placed at the apex of the kyphos. This rotates the spine out of kyphos and into lordosis as well as applying distraction across the vertebrectomy site. These large forceps allow reduction of posttraumatic kyphos or fixed kyphos after anterior and posterior osteotomies are completed. The reduction forceps are designed so the grafts can go around them and the plate can be placed on the vertebral bodies with the reduction forceps still in position.

TECHNIQUE

The ATLP allows a very simple straightforward surgical technique in obtaining a rigid anterior fixation. As with any surgery, preoperative planning is important for successful completion of the operation. Once the decision for anterior decompression and fixation is made, the surgeon then has several options for approach. This would be either a left-sided or a right-sided approach, thoracoabdominal, transthoracic, or retroperitoneal. It is our feeling that for thoracolumbar fractures or thoracolumbar pathology, a right-sided approach is safer and easier. The right-sided approach requires retroperitoneal mobilization of the liver; however, it gives the operator a wider area to work with on the vertebral body without vascular structures. This gives a larger margin of safety for the placement of the ATLP. When doing a lower thoracic fixation, the right side is more desirable for the same reason. However, in the lower lumbar spine it is easier to do a left-sided approach, especially to L5, as the vascular anatomy allows easier mobilization of the vessels. Unfortunately, in the lumbar spine the iliopsoas muscle is a problem and it must be dissected free and mobilized prior to plate placement.

The ATLP may be used to L5 if the iliac artery and vein are dissected anteriorly and retracted. The plate is designed to have a rounded angular shape that allows the plate to be placed on L5 and have the vessels run parallel to the end of the plate. Once the pathologic level is identified, a corpectomy or diskectomy is completed with or without neural decompression (Fig. 22-3). Next, an osteotome is used to square the end plates and make them as parallel as possible. The surgeon may use an autograft, allograft, or cage system. Our current preference is the Moss titanium cage system packed with coral or autologous bone.

Once the appropriate length of the cage has been selected, it is hammered into position across the corpectomy defect

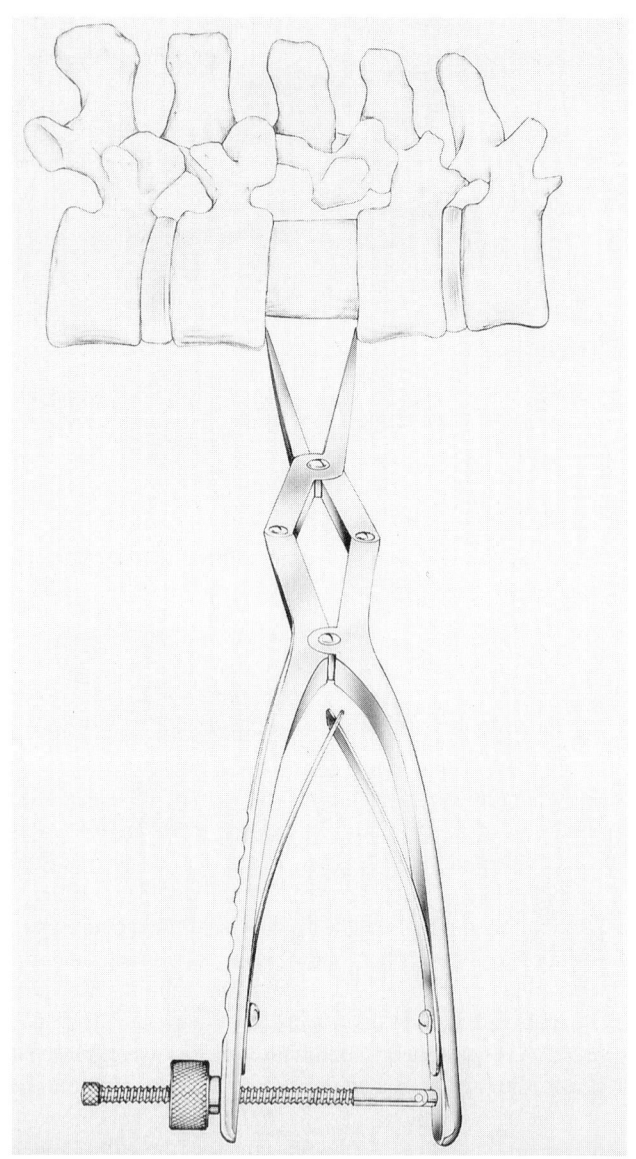

FIG. 22-3. After exposure is obtained and the cord decompressed, the vertebral-body spreader is used to correct the kyphosis and is left in place during insertion of the graft.

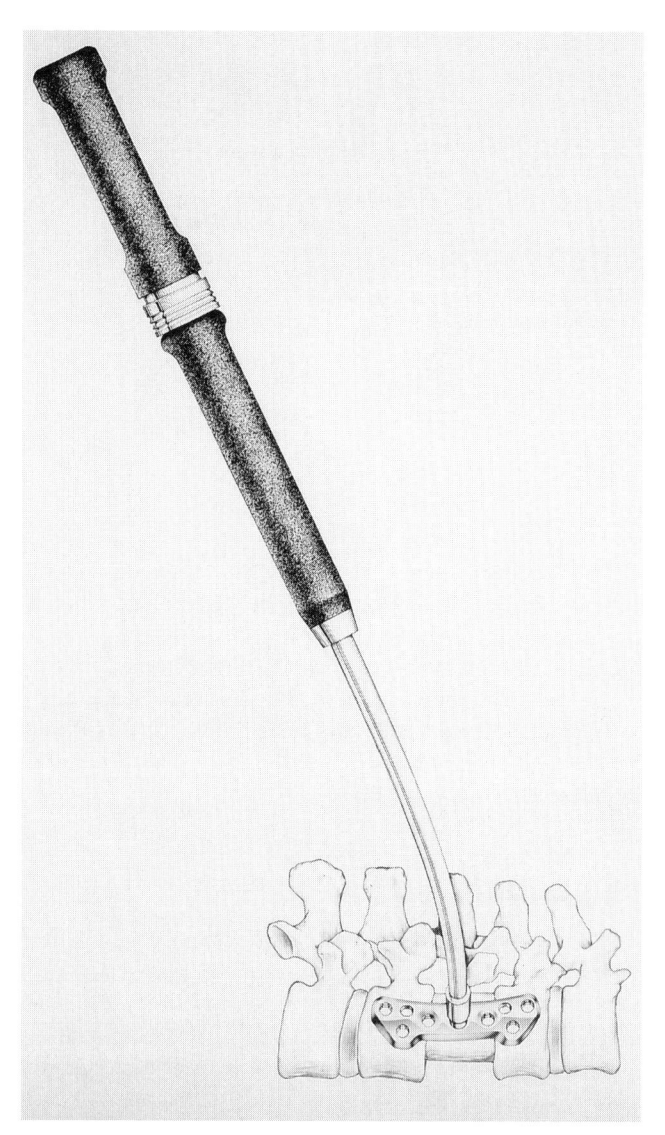

FIG. 22-4. The plate is positioned anterolaterally on the posterior quarter of the vertebral body. The threaded drill guide applicator is used to hold the plate in place and also to screw in the drill guides after the temporary screws have been placed.

with the distractors in place. The distractors add compression across the cage-end plate interface. The appropriate size plate is then selected. The plate must be contained within the vertebral bodies, and the vertebral screws must be at least 5 mm from the end plates. A lateral x-ray film is taken to ensure that the plate is in the appropriate position in the lateral plane (Fig. 22-4). This should be in the posterior quarter of the vertebral bodies. The temporary fixation screws are placed through the spinal DCP guide (Fig. 22-5). The temporary small fragment screws are then placed in a "double DCP" mode. This is done by putting the screws in loosely and tightening each temporary screw against the other, providing additional compression across the graft (Fig. 22-6).

Once secure temporary fixation of the plate has been completed, the permanent fixation screws are placed. It is important to place the posterior screws first. The dedicated drill guides are placed in the plate and drilled with a flexible drill (Fig. 22-7). The drill guides are removed and the 7.5-mm permanent fixation screws are placed at 90 degrees to the plate and locked into position (Fig. 22-8). It is important that the machine threads go completely through the plate and that the screw heads are flush to the plate. If the screws are not flush to the plate, a stress fracture develops and the screws will fail or back out.

Once the posterior screws have been inserted, the temporary screws are removed (Fig. 22-9), and the two anterior screws are placed after drilling with the drill guide (Fig. 22-10). It is imperative that the screw holes are drilled with the dedicated drill guides, as the screws are angle-specific. If the screws are not drilled perfectly within the screw hole, the screws will bind and not set.

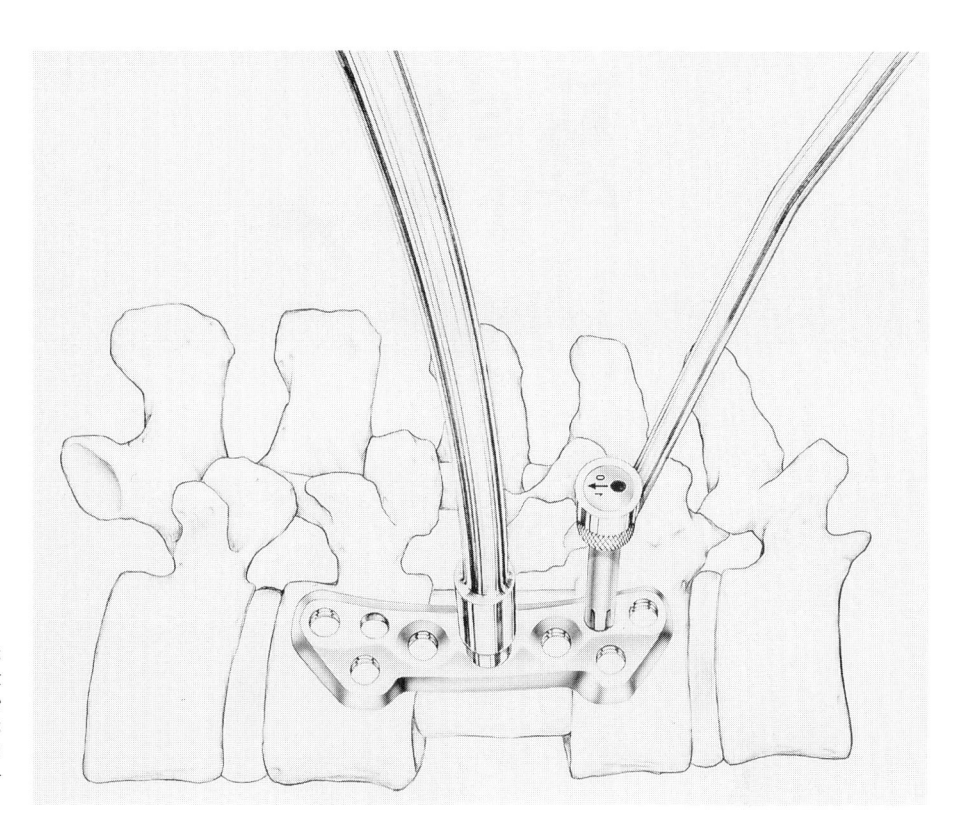

FIG. 22-5. The DCP drill guide has an arrow on the drill barrel that must point toward the graft site to achieve compression. The 2.5-mm drill bit has an automatic stop at 30 mm, which corresponds to the length of the temporary screws.

After the two anterior screws are placed and locked into position (Fig. 22-11), cross-table anteroposterior and lateral films are taken to ensure that the length of the screws is appropriate (Fig. 22-12). These should be as long as possible, engage the far cortex, and be contained within the vertebral body. If the plate is too long or too short the fixation will have a high failure rate. If the plate is a bit long and the screws are too close to the end plate, a 6.5-mm full thread cancellous titanium screw can be used to angle the screw away from the end plate. A single nonlocked screw does not significantly decrease the rigidity of the construct.

With fixation achieved and the x-ray film checked, the patient's wound is closed in a standard fashion and the patient is mobilized in a light brace as quickly as possible. If the permanent fixation screws bind during insertion and cannot be seated completely within the plate, the screw is removed and a new screw is selected. Greater care must be taken for the exact angle to be maintained between the screw and the plate. The most frequent screw to bind is the anterior screw because the abdominal or chest wall has a tendency to push the operator's hand in an angled fashion. Greater care must be taken in placing the anterior screws.

CLINICAL RESULTS

At the time of this writing there have been 25 patients whose deformities have been corrected with the ATLP system. Fifteen patients had burst fractures at the thoracolumbar junction,

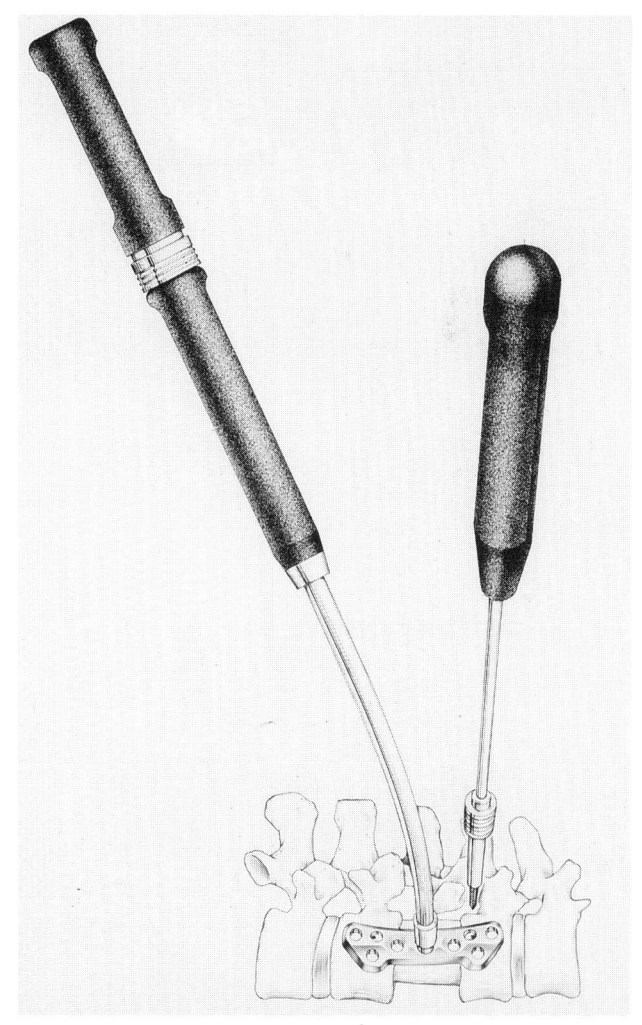

FIG. 22-6. The 4.0-mm titanium cancellous bone screws are inserted through the previously drilled DCP holes.

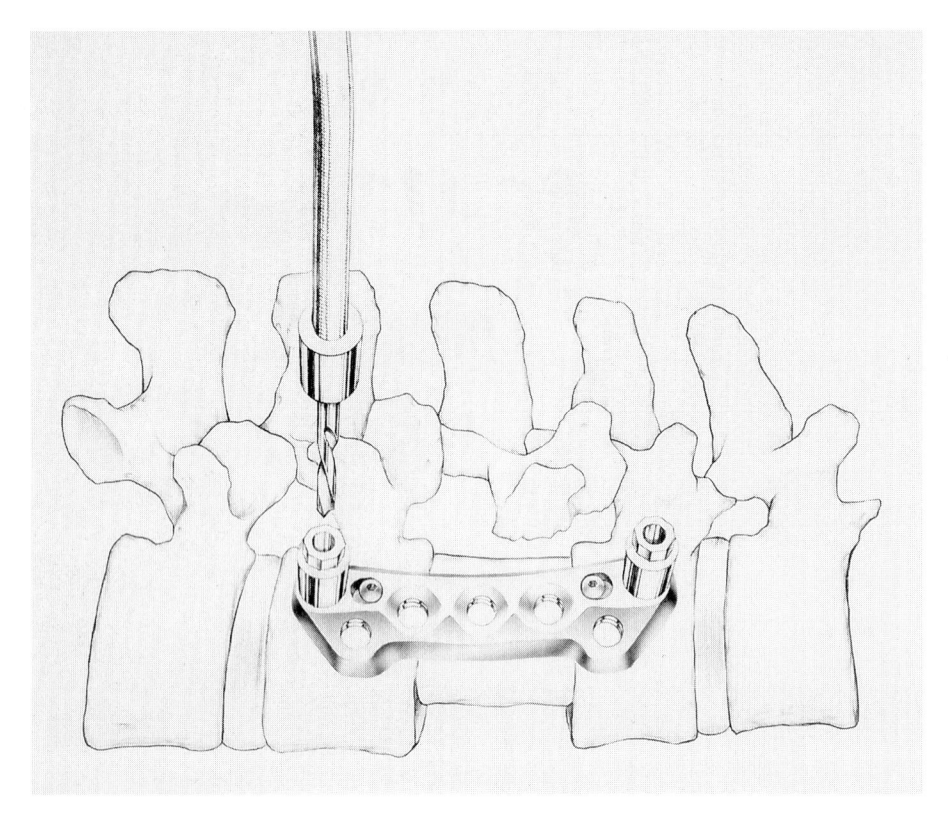

FIG. 22-7. After the drill guides have been screwed in place, the posterior holes are drilled through the drill guides.

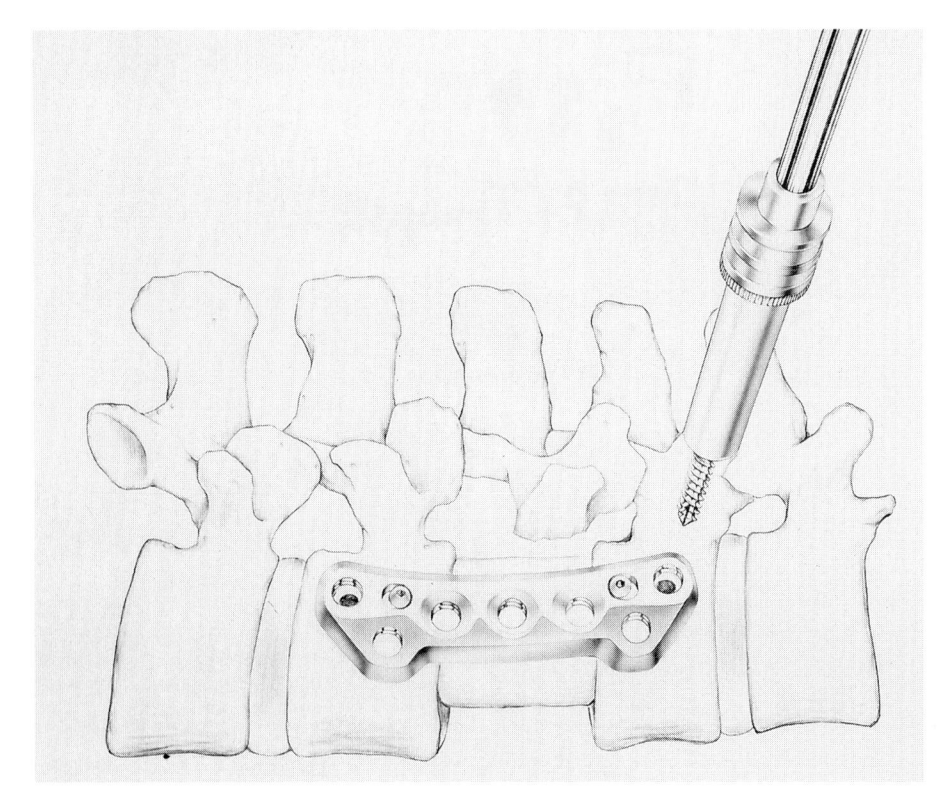

FIG. 22-8. The 7.5-mm titanium anterior spinal locking screws are inserted.

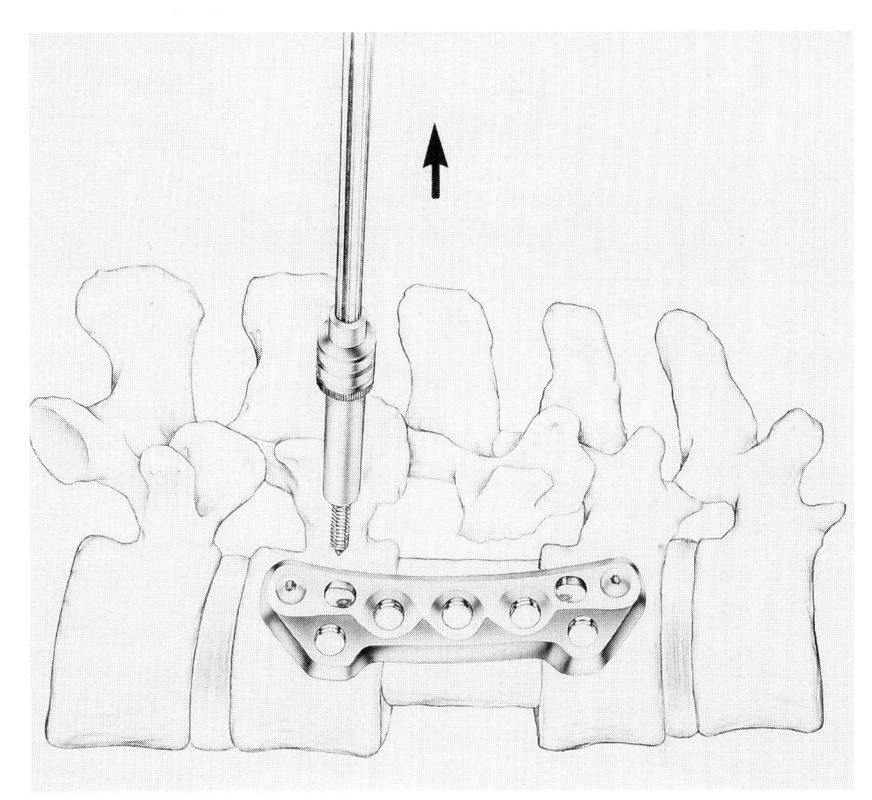

FIG. 22-9. The temporary 4.0-mm titanium cancellous bone screws are removed.

FIG. 22-10. After the drill guides have been screwed in place, the anterior holes are drilled through the drill guides.

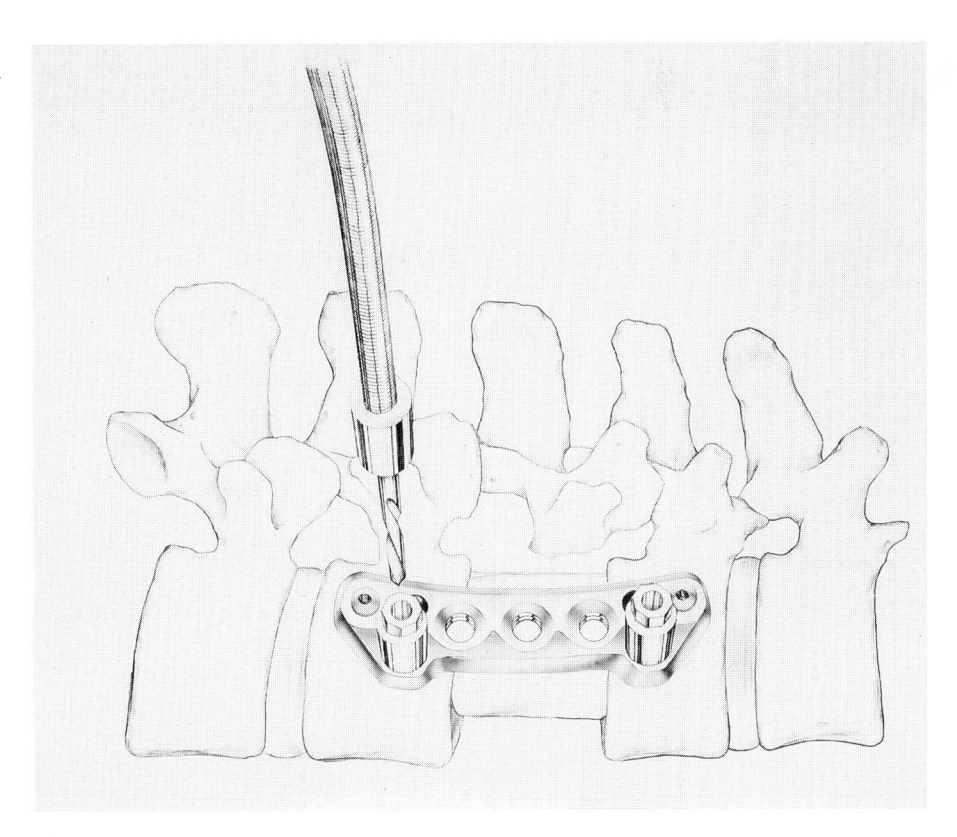

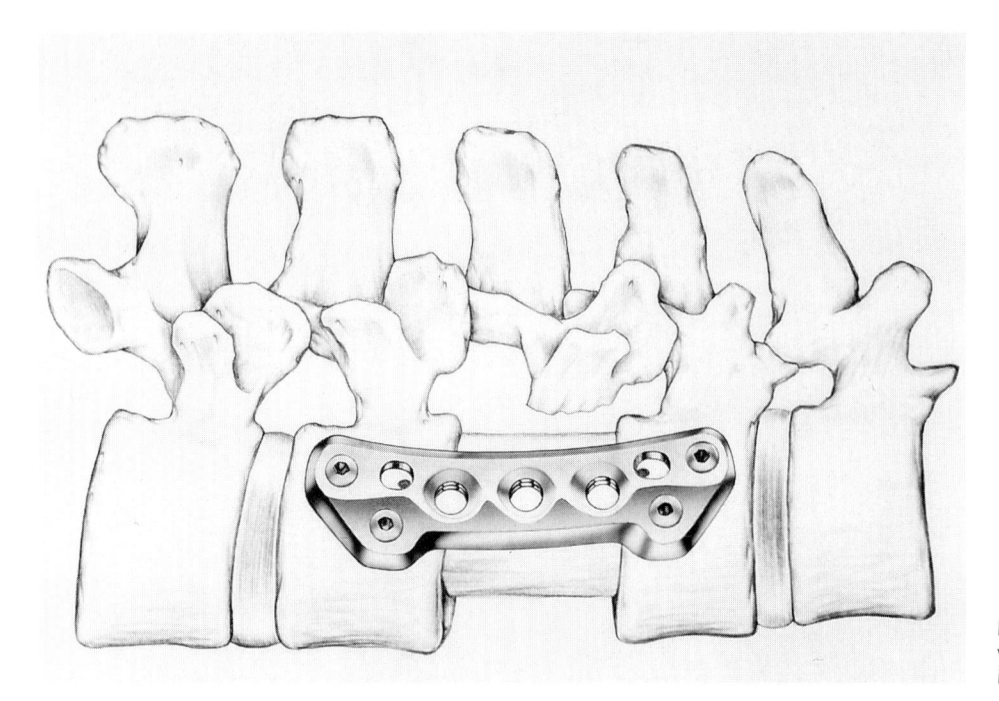

FIG. 22-11. Final view of the plate with all four screws seated securely into the plate.

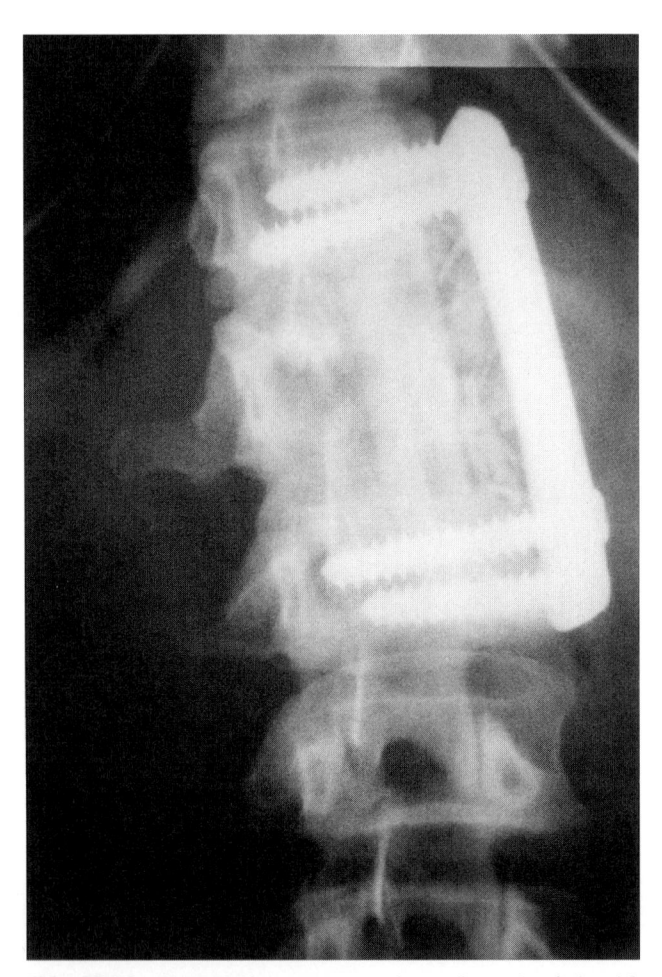

FIG. 22-12. Postoperative anteroposterior radiograph of the AO titanium anterior thoracolumbar locking plate system.

4 patients had metastatic tumors, and the remaining 6 patients had a variety of degenerative pathologies of the spine. Six patients had single-level fusions; 19 patients had double-level fusions. The patients ranged in age from 22 to 78. The average blood loss was 500 ml. Of the 25 patients, 2 died of complications unrelated to the surgery in the perioperative time frame.

The average follow-up at the time of writing was 24 months, and of the remaining 23 patients, 2 had broken screws. These were first-generation screws, which have subsequently been redesigned. The first-generation screw had very short machine threads, which led to a stress riser in the screw. The machine thread design was lengthened, giving a larger cross-sectional area at the plate-screw junction and has solved the screw breakage problem. There was one patient who had a plate that was too long. The screws cut into the end plate and required posterior instrumentation. In one patient, the surgeon became disoriented in the caudal misplacement of the plate, which resulted in violation of the spinal canal by the screw. Fortunately, this did not produce a neurologic deficit; it did require revision, which was accomplished without sequelae. One patient appeared to have lost 5 degrees of correction because of the broken screw and did not require posterior instrumentation. No other complications in this series were related to the implant. After correction of the first-generation screw design, there have been no instrument failures.

SUMMARY

The new AO anterior thoracolumbar locking plate provides a definite technologic advance over conventional and current anterior systems because of its rigidity and ease of insertion. We also feel that the anterior instrumentation designed to go with the implant provides a new level of efficiency in anterior surgery. The biomechanical studies and early clinical experience indicate that the ATLP is a simple, highly rigid implant for anterior spinal stability. The ATLP may be successfully used as a definitive one-stage procedure in many anterior spinal pathologies.

REFERENCES

Aebi, M., Etter, C., Kehl, T., & Thalgott, J. (1987). Stabilization of the lower thoracic and lumbar spine with the internal spinal skeletal fixation system. *Spine, 12,* 544–551.

Aebi, M., Mohler, J., Zach, G., & Morscher, E. (1986). Analysis of 75 operated thoracolumbar fractures and fracture dislocation with and without neurological deficit. *Archives of Orthopaedic and Trauma Surgery, 105,* 100–112.

Been, H.D. (1991). Anterior decompression and stabilization of thoracolumbar burst fractures by the use of the Slot-Zielke device. *Spine, 16,* 70–77.

Black, R.C., Gardner, V.O., Armstrong, G.W.D., O'Neil, J., & St. George, M. (1988). A contoured anterior spinal fixation plate. *Clinical Orthopaedics and Related Research, 227,* 135–142.

Bohlman, H.H., Freeajfel, A., & Dejak, J. (1975). Spinal cord injuries and late anterior decompression of spinal cord injuries. *Journal of Bone and Joint Surgery, American Volume, 57,* 1025–1031.

Bohlman, H.H., & Eismont, E.J. (1981). Surgical techniques of anterior decompression and fusion for spinal cord injuries. *Clinical Orthopaedics and Related Research, 154,* 57–67.

Dunn, H.K. (1984). Anterior stabilization of thoracolumbar injuries. *Clinical Orthopaedics and Related Research, 189,* 116–124.

Gertzbein, D.S., Macmichael, D., & Tile, M. (1982). Harrington instrumentation as a method of fixation in fractures of the spine. *Journal of Bone and Joint Surgery, British Volume, 64,* 526–529.

Haas, N., Blauth, M., & Tscherne, H. (1991). Anterior plating in thoracolumbar spine injuries: Indication, technique, and results. *Spine, 16* (3 Suppl), S100–S111.

Humphries, A.W., Hawk, W.A., & Berndt, K.L. (1959). Anterior fusion of the lumbar spine using an internal fixation device. *Journal of Bone and Joint Surgery, American Volume, 41,* 371.

Jendrisak, M.D. (1986). Spontaneous abdominal aortic rupture from erosion by a lumbar spine fixation device: A case report. *Surgery, 99,* 631–633.

Kaneda, K., Abumi, K., & Fujiya, M. (1984). Burst fractures with neurologic deficits of the thoracolumbar-lumbar spine: Results of anterior decompression and stabilization with anterior instrumentation. *Spine, 9,* 788–795.

Kostuik, J.P. (1983). Anterior spinal cord decompression for lesions of the thoracic and lumbar spine: Techniques, new methods of internal fixation and results. *Spine, 8,* 512–531.

McAfee, P.C., Bohlman, H.H., & Yuan, H.A. (1985). Anterior decompression of traumatic thoracolumbar fractures with incomplete neurological deficit using a retroperitoneal approach. *Journal of Bone and Joint Surgery, American Volume, 67,* 89–104.

McAfee, P.C., Yuan, H.A., & Lasda, N. (1982). The unstable burst fracture. *Spine, 7,* 365–373.

Muller, M.D., Allgower, M., Schneider, R., & Willenegger, H. (1979). *Techniques Recommended by the AO Group: 1979 Manual of Internal Fixation* (2nd ed.) (pp. 304–305). Berlin: Springer-Verlag.

Phillips, D.L., Brick, G.W., & Spengler, D.M. (1988). A comparison of Harrington rod fixation with and without segmental wires for unstable thoracolumbar injuries. *Journal of Spinal Disorders, 1,* 151–161.

Yuan, H.A., Mann, K.A., Found, E.M., et al. (1988). Early clinical experience with the Syracuse I-plate: An anterior spinal fixation device. *Spine, 13,* 278–285.

CHAPTER 23

Methylmethacrylate and Steinmann Pin Stabilization of the Anterior Thoracolumbar Spine

John Shiau
Narayan Sundaresan
Frank Moore
Alfred A. Steinberger

HIGHLIGHTS

Polymethylmethacrylate (PMMA) is an acrylic resin whose development was related initially to research into plastics during the second World War (Fig. 23-1). Since that time, its safe use in surgery has been documented extensively in the literature, although there is still concern about occupational exposure in industrial and health care workers, caused primarily by the liquid monomer (Sharova, Fedotova, Dorofeeve, & Blagodatin, 1993; Wesley & Brinsko, 1992).

Early use of PMMA was restricted to the heat-cured polymer. It was used for plastic procedures in the nose and orbital region, in dental prostheses, in "plombage" using acrylic spheres to collapse the lung in tuberculosis, in orthopedic surgery for anchoring prostheses to bone, in ocular implants, in neurosurgery to repair cranial defects and wrap aneurysms, as well as in otology and urology. Some of the uses, such as plombage have since been abandoned, but others, such as ocular implants, have stood the test of time.

Knight (1959) was the first surgeon to use the self-curing acrylic to stabilize the cervical spine, in rheumatoid arthritis, by molding it as an onlay over the spinous processes and lamina, a use that is accepted even today. In hip prostheses, the earliest surgeons to use self-curing cement were Kiaer and Jansen of Copenhagen (Charnley, 1970). In 1958, Sir John Charnley used self-curing acrylic cement to bond femoral neck prostheses into the femur, and he can properly be regarded as the pioneer of cemented hip arthroplasties (Charnley, 1970, 1961). Most of the orthopedic literature regarding the biomechanical, long-term stability and other properties of bone cement have been obtained primarily from work on cement arthroplasties. In 1967, Scoville, Palmer, Samra, et al. described a technique for vertebral body replacement with PMMA in a patient with lymphoma involving the cervical spine. Although the patient died of pneumonia in the perioperative period, no adverse effect on the spinal cord was seen at autopsy. Since that time there have been numerous reports in the literature describing the use of PMMA for spine surgery, as well analyses of its biomechanical properties and interaction with bone (Chadduck & Boop, 1983; Dunn, 1977; Harrington, 1981; Scoville et al., 1967; Sundaresan, Galicich, Bains, et al., 1984). We have used PMMA fixation for anterior vertebral-body reconstructions following tumor resection for more than 15 years (Sundaresan, Galicich, Lane, et al., 1985), although there is now a tendency to use allografts for vertebral-body reconstruction instead in conjunction with the plethora of spinal instrumentation now available. At present there are numerous uses of PMMA in spine and cranial surgery. It is used in cranioplasties and aneurysm wrapping, for posterior cervical fusion especially in rheumatoid arthritis, in trauma, for replacement of the disk following anterior diskectomies, and for replacement of the vertebral body following corpectomies (Duff, Khan, & Corbett, 1992; Fathie, 1994; Krieg, Clark, & Goetz, 1993). In addition, it is used as an adjunct to screw fixation when the host bone is osteoporotic, and has been injected posteriorly following embolization to replace the vertebral body (percutaneous vertebroplasty) (Cortet, Cotten, Deprez, et al., 1994; Gangi, Kastler, & Dietemann, 1994). In the orthopedic literature, it has been used to maintain fixation in infected bone through the use of antibiotic-impregnated cement, although the commercial variety of antibiotic cement is available only in Europe (Brien, Salvati, Klein, Brause, & Stern, 1993; Dietze & Haid, 1992; Garvin, Evans, Salvati, & Brause, 1994). More exciting future possibilities include the use of cytotoxic drugs in the cement, which allows gradual elution of the antineoplastic drug for treatment of tumors (Wasserlauf, Warshawsky, Arad-Yelin, Mazur, Salama, & Deckel, 1993). There is considerable controversy regarding the use of acrylic constructs in benign disease in spine surgery, but its use in cancer patients is generally accepted. In this review, we focus on its use primarily for replacement of the vertebral body following tumor surgery in the thoraco-lumbar segments.

PHYSICAL CHARACTERISTICS OF PMMA

PMMA monomer is a volatile and flammable liquid with a characteristic, not unpleasant, odor and a boiling point of about 100°C. It polymerizes spontaneously and slowly into a solid resin, a process that is accelerated by exposure to heat or ultraviolet light. To prevent this, an inhibitor, hydroquinone, is used to prevent premature polymerization. To produce rapid polymerization under therapeutic conditions, a catalyst is necessary; this is generally 2% benzoyl peroxide. In the presence of the activator, physical factors such as heat or ultraviolet light can induce polymerization. In the plastic industry, heat is used to produce the commercial varieties of optically translucent PMMA known as Perspex or Lucite.

For the self-curing acrylic currently used in bone cement, polymerization is initiated by a tertiary amine, such as N,N-dimethyl-*p*-toluidine (DPT). It is generally supplied commercially as a powder and a liquid, which when mixed together form a dough that sets into a hard mass as it heats after 5 to 10 minutes. The powder is composed of polymerized PMMA (Fig. 23-1) in a granular form (15%) with methylmethacrylate-Styrene-copolymer (75%) and barium sulfate 10% (this formula pertains to Surgical Simplex P, supplied by Howmedica). The barium sulfate provides radiopacity. The liquid consists of the monomer methylmethacrylate (97.6%) (Fig. 23-1), DPT (2.6%), and hydroquinone 75 ppm.

There are more than 10 commercially marketed forms of PMMA available, although the three most widely used are Simplex P (Howmedica, Rutherford, NJ), Zimmer C (Zimmer, Warsaw, IN), and Palacos R (Richards, Memphis, TN). These are supplied as a package containing the powder and liquid components. Specially designed low-viscosity cements to improve intramedullary penetration and improve shear strength, graphite-reinforced cement to improve fracture toughness, and antibiotic-impregnated cement to treat infected prosthesis are also available (Park, Liu, & Lakes, 1986; Robinson, Wright, & Burstein, 1981).

The speed of the reaction of polymerization following the mixing of the liquid and powder depends on the methods of the manufacturer and also on a number of other factors, including the molecular weight of the polymer, texture, relative proportion of activation and initiator, proportion of liquid and powder, as well as ambient temperature, humidity and the presence of blood. The usual proportion of powder to liquid is 40 g of powder to 20 ml of liquid, but small variations in the volume of liquid can make large changes in the initial viscosity.

Mixing of the powder and liquid can be done in several ways: manual mixing in a bowl, centrifugation, or vacuum mixing with or without precompression. In one study, comparison of manual mixing with other techniques were carried out with 10 cement brands (Hansen & Jensen, 1992). Results revealed that the Simplex brands and low-viscosity cements were the strongest but also the stiffest. Strength in these cements was not improved by any of the vacuum-mixing procedures. Centrifuging was found to be unsuitable for low-viscosity cement. The cements best suited for auxiliary mixing methods such as vacuum mixing or centrifuging were the CMW-1 (a standard-viscosity cement available commercially) and Palacos brands; their strength as well as stiffness was increased. Stiffer cements may possibly increase the risk of crack initiation and crack propagation because of increased stress in the cement mantle. Application of precompression had no additional effect on compressive and bending strengths.

In spine surgery, the cement is mixed either in a bowl or in a plastic mixer available on the market, such as a Sterivac container. The container has a portal that can be attached to suction for the purpose of dissipating the liquid monomer fumes. Systemic toxicity can result from the monomer, and exposure should be minimized (Dahl, Garvik, & Lyberg, 1994; Pinto, 1993; Wade Waters, Baran, Schlosser, Mack, & Davis, 1992). Contact dermatitis can result from contact with the monomer by the hands, and the vapor may also affect soft contact lenses. A single case of carcinoma at the site of

$$a \quad \begin{array}{c} CH_2=C-COOH_2 \\ | \\ CH_2 \end{array}$$

$$b \quad \begin{array}{c} COOH_2 \quad COOH_2 \quad COOH_2 \\ | \quad\quad | \quad\quad | \\ CH_2-C-CH_2-C-CH_2-C- \\ | \quad\quad | \quad\quad | \\ CH_3 \quad\quad CH_3 \quad\quad CH_3 \end{array}$$

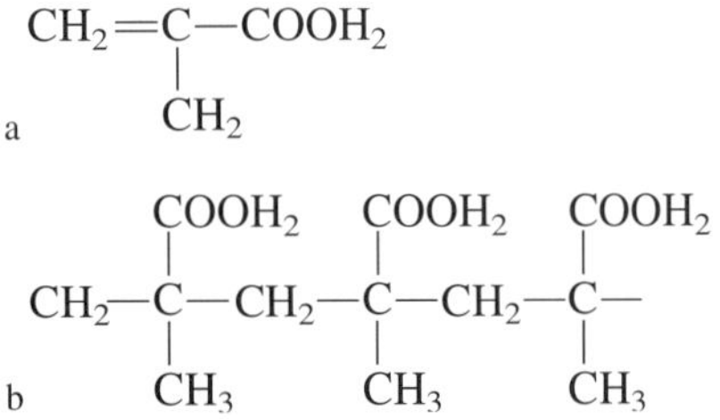

FIG. 23-1. (a) Methylmethacrylate monomer. (b) Polymethylmethacrylate polymer.

plombage thoracoplasty has also been reported. In vitro studies have shown toxic effects of the liquid monomer on leukocytes and endothelial cells, which may explain the intraoperative cardiorespiratory dysfunction and deep venous thrombosis in PMMA fixed joint replacement surgery. Once the liquid and solid are mixed, the mixture should be stirred rapidly and used in several different ways: injected under pressure when still a liquid, molded in place when semisolid, or packed manually by hand when semisolid. We recommend that the liquid be loaded into a 50-ml Toumy syringe and injected when semisolid.

The reaction of polymerization is exothermic. Although the spontaneous generation of heat accelerates the reaction, polymerization of self-curing cement will occur even if the temperature is held down by methods of cooling. If the self-curing cement is held in the hand, it will change from a paste-like consistency to a rubbery consistency after about 4 minutes, with the development of a warm feeling. After the warmth is recognized, it is followed by a sudden rise in temperature, which reaches about 80 to 90% shortly after hardening. However, there is very little heat dissipation to the surrounding tissue in vivo, since both the bone and reinforcing metal rapidly conduct the heat away from nerve and spinal cord. In an experimental study, the effects of polymerization heat and toxicity of polymethylmethacrylate cement was investigated in canine bone (Sturup, Nimb, Kramhoff, & Jensen, 1994). This study found that heat alone had no effect on bone, whereas the combination of polymerization heat and monomer impaired blood perfusion and remodeling, suggesting that heat is of minimal importance for the regeneration process in the cemented bone.

Currently, the major concern regarding methylmethacrylate is related to long-term stability. At present, there are more than 120,000 total hip replacements performed in the United States annually, with the majority using PMMA (Harris & Sledge, 1990). When replacing other joints that bear a heavy load, such as the knee, they are fixed using the acrylic cement as grout. During surgery for joint replacement, PMMA is used in a putty-like form that is packed into the bone before the artificial joint component is inserted. The component is held rigidly in place for 12 to 15 minutes while the PMMA hardens, fixing the implant to bone. Major complications of cemented hip arthroplasties include the loosening of one or more components, nerve damage from surgery, dislocation of the hip, and fracture of the femur. In addition, systemic effects include an increased risk of deep venous thrombosis, deep wound infection, and heterotopic ossification, (Harland, Sharma, & Rosenzweig, 1993).

Although the early results are excellent, the major problem in the long term is the failure of the components to remain fixed, with revision rates approaching 10 to 30% after 10 years (Jasty, Maloney, Bragdon, & O'Connor, 1991). The mechanisms of failure are complex, and may be related to the materials, interface properties, and design of the fixation system. The fixation system consists of the prosthesis, bone cement, and living bone. The major interfaces are the prosthesis-bone cement and the bone cement-bone, which are vulnerable sites for loosening because of interface stress concentration caused by differential properties and possibly poor technique. The order of magnitude difference in elastic modulus between cortical bone (11–17 GPa) and PMMA (2–3 GPa) allows relative motion when subject to the same load. Thus, efforts to increase the modulus of elasticity of the cement closer to cortical bone would theoretically reduce the amount of motion.

In addition, there is lack of bonding between cement and bone. Fixation is achieved as a result of mechanical interlocking between the PMMA and bone trabeculae rather than chemical bonding. One of the characteristic findings is the formation of a fibrous layer between the cement and bone up to 1 mm thick (Coe, Fechner, Jeffers, et al., 1989). In the hip, it has been postulated that this fibrous tissue has a distinct morphologic structure, with a capacity to induce localized resorption of bone and thus result in loosening of the cement from bone (Harris, Schiller, Scholler, et al., 1976). Whitehill and colleagues studied the effects of implanted methylmethacrylate into the posterior canine cervical spine, and noted a thick layer of connective tissue at the bone cement interface (Whitehill, Drucker, McCoig, et al., 1988; Whitehill, Stowers, Fechner, et al., 1987). The tissue was 6 to 8 mm thick, and histologic examination showed that it contained a zone of fibrocytes and plump and teardrop cells within a collagenous matrix. Types I, III, and V collagen were identified by gel electrophoresis.

In the hip, the histologic appearance also included the finding of histiocytes and giant cells, which was attributed to a foreign-body reaction to particles of PMMA. Studies have suggested a synovial-like appearance of the interface membrane. The interface had the potential to absorb bone, mediated by the stimulation by prostaglandin E_2 and subsequent activation of collagenase. It has been postulated that the ability of a bone graft to mature into a solid fusion mass and survive in the vicinity of cement might be jeopardized (Goldring, Jasty, Roelke, et al., 1986).

In another study, Whitehill, Reger, Fox, et al. (1984) studied the evolution of stability in the cervical spine constructs using either autogenous bone graft or PMMA. They noted that immediately after surgery, PMMA constructs had superior stiffness; however, over the next 3 months, the bone constructs had greater stiffness while the PMMA constructs lost stiffness. These reports have been cited as examples of how PMMA constructs lose stability over time, leading to the current recommendation that these constructs should be used only in patients with metastatic cancer whose expected life spans would be less than a year.

It is important to recognize, however, that PMMA used posteriorly is subject to tensile stresses, in which it is relatively weak (28–50 MPA) compared to cortical bone (64–121 MPA) (Park et al., 1986). Used anteriorly it is stronger than cortical bone in resisting axial loads. Estimated compressive strengths range from 76 to 100 MPA (Park et al., 1986; Robinson et al., 1981) and thus it is an excellent material when used to replace the vertebral body.

To improve the mechanical strength, modifications of PMMA include the addition of glass spheres, carbon-graphite, inorganic bone, and phosphates as well as reinforcement with titanium and stainless steel (Topoleski, Ducheyne, & Cuckler, 1995). These alterations will increase the modulus of elasticity of the cement. The two principal methods for improving the fracture resistance of bone cements include porosity reduction and the addition of a reinforcing agent. Porosity reduction increases the fatigue life, but not fracture toughness (Norman, Kish, Blaha, Gruen, & Hustosky, 1995). Fiber reinforcement improves both fracture toughness and fatigue resistance, but fiber incorporation has been difficult. The mechanisms connected with in vivo bone cement failure (i.e., fatigue failure) are not well understood in the clinical setting, but we have not observed fractures of the PMMA constructs in patients followed for 5 years or more.

INDICATIONS

The acrylic and Steinmann procedure is applicable in all cases in which anterior vertebrectomy is carried out and the vertebral body has to be reconstituted. Since many patients with limited life expectancies and others who have failed radiotherapy (RT) are referred for treatment, methylmethacrylate constructs should be considered the reconstructive method of choice (Errico & Cooper, 1993; Harrington, 1988; Lowquet, Thibaut, Thibaut, & Hendricks, 1993; Siegal, Tiqua, & Siegal, 1985). It is inexpensive in comparison to allograft bone and clearly superior in filling large defects when the host bone (e.g., iliac crest) is deficient, as in patients with cancer (Table 23-1).

Although other authors (Harrington, 1988; Siegal, Tiqua, & Siegal, 1985) have recommended the use of PMMA in conjunction with Harrington distraction or Knodt rods, we believe that our technique will suffice in most patients. It is important to recognize that additional posterior fixation may frequently be necessary by virtue of three-column involvement by tumor or because of the extent of vertebral-body resection. In patients with kyphosis secondary to bony collapse, correction of the kyphosis may be performed by using transvertebral screws such as the Z-plate system (Sofamor Danek, Memphis, TN) and keeping the spine under distraction. Once this is done, the methylmethacrylate construct is allowed to solidify and the distraction is released. This allows the methylmethacrylate construct to be held by the Z-plate system, which also provides torsional rigidity.

In patients with spinal metastases who have not received RT, the use of methylmethacrylate constructs allows postoperative RT to be delivered without deleterious effects on the construct. In patients with autografts or allografts, postoperative RT may have to be delayed to allow some incorporation into the host bone before RT can be used. In one review (Townsend, Rosenthal, Smalley, Cozad, Hassanein, 1994), the impact of postoperative radiation therapy and other perioperative factors on outcome after orthopedic stabilization of impending fractures was evaluated; in a series of 64 procedures for stabilization, 35 received adjuvant postoperative RT and 29 patients received surgery. Of the various perioperative variables analyzed, only the use of postoperative RT was found to be associated with achievement of normal function. Thus, in patients with impending, potential, or localized instability, rapid restoration of stability to the spine prior to RT will allow RT to be given postoperatively in patients with spinal metastases.

A major advantage of the PMMA and Steinmann pin technique is that exposure of the spine can frequently be limited to the involved segments and adjacent disks, unlike laterally placed screw systems, which require exposure and dissection of uninvolved vertebrae above and below. Thus, in the thoracolumbar region, this difference may make a substantial difference in morbidity since an extrapleural approach for exposure of the L1 vertebra may suffice for this technique, whereas instrumentation such as the Kaneda or Z-plate requires exposure of three vertebra (T12-L1-L2), potentially increasing the morbidity in elderly or sick patients (Table 23-2).

Furthermore, when tumor recurs and reoperation is required, revision of this system is easier, especially if the tumor has recurred on the opposite side. It is possible to revise and remove the methylmethacrylate constructs from the opposite side, which is not possible with a plate system placed on one side.

The final advantages of this system are its simplicity and widespread availability. Most of the equipment required to

Table 23-1
Indications and Contraindications for Stabilization with Methylmethacrylate and Steinmann Pins

Indications
  Anterior stabilization after anterior vertebrectomy
    Especially useful in cancer patients
      Less expensive than allograft
      Excellent for filling large defects when host bone is deficient
      Stable in face of postoperative radiation therapy
      Ease of revision
  Situations in which a more limited exposure is desired
    Exposure can be limited to involved segments and adjacent disks

Contraindications
  Relative
    Insufficient as sole stabilization technique
      Correction of kyphosis
      Three-column instability
    Situations in which proper Steinmann pin placement may be difficult
      Junctional areas
      Limited exposure
  Absolute
    Infection

Table 23-2
Advantages and Disadvantages of Stabilization with Methylmethacrylate and Steinmann Pins

Advantages
  Exposure limited to involved segments
  Easier revision surgery
  Simple application technique
  Widespread availability

Disadvantages
  Cannot correct preexisting kyphosis
  Requires posterior instrumentation for three-column instability
  May require longer segment fixation in osteoporosis
  Not useful in presence of osteomyelitis

do this procedure is already available in all operating rooms; thus, no special equipment is required to perform these procedures. However, to improve and perfect the technique in difficult cases, specially designed pin holders, drivers, and distracters are available on a custom basis in a specially designed set (Sofamor Danek, Memphis, TN) (Figs. 23-2 and 23-3). In addition, the Steinmann pins made of titanium are also available on a custom basis. Use of the titanium pins allows better postoperative imaging with MRI scans, but this metal is more liable to fatigue fractures. Nevertheless, the ready availability of methylmethacrylate gives this construct an immediate advantage over allograft reconstruction. In our experience the best allograft for resected vertebra is either fresh frozen tibia or femur. However, the required allograft may not always be available when needed. Most hospitals, unless they have specialized storage capacity to keep frozen bone, cannot keep the required allografts available at all times.

However, the use of this technique must be tempered with its limitations. Methylmethacrylate constructs cannot easily be used to correct a kyphosis without additional instrumentation such as transcortical screws. Secondly, it cannot suffice by itself without additional posterior instrumentation if three-column instability is present. If a radical corpectomy is carried out all the way back past the pedicles and facets, a staged posterior procedure may be necessary. In the cervical spine, the small size of the vertebral bodies and frequent involvement of the pedicles and facets generally dictate a combined anterior posterior approach for satisfactory fixation.

We would also not use this technique across junctional areas such as the cervicothoracic or lumbosacral segments, where it might be difficult to place the Steinmann pins in the long axis of the vertebra. In some patients with cancer, the host bone may be markedly osteoporotic. A longer segment of the spine may need to be engaged in such situa-

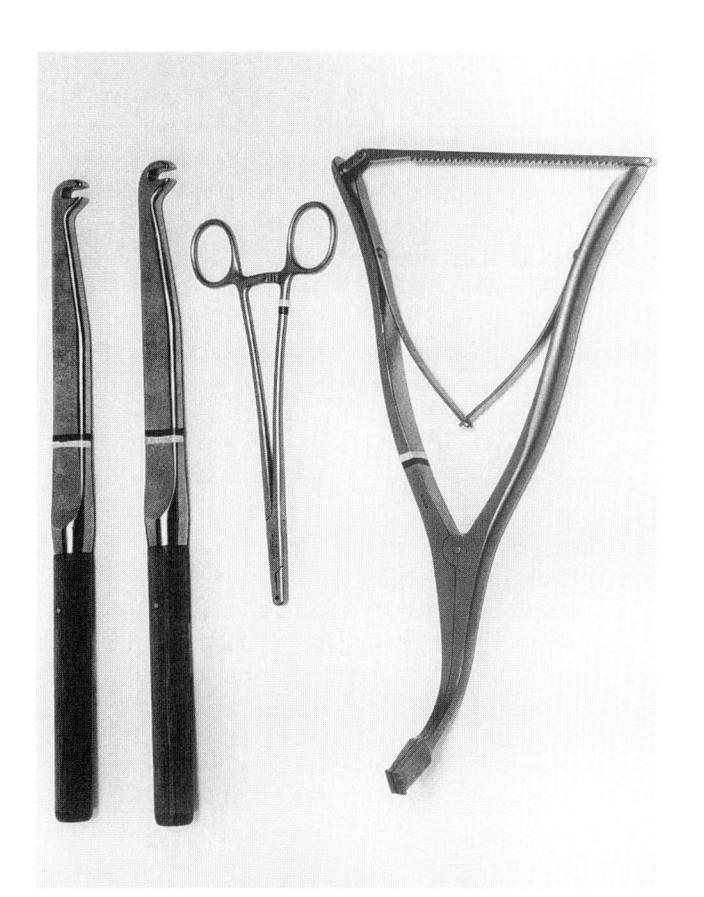

FIG. 23-2. Nonspecialized instruments included in the Steinmann pin insertion set. From left to right, standard pin benders, heavy pin holder, and lamina distractor.

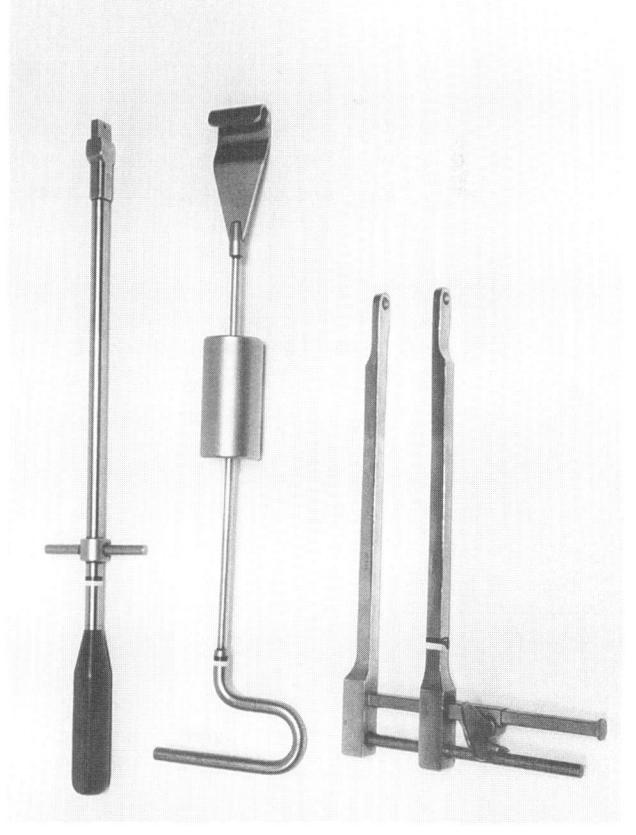

FIG. 23-3. Specialized instruments included in the Steinmann pin insertion set. From left to right, large pin holder, pin driver, and lamina spreader.

tions. If the exposure does not allow sufficient access for pin placement, alternative techniques should be considered; these include the use of interbody devices such as a Harms cage or a polyethylene tube (Errico & Cooper, 1993). We would also not recommend the use of this technique in the presence of infection around the spine although antibiotic impregnated cement fixation is frequently advocated for the treatment of osteomyelitis (Dietze & Haid, 1992; Garvin et al., 1994).

TECHNIQUE

Methylmethacrylate can be used alone or in conjunction with instrumentation. Use of PMMA constructs alone will result in a high incidence of dislodgment, and thus reinforcement either with screws, wires, plates, or an interbody device such as a Harms cage is necessary. In addition, the use of Steinmann pins or a Harms cage increases the fracture stiffness of the construct.

In 1985, we reported the results of a technique using Steinmann pins impacted into the bodies above and below the resected segment to hold the construct in place (Sundaresan et al., 1985). The general principles outlined then are still valid today. In more than 100 patients, an anterior or anterolateral approach was used for the corpectomy. More than 80% of the patients underwent thoracotomy or a thoracoabdominal approach. Prior to surgery, proper patient selection and complete radiologic evaluation by regular x-ray studies, CT scans, and magnetic resonance imaging (MRI) are important. The radiologic demonstration of tumor involvement of the anterior columns, without significant translational deformity, scoliosis, or kyphosis are the ideal findings for this procedure. Certain levels (e.g., the L5 vertebra) may not be amenable for the pin technique.

At present, all operations are performed under general endotracheal anesthesia with the patients positioned in the lateral position on the Olympus bean bag. The choice of side for surgery is based on the radiologic findings of a paravertebral tumor if one is evident. For thoracoabdominal approaches, a left-sided approach is generally used. We generally use the image intensifier with the patient positioned on a radiographic table to outline the skin incision. Additional adjuncts include the cell saver to retrieve blood, use of a level-one transfusion device, and somatosensory evoked potential (SSEP) monitoring. For thoracoabdominal exposures, rib resection of the 10th or 11th rib, as well as detachment of the diaphragm from its costal insertion, is necessary. Double-lumen tubes are usually not necessary at this level, since the lung is generally easily retracted.

The skin incision is generally an oblique incision centered over the appropriate rib. Following the skin incision, cautery is used to divide all the muscles, including the latissimus dorsi and serratus anterior. The rib is stripped off its periosteal attachments with cautery, and dissection is begun at the costochondral junction. Removal of the costal cartilage allows dissection in the subcostal plane. The intercostal nerve and neurovascular bundle is carefully isolated and ligated. The endothoracic fascia and fascia transversalis lie underneath the ribs and are cut. The pleural cavity is then gradually opened. Next, the diaphragm is detached from its costal insertions to the 11th and 12th ribs, while retracting it downward. By gradually retracting the diaphragm downward, the front of the spine is exposed. At this point, the front of the spine is covered by soft tissue, lymphatics, and the sympathetic chain. Underneath lies the crura of the diaphragm and attachments of the psoas major muscle.

The front of the vertebra is cleared by cautery to expose the anterior spine, including the involved body as well as disks above and below. If a paravertebral tumor is present, the correct level may be easily visualized. Otherwise, radiographic confirmation of the correct level should be obtained prior to the vertebrectomy. Initially, the segmental vessels coursing over the midsection of the vertebral body should be identified and clipped. All soft tissues are removed from the spine using rongeurs and cautery. Prior to the vertebrectomy, the disks above and below the level of involvement should be incised and removed with intervertebral disk rongeurs and curettes. The vertebral body is thus isolated.

The vertebrectomy is carried out with osteotomes, rongeurs, and specially designed curettes. If the vertebrectomy is carried out for palliation, the body is generally removed incompletely, leaving a shell of bone on the opposite side. For localized metastasis, and primary tumors, a more radical resection is required. All gross tumor down the dura must be removed, and this generally entails removal of the posterior longitudinal ligament. Brisk bleeding may be encountered during this procedure, which requires control with gentle tamponade and the bipolar current. Once tumor resection is complete, the cavity is packed with sponges while preparations for stabilization are made.

For acrylic fixation to be successful, the disks above and below the resected levels must be completely removed to provide as broad a base for the construct as possible. In our view, failure to provide a broad base of the cortical end plates above and below is a major technical reason for failure of fixation. The end plates should be left intact, without exposing the cancellous bone underneath. A second reason for failure is deficient host bone, either from tumor involvement or the presence of osteoporosis. An osteoporotic bone can be recognized by the ease of penetration of the Steinmann pin as well as toggling when rocked manually.

Steinmann pins are selected from easily available sets, ranging in diameter from $\frac{5}{64}$ to $\frac{12}{64}$ in. Depending on the level, pin diameters of either $\frac{6}{64}$, $\frac{7}{64}$, or $\frac{8}{64}$ in. are chosen. They are cut to appropriate lengths, and this generally means that they must be of sufficient length to engage one vertebral length above and below the level resected. These pins may be smooth or threaded, and are driven in place in the center of the vertebral bodies. To prevent the pins from being driven obliquely, the ends are bent in the shape of a hockey

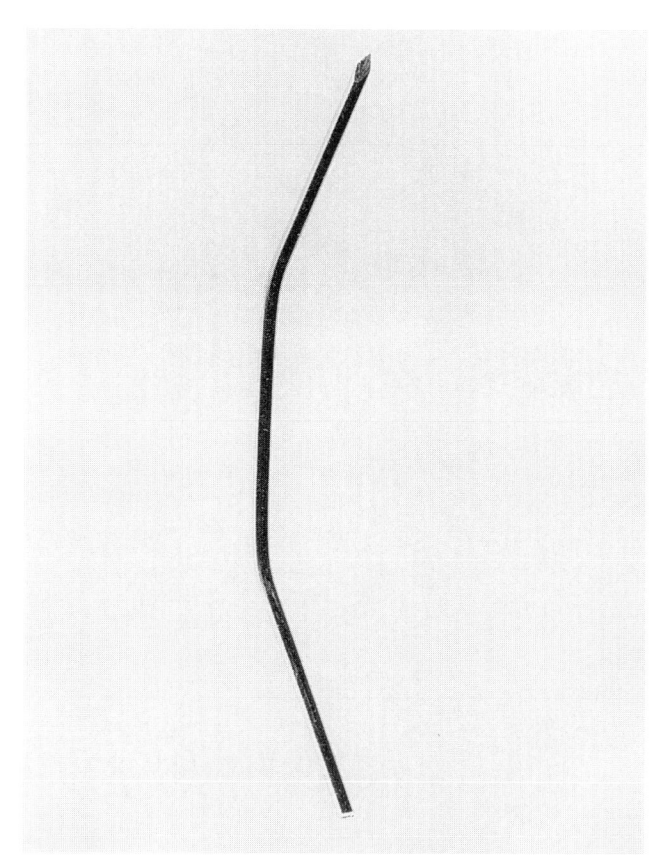

FIG. 23-4. Steinmann pin bent into hockey-stick configuration.

tion, copious saline irrigation is used to dissipate heat. Hemotasis is then checked for, but no attempt is made to pack the epidural space tightly or create a loculated space where blood or fluid may be trapped. Chest tubes are inserted, and the thoracotomy incision is closed in a routine fashion. This technique may be used for multiple levels (Fig. 23-9).

Postoperative care is generally that of a standard thoracotomy procedure. Since this fixation provides immediate stability, patients may be ambulated as soon as possible—within a day or two. Antibiotics and steroids are used routinely in the perioperative period. In patients who have not received prior therapy, postoperative irradiation may be commenced after the wound is healed. Postoperative bracing is not usually required, but a custom prosthesis may be used for patient comfort.

LONG-TERM RESULTS

The value of methylmethacrylate constructs in providing immediate stability, improvement of pain and improvement in

stick (Fig. 23-4). Two strong needle holders, generally those found in median sternotomy sets are used. The pins are driven initially through the upper body the entire distance and then brought back and driven in the reverse direction through the inferior body. We generally use two pins for the fixation. We have developed a special pin holder and pin driver available in the set previously described to enable the pin to be driven accurately (Figs. 23-3 and 23-5). If possible, the pin holes in the vertebral body should be predriven by right-angled drill bits using the Midas Rex or a Hall drill bit. An angled awl may also be used for this purpose.

Once the pins are in position, intraoperative radiography or fluoroscopy may be carried out to confirm their correct position. Proper pin positioning is important; if the exposure is inadequate, the pins may be directed too obliquely and enter the opposite side with the potential for visceral or vascular injury.

After introduction of the pins, methylmethacrylate is mixed, and while still semiliquid, is injected into the cavity with a 50-ml Toumy syringe (Fig. 23-6). The dura is protected with Gelfoam, and the methylmethacrylate is molded away from the dura using Penfield dissectors. It is important to ensure that the cement completely encases the pins (Figs. 23-7 and 22-8). During the heat of polymeriza-

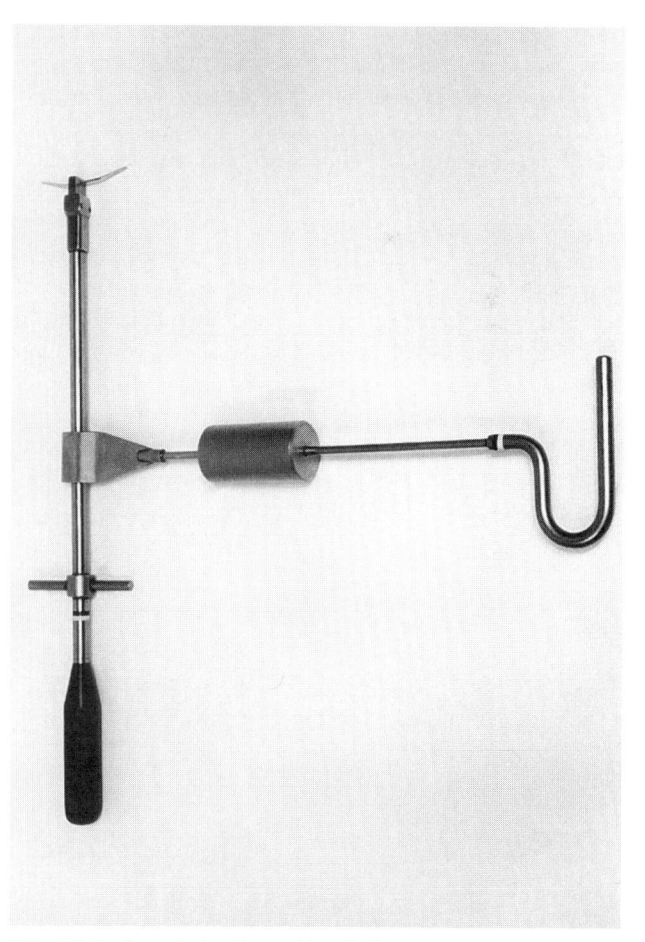

FIG. 23-5. Special pin driver with a Steinmann pin in the large pin holder. The cylindrical weight on the driver is pushed forcefully toward the handle. The resultant force is transmitted to the holder and the pin, thus driving the pin (in this illustration) to the right.

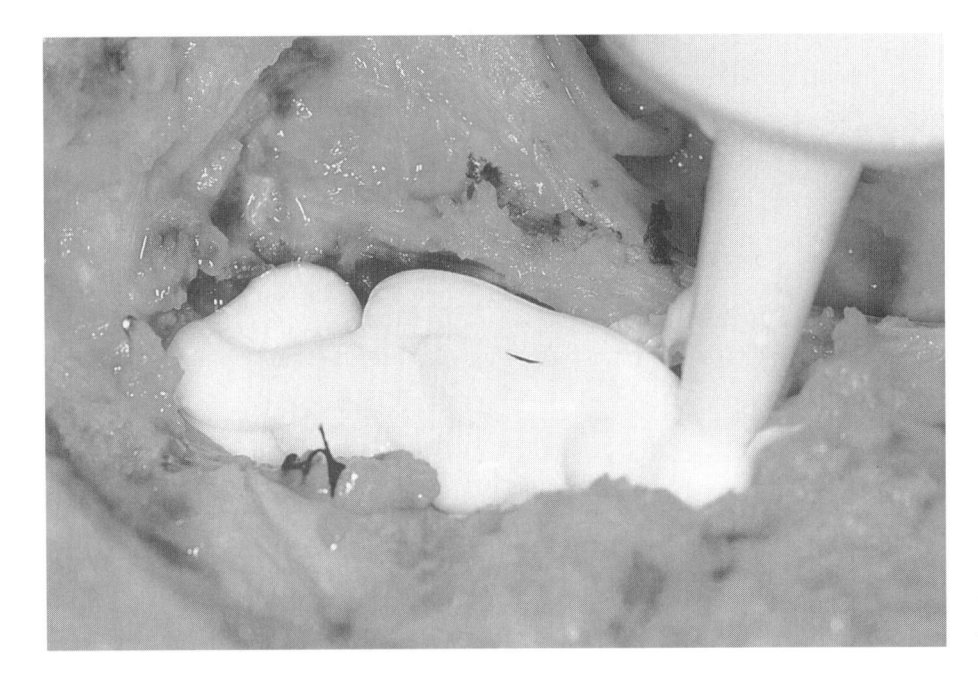

FIG. 23-6. Toumy syringe injecting liquid polymethylmethacrylate into vertebral space.

neurologic deficits is well established by several large series (Harrington, 1981; Lowquet et al., 1993; Sundaresan et al., 1985). Harrington (1988) reported a series of 77 patients who underwent 92 operations for the management of spinal instability and cord compression secondary to metastatic malignancy. Seventy-six patients underwent a one-stage anterior decompression, while five patients had a planned second-stage operation. To maintain spinal alignment, Harrington used a Knodt distraction rod ranging in lengths from 4 to 10 cm. The end plates of the intact vertebral bodies above and below the area of decompression were penetrated using a high-speed bur; this allowed engagement of the hooks. Once the space was distracted, additional decompression and removal of devitalized bone was performed. In addition to the methylmethacrylate reconstruction, additional anterior fusion with bone grafts was used. Excellent postoperative results were noted in 72 of 77 patients, with 5 patients not improving because of failure of fixation. These failures occurred early when Knodt rods were not used to supplement the methylmethacrylate; in two patients, weakness of the vertebra partially involved by tumor resulted in hook pullout. Late loss of stability resulted

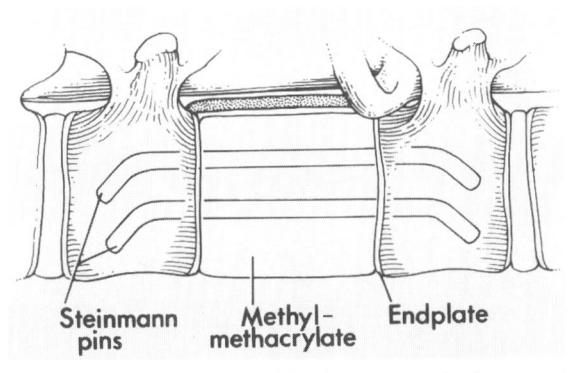

FIG. 23-7. The entire construct. The pins are completely encased by the PMMA. For protection, Gelfoam is placed on top of the dura.

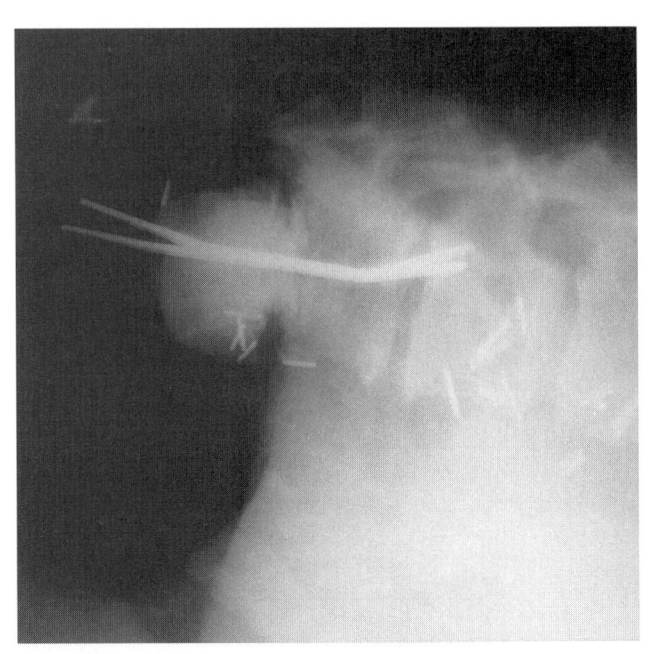

FIG. 23-8. Lateral radiograph of methylmethacrylate and Steinmann pins construct.

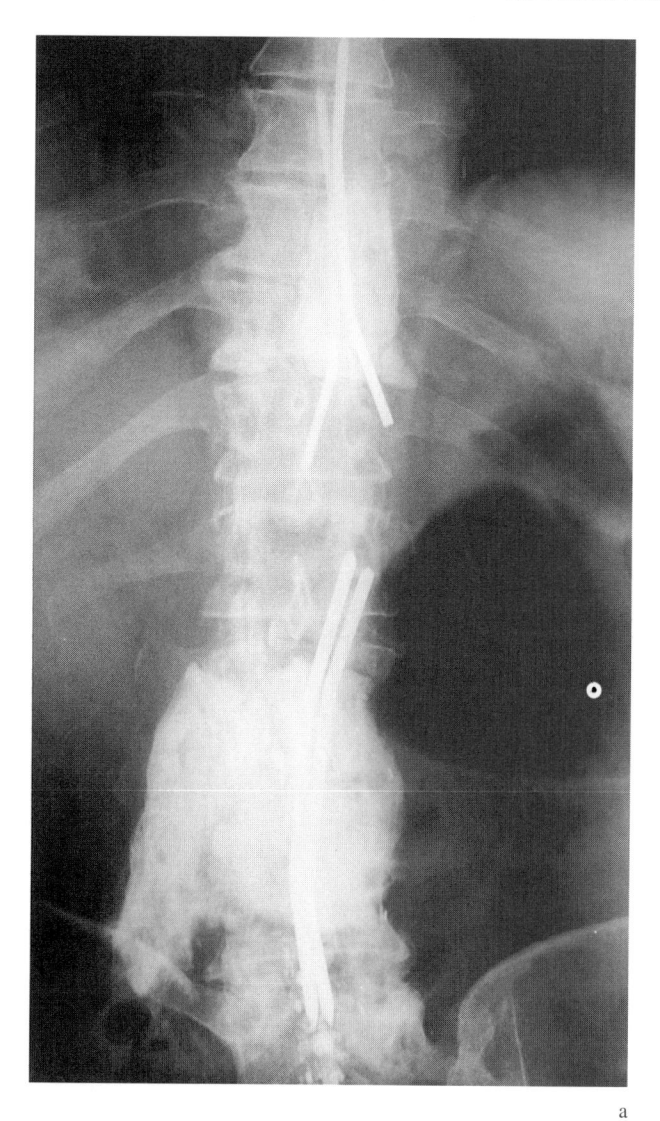

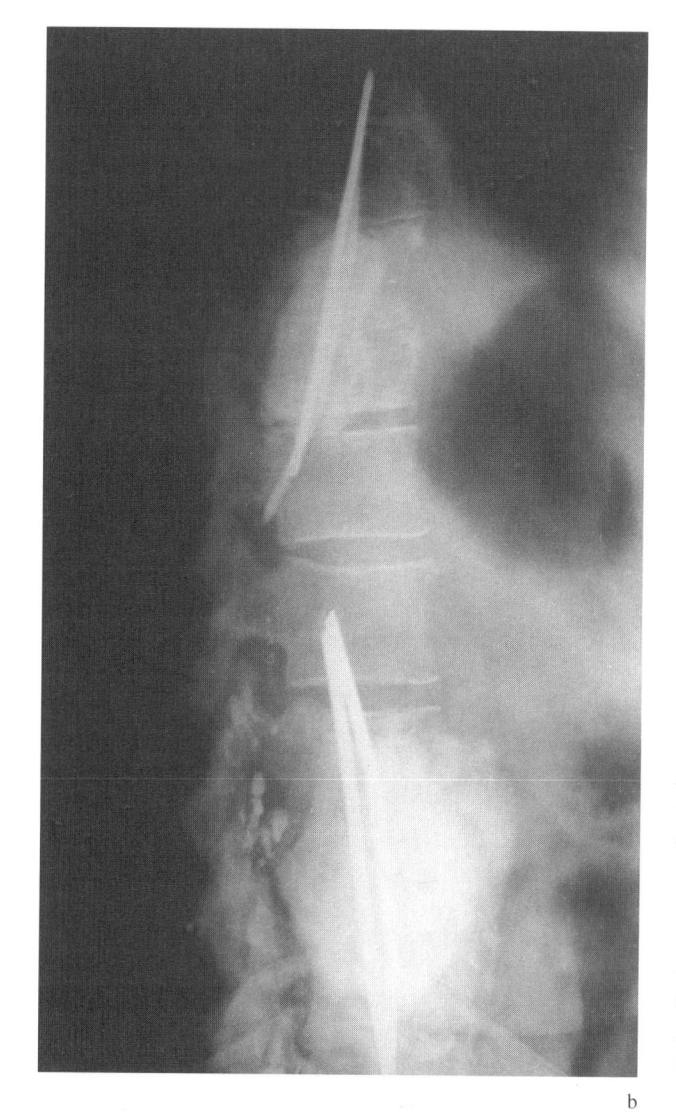

FIG. 23-9. Methylmethacrylate and Steinmann pins stabilization used at both thoracic and lumbar levels. (a) Anteroposterior view. (b) Lateral view.

frequently by the appearance of lytic metastases at other levels. Of the 62 patients with neurologic compromise preoperatively, 52 improved postoperatively. Postoperative radiography done on 10 patients alive at 1 year showed no evidence of motion.

Our experience (Sundaresan et al., 1985) on a larger series of 101 patients showed essentially the same results. More than 80% of patients reported excellent pain relief, while the postoperative ambulation rate was 78%. Of the 23 patients who had received no prior therapy, 90% continued to maintain their ambulatory status until death. A subsequent follow-up study on long-term survivors in a subset of 38 patients who had undergone methylmethacrylate fixation was conducted by retrospective and prospective assessment of long-term survivors (longer than 1 year) with patient interviews and standard flexion-extension x-ray studies (Harrington, 1988) (Fig. 23-10). Over a mean follow-up of 26.5 months, no late loss of stability from PMMA was noted; asymptomatic fracture of the Steinmann pins developed in 3 patients without clinical loss of stability (Fig. 23-11).

The major cause of ongoing pain was tumor recurrence in the adjacent segments. It should be mentioned that postoperative follow-up is greatly facilitated because of the relative lack of artifact in the construct as compared with other instrumentation techniques (Fig. 23-12). The clarity of imaging allows for earlier detection of recurrence. In 8 patients, reoperations were performed to remove recurrent tumor. In all these patients the interface between the host bone and acrylic was removed as a block for histologic study. In all cases, the methylmethacrylate was surrounded by a well-formed pseudocapsule (Fig. 23-13); the interface was

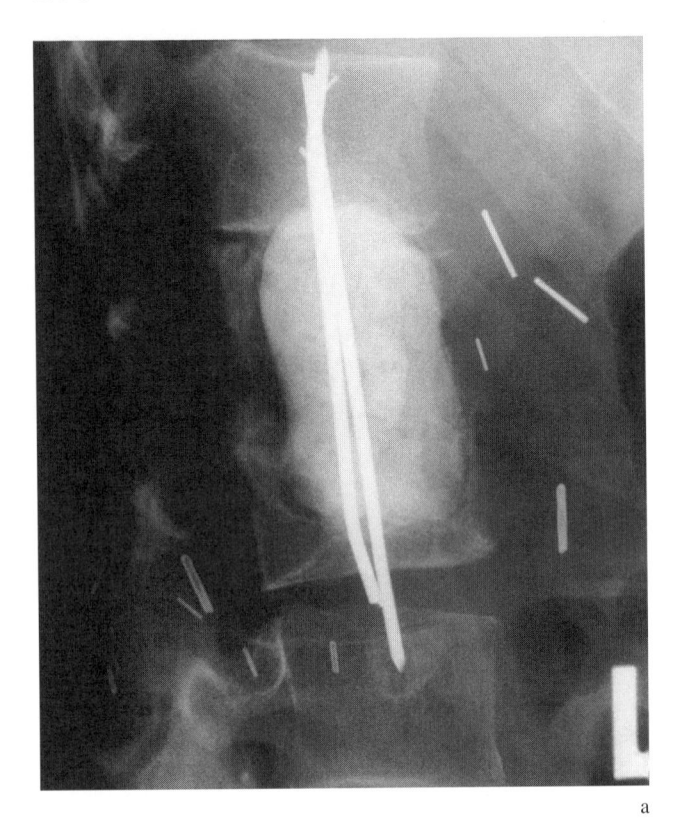

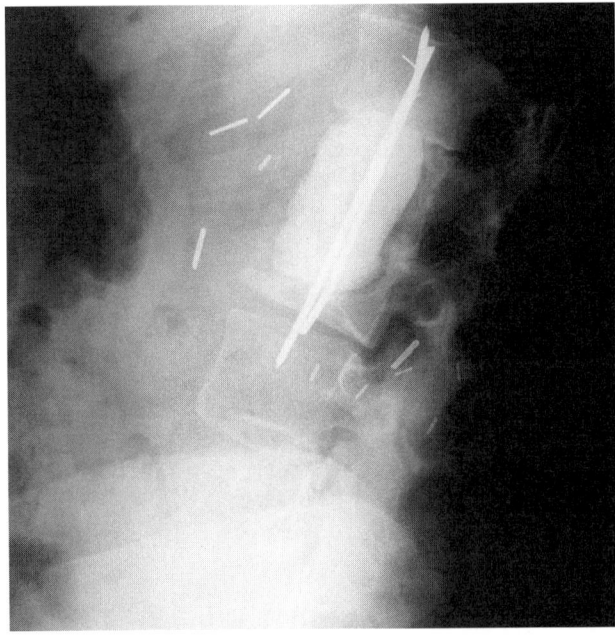

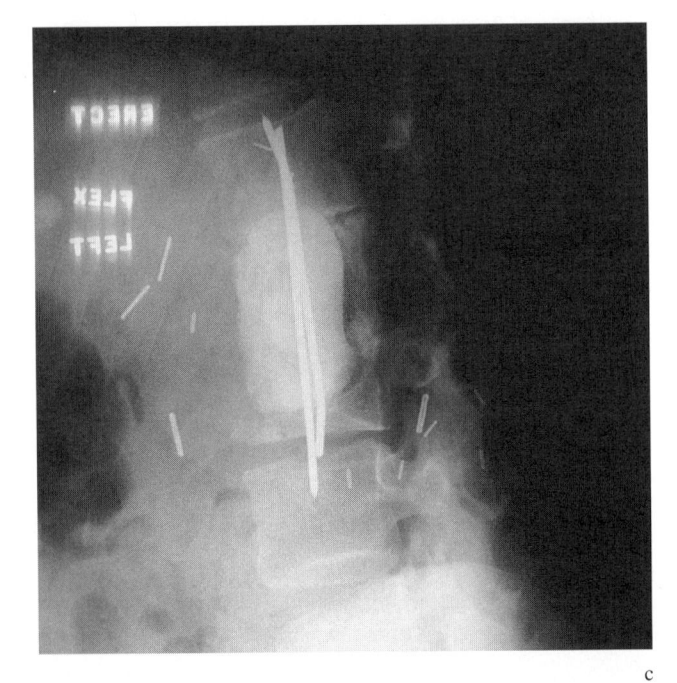

FIG. 23-10. Patient with methylmethacrylate and Steinmann pins construct more than 5 years after stabilization procedure. Radiographs show no instability or collapse. (a) Neutral. (b) Flexion. (c) Extension.

CHAPTER 23 / METHYLMETHACRYLATE AND STEINMANN PIN STABILIZATION   245

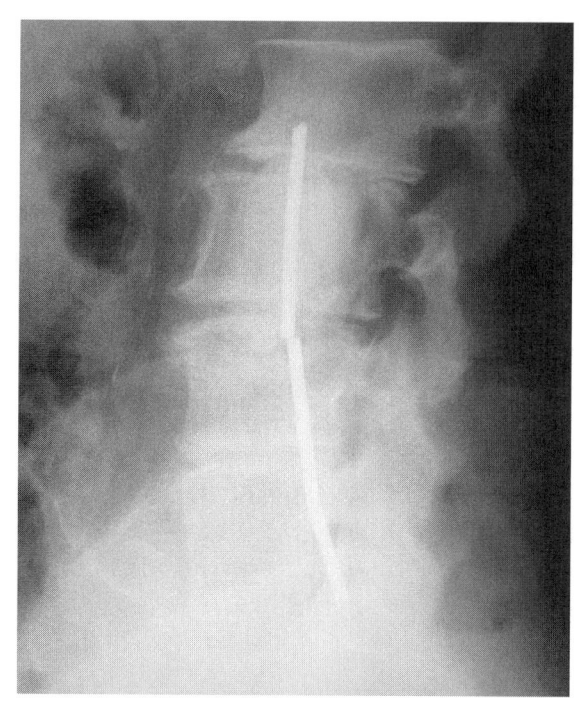

FIG. 23-11. Patient with asymptomatic broken Steinmann pin. The construct itself is intact and has remained stable.

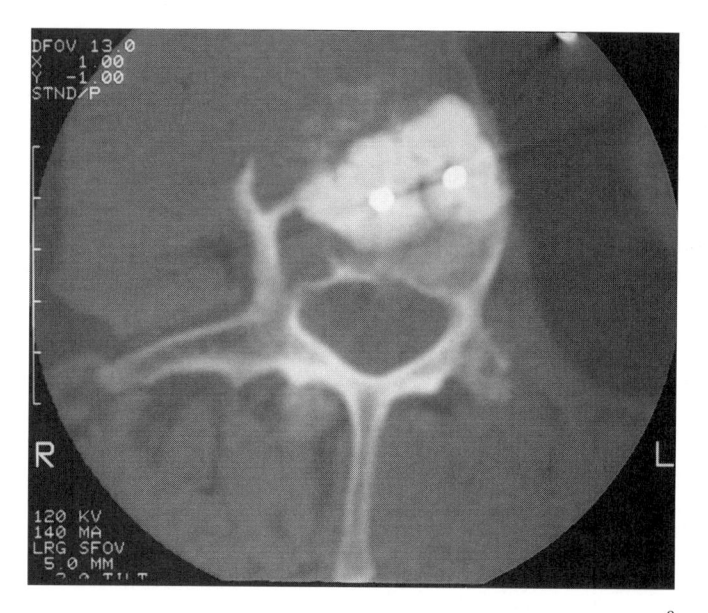

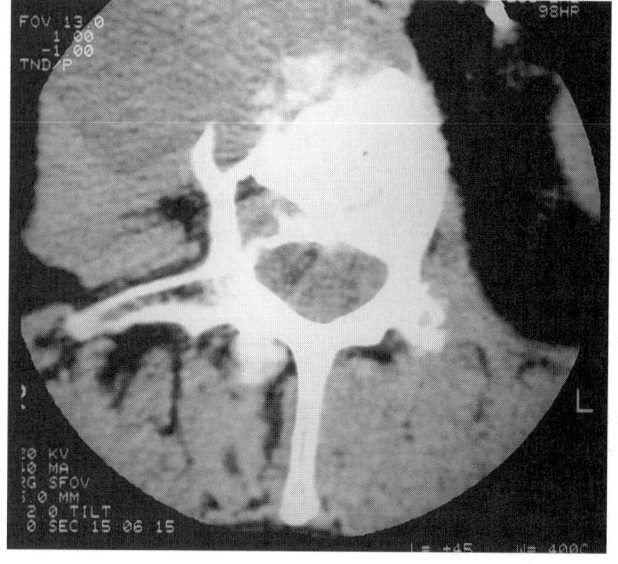

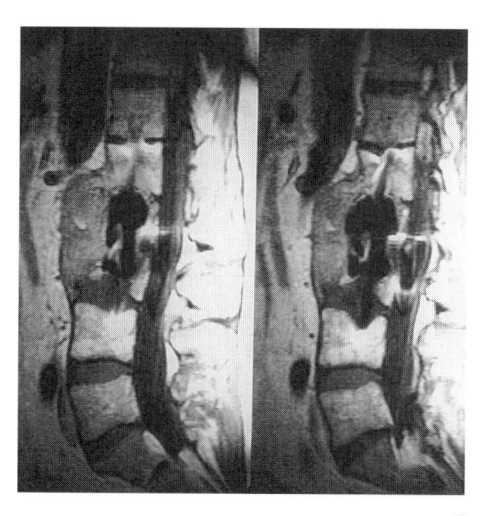

FIG. 23-12. Same patient as in Fig. 23-10. The methylmethacrylate and Steinmann pins technique provides almost an artifact-free image on both CT and MRI. (a) CT bone window. (b) CT soft-tissue window. (c) MRI, T_1-weighted. (d) MRI, T_2-weighted.

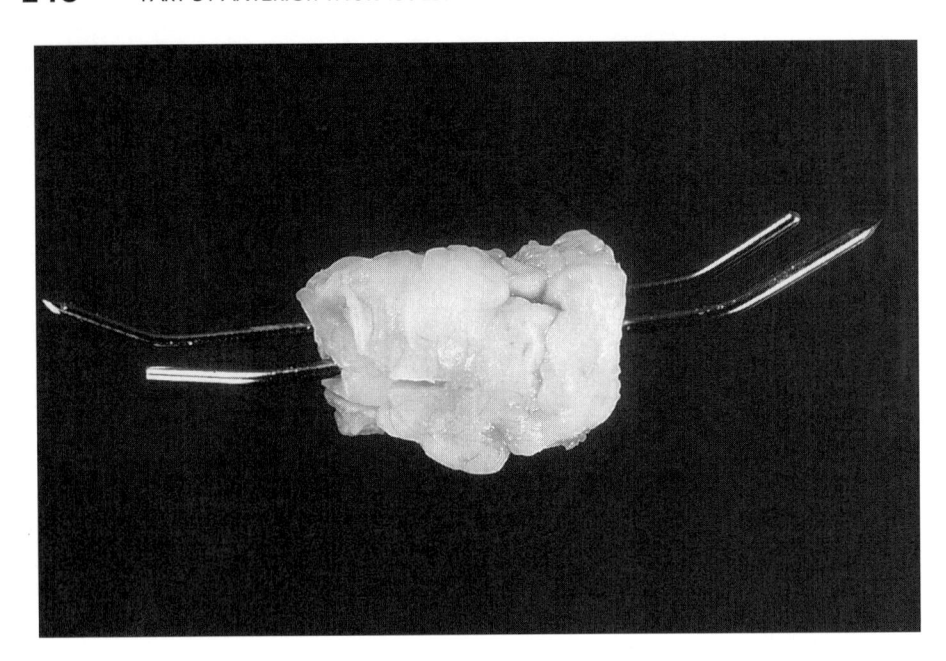

FIG. 23-13. Construct with pseudocapsule formation removed from a patient during reoperation. The construct was found intraoperatively to be stable and intact.

commonly a fibrous membrane with sparse cellularity. Giant cells and macrophages and the formation of a synovial membrane was not seen. These findings are quite different from the histologic findings noted at the interface of cemented arthroplasties (Jasty et al., 1991). For these reasons, we believe that methylmethacrylate constructs are the procedure of choice in the cancer patient regardless of expected longevity.

CONCLUSION

The published experience in long-term stability of methylmethacrylate constructs in the spine for a variety of other benign conditions differs considerably from the experience of McAfee, Bohlman, Ducher, and Eismont (1986) who analyzed 24 selected cases of failures of their cement fixations. Their sweeping recommendations and criticisms of methylmethacrylate constructs are suspect since they based their observations on these failed cases, many of which might well have been the result of poor technique or wrong indications. In a rebuttal, Branch and Kelly (1987) pointed out that their experience in 163 patients with methylmethacrylate fixation, mostly for benign disease, yielded a 96% satisfactory stabilization of the spine. Similar results were noted by Duff et al. (1992). In our experience with this technique in over 200 cases, less than a 5% failure rate was noted; most of these failures were early. We believe that correct patient selection and good surgical technique are as essential in this procedure as in all other cases of spinal instrumentation.

Steinmann pins and acrylic have been used by us for anterior fixation after vertebrectomy in spinal tumors. The appeal of such a construct is its simplicity and ease of application. Methylmethacrylate provides instantaneous fixation and strength when combined with Steinmann pins. In our series, it does not appear to degenerate as do hip replacements and posterior fusions, and it provides permanent fixation and stabilization. Unlike bone grafting, its stability is unaffected by radiotherapy. In the event of recurrence, the construct is relatively easy to remove. These characteristics make it an ideal construct for anterior stabilization in the thoracolumbar spine, especially in the patient with spinal neoplasms who is expected to undergo adjunctive therapy postoperatively or may suffer a recurrence. It is an invaluable technique for any spinal surgeon who must deal with both primary and metastatic disease

ACKNOWLEDGMENT

The authors would like to thank Sofomor–Danek, Memphis, Tennessee for funding a portion of this study by a research grant.

REFERENCES

Branch, C.L., Jr., & Kelly, D.L. (1987). Failure of stabilization of the spine with methylmethacrylate. A retrospective analysis of twenty-four cases [letter]. *Journal of Bone and Joint Surgery, American Volume, 69,* 1108–1110.

Brien, W., Salvati, E.N., Klein, R., Brause, B., & Stern, S. (1993). Antibiotic impregnated bone cement in total hip arthoplasty: An in vivo comparison of the elution properties of tobramycin and vancomycin. *Clinical Orthopaedics and Related Research, 296,* 242–248.

Chadduck, W.M., & Boop, W.C., Jr. (1983). Acrylic stabilization of the cervical spine for neoplastic disease: Evolution of a technique for vertebral body replacement. *Neurosurgery, 13,* 23–29.

Charnley, J. (1970). *Acrylic Cement in Orthopedic Surgery.* Baltimore: William & Wilkins.

Charnley, J. (1961). Arthroplasty of the hip: A new operation. *Lancet, 1,* 1129–1132.

Coe, M.R.K., Fechner, R.E., Jeffers, J.J., et al. (1989). Characterization of tissue from the bone-polymethyl methacrylate interface in a rat experimental mode. *Journal of Bone and Joint Surgery, American Volume, 71,* 863–874.

Cortet, B., Cotten, A., Deprez, X., et al. (1994). Value of vertebroplasty combined with surgical decompression in the treatment of aggressive spinal angioma. *Revue du Rhumatisme. Edition Francaise, 61,* 16–22.

Dahl, O.E., Garvik, L.J., & Lyberg, T. (1994). Toxic effects of methyl methacrylate momomer on leukocytes and endothelial cells in vitro. *Acta Orthopaedica Scandinavica, 65,* 147–153.

Dietze, D.D., Jr., & Haid, R.W., Jr. (1992). Antibiotic impregnated methyl methacrylate in the treatment of infections with spinal instrumentation: Case report. *Spine, 17,* 981–982.

Duff, T.A., Khan, A., & Corbett, J.E. (1992). Surgical stabilization of cervical spinal fractures using methyl methacrylate: Technical considerations and long term results in 52 patients. *Journal of Neurosurgery, 76,* 440–443.

Dunn, E.J. (1977). The role of methyl methacrylate in stabilization and replacement of the cervical spine. *Spine, 2,* 15–24.

Errico, T.J., & Cooper, P.R. (1993). A new method of thoracic and lumbar body replacement for spinal tumors. *Neurosurgery, 32,* 678–680.

Fathie, K. (1994). Anterior cervical diskectomy and fusion with methyl methacrylate. *Mount Sinai Journal of Medicine, 61,* 217–221.

Gangi, A., Kastler, B.A., & Dietermann, J.L. (1994). Percutaneous vertebroplasty guided by a combination of CT and fluoroscopy. *American Journal of Neuroradiology, 15,* 83–86.

Garvin, K.L., Evans, B.G., Salvati, E.A., & Brause, B.O. (1994). Palacos Gentamicin for the treatment of deep periprosthetic hip infections. *Clinical Orthopaedics and Related Research, 298,* 97–115.

Goldring, S.R., Jasty, M., Roelke, M.S., et al. (1986). Formation of a synovial-like membrane at the bone-cement interface. *Arthritis and Rheumatism, 29,* 836–842.

Hansen, D., & Jensen, J.S. (1992). Mixing does not improve mechanical properties of all bone cements: Manual and centrifugation-vacuum mixing compared for 10 cement brands. *Acta Orthopaedica Scandinavica, 63,* 13–18.

Harland, R.W., Sharma, M., & Rosenzweig, D.Y. (1993). Lung carcinoma in a patient with Lucite sphere plombage thoracoplasty. *Chest, 103,* 1295–1297.

Harrington, K.D. (1988). Anterior decompression and stabilization of the spine as a treatment for vertebral collapse and spinal cord compression from metastatic malignancy. *Clinical Orthopaedics and Related Research, 233,* 177–197.

Harrington, K.O. (1981). The use of methyl methacrylate for vertebral body replacement and anterior stabilization of pathological fracture dislocations of the spine due to metastatic malignant disease. *Journal of Bone and Joint Surgery, American Volume, 63,* 36–46.

Harris, W.H., & Sledge, C.B. (1990). Total hip and total knee replacement. *New England Journal of Medicine, 323,* 725–732.

Harris, W.B., Schiller, A.L., Scholler, J.M., et al. (1976). Extensive localized bone resorption in the femur following total hip replacement. *Journal of Bone and Joint Surgery, American Volume, 58,* 612–618.

Jasty, M., Maloney, W.J., Bragdon, C.R., & O'Connor, D. (1991). The initiation of failure in cemented femoral components of hip arthoplaties. *Journal of Bone and Joint Surgery, British Volume, 73,* 551–558.

Knight, G. (1959). Paraspinal acrylic inlays in the treatment of cervical and lumbar spondylosis and other conditions. *Lancet, 2,* 147–149.

Ko, K., & Sundaresan, N. (November, 1991). The long term stability of methyl methacrylate constructs in cancer patients: A follow-up study. Presented to the American Association of Neurological Surgeons, San Francisco, CA.

Krieg, J.C., Clark, C.R., & Goetz, D.D. (1993). Cervical spine arthrodesis in rheumatoid arthritis: A long term follow up. *Yale Journal of Biology and Medicine, 66,* 257–262.

Lowquet, E., Thibaut, R., Thibaut, H., & Hendricks, M. (1993). Surgical treatment of spinal metastases. *Acta Orthopaedica Belgica, 59,* 79–82.

McAfee, P.C., Bohlman, H.H., Ducher, T., & Eismont, F.J. (1986). Failure of stabilization of the spine with methyl methacrylate: A retrospective analysis of 24 cases. *Journal of Bone and Joint Surgery, American Volume, 68,* 1145–1157.

Norman, T.L., Kish, V., Blaha, J.D., Gruen, T.A., & Hustosky, K. (1995). Creep characteristics of hand and vacuum mixed acrylic bone cement at elevated stress levels. *Journal of Biomedical Materials Research, 29,* 495–501.

Park, H.C., Liu, Y.K., & Lakes, R.S. (1986). The material properties of bone-particle impregnated PMMA. *Journal of Biomedical Engineering, 108,* 141–148.

Pinto, P.W. (1993). Cardiovascular collapse associated with the use of methylmethacrylate. *American Association of Nurse Anesthetists Journal, 61,* 603–616.

Robinson, R.P., Wright, T.M., & Burstein, A.H. (1981). Mechanical properties of polymethyl methacrylate bone cement. *Journal of Biomedical Materials Research, 15,* 203–208.

Scoville, W.B., Palmer, A.H., Samra, K., et al. (1967). The use of acrylic plastic for vertebral replacement or fixation in metastatic disease of the spine. *Journal of Neurosurgery, 27,* 274–279.

Sharova, T.G., Fedotova, I.V., Dorofeeva, E.D., & Blagodatin, V.M. (1993). Development, course and late sequelae in workers engaged in organic glass production. *Meditsina Truda I Promyshlennaia Ekologiia, 9–10,* 8–10.

Siegal, T., Tiqua, P., & Siegal, T. (1985). Vertebral body resection for epidural compression in malignant tumors. *Journal of Bone and Joint Surgery, American Volume, 67,* 575–582.

Sturup, J., Nimb, L., Kramhoff, M., & Jensen, J.S. (1994). Effects of polymerization heat and monomers from acrylic cement on canine bone. *Acta Orthopaedica Scandinavica, 65,* 20–23.

Sundaresan, N., Galicich, J.H., Bains, M.S., et al. (1984). Vertebral body resection in the treatment of cancer involving the spine. *Cancer, 53,* 1393–1396.

Sundaresan, N., Galicich, J.H., Lane, J.M., et al. (1985). Treatment of neoplastic epidural cord compression by vertebral body resection and stabilization. *Journal of Neurosurgery, 63,* 676–684.

Topoleski, L.D.T., Ducheyne, P., & Cuckler, J.M. (1995). The effects of centrifugation and titanium fiber reinforcement on fatigue failure mechanisms in polymethylmethacrylate bone cement. *Journal of Biomedical Materials Research, 29,* 299–302.

Townsend, P.W., Rosenthal, H.G., Smalley, S.R., Cozad, S.C., & Hassanein, R.E. (1994). Impact of post-operative radiation therapy and other perioperative factors on outcome after orthopedic stabilization of impending or pathologic fractures due to metastatic disease. *Journal of Clinical Oncology, 12,* 2345–2350.

Wade Waters, I.W., Baran, K.P., Schlosser, M.J., Mack, J.E., & Davis, W.M. (1992). Acute cardiovascular effects of methyl methacrylate monomer: Characterization and modification by cholinergic blockade, adrenergic stimulation and calcium chloride infusion. *General Pharmacology, 23,* 497–502.

Wasserlauf, S., Warshawsky, A., Arad-Yelin, R., Mazur, Y., Salama, R., & Deckel, S. (1993). The release of cytotoxic drugs from acrylic bone cement. *Bulletin/Hospital for Joint Diseases, 53,* 68–74.

Wesley, R.E., & Brinsko, J.D. (1992). Toxicity of methyl methacrylate monomer in orbital and cranial surgery. *Annals of Ophthalmology, 24,* 307–309.

Whitehill, R., Drucker, S., McCoig, J.A., et al. (1988). Induction and characterization of an interface tissue by implanatation of methyl methacrylate cement into the posterior part of the cervical spine of the dog. *Journal of Bone and Joint Surgery, American Volume, 70,* 51–59.

Whitehill, R., Reger, S.I., Fox, E., et al. (1984). The use of methylmethacrylate cement as an instantaneous fusion mass in posterior cervical fusions: A canine in vivo experimental model. *Spine, 9,* 246–252.

Whitehill, R., Stowers, S.F., Fechner, R.E., et al. (1987). Posterior cervical fusions using cerclage wires, methyl methacrylate cement and autogenous bone graft: An experimental study of a canine model. *Spine, 12,* 12–22.

PART 4

Posterior Thoracolumbar Instrumentation

CHAPTER 24

Application of Harrington Rods and the Harri-Luque System for Stabilization of the Thoracolumbar Spine

Brian G. Cuddy
Wade M. Mueller

HIGHLIGHTS

After entering practice in Houston, Texas in the late 1940s, Dr. Paul R. Harrington assumed the care of children with progressive neuromuscular scoliosis resulting from polio. Faced with the problem of stopping the progression of the scoliotic curve, he developed a spinal instrumentation system, employing hooks and rods to achieve spinal fusion and correction of spinal deformities (Harrington, 1988). No bone grafting or fusion techniques were used with his early instrumentation systems, and this led to a high rate of failure with recurrence of the deformity. The development of new instrument design with greater durability, along with the understanding of the need to achieve a solid bone fusion, increased the rate of successful outcomes. It was not until 1958 that Harrington first used posterior instrumentation and fusion for stabilization of a fracture dislocation of the spine (Cotler, Vernance, & Michalski, 1986).

Dr. Harrington introduced his hook and rod system for general use in the early 1960s, and widespread use soon began (Harrington, 1960) (Fig. 24-1). The modern Harrington rod system has undergone numerous modifications over the past 35 years and is frequently used as a comparison when reviewing the design of newer universal spinal instrumentation equipment.

Harrington spinal instrumentation is a system of stainless steel rods and hooks designed to purchase on the posterior elements of the axial skeleton from the first thoracic vertebra to the sacrum. The system is composed of two principle elements: (1) the distraction rod, which is adjusted by the ratchet principle, and (2) the compression rod, which is adjusted by the threaded-rod/and nut principle. It is manufactured by Zimmer, Inc. (Warsaw, IN).

MODIFICATIONS OF THE HARRINGTON SYSTEM

One major modification to improve stability was by Dr. John Moe who designed a square distal hook and a square-ended rod. This change in the system was to increase rotational control with a square peg in a square hole (Fig. 24-2 *a* and *d*) (Denis, Ruiz, & Searles, 1984).

Dr. Charles C. Edwards of Baltimore has made several modifications, including hook design and a rod sleeve system. The Edwards' spinal rod sleeves were designed to fill the potential space between the distraction rods and the anatomic position of the posterior elements. Placement of polyethylene radiopaque sleeves around the rod allow broad surface contact with the posterior element bone, providing an additional loading point when correcting angular deformities (Edwards & Levine, 1986).

Edwards' anatomic hooks were designed with a longer shoe for more secure fixation in the sublaminar position. The shape conforms to the lamina for broad contact surface in the sagittal plane. This design modification is to protect against hook dislodgment by facilitating full-hook seating.

The Edwards sacral fixation device provides fixation directly to the sacrum (Edwards, 1986). The sacral fixation device provides direct fixation by a sacral screw into the thickest portion of the sacrum away from the spinal canal. The screw housing is designed to articulate with a Harrington rod hook providing linkage that accommodates the variation in the lumbosacral angle.

The Harrington compression system was designed to facilitate the application of spinal compression instrumentation. While Harrington distraction rods are efficient in correcting deformity, the compression rods have the ability

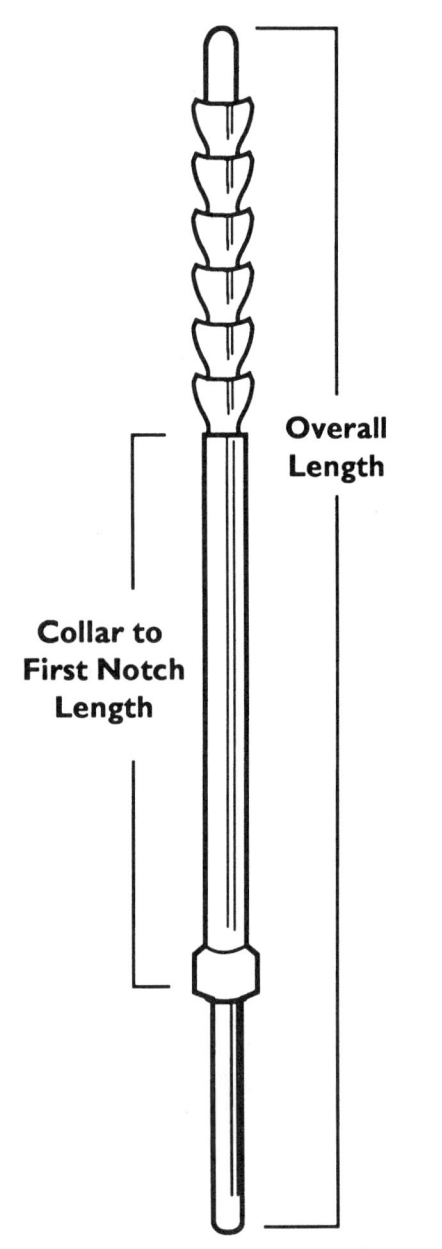

FIG. 24-1. Harrington distraction rods: collar to first notch length (1.2–48.3 cm); overall length (6.1–53.4 cm).

An additional technique has also been used with the Harrington system—the addition of sublaminar wiring or the so-called Harri-Luque technique, referring to the traditional Luque instrumentation with sublaminar wires. This technique combines the Harrington distraction rods with segmental wiring to achieve multiple points of fixation to the spinal column (Fig. 24-3) (Winter, Lonstein, Vanderbrinkik, et al., 1987). The mechanical advantage of this hybrid system has been shown in the laboratory. Wenger, Carollo, Wilkerson, and colleagues (1982) demonstrated the addition of segmental fixation to the Harrington rod system doubled the axial compressive loading to failure in a calf spine model.

IMPLEMENTATION AND USE

Indications for Use

Originally, the Harrington system was indicated in the treatment of idiopathic scoliosis and has been quite safe when used for that application (Renshaw, 1988) (Table 24-1). The Harrington system has several disadvantages including limited derotating ability and loss of lumbar lordosis when using the distraction system in the low lumbar spine (Swank, Mauri, & Brown, 1990) (Table 24-2). As newer universal systems have become available, the Harrington instrumentation system has become less attractive for patients with scoliotic deformity requiring complex reconstructive procedures. Thus, the use is now limited more to single thoracic and thoracolumbar curves that do not require low lumbar fusions.

Harrington constructs continue to be used in the treatment of traumatic disorders. Use of dual distraction fixation in the presence of an intact anterior longitudinal ligament can offer good stability. This application is most useful in injuries with axial displacement or when resistance to axial

to provide stability by means of impaction (Gaines & Leatherman, 1981). The assembly uses multiple hooks that can be placed on a threaded rod, which is smaller than the distraction rod. The Harrington distraction rod was found to be 4.7 times as stiff as the compression rod of the same length (White, Panjabi, & Thomas, 1977). At T11 or above, the hook can be positioned over the transverse process. From T11 caudally, the hook can be placed underneath the lamina as close to the facet joint as can be directed. When using the system for deformity work, three hooks are placed caudad above the apex of the convex side of the curve and three hooks below in a cephalad direction. The compression is formed by tightening the nuts of each hook on the threaded rod, causing the instrumentation to deliver a compressive load.

Table 24-1
Indications and Contraindications for the Use of Harrington Rods

Indications
    Effective distraction of the vertebral column.
    Can restore vertebral height in burst fractures caused by axial loads, provided the posterior longitudinal ligament is intact.
    Most useful where correction of axial displacement or resistance to axial loading is required.
    Relatively easy to apply and to remove.

Contraindications
    If posterior longitudinal ligament has been disrupted, distraction may produce pathologic tension in the spinal cord.
    Very rigid system. Consequently, hook dislocation may occur because of large forces at upper and lower points of fixation.
    Using the rods to correct fractures produced by flexion and compression may cause compression of the spinal cord if the canal has not been surgically remodeled prior to distraction.
    If the anterior longitudinal ligament has been disrupted, rods should not be used, since overdistraction may occur.
    If fusion to the low lumbar spine and lumbosacral junction is required, alternative fixation devices should also be considered.

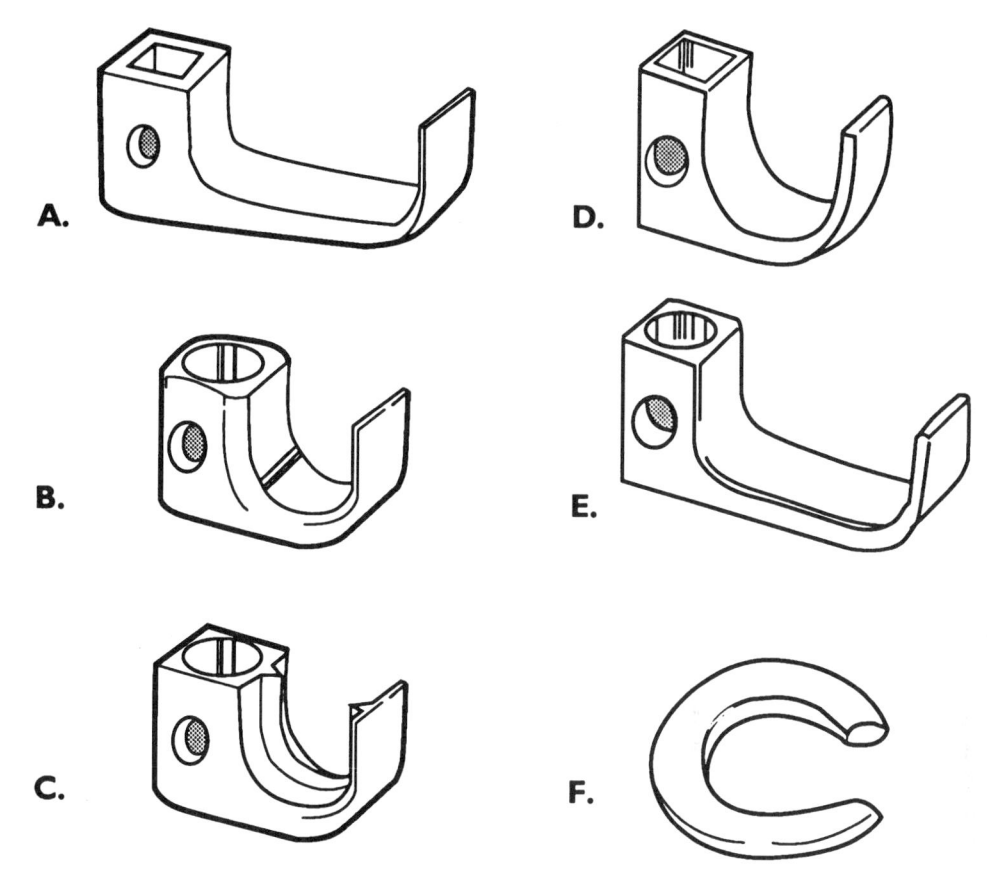

FIG. 24-2. Harrington distraction instrumentation hook selection. (a) Moe square-hole sacro-alar hook. (b) Distraction hook blunt. (c) Distraction hook blunt, ribbed. (d) Moe square-ended hook. (e) Alar hook. (f) C-washer.

loading is required. A combination of effective distraction of the vertebral column and the relatively easy application of the system have been major factors for its use in traumatic injuries.

Although the Harrington distraction system does not prevent axial rotation as well as other systems do, it increases axial torsional stiffness to 150% of normal (White & Panjabi, 1990). Thus because of its relative stiffness the system can be an effective method of correcting posttraumatic kyphotic deformity.

There are several disadvantages to the Harrington system that have made newer universal systems more attractive in the treatment of patients with trauma. The forces of the system are applied directly to the two ends of the construct. The distraction forces are applied maximally and are maintained by a rod-rochet mechanism. The forces are applied in small increments and are limited by the strength of the bony structure in which the hook is attached. The typical limiting factor is the lamina of the thoracic vertebrae, which may fail if the distraction rod has concentrated too great a force in the upper lamina.

The need must be stressed to remodel the spinal canal surgically and to remove any bone fragments causing thecal-sac compression. The use of the distraction rods to cover a fracture site, produced by flexion and compression, may cause compression of the spinal cord if the canal has not been surgically remodeled prior to distraction. Translational injury with anterior longitudinal ligament involvement does not allow the system to be used because of the risk of neurologic injury with distraction. In addition, if the posterior longitudinal ligament has been completely disrupted, distraction can place pathologic tension on the spinal cord.

Table 24-2
Advantages and Disadvantages of the Use of Harrington Rods

Advantages
  Wide familiarity
  Easy application
  Provides good stabilization for axial loads

Disadvantages
  Limited derotating ability
  Flat-back syndrome
  Limited usefulness in translational injuries
  Uses only hooks
  Forces applied directly to two ends of system, sometimes on weak thoracic laminae

Techniques and Placement

Standard Application/Fixation

Harrington distraction rods have a diameter of 0.25 in. (6.4 mm) and range in overall length from 6.1 to 53.4 cm

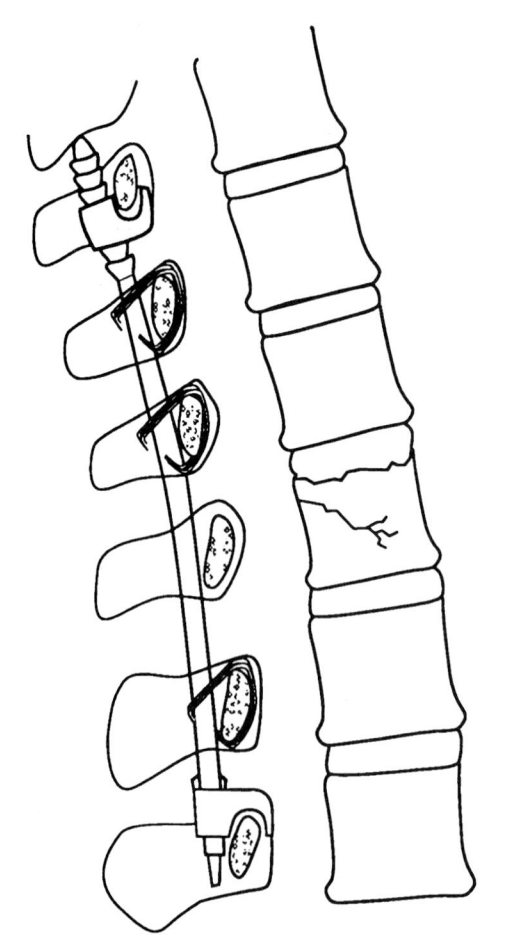

FIG. 24-3. Thoracolumbar fracture with application of Harrington distraction rods with sublaminar wiring. Note three-lamina-above/two-lamina-below construct.

(see Fig. 24-1). The superior end has seven ratchets. The inferior end can be either round or square. The square-end distraction rods and hooks are part of the Moe spinal instrumentation set. For the upper end of the rod, sharp hooks are available to prepare the facet joint purchase site with minimal trauma. These are then replaced with a blunt hook with a triangular rib, to provide added stability, by preventing lateral rotation and drift (see Fig. 24-2, c). Narrow laminar hooks are available for the inferior end. Edwards has a hook design that can also be used; it conforms to the lamina that helps prevent hook dislodgment.

The upper hooks are placed within the facet joint. The curved inferior edge of the facet is removed with a 0.25-inch osteotome, using a slightly oblique cut to prevent the hook from slipping laterally (Fig. 24-4). The sharp hook is grasped in a hook clamp and implanted into a joint with a hook driver. The lower hook is placed beneath the leading edge of a lumbar lamina. (Laminar hooks are not recommended for use in the thoracic region because the relatively wide gap of the hook could permit migration of the hook into the spinal canal). The ligamentum flavum, medial portion of the facet joint, and superior edge of the lamina are removed. Care must be taken not to remove too much of the lamina on which the hook is to be seated as this may cause subsequent weakening of the lamina and failure of the construct.

The hook is grasped with the hook holder, placed beneath the lamina, and held in position if adequately seated. After placement of both superior and inferior hooks the hooks should be inspected to avoid false passage between cortices of the lamina or facets.

The sharp hook is removed from the facet joint and replaced with the blunt upper hook (see Fig. 24-2, b). The rods are contoured in the standard fashion to maintain lordosis at the thoracolumbar junction or kyphosis in the thoracic region. The ratchet end of the rod is passed through the hole in the upper hook until the butt end of the rod is just superior to the lower hook. The rod is withdrawn through the upper hook until the butt end is seated within the hole in the lower hook. The jaws of the Harrington spreader have gaps of slightly dissimilar widths. The jaw with the wider gap is placed against the upper hook and the jaw with the narrower gap against the ratchet. The spreader is then used to push the upper hook toward the superior end of the rod. After distraction has been completed, a C-washer is placed around the rod just below the hook and pinched down with a C-washer clincher to maintain distraction (see Fig. 24-2, f).

This is then repeated for the opposite side. To remove a rod, the jaw with the wider gap is placed against the upper end of the hook, and the narrower end against a more superior ratchet. Spreading the jaws pushes the hook caudally down the rod. This is facilitated by toggling the hook with a hook clamp.

If it is necessary to include the sacrum, laminar fixation is inadvisable, since the sacral lamina is usually not strong enough to take the load, and combination of a thin sacral lamina and narrowed spinal canal increases the possibility of the hooks' injuring the sacral roots. For sacral fixation, alar hooks are used instead of the laminar hook (see Fig. 24-2, e). Also available are the Edwards sacral fixation device, in which a sacral screw is placed in the thickest portion of the sacrum. The screw housing articulates with the hook, providing a linkage that accommodates variations in the lumbosacral angle.

Harri-Luque Technique

The Harri-Luque technique includes passage of sublaminar wires for additional construct stability (see Fig. 24-4). The technique for sublaminar wire passage is described in Chapter 25 on the Luque instrumentation section. Several rod linkage systems are also available to connect the two rods together to share the construct loading forces.

Complications

Instrument failure can occur when the rod breaks or the hooks dislocate. As with all spinal instrumentation procedures the fault may not be with the system but with the preoperative planning and technical errors in its use (McAfee & Bohlman, 1985). An important consideration is the number of levels to instrument so as to decrease the construct failure rate and to lower the number of normal levels above and below the injured site to be included in the construct. In biomechanical studies Purcell, Markoff, and Dawson (1981) showed that hook pullout from the lamina could be prevented by implanting the Harrington hook three levels above the defect and two levels below it. This study and additional biomechanical work provided the basis for the clinical recommendation to span two normal lamina and to place the hook under the third (lamina or pedicle) (Jacobs, Nordwall, & Nachemson, 1982). Below, it is advised to span one normal lamina and place the hook under the second one. This surgical plan requires a larger fusion mass or risks probable irritation and degenerative changes because of immobilizing normal facet joints (Kamanovitz, Arnoczky, Levine, & Otis, 1984). Thus, the "rod-long, fuse-short" approach has certain liabilities. The use of pedicle screw instrumentation is an example of a construct that allows one to immobilize and fuse only one vertebrae above and below the defect and may prove a solution to this problem.

Experimental evaluation of Harrington rod fixation supplemented with sublaminar wire (Harri-Luque) demonstrates improved stabilization in the thoracolumbar fracture dislocations (McAfee, Werner, & Glisson, 1985). Segmental fixation, in addition to improving the stability of Harrington rods, allows improved correction in the sagittal plane with proper rod contouring. The major complication associated with this construct is the risk of neurologic defects following sublaminar passage (see Fig. 24-4). However, the incidence of neurologic injury has been reported to decrease with the surgeon's increasing experience (Turner, Mason, & Webb, 1986).

A well-described complication of the Harrington rod system is the loss of lumbar lordosis and the development of the flat-back syndrome. This occurs with the extension of instrumentation into the lower lumbar segments or sacrum and failure to contour the rods to the normal lordosis. Straight distraction rods inserted posteriorly force the spine into flexion and out of lordosis. This is characterized by the patient presenting with a forward inclination of the trunk with compensatory flexion at the knees and extension of the upper spine to preserve an upright posture. This can result in an awkward gait and is frequently associated with complaints of pain. Aaro and Ohlen (1983) have reported that complaints of pain and stiffness increase after fusion below L3 with Harrington rods. Because of these concerns, the general trend has been not to use the Harrington system in the lower lumbar spine and to consider alternative universal systems that include pedicular fixation.

As with all spinal instrumentation systems, careful surgical techniques and adherence to bone fusion principles to achieve a solid arthrodesis is critical. Erwin, Dickson, and

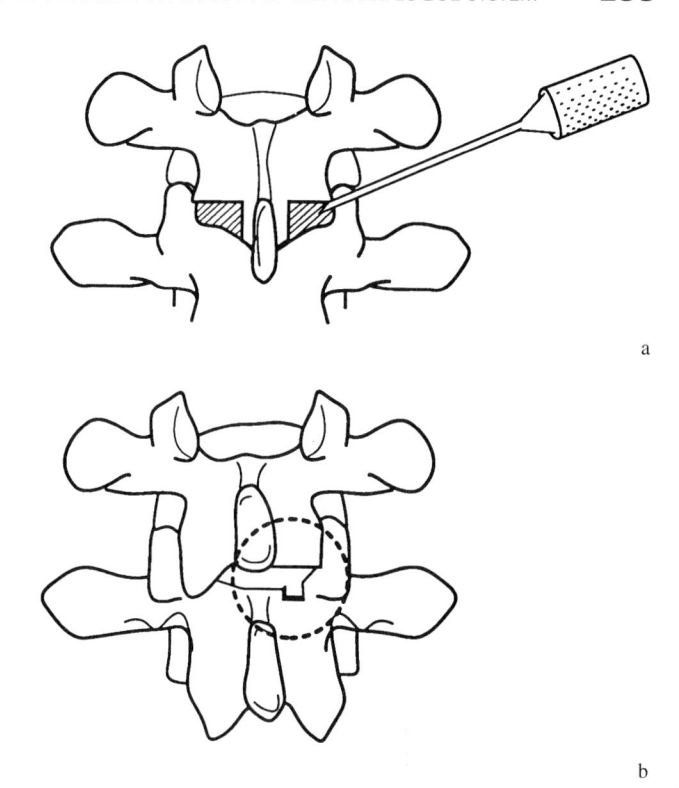

FIG. 24-4. (a) Upper hook placement within the facet joint; the curved inferior edge of the facet is removed with osteotome (cross-hatched area). (b) Lower hook placement beneath the leading edge of lumbar lamina. The ligamentum flavum and superior lamina is removed (square-edged removal).

Harrington (1980) in a review of over two thousand procedures found that the incidence of broken instrumentation was 12.5% in patients without fusion as compared with 2.5% in patients who did have a fusion.

SUMMARY

This chapter reviewed the use of the Harrington instrumentation system and its modifications in the use of spinal trauma and spinal deformity. The system is most useful in situations that destabilize the axial thoracolumbar region. The Harrington system has been shown to be useful in the treatment of idiopathic scoliosis. In the stabilization of the traumatic spine, distraction rods are indicated when the anterior longitudinal ligament is preserved, as in vertical compression fractures. The system is not recommended in translational injuries or in situations in which the spinal canal has not been remodeled after neural compression. There are numerous modifications to the original Harrington distraction rods, each designed to embrace a specific area of possible instrument failure.

Complications with the system tend to be related to improper indications and lack of meticulous fusion techniques. The concepts involved in the Harrington instrumentation system are what many recent universal instrumentation systems are built on.

Although the situations in which to use the Harrington system are fewer today, more recent instrumentation devices continue to be compared to it as a standard of clinical results to be achieved.

REFERENCES

Aaro, S., & Ohlen, G. (1983). The effect of Harrington instrumentation on the sagittal configuration and mobility of the spine in scoliosis. *Spine, 8*, 570–575.

Cotler, J.M., Vernance, J.V., & Michalski, J.A. (1986). The use of Harrington rods in thoracolumbar fractures. *Orthopedic Clinics of North America, 17*, 87–103.

Denis, F., Ruiz, H., & Searls, K. (1984). Comparison between square ended distraction rods and standard round ended distraction rods in the treatment of thoracolumbar spinal injuries. *Clinical Orthopedics, 189*, 162–167.

Edwards, C.C. & Levine, A.M. (1986). Early rod-sleeve stabilization of the injured thoracic and lumbar spine. *Orthopedic Clinics of North America, 17*, 121–145.

Edwards, C.C. (1986). A new method for direct sacral fixation: Rationale and clinical results. *Orthopedic Transactions, 10*, 541–542.

Erwin, W.D., Dickson, J.H., & Harrington P.R. (1980). Clinical review of patients with broken Harrington rods. *Journal of Bone and Joint Surgery, American Volume, 62*, 1302–1307.

Gaines R.W., & Leatherman K.D. (1981). Benefits of Harrington compression system in lumbar and thoracolumbar idiopathic scoliosis in adolescents and adults. *Spine, 6*, 483.

Harrington, P.R. (1960). Surgical instrumentation for management of scoliosis. *Journal of Bone and Joint Surgery, American Volume, 42*, 1448.

Harrington, P.R. (1988). The history and development of Harrington instrumentation. *Clinical Orthopaedics and Related Research, 227*, 3–5.

Jacobs R., Nordwall A., & Nachemson A. (1982). Reduction, stability and strength provided by internal fixation systems for thoracolumbar spinal injuries. *Clinical Orthopaedics and Related Research, 171*, 300.

Kamanovitz N., Arnoczky S.P., Levine D.B., & Otis J.P. (1984). The effects of internal fixation on the articular cartilage of unfused canine facet joint cartilage. *Spine, 9*, 268.

McAfee P.C., & Bohlman, H.H. (1985). Complications following Harrington instrumentation for fractures of the thoracolumbar spine. *Journal of Bone and Joint Surgery, American Volume, 67*, 672.

McAfee P.C., Werner F.W., & Glisson R.R. (1985). A biomechanical analysis of spinal instrumentation systems in thoracolumbar fractures: Comparison of traditional Harrington distraction instrumentation with segmental spine instrumentation. *Spine, 10*, 204–217.

Purcell G.A., Markoff, K.L., & Dawson E.G. (1981). Twelfth thoracic–first lumbar vertebral mechanical stability of fractures after Harrington rod instrumentation. *Journal of Bone and Joint Surgery, American Volume, 63*, 71.

Renshaw, T.S. (1988). The role of Harrington instrumentation and posterior spine fusion in the management of adolescent idiopathic scoliosis. *Orthopedic Clinics of North America, 19*, 257–267.

Swank, S.M., Mauri, T.M., & Brown J.C. (1990). The lumbar lordosis below Harrington instrumentation for scoliosis. *Spine, 15*, 181–186.

Turner, P.L., Mason, S.A., & Webb J.K. (1986). Neurologic complications with segmental spinal instrumentation. *Orthopedic Transactions, 10*, 14.

Wenger, D.R., Carollo, J.J., Wilkerson, J.A., et al. (1982). Laboratory testing of segmental spinal instrumentation versus traditional Harrington instrumentation for scoliosis treatment. *Spine, 7*, 265–269.

White A.A., & Panjabi, M.M. (1990). *Clinical Biomechanics of the Spine.* Philadelphia: J.B. Lippincott.

White A.A., Panjabi, M.M., & Thomas C.L. (1977). The clinical biomechanics of kyphotic deformities. *Clinical Orthopaedics and Related Research, 128*, 8.

Winter, R.B., Lonstein J.C., Vanderbrinkik, et al. (1987). Harrington rod with sublaminar wires in the treatment of adolescent idiopathic thoracic scoliosis. *Orthopedic Transactions, 11*, 89.

CHAPTER 25

Application of Luque Rods and Luque Rectangles for Stabilization of the Thoracolumbar Spine

James P. Hollowell
Dennis J. Maiman

HIGHLIGHTS

Segmental wire fixation of the dorsal spine with steel rods was introduced by Lange in 1902 for the treatment of spondylitis. This earliest fixation was achieved by passing silver wires through the base of the spinous processes and around two 4-mm steel rods. Luque (1982) credits a neurosurgeon, Dr. Javier Verdura, with first performing segmental sublaminar fixation for a fracture dislocation of the cervical spine in 1972. However, Luque popularized the technique and brought it into the mainstream of spinal fixation procedures in the early 1970s, initially for the treatment of scoliosis but soon thereafter applied to essentially all other spinal disorders (Luque, 1986, 1928b, 1982c; Luque, Cassis, & Ramirez-Wiella, 1982; Ogilvie & Millar, 1983; Wenger, Carollo, & Wilkerson, 1982).

Stainless steel rods used for the procedures are either straight, prebent in an L-configuration, or closed rectangles of various lengths and configurations (Dove, 1986, Flatley & Derderian, 1985). These rods are either $\frac{3}{16}$ in. (4.8 mm) or $\frac{1}{4}$ in. (6.4 mm) in diameter and 23.6 in. (60 cm) in length for the straight rod, and 20, 40, and 60 cm in length for the prebent rods, with short leg lengths of 3 or 5 cm (Fig. 25-1). Luque rectangles are 2 cm wide and available in lengths of 4 to 10 cm in 0.5-cm increments and 10 to 50 cm in 1-cm increments. Wires for securing the rods are generally 16-, 18-, or 20-gauge and are available as single-beaded strands, open loops, or closed loops in various lengths. Spools of similar-gauge wire are also available and may represent a significant cost savings. Woven stainless steel cables may also be used for sublaminar rod fixation. They offer some advantages and some distinct disadvantages that will be discussed below. The cost of substituting woven cables for wire may increase the total cost of the implant to the patient over fourfold.

In cases in which cross-linking is desired, rigid plate cross-linking devices are available from Danek Medical Inc. (Memphis, TN). Prebent "HSC unit rods" in a configuration for Galveston fixation are also available from Danek and can be used with standard sublaminar wires, pedicle screws, or any hook configuration.

Luque popularized segmental sublaminar fixation in the 1970s during a period when Harrington distraction devices were nearly the only option for spinal fixation. The Luque segmental devices offered the ability to increase the number of points of fixation and thereby reduce the incidence of failure, provide direct transverse traction at the point of maximal deformity, and reduce the need for postoperative bracing. The subsequent introduction of universal hook/rod fixation devices, which offer many of the same advantages and more, have made segmental laminar fixation an infrequently performed procedure. There are few occasions when this technique would be considered a first choice, but several applications in which sublaminar fixation may provide equivalent results to the more complex, technically demanding, and costly universal systems.

Biomechanical considerations, discussed later, suggest that these devices do not resist axial loads well and therefore should not be used in cases in which compromised anterior column is present. This disadvantage may in part be overcome by procedures that reconstruct the anterior column. In trauma, most surgeons would avoid these devices in axial load and flexion injuries.

Luque devices do prevent axial rotation and rotation about the coronal and sagittal axis, making them suitable for fracture dislocations that maintain axial support of the anterior column. Since this type of fracture is common in ankylosing spondylitis, segmental fixation may be well suited (Trent, Armstrong, & O'Neil, 1988). When ankylosis narrows interlaminar spaces, preventing safe passage of wires, fixation to the bases of the spinous process has been successfully used. In this circumstance placement of pedicle or laminar hooks may be nearly impossible and particularly hazardous.

The most common use of segmental fixation is the correction of scoliosis, especially when fixation to the pelvis is required. While several techniques for sacral-pelvic fixation have been developed, the Galveston technique remains the preferred choice for many. Neuromuscular deformity with marked pelvic obliquity may aggravate pressure ulceration of the buttocks as well as cause imbalance of sitting (Drummond, Guadagni, Keene, Breed, & Narechania, 1984). The Galveston Luque technique is particularly well suited for this application (Table 25-1).

The Galveston technique is also useful when upper sacral tumors leave few options for fixation of the lumbar spine to the pelvis. When fusion is required for rare cases of degenerative disease of the thoracic spine, Luque rods secured to the spinous processes may be preferable to universal instrumentation in terms of safety and cost.

Advantages of Luque instrumentation include the relative ease of application, superior fixation as compared with distraction-type instrumentation, and low cost as compared with universal systems (Table 25-2). The simple Luque sets do not require large inventories and can be used effectively even when experienced scrub technicians are unavailable. Luque rods can be applied in the lateral decubitus position much more easily than pedicle or universal systems, which may be useful when stabilization is required for morbidly obese or pregnant patients. Increased points of fixation may be superior to pedicle fixation or even limited laminar hook fixation in severely osteoporotic spines.

Disadvantages of Luque systems include fixation that is clearly inferior to universal systems in some applications. The technique generally requires longer fixations as compared with certain alternatives such as short segment pedicle fixation or anterior plate fixation. Placement and removal of sublaminar wires entail some neurologic risk, especially by surgeons who are learning the technique (Dove, 1989; Luque, 1982a, 1982c; Wilber, Thompson, Shaffer, Brown, & Nash, 1984).

BIOMECHANICS

Several studies have been performed to compare segmental Luque fixation with other systems, typically Harrington devices. The earliest of these studies was performed by Wenger et al. on cadaveric calf spines, demonstrating that failure of the Luque system occurred outside the instrumented region, unlike the failure of the Harrington distraction devices, which occurred at the bone metal interface (Wenger, Carollo, Wilkerson, Wauters, & Herring, 1982). Axial compression in this model resulted in bending of the paired $\frac{3}{16}$-inch Luque rods at 134 lb. Weiler, Mcneice, and Medley (1986) simi-

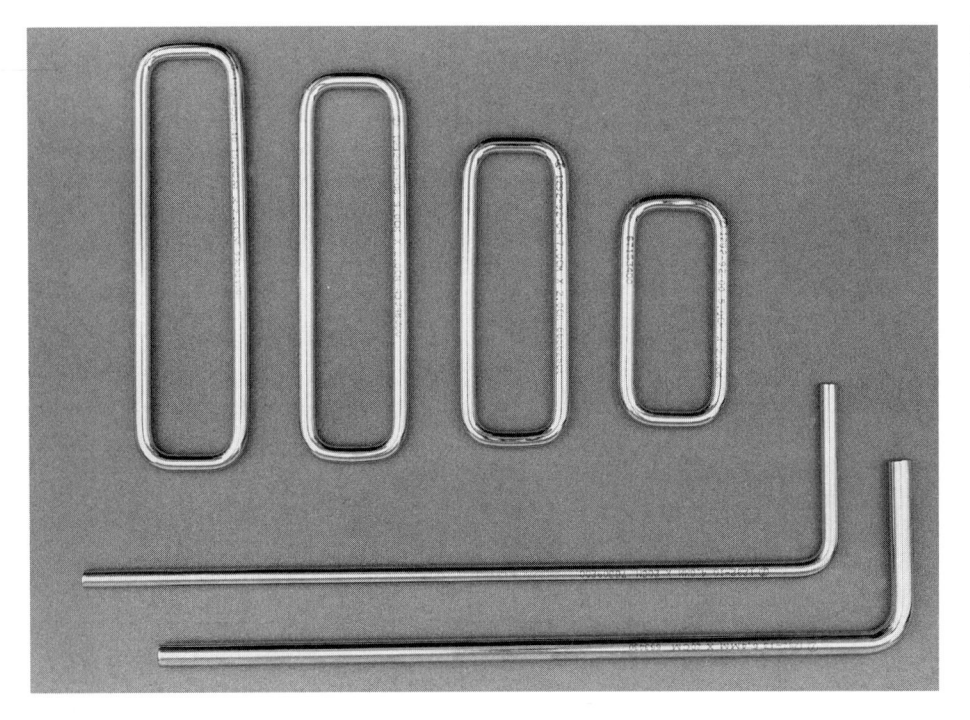

FIG. 25-1. A variety of Luque rectangles and L-rods are available from Zimmer, Inc. (Warsaw, IN).

Table 25-1
Indications and Contraindications for Luque Fixation

Indications
   Tumor/fracture fixation with preserved anterior column
   Fixation of ankylosing spondylitis fractures
   Galveston correction of scoliosis/pelvic obliquity
   Galveston fixation for upper sacral tumors/fractures

Contraindications
   Incompetent anterior column
   Insufficient space to pass sublaminar wires safely

Table 25-2
Advantages and Disadvantages of Luque Fixation

Advantages
   Simple, compact set of instruments and implants
   Luque set easily understood by OR personnel
   Inexpensive, minimal inventory required
   Rapidly, easily installed
   Multiple points of fixation reduces failure
   Can avoid sublaminar wiring by using spinous processes
   May reduce need for post-operative bracing
   Galveston technique provides excellent sacral/pelvic fixation

Disadvantages
   Potential for neurologic injury from sublaminar wires
   Less secure than "universal" segmental fixation
   Relatively long construct required

larly demonstrated the $\frac{1}{4}$-in. rods to increase the buckling load fourfold as compared with the $\frac{3}{16}$-inch rod. Clinical observations of bilateral rod failure with the smaller Luque rods have led to recommendations that the larger $\frac{1}{4}$-inch rods be used for demanding applications, such as correction of large deformities and fractures (Luque, 1986).

McAfee, Werner, and Glisson (1985) compared segmental fixation to distraction instrumentation in human cadaveric spines in several models and concluded that segmental fixation was significantly more stable in rotation than distraction devices but less effective at resisting direct axial loads. These authors concluded in this pre–universal-fixation era that sublaminar-wired distraction devices were most suitable to axial load injuries and segmental Luque devices most suitable to achieve rotational stability in translational injuries. They also noted that the failure in these tests occurred outside the instrumented segment and not at the bone-metal interface, similar to the findings of Wenger et al. (1982).

Nasca, Hollis, Lemons, and Cool (1985) studied segmental Luque fixation and distraction rods on swine spines with cyclical axial compressive loads concluding that Luque L-rods permitted three times as much axial shortening as did the distraction rods. They concluded that these devices should be avoided when axial loads are anticipated. Panjabi, Abumi, Duranceau, and Crisco (1988) studied several fixation systems in a human cadaveric model under physiologic loads and found that Luque rods and rectangles provided better stabilization of lateral bending, flexion, extension and axial rotation than Harrington distraction rods, but noted that none of the devices restored axial stability to that of the normal uninjured spine. This study failed to reveal significant differences between Luque rods and rectangles in the methods tested.

Gurr, McAfee, and Shih (1988) performed nondestructive cyclic studies of several anterior and posterior fixation devices on calf spines. Their studies included a Luque rectangle secured over five levels with 18-gauge sublaminar wires. They determined that the Luque rectangle was the least effective at resisting axial loads when compared to the Harrington distraction device, pedicle rod or plate systems, or anterior plate devices. He found torsional stiffness to be similar to Harrington rods, but less than the intact spine and less than half of the pedicle fixation devices.

Cross-linking devices such as those available from TSRH will convert L-rod configurations into rigid quadrilateral constructs to mimic a Luque rectangle. Ashman, Birth, Bone, Corin, Herring, Johnston, Ritterbush, & Roach (1988) have studied the effect of application of TSRH cross-linking devices to long contoured sublaminar fixation to Luque $\frac{3}{16}$-in. rods in a bovine scolosis model. They found that the addition of the cross-links dramatically increased both axial and torsional stiffness. Their work also compared Luque segmental fixation with $\frac{3}{16}$-in. rods and 18-gauge sublaminar wire in a kyphosis calf model to Wisconsin instrumentation and to cross-linked Cotrel-Dubousset (CD) eight-hook universal fixation. Torsional stiffness was five times greater for CD than for Luque instrumentation, and axial stiffness was twice as great for the CD system. Ashman et al. also studied the Luque rectangle in comparison to Steffee pedicle fixation in a calf spondylolisthesis model at L5, L6, and sacrum. These studies revealed the axial stiffness to be 3 times greater for the Steffee plates, and the torsional rigidity to be 10 times greater for the Steffee plates. Measurements of tensile stress of the Luque $\frac{3}{16}$-in. rods in this kyphotic deformity revealed the rods to be quite susceptible to fatigue failure, again suggesting the use of larger-diameter rods for correction of marked deformity.

Fidler (1986) compared biomechanical properties of 5-mm Luque L-rods, a C-configuration, and wide and narrow closed rectangles in an imitation vertebra model. These studies demonstrated a threefold greater torsional stiffness of the C-configuration or the closed narrow loop compared to the independent L-rods. Further significant stiffness could be achieved by placement of cement around the construct either unilaterally or bilaterally. The cement was able to further reduce slippage of the wires on the Luque rods. These studies confirm that rectangles or C-configuration rods are more effective in resisting rotation. Similarly, rod migration and loss of height of the construct is believed to be improved with these constructs as recommended by Luque et al. (1982). In summary, these and many other studies have found Luque segmental devices to resist axial loads poorly but provide relatively good stabilization of flexion, extension, lateral bending, and axial rotation that surpasses that of Harrington distraction rods but fall far short of pedicle fixation devices or hook-rod universal instrumentation.

Securing the Luque rods through the base of the spinous processes was popularized by Drummond (Drummond, 1992; Drummond, Breed, & Narechania, 1985; Drummond et al., 1984; Drummond & Keene, 1988). The Wisconsin spinal fixation technique he developed includes a single Harrington distraction rod in conjunction with a C-configured Luque rod secured through the base of the spinous process. He has demonstrated that the width at the base of the spinous process is 117% thicker than the adjacent lamina in the thoracic spine and 73% thicker than the lamina in the lumbar region (Drummond et al., 1984). He has also demonstrated that the addition of a small metal disk (Drummond button) to secure the wire to the spinous process increases the pullout strength of the wire to 176 lb, 47% greater than wire alone through the base of the spinous process. However, similar tests with a single loop of wire around the lamina demonstrate failure of 18-gauge wire at 187.5 lb, 16-gauge wire at 225 lb, and 14-gauge wire at 361 lb, resulting in fracture of the lamina (Drummond et al., 1984). These studies suggest that sublaminar fixation is more secure than Drummond button fixation and clearly more secure than simple wiring to the spinous process. Drummond performed further studies comparing the Wisconsin system to paired $\frac{3}{16}$-in. Luque L-rods in calf spines to demonstrate that the Luque system was less stiff but withstood a greater axial load to failure (Drummond et al., 1984). In summary, fixation to the base of the spinous process appears to be an acceptable alternative that is further improved by the use of Drummond buttons. Clinical results have supported the successful use of spinous process fixation (Drummond, 1992).

Wires used for rod fixation are generally 16-, 18-, or 20-gauge used as single or double strands. Single strand 18-gauge wire has a failure rate that exceeds 16-gauge wire, so most avoid the use of single 18-gauge wires. The greater contact area of "doubled" wires improves their resistance to "cut out" in poor bone density and offers excellent strength but does require the passage of twice as many wires. Guadagni and Drummond (1986) have studied several techniques of wire fixation and found that a single symmetrical twist is the preferred technique. Knots and knot twists are more secure but are difficult to perform and may not secure snugly to the rod. A "wire wrap" technique, in which one wire coils around the other, which remains straight, is not sufficient and should be avoided. The "pitch" or tightness of the twist reaches maximal strength at 2 twists per centimeter for 16-gauge wire and 2.5 twists per centimeter for 18-gauge wire. The absolute number of twists required to reach maximal strength is 2. Additional twists do not improve fixation strength (Guadagni & Drummond, 1986; Schultz, Boger, & Dunn, 1985). Crawford, Sell, Ali, and Dove (1989), in similar studies, found that a secondary twist in the already symmetrically twisted wire increases the yield strength of single wire by nearly 40% and more than doubles the yield strength of double-twisted 0.84-mm wire. They also found that decortication of the lamina reduces its resistance to wire pull through by one half in a cadaveric study. They determined that titanium materials are too brittle for sublaminar fixation. Other investigators have emphasized the importance of protecting wires from damage, demonstrating a 63% reduction in fatigue resistance when the diameter of the wire was notched by 1% (Oh, Sander, & Treharne, 1985).

Fixation across the lumbosacral junction has proven to be quite demanding of a device and is associated with a high rate of failure (Balderston, Winter, Moe, Bradford, & Lonstein, 1986; Camp, Caudle, Ashmun, & Roach, 1990). McCord, Cunningham, Shono, Myers, and McAfee (1992) studied 10 different lumbosacral instrumentation systems, including the Galveston technique, in a calf spine model. They found that only when a device extended anteriorly in the pelvis beyond the middle osteoligamentous complex centered at the posterior longitudinal ligament did it significantly improve fixation. This was true of the Isola Galveston configuration and the Isola iliac screws, which demonstrated the highest flexion moment and stiffness at failure of all the devices. They also included a Luque construct that performed poorly under these conditions, questioning its usefulness at the lumbosacral junction. Camp et al. (1990) presented clinical results of different fixation techniques of the lumbosacral junction and biomechanical comparisons. They demonstrated that the Galveston technique with laminar hooks had the greatest flexion moment at failure as compared with bilateral paired sacral screws or iliosacral screw fixation. They reported no clinical failures in the Galveston group, with high rates of device failure in the other two groups in a small series. These studies confirm that the Galveston pelvic fixation technique is a secure technique for lumbosacral fixation that is superior to other currently available techniques.

TECHNIQUES

The techniques discussed below describe spinal fixation with Luque rods. As always, the paramount objective in establishing spinal stability is to achieve solid bone fusion. The surgeon should focus on careful techniques of bone fusion, and should not be distracted by the technical demands of fixation, which are secondary in achieving success in most circumstances. These important techniques of bone fusion will be discussed elsewhere in this book.

Neurologic injuries from the passage of sublaminar wire are more common when wires are passed through the limited free space available between the lamina and the underlying neural tissue. This makes the thoracic cord more vulnerable and the passage of wires at levels adjacent to injured swollen cord more hazardous. Preoperative assessment of canal diameter and available space for wire passage is desirable, especially if stenosis is suspected. While some surgeons prefer to avoid the lower cervical and thoracic regions, others perform sublaminar fixation throughout the entire spine with few complications. Wires should be passed only beneath a single lamina. Early experience has clearly documented the expected increasing complications as multiple levels are included in a single wire (Geremia, Kim, Cerullo, & Calenoff, 1985).

Luque originally described the use of single strands of 18-gauge wire to secure the rods, but later used single 16-gauge wire doubled at the ends of the construct. We have found beaded double 18-gauge wire satisfactory and use this at each level of the fixation. The passage of a beaded closed loop wire does not produce sharp ends until the final wire trimming. Introducing cut wire ends initially produces far too many sharp wires, with a high risk of glove penetration. The use of double gloves during any wiring technique is prudent.

Several studies have considered optimal techniques for wire passage to minimize encroachment into the spinal canal. Zindrick, Knight, Bunch, Miller, Butler, Lorenz, and Behal (1989) studied the depth of sublaminar wire penetration into the neural canal in cadaveric thoracic spines. They found the optimal radius of curvature to be the largest possible radius that permits passage under the lamina. The radius of curvature should be equal to the distance from the inferior lamina of the segment above to the superior lamina of the segment below (Fig. 25-2). Reducing the radius to approximate the width of the lamina increased the penetration of the canal by more than 100%. Partial laminotomies to reduce the width of the lamina further reduced the penetration of the wire, but at the cost of weakening the lamina. A 25% reduction of the laminar width resulted in a 50% reduction of canal penetration. Mathematical models correlated well with their experimental observations.

Goll, Balderston, Stambough, Booth, Cohn, and Pickens (1988) performed similar studies in human cadaveric thoracic spine with direct video imaging of wire penetration. They found that the depth of wire penetration (DOWP) was less with a curvature radius 1.5 × the laminar width as compared with radii equal to or smaller than the laminar width. They demonstrated that central wire passage reduces wire penetration as compared with lateral passage, and removal of the spinous process reduces DOWP only at the thoracolumbar junction but not at other levels. Unlike the findings of Zindrick et al. (1989), they did not find that 25% reduction of laminar width reduced DOWP with central wire passage. They also found that bending the tip of the wire to 45 or 90 degrees resulted in clearly increased DOWP. This study led to the recommendations of central wire passage with spinous processes removal, with radius of curvature greater than laminar width, and the bend at the tip of less than 45 degrees, with no need to reduce laminar width.

When a fixation device must be removed, sublaminar wires may either be cut short and left in place or withdrawn. Several studies have clearly demonstrated significant penetration of the spinal canal when wires are removed. Nicastro, Hartjen, Traina, and Lancaster, 1986 performed cineradi-

FIG. 25-2. Properly configured wire minimizes penetration into canal.

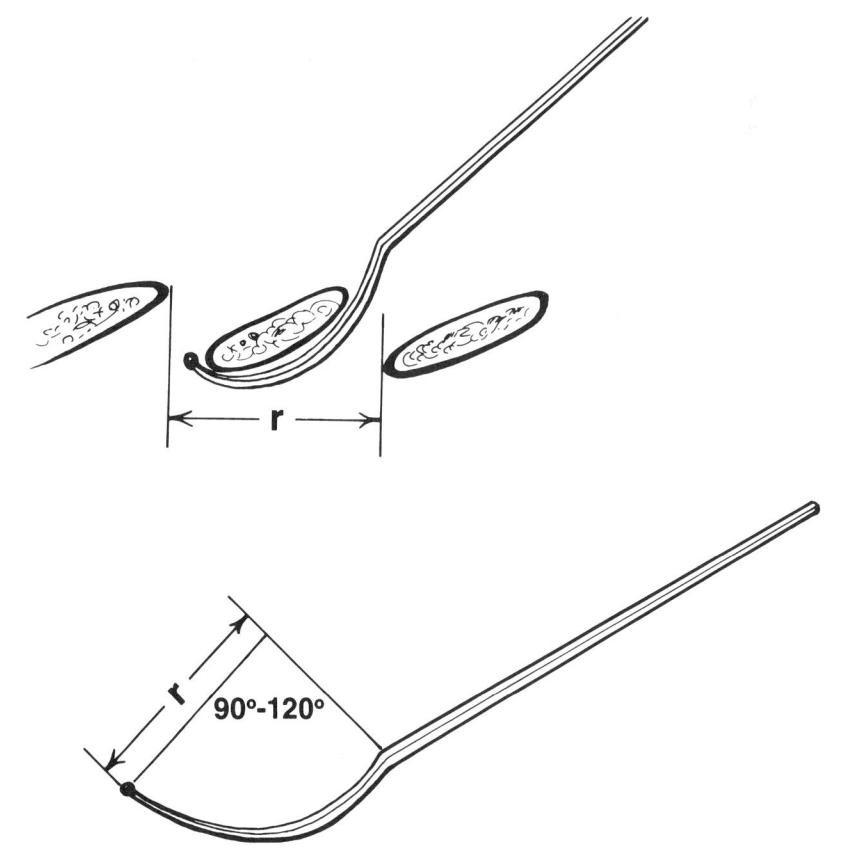

ographic studies in cadaveric human spines of sublaminar wires as they were removed by several techniques. When removed, 45% of the single wires conformed to the lamina, 28% compressed the dura less than 25%, and 27% compressed the dura more than 50%. In two cases, wires penetrated the spinal canal more than 75%. They determined that wires should be cut as short as possible and pulled out as parallel to the lamina as possible. Attempting to "roll" the wire out, or pull double wires together, clearly resulted in greater dural compression.

Schrader, Bethem, and Scerbin (1989) studied removal of wires in a dog model, in which the wires were permitted to scar in place for 10 to 155 days. Cineradiographs of wire removal demonstrated average penetration of 47%, ranging from 17 to 100%. Only one wire conformed to the lamina when removed. Dural laceration occurred in 30% of the animals. They found that longer-duration indwelling wire did not appear to develop protective scarring to improve the safety of wire removal. Histologic examination showed up to 1-mm indentations in the spinal cords in one third of the animals, and evidence of gray and white matter changes of the spinal cord. Coe, Becker, McAfee, and Gurr (1989) also detected histologic changes in the spinal cord of the beagle after sublaminar wire placement, even when the animals appeared to be neurologically intact. Despite these experimental findings, permanent neurologic damage from removal of sublaminar wires is surprisingly rare. Olson and Gaines (1987) reported the removal of 100 wires from 18 patients using a "roll-up" technique without injury. We generally choose to cut the wires short and leave them in place. We have seen no adverse outcomes from this technique.

We prepare the lamina for wire placement by removing the ligamentum flava completely and performing a small laminotomy medially unless a very wide intralaminar space is present (Fig. 25-3). The supraspinous and interspinous ligaments are not routinely disrupted, and the spinous process is not routinely removed. Beaded double 18-gauge wire is passed bilaterally in a cephalad direction configured with a wide radius of curvature as described above, subtending 90 to 120 degrees of arc, without additional curvature of the tip. No resistance to wire passage is tolerated as the bead is kept in contact with the undersurface of the lamina. To prevent the use of excessive force on wire passage, the wire should be held at midshaft, which permits control but prohibits forced entry. If any resistance is encountered, the wire is removed and the sublaminar space is further reevaluated. Removal of additional lamina or ligamentum is often required. Once the wire bead appears it is retrieved with a stout needle holder or a nerve hook and pulled firmly up against the lamina with both hands to prevent encroachment into the canal. Immediately, the tails are crossed over and conformed to the dorsal lamina to prevent inadvertent canal encroachment after release of the wire (Fig. 25-4). It is useful to place the beaded end consistently to one side so that when the Luque device is placed into the wound full of wires, they can easily be sorted into those that go inside and those that go outside the rod.

In circumstances in which rapid fixation is required, the spinous process can be removed to perform a single midline

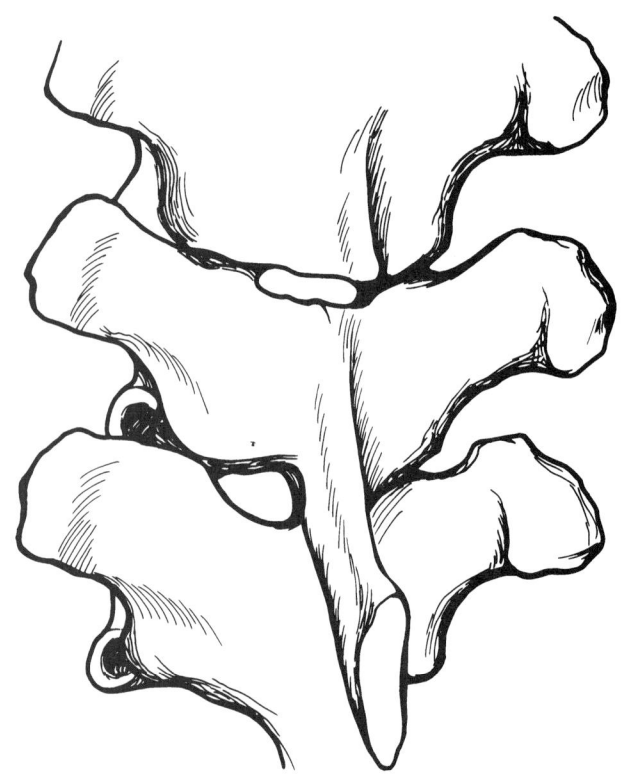

FIG. 25-3. Small bilateral paramedian laminotomies are performed with preservation of interspinous and supraspinous ligamentous structures.

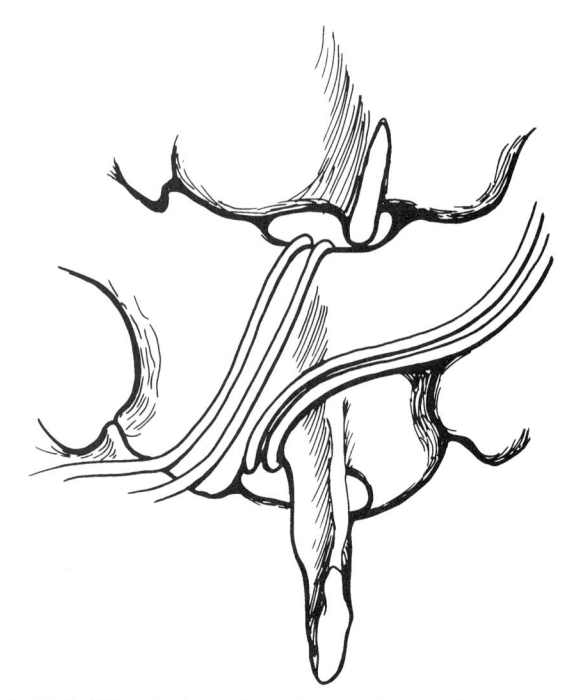

FIG. 25-4. Wires firmly conformed to the dorsum of the lamina prevent inadvertent migration into canal.

laminotomy. This permits rapid passage of doubled Luque wires that can be secured to either side, saving the time required to perform bilateral paramedian laminotomies. Since this requires the disruption of the supraspinous and interspinous ligaments, it is not performed unless speed of fixation becomes important.

Songer, Spencer, Meyer, and Jayaraman (1991) have reported the use of multistranded sublaminar cables in 32 patients without cable failure. If cables are used they can either be passed directly with a rigid lead, or a wire can be passed to place a suture that is used to draw the flexible cable under the lamina. The rigid leads of cables clearly present the same risks to the neural elements on initial passage but may diminish the risk of subsequent migration of a passed but not yet secured wire into the canal. Furthermore, removal of cables would be expected to be safer since they are likely to conform to the lamina when withdrawn. However, no data has clearly demonstrated that the use of cables results in reduced risk to the patient when compared with standard wires.

Either L-rods, C-rods, or closed rectangles may be used. The rods are contoured with the use of a template and extend two or three segments above and below the site of pathology. The shorter limb of the rod should be long enough that it could not rotate into the canal by permitting it to rest on the contralateral facet complex. The short limb should be wired to the opposite rod to reduce rotation (Fig. 25-5). When L-rods are used to reduce kyphotic deformity, the cranial end of one rod and the caudal end of the other rod is initially secured, leaving the opposite ends up off the lamina. Simultaneous downward pressure applies a significant three-point load at the kyphos to reduce the deformity. The remaining wires are then secured. Similarly, a rectangle can be contoured to the expected correction and the wires sequentially tightened until the lamina is opposed to the rod, eventually achieving correction. If the rod is not fully contacting the lamina, fixation is markedly impaired. If L-rods or C-rods are used the supraspinous ligaments may be preserved by passing the rod through a hole in the interspinous ligaments. In some cases it may be necessary to create a notch in the underside of the supradjacent spinous process to accommodate the horizontal limb of the rod. With a laminectomy defect there is the possibility of cord compression due to the overlying rods (Quint & Salton, 1993).

After initial twists are placed in the wires they are cut to 3 to 4 cm in length to facilitate subsequent tightening unless a Luque wire twister (potato hook) is used, which requires the wires to be left at full length. Alternatively, twisting may be performed with a heavy wire twister or a jet twister depending on the surgeon's preference (Fig. 25-6). The wire is sufficiently tight when it no longer can be moved on the rod. Often a subtle color change of the wire indicates maximal tightness beyond which wire failure may occur. After initial tightening, the earlier twists will often loosen as the subsequent wires become more secure. A second or third round of tightening is usually required. Finally the

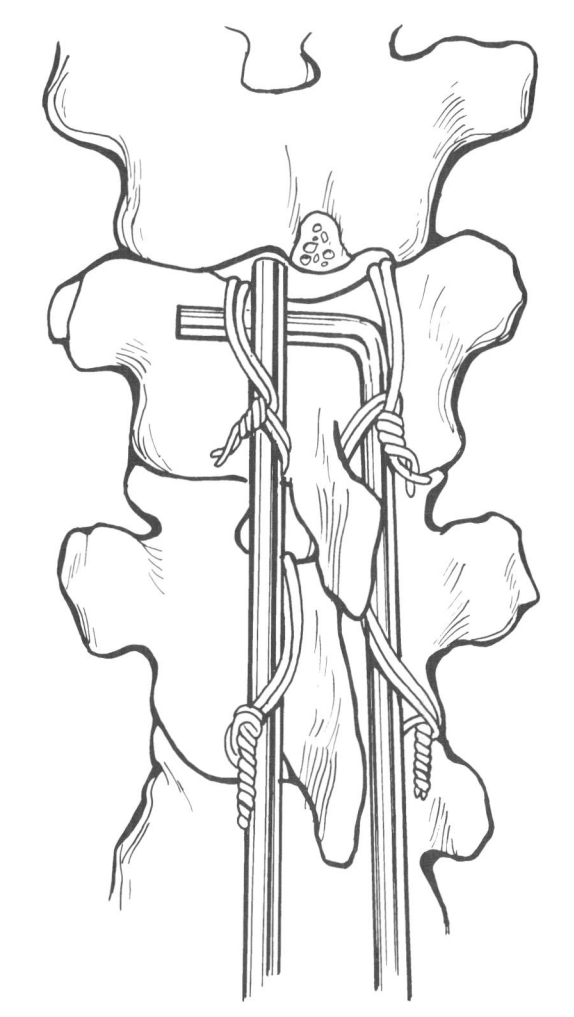

FIG. 25-5. Final secured configuration of rods and wires. Alternatively, horizontal limb of L-rod can be placed immediately beneath cephalad spinous process to reduce migration.

twisted wires are retrimmed to 1 to 2 cm and bent medially (Fig. 25-7).

Fixation to the sacrum requires modified technique. It may not be adequate in many cases unless the Galveston pelvic fixation technique is used. When minimal instability is present, wires may be passed from cephalad to caudad out the first dorsal foramen. Alternatively, or in addition, a hole may be created at the base of the sacral articular facet in a ventrolateral direction toward the sacral alae for an additional wire fixation site. Sacral fixation by these techniques has a higher rate of failure than at other levels of the spine.

The ability to tighten sequentially is complicated by the use of cables. The Songer device will permit sequential tightening if a second crimp is placed on the wire. The first crimping is performed on the outer crimp and a subsequent tightening can be performed with the inner crimp. A small device that temporarily holds the crimp is now available to allow sequential tightening, making the need for the double-crimp technique less common. The Codman cable system permits the disposable tightening handle to remain in place holding

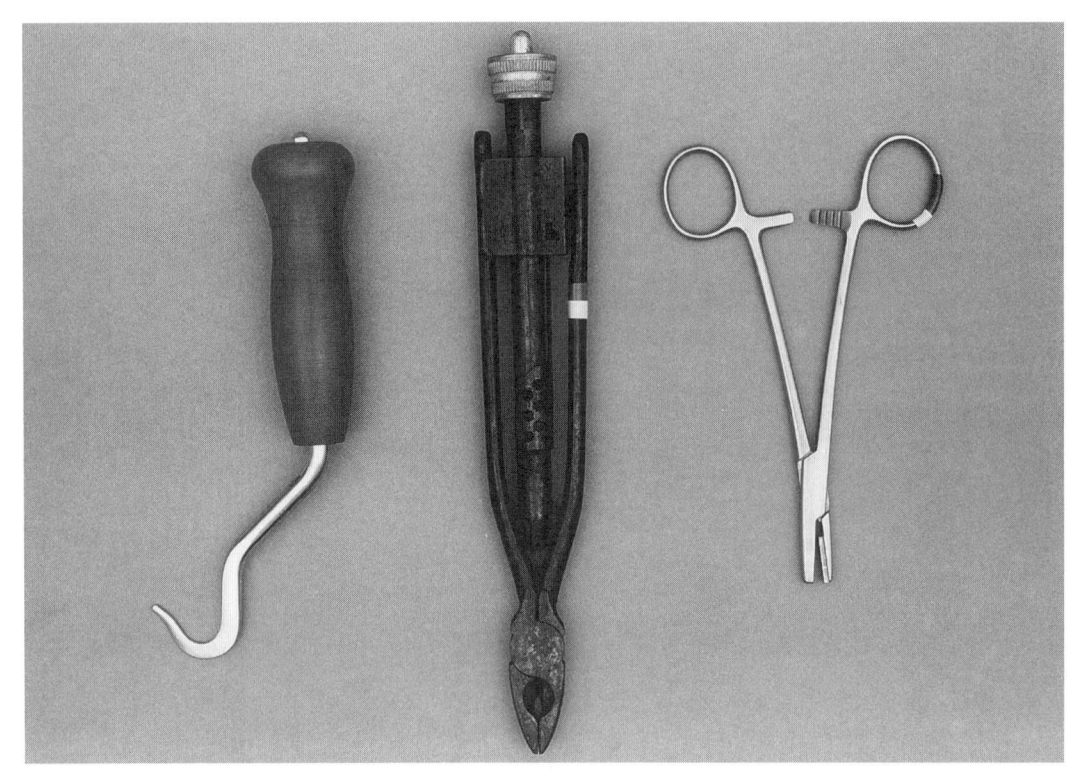

FIG. 25-6. Luque wire twister "potato hook," jet wire twister, or heavy wire twister (*left to right*) may all be used to secure wires effectively.

tension and permitting sequential tightening until finally the crimp is secured. This Codman device presently is available in 0.9-mm-diameter cable, which has a tensile strength of 170 lb—marginal for thoracolumbar fixation. Clinical results are not yet available for this application and it would not be generally recommended. Codman is in the process of developing a larger-diameter cable that is comparable to a Songer cable and should be suitable.

When separate L-rods are used they can be further stabilized to each other by placement of a cross-link device. Texas Scottish Rite cross-link plates can be utilized for this purpose. The plates are placed as with universal fixation systems at either end of the construct. The eyebolts should be installed prior to securing sublaminar wires.

Laboratory investigations and clinical observations have demonstrated that one failure mode of Luque fixation is wires cutting through the lamina (Maiman, Sances, Larson, Myklebust; Chilbert, Nesemann, & Flately, 1985). Nylon and Mersilene bands have been successfully used to secure Luque rods (Crawford, Sell, Ali, & Dove, 1989; Gaines & Abernathie, 1986). They provide a larger contact area with the lamina to prevent wires from cutting through the lamina when bone mineral density is decreased. These devices are not widely used. Failure of Luque sublaminar fixation by wire cutout is not common.

Fixation to the base of the spinous process is a less secure alternative, although favorable clinical experience has been reported by this technique which avoids the risk of sublaminar wires (Fig. 25-8) (Drummond, 1992; Drummond et al., 1984, Drummond & Keene, 1988). The use of Wisconsin "buttons" for fixation to the spinous process improves the security of this fixation significantly (Fig. 25-9). A hole is made at the extreme base of the spinous process with a bone tenaculum or curved awl. Two beaded "Wisconsin" wires are passed in opposite directions through the hole in the bone and then through the third hole in the metallic button. These wires are then twisted down on the Luque rods in a fashion similar to that described for sublaminar wires (Fig. 25-10) (Drummond, 1992; Drummond et al., 1984, Drummond & Keene, 1988).

Generally, dorsolateral, facet, and intertransverse fusion is performed over the full length of the instrumentation. There are occasions when "rod long, fuse short" may be a prudent choice. In these cases it is usually desirable to remove the device after solid fusion has occurred. When this technique is utilized, one should not violate the functional joint capsules when the instrumentation is initially placed. While experimental and clinical evidence suggests that degenerative changes occur within instrumented nonfused segments (Herring & Wenger, 1982; Kahanovitz, Bullough, & Jacobs, 1984), our experience has demonstrated that good clinical results can be obtained using this technique.

Though Luque initially stated that the use of the segmentally wired device made postoperative external orthotics unnecessary, we believe that postoperative bracing is important. Bracing reduces stress on the instrumentation and reminds the patient to avoid applying potentially damaging loads to the device.

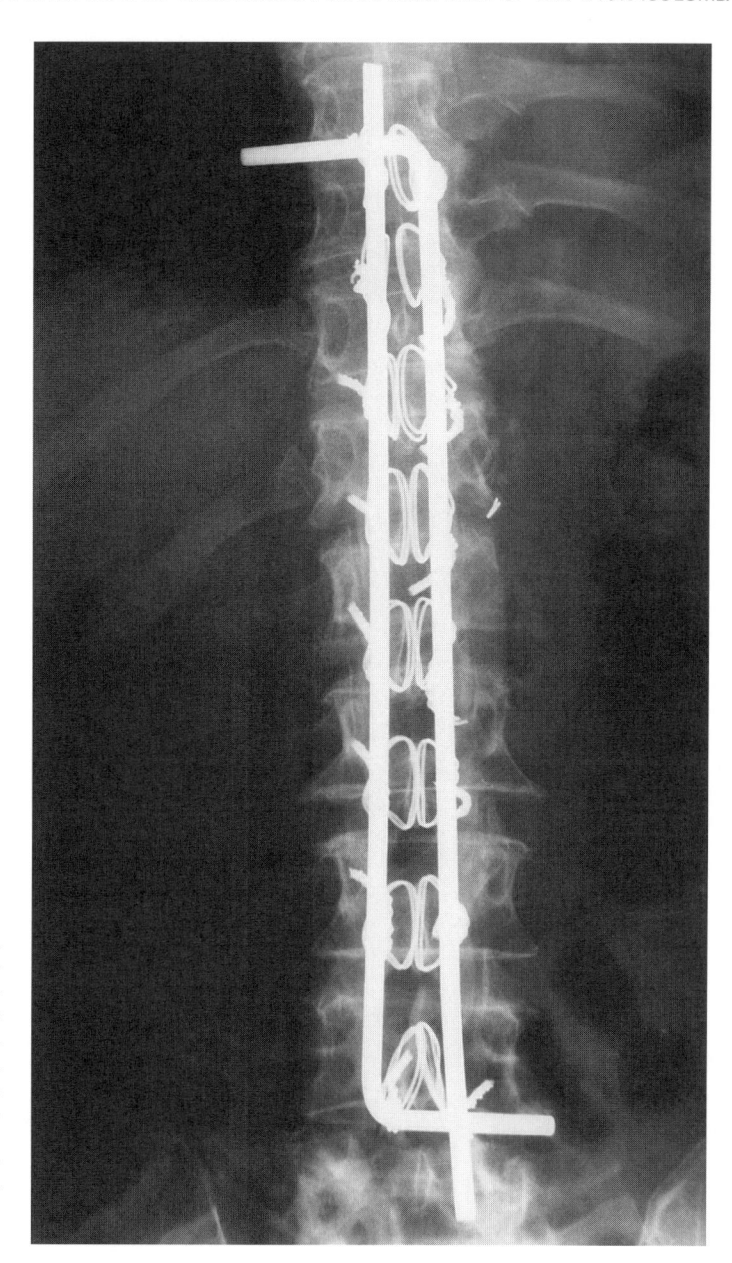

FIG. 25-7. Radiograph from a 65-year-old woman with renal cell cancer presenting with paraparesis and tumor involvement of the L1 vertebral body and ventral canal. She underwent lateral extracavitary ventral decompression with interbody grafting and sublaminar Luque L-rod fixation from T9 to L4. The rod length and horizontal limbs could have been reduced. The patient demonstrated marked neurologic improvement and experienced no complications from the device.

GALVESTON TECHNIQUE OF PELVIC FIXATION

Fixation to the sacrum may be difficult to achieve with traditional application of universal devices. Occasionally, frank instability of the low lumbar spine demands fixation but the sacrum is compromised by tumor or fracture. In these cases, extension of the Luque rods into the pelvis has provided secure fixation. Allen and Ferguson (1984, 1982b, 1979) developed these techniques in the late 1970s initially for the treatment of scoliosis. Many others have reported the successful use of this technique for several pathologic conditions (Boachie-Adjei, Dendrinos, Ogilvie, & Bradford, 1991; Camp et al., 1990; Gau, Lonstein, Winter, Koop, & Denis, 1991; Saer, Winter, & Lonstein, 1990). This technique has the disadvantage of placing instrumentation across the potentially unfused sacroiliac joints, which has been associated with chronic pain (King, 1984).

The posterior iliac crest is exposed by releasing the attachments of the erector spinae from the medial aspect of the iliac crest and the sacrum. The portion of erector spinae inserting into the sacrum can be transected through the ligamentous insertion and later reapproximated at closure. This provides the necessary exposure for insertion of the intraosseous rods. The gluteal muscles are reflected to identify the sacral notch clearly. The entry point for the rod should be 1 to 2 cm rostral to the posterior superior iliac spine. The entry point should be sufficiently anterior on the medial aspect of the crest such that the rod will not project as high as the posterior iliac spine. This is particularly important in thin individuals and in those with compromised sensation to avoid potential erosion of skin overlying prominent hardware. A $\frac{3}{16}$-in. Steinmann pin is introduced into the posterior crest directed 1.5 cm above the sciatic notch to a depth of 6 to 9 cm if possible. The midportion of the sacral notch is about 7 to

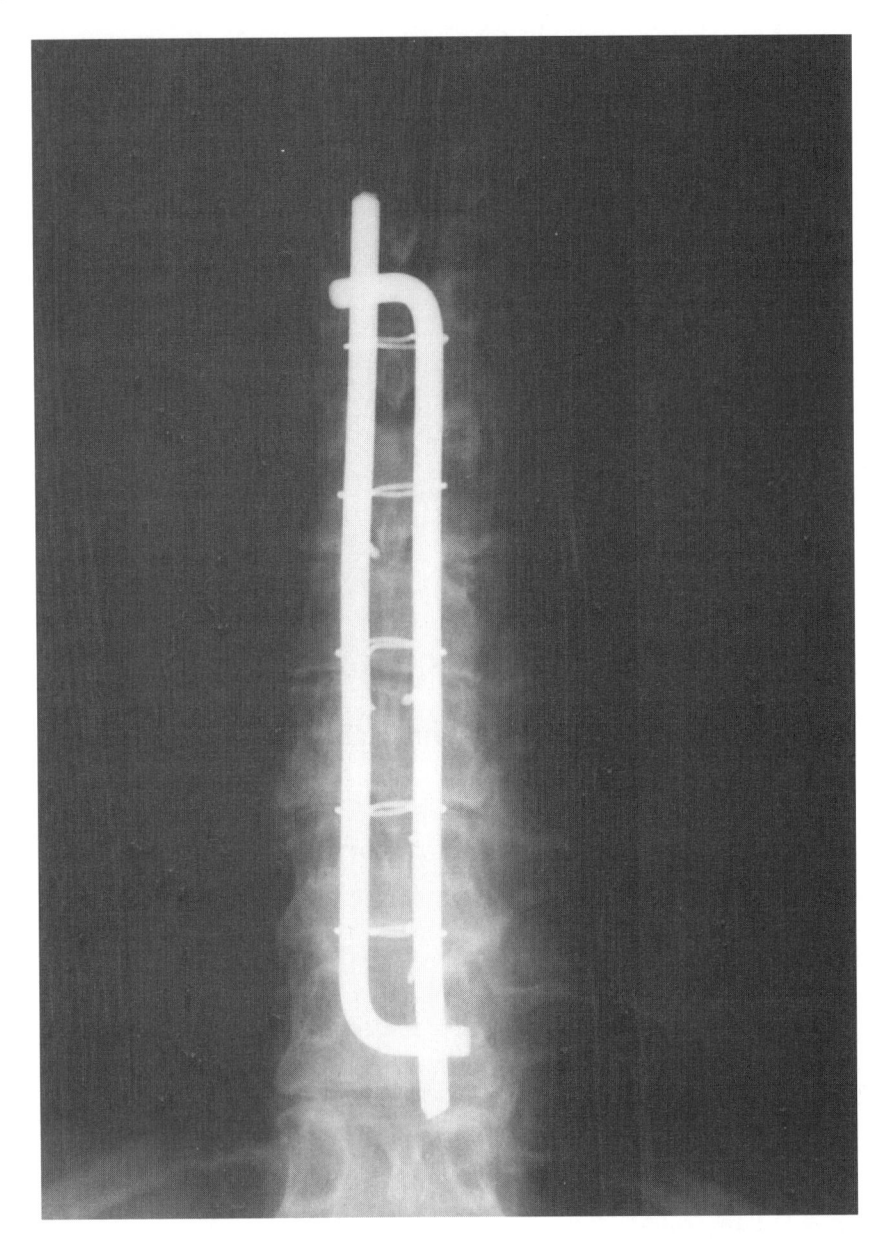

FIG. 25-8. Patient with degenerative disk and joint disease of the midthoracic spine with refractory local pain. Five-level Luque fixation performed through the base of the spinous processes without Wisconsin buttons. Device remained secure and solid fusion was achieved.

8 cm deep, and the acetabulum could be reached by 10 to 11 cm, though the proper trajectory should be above the acetabulum. Proximity to the sacral notch permits buttressing of the rod between the converging cortical tables and adequate length permits entry of the rod into the transverse bar of the ilium. A more superior course traverses a narrower portion of the wing and risks perforation of the pelvis and compromise of fixation. A low trajectory through the pelvis also remains clear of the usual site of iliac bone harvest.

Allen and Ferguson studied the importance of rod placement in a small clinical series (1984). They found that shorter rods less than 6 cm placed higher in the sacrum away from the sacral notch and perforating the pelvis performed poorly. This group had a larger loss of correction, lower fusion rate, and evidence of motion shown by the largest "wiper effect" around the rods. They concluded that the intrapelvic limb should be greater than 6 cm and extend within 1.5 cm of the sacral notch. This produced the least subsequent movement, loss of correction, and failed fusion rate (Fig. 25-11).

Establishing the proper trajectory of this pin may be facilitated by placing the nondominant index finger in the sciatic notch while the pin is advanced. A mallet may be required in particularly dense bone. Perforation of the corticated tables should be avoided. A malleable template is placed within this tract and contoured ventrally to contact immediately the dorsum of the sacrum then turn cephalad to conform to the lumbar lordosis. This double complex curve may be difficult to establish with $\frac{3}{16}$-inch rods and particularly challenging with $\frac{1}{4}$-in. rod material. The use of $\frac{1}{4}$-in. rods permits use of universal laminar hooks or pedicle screws as an alternative to sublaminar wire (Fig. 25-12).

In appreciation of the difficulty of proper rod contouring, Danek has available a "unit rod," which is a prebent $\frac{1}{4}$-inch

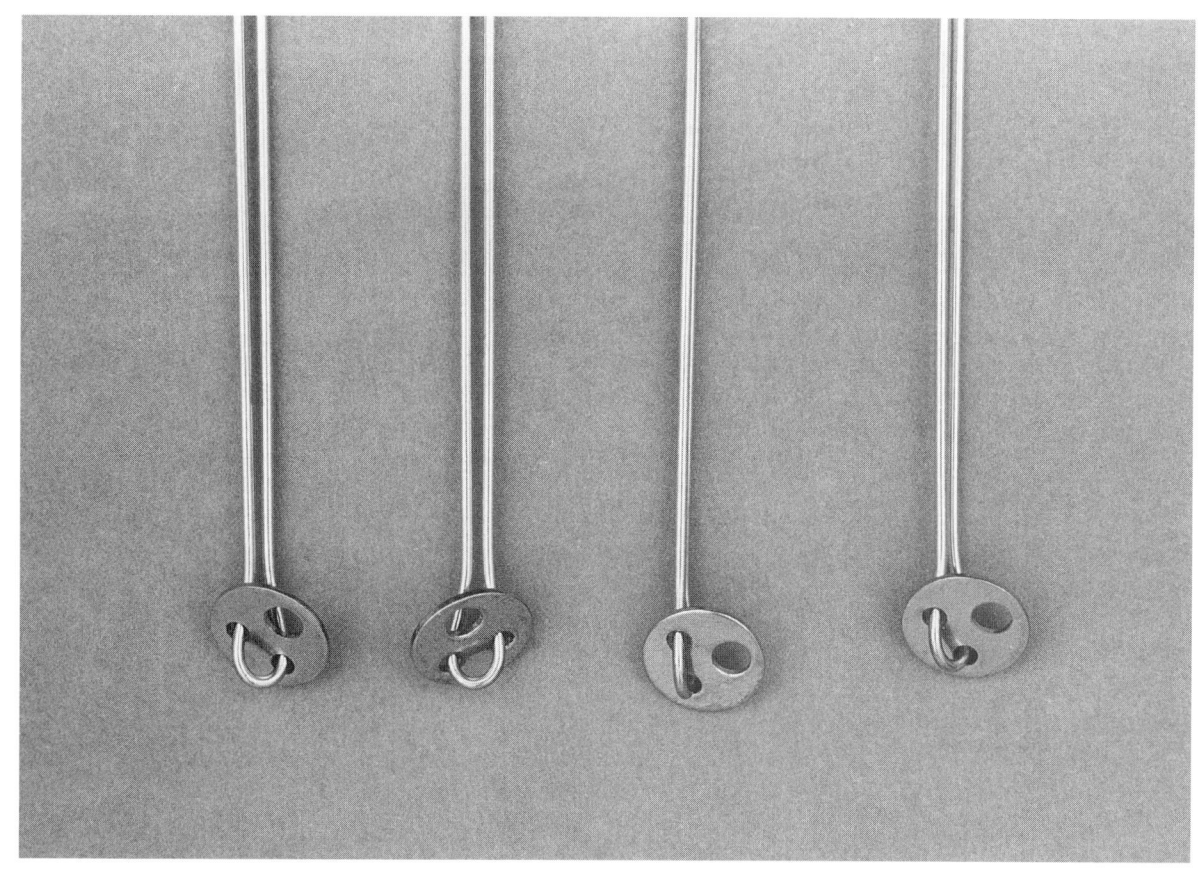

FIG. 25-9. Wisconsin buttons permit the opposite wire to be pulled through the third larger hole in the metallic plate to secure the wires to the base of the spinous process, improving pullout strength.

Galveston configured rod in several sizes (Fig. 25-13). The right- and left-sided rods are connected and may be cut apart to facilitate placement if needed. Minimal modification of these preconfigured rods may greatly reduce the time required on this demanding portion of the procedure. If sublaminar wiring will be used, a short transverse limb should be bent into the cephalad end of the construct similar to the use of the L-rod. Danek transverse connectors may be added to the construct if desired. Heller, Zdeblick, Dunz, McCabe, and Cooke (1993) have studied the addition of cross-links in a calf spine model with anterior and middle column disruption. They were unable to establish significant differences in axial, torsional, or sagittal stiffness with the addition of the cross-links to segmentally secured L-rods. In the same studies they found the imbedding of the rods in methacrylate to improve torsional and sagittal stiffness to that of the intact spine, but axial stiffness remained quite low. One variation of the Galveston technique reported by McCarthy, Dunn, and McCullough (1989) uses the sacral ala as a stout point of fixation in patients requiring this technique but with poor bone quality of the ilium.

CLINICAL RESULTS AND COMPLICATIONS

Neurologic injury with passage of sublaminar wires was initially reported with startling frequency. Rates of cord or root injury have been reported as high as 26% in one early experience of 23 patients, but reduced to 17% and finally 9% in subsequent groups of equal size by the same surgeons (Wilber, Thompson, Shaffer, Brown, & Nash, 1984). Luque (1982c) reported transient sensory deficits occurring in 9%

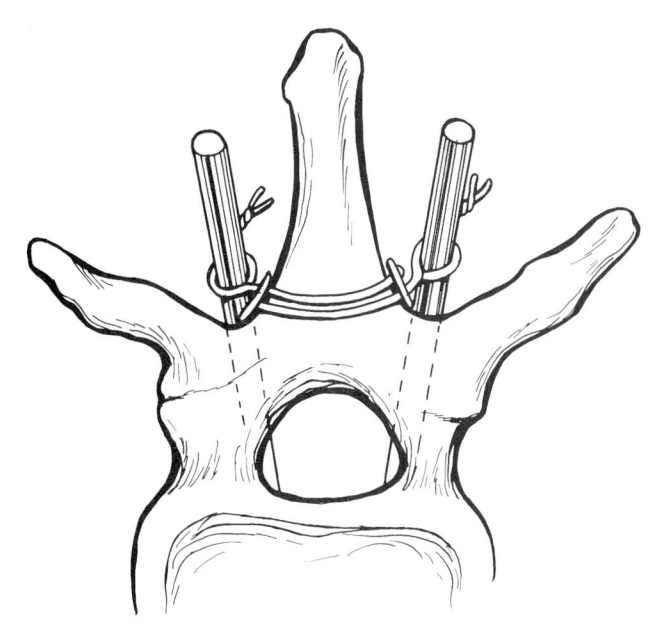

FIG. 25-10. Spinous process wiring utilizing Wisconsin buttons.

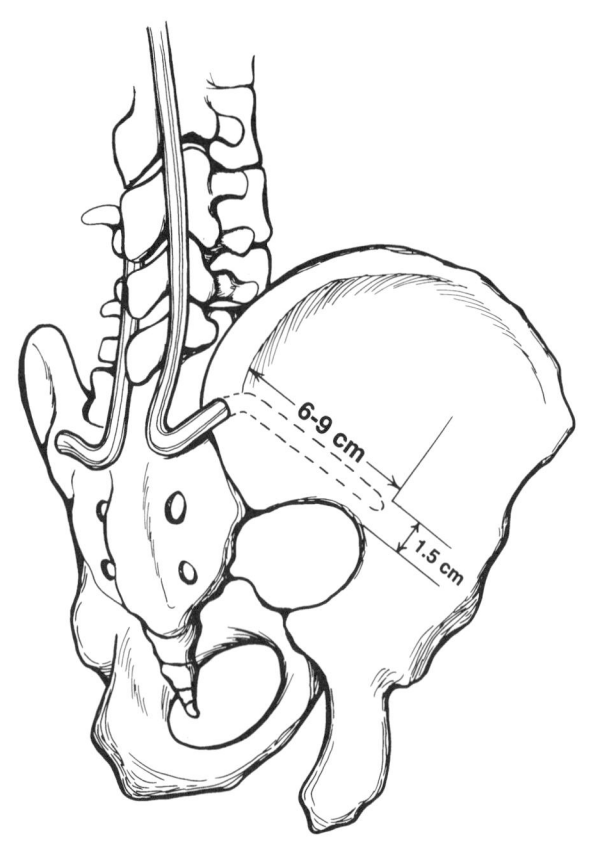

FIG. 25-11. Diagram showing configuration of Galveston rod and intrapelvic course for maximal security.

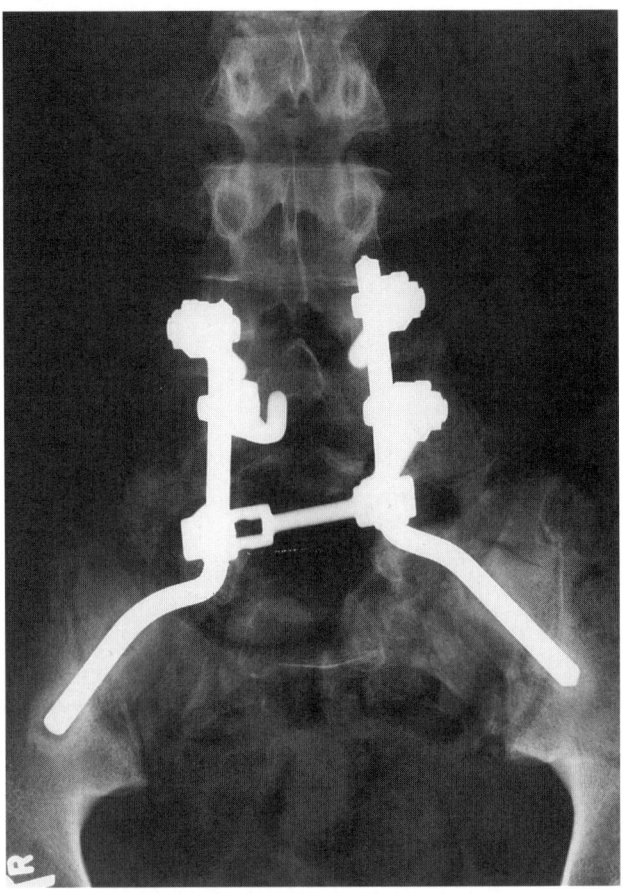

FIG. 25-12. Radiograph one year after pelvic fixation with TSRH rods and cross-link with pedicle fixation to L4 in a 17-year-old patient involved in a motor-vehicle accident who sustained fractures of the L5 vertebral body, pelvic ramus, and upper sacrum. Note the evidence of intrapelvic rod movement on the right as the fixation crosses the unfused sacroiliac joint. The patient is pain-free 18 months after injury.

of 78 patients undergoing scoliosis correction with motor deficits in only 2. Luque (1982a) also reported only 1 neurologic injury in 360 patients undergoing sublaminar segmental fixation for reasons other than scoliosis. More recent series have reported extremely low rates of iatrogenic injury, with several large series free of any significant neurologic deficit (Boachie-Adjei et al., 1991; Boachie-Adjei, Lonstein, Winter, Koop, Vanden Brink, & Denis, 1989; Herndon, Sullivan, Yngve, Gross, & Dreher, 1987; Herring & Wenger, 1982; Kostuik, Errico, & Gleason, 1990; Sasso & Cotler, 1993; Yngve, Burke, Price, & Riddick, 1986). In 1987 the Scoliosis Research Society in a poll of 204 members representing a total of 10,203 spinal procedures, reported an incidence of 1.77% of neurologic injury following sublaminar wire passage. Members of the British Scoliosis Society reported their complications of Luque L-rod and rectangle fixation in 328 patients for the treatment of spinal deformity in 1985 (Dove, 1989). Patients treated with Luque L-rods and rectangles combined suffered neurologic injury with sublaminar wire passage techniques 1.7% of the time. They also noted the fracture of one rod and eight wires. Wires cut out through the lamina in one patient. With few exceptions, neurologic injury has occurred acutely. Bernard, Johnston, Roberts, and Burke (1983) reported on the delayed complications of sublaminar wire breakage in 5 of 69 patients. One patient had new sensory deficit, with myelography demonstrating dural compression. Further surgery resulted in complete recovery. In experienced hands using techniques outlined above, one should expect an extremely low rate of iatrogenic neurologic injury due to sublaminar wire passage at any level of the spine.

Luque (1986) reported rod breakage in 3 of 141 rods, and suggested the use of $\frac{1}{4}$-inch rods instead of $\frac{3}{16}$-inch rods when large loads are anticipated, such as unstable adult fractures or kyphosis. Broom, Banta, and Renshaw (1989) experienced rod breakage in 6 of 74 patients for the correction of marked deformity. The breakage occurred at an average of 44 months and with $\frac{3}{16}$-inch rods in all but one case. Most have found the fracture rate of the smaller rods to be sufficiently low to warrant their routine use. Only in particularly large patients or marked instability do we use the larger $\frac{1}{4}$-in. rods.

Wire breakage is also uncommon, particularly that severe enough to cause failure of the device. Though limited wire breakage often occurs with little clinical consequence, multiple wire fractures may be indicative of failed fusion. In earlier series, wire failure was observed more frequently at the ends of the construct. Common advice was to use double wires at the ends. Luque reported the failure of 27 of 2112

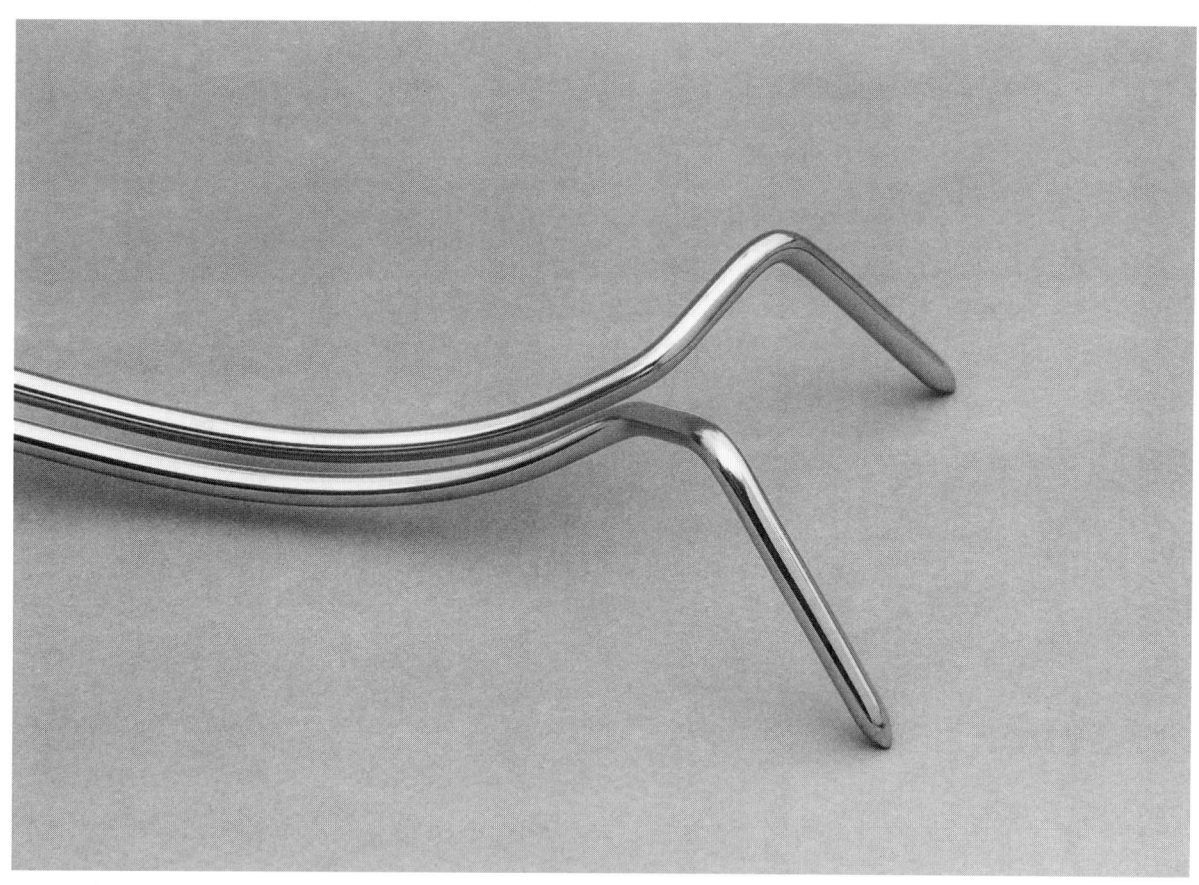

FIG. 25-13. Precontoured Galveston unit rod available from Danek.

single sublaminar wires in a report in 1984. With our use of doubled 18-gauge wires, breakage is distinctly unusual.

Several clinical series have reported the effectiveness of segmental fixation for the treatment of a variety of conditions (Boachie-Adjei et al., 1991, 1989; Broom et al., 1989; Guadagni, Drummond, & Breed, 1984; Herring & Wenger, 1982; Larson & Mueller, 1990; Luque, 1986, 1982b, 1982c; Luque et al., 1982; Ogilvie & Millar, 1983; Saer, Winter, & Lonstein, 1990; Sassa & Cotler, 1993; Trent et al., 1988). Clearly the effectiveness of the device is entirely dependent on the situation in which it was applied. Even when used for demanding severe deformity, maintenance of correction and high rates of fusion are the rule (Saer et al., 1990). Most failures occur when the Luque device is used in an application in which other options would be more appropriate. Sasso and Cotler (1993) compared Luque segmental fixation to Harrington rods and AO pedicle fixation in unstable fractures. They found all three systems poor in maintaining sagittal correction. The Luque system demonstrated an 80% loss of sagittal correction, and a 76% loss of anterior vertebral height which was worse than the other two systems (Sasso & Cotler, 1993). The many other considerable medical and surgical complications of major spinal surgery are similar for segmental sublaminar fixation as for other fixation techniques.

CONCLUSION

Though newer segmental universal fixation devices have largely replaced the Luque segmental techniques, carefully selected applications offer a reasonably simple, less costly alternative for achieving adequate results. In a very few applications such as pelvic fixation or ankylosing spondylitis, Luque segmental fixation may be the procedure of choice. Though early reports emphasized neurologic injury and rod and wire breakage, subsequent experience has demonstrated that these failings were largely technique-dependent and are now easily avoided.

REFERENCES

Allen, B.L., & Ferguson, R.L. (1984). The Galveston technique of pelvic fixation with L-rod instrumentation of the spine. *Spine, 9,* 388.

Allen, B.L., & Ferguson, R. L. (1983). A pictorial guide to the Galveston LRI pelvic fixation technique. *Contemporary Orthopaedics, 7,* 51.

Allen, B.L., & Ferguson, R.L. (1982). The Galveston technique for L-rod instrumentation of the scoliotic spine. *Spine, 7,* 276.

Allen, B.L., & Ferguson, R.L. (1982b). L-rod instrumentation for scoliosis in cerebral palsy. *Journal of Pediatric Orthopedics, 2,* 87.

Allen, B.L., & Ferguson, R.L. (1979). The operative treatment of myelomeningocele, spinal deformity–1979. *Orthopedic Clinics of North America, 10,* 845–862.

Ashman, R.B., Birch, J.G., Bone, L.B., Corin, J.D., Herring, J.A., Johnston, C.E., Ritterbush, J.F., & Roach, J.W. (1988). Mechanical testing of spinal instrumentation. *Clinical Orthopaedics and Related Research, 227,* 113, 1988.

Balderston, R.A., Winter, R.B., Moe, J.H., Bradford, D.S., & Lonstein, J.E. (1986). Fusion to the sacrum for nonparalytic scoliosis in the adult. *Spine, 11,* 824.

Bernard, T.N., Johnston, C.E., Roberts, J.M., & Burke, S.W. (1983). Late complications due to wire breakage in segmental instrumentation. *Journal of Bone and Joint Surgery, American Volume, 9,* 1339.

Boachie-Adjei, O., Dendrinos, G.K., Ogilvie, J.W., & Bradford, D.S. (1991). Management of adult spinal deformity with combined anterior-posterior arthrodesis and Luque-Galveston instrumentation. *Journal of Spinal Disorders, 2,* 131.

Boachie-Adjei, O., Lonstein, J.E., Winter, R.B., Koop, S., Vanden Brink, K., & Denis, F. (1989). Management of neuromuscular spinal deformities with Luque segmental instrumentation. *Journal of Bone and Joint Surgery, American Volume, 71,* 548.

Broom, M.J., Banta, J.V., & Renshaw, T.S. (1989). Spinal fusion augmented by Luque-rod segmental instrumentations for neuromuscular scoliosis. *Journal of Bone and Joint Surgery, American Volume, 71,* 32–44.

Camp, J.F., Caudle, R., Ashmun, R.D., & Roach, J. (1990). Immediate complications of Cotrel-Dubousset instrumentation to the sacro-pelvis. *Spine, 15,* 932.

Coe, J.D., Becker, P.S., McAffee, P.C., & Gurr, K.R. (1989). Neuropathology with spinal instrumentation. *Journal of Orthopaedic Research, 7,* 359.

Crawford, R.J., Sell, P.J., Ali, M.S., & Dove, J. (1989). Segmental spinal instrumentation: A study of the mechanical properties of materials used for sublaminar fixation. *Spine, 14,* 632.

Dove, J. (1989). Segmental wiring for spinal deformity. *Spine, 14,* 229.

Dove, J. (1986). Internal fixation of the lumbar spine. *Clinical Orthopaedics and Related Research, 203,* 135.

Drummond, D.S. (1992). Segmental spinal instrumentation with spinous process wires. In: T.H. Grayson (Ed.). *Spinal Instrumentation* (pp. 105–113). Baltimore: Williams & Wilkins.

Drummond, D., Breed, A.L., & Narechania, R. (1985). Relationship of spine deformity and pelvic obliquity on sitting pressure distributions and decubitus ulceration. *Journal of Pediatric Orthopaedics, 5,* 396–402.

Drummond, D., Guadagni, J., Keene, J.S., Breed, A., & Narechania, R. (1984). Interspinous process segmental spinal instrumentation. *Journal of Pediatric Orthopaedics, 4,* 397.

Drummond, D.S., & Keene, J.S. (1988). Spinous process segmental spinal instrumentation. *Orthopedics, 11,* 1403.

Fidler, M.W. (1986). Posterior instrumentation of the spine. *Spine, 11,* 367.

Flatley, T.J., & Derderian, H. (1985). Closed loop instrumentation of the lumbar spine. *Clinical Orthopaedics and Related Research, 196,* 273.

Gaines, R.W., & Abernathie, D.L. (1986). Mersilene tapes as a substitute for wire in segmental spinal instrumentation for children. *Spine, 11,* 907.

Gau, Y.L., Lonstein, J.E., Winter, R.B., Koop, S., & Denis, F. (1991). Luque-Galveston procedure for correction and stabilization of neuromuscular scoliosis and pelvic obliquity: A review of 68 patients. *Journal of Spinal Disorders, 4,* 399.

Geremia, G.K., Kim, K.S., Cerullo, L., & Calenoff, L. (1985). Complications of sublaminar wiring. *Surgical Neurology, 23,* 629.

Goll, S.R., Balderston, R.A., Stambough, J.L., Booth, R.E., Cohn, J.C., & Pickens, G.T. (1988). Depth of intraspinal wire penetration during passage of sublaminar wires. *Spine, 13,* 503.

Guadagni, J., Drummond, D., & Breed, A. (1984). Improved postoperative course following modified segmental instrumentation and posterior spinal fusion for idiopathic scoliosis. *Journal of Pediatric Orthopedics, 4,* 405.

Guadagni, J.R., & Drummond, D.S. (1986). Strength of surgical wire fixation. *Clinical Orthopaedics and Related Research, 209,* 176.

Gurr, K.R., McAfee, P.C., & Shih, C.M. (1988). Biomechanical analysis of anterior and posterior instrumentation systems after corpectomy. *Journal of Bone and Joint Surgery, American Volume, 70,* 1182–1191.

Heller, J.G., Zdeblick, T.A., Dunz, D.A., McCabe, R., & Cooke, M.E. (1993). Spinal instrumentation for metastatic disease in vitro biomechanical analysis. *Journal of Spinal Disorders, 6,* 17.

Herndon, W.A., Sullivan, J.A., Yngve, D.A., Gross, R.H., & Dreher, G. (1987). Segmental spinal instrumentation with sublaminar wires. *Journal of Bone and Joint Surgery, American Volume, 69,* 851.

Herring, J.A., & Wenger, D.R. (1982). Segmental spinal instrumentation: A preliminary report of 40 consecutive cases. *Spine, 7,* 285.

Kahanovitz, N., Arnoczky, S.P., Levine, D.B., & Otis, J.P. (1984). The effects of internal fixation on the articular cartilage of unfused canine facet joint cartilage. *Spine, 9,* 268.

Kahanovitz, N., Bullough, P., & Jacobs, R.R. (1984). The effect of internal fixation without arthrodesis on human facet joint cartilage. *Clinical Orthopaedics and Related Research,* 189.

King, A.G. (1984). Complications in segmental spinal instrumentation. In: E.R. Luque (Ed.), *Segmental Spinal Instrumentation* (pp. 301–330). Thoroughfare, NJ: Slack.

Kostuik, J.P., Errico, T.J., & Gleason, T.F. (1990). Luque instrumentation in degenerative conditions of the lumbar spine. *Spine, 15,* 318.

Lane, F. (1910). Support for the spondylitic spine by means of buried steel bars, attached to the vertebrae. *American Journal of Orthopedic Surgery, 8,* 344.

Larson, S.J., & Mueller, W. (1990). Segmental fixation of the spine with the Luque rod system. In: N. Sundaresan, H. Schmidek, A. Schiller, & D. Rosenthal (Eds.), *Tumors of the Spine* (pp. 465–472). Philadelphia: W.B. Saunders.

Luque, E.R. (1986). Segmental spinal instrumentation of the lumbar spine. *Clinical Orthopaedics and Related Research, 203,* 126.

Luque, E.R. (1982). The anatomic basis and development of segmental spinal instrumentation. *Spine, 7,* 256.

Luque, E.R. (1982b). The correction of postural curves of the spine. *Spine, 7,* 270.

Luque, E.R. (1982c). Segmental spinal instrumentation for correction of scoliosis. *Clinical Orthopaedics and Related Research, 163,* 192.

Luque, E.R., Cassis, N., & Ramirez-Wiella, G. (1982). Segmental spinal instrumentation in the treatment of fractures of the thoracolumbar spine. *Spine, 7,* 312.

Maiman, D.J., Sances, A., Larson, S.J., Myklebust, J.B., Chilbert, M.A., Nesemann, S.P., & Flately, T.J. (1985). Comparison of the failure biomechanics of spinal fixation devices. *Neurosurgery, 17,* 574.

McAfee, P.C., Werner, F.W., & Glisson, R.R. (1985). A biomechanical analysis of spinal instrumentation systems in thoracolumbar fractures. *Spine, 10,* 204.

McCarthy, R.E., Dunn, H., & McCullough, F.L. (1989). Luque fixation to the sacral ala using the Dunn-McCarthy modification. *Spine, 14,* 281.

McCord, D.H., Cunningham, B.W., Shono, Y., Myers, J.J., & McAfee, P.C. (1992). Biomechanical analysis of lumbosacral fixation. *Spine, 17,* S235.

Nasca, R.J., Hollis, J.M., Lemons, J.E., & Cool, T.A. (1985). Cyclic axial loading of spinal implants. *Spine, 10,* 792.

Nasca, R.J., Lemons, J.M., Walker, J., & Batson, S. (1990). Multiaxis cyclic biomechanical testing of Harrington, Luque, and Drummond implants. *Spine, 15,* 15.

Nicastro, J.F., Hartjen, C.A., Traina, J., & Lancaster, M. (1986). Intraspinal pathways taken by sublaminar wires during removal. *Journal of Bone and Joint Surgery, American Volume, 68,* 1206.

Ogilvie, J.W., & Millar, E.A. (1983). Comparison of segmental spinal instrumentation devices in the correction of scoliosis. *Spine, 8,* 416.

Oh, I., Sander, T.W., & Treharne, R.W. (1985). The fatigue resistance of orthopaedic wire. *Clinical Orthopaedics and Related Research, 192,* 228.

Olson, S.A., & Gaines, R.W. (1987). Removal of sublaminar wires after spinal fusion. *Journal of Bone and Joint Surgery, American Volume, 69,* 1419.

Panjabi, M.M., Abumi, K., Duranceau, J., & Crisco, J.J. (1988). Biomechanical evaluation of spinal fixation devices. II. Stability provided by eight internal fixation devices. *Spine, 13,* 135.

Quint, D.J., & Salton, G. (1993). Migration of Luque rods through a laminectomy defect causing spinal cord compression. *American Journal of Neuroradiology, 14,* 395.

Resina, J., & Ferreira, A. (1977). A technique of correction and internal fixation for scoliosis. *Journal of Bone and Joint Surgery, British Volume, 59,* 159.

Saer, E.H., Winter, R.B., & Lonstein, J.E. (1990). Long scoliosis fusion to the sacrum in adults with nonparalytic scoliosis. *Spine, 15,* 650.

Sasso, R.C., & Cotler, H.B. (1993). Posterior instrumentation and fusion for unstable fractures and fracture-dislocations of the thoracic and lumbar spine. *Spine, 18,* 450.

Schrader, W., Bethem, D., & Scerbin, V. (1989). The chronic effects of sublaminar wires: An animal model. *Orthopedic Transactions, 11,* 106.

Schultz, R.S., Boger, J.W., & Dunn, H.K. (1985). Strength of stainless steel surgical wire in various fixation modes. *Clinical Orthopaedics and Related Research, 198,* 304.

Songer, M.N., Spencer, D.L., Meyer, P.R., & Jayaraman, G. (1991). The use of sublaminar cables to replace Luque wires. *Spine, 16,* S418.

Sullivan, J.A., & Conner, S.B. (1982). Comparison of Harrington instrumentation and segmental spinal instrumentation in the management of neuromuscular spinal deformity. *Spine, 7,* 299–304.

Trent, G., Armstrong, G.W.D., & O'Neil, J.O. (1988). Thoracolumbar fractures in ankylosing spondylitis. *Clinical Orthopaedics and Related Research, 227,* 61.

Weiler, P.J., Mcneice, G.M., & Medley, J.B. (1986). An experimental study of the Buckling behavior of L-rod implants used in the surgical treatment of scoliosis. *Spine, 11,* 992.

Wenger, D.R., Carollo, J.J., & Wilkerson, J.A. (1982). Biomechanics of scoliosis correction by segmental spinal instrumentation. *Spine, 7,* 260.

Wenger, D.R., Carollo, J.J., Wilkerson, J.A., Wauters, K., & Herring, J.A. (1982). Laboratory testing of segmental spinal instrumentation versus traditional Harrington instrumentation for scoliosis treatment. *Spine, 7,* 265.

Wilber, G., Thompson, G.H., Shaffer, J.W., Brown, R.H., & Nash, C.L. (1984). Postoperative neurological deficits in segmental spinal instrumentation. *Journal of Bone and Joint Surgery, American Volume, 66,* 1178.

Yngve, D.A., Burke, S.W., Price, C.T., & Riddick, M.F. (1986). Sublaminar wiring. *Journal of Pediatric Orthopedics, 6,* 605–608.

Zindrick, M.R., Knight, G.W., Bunch, W.H., Miller, M.C., Butler, D.M., Lorenz, M., & Behal R. (1989). Factors influencing the penetration of wires into the neural canal during segmental wiring. *Journal of Bone and Joint Surgery, American Volume, 71,* 742–750.

CHAPTER 26

Utilization of the Texas Scottish Rite Hospital Universal System for Stabilization of the Thoracic and Lumbar Spine

Richard G. Fessler
Michael Sturgill

HIGHLIGHTS

The Texas Scottish Rite Hospital (TSRH) Universal Instrumentation System developed out of attempts to resolve the problem of rod migration, noted particularly during attempted corrections of scoliosis of neuromuscular etiology and cases with pelvis obliquity. Biomechanical testing demonstrated that "locking" the rods together would prevent rod migration, thus the cross-link, which has become one of the trademarks of the TSRH system, was developed for use with the Luque L-rod/sublaminar wire system.

In 1986 the Cotrel Dubousset (CD) system was introduced to the United States. Many of the CD innovations were similar to concepts incorporated into prior experiments performed at the Texas Scottish Rite Hospital and solved several of the problems noted with Harrington and/or Luque systems (e.g., flat-back syndrome from two-point fixation). Therefore, the surgeons at the Texas Scottish Rite Hospital began using the CD system for corrective spinal surgery, but requested the cross-link system as an addition to the CD instrumentation. This request, as well as requests directed toward different hook and screw designs, led to the development of a complete, independent TSRH spinal instrumentation system.

There are several benefits of the TSRH system. First, as with all "universal" systems, it allows for immediate "segmental" stabilization of the spine. This can be accomplished even in the absence of laminae, by using a combination of pedicle screws, pedicle hooks, and transverse process hooks. Second, because it is a "rod" and not a "plate" system, it provides a larger posterolateral surface area for bony fusion. Third, the side-bolt locking assembly and the top-loading system are relatively easy to use. Finally, since all components of the system are fully removable without destroying any component of the system, revision surgery is easier than with previous systems.

This chapter will emphasize use of the TSRH universal instrumentation system. In discussing the use of this system we will first consider indications for instrumentation of the thoracolumbar spine. Thereafter, the specific techniques used with this system will be discussed. Finally, the results and complications of the University of Florida series will be presented.

INDICATIONS

The general indications for fusion and instrumentation of the spine are to (1) provide stability to the unstable spine, (2) prevent injury to neurologic structures, (3) decrease malalignment and deformity, (4) improve the probability of fusion, and (5) decrease long-term pain. The efficacy of spinal instrumentation systems in providing stability, preventing injury, decreasing malalignment and deformity, and improving the probability of fusion has previously been reviewed (Fessler, 1992). Furthermore, the influence of spinal fusion on back versus radicular pain has also previously been discussed (Dickman, Fessler, MacMillan, & Haid, 1992). These topics, therefore, will not be repeated here. This chapter will focus on the indications for stabilization of specific pathologic conditions.

Instability can be associated with various pathologic lesions, such as trauma, tumor, infection, spondylolysis/spondylolisthesis, degenerative spine disease, iatrogenic spinal instability, pseudarthrosis, and deformity. The indications for rigid fixation using TSRH are clear in certain pathologic conditions and less clear, or even controversial, in others. The controversy results from a relative lack of prospective, randomized evaluations, specifically addressing each pathologic condition. Many of these studies are currently underway, or are in the planning stages, thus data from them are not available at time of publication. Therefore, the indications discussed below represent those generally accepted based on the available retrospective data.

Trauma

Table 26-1 compares the classification of instability schemes of Denis (1983) and McAfee (1983) and indicates recommended treatments. In general, it can be seen that trauma that results in injury to two (or three) of three columns (McAfee) or the posterior ligamentous complex (Denis) produces a spinal injury that is sufficiently unstable to require surgical stabilization.

Tumors

Indications for stabilization of spinal tumors are listed in Table 26-2. Primary and metastatic tumors of the spinal column cause pain, instability, deformity, and neurologic deficits. The goals of surgery are to relieve pain, decompress the neural elements, and provide immediate mechanical stability. The approach and fusion technique may be anterior, posterior, or a combination of the two. Since the vertebral body is involved in 85 percent of spinal metastases, the benefit of the anterior approach for adequate decompression and fusion is clear. The definition of instability for tumors of the spinal column follows the three-column theory of Denis (1983).

Infection

Spinal stabilization may be necessary in cases of osteomyelitis in which more than 50% of the vertebral body is eroded, or in which aggressive surgical debridement is expected to produce an unstable spine (Table 26-2). Progressive angulation and new or increasing neurologic deficit are additional indications for instrumentation in spinal infections. Traditionally, however, debridement and stabilization were performed as separate procedures, with a long delay between the two to minimize the possibility of infecting the rods. A recent analysis by Dietze, Fessler, and Jacob (submitted for publication, 1995) has demonstrated that primary reconstruction with TSRH instrumentation for spinal infections can be safely performed, in conjunction with parenteral/oral antibiotics, without further infection of the inserted bone graft or instrumentation material.

Spondylolysis/Spondylolisthesis

The indications for surgery and fusion in spondylolisthesis are persistent pain unresponsive to conservative therapy,

Table 26-1
Classification Schemes of Spinal Instability as Defined by Denis (1983) and McAfee (1983)

Fracture types		Spinal column failure			Assessment of stability	
Denis	McAfee	Anterior	Middle	Posterior	McAfee	Denis
Wedge compression	Wedge compression	F°			Generally stable*	Stable†
Seatbelt-type injury	Chance fracture		F	F	Generally stable‡	Unstable§
	Flexion-distraction injury	F	F	F	Generally unstable	
Burst fracture	Stable burst	F	F		Stable	Unstable‖
	Unstable burst	F	F	F	Unstable	
Fracture dislocation	Translational injury	F	F	F	Unstable	Unstable¶

*Multiple-level wedge compression fractures may require surgical therapy.
†Potential mechanical instability seen with severe wedge fractures. This instability does not acutely threaten the neural elements.
§Potential mechanical instability.
‖Burst fractures are either neurologically unstable or both mechanically and neurologically unstable.
¶Fracture dislocations are both mechanically and neurologically unstable.
‡Unstable if there is facet dislocation, subluxation, or facet fractures.
°Indicates usual column injured for each fracture type.

Table 26-2
Indications for Spinal Stabilization for Tumors and Infections

Tumors
   Loss of anterior and middle column stability resulting from tumor infiltration
      Vertebral collapse, or progressive angulation
      Soft-tissue retropulsion into canal
      Spondylolisthesis or scoliosis
      Previous laminectomy
      New or progressive neurologic deficit
   Iatrogenic instability following vertebrectomy and anterior reconstruction

Infection
   Loss of anterior and middle column stability resulting from destructive inflammatory process
      Vertebral collapse or progressive angulation
      Spondylolisthesis or scoliosis
      Previous laminectomy
      New or progressive neurologic deficit
   Iatrogenic instability following aggressive anterior debridement and anterior reconstruction

Table 26-3
Indications for Fusion and Stabilization of the Spine in Degenerative Disease

Spondylolysis/spondylolisthesis
   Neurologic deficit
   Progressive subluxation
   Persistent pain unresponsive to conservative therapy
Translational instability
   Forward displacement on plain standing x-ray films
   Persistent or recurrent low back pain or claudication
   Relatively preserved disk space
   Minimal bridging osteophyte
   More than 8 degrees of motion on flexion-extension x-ray films
Retrolisthetic instability
   Posterior displacement on plain standing x-ray films
   Deformity increases/decreases during flexion-extension x-ray films
   Lateral recess symptoms
Torsional instability
   Same as translational instability
   Spinous process malalignment
   "Pedicle-to-pedicle" defect
Disk degeneration
   Recurrent disk disruption
   Diskographic disk disruption with reproduction of symptoms
Degenerative scoliosis
   Progressive curve over time on standing x-ray films
   Increasing symptoms of stenosis
   Translation on lateral standing x-ray films
   Rotational deformity
   Potentially destabilizing surgery

progressive subluxation, and neurologic deficit (see Table 26-3). The indications for reduction are slippage greater than 75% and slip angle greater than 45 degrees.

Degenerative Disease

Segmental instability resulting from spinal degeneration is a controversial topic. Although several classification schemes exist, Frymoyer and Selby (1985) have done extensive work to provide a classification scheme that clearly defines the different types of degenerative disease processes, and they recommend criteria for fusion and stabilization. Frymoyer and Selby define segmental instability as a loss of motion segment stiffness such that force applied to that motion segment produces greater displacements than would occur in a normal segment. Frymoyer and Selby divide degenerative disease into two major categories: primary degenerative instability and fixed deformity. Based on clinical, radiographic, and biomechanical data, they further divide primary degenerative instability into translational, retrolisthetic, torsional, disk disruption, and scoliotic degeneration. They subdivide fixed deformity into degenerative spondylolisthesis, fixed retrolisthesis, disk space collapse, and fixed scoliotic deformity. Table 26-3 lists the guidelines recommended by Frymoyer and Selby for stabilization of each of the primary degenerative processes. Indications for fusion in translational instability include: (1) forward displacements on plain standing films, (2) persistent or recurrent low back pain or claudication, (3) relatively preserved disk space, (4) minimal bridging osteophytes, and (5) greater than 8 degrees of motion on flexion-extension x-ray films. Indications for fusion of retrolisthetic instability include: (1) posterior displacements on plain, standing x-ray films, (2) deformity increases/decreases during flexion-extension x-ray films, and (3) lateral recess symptoms. In addition to the same indications as for translational instability, fusion for torsional instability is also recommended for spinous process malalignment, and myelographic "pedicle-to-pedicle" defect. Fusion should be considered for disk degeneration in the presence of recurrent disk herniations and diskographic disk disruption with symptom reproduction. Finally, for degenerative scoliosis, indications for fusion include: (1) progressive curve over time on standing x-ray films, (2) increasing symptoms of stenosis, (3) translation on lateral standing x-ray films, (4) rotational deformity, and (5) potentially destabilizing surgery.

Table 26-4 lists the indications for fusion and stabilization for "secondary" instability. Secondary instability can be divided into four general categories: (1) post–disk excision, (2) postdecompression, (3) postspinal fusion,

Table 26-4
Indications for Fusion and Stabilization for "Secondary" Instability

Instability following:
   Disk excision
      Increasing deformity over time
      Recurrent disk herniation
   Decompressive laminectomy
      Accentuation of preexisting deformity
      Multiple-level decompression in the presence of scoliotic deformity
   Previous fusion
      Progressive degenerative spondylolisthesis
      Symptoms of stenosis
      Pseudarthrosis
         Visible defect on x-ray films
         Relief of symptoms by injection of local anesthetic
         More than 4 degrees of motion on flexion-extension x-ray films
         Recurrent disk herniation

adjacent levels, and (4) postfusion pseudarthrosis. Indications for stabilization following disk excision include increasing deformity over time and recurrent disk herniation. Following decompressive laminectomy, indications for stabilization include accentuation of preexisting deformity and multiple-level decompression in the presence of scoliotic deformity. Indications for stabilization following a previous fusion are progressive degenerative spondylolisthesis, symptoms of stenosis, and pseudarthrosis. Pseudarthrosis is suggested when there is a visible defect on x-ray films, relief of symptoms by injection of local anesthetic into the defect, more than 4 degrees of motion on flexion-extension x-ray films, and recurrent disk herniation.

INSTRUMENTATION

The TSRH universal instrumentation system consists of a series of rods, screws, hooks, and cross-links, with the application devices described below. All components are available in either stainless steel or titanium. All TSRH screws, hooks, and cross-link plates use a "three-point shear clamp" locking mechanism to attach to the spinal rods. Axial and torsional strength in static strength testing has been superior or equal to that of similar systems (Ashman, Herring, Johnston, Lowery, & Sutterlin 1993). Advantages and disadvantages of the TSRH System are listed in Table 26-5.

Rods

Rod strength and fatigue resistance have been enhanced by "shot peening" surface treatment. All rods have hexagonal ends to facilitate rod rotation with a small wrench. Three rod stiffnesses are available: $\frac{3}{16}$ TSRH, $\frac{1}{4}$ flex TSRH, and $\frac{1}{4}$ rigid. The rigid $\frac{1}{4}$-in. rod is similar in stiffness to the Harrington rod. The type of rod selected for use is judged based on an assessment of the stiffness of the deformity, the weight and size of the patient, and the length of time until fusion is anticipated.

Screws

TSRH screws come in two head styles: fixed angle (Fig. 26-1) and variable angle (Fig. 26-2). Outer diameters are 5.5, 6.5, 7.5, and 8.5 mm. Three locking assemblies are available: shear clamp locking eyebolt and nut assembly for the fixed and variable angle screws, a serrated spacer attachment unique to TSRH for the variable-angle screw, and a top-tightening variable-angle screw (Fig. 26-3). Serrations allow angle changes in 6-degree increments, offering many degrees of angulation. Three offset sizes in the eyebolt minimize necessary rod bending by accepting a variable amount of displacement between the rod and the screw. To minimize pullout, all threads have the standard cancellous thread pattern. Because biomechanical data indicate that the shank of the screw is the most prone to fatigue and breakage, TSRH has increased the diameter of this location and tapered the upper threads.

Hooks

TSRH hooks come in various sizes and shapes (large, small, and pediatric) (Fig. 26-4). There are two top configurations—full top and central post. Both use the same eyebolts for connection, and strength is equal in both types of hook-top configurations. Hooks are designed to mirror specific

Table 26-5
Advantages and Disadvantages of TSRH Universal System

Advantages
  Segmental stabilization of spine
  Top-loading or side-loading hooks and screws
  Titanium or stainless steel
  Rod contouring minimized with variable-angle screw
  Relatively fewer number of pieces
  Easily applied, stable cross-link
  Extending or removing systems easily performed
  Improved bone surface for fusion

Disadvantages
  Does not perform reductions in complex scoliosis cases easily
  Top-loading hooks can be difficult to use
  Eye bolts for assembly must be preplanned and applied to rod before connecting to hooks and screws.

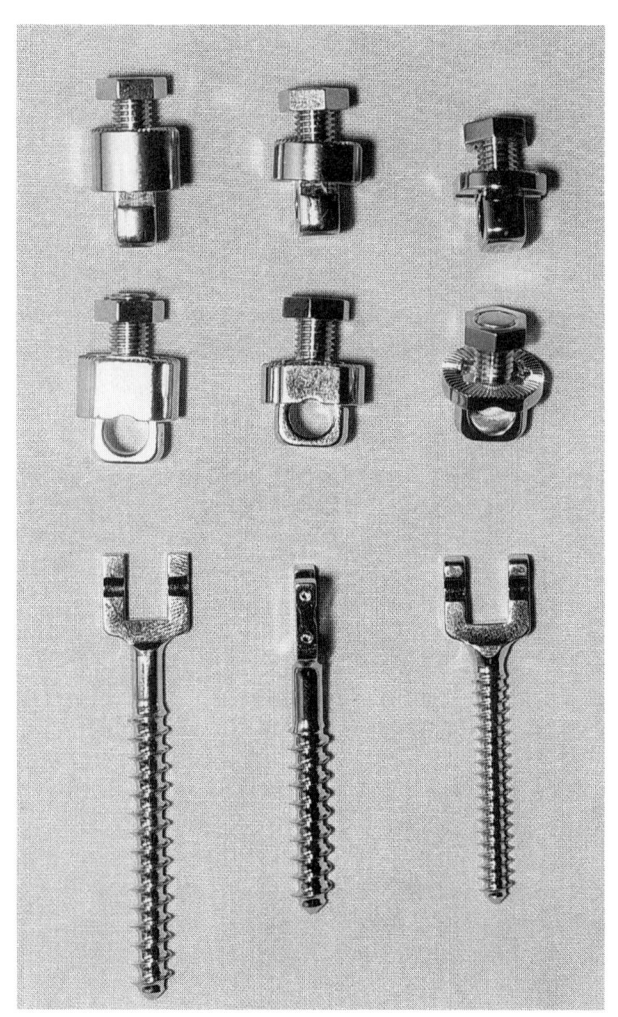

FIG. 26-1. TSRH variable-angle eyebolts of 0, 3, and 6 mm offset for use with variable angle screws (*top*). Examples of TSRH fixed-angle screws, 5.5- and 6.5-mm diameters (*bottom*).

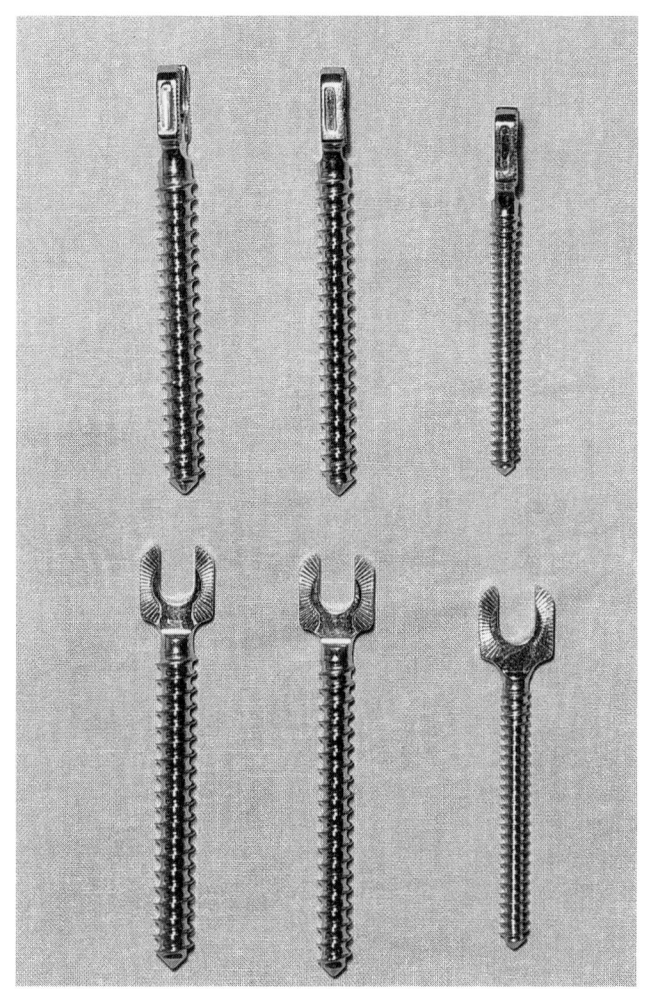

FIG. 26-2. Examples of TSRH variable-angle screws, 5.5-, 6.5-, and 7.5-mm diameters.

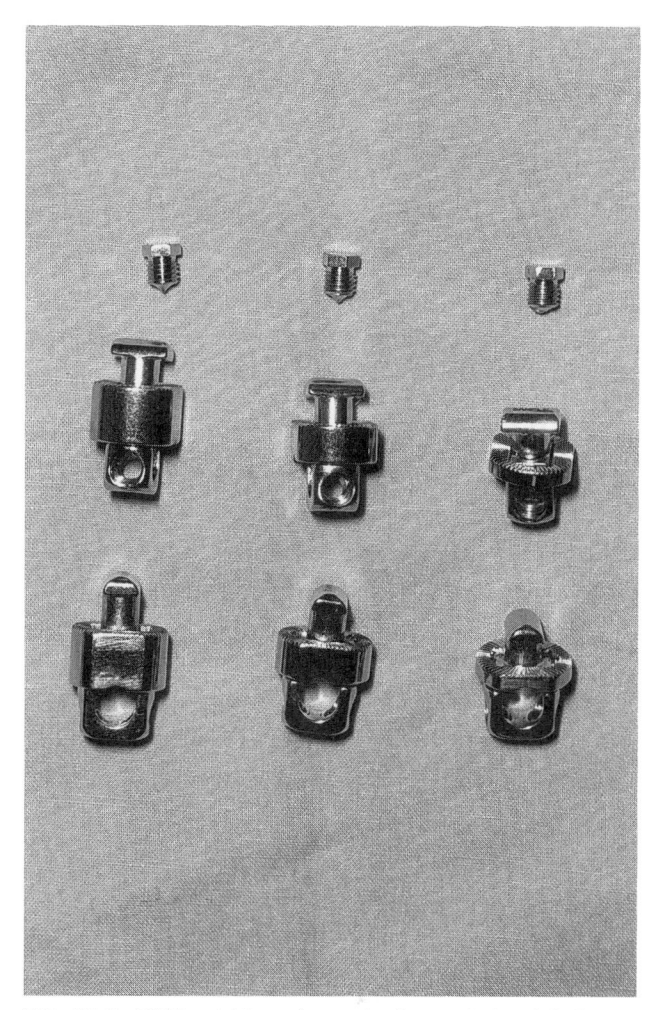

FIG. 26-3. TSRH variable-angle, top-loading eyebolts of 0, 3, and 6 mm offset.

vertebral structures anatomically. Thus, the laminar, pedicle, and transverse process hooks contour to the laminae, pedicles, and transverse processes, respectively. Finally, lumbar laminar hooks come in standard and elevated sizes. Standard (round) laminar hooks are perhaps the most versatile, fitting many aspects of the posterior elements without infringing significantly into the canal. Round elevated hooks allow closer placement to the midline. Cranial and caudal angled hooks are used to attach to lumbar laminae in lumbar claw constructs.

Cross-Links

Axial and torsional forces are more significant than transverse forces between rods. Cross-links prevent rod migration and enhance rigidity of the system (Fig. 26-5). The cross-link uses the same eyebolt locking mechanism as hooks and screws. One-half-inch nuts are used with cross-link plates. This provides a broad, smooth surface, which minimizes sharp edges on areas of skin prominence. Care must taken to ensure that eyebolts for cross-link plates are placed on the rod in the desired position prior to setting all hooks and/or screws. Split eyebolts can be used with cross-link plates if all other hooks and screws are already in place.

The strength of the split eyebolt is comparable to the regular eyebolts. Mechanical testing has demonstrated that two cross-link plates create a construct as rigid as three cross-link plates. One cross-link plate should be located at the superior end of the construct, caudal to the top hook, while the other cross-link is placed at the lower end of the construct above the bottom hook or pelvic fixation instrumentation. Cross-links should not be applied at the point of maximum curve on the rods (due to stress and skin prominence). In short constructs a single cross-link is adequate. Cross-link plates can be bent or torqued about their axis with the cross-link benders.

Instrumentation Application

Instruments used in applying the above hooks, screws and rods are important adjuncts, and a familiarity with their use can be time-saving and important in the quality of the ultimate construct. The TSRH spinal implant system is specific for TSRH implants. Hook holders are designed to ensure a positive attachment to the hooks and screws, and are color coded by size (Fig. 26-6). Eyebolts and rods can be inserted with the hook holders in place. Trial hook holders can be used for site preparation. All, except the transverse process

278 PART 4 / POSTERIOR THORACOLUMBAR INSTRUMENTATION

hook trial, are angled at 30 degrees. The trials can serve as laminar elevators and pedicle finders, but because they are shaped like hooks they are less likely to invade the spinal canal. The minicorkscrew can be used with hooks and screws to reduce the rod downward so that the eyebolt aligns properly with the top of the hook or screw. Excessive force usually means the rod has been poorly contoured. In situ benders are provided but the entire rod can also be easily removed, recontoured, and reapplied.

The three-point shear clamp mechanism provides significant resistance to axial, torsional, and shear forces, as long as the nut is torqued down to 150 in.-lb. Top-tightening screws should be torqued to 100 in.-lb. Several wrenches, (i.e., open and closed face, 10 in. long) are provided to facilitate tightening the nuts. Applying a force of 150 in.-lb can cause the patient to move on the table if the construct is not stabilized. An in situ bender, rod pusher, or vice clamp can be used to secure the rods during final tightening. It is better to overtighten the rod then to undertighten it.

The instrumentation system developed through Texas Scottish Rite Hospital has been demonstrated to be highly versatile in many pathologic conditions. Versatility of the TSRH system can be noted by the ability to build hybrid constructs such as lumbar screws with thoracic or laminar hooks all attached to the same rod. Revision screws and variable-angle screws also add to the versatility. One can also couple a preexisting rod construct to a revision construct through the use of cross-link offset plates or cross-link axial plates. Differing hook sizes, angle screws, and different rod sizes allow for multiple positions in which the rods can be applied.

SURGICAL TECHNIQUE

Techniques for placement of the TSRH system follow general guidelines, but will vary in the design of the construct

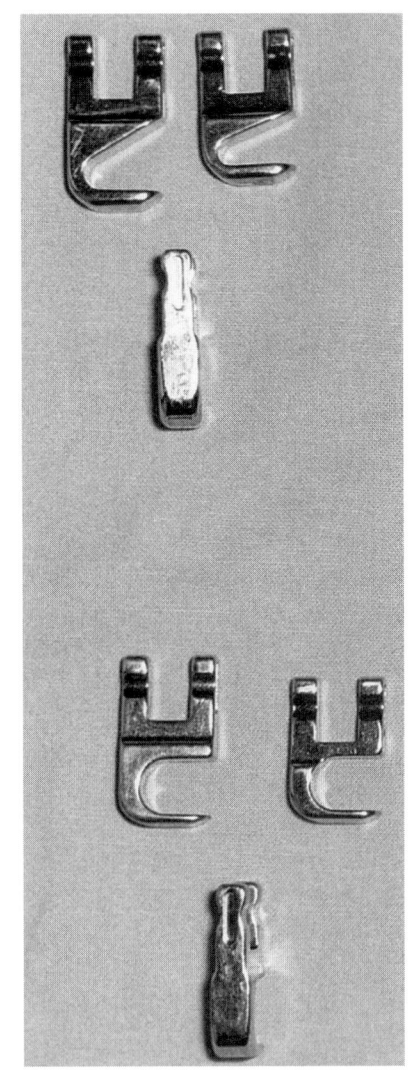

FIG. 26-4. TSRH hook alternatives: *Top*, Thoracic laminar and small thoracic laminar. *Bottom*, Large and elevated laminar hooks.

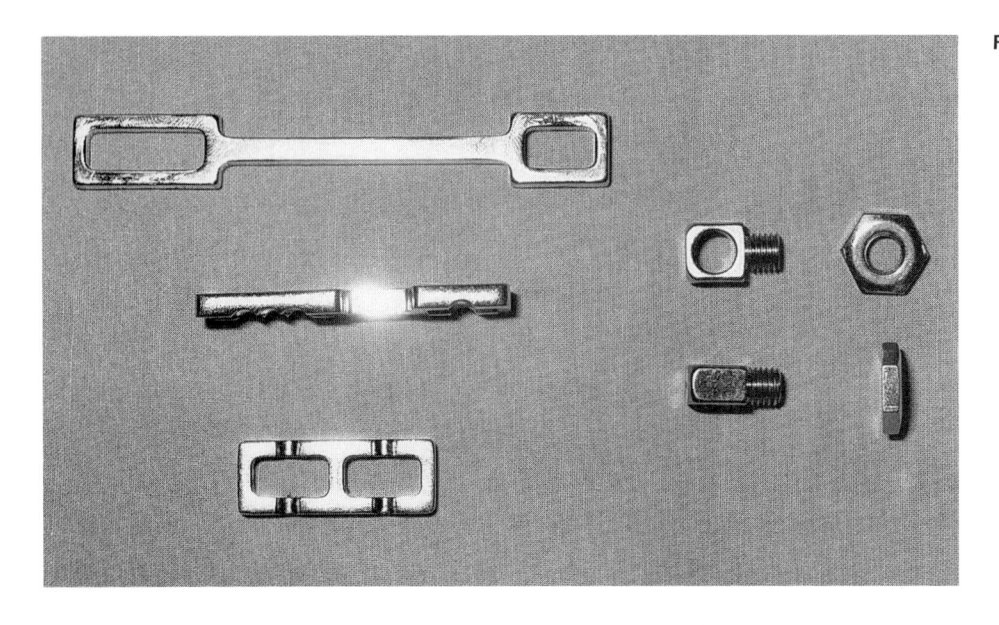

FIG. 26-5. TSRH cross-link assembly.

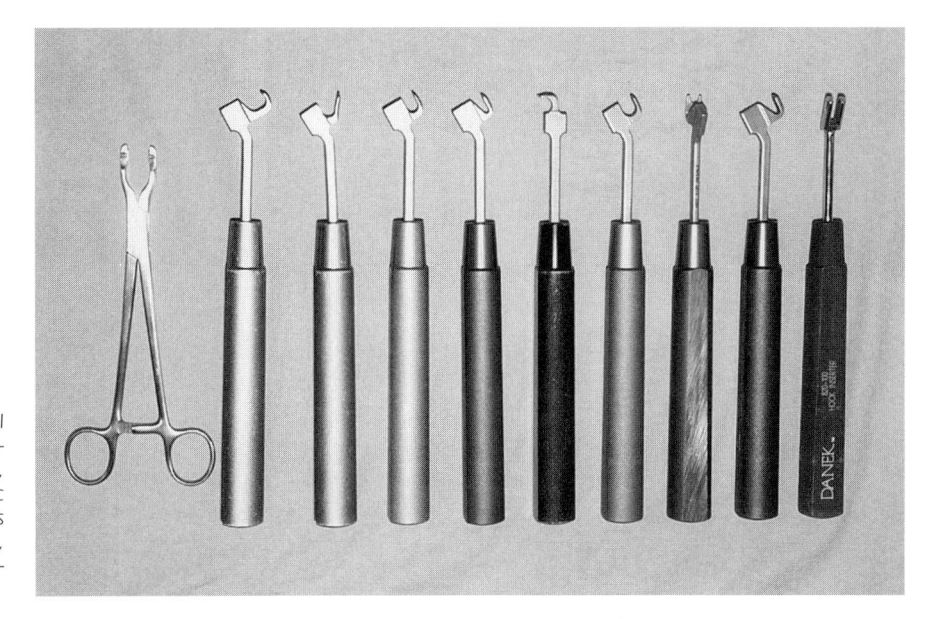

FIG. 26-6. TSRH hook-holder and trial hook inserters. *Left to right,* Cranial angle hook trial, caudal angle hook trial, small laminar hook trial, small thoracic laminar hook trial, transverse process hook trial, large laminar hook trial, pedicle hook trial, large thoracic laminar hook trial, and hook-inserter.

depending on the location of the pathology. For example, pedicle screws are thought to be stronger in the lumbar spine and lower thoracic spine. The pedicles of the midthoracic spine are thought to be too small to accommodate the screws safely. Consequently, hooks are usually used in the mid to upper thoracic spine.

Patient Positioning and Exposure

All patients receive general endotracheal anesthesia, pneumatic compression stockings, and appropriate arterial lines, prior to being turned prone onto the radiolucent operating room table. Prophylactic antibiotics are begun before surgery and continued for 48 hours after surgery. Whenever possible, autologous blood is donated in advance, and a cell saver is used in all cases, unless contraindicated. An adjustable fluoroscopic image intensifier and patient frames or chest rolls are used to permit intraoperative anteroposterior, oblique, and lateral fluoroscopy of the spine. Patients are positioned prone on the operating table, with the thorax supported laterally to avoid epidural venous distention from abdominal compression. An appropriate midline thoracic or lumbar incision is made, extending 2 to 3 in. above and below the segments to be instrumented. Subperiosteal dissection to the lateral tips of the transverse processes of the segments to be fused is performed to maximize available bone surface for fusion. Prior to posterior instrumentation, neural decompression and/or vertebral body reconstruction are performed as indicated.

Pedicle Preparation and Screw Placement

After exposure and decompression of the spine, the external landmarks over the pedicles are identified. Pedicle identification, hole preparation, and screw placement are performed under fluoroscopic guidance.

In the lumbar spine, the external landmark for the pedicle is the intersection of the axial plane through the middle of the transverse process and the sagittal plane through the superior facet (Fig. 26-7). Identification of the facet complex is facilitated by moving the spinous process with a Kocher clamp and then removing the soft tissue from the surface of the superior facet. In the thoracic spine, it is best to rely on fluoroscopy to identify the pedicle.

A Steinmann pin is then placed over this point of intersection and the correct entry position is verified radiographically by orienting the pin along the axis of the central portion of the pedicle. On anteroposterior (or slightly oblique) fluoroscopic images, the pedicle and aligned pin appear as a "bull's eye" or "target sign" within an oval pedicle (Fig. 26-8). The cortical point of intersection can then be entered with either a high-speed drill or Leksell rongeur, and the pin twisted down into the cancellous bone of the pedicle to the desired depth of the vertebral body in preparation for the screw placement. A Steinmann pin with a diameter corresponding to the minor diameter of the screw is used (for example, a $\frac{9}{64}$-in. pin for a 5.5-mm screw or a $\frac{5}{32}$-in. pin for a 6.5-mm screw), and the placement is facilitated by holding the pin with a Jacob chuck. This procedure is repeated at each pedicle, and the final anteroposterior orientation of each pin is assessed fluoroscopically. The progress of pin and screw penetration into the vertebral body is monitored using lateral imaging. This procedure minimizes the possibility of malpositioning any screw.

Sacral screw sites are prepared in a manner similar to this. The external anatomical landmarks differ from the thoracic and lumbar region since the sacrum had no transverse processes. Manipulating the L-5 spinous process helps to identify the L5-S1 facet. Soft-tissue dissection delineates the first dorsal sacral foramina and the osseous

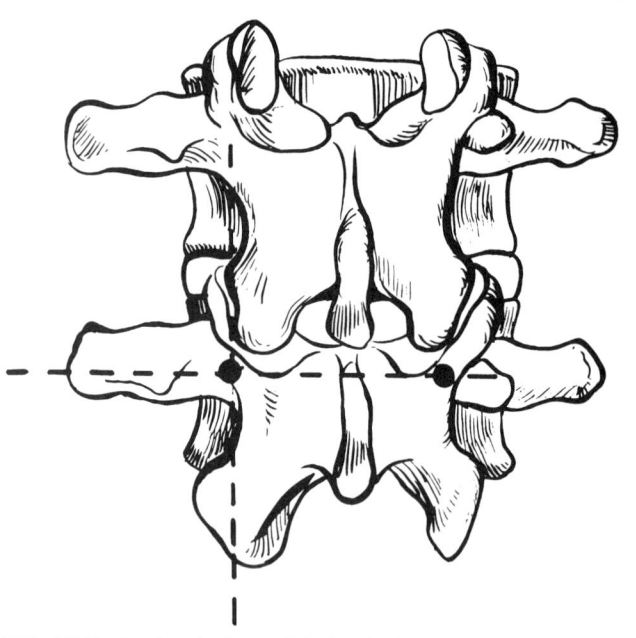

280 PART 4 / POSTERIOR THORACOLUMBAR INSTRUMENTATION

FIG. 26-7. Landmarks for pedicle localization in lumbar spine (see text).

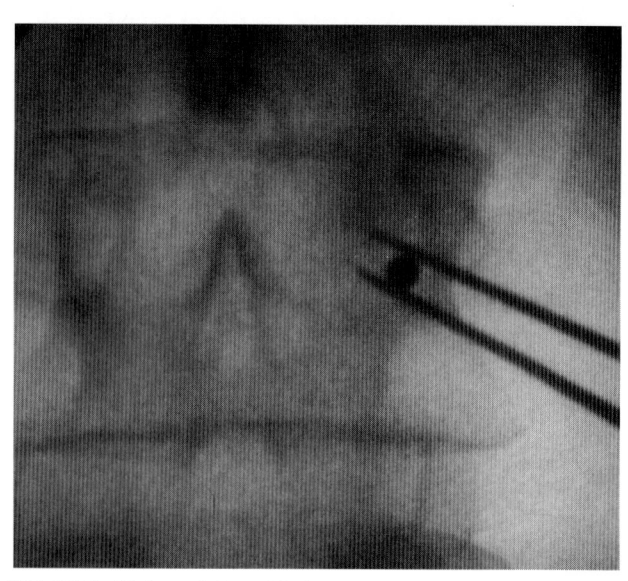

FIG. 26-8. "Bulls-eye" sign of Steinmann pin correctly positioned over pedicle.

recession caudal to the L5-S1 facets. The external landmark for the first sacral pedicle is located at the inferolateral portion of the superior S1 facet (Fig. 26-9). The correct entry sites into the S1 pedicles are fluoroscopically verified.

Each pin is manually positioned parallel to the end plate of the vertebrae; however, penetration into the adjacent disk space should be avoided. This maneuver requires a vertical orientation for the thoracic and lumbar spine and a 30-degree caudal angle for the sacrum. The medial trajectory corresponds to the angle of the pedicles at each level. Penetration of the pin through the hard pedicle into the soft cancellous bone of the vertebral body provides a distinct feel, with a reduction in resistance.

After all pins are placed into the vertebral bodies to create tracks for the screws, the Steinmann pins are removed, and the superficial 5- to 10-mm area of each track is enlarged with a drill or bone awl. This allows the threads of the pedicle screw to engage a purchase on the bone.

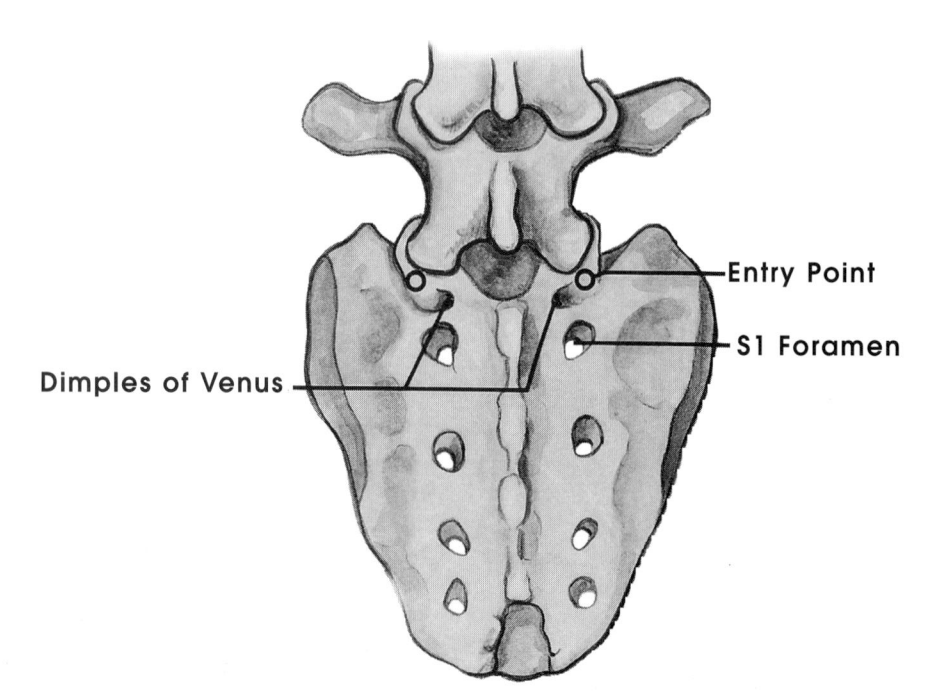

FIG. 26-9. Landmark for pedicle localization in sacrum (see text).

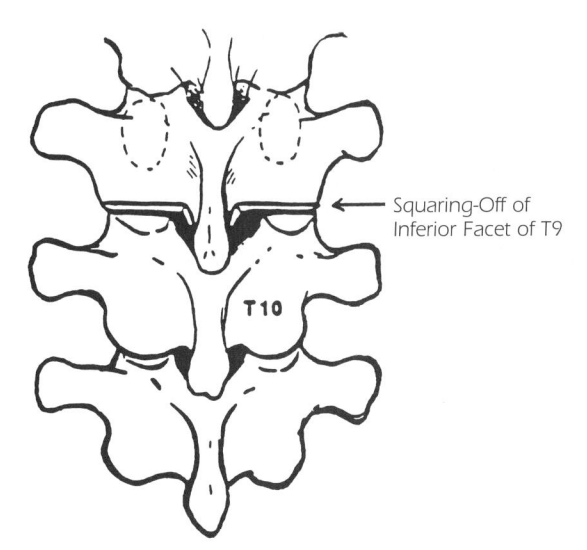

FIG. 26-10. Thoracic facet appropriately prepared for placement of pedicle hook.

Pedicle screw sizes are preselected on the basis of the characteristics of the particular vertebra on computed tomography. The screws are placed into the prepared holes with a trajectory identical to that of the Steinmann pins. Screw purchase is obtained by advancing the screw with a screwdriver, penetrating 70 to 80% of the vertebral body. To avoid injury to the vascular and visceral structures anterior to the vertebral column, the anterior portion of the vertebral body is not penetrated. Throughout the procedure, the progress, depth, and position of the screws is monitored.

Hook Site Preparation and Placement

Hook sites for pedicle screws have the advantage of being mechanically strong while not violating the sublaminar space. The blade of the pedicle hook is bifid. This configuration allows it to "cradle" into the pedicle above. The entrance site for the pedicle hook is through the facet complex, aiming cephalad under the inferior facet of the vertebra above toward the attached pedicle. In order to ensure that the mouth of the hook lies flush against the lamina, it is necessary to "square off" the inferior laminar edge (Fig. 26-10). This can be performed with a small osteotome or a high-speed drill. Only a small amount of the medial inferior laminae should be removed to make certain the hook engages the lamina. Once the inferior laminar edge is removed, the facet joint space is entered with a small freer. The pedicle hook trial is now taken and placed into the facet joint. Care is taken to avoid entering and splitting the lamina above. The pedicle hook trial is advanced cephalad until it engages the pedicle. The trial is manipulated to ensure adequate seating and is then removed. The pedicle hook is then placed into the holder and the pusher placed into the hook. This construct is placed into the pedicle hook site and forced superiorly to engage the pedicle above (Fig. 26-11).

Downward-facing "transverse process" hooks are inserted over the superior edge of the transverse process. This hook position is used primarily as the top half of a "claw" fixation construct at the superior end of the rod. After the transverse process is identified, the superior edge is cleared of soft tissues. A small angled curette is then placed on the anterior surface of the transverse process in a small triangular space. The floor and lateral surface of

FIG. 26-11. Placement of pedicle hook against cephalad pedicle.

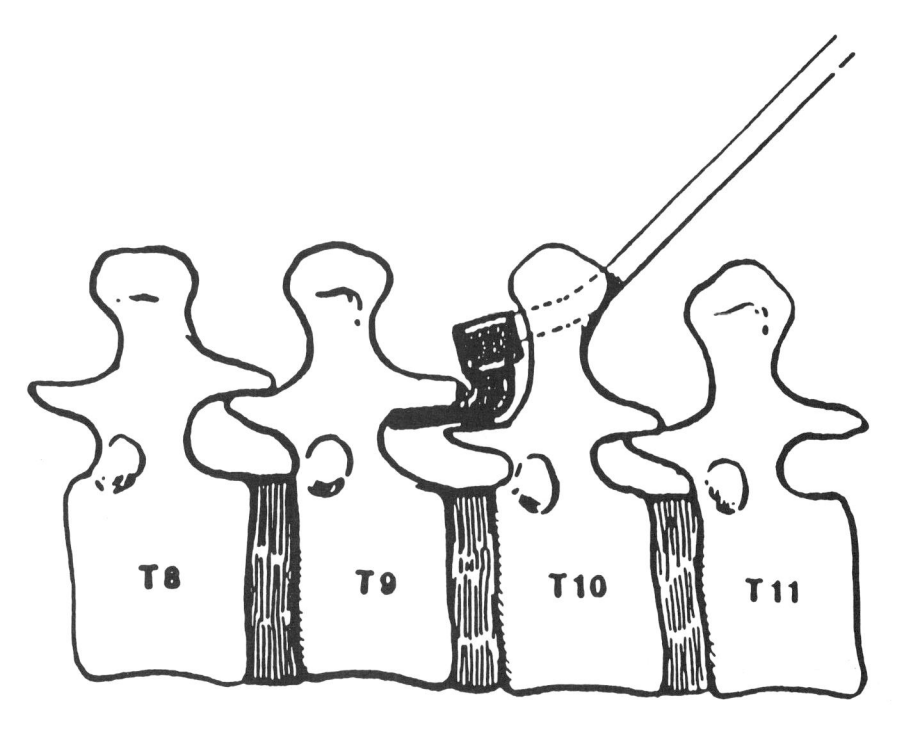

this space is the adjoining rib. It is into this space that the transverse process hook will be placed. The transverse process trial hook is then placed into this triangular space. After firm seating is ensured, the actual transverse process hook is firmly grasped in a hook-holder. With the hook grasped, a hook-pusher is placed in the hook. This combination is used to insert the hook blade into the prepared space (Fig. 26-12).

The thoracic and lumbar laminar hooks can be placed against the inferior or superior edge of the lamina. These positions are used in "claw" constructs in the lumbar spine, and inferiorly facing thoracic laminar hooks can be used in combination with pedicle hooks for a claw in the thoracic spine. The laminar hooks are placed by performing interlaminar laminotomies and slightly widening them laterally. In the thoracic spine it is usually necessary to remove the medial aspect of the superior facets. An angled curette is used to remove the ligamentum from the lamina and sublaminar space. A laminar trial hook is then fitted into the space created. After the laminar hook is grasped with a hook-holder, a hook-pusher is used to insert the hook into position. It may be best to rotate the hook underneath the lamina to avoid dipping it into the spinal canal. The hook purchase should be checked manually.

Construct Assembly

A malleable wire or sterile endotracheal tube stylet is used as a template to approximate the desired rod curvature. The rods are selected, cut to the desired length, and bent to match the contour of the template. An S-shaped curve is used for thoracolumbar rods and a lordotic curve for lumbar or lumbosacral rods. The rods are then connected to the pedicle screws or hooks by attaching the eyebolts to the rods and tightening the nut assemblies.

Final adjustments in rod contour are achieved with in situ rod benders. Hook-holders, corkscrew devices, wrenches, and a variety of other tools help to connect the rods, screws, and hooks. Spinal reductions are performed and instruments can be placed under compression, distraction, or in a neutral position as indicated. Cross-links can then be used to connect the right and left rods as described above. All connections of the screws, hooks, rods, and cross-links are then securely tightened for final fixation.

Fusion Site Preparation and Wound Closure

The fusion site, which extends over the entire length of the instrumentation system, is usually prepared prior to rod placement. After all soft tissue is removed from the surface of the fusion bed, the transverse processes, facet joints, and other bone fusion surfaces are decorticated using a high-speed drill. The articular surfaces of the facet joints are curetted or drilled to remove the cartilage, and cancellous bone grafts are packed into the facets. The rods are then placed and the wound is thoroughly irrigated with bacitracin solution. Cancellous bone and/or cortical matchstick grafts are then placed over the transverse processes and facets for a posterolateral fusion. Autogenous iliac bone is the preferred grafting material. Closed suction drainage systems are then placed and the wound is closed in multiple layers.

Postoperatively, patients with thoracic or lumbar fusions wear an appropriate thoracic or thoracolumbar orthosis for 3 to 6 months. Patients with lumbosacral fusion wear an orthosis with one thigh immobilized. Ambulation is begun within the first few postoperative days, after which progressive rehabilitative therapy is undertaken.

RESULTS

Patient Population

The results of pedicle screw instrumentation in 104 patients who underwent the procedure at the University of Florida between 1987 and 1991 were reported (Dickman et al., 1992). Details of the patient population were reported else-

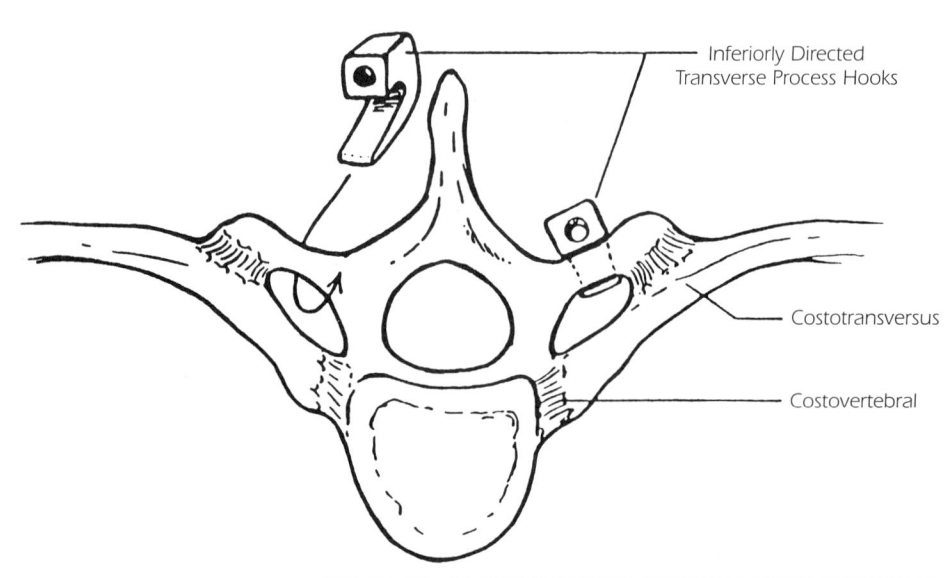

FIG. 26-12. Appropriate position of thoracic transverse process hook.

where and will not be repeated here. The pathologic conditions responsible for their instability were fractures in 28 patients, isthmic or degenerative spondylolisthesis in 29, primary or metastatic neoplasms in 4, vertebral osteomyelitis in 2, and postsurgical instability after operations for spinal stenosis in 26. Approximately two-thirds of these patients had TSRH instrumentation. One third received CD instrumentation.

Neurologic Function and Back Pain

Neurologic improvement occurred in 85 of 96 patients presenting with deficits. In 73 patients with nerve-root or cauda equina compression, 66 experienced improved motor function or resolution of radicular pain; 49 of these patients recovered normal function. Improved motor function or sensation (average recovery, 1.6 Frankel grades) was experienced by 19 of 23 patients with spinal cord or conus medullaris compression; 5 of these patients recovered normal function.

The resolution of back pain was more variable than neurologic recovery. The criteria for evaluation was based on the patients' subjective responses regarding limitations due to their back symptoms. Severe, incapacitating back pain was present preoperatively in the entire patient population. Postoperatively, 20 patients had excellent relief of back pain, 57 had moderate back pain, and 19 had severe, persistent pain.

Fusion Rate

At long-term follow-up examination (10 to 50 months postoperatively), 96% of the patients had osseous union. These patients demonstrated solid, continuous radiographic fusion masses on plain radiographic studies or tomography and had

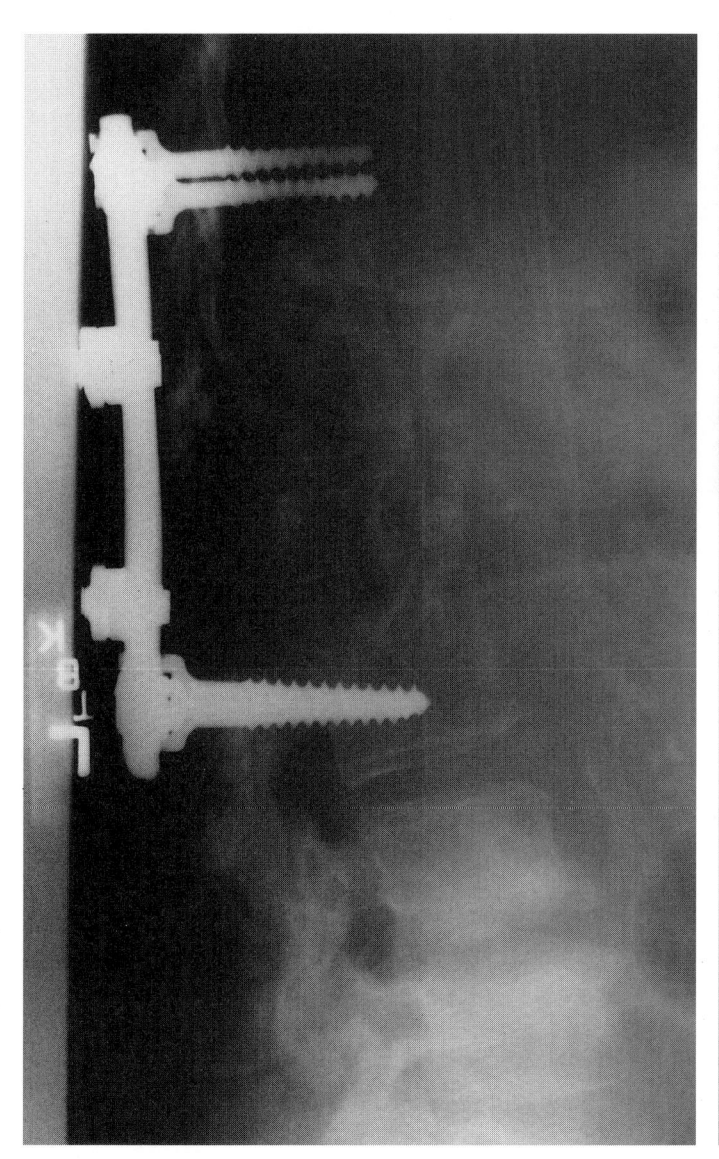

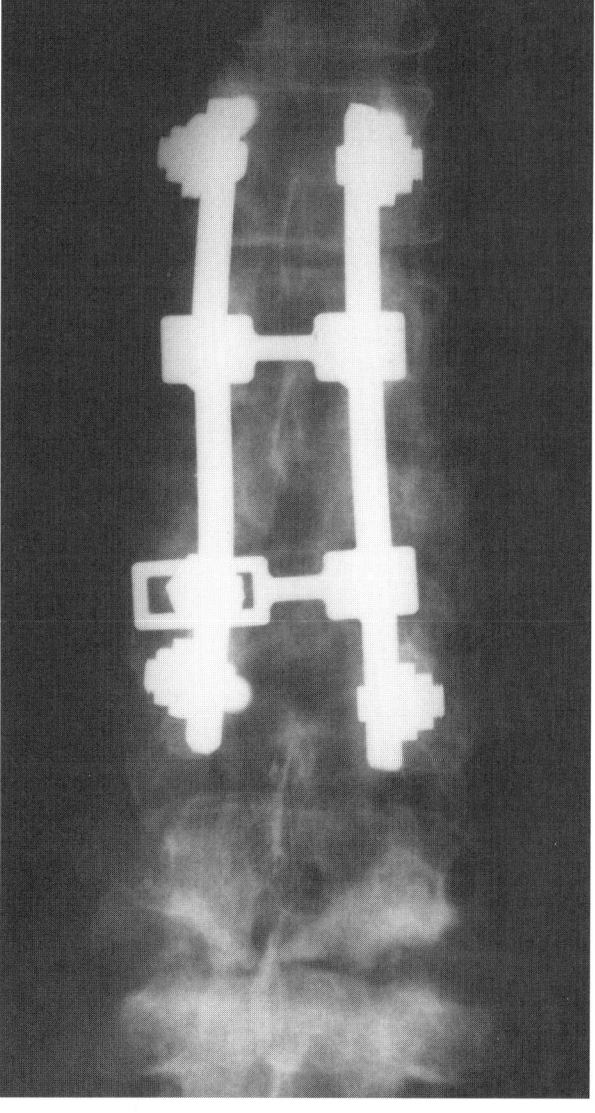

FIG. 26-13. T12 to L3 pedicle screw construct for posterior stabilization following L1-2 vertebrectomy and anterior reconstruction using autologous iliac crest bone graft.

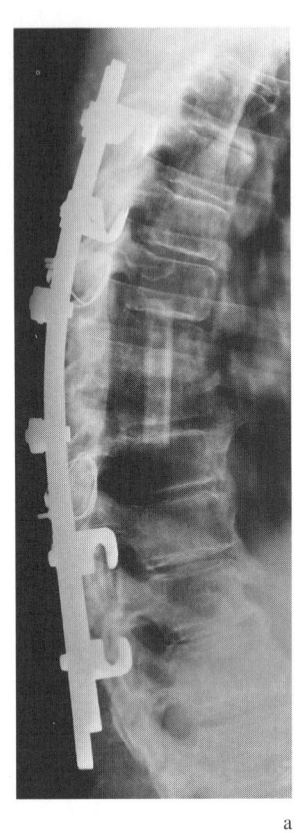

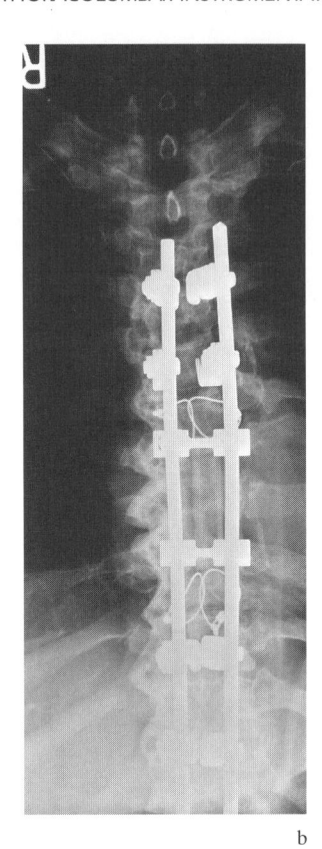

FIG. 26-14. Anteroposterior and lateral x-ray films demonstrate hook construct supplemented with sublaminar cables for T4-12 stabilization following two-level thoracic vertebrectomy and anterior reconstruction using fibular allograft.

no clinical or radiographic evidence of instability. Examples of patients with stabilization using pedicle screws and hooks are provided in Figs. 26-13 and 26-14.

Pseudarthrosis occurred in four patients, three of whom underwent additional surgery for reinstrumentation and fusion, with successful results. The fourth patient refused another operation, and continues to have severe back pain. Factors contributing to nonunion included the use of fresh frozen allograft bone in two patients, prior pseudarthrosis in three, osteoporosis in two, obesity in two, and cigarette smoking in two. Obviously, each of these patients had multiple factors contributing to their pseudarthrosis. Although patients with a prior pseudarthrosis had a higher risk of failure, the 92% fusion rate for this group of patients was excellent after pedicle screw instrumentation.

Correction of Deformity

In the patients with spondylolisthesis, the vertebrae were fused in situ without attempting to correct the spinal deformity. Reduction of spinal deformity was attempted in all other patients, achieving a mean reduction of 14 degrees. Nineteen patients underwent major reductions, which were defined as a correction of 1 cm or more of vertebral body height or a reduction of 30 degrees or more of sagittal angulation. A minor reversal of correction developed in 10 patients during long-term follow-up, with a mean loss of reduction of 2.4 degrees.

COMPLICATIONS

Four patients experienced neurologic complications. Three of these had new postoperative radiculopathy. In one patient, the radiculopathy resolved spontaneously, with no radiographic evidence of root impingement. This transient radiculopathy was attributed to intraoperative root manipulation during foraminotomy. Two cases of radicular deficits occurred secondary to pedicle screw malpositioning and were treated with removal of the offending screw and foraminal decompression. One patient completely recovered; the other had persistent unilateral L5 weakness and numbness 21 months after surgery.

A cauda equina spinal epidural hematoma due to a postoperative coagulopathy developed in the fourth patient with neurologic complications. Although this complication was treated with urgent operative decompression, the patient had residual neurologic dysfunction.

Three wound infections (one superficial and two deep) developed postoperatively. The superficial infection cleared with local wound debridement, packing, and oral antibiotic therapy. The two deep wound infections cleared after open debridement, irrigation, primary closure, and parenteral antibiotic treatment. The instrumentation was not removed in any of these cases, and no recurrent infections developed. Subsequently, all three patients attained a successful arthrodesis.

Other perioperative complications included pneumonia in six patients, urinary tract infection in nine, deep venous thrombosis in three, and a decubitus ulcer in one. Four intraoperative dural tears occurred unrelated to instrument placement; these tears were treated satisfactorily with primary closure of the dural defect. There were no postoperative deaths.

INSTRUMENT FAILURE

Instrument failure eventually developed in 18 cases. Nine patients were asymptomatic with solid fusions and required no therapy. In the other nine patients, the instrument failure was symptomatic or associated with a pseudarthrosis and required operative revision.

Trauma was responsible for two early cases of instrument failure. Both patients fell and dislodged the instrumentation constructs within the first 8 weeks after surgery. These patients required immediate operative revision.

The rods became uncoupled from the screw systems in six patients. Four of these required operative revision, two for instrument prominence and two for pseudarthrosis. No rods bent or broke.

Screws failed in 10 patients, three of whom required reoperation. Among these patients there were nine bent screws, six broken screws, and 10 loose screws, representing an overall 4.8% screw failure rate (25 of 516 screws). Five of the six screws that broke had a narrow diameter (4.5 or 5.0 mm); the other was 7 mm in diameter. Screw breakage was eliminated after the use of narrow-diameter screws was discontinued. No TSRH screws had broken at the termination of follow-up in this group of patients. A variety of screw sizes (5 to 7 mm) bent or loosened. Although the TSRH screws had a lower breakage rate, there were no significant differences in the overall instrument failure rate between the CD and the TSRH systems.

REFERENCES

Ashman, R.B., Herring, J.A., Johnston, C.E., II, Lowery, G.L., Sutterlin, C.E., II (Eds). (1993). *TSRH Universal Spinal Instrumentation,* 1st ed. Dallas, Texas: Hundley and Associates.

Dickman, C.A., Fessler, R.G., MacMillan, M., & Haid, R.W. (1992). Transpedicular screw-rod fixation of the lumbar spine: Operative technique and outcome in 104 cases. *Journal of Neurosurgery, 77,* 860–870.

Dietze, D.D., Fessler, R.G., & Jacob, P.R. (1995). Primary reconstruction for spinal infections. Submitted for publication.

Denis, F. (1983). The three column spine and its significance in the classification of acute thoracolumbar spinal injuries. *Spine, 8,* 817–831.

Fessler, R.G. (1992). Decision making in spinal instrumentation. *Clinical Neurosurgery, 40,* 227–242.

Frymoyer, J.W., & Selby, D.K. (1985). Segmental instability rationale for treatment. *Spine, 10,* 280–285.

Gurr, K.R., McAfee, P.C., & Shih, C.M. (1988). Biomechanical analysis of posterior instrumentation systems after decompressive laminectomy: An unstable calf-spine model. *Journal of Bone and Joint Surgery, American Volume, 70,* 680–691.

McAfee, P.C., Yuan, H.A., Frederickson, B.E., & Lubicky, J.P. (1983). The value of computed tomography in thoracolumbar fractures: An analysis of 100 consecutive cases and a new classification. *Journal of Bone and Joint Surgery, American Volume, 65,* 461–473.

CHAPTER 27

Utilization of the Cotrel-Dubousset Instrumentation System for Stabilization of the Thoracolumbar and Lumbosacral Spine

Paul C. McCormick

Cotrel-Dubousset (CD) instrumentation is the prototypical universal spinal fixation system. Although it was originally developed for the treatment of scoliotic and paralytic deformity, CD instrumentation has been widely used for the management of all types of spinal instability, including trauma and degenerative, neoplastic, congenital, and iatrogenic causes (Cotrel & Dubousset, 1987). Universal spinal instrumentation systems are characterized by a longitudinal rod that is segmentally fixed to the spine via hook or screw anchors (Cotrel, Dubousset, & Guillaumat, 1988). Powerful corrective forces in three planes may be delivered to the spine for deformity correction, graft compression, or spinal canal reconstruction. The secure segmental nature of the fixation provides rigid spinal immobilization. Like other implants, however, internal fixation should be considered as a temporary adjunct to bony arthrodesis. Even the most rigid implant system will eventually fatigue and fail if a solid bony arthrodesis is not achieved. Thus, while the technical aspects of implant application are important, meticulous bone preparation and grafting techniques are essential to a successful clinical result.

SYSTEM COMPONENTS

Rod

The 5- and 7-mm-diameter CD rod is constructed from 316L stainless steel (Fig. 27-1). The rod is stiff but not brittle and may be contoured without a significant loss of mechanical strength. Fatigue fracture of the rod rarely occurs. The CD rod is knurled with diamond-shaped asperites, which allows set screw fixation of the hook or screw implants at any point on the rod. This facilitates deformity correction in all three planes.

Hooks and Screw Anchors

The CD rod is segmentally fixed to the spine via hook and screw anchors. Open and closed body hooks and screws are available (see Fig. 27-1). The rod must be passed through the side of closed body hooks and screws while open body implants allow drop loading of the rod into the implant. Blockers secure the open hooks and screws to the rods (Fig. 27-2). In general, closed hooks and screws are preferable at the ends of a construct, while central anchors are usually open. Laminar, transverse process, or facet hooks are used in the thoracic spine, while only the lamina is used for hook placement at lumbar levels. Laminar hooks may be rostrally or caudally directed over the inferior (i.e., infralaminar) or superior (supralaminar) laminar edge. Facet hooks, characterized by a bifid hook end that may straddle the pedicle, are rostrally directed, while the transverse process hook is caudally directed over its edge. Six- and 7-mm diameter pedicle screws are used at lumbar and sacral levels.

Device for Transverse Traction (DTT)

The $\frac{1}{8}$-in.-diameter threaded DTT rod cross-links the paired CD rods to increase rotational stability significantly (see Fig. 27-1, *d*). Two DTTs are usually applied to establish a continuous rectangular implant, but one or three DTTs may be used for particularly short or long constructs, respectively.

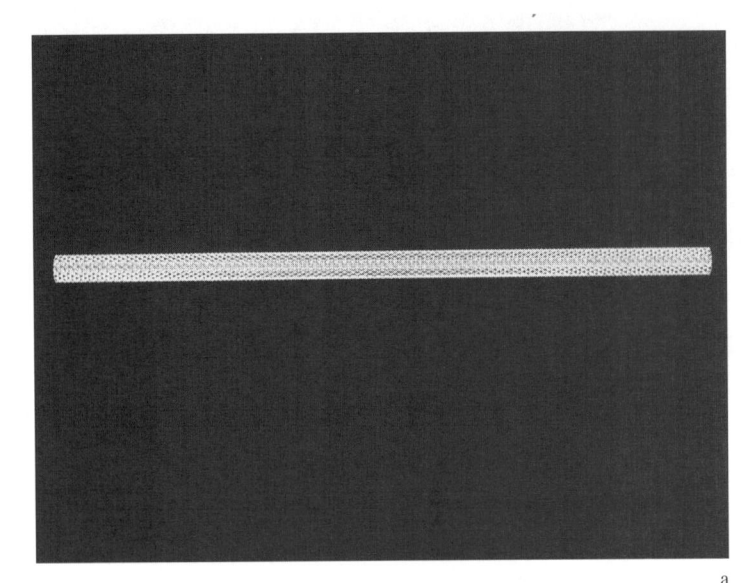

288   PART 4 / POSTERIOR THORACOLUMBAR INSTRUMENTATION

FIG. 27-1. CD components. (a) The 5-cm and 7-mm CD rods are covered with diamond-shaped asperites. (b) A variety of closed and open hook and screw anchors are available. (c) Instrumentation—rod gripper, hook holder, open and closed hook impactors, screwdriver, distractor, compressor, rod bender, in situ bender, and lamina, transverse process, and pedicle dissectors. (d) Device for transverse traction (DTT).

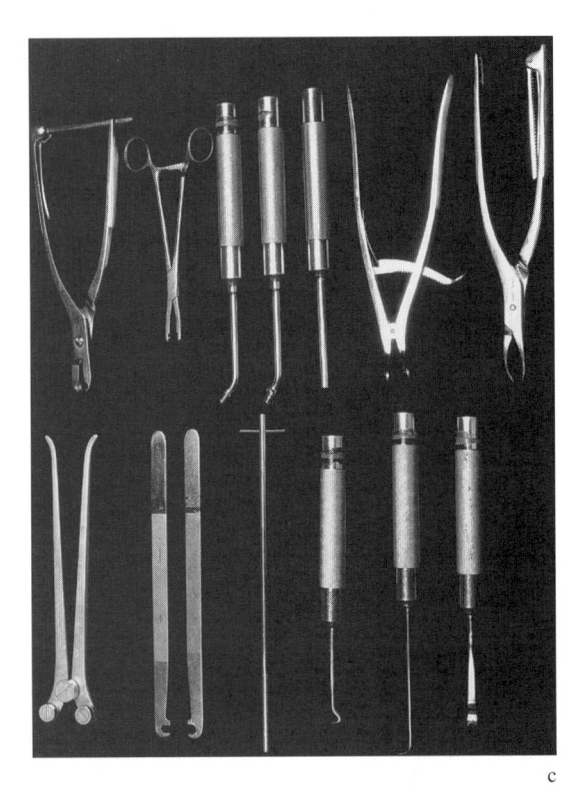

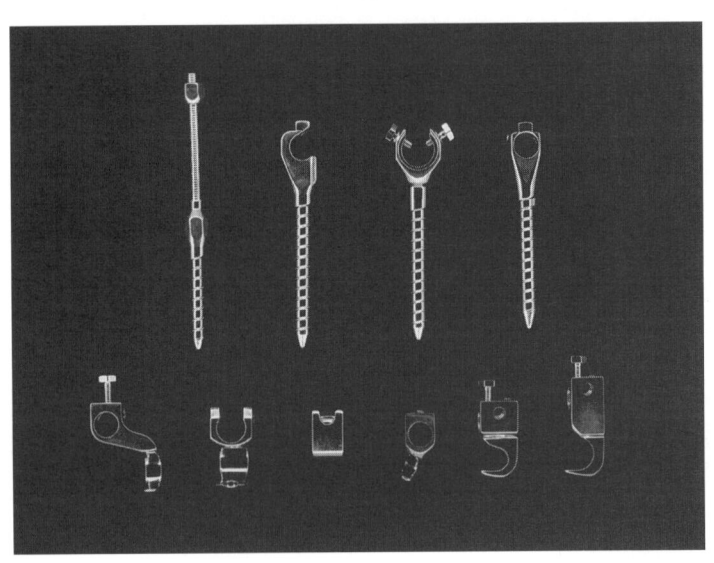

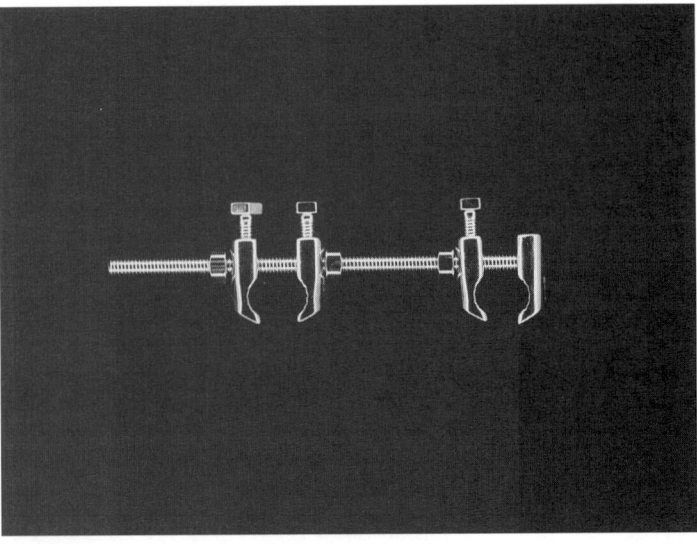

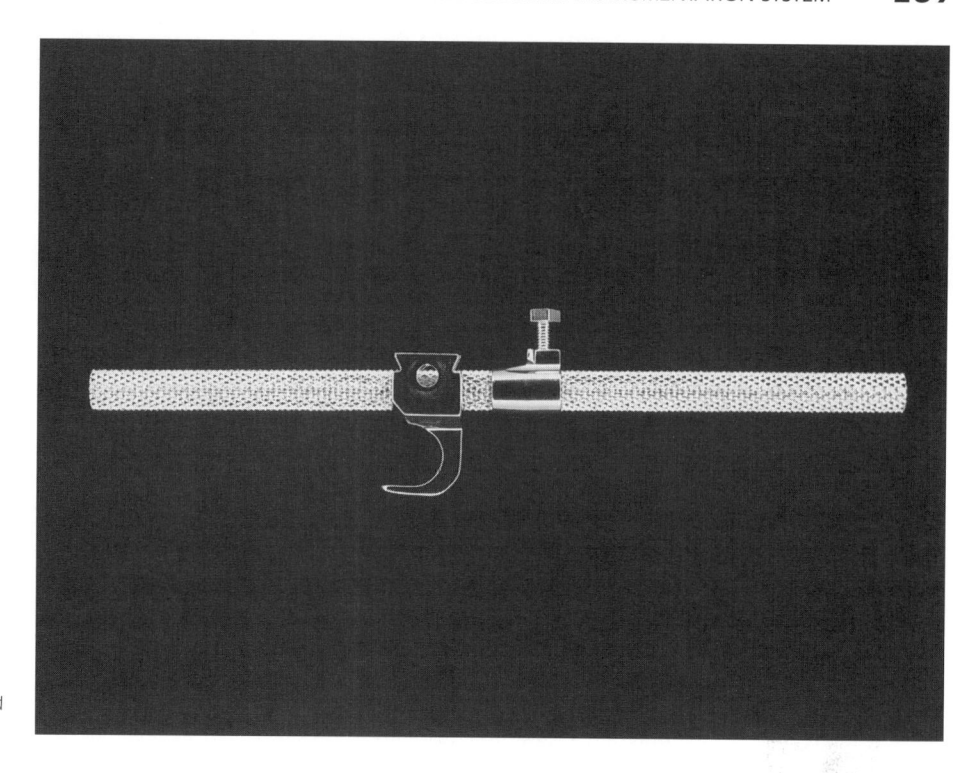

FIG. 27-2. Open anchors are secured to the CD rod with blockers.

Indications

The indications for universal CD instrumentations are broad and essentially include any destabilizing process of the thoracic, lumbar, and lumbosacral, spine (Tables 27-1 and Table 27-2). The versatility of CD and other universal systems allows customization of the implant in terms of length, anchor types and sites, and force application (i.e., compression, distraction) modes for effective management of instability in any plane. Although there are no specific conditions for which CD instrumentation represents the universal implant system of choice, most surgeons tend to use a particular instrumentation system based on experience, personal preference, and implant availability. The versatility of the CD system stems mainly from the wide variety of hook and screw anchors available.

Contraindications

The contraindications to CD instrumentation are relative and can be generalized to all universal instrumentation systems. For example, while implantation of any foreign body in proximation to an active infection should be avoided, spinal implants can be effectively used for stabilization of acute or grossly unstable vertebral osteomyelitis (Fig. 27-3). Severe osteoporosis presents a higher than normal risk of implant-related complications and failure. In these cases, the instrumentation is considerably stronger than the bone, and fixation failure at the anchor-bone interface is common. Long segment fixation to distribute forces over many segments, postoperative bracing, methylmethacrylate pedicle screw supplementation and minimal generated force (i.e., neutral mode) application will reduce the incidence of implant failure in these patients.

Significant loss of anterior column stability, particularly in the axial (weight-bearing) plane, can stress posterior

Table 27-1
Indications and Contraindications for Cotrel-Dubousset Instrumentation

Indications—spinal instability due to:
  Trauma
    Fracture
    Dislocation
  Neoplasia
  Iatrogenic causes
    Postsurgical
  Degenerative causes
    Spondylolisthesis
    Degenerative disk disease
  Idiopathic causes
    Scoliosis
    Spondylolisthesis
  Congenital causes
    Paralytic deformity
    Scoliosis
    Spondylolisthesis
  Infection

Contraindications
  Absolute
    Absence of spinal instability
  Relative
    Infection
    Severe osteoporosis
    Significant anterior column instability
    Cervical fixation requirement

Table 27-2
Advantages and Disadvantages for Cotrel-Dubousset Instrumentation

Advantages
   Prototypical universal system
   Rigid three-dimensional fixation
   Wide variety of rod, hook, and screw designs
   Knurled rods

Disadvantages
   Extensive rod contouring necessary
   Set screw design requires destruction of previous construct for revision, or drilling metal to remove construct
   Multiple pieces can be confusing

universal instrumentation and lead to fixation failure. In cases in which instability exists only or primarily in the anterior column, consideration should be given to anterior surgical decompression and stabilization or supplementation of posterior universal instrumentation with an anterior interbody strut graft. Instability at the cervicothoracic junction poses significant problems for universal systems that are not designed for cervical spine fixation. Nevertheless, small specialized CD cervical hooks are available for fixation to the cervical lamina. Great care must be taken not only with hook placement but also with rod passage to avoid cervical spinal cord injury.

Techniques

General Considerations

The technique of CD implantation is challenging and associated with a steep learning curve. Its application is facilitated considerably by careful preoperative planning. Most importantly, the role of the implant is individually determined, based on the understanding of the mechanics of the underlying destabilizing process and the capabilities of the implant system. A preoperative construct design that diagrams the location, type, and direction of the anchors provides a useful formulation of the operative objective.

The specific construct design depends on the location and severity of spinal instability as well as on the operative objective. Above all, there should be secure rigid fixation above and below the unstable spinal segments. This is best achieved with an apposing paired hook-claw configuration or screw at either end of the construct. Further, while it is preferable to minimize the number of instrumented motion segments, especially in the lumbar spine, a longer implant may be required either to increase the mechanical advantage or to distribute forces more diffusely in patients with gross instability and/or severe osteoporosis, respectively. Degenerative lumbar instability, for example, can usually be effectively managed with short segment pedicle fixation, while severe thoracic or thoracolumbar fractures and/or dislocations necessitate longer implants to secure fixation (Fig. 27-4).

In the thoracic spine paired hooks in an apposing claw configuration provides a particularly secure fixation point

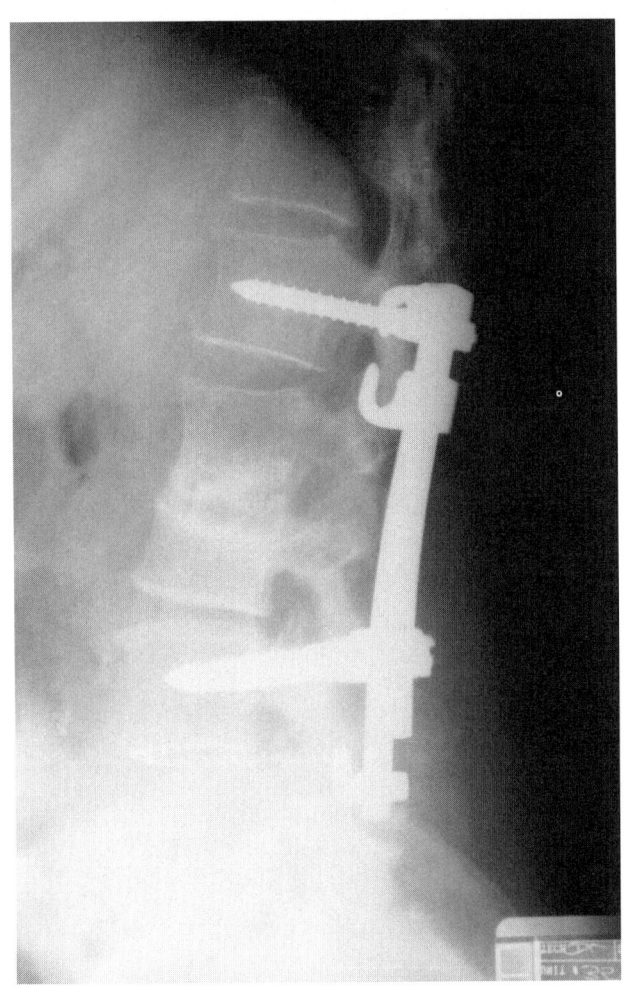

FIG. 27-3. Postoperative lateral radiograph following CD instrumentation of grossly unstable L2-3 osteomyelitis in a patient who had previously undergone laminectomy. The use of pedicle screws allows short segment lumbar instrumentation. Infralaminar hooks help secure the screws.

(Fig. 27-4). Claws are especially useful at the ends of a construct. They may be configured over adjacent lamina (laminolaminar), pedicle (facet)-transverse process (pediculotransverse), or pedicle-lamina (pediculolaminar). While a pediculotransverse claw avoids spinal canal hook placement, it is not as strong as a laminolaminar claw. It may not be possible to use a pediculotransverse claw at lower thoracic levels because of the small sagittally oriented transverse process and facet joints. Laminar claws may also be used in the lumbar spine. The large size of the lumbar lamina usually allows a single-level claw. Unpaired intermediate hooks are used primarily to increase segmental fixation sites or for the delivery of localized force.

Pedicle screws are the preferred anchor in the lumbar spine, especially at lower lumbar and lumbosacral levels. Secure rigid fixation of both anterior and posterior columns with pedicle screws minimizes the number of instrumented lumbar segments and allows more efficient deformity correction. Placement of an infralaminar hook may help 'shield' the pedicle screw and prevent late screw failure (see Fig. 27-3).

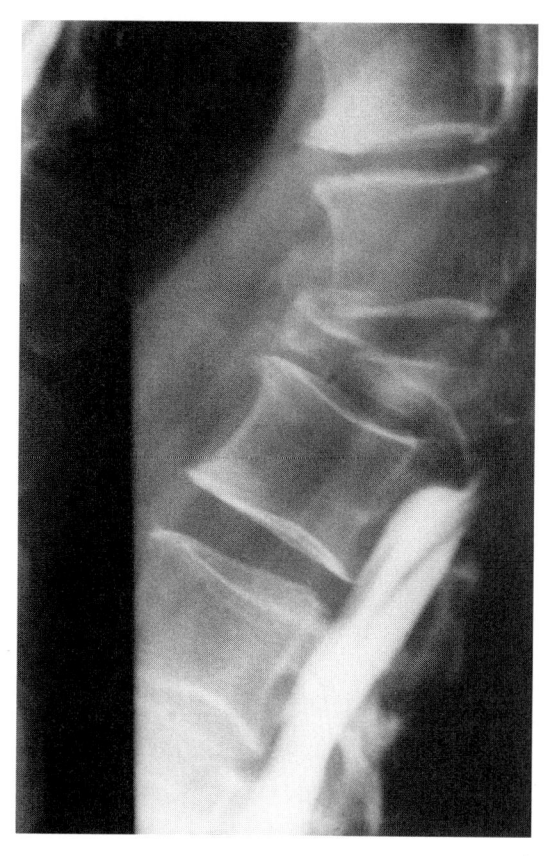

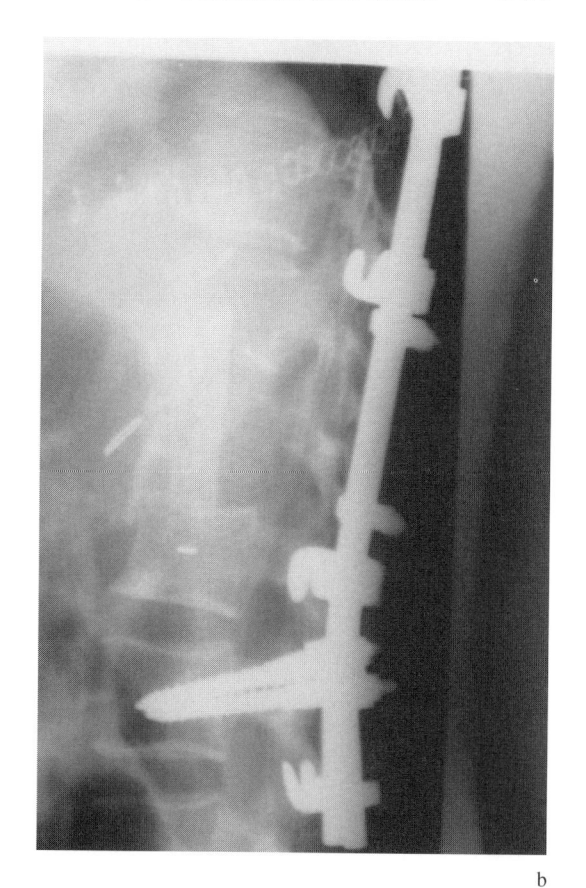

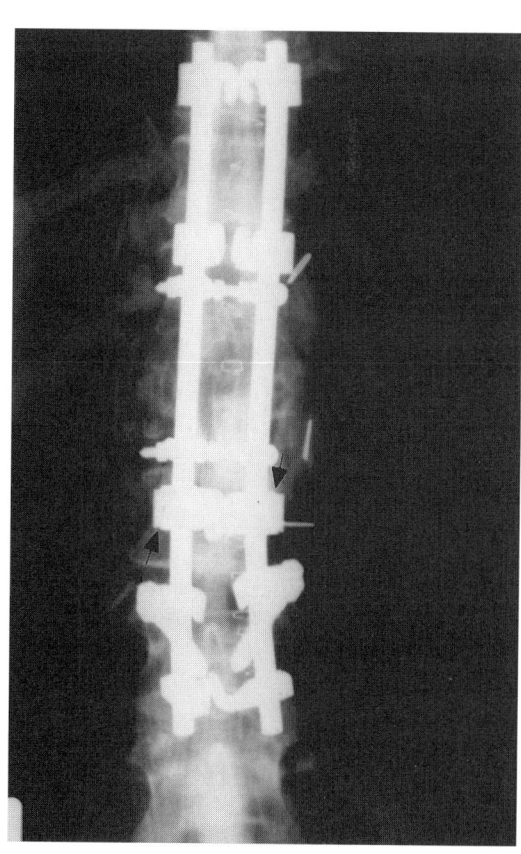

FIG. 27-4. (a) Lateral radiograph demonstrates L1 flexion-compression fracture with significant anterior and posterior column instability as evidenced by loss of vertebral-body height and significant kyphotic deformity, respectively. Lateral (b) and anteroposterior (c) radiographs following combined anterior decompression and interbody strut graft reconstruction and posterior stabilization with CD rods and onlay graft shows restoration of spinal canal, vertebral-body height, and sagittal alignment. Note bilateral thoracic claw. Intermediate open supralaminar hooks allow distraction for restoration of vertebral body height (arrows). A double-threaded pedicle screw and infralaminar hook provided a "lordosing" corrective force at the lower end of the construct.

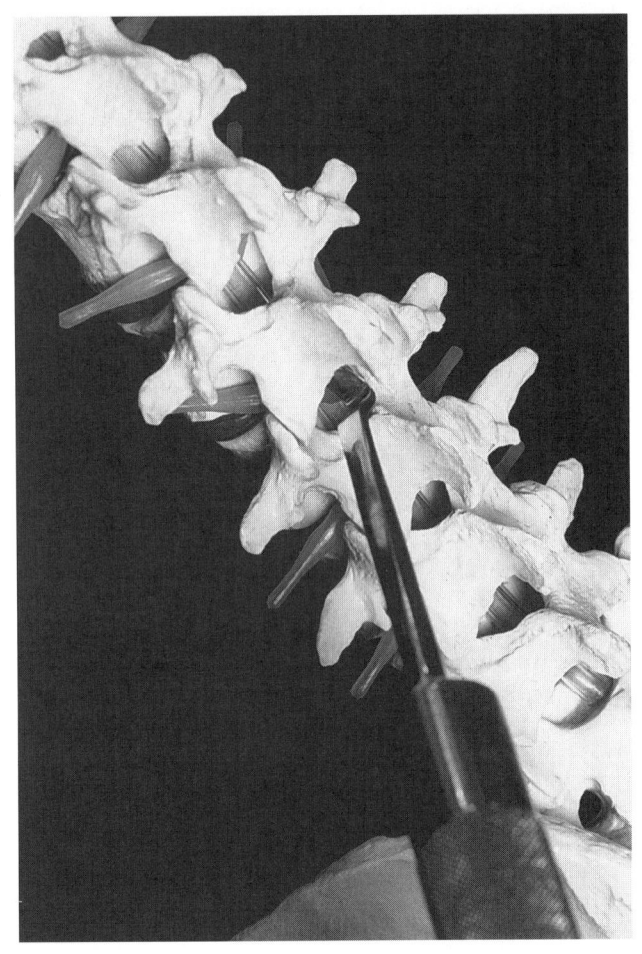

FIG. 27-5. Preparation of lamina with laminar dissectors for infralaminar hook.

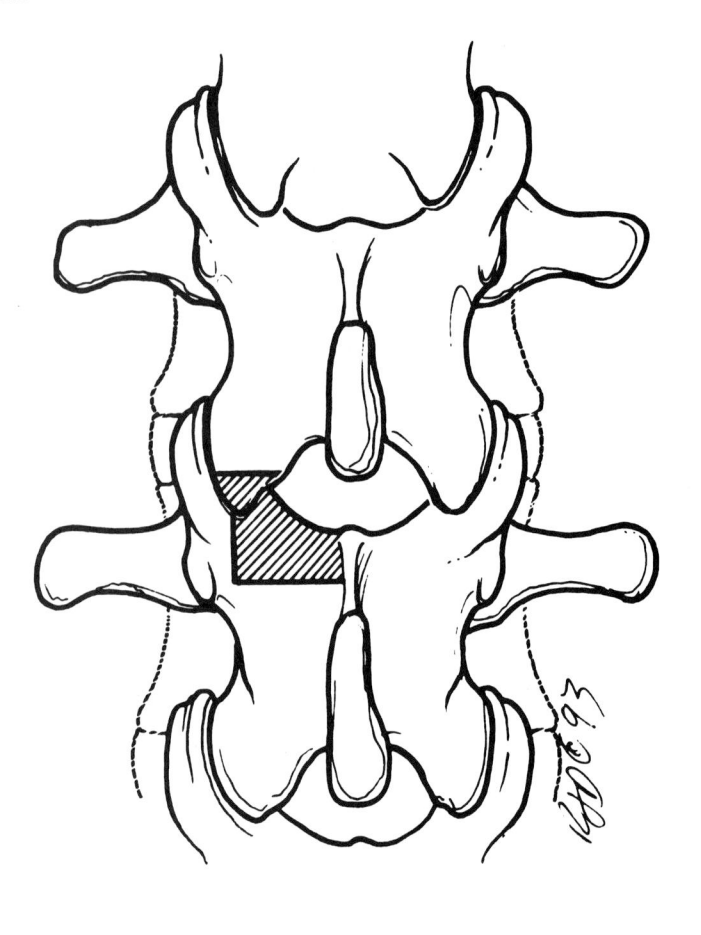

FIG. 27-6. A supralaminar hook requires a small interlaminar laminotomy (shaded). A slight medial facetectomy may be required in the lumbar spine.

Anchor Site Selection and Preparation

Lamina.
Infralaminar. Rostrally directed infralaminar hooks are used in the thoracic and lumbar spine. Lamina preparation of these hooks usually requires only detachment of the ligamentum flavum from the inferior lamina surface. This is achieved with a curved laminar dissector, which is directed forward on the undersurface of the lamina until it engages the inferior lamina edge (Fig. 27-5).

Supralaminar. Laminar preparation for an inferiorly directed supralaminar hook requires a small interlaminar laminotomy with removal of the intervening ligamentum flavum (Fig. 27-6). The hook should be inserted by rotation about the arc of the hook to facilitate placement and minimize spinal canal hook intrusion.

Facet (Pedicle) Hooks

Facet (pedicle) hooks are used only in the thoracic spine. These specialized hooks have a bifid shoe, which is meant to engage the inferior pedicle margin. Placement of these hooks is frequently not possible at the lower thoracic (T10 to T12) level because of a more sagittal facet orientation. Preparation of the facet for hook placement requires removal of the inferior $\frac{1}{8}$-in. inferior facet (Fig. 27-7). Just enough of the facet is removed to expose the joint cartilage. This accurately identifies the joint's location and avoids the common error of lateral misplacement of the facet hook. This is easily avoided if the facet cartilage is visualized prior to hook placement. Preparation of the facet for hook placement is achieved with a bifid joint dissector, which is advanced into the joint until the pedicle is engaged. The facet hook is then rolled into the joint along the arc of the hook shoe.

Transverse Process

The transverse processes are used for hook placement in the thoracic spine. Hook placement may not be possible in the lower thoracic spine because the transverse processes become smaller in size and more vertically oriented. Usually only

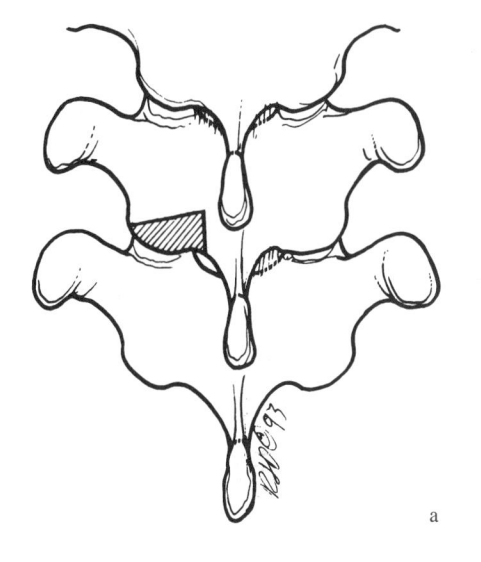

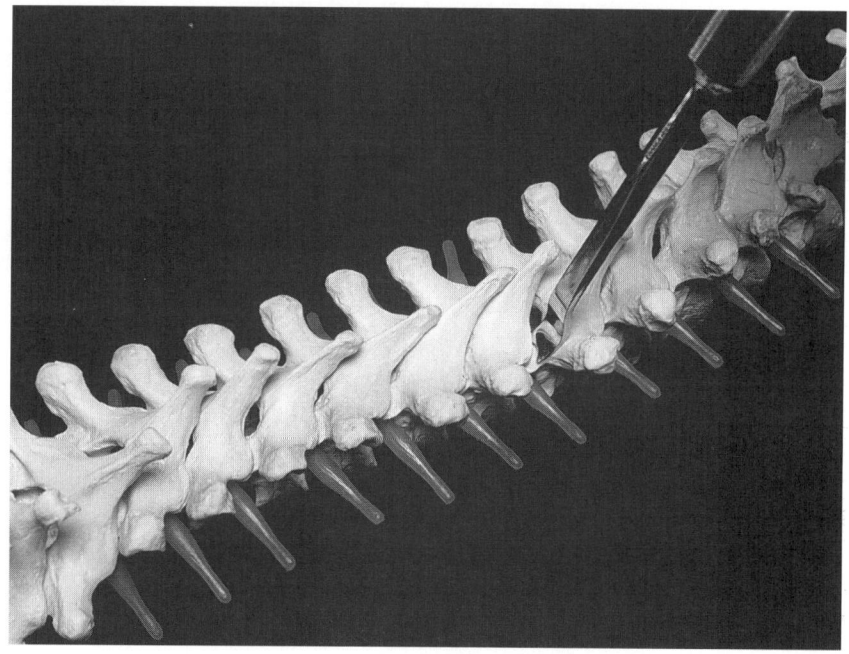

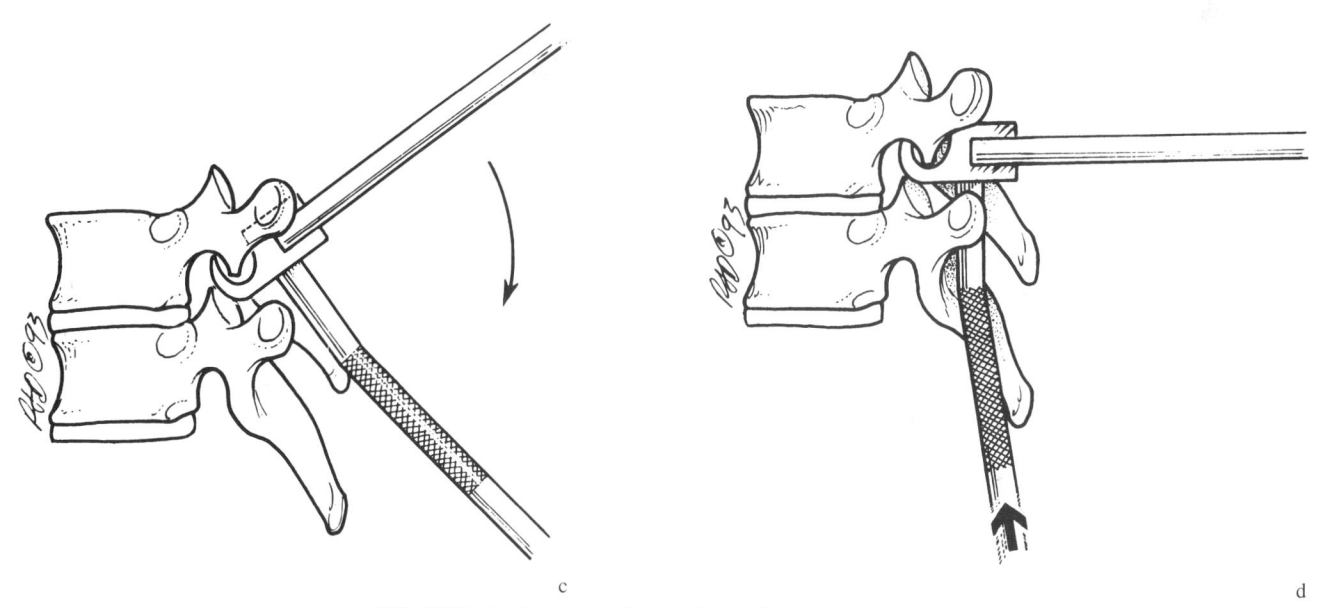

FIG. 27-7. (a) Removal of the tip of the inferior facet exposes the articular cartilage for facet hook placement. (b) The facet is engaged with a facet (pedicle) dissector. (c and d) The facet (pedicle) hook is inserted with a gentle rotation about the arc of the hook.

caudally directed hooks are placed over the superior edge of the transverse process. Transverse process preparation is achieved with a transverse process elevator, which is inserted with an arcing motion over the superior surface of the transverse process (Fig. 27-8). The sharp edge of the dissector divides the costotransverse ligaments to allow hook placement.

Pedicle

A variety of methods are available for pedicle-screw placement. The author uses pedicle fixation only in the lumbar and sacral spine. An entry point at the base of the transverse process and superior facet is preferred (Fig. 27-9). A small

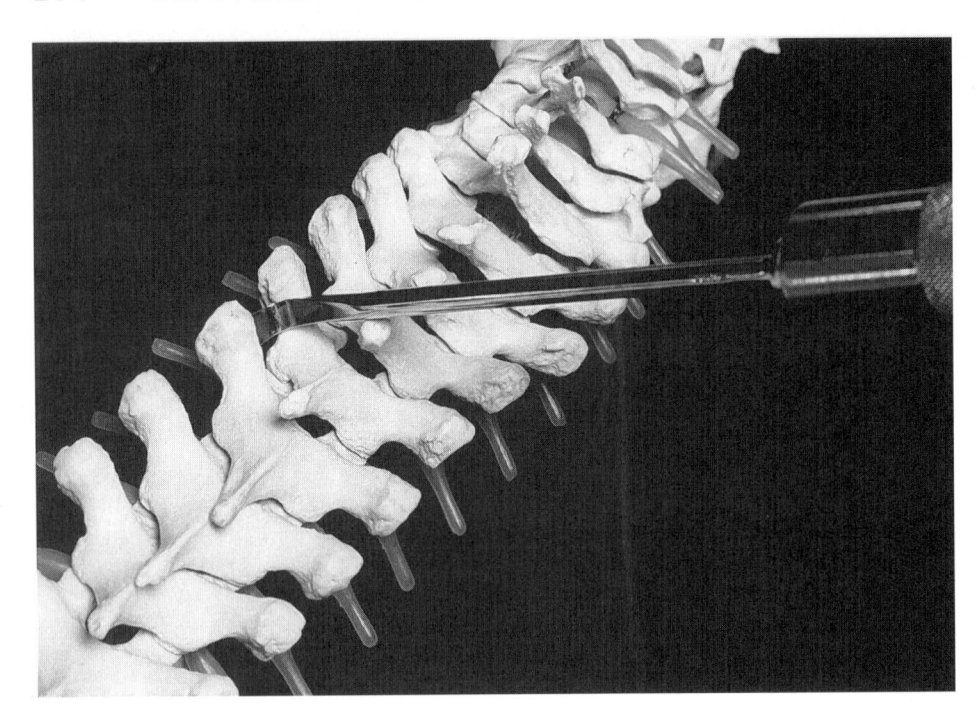

FIG. 27-8. A transverse process dissector sharply divides the costotransverse ligaments for transverse process hook placement.

ridge of cortical bone is removed to allow initial pedicle penetration with an awl. A small curette is then advanced into the vertebral body, with a lateral to medial angulation that increases from 0 to 10 degrees at upper lumbar levels to 25 degrees at L5 and S1. Radiopaque pins are then placed into the pedicle holes and placement is confirmed with fluoroscopy or biplanar films. The appropriate diameter and length screw is then inserted following tapping of the screw hole. In general, 6-mm-diameter screws are used in the upper lumbar (L1 to L4) spine, while 7-mm screws are placed at L5 and S1. The depth of screw penetration is 50 to 75% of lumbar vertebral body sagittal diameter. Bicortical purchase is preferred in the sacrum.

Rod Placement

Rod placement is the most difficult aspect of CD implantation because of the nearly matched diameters of the rod and anchor apertures. Sequential rod engagement through each anchor progressively limits rod adjustments for passage through the remaining anchors. Rod placement can be facilitated by several techniques. First, only the minimal amount of anchors needed to achieve secure fixations should be used. While closed anchors are preferred at either end of the construct, open anchors are used at intermediate sites. Secondly, adjacent anchors should be selected to allow their apertures to be lined up in the same plane. This avoids acute rod angulations, which are difficult to pass.

Rod length and contour are also important. The rod should only extend about 1 cm beyond the end anchors. Rod contour must be precise. In general, rod bending should be gradual and evenly distributed over the length of the curve; acute angulations complicate rod passage. A pliable rod template should be used to determine the appropriate length and contour prior to rod passage.

CD placement may be further facilitated by other technical maneuvers performed prior to rod placement. First, the set screws are removed from the anchors to avoid inadvertent aperture intrusion, which can block rod passage. Secondly, holders are placed on all hook anchors to allow stabilization and minor angular adjustments of the hook during rod placement. Third, the appropriate number and direction of blockers are confirmed.

Passage of the rod through the anchor apertures is sequentially accomplished. The rod is usually overpassed through either the upper or lower anchor apertures to bring the other end of the rod beyond the most central closed anchor. The rod is then brought back and passed through the remaining anchors. The rod is advanced with short, jerky rotating movements but should never be forced. Gentle toggle of the hook holders prevents rod-anchor impingement and facilitates rod passage. Axially directed compressive or distractive forces can be delivered to the spine through the hook and screw anchors. Alternatively, correction of a nonrigid deformity (e.g., kyphosis, scoliosis) can be achieved with three-point bending or in situ rotation of a rod that has been prebent to the desired contour.

Rod fixation to the anchors is achieved with set screws. Hooks should be firmly seated prior to set-screw tightening.

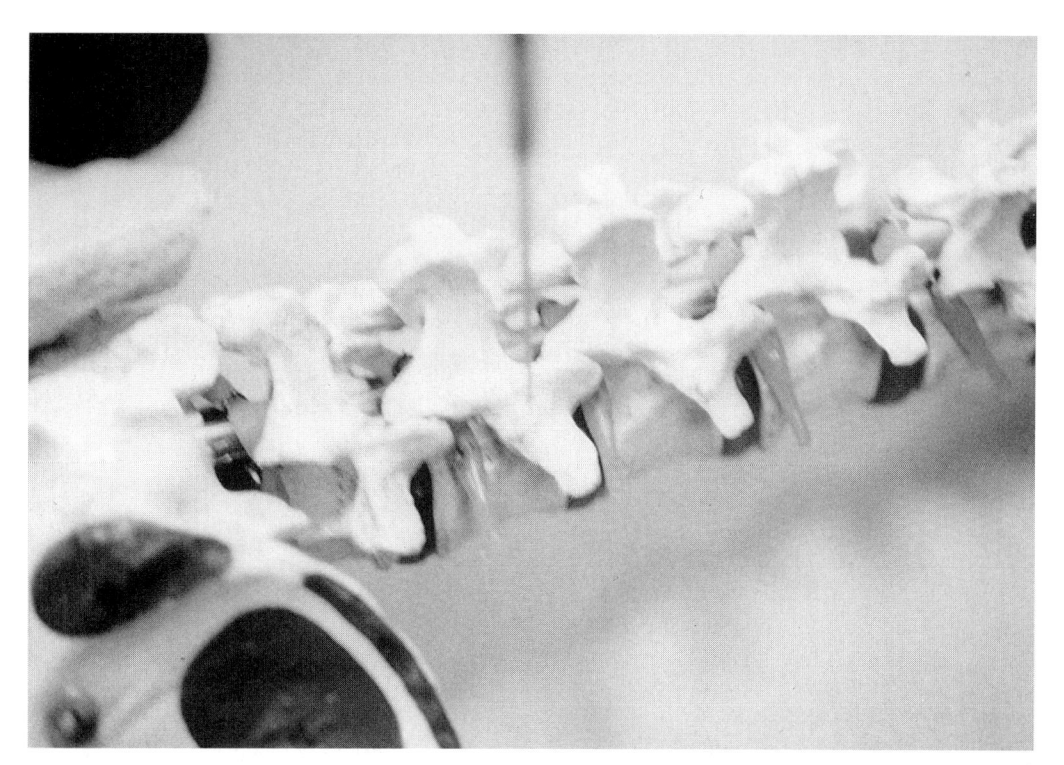

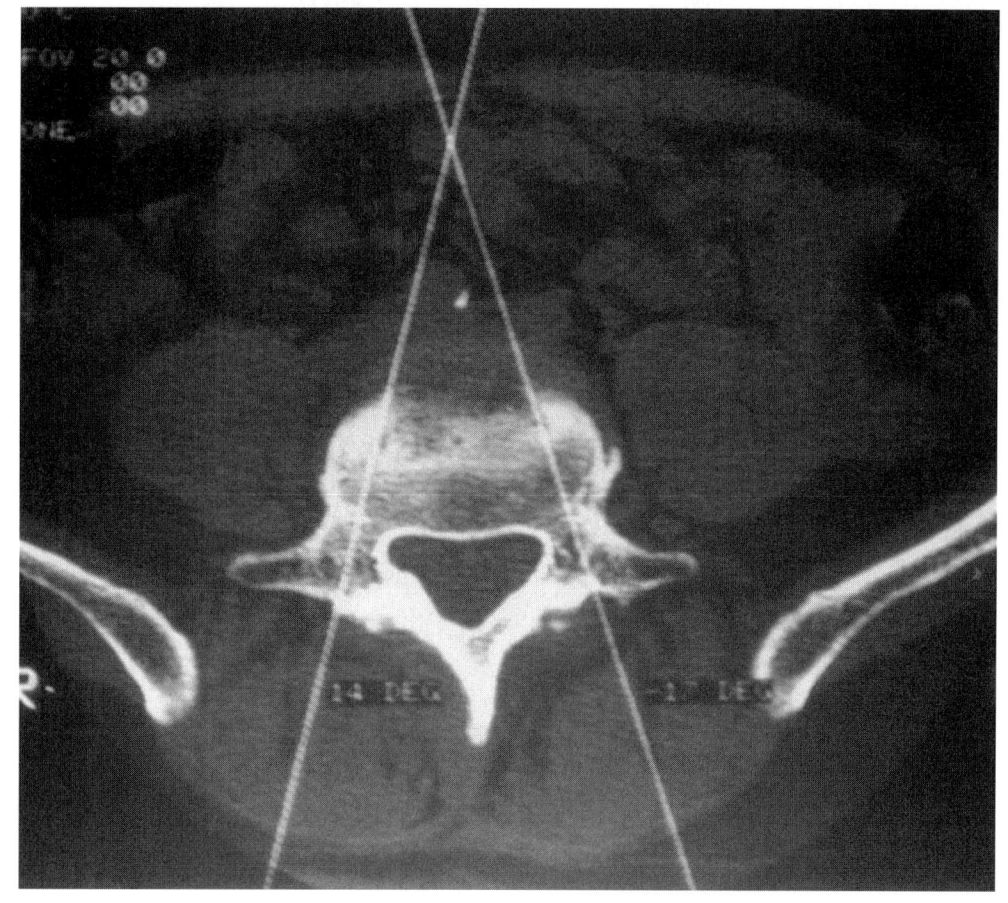

FIG. 27-9. (a) Pedicle insertion point at junction between the transverse process and superior facet. (b) Note medial angulation of pedicle axis at the L5 level.

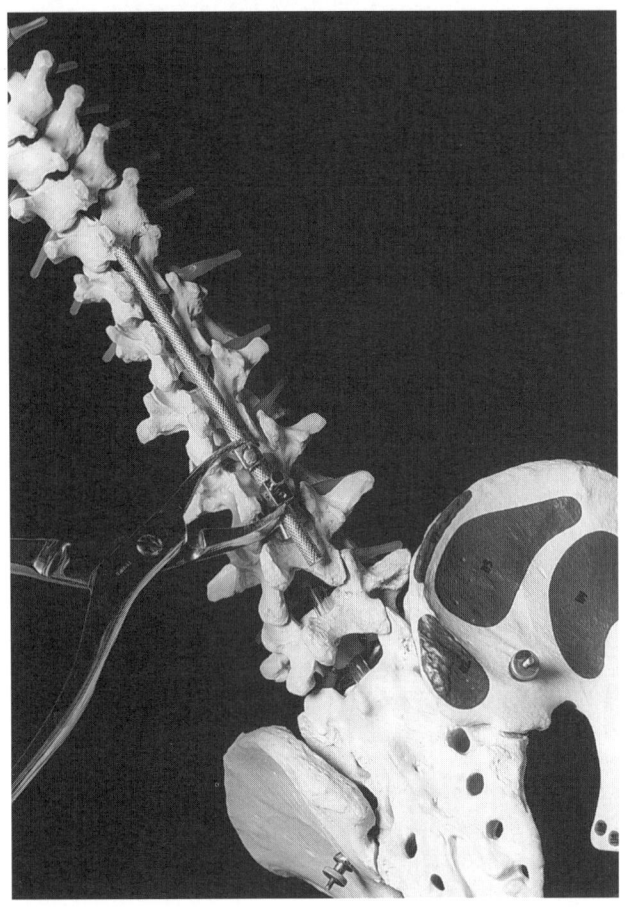

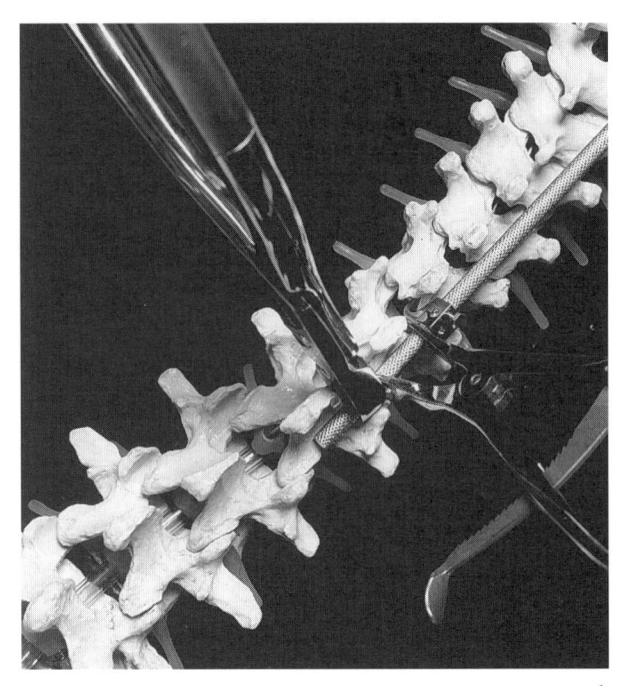

FIG. 27-10. (a) The claw is compressed prior to set screw fixation. (b) A distractor is utilized to fully seat a solitary hook. Localized distraction or compression may be achieved between the solitary hook and a secured anchor-rod site.

Claw components are compressed simultaneously while solitary hooks may be seated with a hook impactor or compression-distraction against a rod holder (Fig. 27-10). The set screws are tightened until the screw head breaks off. All available set-screw placement sites should be used to prevent loosening at the anchor-rod interface.

DTTs are then applied to either end of the construct. They are secured to the rods with threaded nuts and set screws. Bone graft is then placed over the previously decorticated exposed posterior spinal elements. The wound is closed in layers. Early mobilization is encouraged in the postoperative priod. The author prefers 3-month postoperative immobilization with a molded brace. A thigh extension (i.e., spica) is used for fusions that incorporate the lumbosacral junction.

REFERENCES

Cotrel, Y., & Dubousset, J. (1987). A new technique of spine fixation by a posterior approach in the treatment of scoliosis. *Revue de Chirurgie Orthopedique et Reparatrice de L'Appareil Moteur 70,* 489–494.

Cotrel, Y., Dubousset, J., & Guillaumat, M. (1988). New universal instrumentation in spinal surgery. *Clinical Orthopaedics and Related Research 227,* 10–23.

CHAPTER 28

Utilization of the Compact Cotrel-Dubousset System for Stabilization of the Thoracolumbar and Lumbar Spine

Philippe Gillet

HIGHLIGHTS

In the early 1980s, Harrington rods with laminar hooks, Luque rods with sublaminar wires and Roy-Camille plates with pedicular screws represented the classic spine instrumentations available in most countries. In 1983, a revolutionary instrumentation developed by Yves Cotrel and Jean Dubousset was used in Paris for the first time to treat an idiopathic scoliosis. The Cotrel-Dubousset instrumentation has, during the past 12 years, gained wide popularity in the treatment of various spine disorders and initiated the development of a great number of new systems, which greatly improved the management of spine instability. The original CD instrumentation, designed to treat scoliotic deformations, has been used widely to treat traumatic conditions of the thoracic and lumbar spine, degenerative diseases, spondylolisthesis, and tumors. It presented a number of disadvantages, though, when used in these indications. Among these are an unnecessary great number of vertebral implants and ancillary instruments and a permanent rod-implant locking system, making instrumentation removal a challenge.

To meet the specific needs of thoracolumbar, lumbar, and lumbosacral surgery, a new version of CD instrumentation was developed: the compact Cotrel-Dubousset (CCD) instrumentation (Table 28-1). Its aim was to offer a limited but still sufficient number of instruments and implants, making it also more easy to use by the spine surgeon not surrounded by a highly trained team. A system of rods meeting the specific biomechanics of the low back and an improved locking system enabling easy removal if desired were made available. Postoperative bracing was to remain exceptional, as with the original CD instrumentation.

With other hospitals in France, our Orthopaedic Department was selected to evaluate this new instrumentation during 2 years before it would be made commercially available. The first implantation of a CCD instrumentation was performed in the Liège University Hospital, Belgium, on June 20, 1990. We acquired our experience with the system with 107 patients, who have follow-ups of 3 to 5 years at the time of writing.

DESCRIPTION OF THE SYSTEM

The specifications listed below are those of the hardware available in Europe at the time of writing (Cotrel, 1992); other implants may be available in the United States (e.g., different hooks and different lengths or diameters of screws). The reader should refer to the manufacturer for availability in his or her own country (Sofamor-Danek, Rang-Du-Fliers, France).

All the vertebral implants and rods are made from 316L stainless steel but can be made from titanium on special request. We have experience only with stainless steel implants.

The Rods

As in the original CD instrumentation, the rods are covered by a great number of diamond-shaped knurls, their height being reduced to 0.2 mm, the core diameter of the rod is

Table 28-1
Indications and Contraindications for CCD Instrumentation

Indications
    Degenerative spine disease between T12 and S1
    Stabilization of unstable thoracolumbar, lumbar and lumbosacral spine in trauma, tumor or previous surgery
    Correction and stabilization of spondylolisthesis, transverse dislocation, scoliosis and kyphosis

Contraindications
    Severe osteoporosis
    Anterior column destruction may require anterior strut grafting to avoid implant failure

hence enlarged (Fig. 28-1). Rods are available in 5-, 6-, and 7-mm diameters and in hyperquenched or cold rolled metal. The reference rod is the 6-mm hyperquenched rod. In comparison, the 5-mm rods have a stiffness of 48% and the 7-mm rods of 140%. Cold rolled rods offer 150% resistance to permanent deformation compared to hyperquenched rods by offering an increased elastic range thanks to the mechanical characteristics of cold-rolled metal (Cotrel, 1992; Sofamor, 1993).

Vertebral Implants

Hooks

Offset hooks are available to facilitate alignment with pedicular screws. They have a closed body and are intended to be used at the end of the instrumentation when desired. On the U.S. market, a greater number of hooks should be available, with both closed and open bodies; we have no personal experience with these latter hooks, which are not available on the European market, where pedicular screwing is increasingly popular.

Lumbar and Sacral Pedicle Screws

Lumbar screws are available in two diameters (5 and 6 mm) and three lengths (35, 40, 45 mm). The core diameters of the 5 and 6 mm screws are 3.5 and 4.5 mm. The thread depth is small, 0.75 mm, so that the core diameter is favored to withstand bending forces. Resistance against screw pullout is obtained by convergent pedicular screwing and transversal cross-linking of the rods creating a triangular construct in the vertebra (Fig. 28-2). All the screws have a smooth, extended neck (10-mm length, 5- or 6-mm diameter) also designed to offer better resistance to bending forces by avoiding the change of core diameter occurring at the level of the introduction point of the screw in the vertebra (Fig. 28-3). All the lumbar pedicle screws are of the open body type to favor easy placement of the rod.

Sacral screws have a 7-mm outer diameter and are available in 35, 40, and 45 mm lengths, the core diameter is 4.5 mm and the thread depth 1.25 mm. All have an extended neck and are available with a closed or open body. The greater thread depth is intended to offer better pull-out resistance in the soft cancellous bone of the sacrum. The closed body implant is less cumbersome in slender patients.

Sacral Chopin Block

This implant offers the possibility, while aligning the rod with a single open body implant, to obtain a double screw fixation in divergent directions to reinforce sacral anchoring. Specific 7-mm-diameter screws with a sacral type thread are to be used (length, 35 to 60 mm). An iliac extension device enables the surgeon to improve the fixation with a third long sacral type screw in the iliac wing.

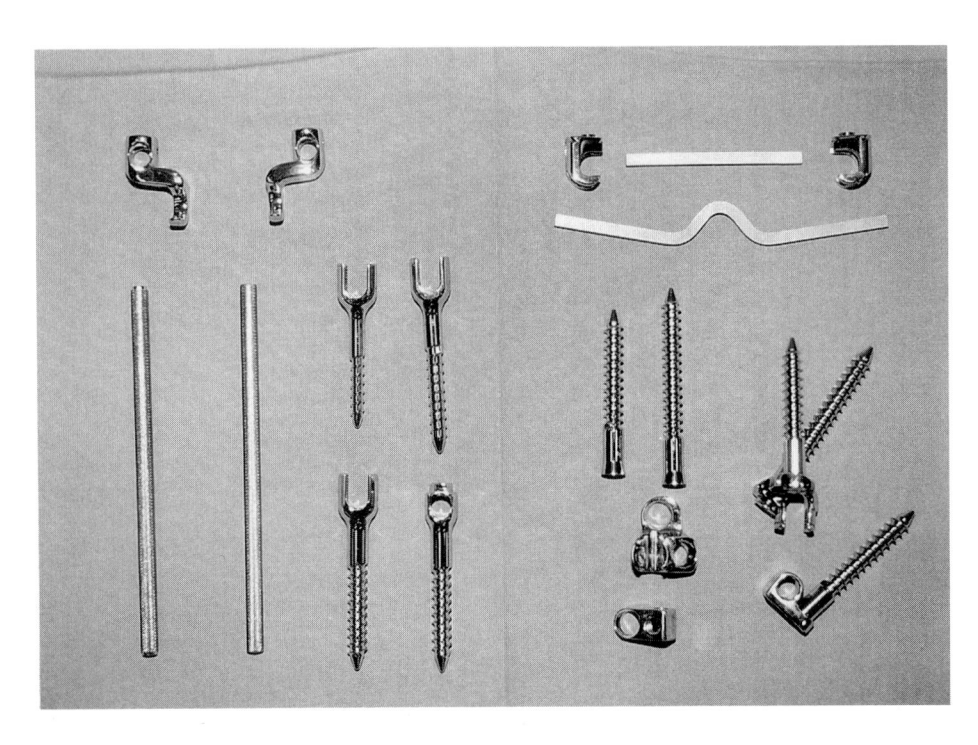

FIG. 28-1. CD implants. *Left to right,* offset hooks, rods, open and closed pedicle and sacral screws, transverse linking device with example of custom made shape of the bar, and Chopin blocs with iliac extension and screws.

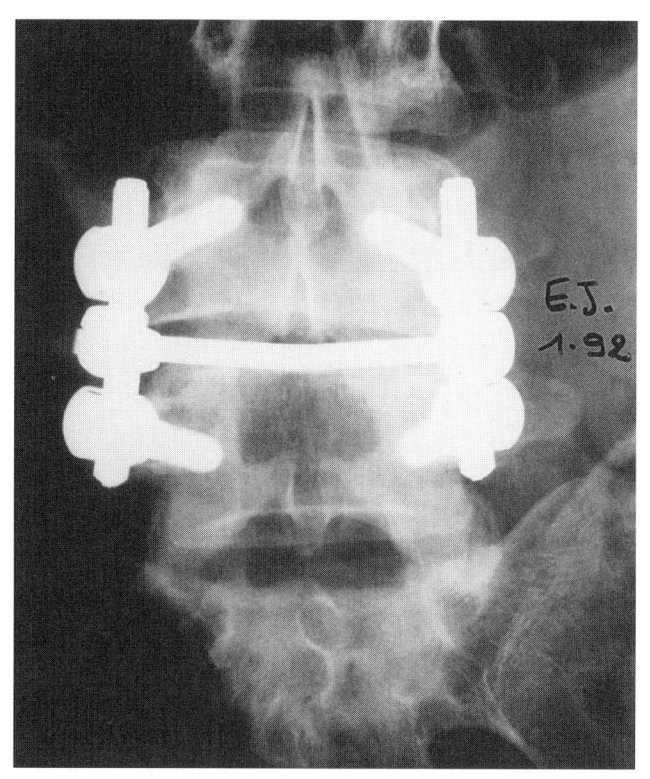

FIG. 28-2. Example of convergent pedicle screw placement in a short segmental fusion for degenerative disk disease.

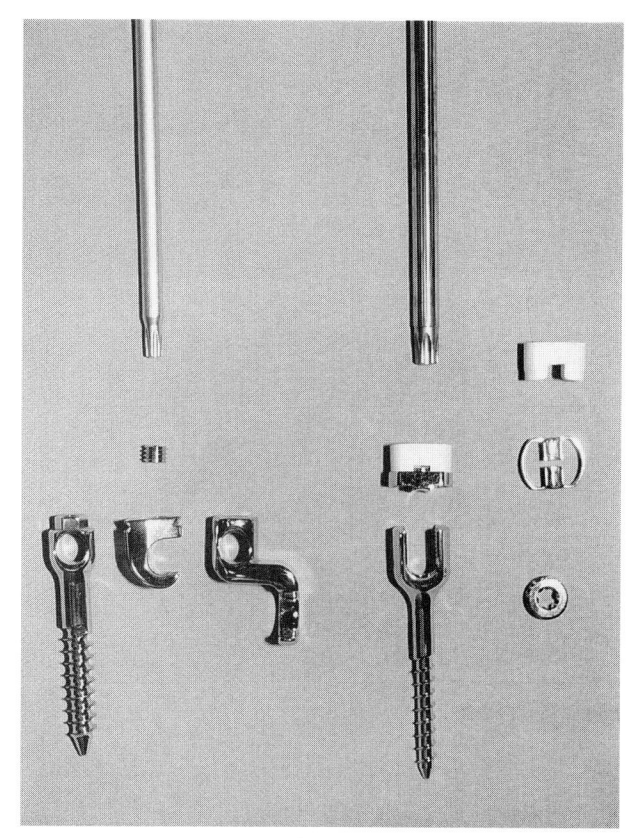

FIG. 28-3. Locking devices. *Left,* for closed-body implants; *right,* for open-body implants.

Rod-Implant Locking Devices

Two rod-implant locking devices are available depending on the type of implant: closed or open body (Fig. 28-3). Both have the common feature of being easily unlocked for intentional removal of the instrumentation if necessary.

Closed-body offset hooks and sacral screws are equipped with a 6-mm threaded plug. When tightened against the rod, this locking device resists to 2515 N axial loading before sliding; in comparison the older CD locking system withstands 1600 or 2100 N depending on the use of one or two locking screws (Cotrel, 1992; Sofamor, 1993).

Open body implants (pedicle and sacral screws, sacral blocks) are equipped with a set of two components: a 10-mm threaded plug and a washer that enhances the contact with the rod and prevents opening of the open body rims. This locking device withstands 2400 N load before slipping. After tightening the plug against the rod, the washer can be crushed against the threaded plug to prevent spontaneous unscrewing. A silicone piece holds the washer and the threaded plug together to offer single-hand manipulation of the device with the T-wrench; it is discarded after use.

Transverse Linking Device (TLD)

The TLD is composed of a rectangular section bar and a pair of hooks with a closed-body-type locking device. The rigidity of the TLD is increased threefold in torsion and ninefold in axial loading as compared with the original CD instrumentation transverse traction device.

INSTRUMENTS

See Figures 28-4 and 28-5 for CCD instruments.

Screwdrivers

A screwdriver for open screws and a screwdriver for closed-body screws permit single-hand gripping and insertion of the implants. The other hand remains free to use another instrument if desired.

Universal Implant Holder

The implant holder is usually used for the manipulation of laminar or TLD hooks but may also be used for open screws or Chopin blocks.

Rod Holder and Rod Gripper

A small clamp is used for the quick manipulation of the rods and TLD bars when the necessary bending and length are measured in the operative field. A strong vice-grip is used for the insertion of the rods and the rotation of these to obtain correction of scoliotic deformities. It is mandatory to hold the rod firmly with the rod-gripper while tightening the blocking systems of the open and closed body implants to ensure reliable fixation.

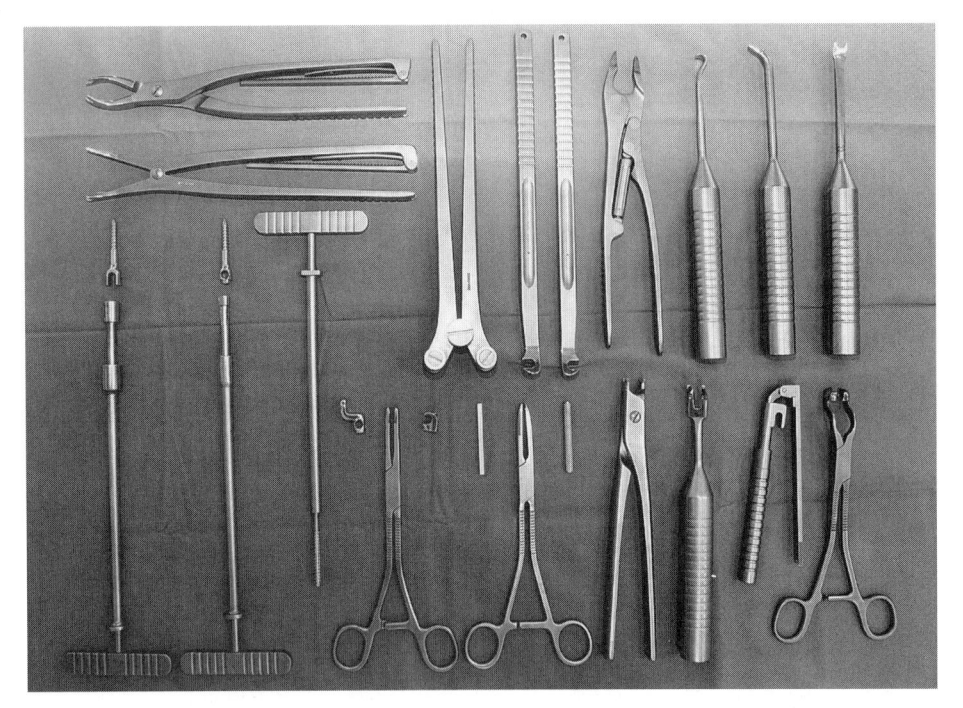

FIG. 28-4. CCD instruments, clockwise from upper left: distraction and compression forceps, French bender and bending irons, rod gripper, laminar elevator, hook and rod pushers, offset introducer forceps and articulate rod pusher, rod introducer lever, blocking forceps, rod and TLD bar holder, universal implant holder, tap, and screwdrivers for closed and open screws. (The locking wrenches are shown in Fig. 28-3.)

Locking Wrenches

A small and a large locking wrench are available to tighten the locking devices of the closed and open implants. Both locking wrenches can be used single-handedly, leaving the other hand free to grip the rod while tightening the device. It is important never to use the locking device to align the rod with the implant or to make a correction of deformity; the locking device must be fixed while the rod is well secured in the bottom of the groove of the open-body implants with one of the reduction instruments described below. Nonobservance of this rule will lead to unreliable fixation and loosening.

Correction Instruments

A French rod bender and in situ bending irons are available to bend the rods and TLD bars according to the anatomy and the desired amount of correction (Fig. 28-6). A compression forceps and a spreading forceps are used

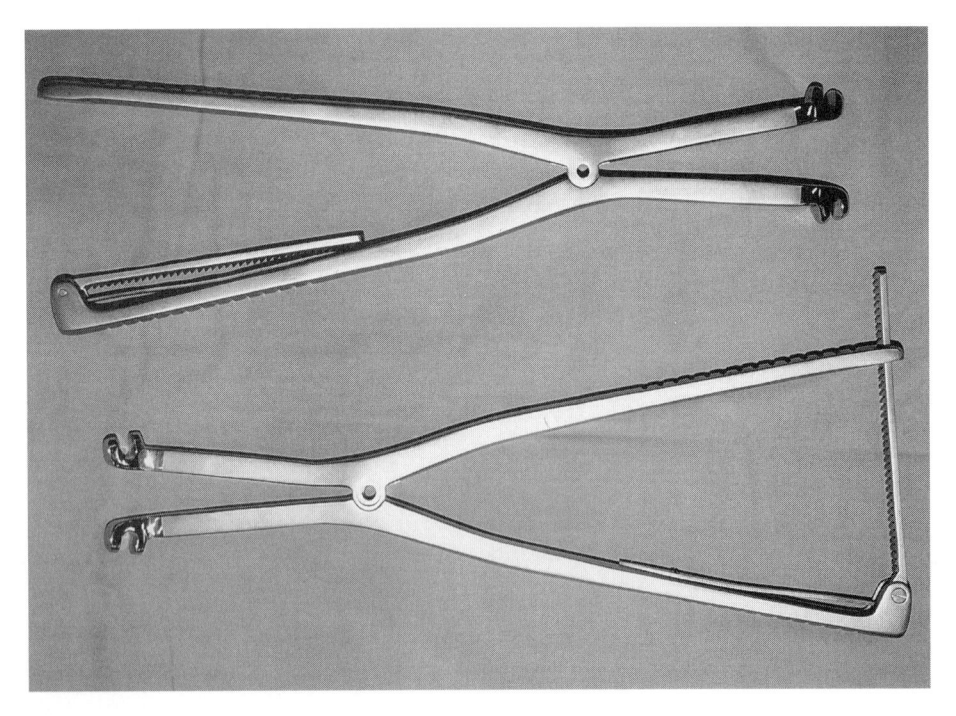

FIG. 28-5. Coupled rod bending irons (not part of the standard set of instruments).

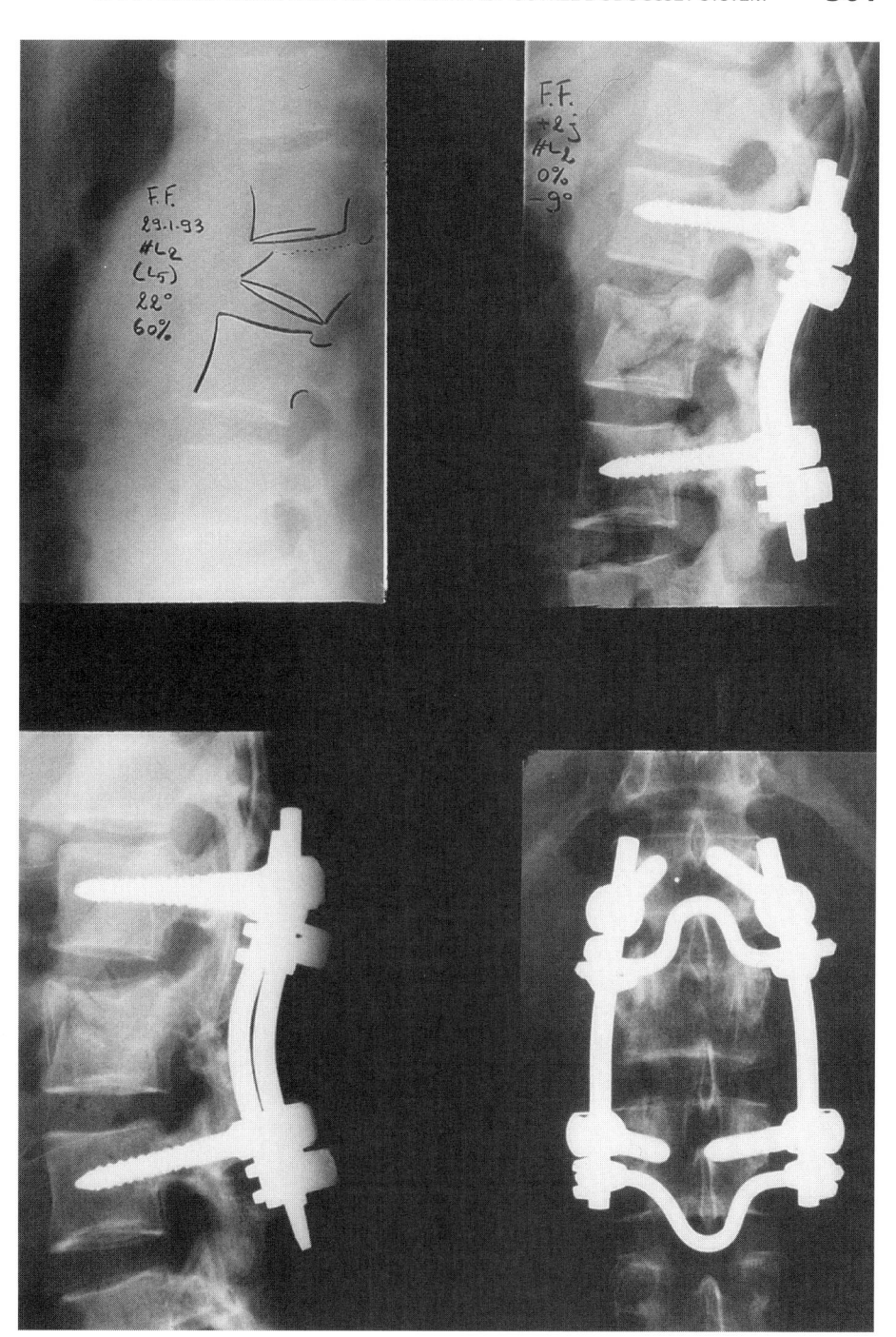

FIG. 28-6. Original short segmental construct reinforced by transverse linking devices taking support from the spinous processes. Postoperative and 8-month follow-up roentgenograms of burst type II fracture of L2 of a 30-year-old woman who wore a Jewett brace for 3 months show no loss of correction. Correction was obtained thanks to minimal distraction prior to in situ contouring of the rods with the coupled rod bender.

to perform distraction or compression between two vertebral implants. The rod gripper enables rotation of the rods. A rod pusher, a rod introducer lever, and an articulated rod pusher combined with an offset introducer forceps can be used to align the rods with the body of the open-body implants. This is useful for the correction of, for example, spondylolisthesis, and is mandatory to ensure perfect alignment of the rod in the bottom of the groove of the open-body implant before tightening the locking plug.

Miscellaneous Instruments

A laminar elevator is used to prepare the fitting of laminar hooks. A hook pusher can be used in conjunction with the implant holder to fit a hook and is also useful to maintain the alignment of the sacral block while inserting the S1 pedicle screw and the divergent screw; while introducing the latter, there is indeed a tendency to rotate the sacral block if it is not held. A blocking forceps is used to crush the washer of the open-body locking device against the threaded plug in order to prevent spontaneous unscrewing; this does not prevent intentional dismantling with the locking wrench. A tap is available for the sacrum.

SURGICAL TECHNIQUE AND USEFUL HINTS

Pedicle-Screw Placement

Insertion of pedicle screws from L1 to S1 is made with 10 to 20 degrees of convergence to take advantage of the greatest diameter of the pedicle and the greater anteroposterior length of the vertebra. In the sagittal plane, the tip of the screw should not be more anterior than the junction of the first and second quarters of the vertebral body, otherwise, violation of the anterior cortex and lesion to the aorta or vena cava is possible. The introduction point of the screw is situated on a little bony crest joining the upper articular facet and the basis of the transverse process; this is at the crossing-point of a horizontal line aligned with the transverse processes and a vertical line aligned with the facet joints. The entry point is prepared with a rongeur to remove the cortical bone; the direction of the pedicle is searched with an awl or 3-mm curette, guided by its cortical walls; the pedicle is further prepared either with the curette or with a 3.2-mm hand drill; the length of the cortex of the pedicle or vertebral body is probed with a depth gauge to avoid violating the cortex. (Its usual length is 40 or 45 mm.) We strongly advise against the use of power instruments, since feeling the resistance of cancellous and cortical bone would be impossible, leading to frequent false tracking. The use of 6-mm screws is strongly recommended since they resist more against bending than 5-mm screws; in our experience 6-mm-diameter screws can, with only rare exceptions, always be inserted from L1 to L5; in the S1 pedicle, 7-mm screws should be used; in T11 and T12, 5-mm screws must sometimes be used and a more sagittal fitting of the implant is necessary because the anatomical direction of the pedicles at those levels is less oblique than at the lower lumbar levels; the anteroposterior length is hence shorter and 40-mm length screws are to be selected in many cases. If using screws in the treatment of fractures while making a short instrumentation, taking purchase in only one vertebra above and below the fracture, 6-mm screws must be selected, 5-mm screws will always bend in such conditions where bending torque can be tremendous; if the pedicles are too thin, accepting only 5-mm-diameter implants, protection against bending and loss of correction must be ensured by complementing the construct with hooks or screws on the second vertebrae (Argenson or Jackson's frames) (Argenson, Lovet, Cambas, Griffet, & Barraud, 1989; Ebelke, Jackson, Hess, & McManus, 1992).

Sacral Screw and Chopin Block Placement

Placement of an S1 pedicle screw is best performed after removal of the inferior articular process of L5, which gives a clear view of the anatomical landmarks. The entry point is situated on a little crest, just below the articular cartilage of the S1 facet and lateral to a little dimple. The awl, curette, or hand drill is aimed to the sacral end plate, where strong bone is available; the end plate may be penetrated, offering even better purchase. A second screw can be placed with a 30- to 45-degree divergence about 7 mm distal to the S1 pedicle screw; the entry point is about 7 to 10 mm more lateral so that the bodies of the two screws will be well aligned, permitting easy introduction of the rod in both implants. We personally recommend the use of closed-body sacral screws.

The placement of a sacral block is similar with regard to the fitting of the S1 pedicle screw. While inserting the divergent screw, one has to make sure that tilting of the block does not occur; placement of a rod aligned with the lumbar implants and the sacral block can be of help in ensuring ideal placement.

Hook Placement

Proper placement of a supralaminar hook requires incision and removal of the ligamentum flavum and resection of a few millimeters of the upper lamina to ensure safe introduction of the hook without compressing the spinal cord or cauda equina. It is also often necessary to remove the medial aspect of the articular facets to have enough room for the placement of two adjacent hooks—to avoid overlapping of the blades and neurologic compromise. This leads, unfortunately, to some weakening of the junction between the instrumented and the normal spine.

Placement of infralaminar hooks is usually easy and can be performed between the lamina and the insertion of the ligamentum flavum; since the anteroposterior diameter of the spinal canal is greater at the distal aspect of the lamina than at the proximal aspect, neurologic compromise is less likely.

Rod Placement and Correction of Deformities

Prebending of the rod can both accommodate the actual alignment of the spine and serve as a guide to correct a deformation by realigning the vertebrae on the rod by the use of the vertebral implants and the specific instruments. The corrective maneuvers must always be smooth and avoid excessive use of the anchoring sites of the implants, which could lead to loosening and less than optimal stability as an end result. With the use of the different instruments listed above, it is possible to correct spondylolisthesis, transversal dislocations, scoliosis, and kyphotic deformities. An adequate degree of freedom of the various vertebra must first be obtained by sectioning ligamentous or capsular tethers and removing ankylosing osteophytes or articular processes. The desired amount of correction must not jeopardize neurologic structures, and one must be aware that total correction of deformities can be impossible to obtain, especially in a degenerative spine.

IMPORTANT NOTE ABOUT THE CORRECT FITTING OF THE ROD-IMPLANT LOCKING DEVICES

As has already been stressed, the rod-implant blocking sets may not be used to correct any malalignment between the rods and the vertebral implants. This would lead to a loose fixation and failure of the instrumentation. Any tilt of the rod in regard to the groove of the open-body implant must be corrected—for example, with the articulated rod pusher. While fitting the blocking sets with the T-wrench, the rod must be firmly held by a rod gripper; otherwise the power of the T-wrench could mobilize the spine and give the illusion of solid fixation, which would not be the case. It is also advisable to check the fixations a few minutes later and once more before wound closure, this rule is well known by all orthopedic surgeons who use plates and screws in internal fixation of fractures. All the loosenings of CCD instrumentations of which we are aware can be attributed to less then optimal fitting of the plugs. In our experience, only one dislodgment of a locking plug was found among more than 700 open-body screws or sacral blocks.

PLACEMENT OF THE TRANSVERSE LINKING DEVICES

The hooks of the TLD may be placed laterally or medially according to local anatomy. They must be perfectly perpendicular to the rods, and bending of the transverse bar is often required.

By bending the transverse bar it is possible to obtain additional stability of the construct thanks to a support on the spinous processes (e.g., in spinal fractures) (Gillet, 1992b) (Fig. 28-6).

One or more TLDs are placed to improve the rigidity of the construct according to its length.

CLINICAL EXPERIENCE

We have operated on 107 patients with the CCD from June 1990 to September 1992. Follow-ups range from 2 to 5 years.

CCD in Trauma

The thoracolumbar level was involved in 13 of 19 cases. The instrumentation was generally of the short segmental type, since this gave us satisfactory functional results with the original CD84 instrumentation (Gillet, Meyer, Fatemi, & Lemaire, 1991).

Sitting or standing was allowed on the second postoperative day, a Jewett brace was prescribed for 10 weeks, and anterior bending was prohibited. The brace could be taken off during showering provided bending was avoided. The hospital stay, when there was no neurologic compromise, was often as short as 1 week after surgery.

Return to normal everyday life, including domestic work, was obtained in all but 2 of 15 neurologically intact patients; 1 reports persistent local pain (compensation case), the other is impaired by a complicated open tibial fracture, but his spine is pain-free. Eight of 10 working patients could return to work; 1 could not because of local pain (see above), another recovered insufficiently from a Frankel grade C to a grade B lesion.

Implant removal had to be performed in 12 patients. In 5, implant removal was intended from the beginning since instrumentation was performed without bone fusion or while the bone graft was one segment shorter than the instrumentation. The other 7 patients required removal because of local discomfort; all these patients were very slender; pain was localized at the level of the thoracolumbar junction in 6 and at the sacral level in 1.

One rod fracture occurred above an L4 distal screw 4.5 months after surgery. This patient presented with an L3 burst fracture plus L4-5 and L5-S1 disk disease; he was treated by L2-5 instrumentation without bone fusion. There was no loss of correction and no pain related to the rod fracture. The use of cold rolled rods, which have a greater elastic range and a higher elastic limit than hyperquenched rods, could possibly have avoided this rod failure due to overloading by lack of arthrodesis. However, because of their remarkable elastic properties, cold rolled rods are difficult to bend in situ, we recommend, if such rods are chosen, to make the fracture reduction with hyperquenched rods using distraction and in situ bending of the rod with our coupled rod bender (see Fig. 28-6), then replace each rod by prebent cold rolled rods.

Good functional results could be obtained using short segmental fixation with the original CD instrumentation (Cotrel, 1992) but we have seen, as pointed out by other authors (Argenson et al., 1989; Ebelke et al., 1992), some loss of correction on the postoperative x-ray films after 3 months. However, the radiologic loss of correction was moderate and was not associated with poor clinical outcome. It occurred if severe wedging was present initially and particularly if reduction was not complete in the sagittal plane. Since radiologic results with short segmental fixation using the CD84 implants were less satisfactory then the clinical outcome, an original frame (Gillet, 1992b) has been used with the CCD to avoid, if possible, such loss of correction, taking advantage of a more rigid transverse linking device, bent in a "moustache" shape to gain additional support from the spinous process of the vertebra in which the pedicular screws are anchored (see Fig. 28-6). Short-term results are favorable.

CCD in Spondylolysis with and Without Spondylolisthesis

Thirty-five patients presenting with L4 or L5 spondylolysis with or without slip underwent surgery; 30 had lumbar or lumbosacral instrumentation, with posterolateral fusion in 24 and posterior lumbar interbody fusion in 6 (Fig. 28-7). The Gill procedure was used in 29 patients; 3 had isthmic

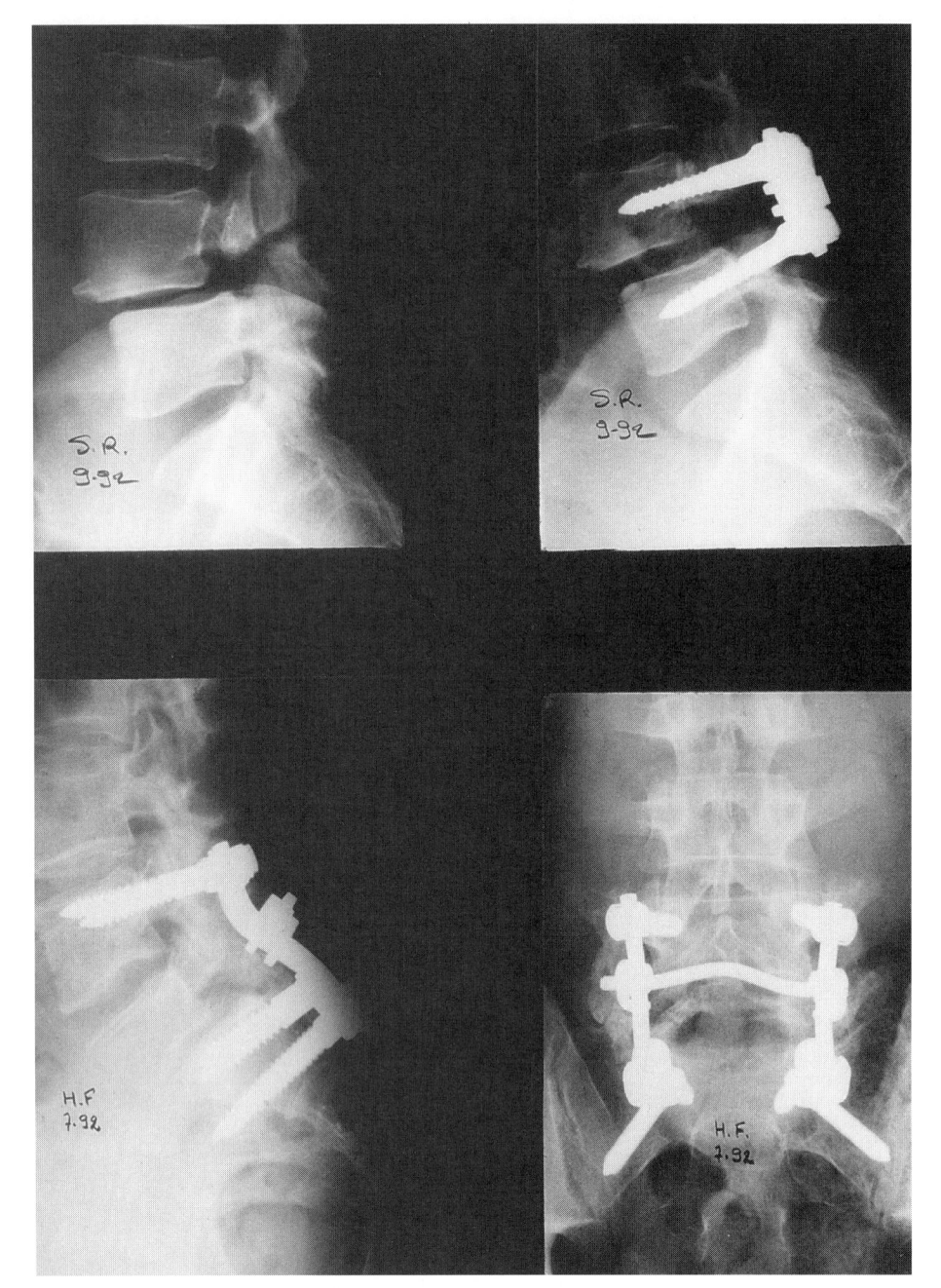

FIG. 28-7. Posterior lumbar interbody fusion and posterolateral fusion in patients with spondylolysis who underwent CCD fixation and wore no brace.

reconstruction with instrumentation by an original V-frame (Fig. 28-8); 2 patients had isthmic reconstruction with temporary fixation of L4-5 by a short construct.

Walking was encouraged on the second postoperative day, the hospital stay ranged from 7 to 10 days, and no brace was worn. Excessive hip flexion was avoided, but this advice was rarely respected for more then a few weeks because there was early pain relief and the patients wore no external support to remind them of the fusion procedure.

Pain-free everyday life was the end result in 75% of the patients, 10% describe themselves as only slightly impaired, and 15% describe residual pain. Four patients had an obvious failure of the procedure, which will be described below; 85% of previously working patients returned to work, 25% of them to a lighter job.

Implant removal was performed in three cases because of muscle irritation at the sacral level.

Five patients had complications. One had loosening of the upper L4 left locking nut between 6 weeks and 3 months; punching of the ring had been forgotten. Surprisingly, the patient was pain-free at 6 months, and the bone graft seemed fused. Another patient had broken 6-mm diameter screws at the sacral level. This patient showed reckless behavior and was involved in a scuffle 6 weeks after the operation. This is the only patient in whom implant failure, which could have been avoided, was related to a bad clinical outcome.

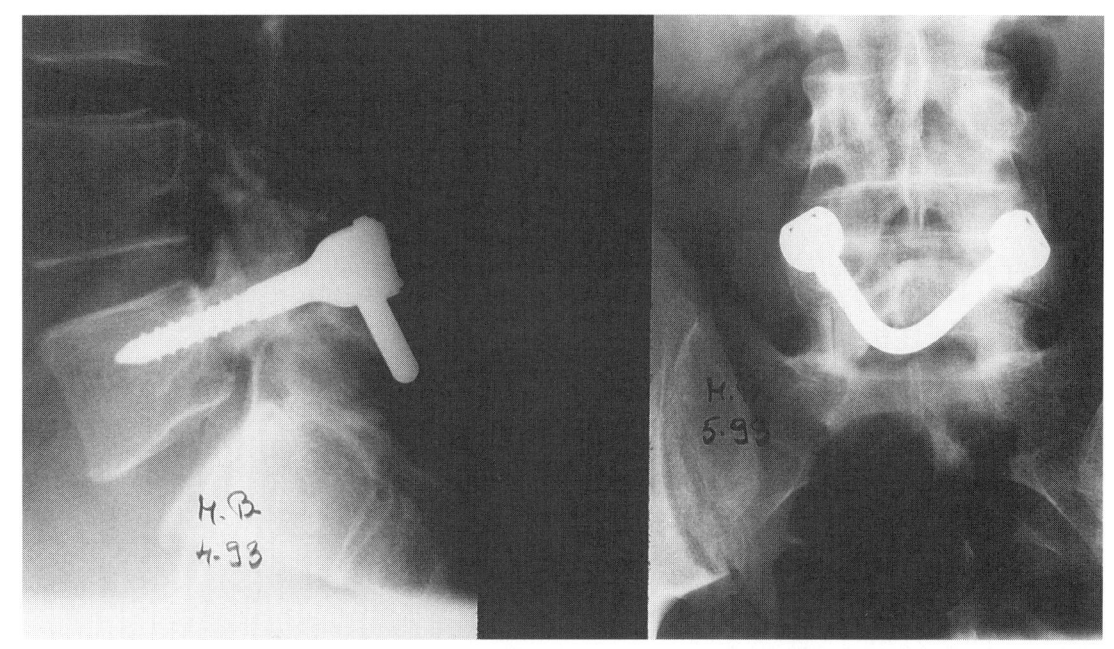

FIG. 28-8. Original isthmic reconstruction with CCD instrumentation using pedicle screws at the involved level and a V-shaped rod taking support from the posterior arch on both laminae and under the spinous process.

Nonunion developed in one patient under a previously fused thoracic and lumbar scoliosis; a complementory hip spica should probably have been used. The two patients who underwent isthmic reconstruction with temporary short segmental fixation had unilateral nonunion due to unsufficient stabilization of the posterior arch with the DLT, the original V-shaped rod design was hence used.

CCD in the Degenerative Spine

Fifty-one patients suffering from degenerative disease underwent fusion with instrumentation: lumbar, lumbosacral, one or multiple levels, with correction of degenerative scoliosis (Fig. 28-9) or spondylolisthesis and with laminectomy or diskectomy in most cases.

As in spondylolysis, early sitting and walking was possible, depending on the length of the fusion and the age and general condition of the patient. No brace was worn. Hospital stay (1 to 2 weeks) varied according to the patient's age and general status rather than to the length of the instrumentation.

Twenty-nine patients recovered a pain-free spine, 16 described themselves as greatly but incompletely improved, 6 were disappointed with the end result (4 one-level fusions, 1 two-level L3-5 fusion [control roentgenograms were not relevant in these disappointed patients], 1 infection). Ten patients of 13 returned to work, 2 of them to a lighter job. Implant removal had to be performed in three patients because of muscle irritation at the sacral level.

Complications occurred in three cases. One patient had a short L3-4 kyphosis after diskectomy and laminectomy for herniated disk and congenital spinal stenosis; maybe posterior lumbar interbody fusion (PLIF) should have been elected instead of posterolateral fusion. One patient treated for degenerative scoliosis showed a bad sacral bone stock, and unilateral divergent Chopin block screw loosening was observed at 6 weeks; bone fusion was obtained and a pain-free spine was the end result. The divergent screw was too short and did not take purchase in the anterior cortex. Severe infection developed in one patient after a difficult multiple-level procedure, and the instrumentation had to be removed. A nonunion was the end result, with persistent back pain, but the infection was cured.

CCD in Pott's Disease

One case of Pott's disease was treated with CCD. The patient had undergone laminectomy elsewhere. He was admitted with a spondylolisthesis and a large abcess reaching the subcutaneous tissues and was bedridden because of pain. Treatment included chemotherapy, drainage, interbody fusion with bone paste through the fistula and short L4-5 fixation. No complementary brace could be worn because of the patient's corpulence. The spine was pain-free at 4 weeks and the patient was able to climb on his roof at 5 months after surgery. The spine remained stable and fusion was obtained, the instrumentation was well tolerated and has not been removed, and both infection and instability were cured.

CCD in Tumors of the Spine

The use of CCD in the treatment of tumors (Fig. 28-10) proved satisfactory in four cases of spinal metastasis. Early pain relief and mobilization without a brace were obtained,

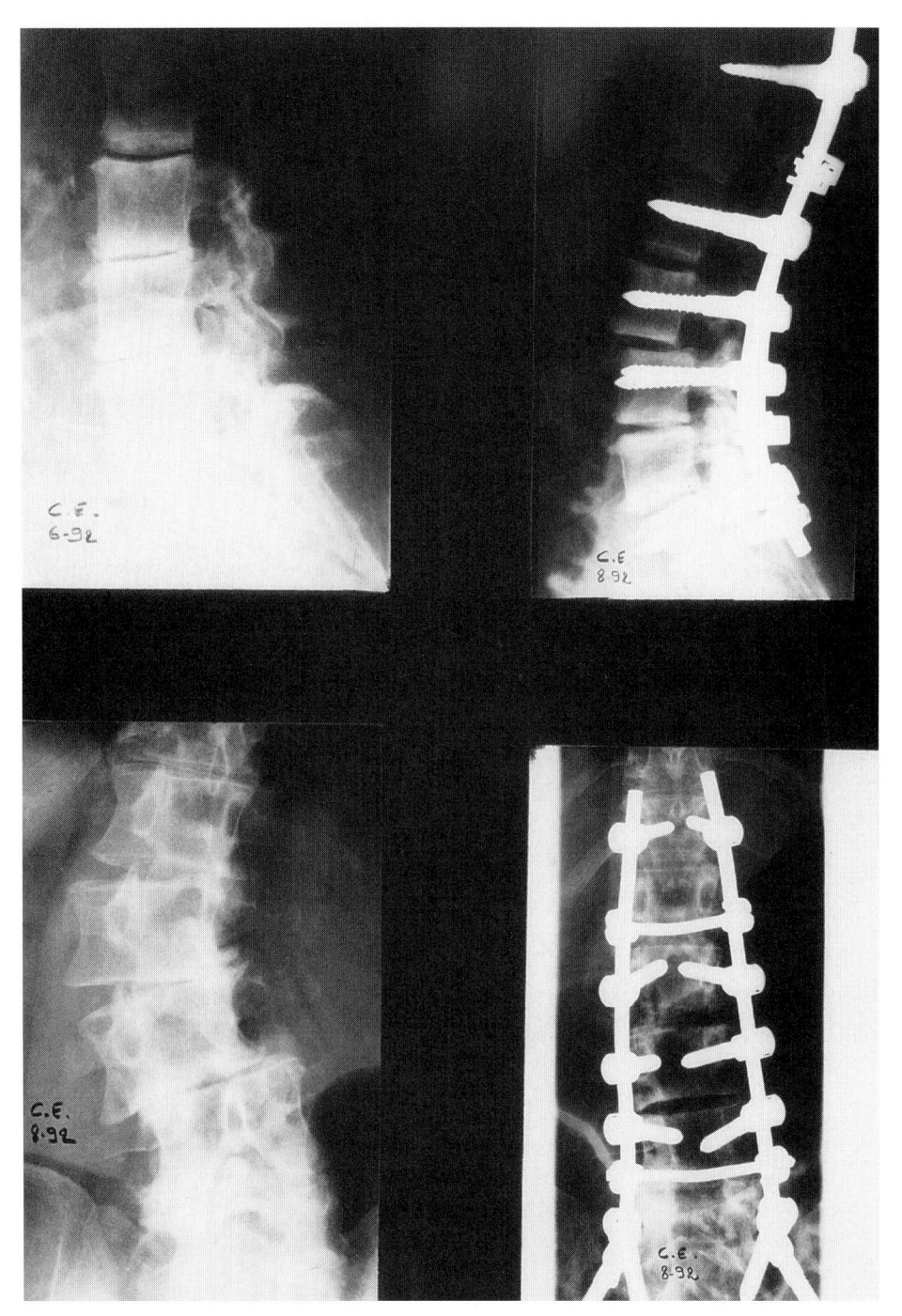

FIG. 28-9. Degenerative scoliosis with spinal stenosis. Restoration of normal spinal alignment in the sagittal and frontal plane with the instrumentation, laminectomy, and posterolateral bone fusion.

which were the functional goals in these cases in which comfort is all we can hope for and offer.

One patient was a 50-year-old woman with multiple-level metastasis from T10 to S1. At L3 there was neurologic compromise of the left root requiring posterolateral decompression. The spine had to be stabilized from the thoracic region to the pelvis, and sacral fixation was weak. We used a mixture of CD and CCD implants: long CD rods from the T8 to the S1 levels, CD hooks at the thoracic level, CCD screws at the lumbar and sacral levels, short CD rods supplementing this fixation with Galveston type fixation in the pelvis, and linkage to the longer rods with dominos. CCD screws can be perfectly fixed on CD rods; however, CD implants cannot be fixed in a reliable manner on CCD rods because of the thinner shape of the diamond points.

CONCLUSIONS

Since the availability of the CCD implants and instruments, all the patients who needed lumbar instrumentation for instability could be treated with the CCD. There has been no

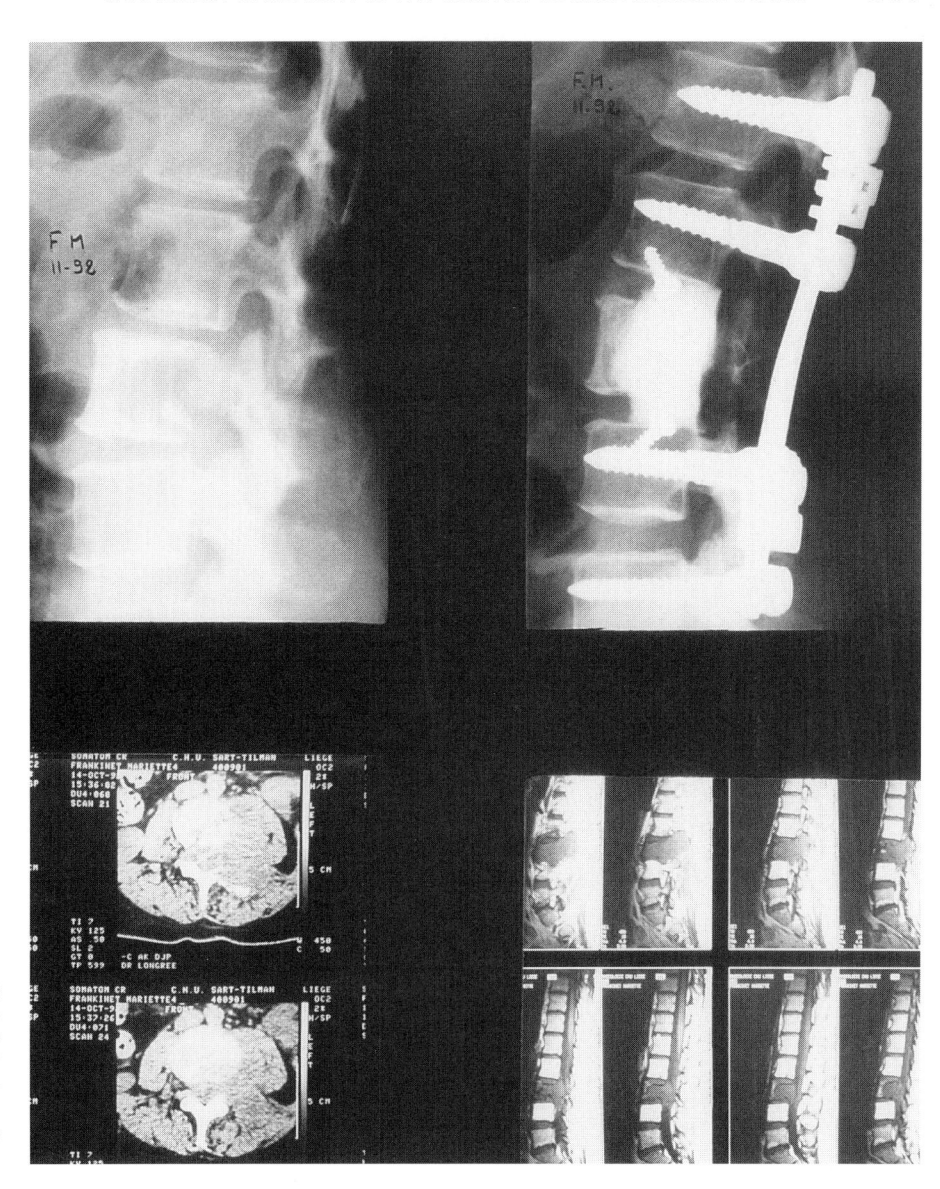

FIG. 28-10. L3 metastasis of breast cancer. Posterolateral decompression of the nerve root, reconstruction of the vertebral body with bone cement and two levels above–two levels below instrumentation using pedicular screws. Early walking and pain relief were achieved, and no brace was worn.

need for another instrumentation (Table 28-2). The correction of deformities, when desired, was obtained. The different rod-introducing levers and rod in situ bending irons and the large choice of sacral fixation were particularly appreciated. The complications that occurred were surgeon-related and could have been avoided by a better choice of implants, surgical indication, or procedure; they were probably the result of an unavoidable learning curve.

After more than 5 years of use of the CCD we think that it has gained a privileged place in the treatment of the lumbar and lumbosacral diseases that require instrumentation. The use of the CCD instrumentation can be contemplated in all unstable conditions of the spine, traumatic or not, from T11 to L5. Since the CD and the CCD instrumentations can be linked together if necessary, it widens possible indications to combined lesions of the thoracic and lumbar spine.

Since 1995, a CCD2 instrumentation has been introduced, it is intended to replace the instrumentation described above. Only slight differences exist with the first CCD instrumentation and they are the results of improvements in design. The CCD2 instrumentation has the same indications and is used exactly in the same way as its predecessor.

Table 28-2
Advantages and Disadvantages of CCD Instrumentation

Advantages
  Limited number of instruments
  Improved locking system enabling easy removal
  Double sacral screw fixation possible
  Improved transverse linking device

Disadvantages
  Difficult to fit rod correctly in open-body screw implant

REFERENCES

Argenson, C., Lovet, J., Cambas, P.M., Griffet, J., & Barraud, O. (1989). Osteosynthesis of thoraco-lumbar spine fractures with Cotrel-Dubousset instrumentation. *Proceedings of the 5th Groupe International Cotrel Dubousset* (pp. 75–82). Montpellier, France: Sauramps Médical.

Cotrel, Y., Dubousset, J., & Guillaumat, M. (1988). New universal instrumentation in spinal surgery, *Clinical Orthopaedics and Related Research, 227,* 10–23.

Cotrel, Y. (1992). Compact Cotrel-Dubousset instrumentation, Proceedings of the 8th international congress on CD instrumentation (pp. 111–130). Montpellier, France: Sauramps Médical.

Ebelke, D.K., Jackson, R.P., Hess, W.F., & McManus A.C. (1992). CD pedicle instrumentation for improved burst fracture fixation and reduction with in situ extension contouring of the rods. *Proceedings of the 8th Groupe International Cotrel Dubousset* (pp. 45–58). Montpellier, France: Sauramps Médical.

Gillet, P., Meyer, R., Fatemi, F., & Lemaire, R. (1991). Interêt des osteosynthèses courtes avec fixations pédiculaires dans le traitement des fractures instables du rachis dorso-lombaire: Étude biomécanique et résultats cliniques actuels. *Acta Orthopaedica Belgica, 57* (Suppl. 1), 177–183.

Gillet, P. (1992a). Preliminary results with the new CCD instrumentation for the lumbar and lumbosacral spine. *Proceedings of the 8th Groupe International Cotrel Dubousset* (pp. 161–166). Montpellier, France: Sauramps Médical.

Gillet, P. (1992b). Usefullness of the DDT n*3 in trauma to prevent pedicular screw bending and loss of correction. *Groupe International Cotrel Dubousset News, 3,* 4.

Sofamor* Spine Division, Compact Cotrel-Dubousset Surgeon's Documentation, Sofamor France, 1993.

Steib, J.P., Bogorin, J., Lang, G., & Kehr, P. (1992). Own experience with the CCD. *Proceedings of the 8th Groupe International Cotrel Dubousset* (pp. 167–170). Montpellier, France: Sauramps Médical, 1992.

CHAPTER 29

Dynalok Fixation System

Stephen E. Heim
Douglas L. Johnson

HIGHLIGHTS

The Dynalok Fixation System (Danek Group Inc., Memphis, TN) evolved out of early clinical experiences with the spinal instrumentation systems of the early 1980s (Bernhardt, Swartz, Clothiaux, Crowell, & White, 1992; Heim & Luque, 1992; Kaneda, Kazama, Satoh, et al., 1986; Johnston, Ashman, Baird, & Allard, 1990; Zindrick, 1991; Dekutoski, Conlan, & Salciccioli, 1993). In North America, the initial phase of pedicular instrumentation systems developed at a time when the concepts of load sharing and load bearing were the "hot topics" in bone healing. Load-sharing instrumentations would carry a portion of the stress applied to the bony segment, whereas load-bearing instrumentations would divert the stress applied away from the bony segment spanned. Understandably, two design rationales for spinal instrumentation arose—semiconstrained (load sharing) and fully constrained (load bearing). The initial semiconstrained systems were exemplified by the Luque plate screw and the Synthes plate screw systems. The initial Steffee plate-screw system was a example of the fully constrained systems of the time. Each type of system had relative merits and problems.

Semiconstrained instrumentation systems, in general, provided an increased flexibility and ease of use for the surgeon because the screws were able to be angled individually relative to the plate as well as in relation to adjacent screws. Furthermore, because the screws were not rigidly fixed to the plate, internal construct stresses were minimized as compared with fully constrained systems. This feature resulted in a somewhat lower comparative instrumentation failure rate. Lastly, the load-sharing characteristic of such systems would tend to minimize stress shielding of the fusion mass (Esses & Moro, 1993; Farey, McAfee, Gurr, & Randolph, 1989; Goel, Lim, et al., 1991; Johnston, Ashman, Baird, & Allard, 1990; Lipscomb, Grubb, & Talmage, 1989; McAfee, Farey, Sutterlin, et al., 1989; Soshi, Shiba, Kondo, & Murota, 1991).

Fully constrained instrumentation systems, on the other hand, were much more effective in restoring the stability of a grossly unstable spinal segment than were their load-sharing counterparts (An, Simpson, Ebrahaim, et al., 1992; Cooper, Errico, Martin, Crawford, & DiBartolo, 1993; Doerr, Montesano, Burkus, & Benson, 1991; Goel, Lim, et al., 1991; Krag, 1991; Sasso & Cotler, 1993; Zindrick, 1991). However, as a result of the fully constrained nature of these systems the technique of implantation was significantly more difficult. If a perpendicular bolt-plate interface was not present, the fixation was compromised and the internal stresses within the construct were increased. This resulted in a significant incidence of instrumentation fatigue failure. As the importance of proper technique became recognized and the design of implants improved, the incidence of such fatigue failures was able to be diminished (Ashman, Johnston, & Corin, 1990; Boss, Marchesi, & Aebi, 1992; Carson, Duffield, Arendt, Ridgely, & Gaines, 1990; Davne & Myers, 1992; Kabins, Weinstein, & Spratt, et al., 1992; Krag, 1991; Mattheck, Bethge, Erb, & Blomer, 1992; McAfee, Weiland, & Carlow, 1991; Rosen, 1991; Ruland, McAfee, Warden, & Cunningham, 1991; Yamagata, Kitahara, Minami, et al., 1992).

In time, as data became available regarding outcomes in the use of the various spinal instrumentation systems it became apparent that fusion rates seemed to be increased over noninstrumented fusions (Bernhardt, Swartz, Clothiaux, Crowell, & White, 1992; Cotler & Cotler, 1990; Dickman,

Fessler, MacMillan, & Haid, 1992; Farey, McAfee, Gurr, & Rudolph, 1989; Grubb & Lipscomb, 1992; Johnston, Ashman, Baird, & Allard, 1990; Sano, Yokokura, Nagata, & Young, 1990; Steinmann & Herkowitz, 1992; Van Horn & Bohnen, 1992; Watkins, 1992; West, Bradford, & Ogilvie, 1991b; Zdeblick, 1992). More recently, Zdeblick (1992) studied the success rates of noninstrumented fusions versus fusions using semiconstrained or fully constrained instrumentation systems. In a prospective, randomized study of lumbar fusion he was able to demonstrate a 65% fusion rate in the noninstrumented group as compared with an 81% fusion rate in the semiconstrained group and a 97% fusion rate in the fully constrained group. In view of the improved fusion success rate documented using a fully constrained pedicular spinal instrumentation system, it is also of particular importance to note that the theoretical stress-shielding effect of a load-bearing construct has not been demonstrated to have any apparent clinical significance (Farey, McAfee, Gurr, & Randolph, 1989; Goel, Lim, et al., 1991; Johnston et al., 1990; McAfee, Farey, Sutterlin, et al., 1989).

The Dynalok Fixation System was designed with these early lessons in mind. Indications and contraindications for its use are listed in Table 29-1. The actual design criteria included the goals of

1. system modularity to permit the use of fully constrained, semiconstrained, or hybrid constructs;
2. adjustability of plate cross-bridges to allow optimal flexibility in bolt and screw placement; and
3. reduction of the incidence of implant failure by improving the construct strength and fatigue characteristics and avoiding internal stress concentrations.

SYSTEM BIOMECHANICS

The development of the Dynalok system as a new entity allowed the design engineers to study the types of instrumentation failures that had become apparent with the systems designed initially in the 1980s (Ashman, Johnston, & Corin, 1990; Boos, Marchesi, & Aebi, 1992; Carson, Duffield, Arendt, Ridgely, & Gaines, 1990; Heim & Luque, 1992; Kabins, Weinstein, Spratt, et al., 1992; Mattheck, Bethge, Erb & Blomer, 1992; McAfee, Weiland, & Carlow, 1991; West, Bradford, & Ogilvie, 1991a; Zucherman, Hsu, et al., 1992). With the mechanisms of these failures in mind, particular attention was paid to the bolt-plate interface, the bolt design itself, and the stress distribution at the nut-bolt interface. As the overall strength of a bolt varies exponentially with the minor diameter, a slight increase in this dimension results in a significant improvement in the strength (Fig. 29-1). In addition, the increased minor diameter allows the Dynalok bolts to be cannulated for implantation safety. Furthermore, a conical minor diameter has the effect of avoiding stress concentration at the important bolt shaft–thread junction, as well as placing a more "cortical" bolt design in the cortical pedicle and a more "cancellous" bolt design in the cancellous vertebral body. Lastly, the implementation of the Spiralock thread design in the nut-bolt interface vastly improves the stress distribution at this important junction (Fig. 29-2). The overall effect of these design features is demonstrated in Fig. 29-3, which indicates construct stiffness and fatigue life. Figure 29-3 includes the data on Dynalok titanium implants as well. In order to maintain the construct fatigue life, additional modifications to the design were made in recognition of the inherently different metallurgical characteristics of titanium as compared with stainless steel.

Dynalok System Instruments

Figure 29-4 shows the instruments that comprise the Dynalok system. At this point only the key instruments will be discussed. The "Surgical Technique" section of this chapter includes a step-by-step description of the Dynalok instruments in their general order of use. One key point to mention, however, is the fact that the Dynalok instruments and implants are cannulated to allow use of guiding K-wires for improved safety of implantation.

Table 29-1
Indications and Contraindications to the Use of the Dynalok Fixation System*

Indications
    Trauma
    Tumor
    Spondylolysis/spondylolisthesis
    Segmental instability
    Painful motion segment
    Internal disk disruption

Contraindications
    Scoliosis/sagittal plane deformity
    Developmentally inadequate pedicles
    Active infection
    Profound osteopenia

*(An, Simpson, Ebraheim, et al., 1992; Coe, Warden, Herzig, & McAfee, 1990; Cooper, Errico, Martin, Crawford, & DiBartolo, 1993; Cotler & Cotler, 1990; Doerr, Montesano, Burkus, & Benson, 1991; Esses & Moro, 1993; Grob, Scheier, et al., 1991; Grubb & Lipscomb, 1992; Haid & Dickman, 1993; Heim & Luque, 1992; Herkowitz & Kurz, 1991; Kaneda, Kazama, Satoh, et al., 1986; Kim, Denis, Lonstein, & Winter, 1990; Konogi & Hasue, 1991; Lenke, Bridwell, et al., 1992; Linson & Williams, 1991; Markwalder, 1993; North, Campbell, et al., 1991; Ohmori, Suzuki, & Ishida, 1992; Postacchini & Cinotti, 1992; Rimoldi, Zigler, Capen, & Hu, 1992; Salib & Pettine, 1993; Sano, Yokokura, Nagata, & Young, 1990; Sasso & Cotler, 1993; Satomi, Hirabayashi, Toyama, & Fujimura, 1992; Steinmann & Herkowitz, 1992; Weatherley, Mehdian, & Berghe, 1991; Wetzel & LaRocca, 1992; Wittenberg, Shea, Lee, White, & Hayes, 1991; Zindrick, 1987; Zindrick, 1991; Zucherman, Hsu, et al., 1992).

CALCULATED BOLT/SCREW STRENGTH
(Section Modulus)

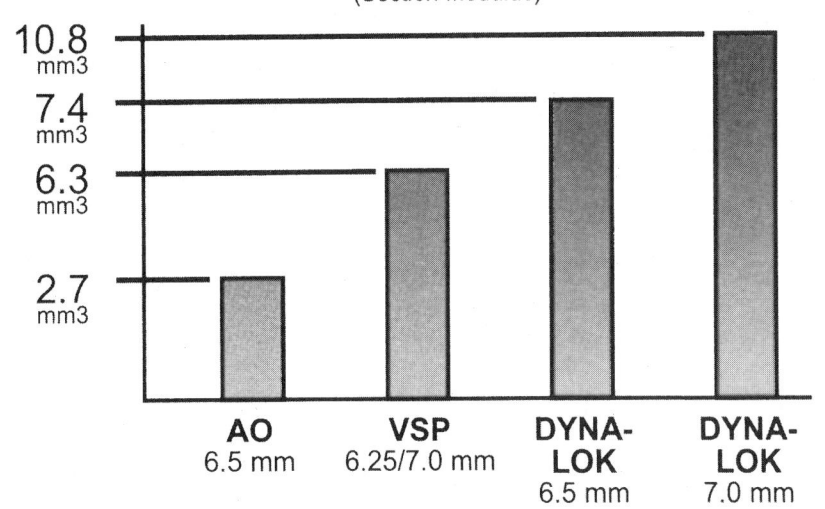

AO 6.5 mm	2.7 mm3
VSP 6.25/7.0 mm	6.3 mm3
DYNA-LOK 6.5 mm	7.4 mm3
DYNA-LOK 7.0 mm	10.8 mm3

FIG. 29-1. Comparative bolt diameter versus strength.

The blunt tip guiding K-wires included in the system are 9 cm in length. The blunt tip design and the flexible nature of the K-wires decreases the risk of penetration of a pedicular cortex in the process of pedicle sounding. The K-wire inserter is used to advance the wires along the pedicle. A friction lock design permits rapid adjustment of the K-wire length during insertion. A direct-read depth gauge is then employed to determine the appropriate-length bolt for insertion by measuring the visible portion of the K-wire.

A straight-tip pedicular sound is also included for direct pedicle entrance. This is not necessary to use prior to the steps of tapping or bolt insertion if the cannulated technique is used. However, some surgeons may prefer a technique of direct pedicle sounding rather than the K-wire–guided technique.

All taps and screwdrivers feature a removable shaft that inserts into a ratcheting handle—either straight or T-shaped. This ratcheting feature significantly increases the ease of use of the taps and screwdrivers.

The deflection beam torque wrench allows accurate nut tightening. This is used as a socket wrench, which passes over a screwdriver (back-up screwdriver) engaging the bolt on which the nut is being tightened. The back-up screwdriver also has a short area of threads along its shaft. These serve the purpose of allowing the surgeon to stack a series of nuts on the shaft and initially apply these nuts to each of the bolts rapidly.

A distractor is also included in the set, permitting simultaneous bolt distraction and tightening as indicated by the clinical pathoanatomy.

Dynalok System Implants

Examples of the Dynalok plate, bolt, screw, plate ring, T-bolt, and cross-link are shown in Fig. 29-5. The implants are available in either stainless steel or titanium. Extensive bioengineering design features have been used to limit the incidence of implant fatigue. These design features were modified further to produce the implants from titanium, because of the different metallurgical properties of stainless steel and titanium. These features have been shown to succeed biomechanically (see Fig. 29-3).

The Dynalok instrumentation system includes plates, bolts, and screws in a wide variety of sizes. The plates feature a double-scalloped design for the creation of a stable bolt-plate interface. This scalloping is identical top and bottom, so there is actually not a top or bottom to the plates before they have been contoured. The open longitudinal slot of the plate allows the surgeon to place the bolts as determined by patient anatomy, with no limitations of plate design by internal cross-bridges. The plate rings serve the purpose of a cross-bridge and are placed adjacent to each bolt. They are, however, fully adjustable in their location. Plates are available in lengths from 4 to 12 cm, in 1-cm increments, as well as in 14 and 16 cm lengths.

The bolts feature a conical minor diameter, cannulated design. They are available in 6.5-, 7.0-, 7.5-, and 8.5-mm diameters. Lengths vary in 5-mm increments ranging from 30 to 45 mm for the 6.5-mm bolts; 35 to 50 mm for the 7.0-mm bolts; 35 to 55 mm for the 7.5-mm bolts; and 30 to 45 mm for the 8.5-mm bolts. Reduction bolts are also available for the reduction of anterior vertebral displacements if clinically indicated. Constructs formed with the bolts create a rigid biomechanical construct. In such constructs a 90-degree bolt-plate interface is required. This may be obtained most readily by proper plate contouring; however, in some instances where the contouring is difficult 4-mm spacers or 15-degree wedges are used (see "Surgical Technique").

The screws are similar to the bolts in that they also feature a conical minor diameter, cannulated design. Available diameters are 5.5 and 6.5 mm. Lengths range from 35 to

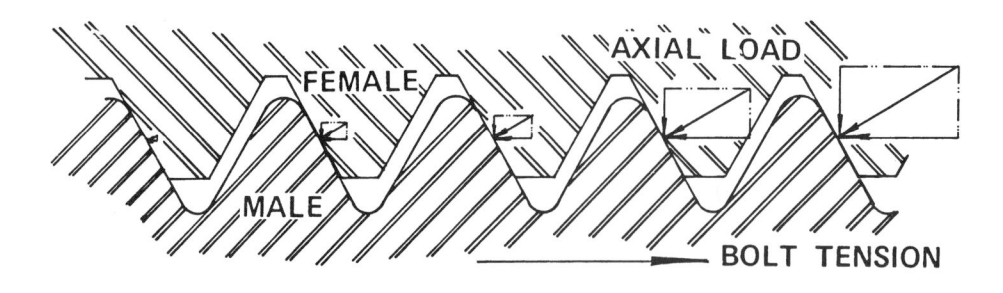

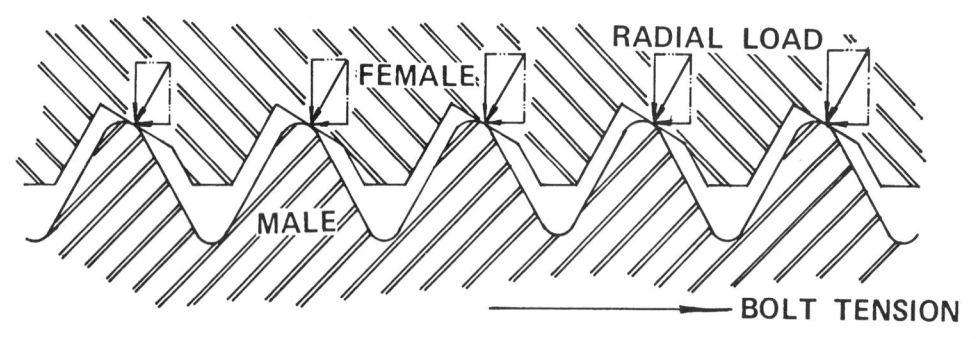

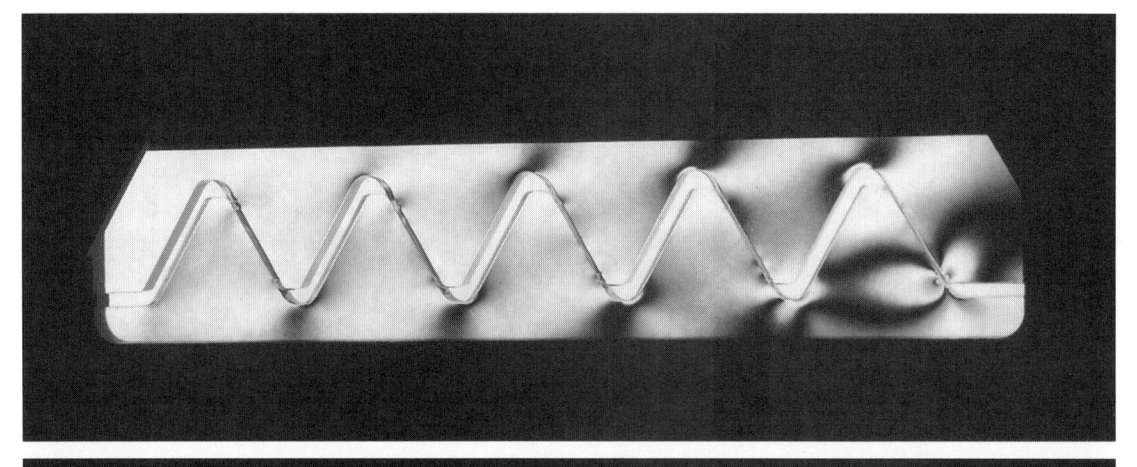

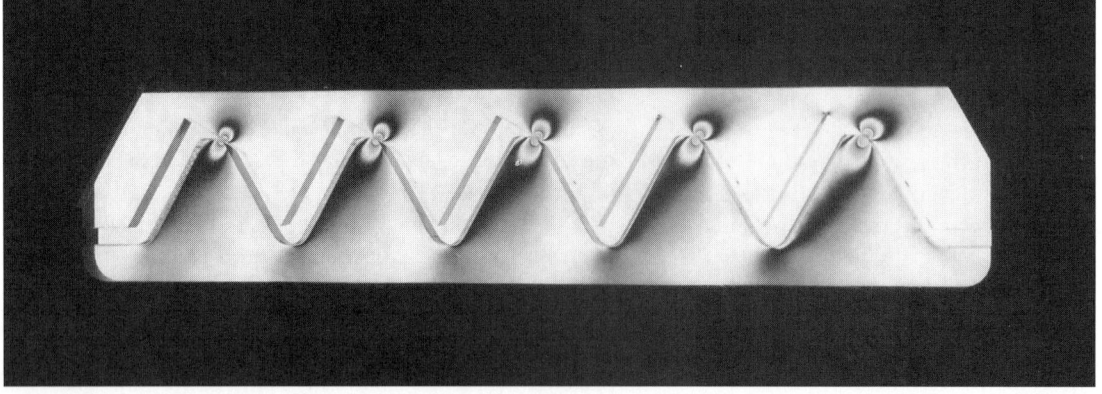

FIG. 29-2. Spiralock Thread Form (Detroit Tool Industries) produces a much more even distribution of stress at the nut-bolt interface. The schematic (a) demonstrates the principle behind the design; while the photoelastic analysis picture (b) demonstrates the true effectiveness of the design. (*Photoelastic analysis picture courtesy of the Kaynar Division of Microdot, Inc.*)

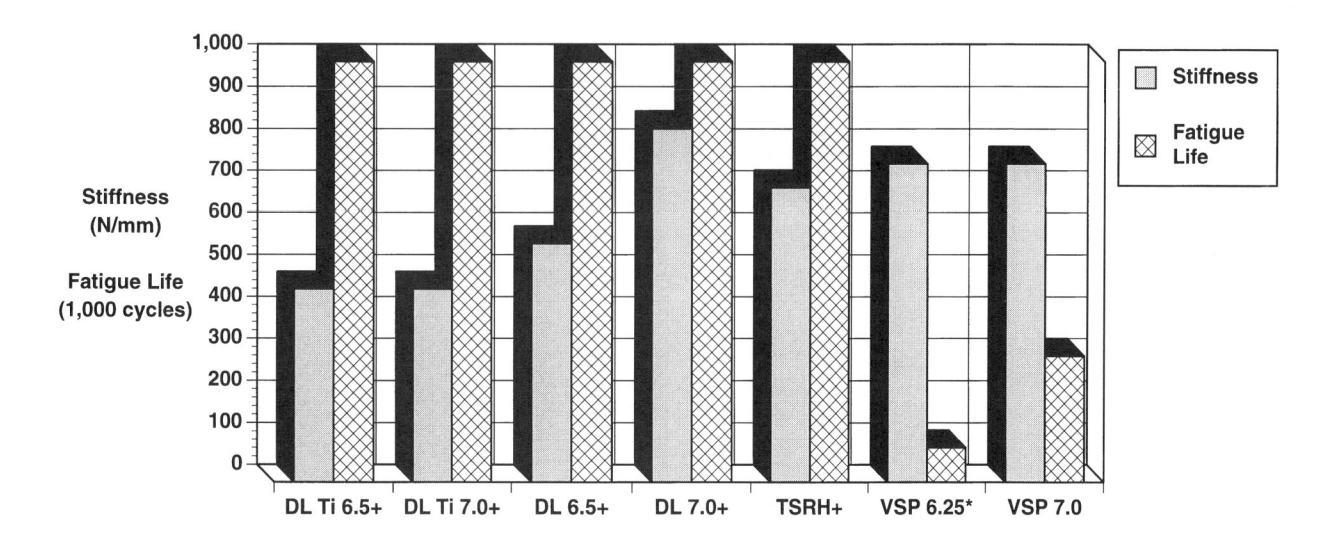

STIFFNESS AND FATIGUE

FIG. 29-3. Comparative construct stiffness and fatigue lifes. Note the demonstrated relative stiffness and fatigue characteristics of the titanium Dynalok construct.

* Not yet retested since material change.
+ No failure experienced in fatigue tests.

---

45 mm for the 5.5-mm screws, and 35 to 50 mm for the 6.5-mm screws. The system design allows up to 15 degrees of medial-lateral and 30 degrees of craniocaudal angulation of the screws relative to the plate. This is useful in multisegment constructs, in which suboptimal bolt placement may result in nonlinear alignment of the bolts and, thereby, difficulty in plate application. Substitution of a screw, with its inherently greater degree of freedom relative to the plate, for an intermediate bolt may allow for the "indiscretions" of the initial bolt placement technique. More importantly, this degree of freedom in the screw-plate interface is very useful in the reduction step of a high-grade spondylolisthesis in

FIG. 29-4. Dynalok instrument tray.

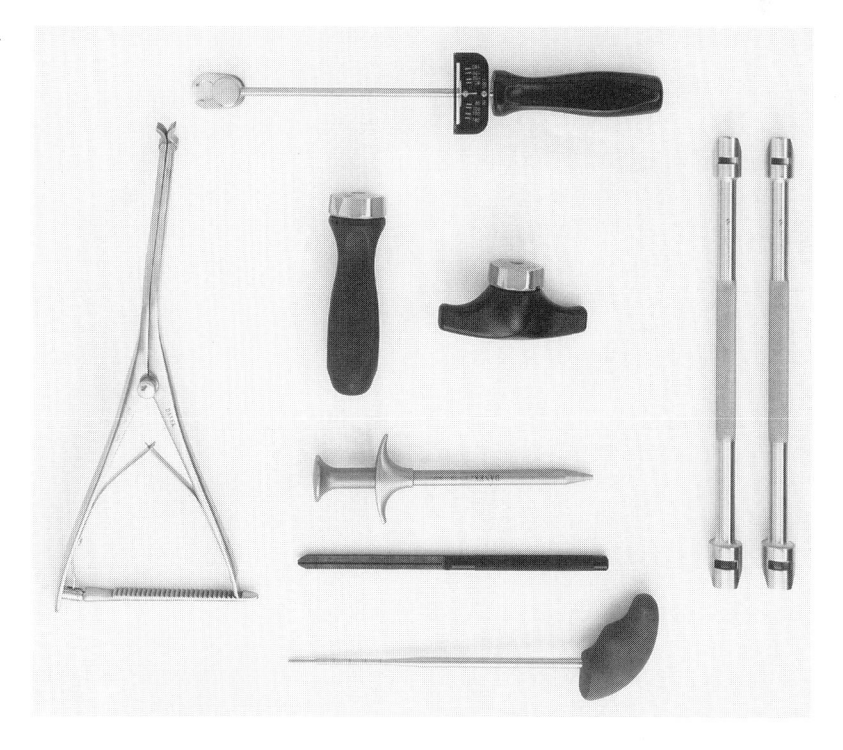

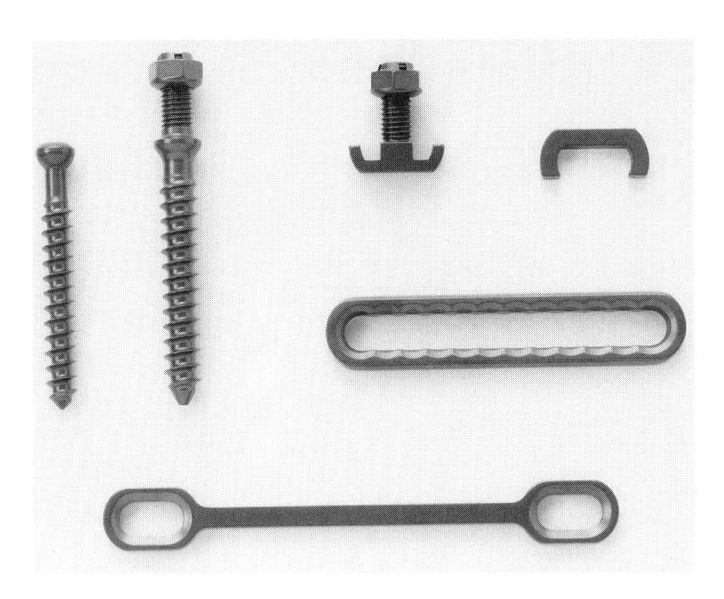

FIG. 29-5. Dynalok plate, bolt, screw, plate ring, T-bolt, and cross-link.

which the craniocaudal angle of the pedicle will change relative to the plate. A rigid implant in this step of reduction will result in excessive bone-implant stress, increased internal construct stress, and/or partial blockage to reduction (Fig. 29-6).

The Dynalok system also allows cross-linkage for increased construct rigidity. Cross-links may be applied in a bolt-to-bolt manner, thereby rigidly and directly triangulating a pair of bolts. They may also be applied in a plate-to-plate fashion, using T-bolts. The T-bolts are applied from the undersurface of a plate and held in position by screw on handles while the plate is being manipulated or inserted. The T-bolts also serve a "plate-closing" purpose and substitute for a plate ring at the level to which they are applied. The Dynalok cross-links are readily contoured with the bending irons included in the set and are available in five sizes.

Titanium versus Stainless Steel Spinal Implants

Since surgeons first began attempting to fuse the spine, one burning question has persisted—Is it fused? The efficacy of spinal instrumentation in increasing the success rate of spinal fusion has become apparent (Cotler & Cotler, 1990; Dickman et al., 1992; Johnston et al., 1990; Sano et al., 1990; Zdeblick, 1992). Furthermore, the success of fusion has been demonstrated in a randomized, prospective study by Zdeblick (1992) to be increased with rigid constructs (97%) over that obtained with semirigid constructs (81%) and uninstrumented fusions (65%). The theoretical concerns of stress shielding of the fusion mass have not been borne out clinically (Farey et al., 1989; Goel et al., 1991; Johnston et al., 1990; McAfee et al., 1989).

The determination of fusion success has generally been a radiographic exercise. In the past, when noninstrumented fusions were the norm, flexion-extension radiographs, tomograms, and/or computed tomographic (CT) scans were used (Brodsky, Kovalsky, & Khalil, 1991) in the assessment of fusion. However, with the rigidity of current implants, flexion-extension radiographs are no longer useful, and both tomography and CT imaging are greatly limited by the degree of metallic artifact present with stainless steel implants. Furthermore, the ability to image the spinal canal by way of CT scan or magnetic resonance imaging (MRI) is similarly limited to a great extent by this same artifact (Ebraheim, Savolaine, Stitgen, & Jackson, 1992). It is in the ability to image the spine that titanium has its greatest advantages over stainless steel as an implant material. An additional advantage of titanium is that of being an "unfriendly electrobiologic surface" to bacteria. Figure 29-7 demonstrates the axial and reconstructed sagittal and coronal CT scan images obtained in patients with the Dynalok Titanium Instrumentation System. These images were obtained 10 weeks postoperatively to assess early fusion progression and to decide whether to discontinue postoperative bracing and progress to rehabilitation. In Fig. 29-8 the axial and sagittal MRI images as well as the axial myelogram–CT images are shown for a patient treated with L5-S1 fusion (spondylolytic spondylolisthesis with back and leg pain) in whom recurrent leg pain developed after a separate injury, approximately 9 months postoperatively. The clarity with which the spinal canal can be visualized and the ability to see the early bony incorporation extending up to the undersurface of the plate is truly impressive. It is the authors' opinion that the titanium implants greatly improve the ability to evaluate the incorporation of the fusion mass as well as the ability to image the spinal canal. The imaging of the spinal canal is of great benefit in cases in which residual or recurrent radicular symptoms are present as well as in cases in which tumor is involved.

The so-called down side of titanium as an implant material is mainly that it is more "manufacturing sensitive" as compared with stainless steel. The manufacturer must be particularly stringent in the selection of core material and the final finishing process in order to ensure an implant of appropriate biomechanical characteristics. The system implants are actually an alloy of titanium (Ti 6Al-4V). For

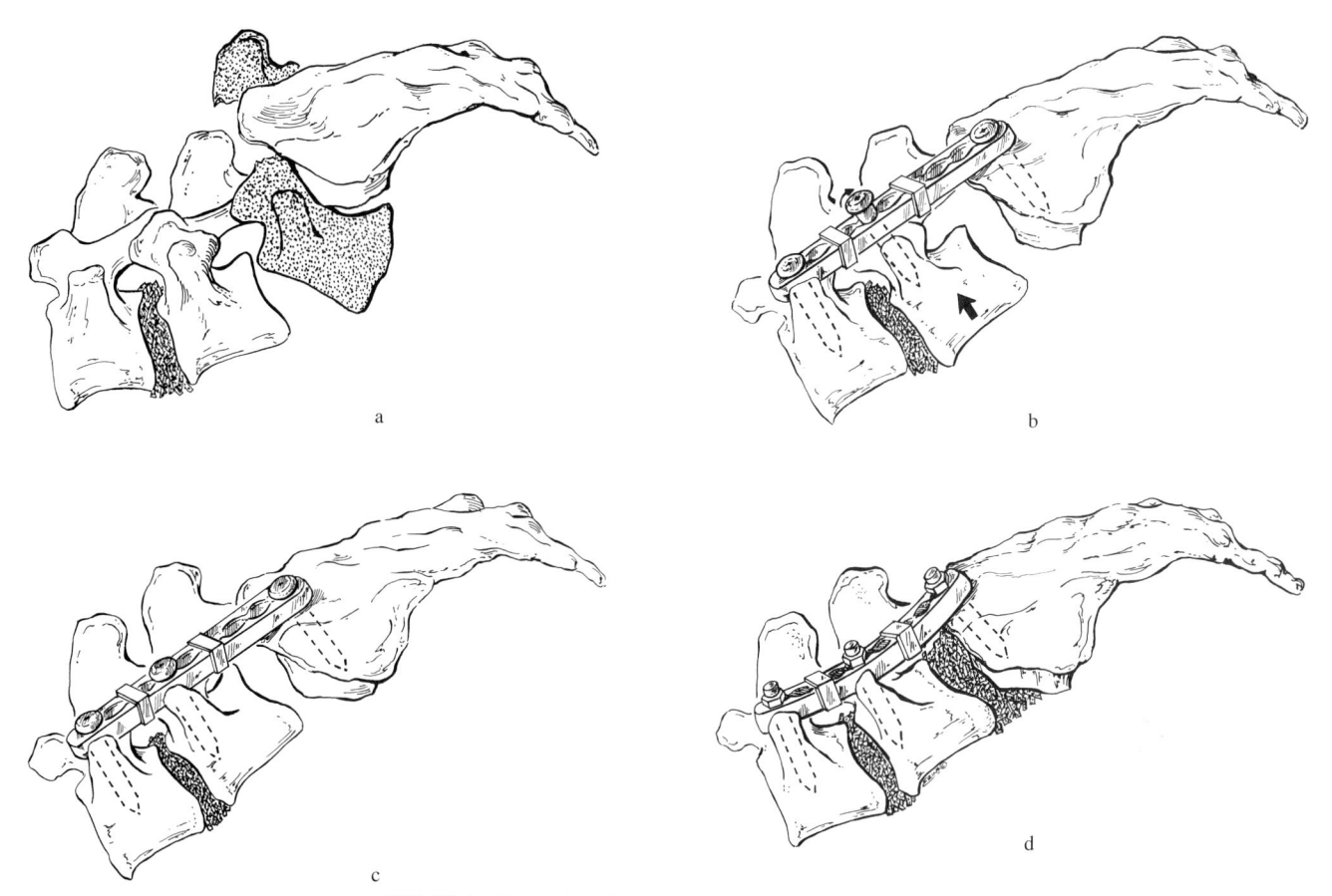

FIG. 29-6. The option of either semiconstrained or fully constrained constructs with the Dynalok Fixation System has led to the development of a system specific spondyloptosis reduction sequence. (a) The vertebral body of L5 is resected anteriorly, and used to bone graft the L3-4 disk space. (b) The remaining posterior elements of L5 are resected. The screws are then inserted at L3 and S1, through a straight Dynalok plate. (c) A 6.5-mm screw is then inserted through the plate into the L4 pedicle. With gentle distraction applied to the spine, the L4 screw is slowly tightened, drawing the spine into a reduced position. This is done gradually, with careful monitoring of the thecal sac and individual nerve roots. (d) With the spine reduced and under slight distraction, the L4-S1 interval is grafted. The construct is then switched to a fully constrained construct (with the plates being contoured at this point) one side at a time. The neural elements are again carefully evaluated for any evidence of impingement or tension/compression. The authors use dermatomal evoked potentials during such procedures.

this particular alloy of titanium, the processing options for implant production are readily available, therefore the manufacturing costs are not inordinate. Pure titanium and the medical-grade alloy Ti 6Al-4V possess excellent corrosion resistance, actually surpassing that of stainless steel in the human body. Additional bioengineering design features also must be used because of titanium's greater notch sensitivity and crack propagation tendencies as compared with stainless steel—this being one of the key considerations in the surgeon's decision to use a particular titanium implant system. The biomechanical testing of the Dynalok Titanium System constructs demonstrates that these factors are not insurmountable (see Fig. 29-3).

SURGICAL PLANNING

The most important factor in an optimal surgical procedure is that of appropriate surgical planning (McGuire, 1992; Murtagh & Arrington, 1992; Nugent & Dawson, 1993; Ono, Shikata, Shimizu, & Yamamuro, 1992; Reich, Kuflik, & Neuwirth, 1993; Yoganandan, Pintar, Maiman, Reinartz, et al., 1992; Zdeblick, Smith, Warden, Eng, & McAfee, 1991). While patient selection and a discussion of the levels for fusion are beyond the scope of this chapter, certainly a consideration in terms of instrumentation options is important. In particular, is a plate system indicated in the treatment of the individual patient's pathoanatomy? Our goal should be one of applying select treatment options as indicated by the individual clinical situation, rather than one of becoming a master of one system and making it address all clinical problems. In terms of plate-screw systems, in general, significant sagittal deformities of the spine (i.e., scoliosis) are more appropriately addressed via rod-hook-screw systems such as the TSRH system. Virtually all other clinical entities requiring lumbar pedicular fixation are able to be treated readily by the Dynalok system (Table 29-2).

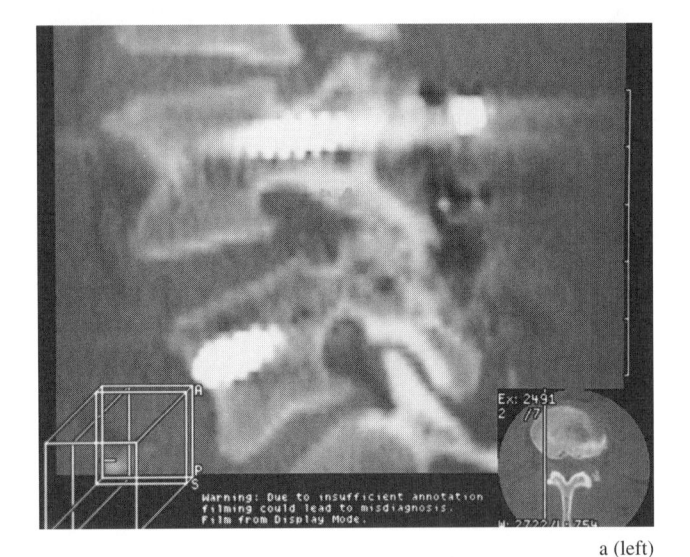

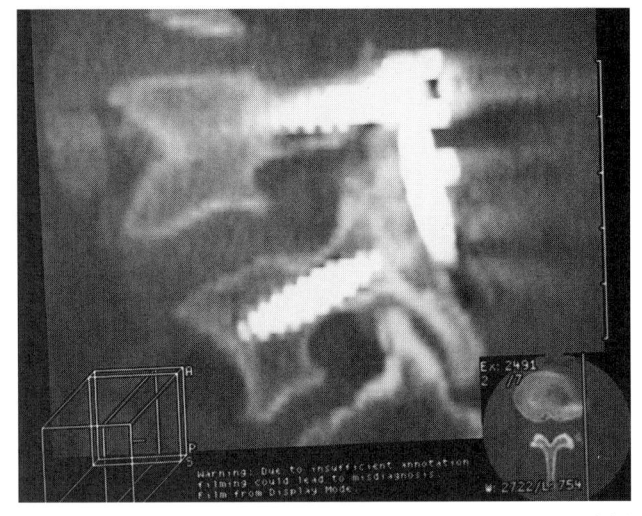

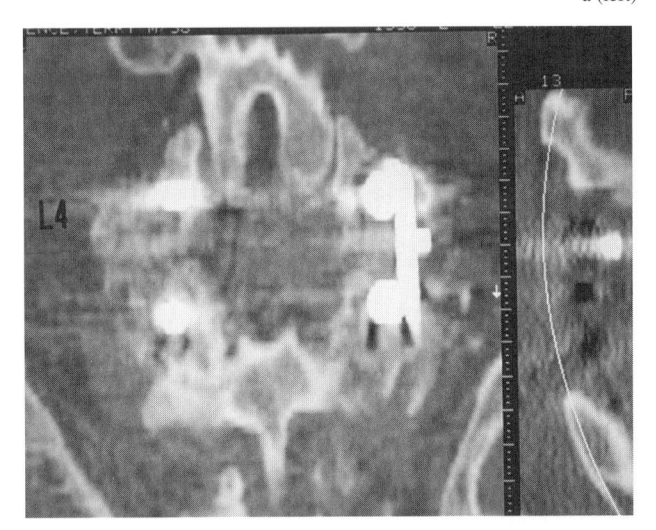

FIG. 29-7. (a) Sagittally reconstructed CT scan 12 weeks after fusion. The early incorporation of the facet joints is apparent in the image on the left. The lack of limiting artifact is seen in the image on the right, where the graft material is clearly evident to the undersurface of the plate. (b) Coronal reconstruction of a CT scan 12 weeks after fusion. This image allows the surgeon to evaluate the graft clearly for maturation of the fusion, as well as the possibility of graft resorption. Note the lack of significant metallic artifact.

Table 29-2
Advantages and Disadvantages of the Use of the Dynalok Fixation System

Advantages
  System modularity
  Plate ring adjustability of placement
  Titanium implant availability
  Low profile
  Cannulated, top-loading design
  Favorable construct strength and fatigue characteristics
  System ability to "cross over" with the TSRH system

Disadvantages
  Not readily adaptable to sagittal plane deformities
  Inability to place sacral alar bolts

Incision

The most commonly used surgical approach to the thoracolumbosacral spine is the midline approach. While this is satisfactory in the majority of clinical instances and for most instrumentation systems, some spines may be more readily exposed via the bilateral paravertebral approach popularized by Wiltse (1973). A fairly common example of a situation in which the paravertebral approach can be helpful is the very large, heavily muscled patient in whom a midline decompression is not required. In these patients, if a standard midline approach is used it may be very difficult to gain sufficient lateral exposure to obtain an ideal triangulated screw insertion angle.

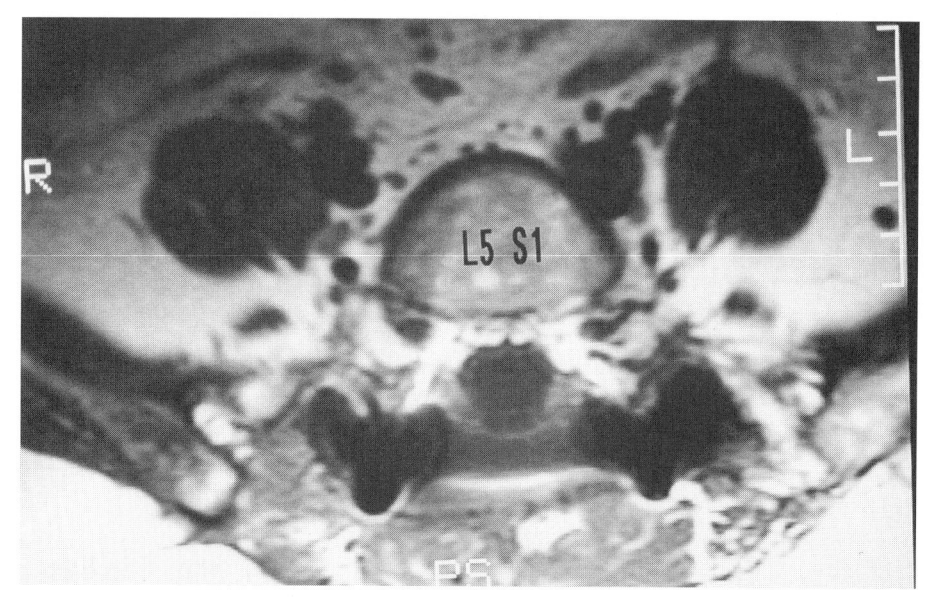

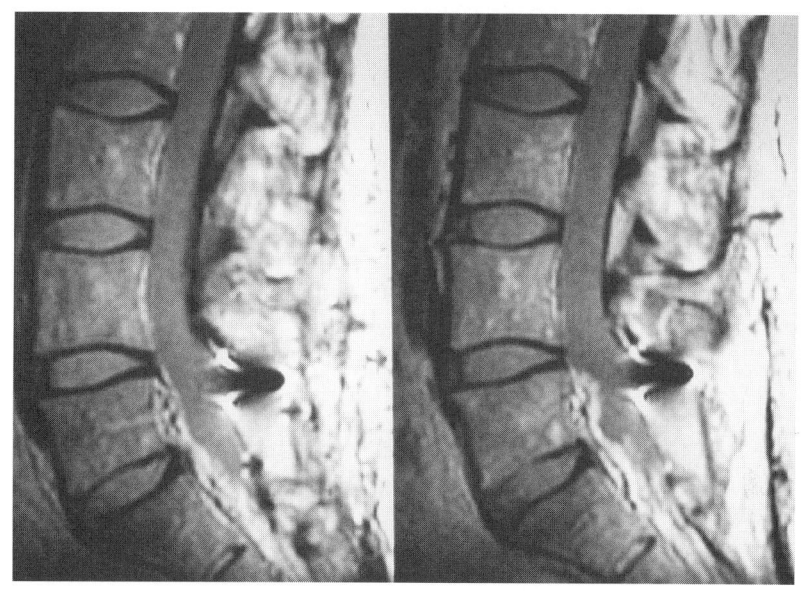

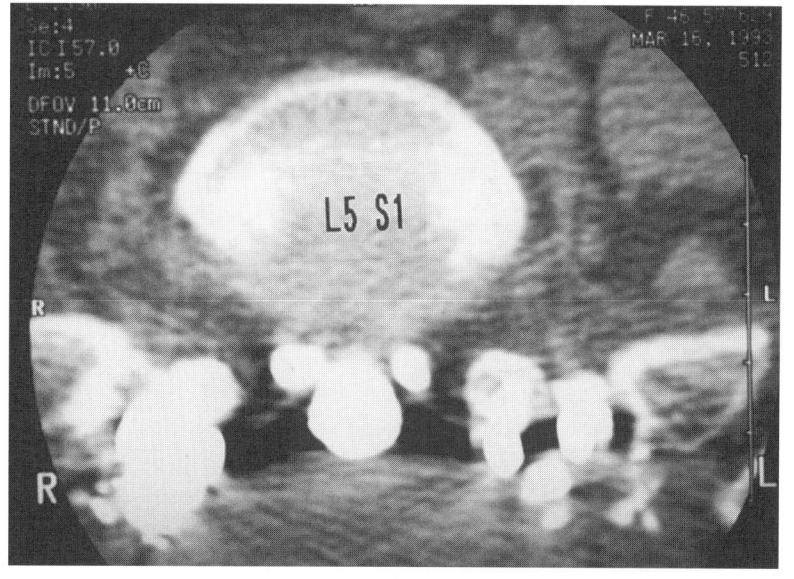

FIG. 29-8. Titanium implants produce little artifact on MRI evaluation. Axial and sagittal MRI, as well as post-myelogram CT scan images are shown.

Screw Insertion Technique

Once the surgical approach is elected, the surgeon needs to have a plan for the technique of screw insertion that is appropriate. The two standard pedicle screw placement techniques are those of Roy-Camille and Weinstein (1970). The Roy-Camille (1986) technique is a straight ahead (sagittal plane) approach, while the Weinstein technique is an oblique (triangulated) approach. Weinstein, Spratt, et al. (1988) studied the two techniques in cadavers as applied by experienced spinal surgeons. The techniques were used from the thoracolumbar junction to the sacrum, the specimens sectioned, and the accuracy of screw placement determined for each technique by level. As might be expected anatomically, the straight-ahead technique of Roy-Camille was the most accurate from T11 to L2, where the pedicles are relatively narrow and sagittal in their orientation, whereas the triangulated technique of Weinstein was the safer from L3 to S1—the vertebral levels with broader, obliquely oriented pedicles.

Beyond the purely anatomical factors in the selection of the appropriate pedicle insertion technique, there are additional advantages of the Weinstein technique. First, the triangulation of screws/bolts is quite effective in optimizing construct stability and resistance to pullout (Carson et al., 1990; Goel et al., 1991; Krag, 1991). Second, the more lateral site of entry employed in the Weinstein technique keeps the cephalad end of the instrumentation lateral to the mobile inferior facet process of the unfused segment at the upper end of the construct. The risk of impingement and subsequent pain in the upright position or extension of the spine is thereby avoided.

In short, the triangulated technique of Weinstein is safer from L3 to S1 and offers the further benefits of improved biomechanics and preservation of the adjacent, unfused facet joints. Roy-Camille's technique is safer from T11 to L2 and in general is dictated more by the regional anatomy.

The last statement leads to the next point of consideration in preoperative planning of pedicular instrumentation—namely, the assessment of pedicular size in the particular patient. Several extensive studies (Banta, King, Dabezies, & Liljeberg, 1989; Bernard & Seibert, 1992; Ferree, 1992; Misenhimer, Peek, Wiltse, & Rothman, 1987; Zindrick, 1987) have demonstrated very effectively the average pedicular dimensions by level. However, the studies also elucidate a potentially more important point—that of the significant variance that exists from these average dimensions. Therefore, in the process of preoperative planning the surgeon must consider the individual patient's pedicular anatomy both in terms of size and in regard to the medial-lateral orientation of the pedicles. In terms of pedicular size, one attempts to place the largest-diameter screw/bolt that is safely accommodated by the pedicle. The medial-lateral orientation of the pedicle provides information on the appropriate angles for screw/bolt insertion at each level. Both the pedicle size and the orientation are effectively demonstrated by a preoperative CT scan (3-mm sections).

SURGICAL TECHNIQUE

Exposure

In the preoperative holding area, an appropriate prophylactic antibiotic is given intravenously. The patient is then taken to the surgical suite and anesthetized and an indwelling urinary catheter is placed. The patient is carefully turned prone and positioned, ensuring there is no undue pressure on the bony prominences, breasts, genitalia, or the neurovascular structures. The back is prepared and draped in a sterile manner. The skin is then incised (we will assume a midline approach for the purposes of this discussion) and sharp dissection is carried down to the lumbodorsal fascia. Hemostasis is obtained with electrocautery and the paravertebral muscles are elevated subperiosteally from the posterior elements. Hemostasis is again obtained using electrocautery.

At this point a radiopaque marker is applied to a spinous process and a cross-table radiograph is obtained, verifying spinal levels. This film will also provide the demonstration of the craniocaudal orientation of the pedicles to be instrumented. If the Trendelenberg tilt of the table is changed, another radiograph should be obtained in order to reverify the orientation of the pedicles. The medial-lateral plane of the pedicles will have been determined preoperatively with a CT scan. After delineating the spinal levels it is recommended that the appropriate spinous process be marked with a small notch using a rongeur.

The exposure is now continued laterally to the tips of the transverse processes of the vertebral levels to be fused. The lateral aspect of the facet joints at each level is also exposed subperiosteally. In the process of exposing the pars interarticularis and/or the lateral aspect of the facet joints the surgeon will encounter the facet branch of the segmental lumbar artery and corresponding vein. Most often this may be readily cauterized by bending the tip of the cautery pencil and applying it along the lateral aspect of the facet joint. Care should be taken to avoid extending anteriorly to the plane of the transverse process/transversalis fascia, where injury may occur to the exiting lumbar nerve root. Exposure of the lateral aspect of the facet joint, at the levels to be fused, is indeed important in optimizing the surface area for bone grafting. In fact, it has been estimated that this additional bony surface increases the surface area for fusion by as much as 30%.

If difficulty is encountered in retraction of the paravertebral musculature, proximal and/or distal extension of the midline exposure may be helpful. In order to minimize intraoperative blood loss, the judicious use of packing sponges in any areas not being worked on at that time is strongly recommended. At this point the self-retaining retractors are reapplied for the decompression and stabilization portions of the procedure. It is suggested that one carefully consider the type of retractors to be used, both in terms of the possible ischemic effect that may result from their rather lengthy application, and in terms of the potential for many of the larger, bulky retractors to limit the surgeon's ability to work through as an oblique pedicle approach angle. This latter effect may result in suboptimal triangulation of the screws/bolts and an increased risk of lateral penetration of the vertebral body or pedicle. The authors prefer a lighter retractor, which decreases each of these risks, although will in general require more frequent readjustment. Examples are the Adson-Beckman and Oberhill retractors.

At this time the wound is irrigated with antibiotic saline and hemostasis again verified. The bony surfaces are further debrided of any remaining soft tissue and any indicated decompression is performed. After the decompression it is recommended that any exposed dura mater be covered with thrombin-soaked Gelfoam to prevent desiccation during the remainder of the procedure.

Pedicle Preparation—General

Having cleared any remaining soft tissue from the posterior elements, the bony landmarks of the pedicle are identified (Farcy, Rawlins, & Glassman, 1992; George, Krag, et al., 1991; Hu & Wilber, 1992; Krag, Van Hal, & Beynnon, 1989; Licht, Rowe, & Ross, 1992; Skinner, Maybee, Transfeldt, Venter, & Chalmers, 1990; Weinstein, Rydevik, & Rauschning, 1992; Wu, Liang, Pai, Au, & Lin, 1990). As discussed in the section on screw insertion technique, the most appropriate approach is determined. The pedicle entry site for Weinstein's technique is located at the intersection of the midpoint of the base of the transverse process and the lateral aspect of the corresponding facet joint. The entry site for Roy-Camille's technique is 1 mm below the tip of the inferior facet joint at its middle. This site also corresponds to the midpoint of the base of the transverse process line.

Once the entry point is identified, the dorsal cortex is penetrated with the awl or with a 4-mm carbide bur. For safety, the authors prefer not to drill the pedicle. Utilizing the cannulated technique for the Dynalok system, the blunt-tipped K-wires are now inserted with the K-wire driver. The medial angle and the craniocaudal angle of approach for each pedicle has been determined by the preoperative CT scan and the positioning lateral radiograph, respectively.

With the K-wires in place, cross-table lateral and anteroposterior (AP) radiographs are obtained to verify the position and angle of the K-wire relative to each pedicle and the depth of K-wire insertion. The K-wire should extend to 50 to 75% of the depth of the vertebral body (Krag, Van Hal, & Beynnon, 1989). If the depth is suitable, the direct-read depth gauge is used to determine the length of the bolt to be placed at each level. While this radiograph is being developed the authors harvest the iliac crest bone graft.

If the surgeon prefers a noncannulated technique, the speed shift pedicle sound is used to open each pedicle after the dorsal cortex has been penetrated (George, Krag, et al., 1991). The authors place the Dynalok K-wires into the pedicles on the patient's right, and a slightly larger threaded K-wire into the pedicles on the left. A single lateral radiograph is then obtained to check the K-wire positions and angles. The different appearance of the wires allows one to know which K-wire is on the right and which is on the left, with a single x-ray film. Once these factors are determined the K-wires are removed.

When obtaining the verification radiographs, it is important that the film be centered on the middle of the spinal segment being instrumented to avoid parallax. Oblique fluoroscopy can also be useful particularly in revision cases, in which the bony landmarks can be very obscured.

The pedicles are then tapped. The tap size corresponds to the diameter of the bolt or screw to be inserted, except in patients with osteopenia, in whom a one-size-smaller tap is used. Weinstein et al. (1988) and others have documented the inaccuracy of standard AP/lateral radiographs in ensuring an intrapedicular placement. Therefore, it is of paramount importance that the tapped pedicles be palpated to verify the absence of bony cortical penetration. This is performed with the ball-tipped Holt probes—each quadrant of each pedicle is checked. If a defect is suspected, further investigation is prudent via a laminotomy if medial, inferior, or superior penetration is a concern.

Decortication

Unfortunately, it is apparent that with the greater technical demands of the increasingly sophisticated spinal instrumentation systems there seems to be less consideration of the importance of a meticulous decortication and grafting during a fusion procedure. The experiences since the early 1900s have accurately shown the significance of this step. Fig. 29-9

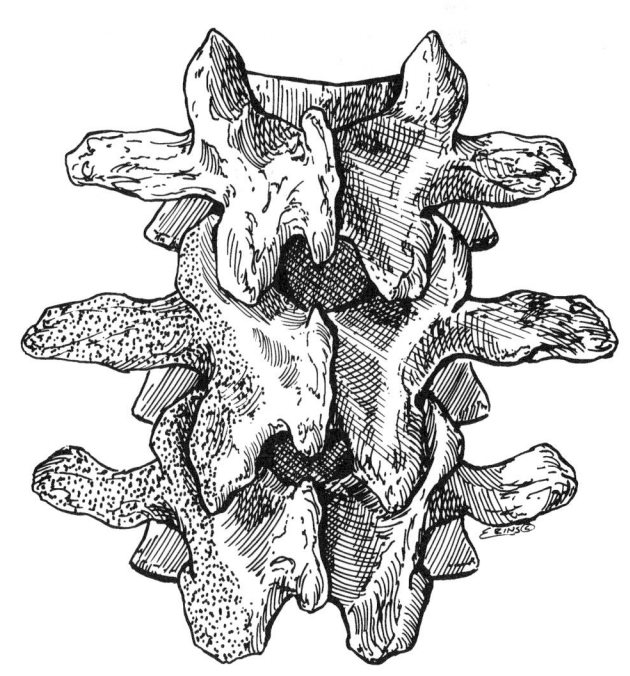

FIG. 29-9. Surfaces for decortication include the transverse processes, the lateral aspect of the facet joints, the facet articular surfaces, and the remaining lamina of the levels to be fused.

demonstrates the surfaces to be included in the decortication and subsequent bone graft application. These include the relevant transverse processes, lateral aspect of the facet joints, the facet articulation itself, pars interarticularis, remaining lamina, and the sacral ala (if fusing to the sacrum).

It is strongly recommended that decortication be performed prior to the insertion of any implants. If attempted after bolt insertion there is simply a degree of obstruction for decortication of all available surface area. This would result in an unacceptable technical compromise of the fusion success rate. Decortication may be performed by way of rongeurs, gouges, and/or cutting burs. The authors prefer a cutting bur and carefully preserve the bone slurry that results. This slurry is concentrated over the transverse processes and lateral aspect of the facet joints with additional graft being added later.

Dynalok Construct Insertion

The spine has now been suitably prepared for construct insertion. In the Dynalok system, the minor diameter of the bolts is greatest, and unchanging in the 7.0- to 8.5-mm bolts. Therefore, biomechanically the strength will be greater for these bolts (see Fig. 29-3) than the 6.5-mm bolts. Based on the preoperatively determined pedicle sizes, an attempt is made to use the largest-diameter bolt that can be safely placed within the pedicle, not to exceed approximately 85% of the pedicle diameter.

The selected Dynalok bolt is then inserted with the rachet handle screwdriver. The first bolt inserted should be the most cephalad within the construct. Next the caudalmost bolt is inserted. The bolts are inserted to a point at which the bolt flange rests on the bony surface at the pedicle entry site.

The plate template is then used to determine the appropriate plate length as well as to guide the contouring of the selected plate. Contouring is performed with the plate benders, with a goal of restoring lumbar lordosis and forming a 90-degree bolt plate junction at each level.

For multiple-level constructs, the contoured plates are then set over the two end bolts initially placed. The awl, or a carbide bur, is then used through the plate to mark the optimal pedicle entry sites for the intermediate levels. These optimized sites should correspond accurately with the anatomical area for pedicle entry. The plates are then removed and each of these intermediate pedicles are sounded and tapped employing the techniques previously described (Fig. 29-10).

The intermediate pedicle bolts are then inserted. The templating technique described results in a truly colinear bolt placement for multiple-level constructs, and the previously contoured plates should be readily applied. The bolt-plate junctions should be 90 degrees at each level. If this is not the case, further contouring or the placement of 15-degree wedges or 4-mm spacers on the bolt flange may be used to create this 90-degree interface. If an appropriate bolt-plate junction is not established, later loss of the rigidity of this level may occur, as illustrated in Fig. 29-11. If either the 15-degree wedges or the 4-mm spacers are necessary, the concave surface of each should face down onto the bolts.

Once a 90-degree bolt-plate junction is established at each instrumented level the plates are again removed. The wound is then copiously irrigated with antibiotic saline solution. The autogenous iliac crest bone graft, which has been morselized, is then placed over all decorticated surfaces and tapped into the relevant, prepared facet joints.

Plate rings (and/or T-bolts) are applied to the plates. There should be either a plate ring or a T-bolt on each side of all intermediate bolts. At levels at which the heads of the bolts are close to one another the plate rings may be placed on the underside of the plate. A small notch may need to be fashioned in the vertebral cortex to accommodate such an inverted plate ring.

The contoured plates (with plate rings and/or T-bolts) are then reapplied. The Dynalok nuts are placed with the nut starter onto each bolt, except where a bolt-to-bolt cross-link is desired. Bolt-to-bolt cross-linkage is not possible at levels at which a wedge or a spacer has been required. Cross-linkage is recommended, space permitting. At this time, the appropriate length Dynalok cross-link is selected. It is then contoured so that each end sits flush on the corresponding plate when inserted. The cross-link is applied in either a bolt-to-bolt or a plate-to-plate (using T-bolts) configuration. The nuts are applied over the cross-links.

The Dynalok nuts are then tightened to 120 in.-lb with the back-up screwdriver/ratchet T-handle to apply a neutralizing counterclockwise force to the bolt. This ensures that the nut is truly tightened onto the bolt and spinning of the bolt does not occur. The initial tightening is performed with the speed wrench and the final torque with the deflection beam torque wrench.

Based on the particular patient's pathoanatomy, if distraction is desired it is obtained at the time of nut tightening. The distractor is positioned between the bases of the socket wrenches as they engage the nuts. The indicated amount of distraction is produced and the nuts tightened.

Any remaining bone graft is placed through and around the construct. Frayed or dusky paravertebral muscle is debrided and hemostasis again ensured. Closed system drains are inserted and a meticulous, interrupted closure is performed in layers.

AUTHORS' POSTOPERATIVE PROTOCOL

Patient-controlled analgesia, intermittent compression stockings, low-molecular-weight heparin, aggressive incentive spirometry, and a urinary catheter are typically used in the immediate postoperative period. Unless limited by a postanesthetic effect, patients are mobilized at their bedside the evening of surgery. A custom, front opening thoracolumbosacral orthosis is used for the first 12 weeks following surgery. Generally, the urinary catheter, operative drains, and patient-controlled analgesia are discontinued on the second postoperative day. A low dose of diazepam has

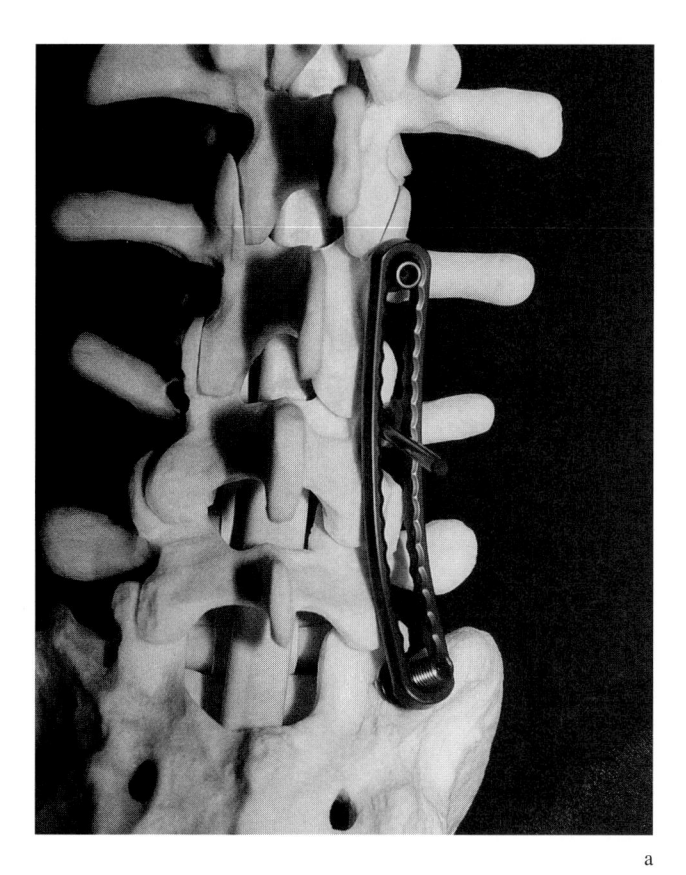

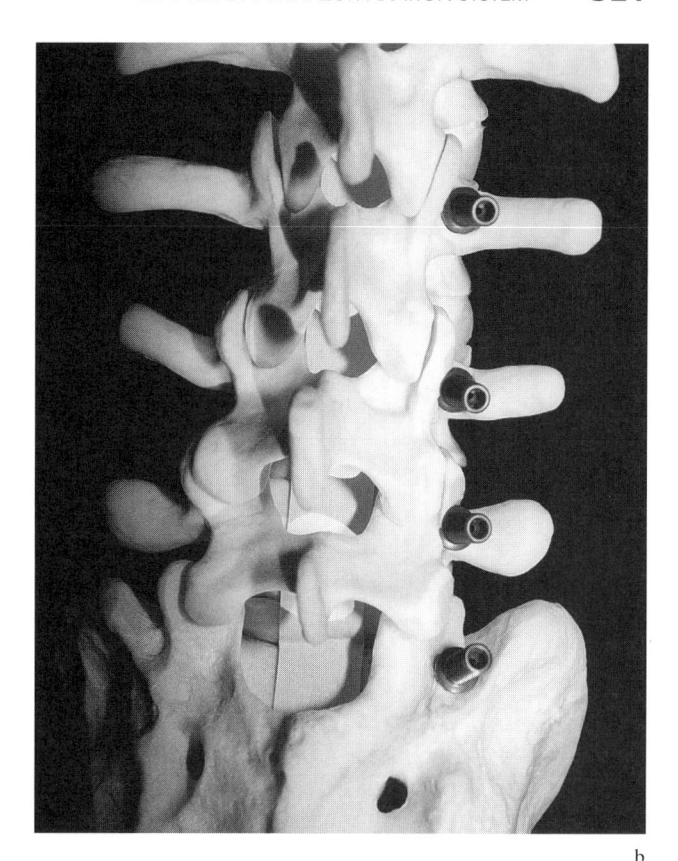

FIG. 29-10. Templating technique for multiple-level bolt placement. (a) The bolts are placed at the upper and lower vertebrae within the construct. The plate of appropriate length is selected, contoured, and set over the end bolts. The optimal pedicle entry sites for the intermediate levels are then marked, the plate removed, and the intermediate pedicles sounded and tapped. (b) The intermediate bolts are placed.

been found to be quite effective in allowing earlier mobilization and switch over to oral analgesics.

At the time of discharge from the hospital, patients are instructed to increase their ambulation progressively, to shower but not submerge the incision under water (i.e., bath or hottub), wear the TLSO (thoracolumbar sacral osthiosis) when upright, not to lift more than 5 lbs or perform bending/twisting activities, not to drive, and to take one aspirin twice daily with meals (unless medically contraindicated) (Axelsson, Johnsson, & Stromqvist, 1992; Rask & Dall, 1993). In smokers, the authors are routinely using a pulsed electromagnetic field stimulator (Spinal-Stim, AME) (Di Silvestre & Savini, 1992). At the first postoperative office visit, radiographs are obtained and patients are instructed to increase their ambulation further. They may also begin swimming for exercise. Now that we are primarily using titanium implants, a CT scan is scheduled for 12 weeks postoperatively. This is ordered for the instrumented levels as a 1.5-mm section, sagittally and coronally reformatted study. This has been particularly helpful in demonstrating early fusion mass incorporation and ruling out graft resorption.

Twelve weeks after surgery the orthosis is discontinued if early graft incorporation is demonstrated on the CT scan, and physical therapy is begun for rehabilitation. Patients are instructed to increase their home activities parallel to their level of performance in therapy. Heavy physical laborers will typically progress into work-hardening after approximately 6 weeks of rehabilitation.

DYNALOK-TSRH SYSTEM CROSSOVER: THE OFFSET CONNECTOR SET

The Offset Connector Set (Danek Group Inc.) has been developed to offer improved surgical options to the users of either the TSRH or Dynalok system. This set is a separate system including titanium and stainless steel components allowing the crossover between these implant systems. The set includes a series of connectors that mate Dynalok bolts to TSRH rods. This system crossover greatly increases the surgeon's intraoperative options for each individual implant type. For example, in a multiple-level construct using the Dynalok implants, if a nonlinear bolt placement occurs plate application may be difficult. The surgeon may address this situation in one of three ways: (1) remove an intermediate bolt; (2) switch a nonlinear intermediate bolt to a screw for semiconstrained fixation of that particular level, though still aiding in the construct stress distribution; or (3) switch to a

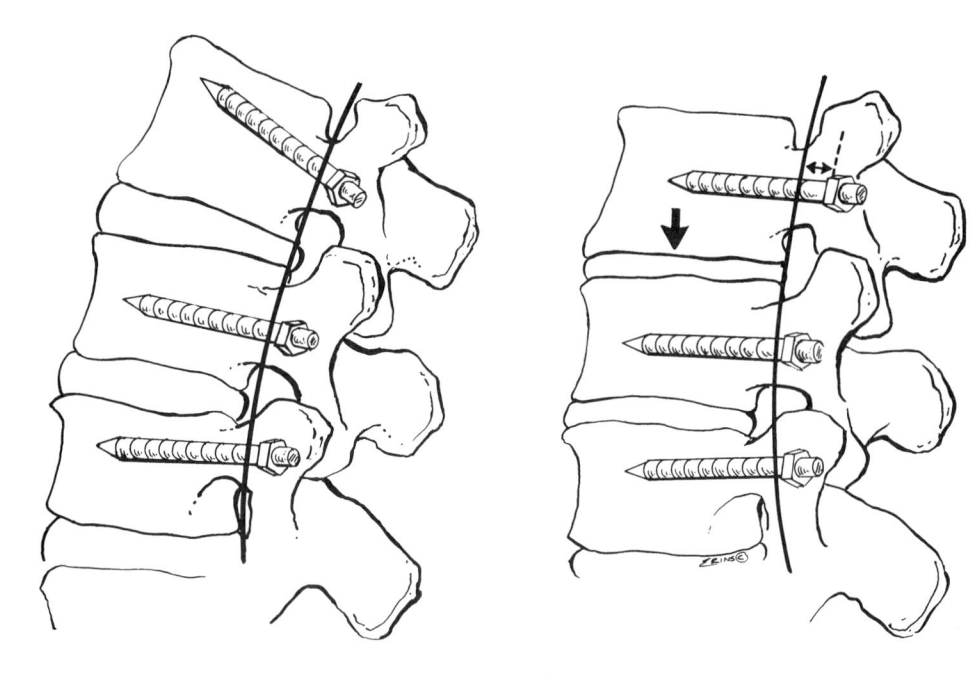

FIG. 29-11. Failure to create a stable bolt-plate interface may result in the loss of construct rigidity at that level. A stable bolt-plate interface is 90 degrees, being obtained by plate contouring or the use of a 4-mm spacer or a 15-degree wedge.

stainless steel or titanium rod connecting to the previously placed bolts via the offset connector set.

Furthermore, the availability of the Offset Connector Set allows the surgeon to salvage broken or stripped TSRH screws using Dynalok bolts, thereby obviating the need to carry wider sizes of the TSRH screws routinely.

EARLY CLINICAL EXPERIENCE WITH THE DYNALOK FIXATION SYSTEM

Early clinical experience with the Dynalok system has been favorable. To date, we have implanted the stainless steel version in 63 patients from September 1991 to December 1992, and the titanium version in 36 patients from October 1992 to the present. During the initial development of the system it was recognized that it was possible for nuts, on tightening, to spin the bolt. This would result in incomplete torque application to the nut. In our initial series of patients (stainless steel implants) we found three instances (three nuts in two patients) in which nut loosening was evident. These patients were all women with osteopenia. This led to the development of the deflection beam torque wrench and back-up screwdriver, which acts to engage the bolt directly during nut tightening, to provide a neutralizing counterclockwise force to the bolt. Since this technical modification has been adapted, we have experienced only one further instance of a nut backing off. This is thought to have occurred as a result of the failure to create a 90-degree bolt-plate junction at the time of surgery (see Fig. 29-11). Such a technical lapse may result in the subsequent axial loads of weight bearing, causing a slight shift in the bolt-plate interface. This may result in the loss of a full contact fit and nut loosening. The nuts have now been modified to a locking design, thereby avoiding loosening or disengagement.

Having begun to use the Dynalok system in September 1991 the authors have not been able to demonstrate any frank pseudarthroses, though the follow-up is not yet long enough to be complete in this evaluation. However, it is thought that the clarity of the images of the fusion mass with a reconstructed CT scan for the titanium implants greatly improves our ability to evaluate bony healing. This will serve well in the future long-term follow-up of these patients.

The only true intraoperative complication was that of spinning of the bolt on nut tightening, as discussed above. Perioperatively, we have experienced two iliac crest graft site seromas, three urinary tract infections, one deep venous thrombosis, and two instances of delayed wound healing (without clinical infection). There have been no dural tears, neurologic injuries, or deep infections. To date there have been no failures of the hardware.

In view of the ease of use of the system with its top-loading design, the option of the cannulated implantation technique, the favorable system biomechanics, and particularly the titanium imaging capabilities the Dynalok Fixation System is thought by the authors to be a state-of-the-art system with wide applicability. As our clinical experience has increased, we have gained a greater understanding of how to work with the system and its many options. Out of this experience we have found the option of a semiconstrained construct to be particularly beneficial in the treatment of high-grade spondylolisthesis or spondyloptosis. Figure 29-6 demonstrates the basic technique we have utilized in such cases. The development of the Offset Connector Set further enhances the attractiveness of system.

REFERENCES

An, H.S., Simpson, J.M., Ebraheim, N.A., et al. (1992). Low lumbar burst fractures: Comparison between conservative and surgical treatments. *Orthopedics, 15,* 367–373.

Ashman, R.B., Johnston, C.E., & Corin, J.D. (February 1990). Pedicle screw-plate junction: Susceptibility to fatigue fracture. Presented at the 36th Annual Meeting of the Orthopedic Research Society, New Orleans, LA.

Axelsson, P., Johnsson, R., & Stromqvist, B. (June, 1992). Effect of lumbar orthosis on intervertebral mobility: A roentgen sterophotogrammetric analysis. *Spine, 17,* 678–681.

Banta, C.J., II, King, A.G., Dabezies, E.J., & Liljeberg, R.L. (1989). Measurement of effective pedicle diameter in the human spine. *Orthopedics, 12,* 939–942.

Bernard, T.N., & Seibert, C.E. (1992). Pedicle diameter determined by computed tomography: Its relevance to pedicle screw fixation in the lumbar spine. *Spine, 17,*(6 Suppl), S160–S163.

Bernhardt, M., Swartz, D.E., Clothiaux, P.L., Crowell, R.R., & White, R.R., III. (1992). Posterolateral lumbar and lumbosacral fusion with and without pedicle screw internal fixation. *Clinical Orthopaedics and Related Research, 284,* 109–115.

Brodsky, A.E., Kovalsky, E.S., & Khalil, M.A. (1991). Correlation of radiologic assessment of lumbar fusions with surgical exploration. *Spine, 16*(6 Suppl), S261–S265.

Boos, N., Marchesi, D.G., & Aebi, M. (1992). Survivorship analysis of pedicular fixation systems in the treatment of degenerative disorders of the lumbar spine: A comparison of Cotrel-Dubousset instrumentation and the AO internal fixator. *Journal of Spinal Disorders, 5,* 403–409.

Carson, W.L., Duffield, R.C., Arendt, M., Ridgely, B.J., & Gaines, R.W., Jr. (1990). Internal forces and moments in transpedicular spine instrumentation. The effect of pedicle screw angle and transfixation—the 4R-4bar linkage concept. *Spine, 15,* 893–901.

Coe, J.D., Warden, K.E., Herzig, M.A., & McAfee, P.C. (1990). Influence of bone mineral density on the fixation of thoracolumbar implants: A comparative study of transpedicular screws, laminar hooks, and spinous process wires. *Spine, 15,* 902–907.

Cooper, P.R., Errico, T.J., Martin, R., Crawford, B., & DiBartolo, T. (1993). A systematic approach to spinal reconstruction after anterior decompression for neoplastic disease of the thoracic and lumbar spine. *Neurosurgery, 32,* 1–8.

Cotler, J.M., & Cotler, H.B. (1990). *Spinal Fusion: Science and Technique.* New York: Springer-Verlag.

Davne, S.H., & Myers, D.L. (1992). Complications of lumbar spinal fusion with transpedicular instrumentation. *Spine, 17*(6 Suppl), S184–S189.

Dekutoski, M.B., Conlan, E.S., & Salciccioli, G.G. (1993). Spinal mobility and deformity after Harrington rod stabilization and limited arthrodesis of thoracolumbar fractures. *Journal of Bone and Joint Surgery, American Volume, 75,* 168–176.

Dickman, C.A., Fessler, R.G., MacMillan, M., & Haid, R.W. (1992). Transpedicular screw-rod fixation of the lumbar spine: operative technique and outcome in 104 cases. *Journal of Neurosurgery, 77,* 860–870.

Di Silvestre, M., & Savini, R. (1992). Pulsing electromagnetic fields (PEMFs) in spinal fusion preliminary clinical results. *Chirrurgia Degli Organi Di Movimento, 77,* 289–294.

Doerr, T.E., Montesano, P.X., Burkus, J.K., & Benson, D.R. (1991). Spinal canal decompression in traumatic thoracolumbar burst fractures: posterior distraction rods versus transpedicular screw fixation. *Journal of Orthopedic Trauma, 5*(4), 403–411.

Ebraheim, N.A., Savolaine, E.R., Stitgen, S.H., & Jackson, W.T. (1992). Magnetic resonance imaging after pedicle screw fixation of the spine. *Clinical Orthopaedics and Related Research, 279,* 133–137.

Esses, S.I., & Moro, J.K. (1993). The value of facet joint blocks in patient selection for lumbar fusion. *Spine, 18,* 185–190.

Esses, S.I., & Moro, J.K. (1993). Intraosseous vertebral body pressures. *Spine, 17*(6 Suppl), S155–S159.

Farcy, J.P., Rawlins, B.A., & Glassman, S.D. (1992). Technique and results of fixation to the sacrum with iliosacral screws. *Spine, 17*(6 Suppl), S190–S195.

Farey, I.D., McAfee, P.C., Gurr, K.R., & Randolph, M.A. (1989). Quantitative histological study of the influence of spinal instrumentation on lumbar fusions: a canine model. *Journal of Orthopedic Research, 7,* 709–722.

Ferree, B.A. (1992). Morphometric characteristics of pedicles of the immature spine. *Spine, 17,* 887–891.

George, D.C., Krag, M.H., et al. (1991). Hole preparation techniques for transpedicular screws: Effect on pull-out strength from human cadaveric vertebrae. *Spine, 16,* 181–184.

Goel, V.K., Lim, T.H., Gwon, J. (1991). Effects of rigidity of an internal fixation device: A comprehensive biomechanical investigation. *Spine, 16*(3 Suppl), S155–S161.

Grob, D., Scheier, H.J., Dvorak, J., et al. (1991). Circumferential fusion of the lumbar and lumbosacral spine. *Archives of Orthopedic and Trauma Surgery, 111,* 20–25.

Grubb, S.A., & Lipscomb, H.J. (1992). Results of lumbosacral fusion for degenerative disc disease with and without instrumentation: Two and five-year follow-up. *Spine, 17,* 349–355.

Haid, R.W., Jr., & Dickman, C.A. (1993). Instrumentation and fusion for discogenic disease of the lumbosacral spine. *Neurosurgery Clinics of North America, 4,* 135–148.

Heim, S.E., & Luque, E.R. (1992). Danek plate and screw system. In: D.M. Arnold, & J.E. Lonstein (Eds.), *State of the Art Reviews—Spine: Pedicle Fixation of the Lumbar Spine.* (pp. 201–232). Philadelphia, PA: Hanley and Belfus.

Herkowitz, H.N., & Kurz, L.T. (1991). Degenerative lumbar spondylolisthesis with spinal stenosis. A prospective study comparing decompression and decompression with intertransverse process arthrodesis. *Journal of Bone and Joint Surgery, American Volume, 73,* 802–808.

Hu, R., & Wilber, R.G. (1992). Drill sleeve for pedicle screw fixation. *Orthopedic Review, 21,* 783–787.

Johnston, C.E., II, Ashman, R.B., Baird, A.M., & Allard, R.N. (1990). Effect of spinal construct stiffness on early fusion mass incorporation: Experimental study. *Spine, 15,* 908–912.

Kabins, M.B., Weinstein, J.N., Spratt, K.F., et al. (1992). Isolated L4-5 fusions using the variable screw placement system: unilateral versus bilateral. *Journal of Spinal Disorders, 5,* 39–49.

Kaneda, K., Kazama, H.J., Satoh, S., et al. (1986). Follow-up study of medial facetectomies and posterolateral fusion with instrumentation in unstable degenerative spondylolisthesis. *Clinical Orthopaedics and Related Research, 203,* 159–167.

Kim, S.S., Denis, F., Lonstein, J.E., & Winter, R.B. (1990). Factors affecting fusion rate in adult spondylolisthesis. *Spine, 15,* 979–984.

Krag, M.H., Van Hal, M.E., & Beynnon, B.D. (1989). Placement of transpedicular vertebral screws close to the anterior vertebral cortex: Description of methods. *Spine, 14,* 879–883.

Krag, M.H. (1991). Biomechanics of thoracolumbar spinal fixation: A review. *Spine, 16*(3 Suppl), S84–S99.

Kunogi, J., & Hasue, M. (1991). Diagnosis and operative treatment of intraforaminal and extraforaminal nerve root compression. *Spine, 16,* 1312–1320.

Lenke, L.G., Bridwell, K.H., Bullis, D., et al. (1992). Results of in situ fusion for isthmic spondylolisthesis. *Journal of Spinal Disorders, 5,* 433–442.

Licht, N.J., Rowe, D.E., & Ross, L.M. (1992). Pitfalls of pedicle screw fixation in the sacrum: A cadaver model. *Spine, 17,* 892–896.

Linson, M.A., & Williams, H. (1991). Anterior and combined anterior-posterior fusion for lumbar disc pain: A preliminary study. *Spine, 16,* 143–145.

Lipscomb, H.J., Grubb, S.A., & Talmage, R.V. (1989). Spinal bone density following spinal fusion. *Spine, 14,* 477–479.

Markwalder, T.M. (1993). Surgical management of neurogenic claudication in 100 patients with lumbar spinal stenosis due to degenerative spondylolisthesis. *Acta Neurochirurgica, 120*(3–4), 136–142.

Mattheck, C., Bethge, K., Erb, D., & Blomer, W. (1992). Successful shape optimisation of a pedicular screw. *Medical and Biological Engineering and Computing, 30,* 446–448.

McAfee, P.C., Weiland, D.J., & Carlow, J.J. (1991). Survivorship analysis of pedicle spinal instrumentation. *Spine, 16*(8 Suppl), S422–S427.

McAfee, P.C., Farey, I.D., Sutterlin, C.E., et al. (1989). 1989 Volvo Award in Basic Science Device-related osteoporosis with spinal instrumentation. *Spine, 14,* 919–926.

McGuire, R.A., Jr. (1992). A method for removal of broken vertebral screws. *Orthopedic Review, 21,* 775–776.

Misenhimer, G.R., Peek, R.D., Wiltse, L.L., & Rothman, S.L. (1987). Anatomic analysis of pedicle cortical and cancellous diameter as related to screw size. *Spine, 14,* 367.

Murtagh, F.R., & Arrington, J.A. (1992). Computer tomographically guided discography as a determinant of normal disc level before fusion. *Spine, 17,* 826–830.

North, R.B., Campbell, J.N., et al. (1991). Failed back surgery syndrome: 5-year follow-up in 102 patients undergoing repeated operation. *Neurosurgery, 28,* 685–690.

Nugent, P.J., & Dawson, E.G. (1993). Intertransverse process lumbar arthrodesis with allogenic fresh-frozen bone graft. *Clinical Orthopaedics and Related Research, 287,* 107–111.

Ohmori, K., Suzuki, K., & Ishida, Y. (1992). Translamino-pedicular screw fixation with bone grafting for symptomatic isthmic lumbar spondylolysis. *Neurosurgery, 30,* 379–384.

Ono, K., Shikata, J., Shimizu, K., & Yamamuro, T. (1992). Bone-fibrin mixture in spinal surgery. *Clinical Orthopaedics and Related Research, 275,* 133–139.

Postacchini, F., & Cinotti, G. (1992). Bone regrowth after surgical decompression for lumbar spinal stenosis. *Journal of Bone and Joint Surgery, British Volume, 74,* 862–869.

Rask, B., & Dall, B.E. (1993). Use of the pantaloon cast for the selection of fusion candidates in the treatment of chronic low back pain. *Clinical Orthopaedics and Related Research, 288,* 148–157.

Reich, S.M., Kuflik, P., & Neuwirth, M. (1993). Translaminar facet screw fixation in lumbar spine fusion. *Spine, 18,* 444–449.

Rimoldi, R.L., Zigler, J.E., Capen, D.A., & Hu, S.S. (1992). The effect of surgical intervention on rehabilitation time in patients with thoracolumbar and lumbar spinal cord injuries. *Spine, 17,* 1443–1449.

Rosen, C.D. (1991). Complications of pedicle screw fixation. *Spine, 16,* 599.

Roy-Camille, R., Roy-Camille, M., Zemealenacre, C. (1970). Pedicle screws for spinal fixation. *Press Med., 78,* 1447–1448.

Roy-Camille, R., Saillant, G., & Mazel, C. (1986). Internal fixation of the lumbar spine with pedicle screw plating. *Clinical Orthopaedics, 203,* 7–17.

Ruland, C.M., McAfee, P.C., Warden, K.E., & Cunningham, B.W. (1991). Triangulation of pedicular instrumentation: A biomechanical analysis. *Spine, 16*(6 Suppl), S270–S276.

Salib, R.M., & Pettine, K.A. (1993). Modified repair of a defect in spondylolysis or minimal spondylolisthesis by pedicle screw, segmental wire fixation, and bone grafting. *Spine, 18,* 440–443.

Sano, S., Yokokura, S., Nagata, Y., & Young, S.Z. (1990). Unstable lumbar spine without hypermobility in postlaminectomy cases: Mechanism of symptoms and effect of spinal fusion with and without spinal instrumentation. *Spine, 15,* 1190–1197.

Sasso, R.C., & Cotler, H.B. (1993). Posterior instrumentation and fusion for unstable fractures and fracture-dislocations of the thoracic and lumbar spine: A comparative study of three fixation devices in 70 patients. *Spine, 18,* 450–460.

Satomi, K., Hirabayashi, K., Toyama, Y., & Fujimura, Y. (1992). A clinical study of degenerative spondylolisthesis: Radiographic analysis and choice of treatment. *Spine, 17,* 1329–1336.

Skinner, R., Maybee, J., Transfeldt, E., Venter, R., & Chalmers, W. (1990). Experimental pullout testing and comparison of variables in transpedicular screw fixation: A biomechanical study. *Spine, 15,* 195–201.

Soshi, S., Shiba, R., Kondo, H., & Murota, K. (1991). An experimental study on transpedicular screw fixation in relation to osteoporosis of the lumbar spine. *Spine, 16,* 1335–1341.

Steinmann, J.C., & Herkowitz, H.N. (1992). Pseudarthrosis of the spine. *Clinical Orthopaedics and Related Research, 284,* 80–90.

Van Horn, J.R., & Bohnen, L.M. (1992). The development of discopathy in lumbar discs adjacent to a lumbar anterior interbody spondylodesis: A retrospective matched-pair study with a postoperative follow-up of 16 years. *Acta Orthopaedica Belgica, 58,* 280–286.

Watkins, R. (1992). Anterior lumbar interbody fusion surgical complications. *Clinical Orthopaedics and Related Research, 284,* 91–98.

Weatherley, C.R., Mehdian, H., & Berghe, L.V. (1991). Low back pain with fracture of the pedicle and contralateral spondylolysis: A technique of surgical management. *Journal of Bone and Joint Surgery, British Volume, 73,* 990–993.

Weinstein, J.N., Spratt, K.F., et al. (1988). Spinal pedicle fixation: Reliability and validity of roentgenogram based assessment and surgical factors on successful screw placement. *Spine, 13,* 1012–1018.

Weinstein, J.N., Rydevik, B.L., & Rauschning, W. (1992). Anatomical and technical considerations of pedicle screw fixation. *Clinical Orthopaedics and Related Research, 284,* 34–46.

West, J.L., III, & Anderson, L.D. (1992). Incidence of deep venous thrombosis in major adult spinal surgery. *Spine, 17*(8 Suppl), S254–S257.

West, J.L., III, Bradford, D.S., & Ogilvie, J.W. (1991a). Complications of the variable screw plate pedicle screw fixation. *Spine, 16,* 576–579.

West, J.L., III, Bradford, D.S., & Ogilvie, J.W. (1991b). Results of spinal arthrodesis with pedicle screw-plate fixation. *Journal of Bone and Joint Surgery, American Volume, 73,* 1179–1184.

Wetzel, F.T., & LaRocca, H. (1992). The failed posterior lumbar interbody fusion. *Spine, 16,* 839–845.

Wiltse, L.L. (1973). The paraspinal sacrospinalis splitting approach to the lumbar spine. *Clinical Orthopaedics and Related Research, 91,* 48.

Wittenberg, R.H., Shea, M., Lee, K.S., White, A.A., III, & Hayes, W.C. (1991). Importance of bone mineral density in instrumented spine fusions. *Spine, 16,* 647–652.

Wu, S.S., Liang, P.L., Pai, W.M., Au, M.K., & Lin, L.C. (1990). Spinal pedicular finder for transpedicular screw fixation—Design and early clinical result. *Proceedings of the National Science Council, Republic of China–Part B Life Sciences, 14*(4), 209–216.

Yamagata, M., Kitahara, H., Minami, S., et al. (1992). Mechanical stability of the pedicle screw fixation systems for the lumbar spine. *Spine, 17*(3 Suppl), S51–S54.

Yoganandan, N., Pintar, F., Maiman, D.J., Reinartz, J., et al. (1993). Kinematics of the lumbar spine following pedicle screw plate fixation. *Spine, 18,* 504–512.

Zdeblick, T.A., Smith, G.R., Warden, K.E., Eng, M.B., & McAfee, P.C. (June, 1991). Two-point fixation of the lumbar spine: Differential stability in rotation. *Spine, 16*(6 Suppl), S298–S301.

Zdeblick, T.A. (February, 1992). A prospective, randomized study of lumbar fusion. Presented at the American Academy Orthopedic Surgeons Meeting, San Francisco, CA.

Zindrick, M.R. (1991). The role of transpedicular fixation systems for stabilization of the lumbar spine. *Orthopedic Clinics of North America, 22,* 333–344.

Zindrick, M.R. (1987). Analysis of the morphometric characteristics of the thoracic and lumbar pedicles. *Spine, 12,* 160–166.

Zucherman, J., Hsu, K., Picetti, G., III, et al. (1992). Clinical efficacy of spinal instrumentation in lumbar degenerative disc disease. *Spine, 17,* 834–837.

CHAPTER 30

Utilization of the Simmons Plating System for Stabilization of the Spine

James W. Simmons

HIGHLIGHTS

The Simmons plating system (Smith and Nephew Spine, Memphis, TN) was designed to enhance decompression and stabilization of the spine. Although applicable for spinal stabilization with placement of bone graft material in any of a number of fusion techniques—posterolateral (intertransverse), anterior lumbar interbody fusion (ALIF), and posterior lumbar interbody fusion (PLIF)—in our center it has been incorporated most frequently into our technique for PLIF.

The Simmons plating system is comprised of plates, washers, locking nuts, cannulated bolts, and cannulated screws. The various components of the system are shown in Fig. 30-1.

The system was designed to maximize the attributes of versatility, stability, and simplicity. The versatility of the system is manifested by the range of sizes and diameters of system components: three diameters of bolts, two diameters of screws, four lengths of bolts and screws, standard washers, contoured washers, oblique washers, wide-radius washers, and offset bolts in varying lengths and diameters with a locking nut. This wide selection allows for variable placement of the bolts and screws without placing undue stress on the pedicle. Plates also come in various lengths that can be adapted to the number of segments instrumented.

Stability of the system is manifested by the ability to vary the extent of constraint of the construct. A Spiralock nut is included in the system and allows for very secure fixation of the washer and plate to the bolt. Along with stability of constructs, however, a built-in capacity for micromotion is inherent in the system through the wide radius of the bolt-plate interface. Thus, the degree of constraint of the system can be varied according to the surgeon's preference or the requirements of a particular case, ranging from an all-screw construct as a relatively unconstrained application to the all-bolt and cross-plate construct, which affords a high degree of constraint (Fig. 30-2).

Simplicity of the system is accommodated through component adaptations that make application as simple as possible. Bolts are precut for ease of placement. Screws and bolts are cannulated for ease of use by surgeons who prefer cannulation. (Cannulation reduces the strength of the bolts only by 3.8%.) The instruments provided for placement of the system are cannulated and scored. Finally, the locking nut is simply designed and thus easy to apply.

Special attention has been given to design of the bolt and screw and the accompanying Spiralock nut to reduce occurrences of the most frequently reported fixation failures. The tapered shank of the bolt increases the overall bolt strength and eliminates the stress-riser effect at the most common point of breakage in other systems. The bolts and screws are of a large minor diameter with a relatively decreased pitch of threads, with the effect that the strength of the bolt and screws is increased without diminishing pullout strength. Stress-shielding and bolt fatigue are avoided by the large radius at the bolt-plate interface which allows micromotion. The Spiralock nut is a self-locking device requiring 75 inch-pounds of torque for final securing of the system, but the nut can be tightened and loosened as needed without diminishing the self-locking effect.

It was noted through biomechanical testing that the Simmons plating system demonstrated a lower bending strength than three other plating systems (Cunningham, Sefter, et al., 1993). Static strength of a construct is dependent on the material properties and geometry of the individual system components; the Simmons plating system was designed to provide as low a profile as possible. The Simmons plate is 4 mm thick and can be bent intraoperatively to accommodate changes in spinal geometry. There is no report of plate breakage or additional bending in vivo. A clinical investigational device exemption (IDE) study involving 413 patients revealed five screw/bolt breakages. These breakages resulted from fatigue fracture or external trauma and therefore the static bending strength of the system has not been shown to be clinically relevant. Construct flexibility and stiffness also were determined in the study. It was noted that the Simmons system was less stiff, and therefore more flexible, than the other plating systems. The optimal stiffness necessary for a spinal construct is not known. While it is necessary for a system to provide adequate spinal stability, excessive stiffness may result in stress shielding. This was taken into consideration in the design of the Simmons plating system. Micromotion was intentionally built into the system at the bolt-plate interface, not only to decrease stress-shielding effects, but also to increase bolt fatigue strength.

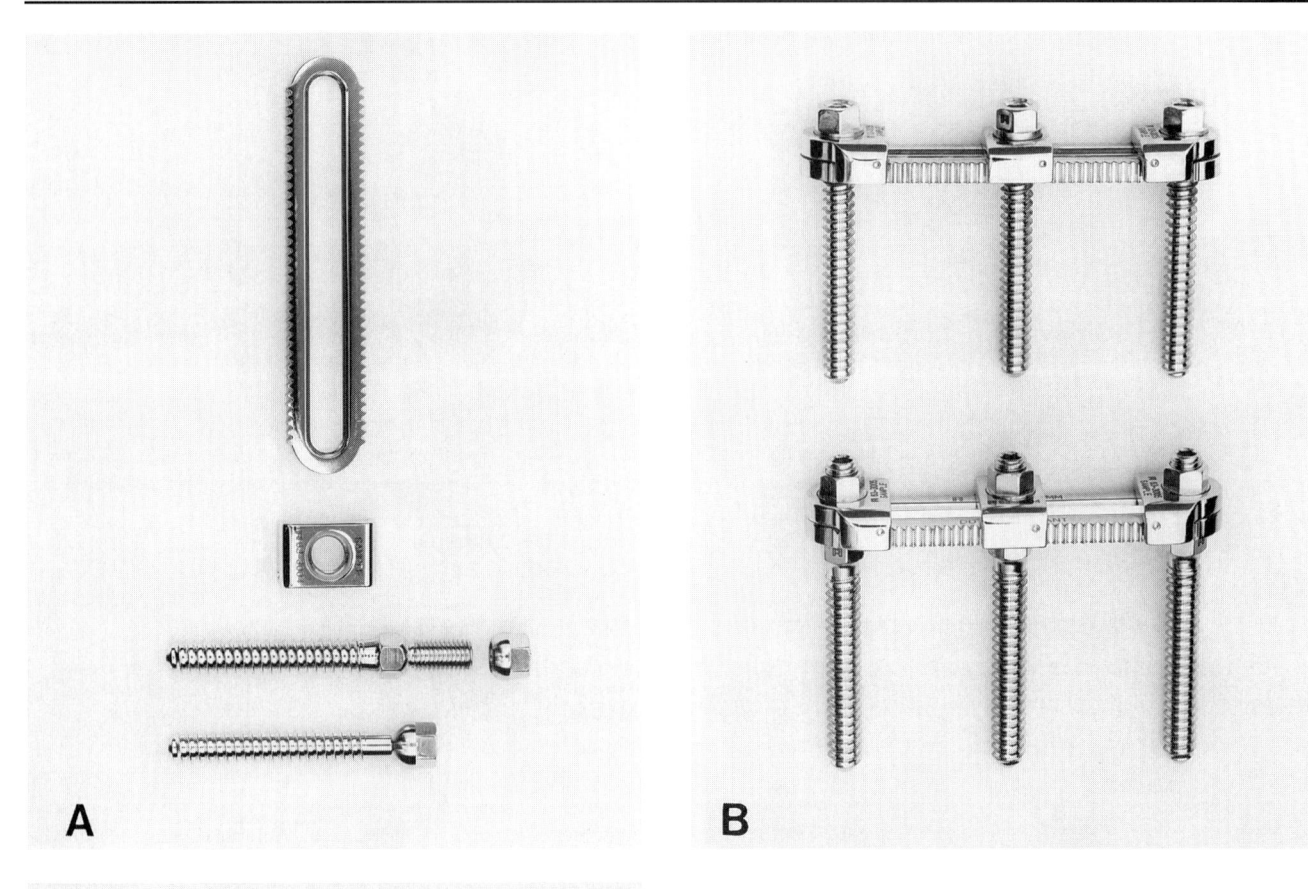

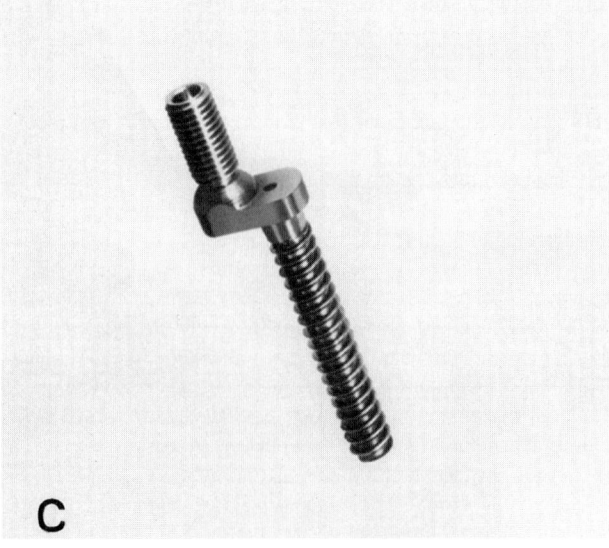

FIG. 30-1. Components of the Simmons plating system. (a) *Top to bottom*, Plate, washer, bolt with Spiralock locking nut, screw. (b) *Top*, Assembled screw construct. *Bottom*, Assembled bolt construct. (c) Offset bolt.

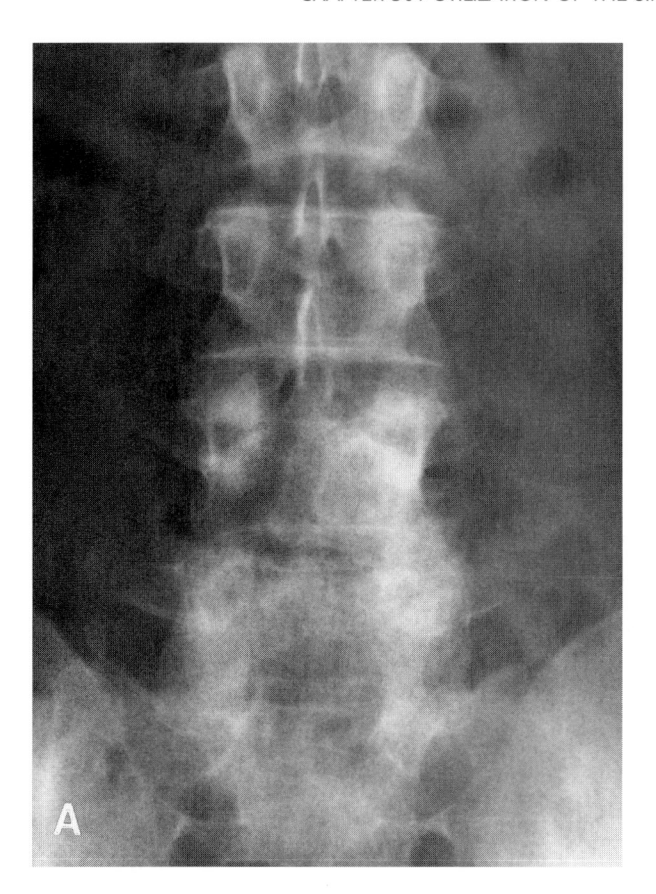

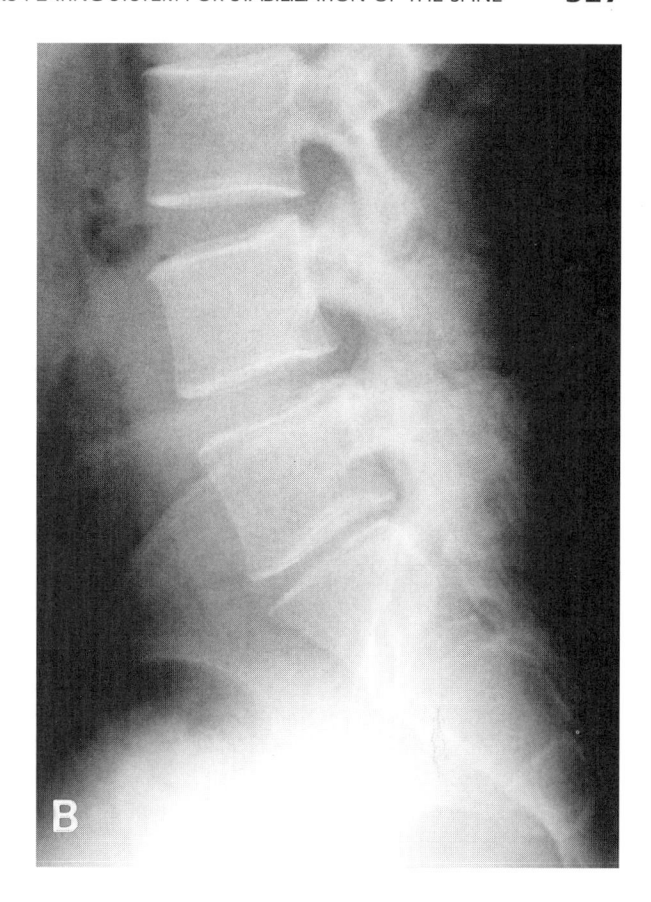

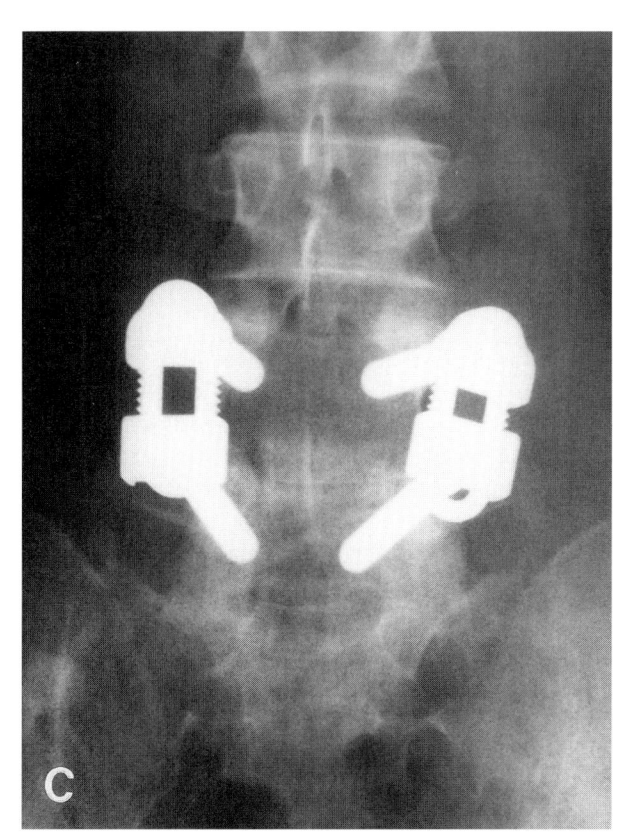

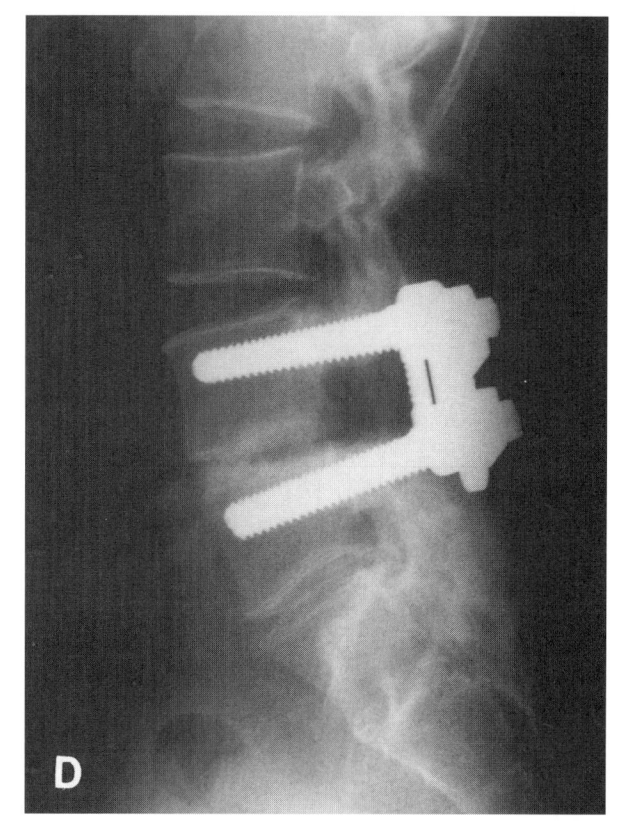

FIG. 30-2. (a to d) Preoperative and postoperative radiographs of a 36-year-old male with a previous L5 to S1 lateral fusion and subsequent deterioration of the L4 segment requiring extensive decompression and stabilization with the bolt-plate construct and body-to-body fusion.

INDICATIONS AND ADVANTAGES

The Simmons system is indicated when spinal fusion becomes necessary in the treatment of a number of spinal abnormalities, or a combination of them, causing a clinical presentation of incapacitating low back pain with or without sciatica that is unresponsive to conservative treatment. Pain may be secondary to abnormalities of the motion segment (Table 30-1). These spinal abnormalities include degenerated disk, disk prolapse, disk herniation, spinal stenosis, postlumbar laminectomy-diskectomy syndrome, spondylolysis, spondylolisthesis, failed back-surgery syndrome, and pseudarthrosis. Although appropriate for a wider range of fusion techniques, PLIF with instrumentation has been cited by some investigators (Lin, 1982) as the most biomechanically satisfying stabilizing procedure, and it is our preference.

At our center we consider indications for PLIF (Simmons, 1991) to be a combination of pathophysiologic, functional, and lifestyle requirements: (1) Spinal stenosis unresponsive to nonoperative measures, particularly subarticular or foraminal stenosis requiring partial or complete facetectomy; (2) Segmental instability unresponsive to nonoperative measures (primary sagittal or rotational instability may be difficult to quantify or define); (3) Diskogenic disease unresponsive to job or activity modification, including chemically induced disk pain.

Improvements in posterior spinal fixation instrumentation, especially those incorporating pedicle screws, has brought reconsideration of PLIF in the 1980s after a limited following by U.S. surgeons in previous decades (Christoferson & Selland, 1975; Cloward, 1953; Collis, 1985; Lin, 1977; Ma, 1985; Wiltberger, 1957). Advantages of PLIF with instrumentation (Table 30-2) include formation of three-column stability, with allowance for wider decompression, prevention of graft dislodgment, and improved fusion rate. Instrumented PLIF affords biomechanical advantages, including load sharing and graft protection, while disk height and interpedicular distance are maintained by the instrumentation. This, in turn, allows earlier patient mobilization, shorter hospital stays, freedom from brace requirements, and earlier return to work and activities of daily living.

CONTRAINDICATIONS AND DISADVANTAGES

Contraindications to the performance of PLIF with Simmons plating system instrumentation (see Table 30-1) include conditions that contraindicate any technique of spinal fixation, that is, systemic infection or infection of spinal elements and severe osteopenia. The plating systems are difficult to use for idiopathic scoliosis and severe degenerative scoliosis. These problems, however, are difficult to treat using any system (see Table 30-2).

The decision to proceed to internal fixation and fusion should be made relating to the anatomic structure involved, the lesion, the morphologic changes, instability, and extent of neurologic involvement. Also, the surgeon must recognize the need to distinguish between instability and physiologic hypermobility of the spine. Even normative values of intervertebral mobility in asymptomatic patients may present ranges of translation that exceed the criteria for pathologic instability (Knutsson, 1944; Posner & White, 1982). Therefore, the need to correlate clinical with radiographic findings must be emphasized.

PLIF TECHNIQUE WITH SIMMONS PLATING SYSTEM INSTRUMENTATION

The patient is placed in a prone position on the spinal table, allowing for abdominal dependence and C-arm positioning. An exception to this positioning is for patients with spondylolisthesis and other patients who require extensive decompression. Routine use is made of hypotensive anesthesia, the cell saver, and autologous blood transfusion. In addition, prophylactic antibiotics for both gram-negative and gram-positive bacteria are given preoperatively. Antiembolus stockings with sequential gradient pumps are used intraoperatively.

A wide laminectomy with Kerrison rongeurs and osteotomes is performed. Posterior elements are exposed by careful soft-tissue dissection. Exposure of the site is afforded by removal of the ligamentum flavum of the affected segment. Lateral imaging with C-arm fluoroscopy is done to confirm position and provide reference for subsequent placement of pedicle bolts. Pedicles are broached with care to probe at the angle of the pedicle corresponding to that shown

Table 30-1
Indications and Contraindications for Spinal Fusion with the Simmons Plating System

Indications
  Diagnostic categories
    Degenerated disk
    Disk protrusion
    Disk herniation
    Spinal stenosis
    Postlumbar laminectomy-diskectomy syndrome
    Spondylolisthesis with or without spondylolysis
    Failed back-surgery syndrome
    Pseudarthrosis
  Clinical indicators (combination of pathophysiologic, functional, and lifestyle indicators)
    Spinal stenosis unresponsive to nonoperative measures, particularly subarticular or foraminal stenosis requiring partial or complete facetectomy
    Segmental instability unresponsive to nonoperative measures, if radiographically definable (primary sagittal or rotational instability may be difficult to quantify or define)
    Diskogenic disease unresponsive to job or activity modification, including chemically induced disk pain
Contraindications
  Systemic infection
  Infection of spinal elements
  Severe osteopenia
  Idiopathic scoliosis
  Severe degenerative scoliosis

Table 30-2
Advantages and Disadvantages of PLIF with Simmons Plating System Instrumentation

Advantages
   Formation of three-column stability
   Allowance for wider decompression
   Prevention of graft dislodgment
   Improved fusion rate
   Design advantages
      Wide range of component sizes
      Wide range of construct sizes and configurations
      Ease of use of components (cannulated bolts and screws, bolts are precut, Spiralock self-locking nut capable of repeated loosening and tightening)
      Enhanced strength (large radius at the bolt-plate interface, tapered bolts, large minor diameters of screws and bolts, decreased thread pitch)
   Biomechanical advantages
      Load sharing
      Graft protection
      Maintenance of disk height and interpedicular distance while awaiting physiologic fusion mass development
   Patient outcome advantages
      Earlier mobilization
      Shorter hospital stays
      Freedom from brace requirements
      Earlier return to work and/or activities of daily living

Disadvantages
   Difficult to use in idiopathic scoliosis
   Difficult to use in severe degenerative scoliosis
   Number of spinal segments that can be simultaneously instrumented limited by size of pedicles

on the lateral roentgenogram. Each pedicle is probed in turn. On completion of preparation of the bed (if an intertransverse process fusion is being performed) and probing of all pedicles to be included in the fixation, assisted by fluoroscopic imaging, the pedicles are tapped. The bolts are then placed. The bolts at S1 engage the promontory. Thereafter, the appropriate plates are selected and bent to maintain the lumbar lordosis. The plate is fixed on the bolts with the system's washer and locking nut mechanism.

Subsequent to placement of instrumentation, if the PLIF technique is undertaken, the intervertebral disk is approached and a radical diskectomy is performed to include the lateral disk, midline annulus, and posterior longitudinal ligament. Osteotomes, pituitary rongeurs, Scoville curettes, and a posterior longitudinal ligament resector are all used to achieve a total diskectomy.

End plate preparation is critical to secure graft fit and incorporation. The disk space is thoroughly cleared with curettes and the disk removed to the lateral and anterior edges of the annulus. Visualization is aided through the use of a lamina spreader. A punch or osteotomes are employed to obtain a bleeding surface of the end plates for bone plugs. The anterior portion of the end plates is petaled. Chips of the posterior lamina are then placed anteriorly and impacted.

A disk spacer is placed unilaterally if the plates have not been positioned. An appropriately sized and contoured iliac crest bone plug is impacted on the contralateral side. The bone plugs may be bicortical or tricortical, allograft or autograft. After the local autogenous chips are impacted anteriorly in the disk space, the bone plugs are then inserted (creating a composite graft if allograft plugs are used). Next, the spacer is removed and a second bone plug is inserted. Puka chisels are used to "walk" the bone blocks to the midline. In most cases, three to four bone blocks are comfortably accommodated in the intervertebral disk space. The bone plugs should be impacted 2 to 4 mm below the posterior border of the vertebral body. An alternative to the bone blocks is placement of autogenous chips, if there are enough to fill the disk space.

The nerve roots are inspected for any residual impingement. After pulse lavage irrigation with a bacitracin solution, with the dura covered with a gauze sponge, a fat graft is placed between the dura and the PLIF plugs and posterior to the dura. A sheet of Gelfoam is used if fat is not available. A large Hemovac drain is placed in the wound and the wound is closed. A pressure dressing is placed over the wound.

Figure 30-3 shows the Simmons plating system in place after an instrumented PLIF in a 51-year-old man.

SPECIAL TIPS FOR SUCCESSFUL USE OF THE SIMMONS PLATING SYSTEM

Tapping of the pedicles is aided by Simmons instrumentation. The pedicle tap has a quick-release T-handle and is scored. A sleeve is used with the tap; the sleeve takes up very little space and allows tapping without damage to the surrounding soft tissue (muscles, capsule, etc.). The position of the top of the sleeve on the scored tap allows for determination of the depth of the tap within the vertebral body.

Integrity of pedicle walls is mandatory for safe use of the system. Every effort is made to ensure that the walls of the pedicle remain intact. The flexible sound is used to "feel" the inner walls of the pedicle. The outer walls of the pedicle are visualized or felt with an instrument. The "suck test," performed by suctioning the pedicle and observing for reappearance of fluid on the outside of the pedicle helps to ensure that the pedicle remains intact.

Determining the pedicle entry site and the direction of the pedicle can be very difficult. Lateral fluoroscopy is used to assist in locating the pedicle in an axial plane. Using an anatomical landmark such as the mamillary body of the lateral facet, the transverse process, and the ridge of the pars interarticularis, the entrance point can usually be identified prior to removing the cortex over the entrance to the pedicle. The pedicle can be entered with the rigid sound (gearshift) or the 2-mm guide wire. Placement of these instruments is assisted with lateral fluoroscopy.

Placement of the screws, bolts, and nuts is controlled by fixing the screws, bolts, and nuts to the wrench with a stabilizing bar. If a laminectomy has been performed, the dura must be protected while tapping and placing the screws and bolts in the pedicle. A Cobb elevator or a malleable

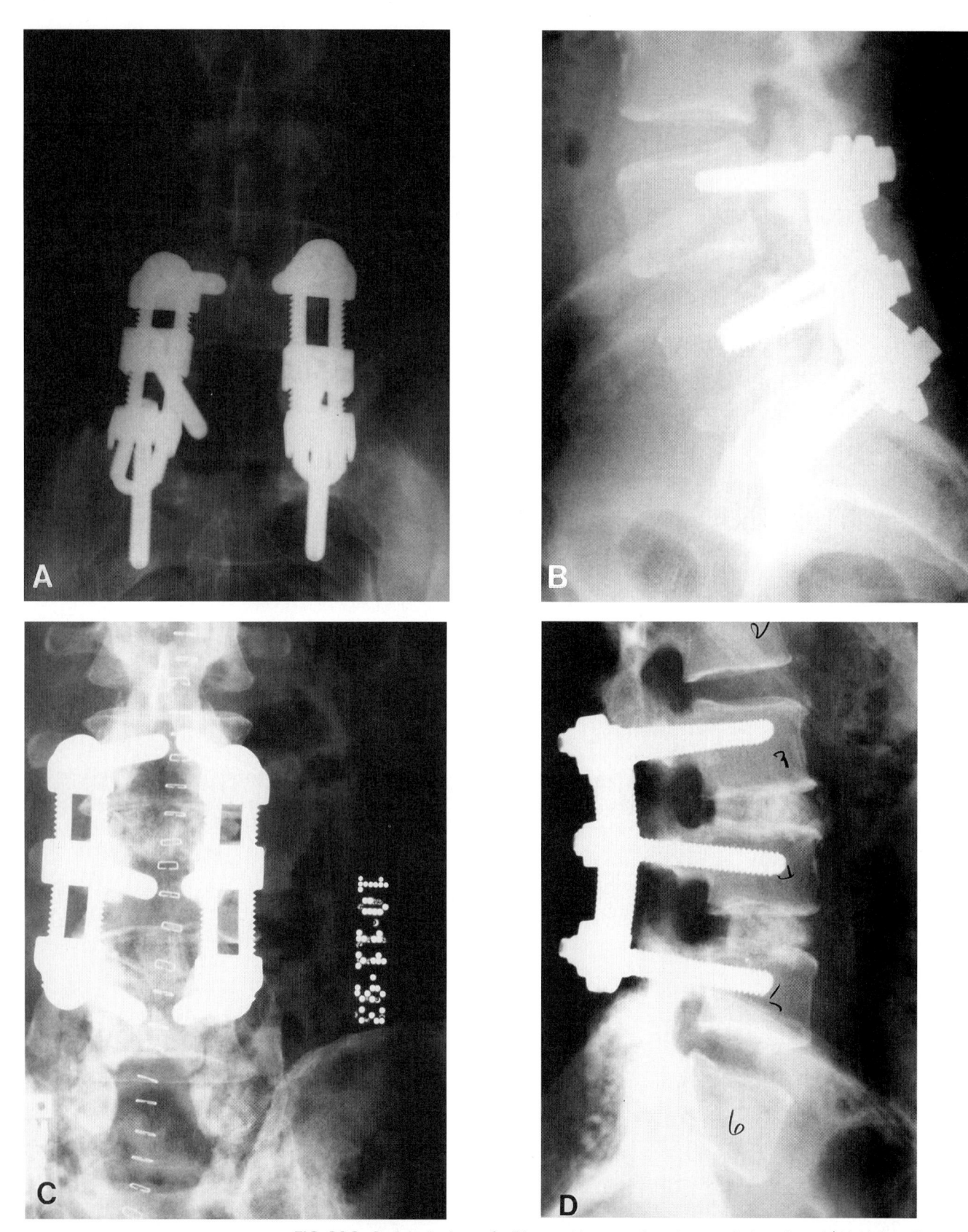

FIG. 30-3. Radiologic views of a 51-year-old man undergoing two fusions. (a and b) Initially, a Simmons all-screw plate construct fixation of the L5 and L6 segments was performed (there are six lumbar vertebrae with lumbarization of S1). Painful segments subsequently developed at L3 and L4, which was confirmed on diskography. The all-screw construct was removed, revealing good stability and consolidation of the lateral fusion. (c and d) This was followed by decompressive laminectomy and foraminotomy with diskectomy and PLIF wherein autogenous chips were placed anteriorly and allograft plugs posteriorly. The L3 and L4 segments were instrumented with a Simmons all-bolt/plate construct.

retractor is placed against the pedicle and over the dura to prevent dural injury.

The bolts have a hex hole at the top in which the hex wrench can be placed for control of the bolt while tightening the nut or changing the depth of the bolt in the vertebra, even with the plate and washer in place. Because of the high level of strength of the bolt, it is not necessary to place the bolt completely within the pedicle. This allows for adjustment of the bolt to the plate as well as allowing for a change in height of the plate above the facets.

When bending the plate with an accentuated lordosis of 25 degrees or more, by measuring the distance between the teeth on the concave side of the bent plate, the teeth of the plate may approximate, making it difficult to place the washer on the plate. However, by putting the washer in place while bending the plate, the teeth will not approximate. It is seldom necessary to bend the plate to that extent, and with the sagittally oriented washers, the bend in the plate does not have to be at an acute angle.

The cannulated torque wrench allows for tightening of the nut onto the bolt while stabilizing the bolt with the hex wrench placed through the cannula of the torque wrench. With the cannulated torque wrench lock nut in the open position, the Spiralock nut is torqued to 75 in.-lb. Thereafter, by simply closing the torque wrench lock nut, slightly more torque can be placed on the nut, if desired.

Segmental compression and distraction can be obtained by engaging the washer at one end of the plate, locking it in place, while leaving the washer of the next segment loose on top of the plate and held in place loosely by a Spiralock nut. Following distraction or compression, the washer is turned 90 degrees and the teeth engaged on the plate followed by tightening of the nut.

Reduction of spondylolisthesis can be obtained by using the mechanical advantage of the screw within the body of the vertebra, tightening the bolt with the hex wrench, thus pulling the vertebra to the plate that has been fixed to the pedicle below.

Placement of the S1 bolt is done in a fashion to use the promontory of the sacrum, using the strength of the promontory to enhance the stability of the S1 bolt.

Misalignment of the pedicle hole can be remedied by using the offset bolt to redirect the bolt to the plate and washer. To minimize the failure of the pedicle, close attention needs to be paid to the strength of the bone. The instrumentation using the offset bolt and the various washers will decrease the stress on the pedicle, minimizing occurrences of fracture and the stress-shielding effect.

Placement of graft material is readily accommodated by the system, whether a PLIF, ALIF, posterolateral technique, or combination of techniques is employed. When doing the PLIF, the profile of the plate is such that the PLIF can be done without obstruction. When doing the lateral gutter fusion, the capability of having the hex hole in the bolt, allowing the plate to be raised and lowered while in place, gives the advantage of placing the lateral fusion and then positioning the plate following placement of the fusion, if indicated. When doing a 360-degree fusion, the plates can be easily placed using the midline approach or the Wiltse lateral approach to the pedicles.

Removal of the hardware is made simple with the hex hole in the top of the bolt, allowing for stabilization of the bolt while the nut is being removed.

RESULTS

No universally accepted standards exist to measure results after spinal fusion. Investigators report results based on presence or absence of radiographic evidence of solid union, although such a parameter does not necessarily reflect long-term postoperative spinal stability. Stability may indeed be afforded by fibrous union as well as by bony union.

Fusion rates with PLIF have been reported by several investigators. Cloward (1985) reported 92% with successful fusion; Lin (1985) reported 88%; and Ma (1985) reported 85% rates of solid union. Our fusion rate of 91% using PLIF without instrumentation has been reported previously (Simmons, 1985; 1980).

A formal clinical study of the Simmons implant in conjunction with PLIF is in progress and data await statistical analysis. However, a few reports of rates of fusion experienced by other investigators using pedicle instrumentation with PLIF have been published. Steffee and Sitkowski, employing PLIF technique with plates, reported in 1988 a 100% rate of solid union. Stonecipher and Wright (1989), employing PLIF technique with facet screws, also reported a 100% rate of solid union. Brantigan, Steffee, Kepler, and associates (1992) have described their use of a plating system in association with the PLIF technique. Although they do not report fusion rates with their group of 501 patients, they report their criteria for determining failure of their lumbar procedures (regardless of the presence of solid fusion): failure to reduce degenerative deformity, failure to decompress the neural structures adequately, and failure to restore disk space height. They find that for patients in whom the procedure is indicated, the instrumented PLIF procedure enables them to carry out wide and destabilizing decompressions and reduction of deformities while reestablishing firm posterior support in anatomic alignment.

COMPLICATIONS

All spine surgery carries the risks of blood loss, epidural bleeding, nerve-root injury, intraabdominal vascular injury, pseudarthrosis, instability, graft resorption, infection, epidural scar, arachnoiditis, dural tears, graft retropulsion, and adjacent-level degeneration. In one study of more than 1000 lumbar spine operations, the overall complication rate was in excess of 20%, with reoperations and fusion operations showing significantly higher rates of complications than primary operations or laminectomy alone (Smith, 1993).

Complications implicated particularly after PLIF include nerve-root injury, epidural scar, dural tears, graft retropulsion, and adjacent-level degeneration (Cotler & Star, 1990; Lin, 1985; Ma, 1985; Macnab & Dall, 1971).

Nerve-root injury can be avoided by careful decompression and retraction. Having sufficient lateral disk exposure with ample facetectomy protects the exiting and traversing nerve roots at the time of graft impaction.

Epidural scarring has been particularly troublesome with PLIF, although the addition of pedicle fixation prevents excessive neural traction from epidural scar mass. Fat grafting, gentle retraction, and consistent hemostasis can reduce the occurrence of epidural scarring.

Graft retropulsion is problematic with PLIF. Careful end plate shaping, graft sizing, and countersinking of graft material should prevent this complication. The addition of pedicle fixation to the PLIF procedure has reduced its occurrence.

The stability afforded to the segment operated on has been implicated in degeneration of adjacent levels. Appropriate preoperative examinations, including awake diskography, are aids in predicting this risk. It is important to spare the facets adjacent to the fused segment to avoid subsequent degeneration of adjacent levels.

It should be noted that most of the complications related to spinal surgery occur as a result of the surgery itself, not the utilization of the pedicle for fixation. The problems of blood loss, nerve-root injury, intraabdominal vascular injury, pseudarthrosis, graft retropulsion, infection, epidural scar, arachnoiditis, dural tears, and graft displacement all occur with spinal surgery without, as well as with, instrumentation.

The problems that are unique to the use of the pedicle for fixation are relatively few. The primary problem is screws or bolts breaking out of the pedicle and causing injury to the neural elements. Postoperative problems such as stress shielding, bolt or screw loosening, and bolt or screw breakage are problems unique to the use of the pedicle for fixation. However, these problems have no greater occurrence than does the failed back-surgery syndrome, which complicated surgical outcome prior to the use of the pedicle for spinal fixation.

REFERENCES

Brantigan, J.W., Steffee, A.D., Keppler, L., et al. (1992). Posterior lumbar interbody fusion technique using the variable screw placement spinal fixation system. In: D.M. Arnold & J.E. Lonstein (Eds.), *Pedicle Fixation of the Lumbar Spine. Spine: State of the Art Reviews* (pp. 175–200). Philadelphia, Hanley & Belfus.

Christoferson, L.A., & Selland, B. (1975). Intervertebral bone implants following excision of protruded lumbar discs. *Journal of Neurosurgery, 42,* 401.

Cloward, R.B. (1985). Posterior lumbar interbody fusion updated. *Clinical Orthopaedics and Related Research, 193,* 16.

Cloward, R.B. (1953). The treatment of ruptured lumbar intervertebral disc by vertebral body fusion: Indications, operative technique, after care. *Journal of Neurosurgery, 10,* 154.

Collis, J.S. (1985). Total disc replacement: A modified posterior lumbar interbody fusion. *Clinical Orthopaedics and Related Research, 193,* 64.

Cotler, J.M., & Star, A.M. (1990). Complications of spinal fusion. In: J.M. Cotler, H.B. Cotler (Eds.), *Spinal Fusion: Science and Technique.* (pp. 361–387). New York: Springer-Verlag.

Cunningham, B.W., Sefter, J.C., et al. (1993). Static and cyclical biomechanical analysis of pedicle screw spinal constructs. *Spine, 18,* 1677.

Knutsson, F. (1944). The instability associated with disc degeneration in the lumbar spine. *Acta Radiologica, 25,* 593.

Lin, P.M. (1985). Posterior lumbar interbody fusion technique: Complications and pitfalls. *Clinical Orthopaedics and Related Research, 193,* 90.

Lin, P.M. (1982). *PLIF: Biomechanical Principles and Indications* (p. 3). Springfield, MO: Charles C. Thomas.

Lin, P.M. (1977). A technical modification of Cloward's posterior lumbar interbody fusion. *Neurosurgery, 1,* 118.

Ma, G.W. (1985). Posterior lumbar interbody fusion with specialized instruments. *Clinical Orthopaedics and Related Research, 193,* 57.

Macnab, I., & Dall, D. (1971). The blood supply of the lumbar spine and its application to the technique of intertransverse lumbar fusion. *Journal of Bone and Joint Surgery, British Volume, 53,* 628.

Posner, I., & White, A.A., III, et al. (1982). A biomechanical analysis of the clinical stability of the lumbar and lumbosacral spine. *Spine, 7,* 374.

Simmons, J.W. (1991). Posterior lumbar interbody fusion. In: J.W. Frymoyer (Ed.), *The Adult Spine: Principles and Practice* (pp. 1961–1987). New York: Raven Press.

Simmons, J.W. (1985). Posterior lumbar interbody fusion with posterior elements as chip grafts. *Clinical Orthopaedics and Related Research, 193,* 85.

Simmons, J.W. (1980). Posterior interbody fusions. Presented at the Seventh Annual Meeting of the International Society for the Study of the Lumbar Spine, New Orleans.

Smith, G.J. (1993). Complications of lumbar spine surgery. Presented at the 8th Annual Meeting, North American Spine Society, San Diego, CA.

Steffee, A.D., & Sitkowski, D.J. (1988). Posterior lumbar interbody fusion and plates. *Clinical Orthopaedics and Related Research, 227,* 99.

Stonecipher, T., & Wright, S. (1989). Posterior lumbar interbody fusion with facet-screw fixation. *Spine, 14,* 468.

Wiltberger, B.R. (1957). The dowel intervertebral-body fusion as used in lumbar-disc surgery. *Journal of Bone and Joint Surgery, American Volume, 39,* 284.

CHAPTER 31

Utilization of the Rogozinski Spinal Rod System for Stabilization of the Lumbosacral and Thoracolumbar Spine

Chaim Rogozinski
Abraham Rogozinski
William C. Watters, III

HIGHLIGHTS

The Rogozinski spinal rod system (Smith and Nephew Spine, Memphis, TN) was designed in response to what the developers saw as deficiencies or problems of other systems for spinal stabilization—problems compounding the inherent difficulties in performing spinal surgery. A system that addressed the problems of variability in spinal anatomy and variability of applications was the primary goal. Such a system would conform to spinal anatomy without the need for surgeons to alter anatomy to conform to the system. It would be a simple, modular internal fixation device requiring only simple tools to make it work. Finally, it would be sufficiently strong to enhance arthrodesis. First implanted in a patient in 1988, the Rogozinski system has been implanted in the lumbosacral spine by the authors in more than 200 cases. Various spinal surgery centers throughout the United States have employed the system for lumbosacral and thoracolumbar spine stabilization procedures since 1990. The system has been used to accompany posterolateral spinal fusion as well as interbody fusion (posterior and anterior).

SYSTEM COMPONENTS

The system inventory (Fig. 31-1) includes rods, pedicle screws, hooks, couplers, set screws, and cross-bars. System implants are comprised of screws/hooks attached to bilateral rods linked by cross-bars at each level, forming a quadrilateral or ladder-shaped configuration.

In the case of pedicle screw fixation, screws are placed bilaterally in the central axis of the pedicles to avoid preloading of forces on the screws (Abumi, Panjabi, & Duranceau, 1989; Arnold & Wiltse, 1992; George, Krag, Johnson, et al., 1991; Krag, Weaver, Beynnon, et al., 1988; Rulan, McAfee, Warden, et al., 1991; Zindrick, Wiltse, Widell, et al., 1986). Screws are connected independently to the rods via various-sized cross-bars, thus eliminating the need to align screws in the sagittal plane (Fig. 31-2).

Hooks may be used alone or in pairs to "sandwich" laminae above and below. Also, they are used as a double anchor in the sacrum along with sacral pedicle screws. Hooks are closed with modified cross-bars called hook-bars.

Finally, the bilateral rods are connected by cross-bars to enhance rigidity of the construct to withstand torsional stresses on the implant and to increase pullout strength significantly (Fig. 31-3).

The system is designed to provide a top-loading construct. Screws are seated within an open-backed coupler and hooks are themselves open-backed to facilitate ease of insertion and construction of the implant. Only when the surgeon is satisfied with placement of hooks and screws is rod attachment performed and the implant completely assembled and tightened down with torquing of set screws.

BIOMECHANICAL CONSIDERATIONS

Two types of systems for pedicular arthrodesis are currently available: those employing rods and those employing plates. Rods were chosen for the Rogozinski system because: (1) rods were deemed more versatile, less constrained. Rod systems allow optimal pedicle screw placement and contouring of the construct in multiple planes

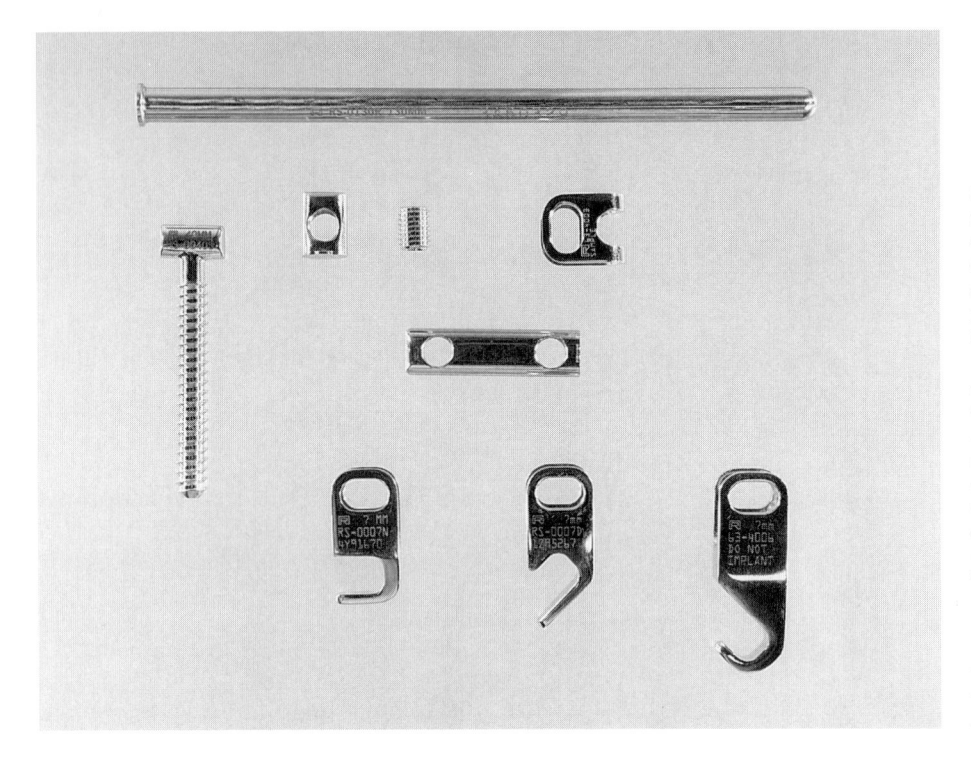

FIG. 31-1. System components—rods, hooks, pedicle screws, cross-bars, couplers, set screws. Rods (*top*) are smooth, measure 6.4 mm in diameter, and are flared at one end. They are supplied in lengths of 50 to 300 mm in 10- or 20-mm increments. Hooks (*bottom*) are supplied in 7- and 11-mm aperture sizes with three hook designs—up-angle, down-angle, and neutral. Pedicle screws (*left*) are supplied in lengths from 35 to 60 mm in 5-mm increments, and in three sizes—6.4 mm major with a 4.8-mm minor diameter, 5.5-mm major with a 4.8-mm minor diameter, and 7.0-mm major with a 5.4-mm minor diameter. Cross-bars (*center*) are supplied in 10- to 55-mm lengths in 3-mm increments. Couplers (*below rod, right*) are used for seating pedicle screws for connection to rods, and set screws (*below rod, left*) are used to secure cross-bars.

(Pool & Gaines, 1992). (2) Rigid rods, rather than malleable rods, were chosen for the Rogozinski system. The advantage of a rigid rod system is its capability to reduce and correct deformity (Kornblatt, Casey, & Jacobs, 1986; Krag, Beynnon, Pope, et al., 1986; Ogilvie & Schendel, 1986). Disadvantages of rigid arthrodesis systems are stress-shielding and osteopenia, as shown in canine (McAfee, Farey, Sutterlin, et al., 1989; Smith, Hunt, Asher, et al., 1991) and goat (Johnston, Ashman, Baird, et al., 1990) models, wherein constructs were determined to be excessively rigid. However, stress-shielding and osteopenia have not been encountered clinically with the Rogozinski system; indeed, the highest fusion rates have been seen in the more rigid constructs, those employing segmental pedicle screw fixation. Others have reported the virtue of construct rigidity, as well, with other instrumentation systems (Dickman, Fessler, MacMillan, et al., 1992; Pool & Gaines, 1992). (3) Rod systems are generally less bulky and retain a more medial profile than plate systems, thus affording a more ample field for bone graft.

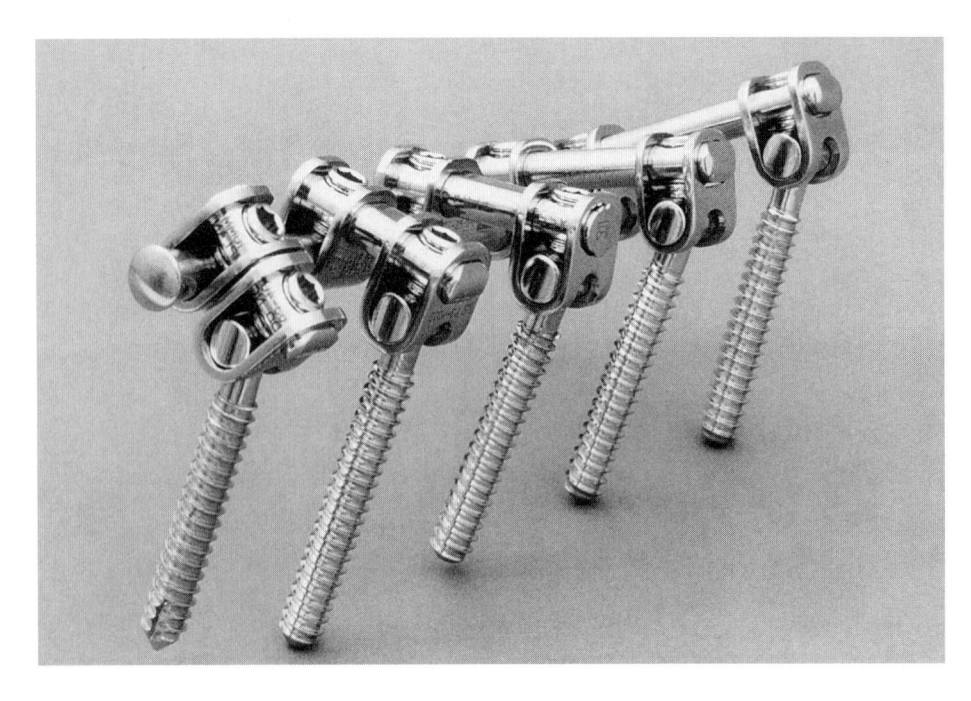

FIG. 31-2. This model demonstrates the degree of freedom allowed by the various combinations of cross-bars and variable pedicle screw trajectory within the coupler. This allows the surgeon the flexibility to perform independent placement of each pedicle screw to accommodate a patient's anatomy rather than the instrumentation's.

permobility, instability, or deformity of the spine (Table 31-1). A number of diagnoses fall within this category: degenerative disk disease, facet arthropathy, pseudarthrosis of previous fusions, spondylolisthesis, and scoliosis. Typically, patients are referred because of mechanical instability of the spine in combination with persistent pain despite treatment trials of at least 6 months and because of the failure of other methods of fixation.

Although we have not used the system for other applications in our center, it is indicated also for stabilization of the spine in the presence of trauma, fracture, and tumor resection (Table 31-2).

The Rogozinski spinal rod system bears an FDA 510K approval for hybrid or all-hook constructs; use of pedicle screws at levels other than the sacrum is under investigation.

Contraindications

The Rogozinski system is contraindicated in patients with metabolic etiologies of spinal degenerative changes (see Table 31-1). Presence of advanced osteoporosis precludes use of the system. Immunologic factors contraindicating surgery include sensitivity to implant materials and immunosuppressive conditions. Infection of spinal elements unresponsive to antibiotic treatment or infection of associated structures or systemic infection all are contraindications to use of the system. Patients who cannot or will not comply with recommendations to discontinue smoking or drug and alcohol abuse are unlikely to have a positive outcome after spinal arthrodesis surgery. Patients in our series who are considered for surgical arthrodesis undergo extensive preoperative isokinetic and psychological testing. Those who require treatment for psychiatric disorders receive appropriate referrals. Those who exhibit symptoms compatible with depression secondary to back injury and associated

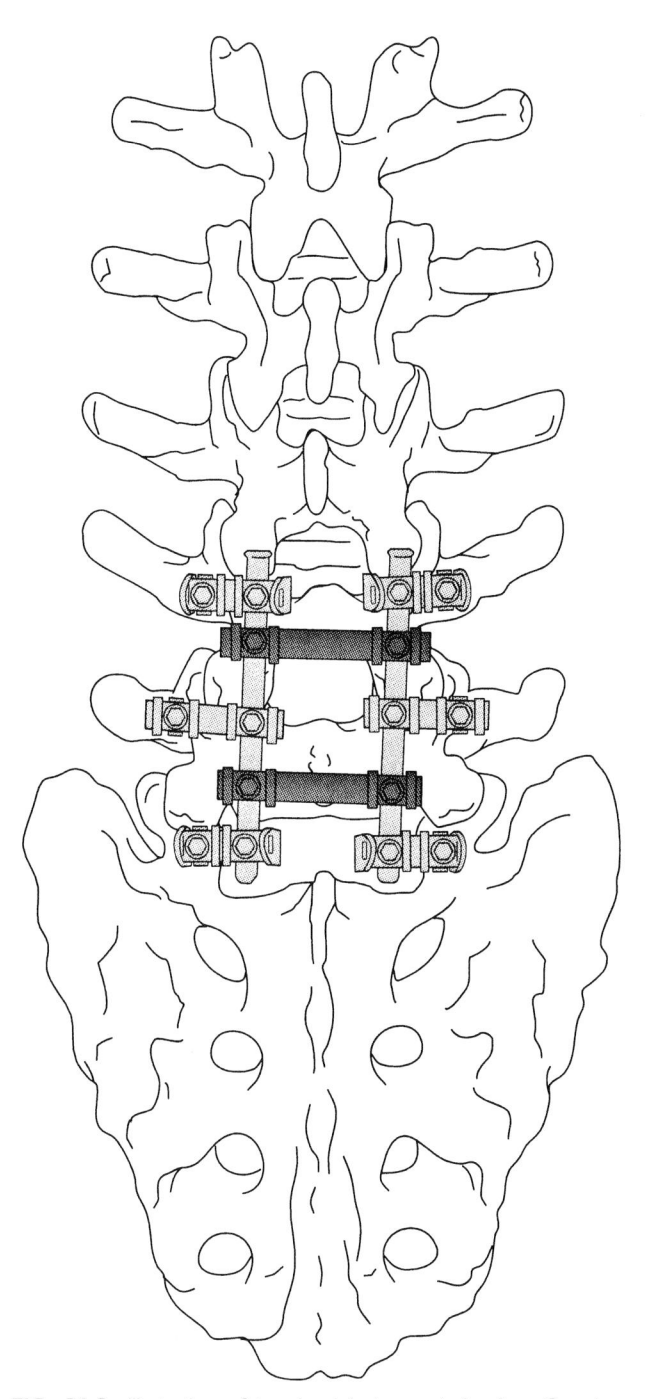

FIG. 31-3. Illustration of two-level instrumented spine. Cross-bars connect the bilateral rods to provide a ladder-shaped configuration that increases pullout strength and enhances rigidity of the construct to withstand torsional stresses.

Studies continue to affirm the use of heavier rods and cross-connection of double rods to afford sufficient construct stiffness to enhance fusion (Johnston et al., 1990; Johnston, Welch, Baker, et al., 1992).

USE IN THE LUMBOSACRAL SPINE

Indications

The Rogozinski system is indicated whenever internal fixation is desired for spinal arthrodesis to correct chronic hy-

Table 31-1
Indications and Contraindications for Use of the Rogozinski Spinal Rod System

Indications
  Hypermobility or instability of the spine
    Degenerative disk disease
    Spinal stenosis
    Postlaminectomy syndrome
    Spondylolisthesis
    Pseudarthrosis after previous fusion or decompression
  Correction of deformity
    Scoliosis
    Tumor resection
  Trauma
    Fracture

Contraindications
  Metabolic diseases of bone
  Osteoporosis
  Infection—local or systemic
  Immunosensitivity to components
  Immunosuppressive conditions
  Psychiatric conditions
  Noncompliance with medical recommendations regarding alcohol and drug (including tobacco) cessation

Table 31-2
Advantages and Disadvantages of the Rogozinski Spinal Rod System

Advantages
    Provides multiplane stability
    Stabilizes the screw torsionally
    Offsets the construct to maximize graft bed
    Spares the nonfused facet
    Minimizes differences between the screw major and minor diameters
    Provides ability to connect three or more points without preloading
    Accommodates for screw convergence
    Allows dorsal application of components
    Provides ability to reconfigure the construct intraoperatively
    Allows ease of retrieval
    Eliminates the need for postoperative immobilization
    Achieves multiplane correction of deformity
    Conforms to anatomy with minimal alterations of anatomy to fit construct
    Fewer tools required for implantation
    Top-loading
    Universal hook and screw systems
    Easy alignment and attachment of screw to rod

Disadvantages
    Creates increased dead space (as is true in all systems with cross-connectors)
    Requires more operative time than uninstrumented fusions
    Limits postoperative imaging of site following instrumentation
    Multiple couplers and set screws increase fiddle-factor

disability or chronic pain may be reconsidered for surgical arthrodesis after appropriate treatment and evidence of symptom resolution.

Surgical Criteria and Patient Selection

Adult patients with persistent back pain alone or back pain in combination with leg pain may be considered. However, before surgery is contemplated, rigorous attempts at conservative treatment must be undertaken for a period of at least 6 months; in many cases, conservative treatment is attempted for a year or more. Conservative treatment includes physical therapy and reconditioning, judicious use of selected analgesics, use of nonsteroidal antiinflammatory drugs, and epidural steroid and trigger point injections. Thoracolumbosacral orthoses may be tried when indicated.

Patients whose pain and physical limitations remain unacceptable to them after an extended period of conservative treatment and who request consideration for surgery are referred for base-line isokinetic testing and extensive psychological evaluation. Patients who smoke are required to discontinue smoking before surgery. Smoking cessation is confirmed by preoperative serial carboxyhemoglobin levels titrated for urban- or rural-dwelling populations, as determined by area demographics.

Findings of limitations of range of motion, pain, and neurologic impairment are documented and when possible quantified. Patients are queried about bowel and bladder function, sexual impairment, or cauda equina syndrome.

Patients respond to questionnaires to rate their pain (10-point scale) and level of impairment (modified Oswestry scale) for comparison with postoperative levels as an aid to evaluating clinical outcome.

Preoperative Radiologic Evaluation

All patients are evaluated by plain x-ray films and magnetic resonance imaging (MRI) of the lumbar spine. Gadolinium-enhanced studies are obtained in patients who have undergone previous operation. Provocative diskography and computed tomographic (CT) scans are performed in most patients; those whose pathology warrants further investigation have at least one additional study performed from among the following: myelography, bone scans, stress films, selected nerve-root blocks, and electromyography/nerve conduction studies.

OPERATIVE TECHNIQUE

General Exposure for Posterior Lumbosacral Fusion

Our technique for a three-level instrumentation (L3 to S1) using pedicle screws is described. Participants in an AAOS (American Academy of Orthopaedic Surgeons) summer institute (American Acadency of Orthopaedic Surgeons, 1988) have recommended direct visualization of the pedicle by limited decompression. This is our preference, and this technique is presented.

Patients are positioned on an Andrews frame. Thermal blankets are placed over the head, upper thoracic region, and arms. Draping includes a self-adhesive plastic hip drape that acts as a greenhouse to contain body heat and moisture. A midline incision is made and extends one-and-one-half levels proximal and distal to the anticipated fusion level. (This length allows lateral retraction of the wound so that an adequate convergent angle can be applied on the pedicle screw trajectory.)

A lateral roentgenogram is taken to establish the degree of lordosis on the frame and to confirm operative levels. The resultant roentgenogram is used to establish the cephalad-caudad tilt of the pedicles in the sagittal plane. The superior end plates' inclination closely parallels this axis in the sagittal plane during pedicle preparation.

Dissection proceeds laterally and subperiosteally to the tip of the transverse process and is carried initially extracapsularly to the facet joints. Complete capsulectomies are then performed at the intervertebral levels to be incorporated in the fusion. This allows better control of capsular bleeders and minimizes blood loss. Prior to capsulectomy, the paraspinal muscles have been mobilized laterally off the intertransverse fascial ligament. Once adequate exposure has been obtained, retraction of the soft tissue is achieved using very large Gelpi-type retractors to avoid foreshortening the wound or compromising paraspinal muscular blood flow. Any work within the canal, such as bony decompression or disk exploration, is undertaken as needed.

Technique for Pedicle Screw Instrumentation

After completing the exposure, attention is directed at visualization of the pedicles in preparation for instrumentation. Small bilateral laminotomies are performed at each instrumented level. This is achieved by first elevating the ligamentum flavum in a subperiosteal manner off the margins of the laminae. Positioning the lamina spreader may facilitate this. Thereafter, the dura is visualized, and a Kerrison rongeur is used over cottonoid pledgets. The laminotomy is lateralized to the medial wall of the pedicle by unroofing the subarticular recess.

With the medial wall of the pedicle exposed, the exiting nerve root and dural sac are retracted medially to allow better visualization of the pedicle. The entry point into the pedicle is determined by palpating the superior, medial, and inferior wall of the pedicle from within the canal by the use of a right-angle nerve hook (Fig. 31-4). Once done, the superior and inferior margins of the pedicle are marked on the pars and facet region with electrocautery. The nerve hook is used as a stylus within the canal to determine the widest pedicle diameter at the point at which the medial wall is most convex. This should correspond to the equator of the pedicle, and thus is the optimal location for initiating entry (Fig. 31-5). At this point, with three sides of the pedicle visualized, the entry point is established. (The relationship of the transverse process to its adjoining facet provides additional visual cues and guidance.)

A high-speed bur is used to decorticate the bone overlying the anticipated entry point in the central axis of the pedicle. (Fig. 31-6, a). The pedicle probe (Fig. 31-6, b) is then advanced into this opening. The intraoperative lateral roentgenogram is used to guide the cephalad-caudad trajectory in the sagittal plane. Pedicle convergence angle and depth are ascertained from preoperative MRI or CT scan films. Typically, the probe is driven 20 to 25 mm to cannulate the pedicles completely.

One of the advantages of the open pedicle technique is the ability to perform the following confirmatory tests to evaluate the possibility of cutout into the canal through the pedicle: (1) The medial pedicle wall is directly visualized as described above, and (2) a "suck" test is performed, wherein a small neurosucker is placed into the cannulated pedicle and the blood fluid level is observed within the laminotomy. Normal saline may be placed within the canal if the field is dry. If suction fails to evacuate the fluid (blood or saline), the test is deemed negative (that is, the pedicle walls are deemed intact adjacent to the canal). A reamer is then placed into the pedicle and driven to approximately 50% of the vertebral-body depth, as guided by the intraoperative lateral roentgenogram. The reamer trajectory and integrity of the lateral wall of the pedicle and vertebra are palpated with a flexible pedicle feeler probe to perform a "four-quadrant" test. If the trajectory is acceptable, a calibrated x-ray guide pin is placed into the pedicle to the depth of the reamer, usually 30 to 40 mm (Fig. 31-7). The bore is plugged with a small pledget to tamponade back bleeding.

Once each pedicle is prepared and marked, a repeat lateral roentgenogram is taken to reconfirm trajectory and depth of the pedicle markers. If the guide wire position and trajectory within the pedicle are radiographically acceptable, each pedicle marker is removed and an equal-length screw is chosen for later application. To determine optimal screw length (Fig. 31-7, a): (1) the depth of penetration of the guide wire is determined from lateral roentgenograms. (2) The optimal screw depth should be between 50–75% penetration into the vertebral body. Anterior cortical purchase is unnec-

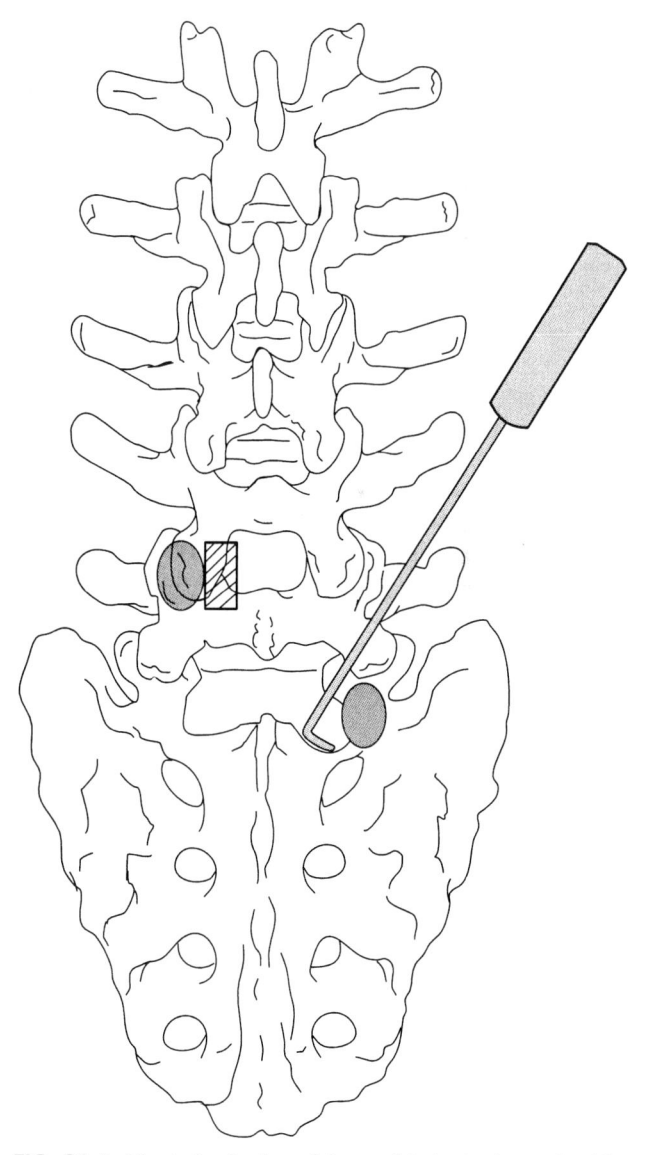

FIG. 31-4. Direct visualization of the pedicle by laminotomies. The shaded areas represent the underlying pedicle; the striped area represents the area to undergo laminotomy. Direct visualization of L5 will be assisted by laminotomy of the striped area. At S1, a laminotomy has already been performed and a nerve hook is used to palpate the inferior wall of the pedicle.

PEDICLE

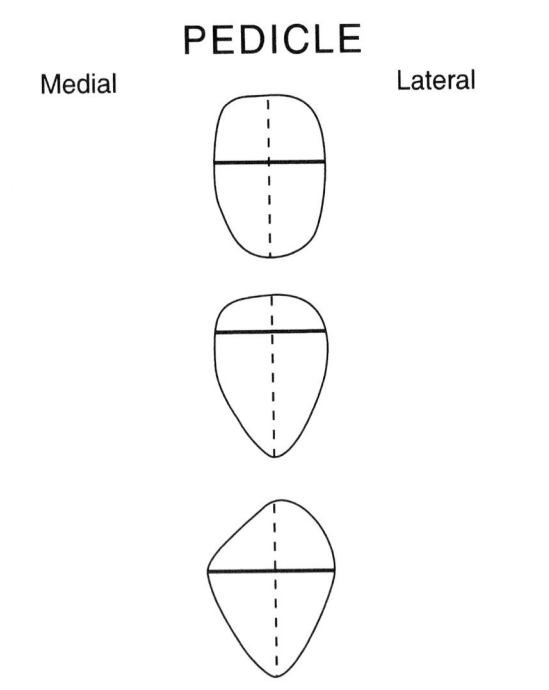

Medial ── Lateral

FIG. 31-5. Various pedicle shapes in cross-section. The solid line represents the pedicle equator, which is the widest portion of the pedicle. Note that this is not necessarily the point midway between the superior and inferior extent of the pedicle.

essary. (3) From the guide wire length, the surgeon can add or subtract length to achieve the tip position within the desired quadrant. Once the appropriate depth is determined, the surgeon should add an extra 5 mm to the calculation so that the screw head sits proud. At this length, the screw head is not impinging on the most cephalad facet joint. But in the more caudad screws, maintaining the screw head proud by 5 mm ensures that the screw head and rod are level. This adjustment maintains a top-loading application of set screws (Fig. 31-7, b).

An instrument nurse records the depth of guide wire penetration and then the size and length of each screw at each vertebral level. Each pedicle is then tapped to an appropriate depth. The bore is again plugged with pledget to maintain hemostasis (and assist in easier identification of the prepared pedicles after decortication).

With pedicle preparation completed, decortication is undertaken prior to insertion of any implants. This allows more aggressive decortication and easier access to bone surfaces for decortication. Decortication is performed aggressively to include the transverse process, the facet, and the pars region of each level. We prefer to use Capener gouges and a large cup curette that works well to "banana peel" the transverse process to expose the cancellous portion. The facets at the

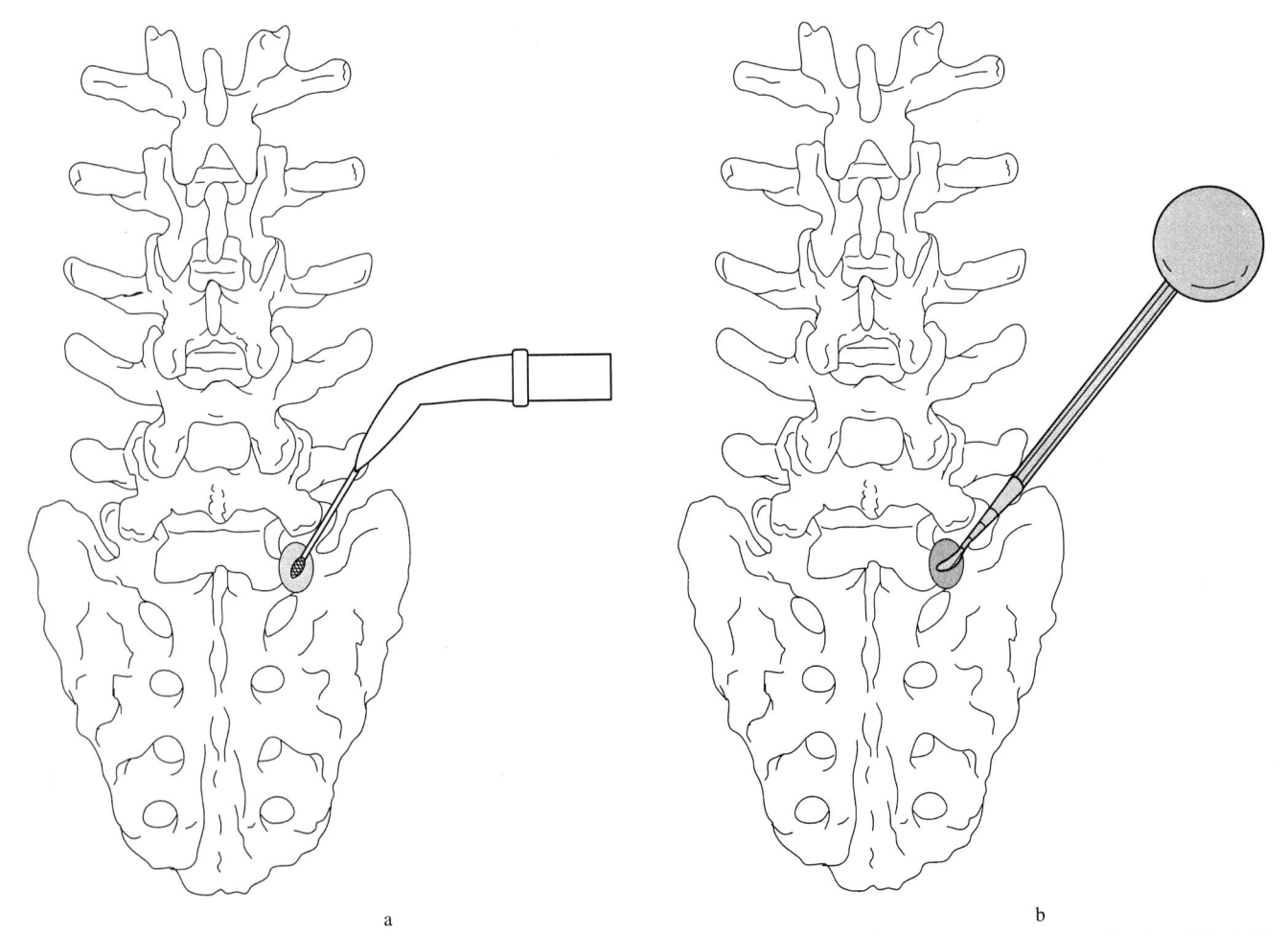

a b

FIG. 31-6. (a) A high-speed bur is used to decorticate the bone overlying the anticipated entry point (*shaded area*). (b) A pedicle probe is then advanced into the decorticated area, into the entry hole.

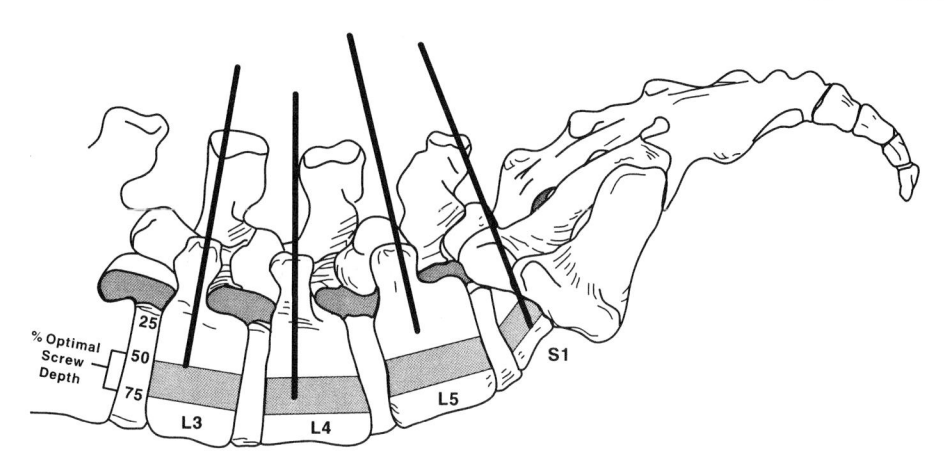

FIG. 31-7. Screw length determination. (a) (1) The depth of penetration of the guide wire is determined from lateral roentgenograms. (2) The optimal screw depth should be between 50 and 75% penetration (shaded area) into the vertebral body. (3) From the guide wire depth of penetration (see Screw Length Selection table below), the surgeon can add or subtract length to achieve the tip position within the desired quadrant. (b) With 5 mm of threads proud, the T-head of the rear screw is raised to a level more even with the rod, with the result that the cross-bar is connected in the desirable horizontal position, allowing top-loading of set screws. In the case shown, an extra 5 mm of nonengaged screw in the sacrum ensures top-loading application of set screws. The desirable top-loading angle, in comparison to the undesirable side-loading angle, is shown in the inset.

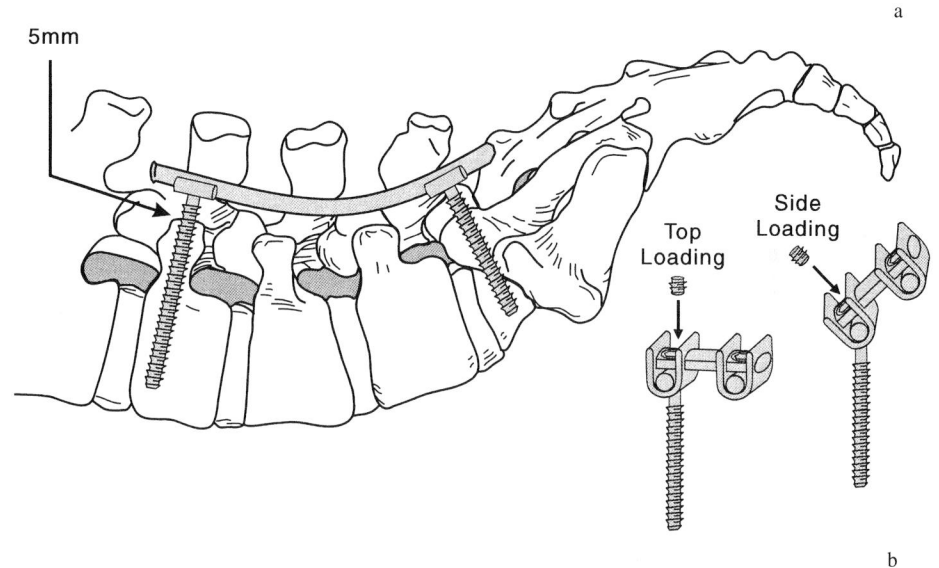

Screw Length Selection

	L3	L4	L5	S1
Guide wire depth (mm)	35	40	30	30
Optimal screw depth (mm)	40	40	40	30
Optimal screw length (add 5 mm)	45	45	45	35

fusion level interspaces are osteotomized obliquely in the frontal plane to allow incorporation of facets into the arthrodesis. Bony remnants are discarded. The ala of the sacrum is osteotomized axially with the anterior bony and soft-tissue attachment intact. It is flipped into the L5-S1 interspace. Following decortication, cancellous graft (previously removed from the iliac crest) is packed into the prepared fusion bed. Only half of the total graft material is used initially. The spinous process at the fusion levels can be removed and the bone used to increase graft volume.

Pedicle screws are readied for insertion (Fig. 31-8). The prepared pedicles are found by following the cottonoid

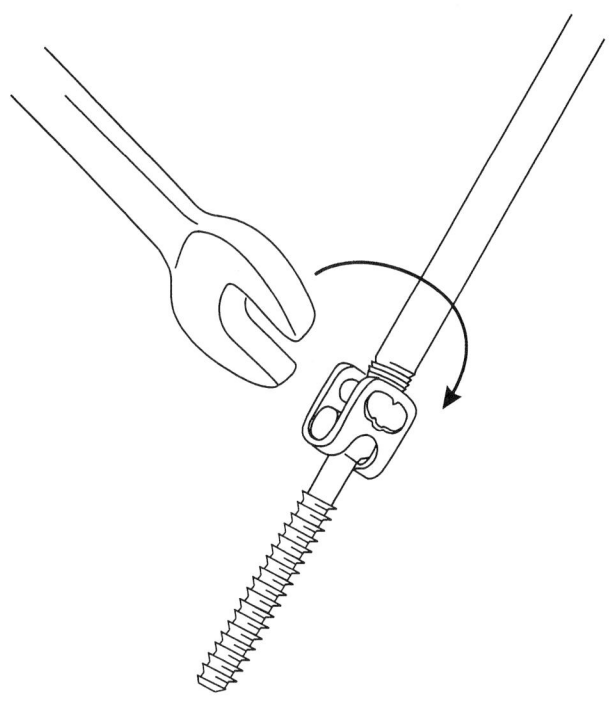

FIG. 31-8. A pedicle screw in the coupler, ready for insertion in the pedicle.

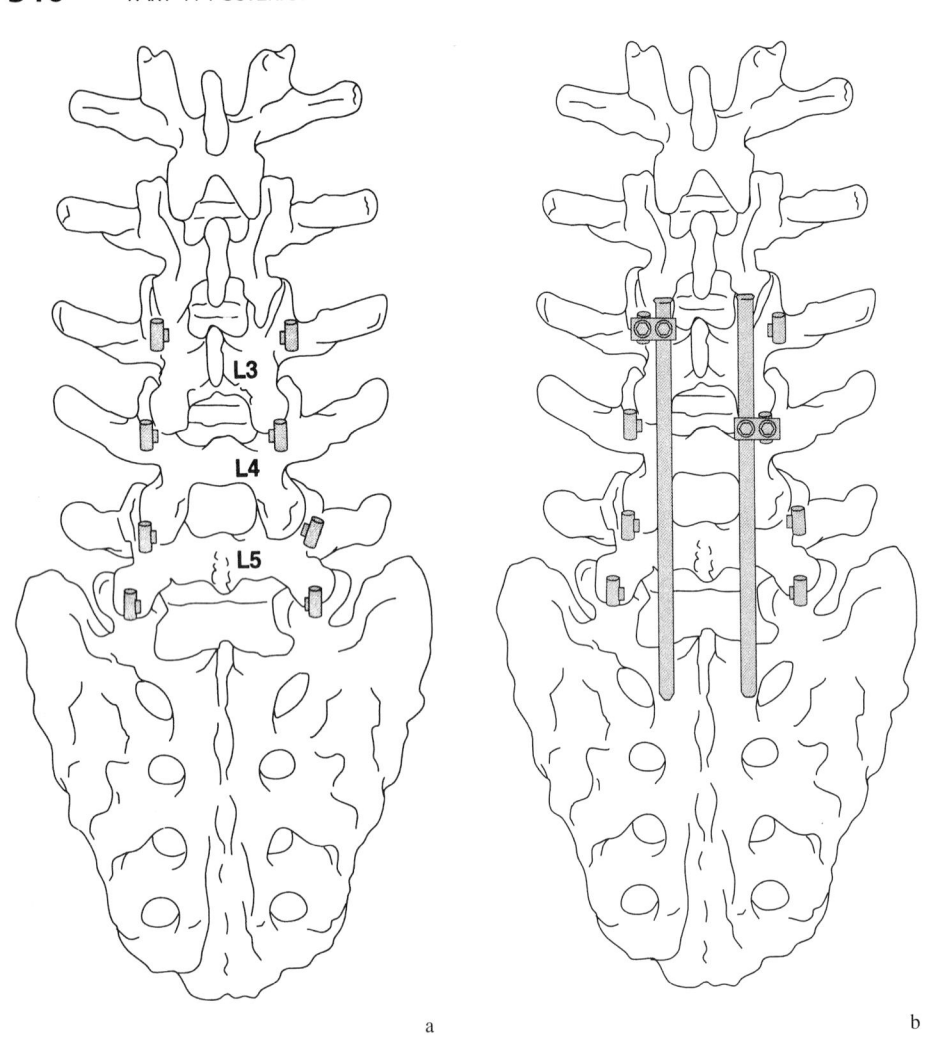

FIG. 31-9. (a) T-heads in position prior to placement of rods and crossbars. (T-heads would normally be positioned in a coupler at this point but are deleted here to better highlight positioning of pedicle screw heads.) The screw in L3 on the left is the most medial and will thus be the first point of attachment to the left rod. On the right, L4 is the most medial and should be the first rod attachment site. Always use the 10-mm cross-bar (shortest possible) to begin rod attachment to this most medial screw. Note also that the right L5 pedicle screw is malrotated and should be adjusted. (b) The rod on the left is first attached to L3 followed by attachment of the rod on the right to L4. (As described in a, the screws in L3 on the left and L4 on the right are the most medial and thus are the first attached to the rods on their respective sides.)

strings and removing them sequentially followed by placement of the screws. Not all screw threads will be engaged. This allows the T-head of the most cephalad pedicle screw to sit above the nonfused facet, thereby sparing injury to that joint. On placement of all pedicle screws and alignment of the T-head with the long axis (Fig. 31-9, a), the appropriate length rods are selected and contoured symmetrically for lordosis. Only one rod is inserted at a time. The fixation is begun with the smallest transverse cross-bar loosely premounted in a lateral direction on the rod. This cross-bar is then inserted into the coupler of the most medially based pedicle screw, regardless of its corresponding vertebral level. (All other screws are more lateral, and there is an infinite variety of cross-bar sizes to span the rest of the construct.) The rod is maintained parallel to the long axis. The set screw is placed over the lateral hole of the cross-bar within the pedicle screw coupler; the set screw is advanced only halfway. The remainder of the ipsilateral pedicle screws are attached to the rod in any sequence via couplers and variable-length transverse crossbars (Fig. 31-9, b). (All cross-bars should be oriented with the dimple or notch in the dorsal position.) The process is repeated on the contralateral side, again beginning with the most medial pedicle screw as the initial rod attachment site. We keep the system very loose or "sloppy" at this point, engaging only half of the threads of the set screws. A caliper is used to measure the distance between rods and to assist in the choice of an appropriate-length cross-bar to connect the bilateral rods (Fig. 31-10). A minimum of two transverse cross-bars are used, forming a ladder configuration. The cross-bars are placed as far apart as possible. We use and recommend a 3- to 5-mm overhang of the rod distal to the last coupler to ensure proper containment within the coupler. Set screws are tightened provisionally with a hex screwdriver with simultaneous counterclockwise stabilization of the construct via a rod holder.

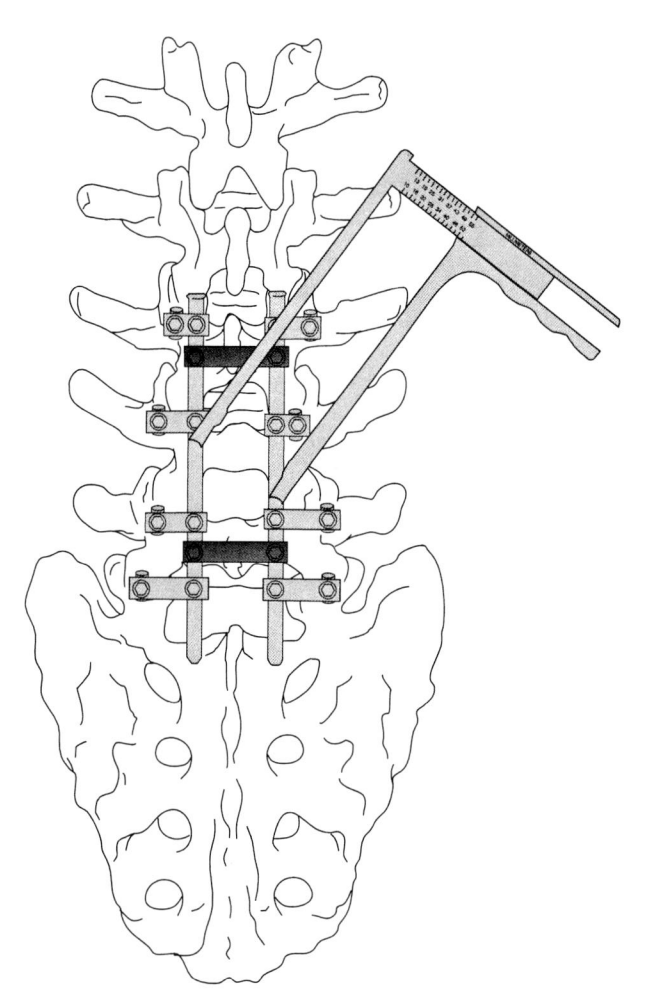

FIG. 31-10. A caliper is used to measure the distance between rods before cross-bars are added. At least two cross-bars are used in each construct to ensure maximal construct rigidity.

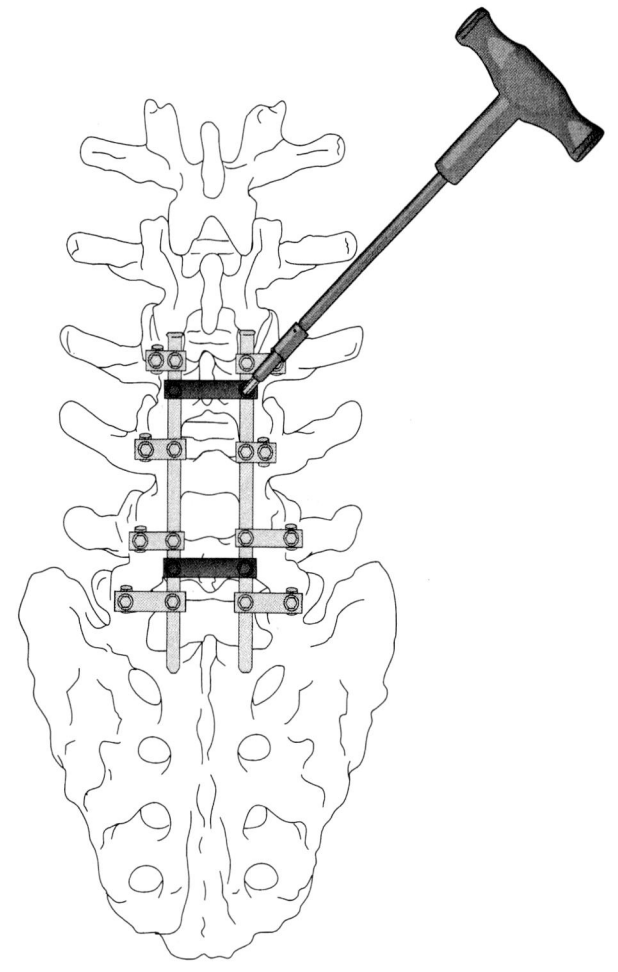

FIG. 31-11. Final tightening of the construct is performed by torquing set screws with a torque wrench preset at 50 in.-lb of torque.

It should be noted that as the construct is assembled, the surgeon has at no time had to alter pedicle screw placement to accommodate design constraints of the device.

Final tightening of set screws is performed with a torque wrench preset to apply 50 in.-lb of torque (Fig. 31-11). The remainder of the graft material is impacted into both gutters.

Any structural correction required should be effected after provisional tightening and final torquing. For example, often a disk space collapse occurs because of degeneration with secondary foraminal stenosis. We apply distraction at these collapsed levels to reconstitute foraminal height and physiologically effect a foraminotomy. By employing this method, as described by Edwards (1992), an "indirect decompression" can be effected rather than a more radical decompression.

At this juncture, 0.5 mg of preservative-free morphine is injected into the subarachnoid space for postoperative pain control. A 27-gauge needle is used and is placed at a more proximal level than that laminotomized to reduce the possibility of subsequent dural leak. A deep drain is inserted and the wound is closed in layers.

Patients are mobilized out of bed on the first postoperative day. They do not receive postoperative corsets, braces, or orthoses.

The above technique employs an all-screw pedicle attachment (Fig. 31-12). Use of the Rogozinski spinal rod system as a hybrid application of screws and hooks has been described elsewhere (Rogozinski & Rogozinski, 1992).

Results

In a review of our own clinical results with the system, we have found that in 150 cases with an average follow-up pe-

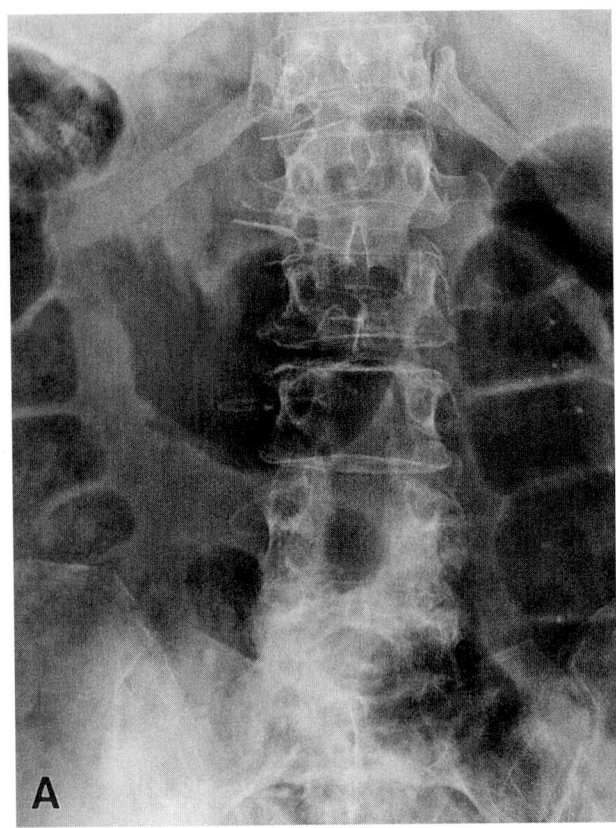

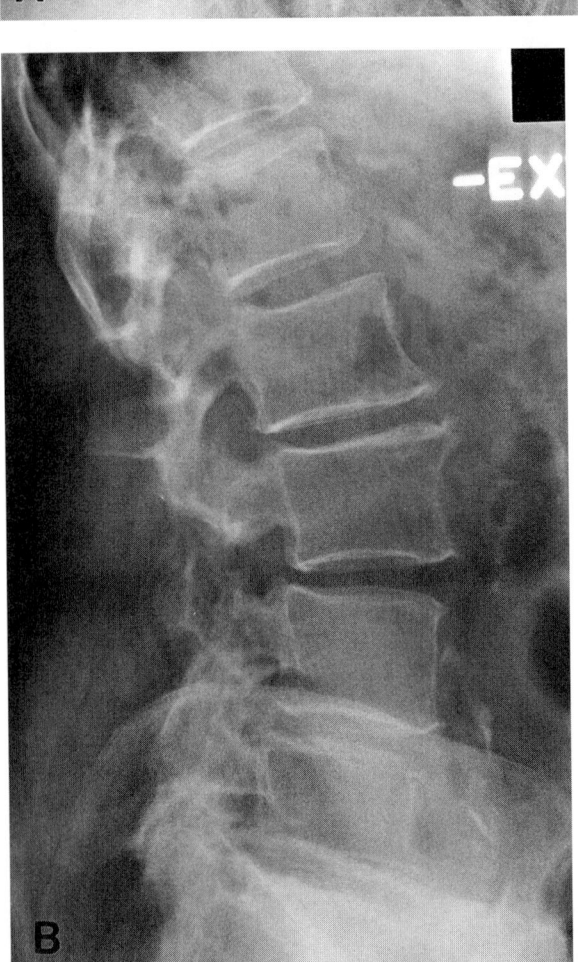

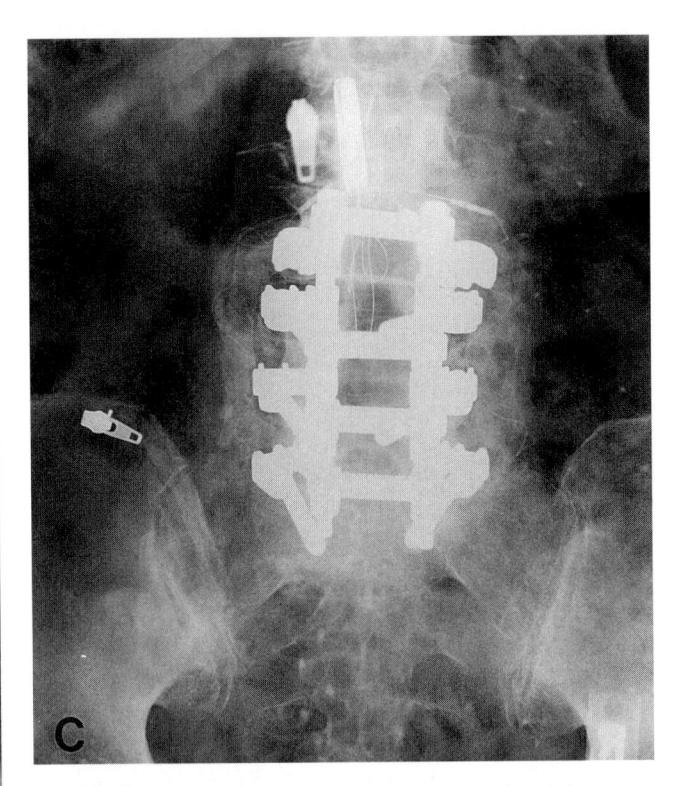

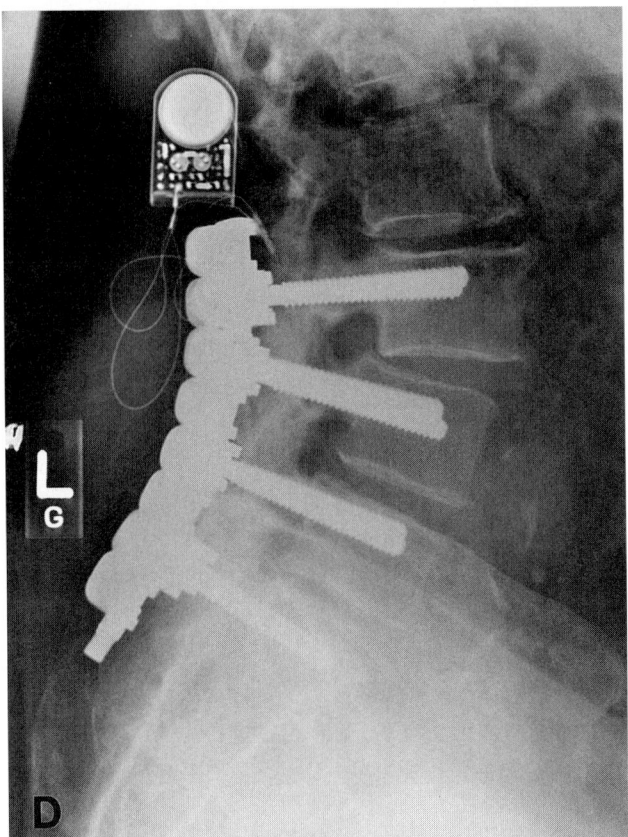

FIG. 31-12. The technique is demonstrated in the following case. A 67-year-old woman presented with progressive low back pain and persistent neurogenic claudication following two previous decompressive laminectomies of L3 to L5. (a and b) The presenting roentgenograms demonstrate the wide decompression and associated mild spondylolisthesis of L3 to L4 and L4 to L5. Iatrogenic pars defects were present on oblique films and stress views confirmed segmental instability. (c and d) Six months postoperatively, films reveal a solid-appearing posterolateral fusion with Rogozinski spinal rods in place from L3 to S1. Clinically, the patient reports complete relief of low back and leg pain with return to a normal level of activities and function.

Table 31-3
Clinical Results in 60 Cases of Lumbosacral Fusion Using Pedicle Screws

Patient profile
   Average age: 38.6 years (range, 21–59)
   Gender: 38 male, 22 female
   Average blood loss: 461 ml (range, 175–1500)
   Insurance status: 52 worker's compensation; 8 privately insured
Overall fusion rate
   54 cases solid union (90%)
   6 cases nonunion (10%)
Fusion rate by level
   One level: 29 solid union (97%); 1 nonunion
   Two levels: 23 solid union (85%); 4 nonunion
   Three levels: 1 solid union (50%); 1 nonunion
   Four levels: 1 solid union (100%)
Patient-reported pain relief at one year: 10-point scale
   (Average % improvement or decline, preoperatively and postoperatively)
   Patients with solid union: +20.4% improvement
     (range, −2 to +100)
   Patients with nonunion: +16% improvement
     (range, 0 to +50)
Rate of return to work
   Patients with solid union
     45% at full or modified activity
     38% cleared to return; looking for work
     18% disabled or not seeking work
   Patients with nonunion
     66% at full or modified activity
     0   cleared to return
     33% disabled or not seeking work

riod of 98 weeks, use of the Rogozinski system accompanied by bone graft has produced solid union as follows: 90% in constructs using pedicle screws; 84% using screw/hook combinations (so-called hybrid constructs); 94% of combined simultaneous anterior-posterior fusion; and 56% using all-hook constructs. As clinical results with the Rogozinski system were observed over time, several adjustments were made in our application of the system: we have abandoned use of all-hook constructs. We prefer pedicle screw fixation of constructs, and, when indicated, pedicle screw attachment posteriorly in combination with freeze-dried dowel grafts anteriorly.

Clinical results in 60 cases of posterolateral fusion using pedicle screws with a minimum of 52 weeks follow-up are shown in Table 31-3. Solid union, as evidenced by trabeculation of bone graft across the operative levels and absence of motion on stress films, occurred in 54 of 60 cases (90%) overall.

Complications

No deep infections have occurred in our series employing this technique. Fixation failure occurred in one early case when the rod was cut too short and slipped free of its attachment. It is recommended that rods be cut to extend 3 to 5 mm distal to the last coupler to prevent such disengagement. No other fixation failures occurred; there were no occurrences of fatigue failure, component fracture, pedicle fracture, or screw pullout. In one case, a patient suffered a neurologic sequela when a preexisting Grade 4 to 5 foot-drop was found to have dropped a grade in the course of postoperative follow-up.

USE IN THE THORACOLUMBAR SPINE

We have used the Rogozinski spinal implant for internal fixation of thoracolumbar burst fractures. The choice of treatment options in the care of thoracolumbar fractures is one of the most challenging decisions in contemporary spinal surgery. The decision process is highly complex, fraught with uncertainty, and beyond the scope of this chapter to describe in detail (Bohlman, 1985; Denis, 1983; Denis, Armstrong, Searls, et al., 1984; Esses, Botsford, & Kostuik, 1990; Gertzsbein, 1992; Gertzsbein & Court-Brown, 1989; Jacobs, Asher, & Snider, 1980; Rimoldi, Hu, Ziegler, et al., 1992; Weinstein, Collato, & Lehmann, 1988). When the surgeon has decided that the patient would benefit from operative intervention with internal fixation, this decision has been made with several stated and implied goals. The stated goals of internal fixation of the spine are to restore the premorbid anatomy to the greatest degree possible, to stabilize the spine rigidly, to prevent future deformity, and to promote early mobilization of the patient. Implied in this type of treatment is the prevention of further neurologic deterioration and, with much less certainty, a hope for the reversal of some of the neurologic loss already present.

The gold standard for the treatment of thoracolumbar burst fractures has been posterior fusion augmented with Harrington rod instrumentation applied in distraction. The best results have been achieved with the "rod long and fuse short" technique (DeKutoski et al., 1993). In this technique, the rods are placed three levels above and two levels below the fracture. The rods are then distracted in an attempt to reduce the fracture by pulling the intact posterior longitudinal ligament against the fracture fragments. A short fusion is then applied from one level above to one level below the fractured level. Posterior decompression at the fracture site is at the surgeon's discretion. At the completion of fracture and fusion healing, the rods can be removed, minimizing the loss of segmental motion as a result of fracture treatment. Numerous studies over the past two decades have been published testifying to the utility of this approach (Bryant & Sullivan, 1983; Cotler, Vernace, & Michalski, 1986; DeKutoski, Conlan, & Salciccioli, 1993; Dickson, Harrington, & Erwin, 1978; Flesch, Leider, Erickson, et al., 1977; Purcell, Markolf, & Dawson, 1981; Svensson, Aaro, & Ohlen, 1984; Willen, Lindahl, Irstam, et al., 1984).

Despite the success of Harrington rods in the treatment of thoracolumbar burst fractures, this technique has limitations (Ferguson & Allen, 1982; McAfee, Werner, & Glisson, 1985). Simple rods alone merely distract the fragments and even if contoured with Edwards sleeves, correction of kyphosis is difficult. Secondly, hook-rod systems require invasion of the spinal canal to achieve fixation on the lamina with the attendant risk to neural structures. Finally, to

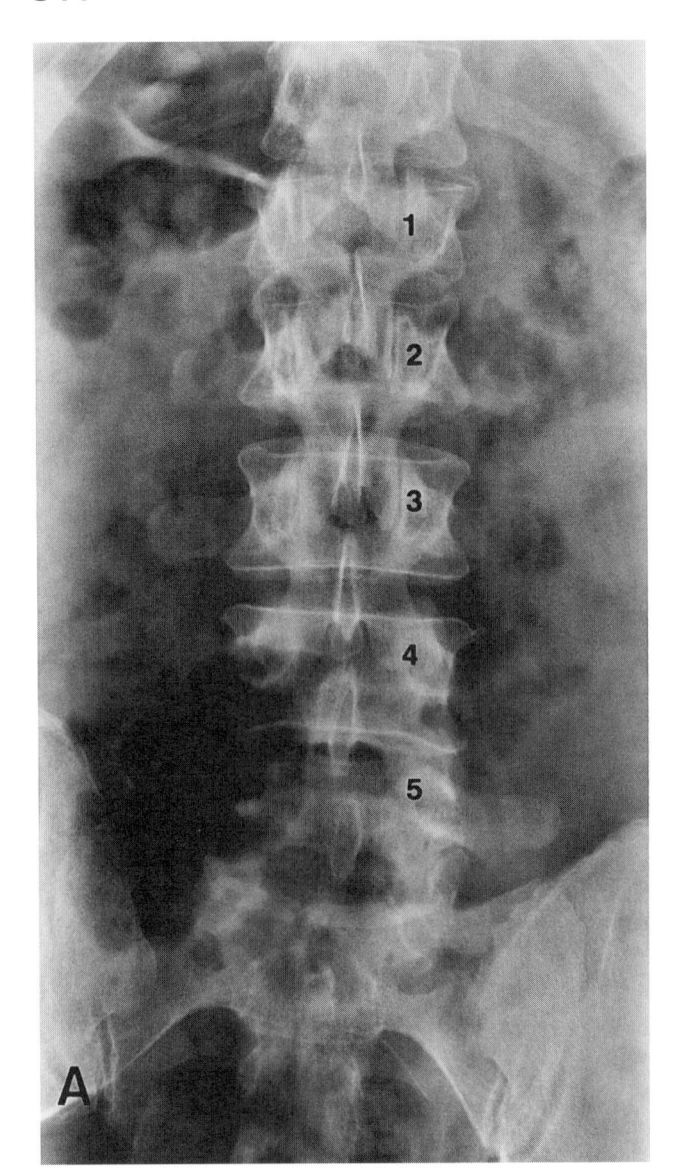

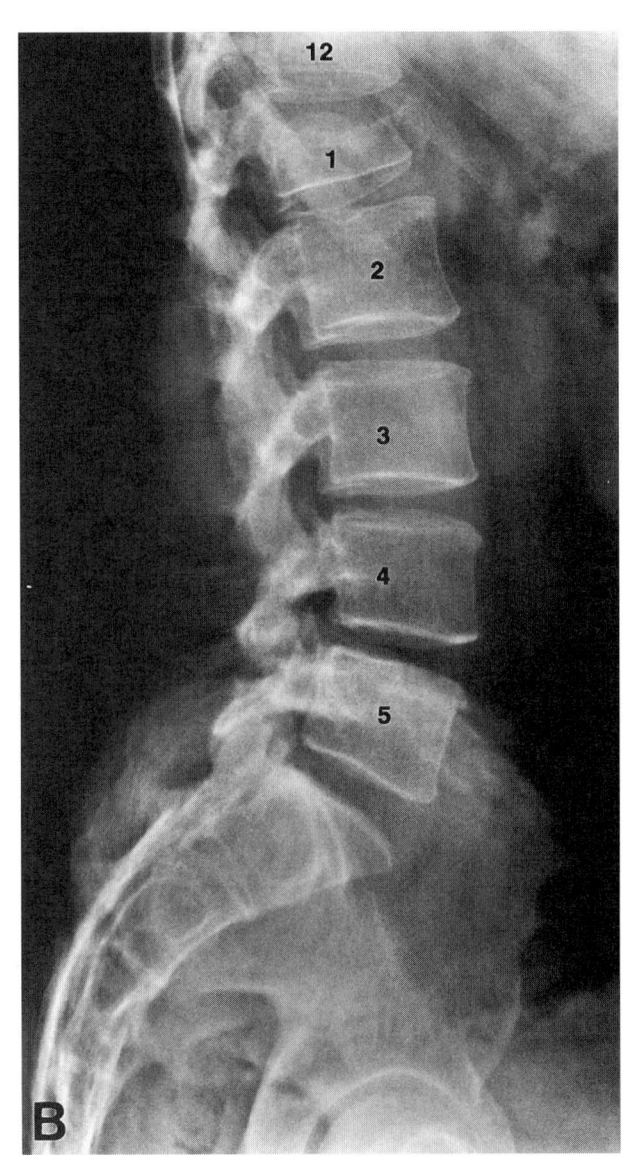

FIG. 31-13. (a and b) Anteroposterior and lateral roentgenograms of a patient with a burst fracture of L1.

achieve the desired minimal loss of segmental motion after fracture healing, an additional operation is required to remove the rods.

The advent of successful pedicle screw devices has eliminated the above limitations to the use of internal fixation in the treatment of thoracolumbar burst fractures (Dick, 1987; Dick, Kluger, Magerl, et al., 1985; Ferguson & Allen, 1982; McNamara, Stephens, & Spengler, 1992; Roy-Camille, Saillant, & Mazel, 1986; Steffee, Biscup, & Sitkowski, 1986). By securing the fixation device through the pedicle and into the vertebral body, no intrusion into the spinal canal is necessary for fixation. Furthermore, particularly with cross-linked implants such as the Rogozinski device, the rigidity is sufficient that only immobilization one level above and one level below the fracture is required. This minimizes the loss of segmental motion and eliminates the necessity for a further operation for implant removal.

Technique in Fractures in Situ

Figure 31-13 shows a burst fracture of L1 in a 5-ft 10-in., 260-lb man who presented to us in transfer from another hospital with increasing back pain after 2 weeks' treatment with bed rest. This patient had sustained his fracture by falling 15 ft from a roof. Although neurologically intact, his CT scan (McAfee, Yuan, Fredrickson, et al., 1983) demonstrated a moderate amount of spinal canal compromise and showed the lesion to be a two-column fracture (Fig. 31-14). Because this patient was quite obese and had an unstable fracture, we felt the risk for future deformity was great. Because 2 weeks had elapsed after injury, the probability of reducing the fracture was remote. We therefore elected to perform an internal fixation and fusion in situ (Fig. 31-15). The patient was asymptomatic, and the fracture healed in 3 months.

CHAPTER 31 / UTILIZATION OF THE ROGOZINSKI SPINAL ROD SYSTEM   345

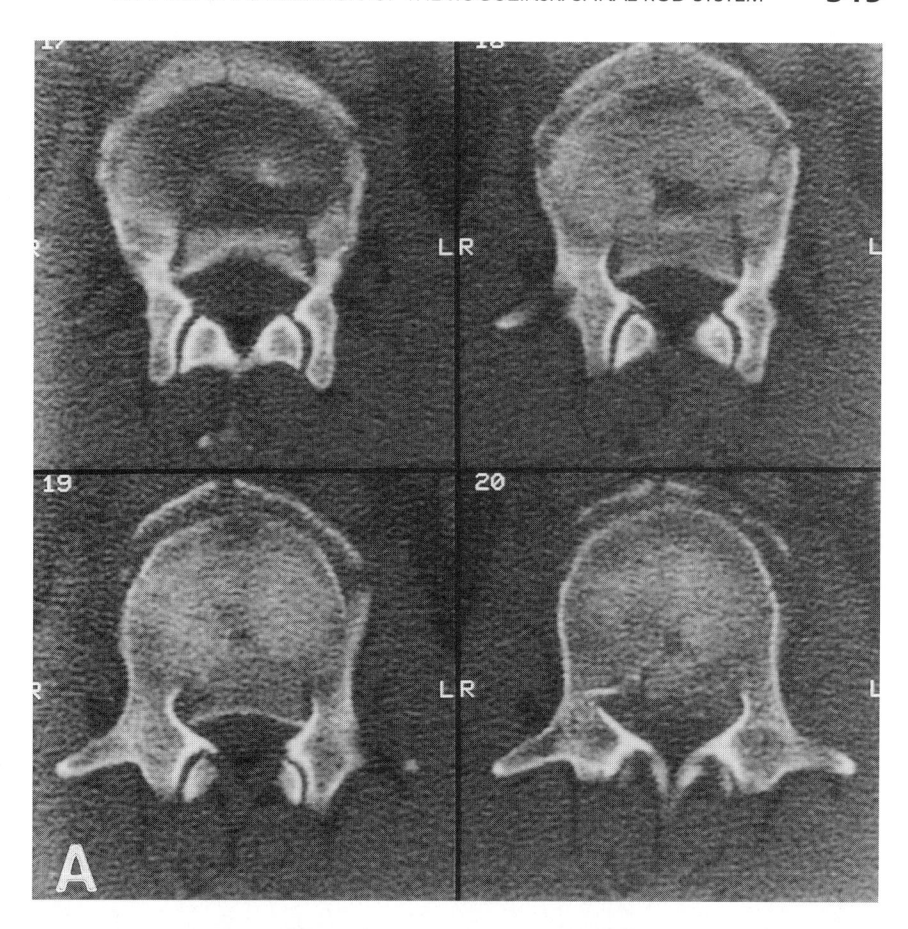

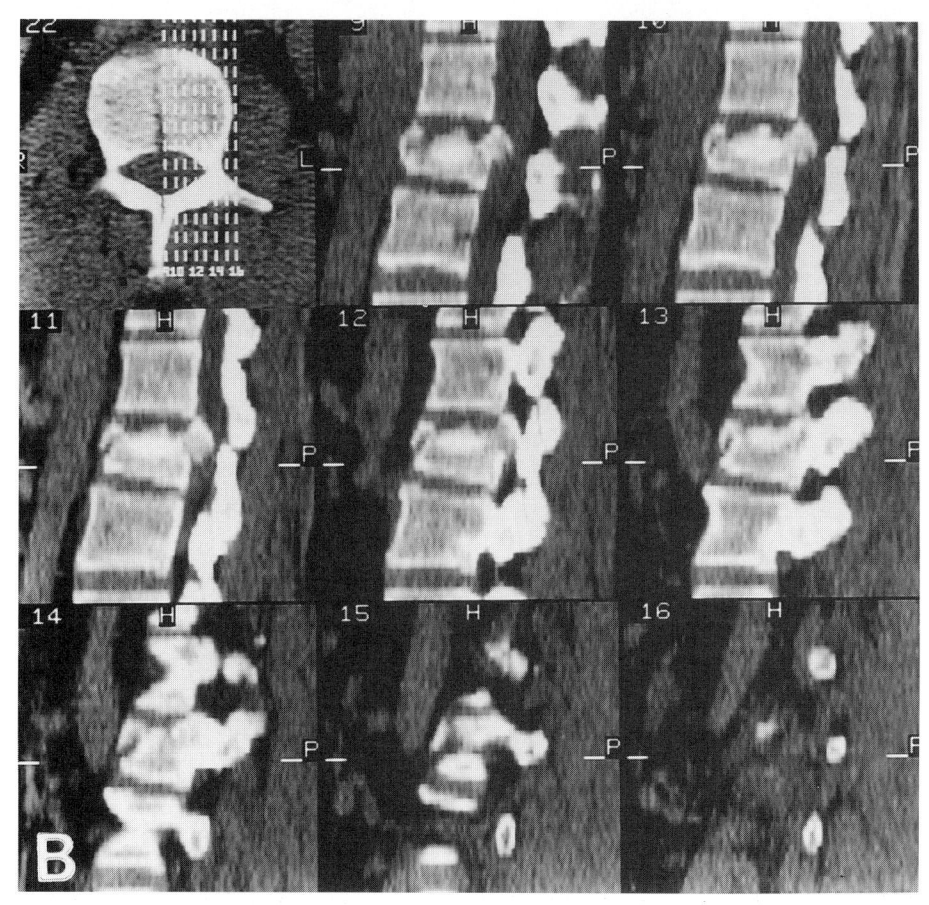

FIG. 31-14. (a and b) CT scans of the patient presented in Fig. 31-13, demonstrating a moderate amount of spinal canal compromise in the presence of a two-column fracture.

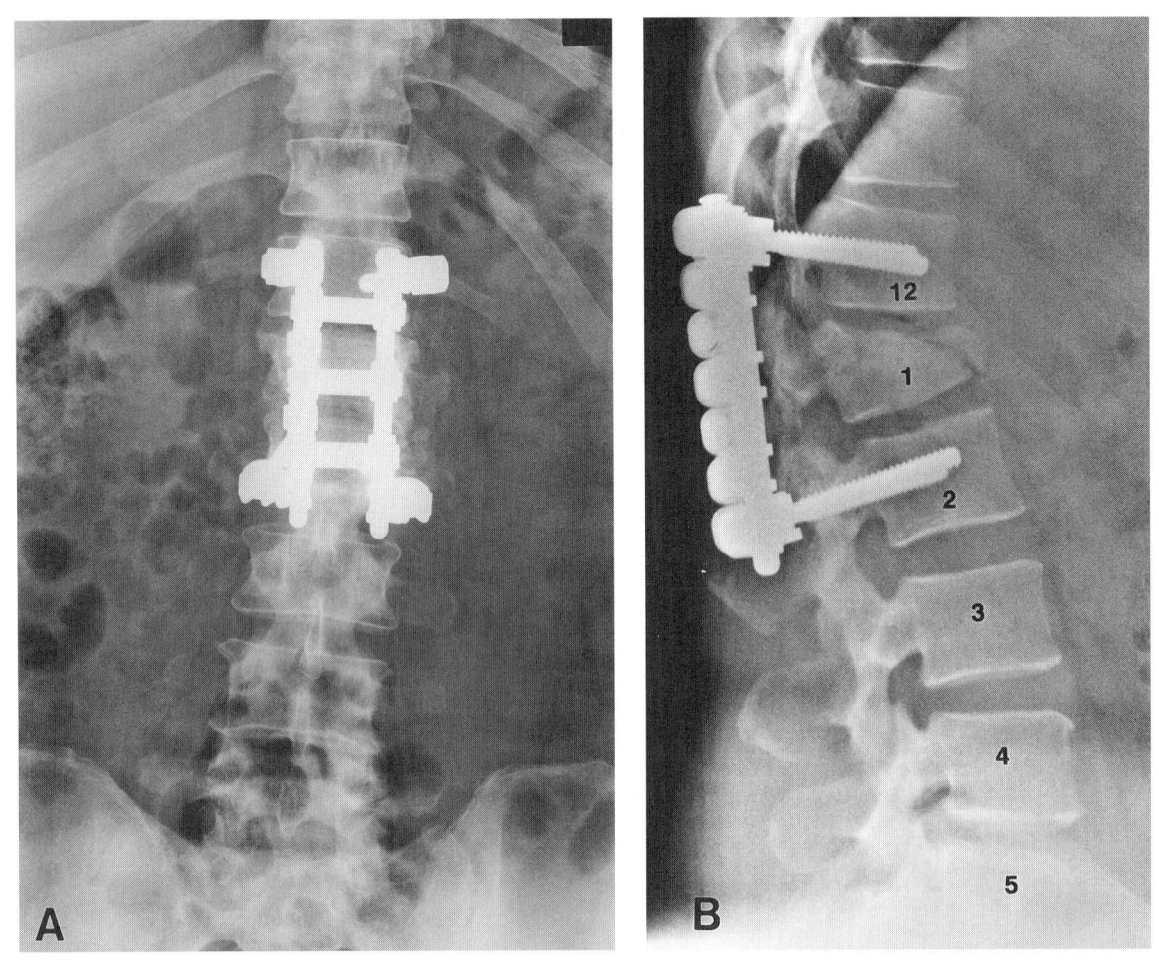

FIG. 31-15. (a and b) Anteroposterior and lateral roentgenograms of the patient presented in Figs. 31-13 and 31-14 after internal fixation and fusion in situ using the Rogozinski spinal rod system.

Figure 31-16 shows the roentgenograms of a 30-year-old woman who was involved in an automobile accident. A fracture dislocation of T12 on L1 was not recognized by her treating physicians, and she was discharged from the emergency room with low back pain and no neurologic changes. Her back pain persisted and worsened over the next 2 months, at which time she presented to us for evaluation. Her CT scan (Fig. 31-17) demonstrates the "empty facet" sign characteristic of this injury. MRI showed no evidence of significant disk disruption, but her routine roentgenograms documented continued collapse of her disk space. The decision to operate was made to alleviate the patient's pain, because significant future deformity was unlikely. At operation, reduction of the dislocation required osteotomy of the fractured facet joints bilaterally, rendering them unstable. The reduction, therefore, was followed by internal fixation and fusion from T12 to L1. The patient was asymptomatic within 6 weeks of surgery with fusion present at 3 months (Fig. 31-18).

Technique in Acute Fractures

In the presence of acute injury, within the first few days after a burst fracture, the fracture can be significantly reduced and fixated by the posterior approach using the Rogozinski spinal system. The resulting short fusion will minimally affect spinal mobility when the fracture is healed. The technique for reduction is straightforward, as shown in Fig. 31-19. After the patient has been carefully positioned on the spinal frame, a portable lateral roentgenogram of the fracture site is obtained to demonstrate any change in the fracture position and to confirm the orientation of the pedicles above and below the fracture. In this technique, it is critical to place the screws directly down the pedicle above and below the fractured vertebra. This will require placing the screws in what appears to be an inappropriate and nonanatomic orientation because of the kyphotic deformity that often occurs as a result of a two-column vertebral fracture (Fig. 31-19, *a*).

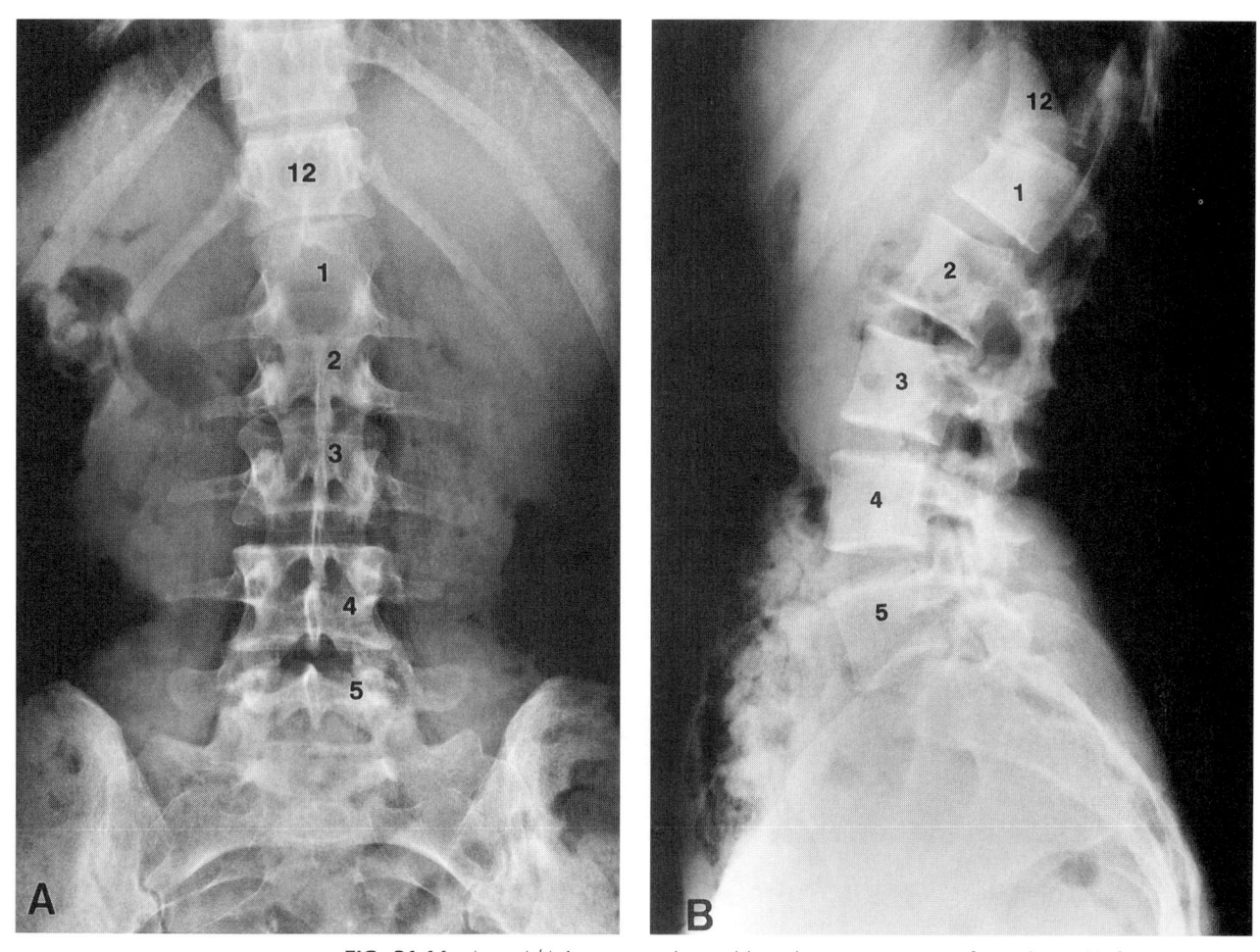

FIG. 31-16. (a and b) Anteroposterior and lateral roentgenograms of a patient with fracture dislocation of T12 on L1 after an automobile accident. The spinal lesion was not diagnosed in the emergency room and remained untreated for 2 months.

It must be noted that as one views the spine from the sacrum on up through the thoracic spine, the diameter of the pedicles decreases on average. Thus, the lower thoracic pedicles (T9–T12) average only 6.6 mm in diameter, with a standard deviation of 1.8 mm. The diameter of the standard Rogozinski screw is 6.4 mm, but there is a 5-mm-diameter version available as well, and this screw should be strongly considered in the thoracic spine. Even this smaller 5-mm screw, however, will be too large for 16% of the pedicles above T12, making CT assessment of the lower thoracic pedicles mandatory before consideration is given to the use of any pedicle system. The average pedicle size above T6 is so small (4.5 ± 1.1 mm) that one should not even consider a pedicle system (Scoles, Linton, Latimer, et al., 1988; Zindrick, Wiltsek, Doorik, et al., 1987).

Performing a laminectomy at the affected level will facilitate screw placement by allowing direct visualization of the pedicles above and below the fracture (Fig. 31-19, b).

When the screws have been placed, intraoperative roentgenograms are repeated to confirm appropriate intrapedicular placement of the screws in the perpendicular axis of the pedicle and vertebral body. After good screw placement is confirmed, the interpedicular distance is measured. A rod 30 to 40 mm longer than this distance is selected to allow for the increase in interpedicular distance that will occur with distraction and reduction of the fracture. Using small guide wires placed down the cannula in the screws above and below the fracture site, the angle of deformity is measured with a goniometer (Fig. 31-19, c). To this number in degrees is added an additional 20 degrees, 10 degrees for the 5-degree cephalad/caudad looseness in the screw-connector interface above and below the fracture, and 10 degrees for overcorrection of the kyphosis. The total number of degrees is then contoured into each of the rods.

Because of the flexibility of the linkage system, a hyperlordosed rod can easily be applied to both the screws

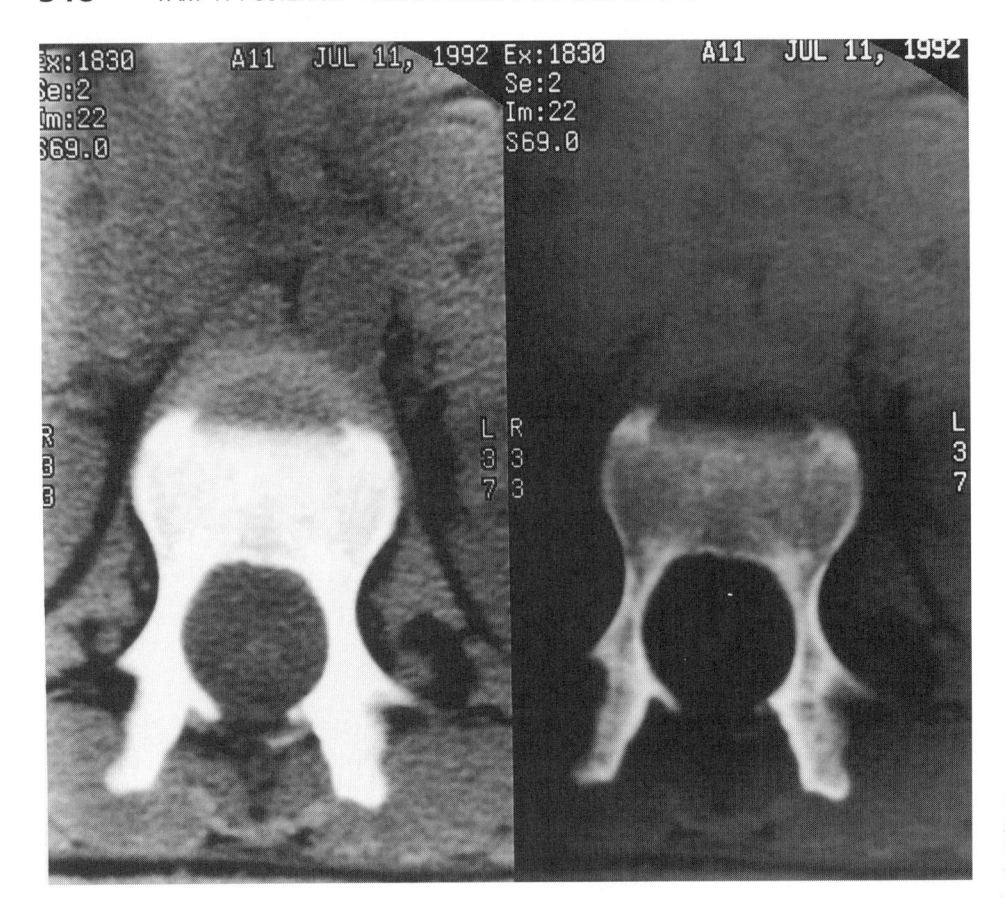

FIG. 31-17. CT scans of patient presented in Fig. 31-16, demonstrating the "empty facet" sign characteristic of fracture dislocation injury.

without a struggle (Fig. 31-19, *d*). After the rods are appropriately and loosely attached, reduction and distraction can be accomplished simultaneously. This is done by applying the rod distractor on the rod between the two couplers and distracting until resistance is met. In a large patient, if the interpedicular distance exceeds the range of the distractor, several couplers with hook-bars can be attached to the rods loosely and distraction with reduction can be accomplished in the same fashion (Fig. 31-19, *e*). The additional couplers and hook-bars are then removed. If two distractors are available at the time of reduction, bilateral distraction can be carried out simultaneously. If only one distractor is available, it is best to distract partially on only one side, temporarily lock the two set screws, distract further on the opposite side, lock and return to the first side. These procedures are alternated until full reduction is completed.

At the completion of reduction, the canal can be palpated through the laminectomy site to verify reduction. A roentgenogram is obtained to demonstrate the completeness of the reduction. When reduction is accomplished, all set screws are tightened to 50 in.-lb of torque and the system is cross-connected with two cross-bars for maximal rigidity (Fig. 31-19, *f*). If desired, bone graft can be packed down the pedicles of the fractured vertebra to help restore and maintain vertebral height. The wound is then pulse-lavaged with 3 liters of double-antibiotic wash to minimize the risk of infection and closed over medium Hemovac drains to avert hematoma formation.

The above technique is demonstrated in the following case. A 42-year-old roofer fell from a height of 17 ft, sustaining a vertical load injury to his lumbar spine. Physical examination demonstrated loss of sensation and motor function below the knees and poor rectal tone. The CT scan shown in Fig. 31-20 demonstrates a three-column fracture with approximately a 70% canal encroachment at L1. The decision to operate on this three-column fracture was made on the basis of presence of gross instability, the desire to protect the patient from further neurologic deterioration, and the anticipation of a rapid remobilization.

Intraoperative roentgenograms (Fig. 31-21) demonstrate the fracture position with Rogozinski screws in the pedicles of the vertebra below. At the completion of distraction and reduction, intraoperative roentgenograms (Fig. 31-22) show excellent apparent realignment of the vertebral fragments.

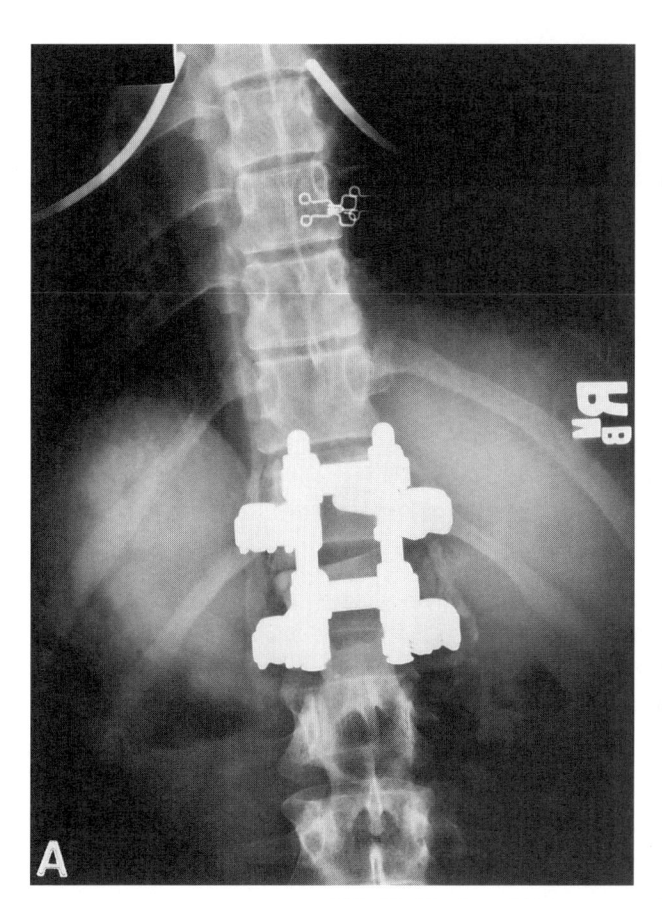

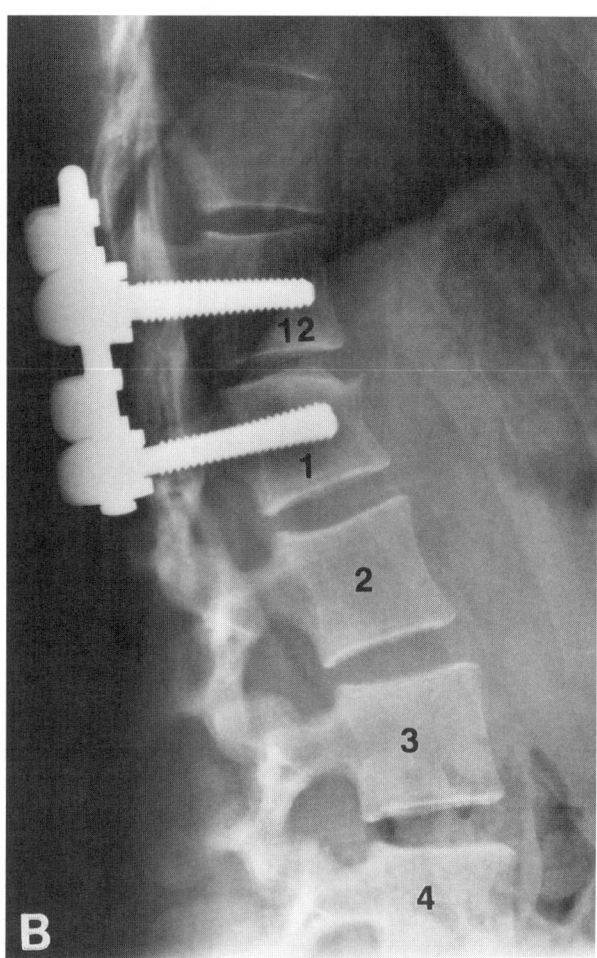

FIG. 31-18. (a and b) Anteroposterior and lateral roentgenograms of the patient presented in Figs. 31-16 and 31-17 after reduction of the dislocation and internal fixation and fusion from T12 to L1.

A CT scan several days postoperatively (Fig. 31-23) shows good restoration of canal diameter.

Postoperatively, we place our patients in a molded thoracolumbar plastic orthosis and begin rehabilitation immediately or as soon as the patient's general condition allows. The orthosis is used primarily as a load-sharing device when the implant is used over a short distance at these higher lumbar levels. Successful fusion can be anticipated in 3 to 6 months.

Conclusions

There are, of course, indications for an anterior approach or a combined anterior-posterior approach for thoracolumbar burst fractures. When the decision is made, however, for a posterior approach with internal fixation, the Rogozinski spinal implant meets the goals of rigid internal fixation and fusion in the treatment of thoracolumbar fractures. The premorbid anatomy is reestablished well and rigidly fixated while the risk of future deformity is minimized during the period of early remobilization.

DISCUSSION

As with any arthrodesis instrumentation, use of the Rogozinski spinal rod system is recommended only after hands-on training has been completed and the appropriate techniques mastered by the surgeon. Instrumentation is not a substitute for meticulous surgical technique. However, in experienced hands we feel the Rogozinski system enhances fusion results and patient outcome, reduces the circumstances that spawn complications, and offers a consistent intraoperative experience.

One of the most significant benefits of the system is the capacity for pedicle screw placement down the central axis of the pedicle. Because the system is designed always to allow the pedicle screw to be attached to the rod regardless of

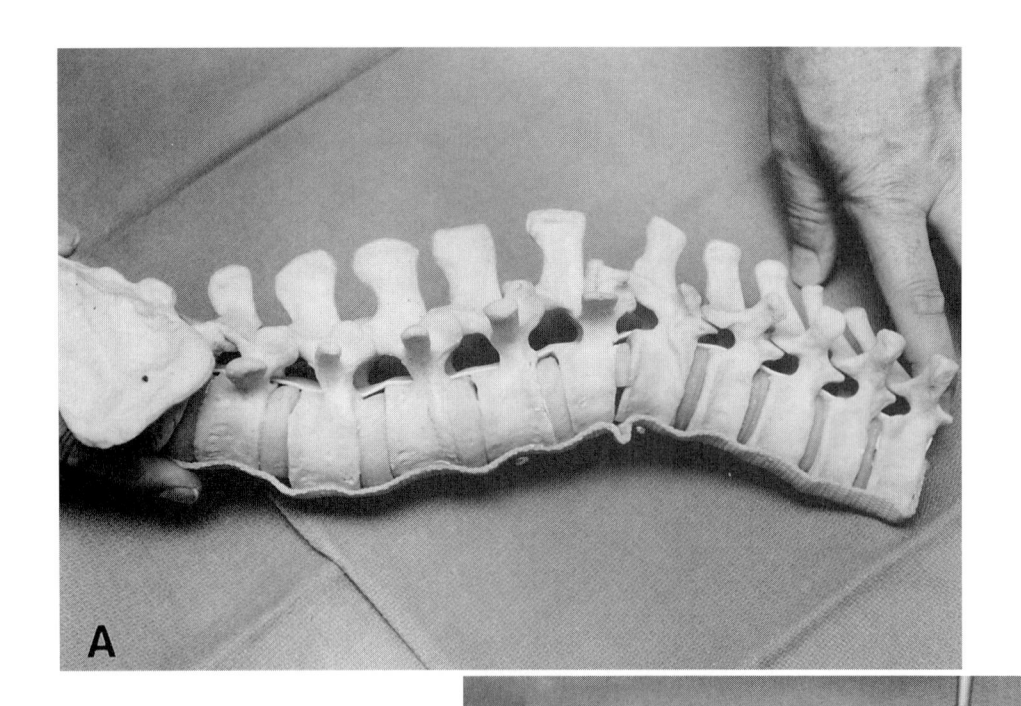

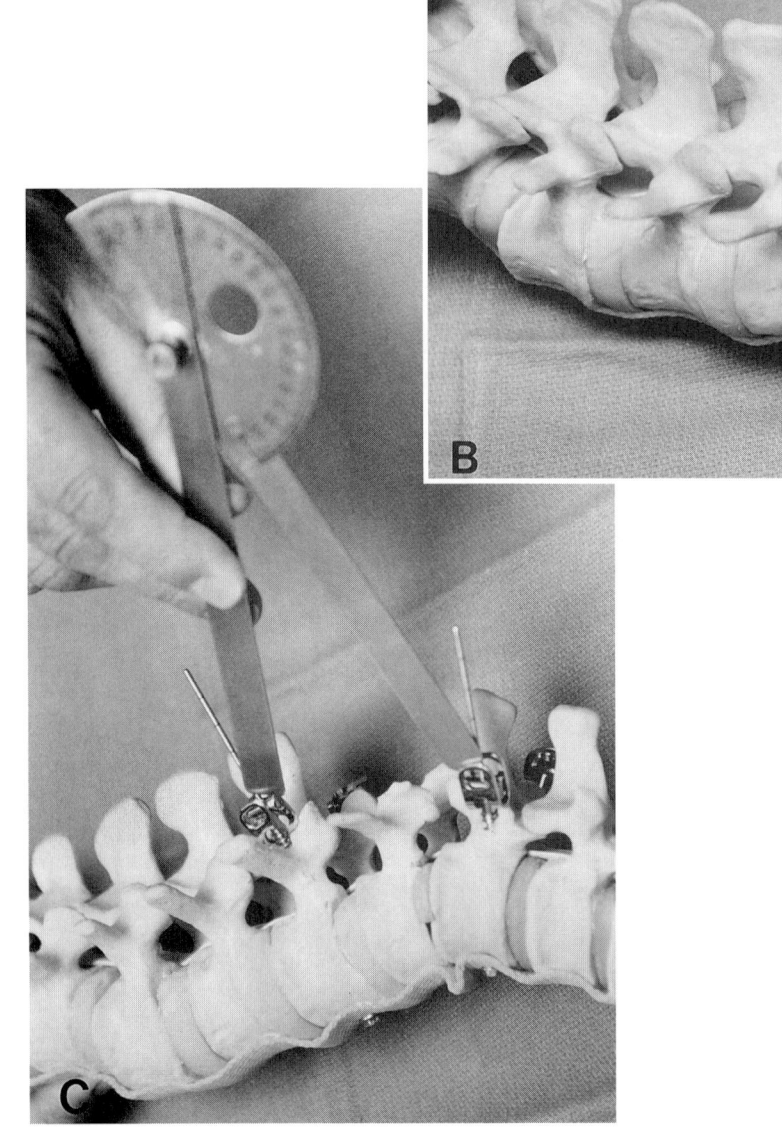

A

B

C

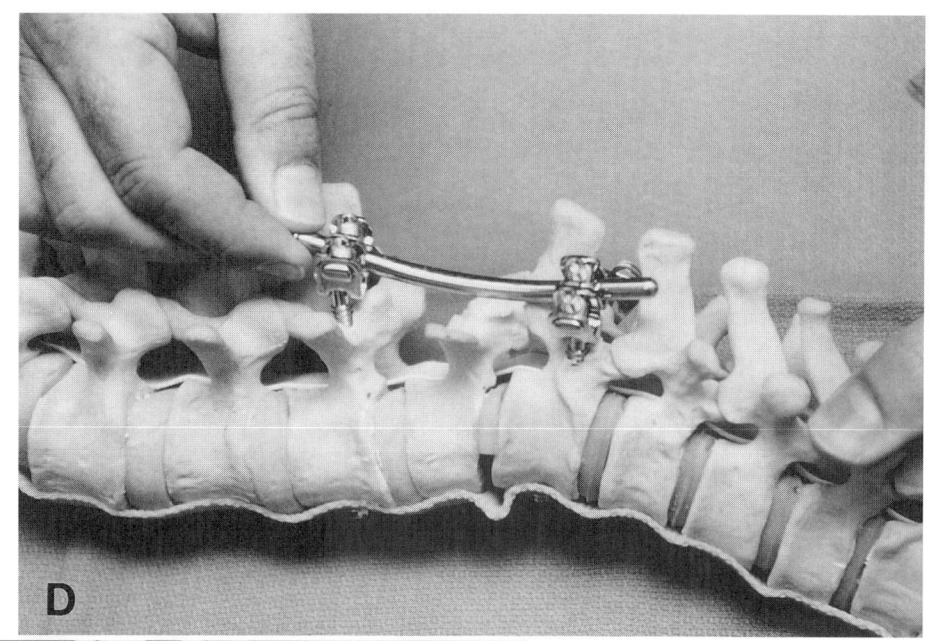

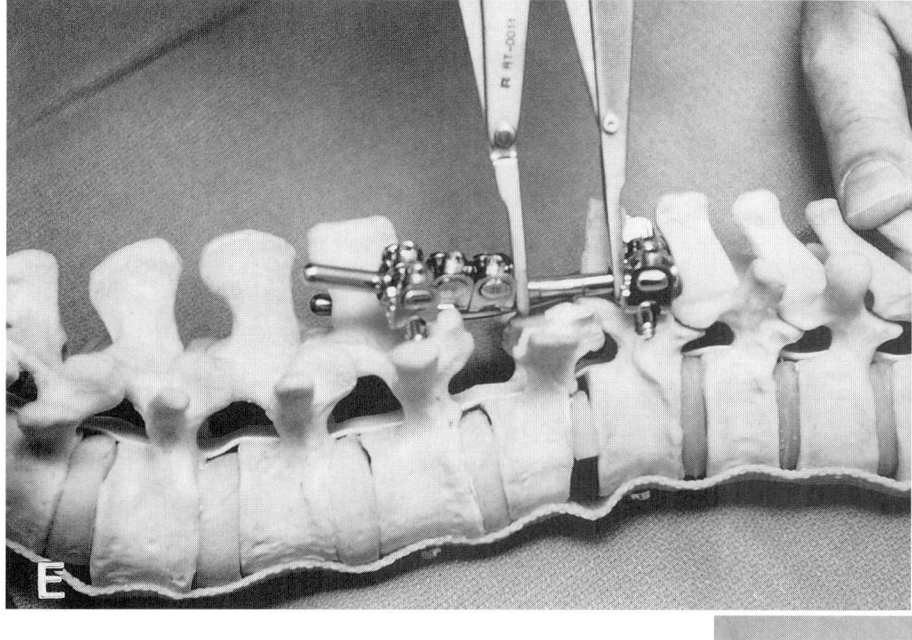

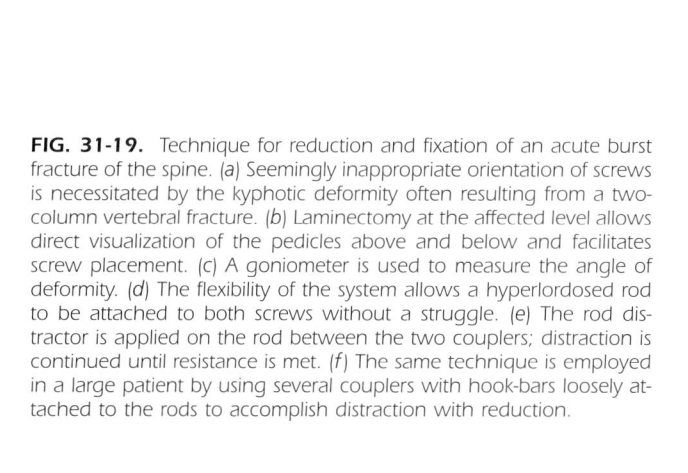

FIG. 31-19. Technique for reduction and fixation of an acute burst fracture of the spine. (a) Seemingly inappropriate orientation of screws is necessitated by the kyphotic deformity often resulting from a two-column vertebral fracture. (b) Laminectomy at the affected level allows direct visualization of the pedicles above and below and facilitates screw placement. (c) A goniometer is used to measure the angle of deformity. (d) The flexibility of the system allows a hyperlordosed rod to be attached to both screws without a struggle. (e) The rod distractor is applied on the rod between the two couplers; distraction is continued until resistance is met. (f) The same technique is employed in a large patient by using several couplers with hook-bars loosely attached to the rods to accomplish distraction with reduction.

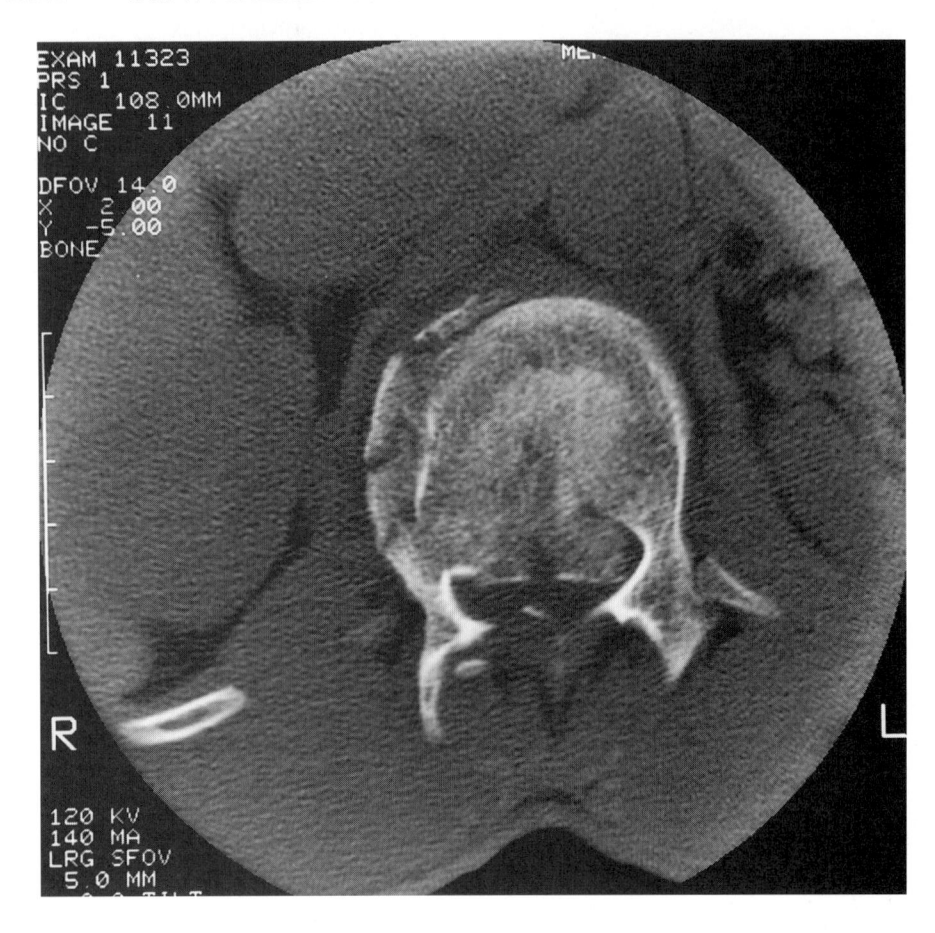

FIG. 31-20. CT scan of a patient who sustained a vertical load injury after a fall from a roof. The scan demonstrates a three-column fracture with an approximately 70% canal encroachment at L1.

its location relative to other pedicles, it avoids the scenario in which the surgeon must become a "fencepost digger" to ensure alignment of pedicle screws.

The system continues to undergo refinements as we seek wider applications and higher levels of patient acceptability and therapeutic outcomes. Currently, the system is undergoing modifications for use in pediatrics, especially pediatric scoliosis. Also, we continue to explore its use in anterior fixation applications. New materials are being tested; both metals and polymer plastics show promise of possessing strength and rigidity without the attendant radiographic limitations.

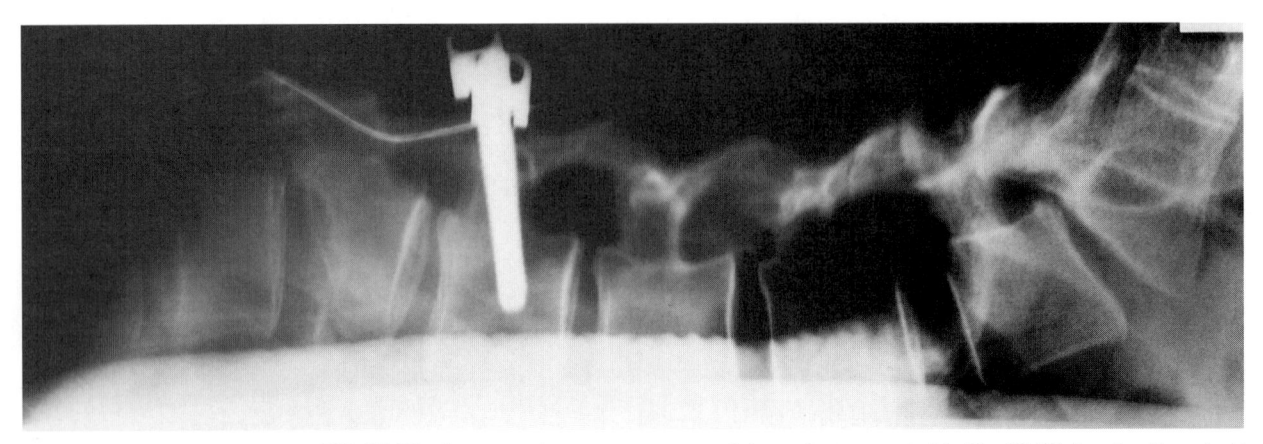

FIG. 31-21. Intraoperative roentgenogram of the patient presented in Fig. 31-20 showing Rogozinski screws in the pedicle of the vertebra below the fracture level.

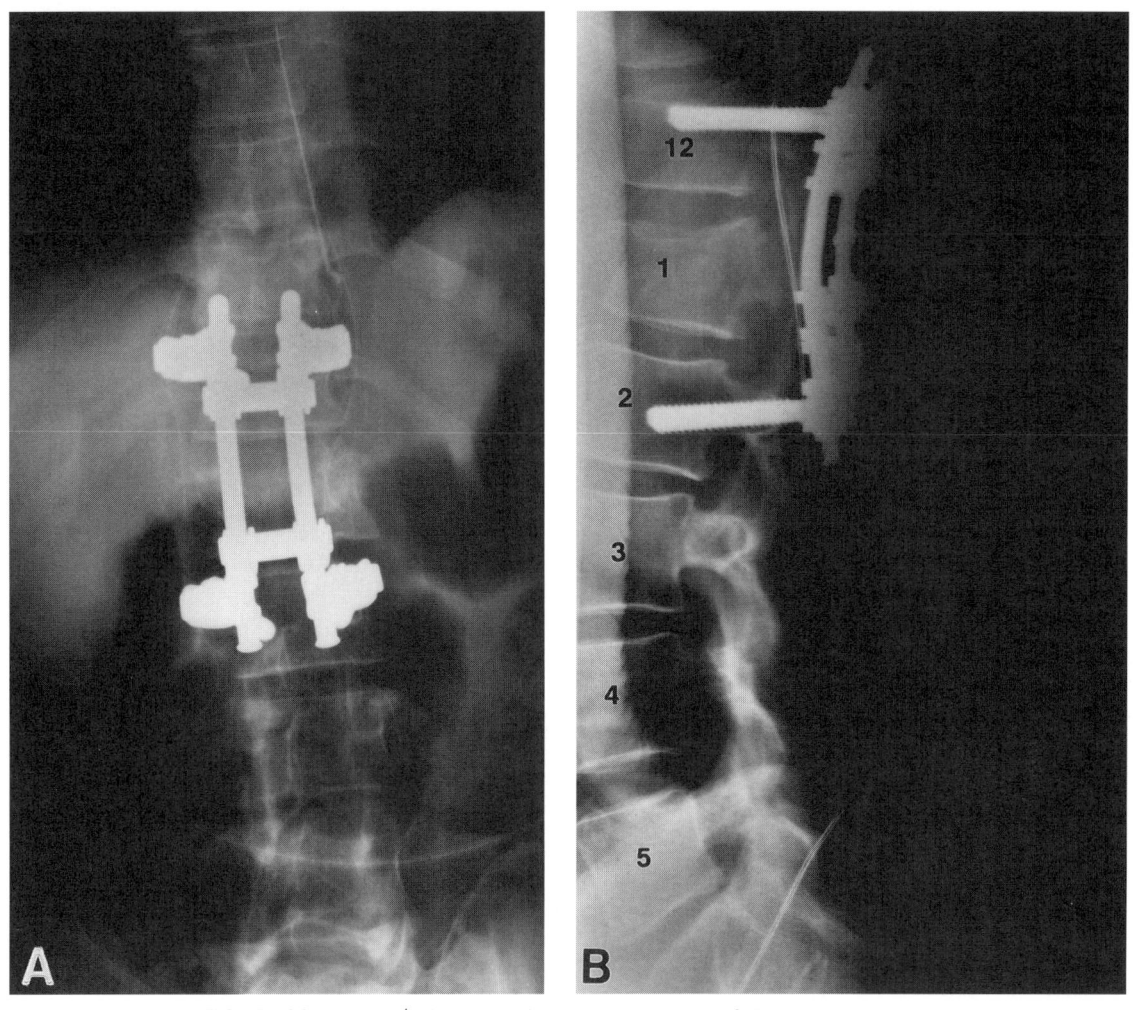

FIG. 31-22. (a and b) Intraoperative roentgenograms of the patient presented in Figs. 31-20 and 31-21 after completion of distraction and reduction of the fracture with excellent apparent realignment of the vertebral fragments.

FIG. 31-23. CT scan of the patient presented in Figs. 31-20, 31-21, and 31-22 several days postoperatively showing good restoration of canal diameter.

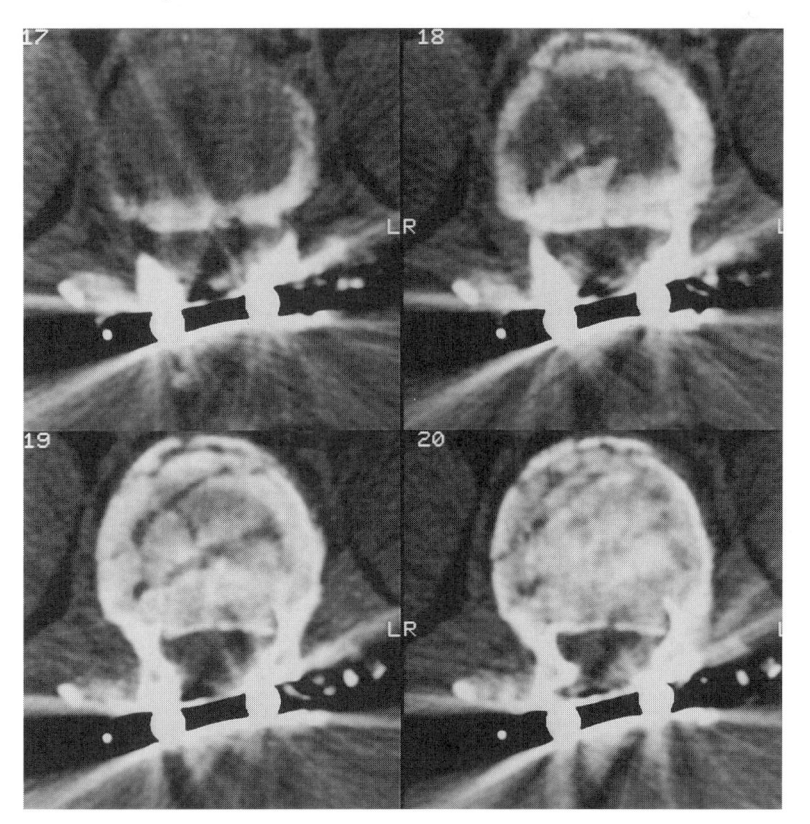

353

REFERENCES

Abumi, K. Panjabi, M.M., & Duranceau, J. (1989). Biomechanical evaluation of spinal fixation devices. Part III. Stability provided by six spinal fixation devices and interbody bone graft. *Spine, 14,* 1249.

American Academy of Orthopaedic Surgeons (1988). AAOS summer institute. San Diego, CA.

Arnold, D.M., & Wiltse, L.L. (1992). The Wiltse system of internal fixation for the lumbar spine. In: D.M. Arnold & J.E. Lonstein (Eds.), *Spine: State of the Art Reviews* (pp. 55–82). Philadelphia: Hanley & Belfus.

Bohlman, H.H. (1985). Treatment of fractures and dislocations of the thoracic and lumbar spine. *Journal of Bone and Joint Surgery, American Volume, 67,* 165.

Bryant, C.E., & Sullivan, J.A. (1983). Management of thoracic and lumbar spine fractures with Harrington distraction rods supplemented with segmental wiring. *Spine, 8,* 532.

Cotler, J.M., Vernace, J.V., & Mickalski, J.A. (1986). The use of Harrington rods in thoracolumbar fractures. *Orthopedic Clinics of North America, 17,* 87.

DeKutoski, M.B., Conlan, E.S., & Salciccioli, G.G. (1993). Spinal mobility and deformity after Harrington rod stabilization and limited arthrodesis of thoracolumbar fractures. *Journal of Bone and Joint Surgery, American Volume, 75,* 168.

Denis, F. (1983). The three column spine and its significance in the classification of acute thoracolumbar spinal injuries. *Spine, 8,* 817.

Denis, F., Armstrong, G.W., Searls, K., et al. (1984). Acute thoracolumbar burst fractures in the absence of neurologic deficit: A comparison between operative and nonoperative treatment. *Clinical Orthopaedics and Related Research, 189,* 142.

Dick, W. (1987). The "fixateur interne" as a versatile implant for spine surgery. *Spine, 12,* 882.

Dick, W., Kluger, P., Magerl, F., et al. (1985). A new device for internal fixation of thoracolumbar and lumbar spine fractures: The "Fixateur Interne." *Paraplegia, 23,* 225.

Dickman, C.A., Fessler, R.G., MacMillan, M., et al. (1992). Transpedicular screw-rod fixation of the lumbar spine: operative technique and outcome in 104 cases. *Journal of Neurosurgery, 77,* 860.

Dickson, J.H., Harrington, P.R., & Erwin, W.D. (1978). Results of reduction and stabilization of the severely fractured thoracic and lumbar spine. *Journal of Bone and Joint Surgery, American Volume, 60,* 799.

Edwards, C.C. (1992). The Edwards modular system for three-dimensional control of the lumbar spine. In: D.M. Arnold & J.E. Lonstein (Eds.), *Spine: State of the Art Reviews* (p. 239). Philadelphia: Hanley & Belfus.

Esses, S.I., Botsford, D.J., & Kostuik, J.P. (1990). Evaluation of surgical treatment for burst fractures. *Spine, 15,* 667.

Ferguson, R.I., & Allen, B.L., Jr. (1982). The evolution of segmental spinal instrumentation in the treatment of unstable thoracolumbar spine fractures. *Orthopedic Transactions, 6,* 346.

Flesch, J.R., Leider, L.L., Erickson, D.L., et al. (1977). Harrington instrumentation and spine fusion for unstable fractures and fracture-dislocations of the thoracic and lumbar spine. *Journal of Bone and Joint Surgery, American Volume, 59,* 143.

George, D.C., Krag, M.H., Johnson, C.C., et al. (1991). Hole preparation techniques for transpedicle screws: Effect on pull-out strength from human cadaveric vertebrae. *Spine, 16,* 181.

Gertzsbein, S.D. (1992). Classification of thoracic and lumbar fractures. In: S.D. Gertzsbein (Ed.), *Fractures of the Thoracic and Lumbar Spine* (pp. 25–57). Baltimore: Williams & Wilkins.

Gertzsbein, S.D., & Court-Brown, C.M. (1989). Rationale for the management of flexion-distraction injuries of the thoracolumbar spine based on a new classification. *Journal of Spinal Disorders, 2,* 176.

Jacobs, R.R., Asher, M.A., & Snider, R.K. (1980). Thoracolumbar spine injuries: a comparative study of recumbent and operative treatment in 100 patients. *Spine, 5,* 463.

Johnston, C.E., II, Ashman, R.B., Baird, A.M., et al. (1990). Effect of spinal construct stiffness on early fusion incorporation: experimental study. *Spine, 13,* 908.

Johnston, C.E., Welch, R.D., Baker, K.J., et al. (September 1992). Effect of spinal construct stiffness on short segment fusion mass incorporation. Proceedings of the Scoliosis Research Society Meeting, Kansas City, MO.

Kornblatt, M.D., Casey, M.P., & Jacobs, R.R. (1986). Internal fixation in lumbosacral spine fusion: A biomechanical and clinical study. *Clinical Orthopaedics and Related Research, 203,* 141.

Krag, M.H., Beynnon, B.D., Pope, M.H., et al. (1986). Internal fixator for posterior application to short segments of the thoracic, lumbar, or lumbosacral spine. *Clinical Orthopaedics and Related Research, 203,* 75.

Krag, M.H., Weaver, D.L., Beynnon, B.D., et al. (1988). Morphometry of the thoracic and lumbar spine related to transpedicular screw placement for surgical spinal fixation. *Spine, 13,* 27.

McAfee, P.C., Farey, I.D., Sutterlin, C.E., et al. (1989). Device-related osteoporosis with spinal instrumentation. *Spine, 14,* 909.

McAfee, P.C., Werner, F.W., & Glisson, R.R. (1985). A biomechanical analysis of spinal instrumentation systems in thoracolumbar fractures: Comparison of traditional Harrington distraction instrumentation with segmental spinal instrumentation. *Spine, 10,* 204.

McAfee, P.C., Yuan, H.A., Fredrickson, B.E., et al. (1983). The value of computed tomography in thoracolumbar fractures: An analysis of one hundred consecutive cases and a new classification. *Journal of Bone and Joint Surgery, American Volume, 65,* 461.

McNamara, M.J., Stephens, G.C., & Spengler, D.M. (1992). Transpedicular short-segment fusions for the treatment of lumbar burst fractures. *Journal of Spinal Disorders, 5,* 183.

Ogilvie, J.W., & Schendel, M. (1986). Comparison of lumbosacral fixation devices. *Clinical Orthopaedics and Related Research, 203,* 120.

Pool, H.A., & Gaines, R.W. (1992). Biomechanics of transpedicular screw spinal implant systems. In: D.M. Arnold & J.E. Lonstein (Eds.), *Spine: State of the Art Reviews* (pp. 27–44). Philadelphia: Hanley & Belfus.

Purcell, G.A., Markolf, K.L., & Dawson, E.G. (1981). Twelfth thoracic-first lumbar vertebral mechanical stability of fractures after Harrington-rod instrumentation. *Journal of Bone and Joint Surgery, American Volume, 63,* 71.

Rimoldi, R.L., Hu, S.S., Ziegler, J.E., et al. (1992). The effect of surgical intervention on rehabilitation time in patients with thoracolumbar and lumber spinal cord injuries. Presented at the American Academy of Orthopaedic Surgery meeting, Washington, DC.

Rogozinski, C., & Rogozinski, A. (1992). The Rogozinski spinal rod system: A new internal fixation of the spine. In: D.M. Arnold & J.E. Lonstein (Eds.), *Spine: State of the Art Reviews* (p.107). Philadelphia: Hanley & Belfus.

Roy-Camille, R., Saillant, G., & Mazel, C. (1986). Internal fixation of the lumbar spine with pedicle screw plating. *Clinical Orthopaedics and Related Research, 203,* 7.

Rulan, C.M., McAfee, P.C., Warden, K.E., et al. (1991). Triangulation of pedicular instrumentation: A biomechanical analysis. *Spine, 16* (6 Suppl), 5270.

Scoles, P.V., Linton, A.E., Latimer, B., et al. (1988). Vertebral body and posterior element morphology: The normal spine in middle life. *Spine, 13,* 1082.

Smith, K.R., Hunt, T.R., Asher, M.A., et al. (1991). The effect of a stiff spinal implant on the bone-mineral content of the lumbar spine in dogs. *Journal of Bone and Joint Surgery, American Volume, 73,* 115.

Steffee, A.D., Biscup, R.S., & Sitkowski, D.J. (1986). Segmental spine plates with pedicle screw fixation: A new internal fixation device for disorders of the lumbar and thoracolumbar spine. *Clinical Orthopaedics and Related Research, 203,* 45.

Svensson, O., Aaro, S., & Ohlen, G. (1984). Harrington instrumentation for thoracic and lumbar vertebral fractures. *Acta Orthopaedica Scandinavica, 55,* 38.

Weinstein, J.N., Collato, P., & Lehmann, T.R. (1988). Thoracolumbar "burst" fractures treated conservatively: A long-term follow-up. *Spine, 13,* 33.

Willen, J., Lindahl, S., Irstam, L., et al. (1984). Unstable thoracolumbar fractures: A study by CT and conventional roentgenology of the reduction effect of Harrington instrumentation. *Spine, 9,* 214.

Zindrick, M.R., Wiltse, L.L., Widell, E.H., et al. (1986). A biomechanical study of intrapeduncular screw fixation in the lumbosacral spine. *Clinical Orthopaedics and Related Research, 203,* 99.

Zindrick, M.R., Wiltse, L.I, Doorik, P., et al. (1987). Analysis of the morphometric characteristics of the thoracic and lumbar pedicles. *Spine, 12,* 160.

CHAPTER 32

The AMS Reduction Fixation System

Mark N. Hadley
Benjamin H. Fulmer

HIGHLIGHTS

A variety of instrumentation systems have been developed and employed in the treatment of thoracolumbar and lumbosacral spinal instability (Aebi, Etter, Kehl, & Thalgott, 1987; Bryant & Sullivan, 1983; Chang, 1990; Chang & McAfee, 1989; Dick, Kluger, Magerl, Woesdorfer, & Zach, 1985; Jacobs, Nordwall, Nachemson, & Perren, 1984; Krag, 1991; Roy-Camille, Saillant, & Mazel, 1986). The reduction fixation (RF) system manufactured by AMS Incorporated of Hayward, California, is one such system. Relying on U-shaped cancellous bone screws and threaded 8-mm-diameter longitudinal rods, the RF system provides the advantage that it is both a reduction device and an internal fixation device (Chang, 1990; Chang & McAfee, 1989; Fredrickson, Edwards, Rauschning, Bayley, & Yuan, 1992). Using bone screws of four different angles—0, 5, 10, and 15 degrees—between the U-shaped screw head and the shank of the screw, secured to the threaded rod with paired washers, the RF system provides symmetric lordotic distraction to reduce fracture deformity and restore anatomic height and alignment (Fig. 32-1). It provides rigid internal fixation as an adjunct to spinal fusion in patients with two- to three-level vertebral instability/deformity from T10 through the sacrum.

DESCRIPTION OF THE RF SYSTEM COMPONENTS

The RF system has six basic components, which are used to create the specific internal fixation construct required to provide distraction, reduction, and compression as needed to create translational stability and rigid fixation.

RF Screws

The RF screws are offered in three designs (angled, threaded transpedicular, and self-locking) to accommodate the anatomical and biomechanical requirements routinely encountered in the reduction and fixation of traumatic or degenerative spinal abnormalities from T10 through S1.

The angled pedicle screws are designed to permit controlled application of corrective forces to produce kyphosis, lordosis, distraction and compression. The screws are offered in four angles—0, 5, 10, and 15 degrees (Fig. 32-2). This measurement is the degree of angle between the U-shaped screw head and the shank of the screw. Each angled screw is offered in five diameters, from 5.75 to 7 mm, and four lengths, ranging from 35 to 50 mm. Versatility in screw diameter, length, and angle provide for the variances in sizes required to meet a broad patient population. The U-shaped head of the screw, with a flat and concave side, prevents unwanted rotation of the screw within the pedicle, yet provides for the application of corrective forces to control the vertebrae in all planes.

The RF transpedicular bone screw is offered in three lengths, ranging from 40 to 50 mm, and provided in 6.25- and 6.50-mm diameters (Fig. 32-3). An integrated hexagonal nut is located at the proximal end of the cancellous threaded section of the screw, which is used to insert the self-tapping screw into the vertebral pedicle.

The RF 6-mm self-locking screws are offered in five lengths, ranging from 25 to 45 mm (see Fig. 32-3). Self-locking screws are designed with two sets of threads. The distal cancellous threads provide secure fixation in the pedicle and the vertebral body, while the proximal threads lock

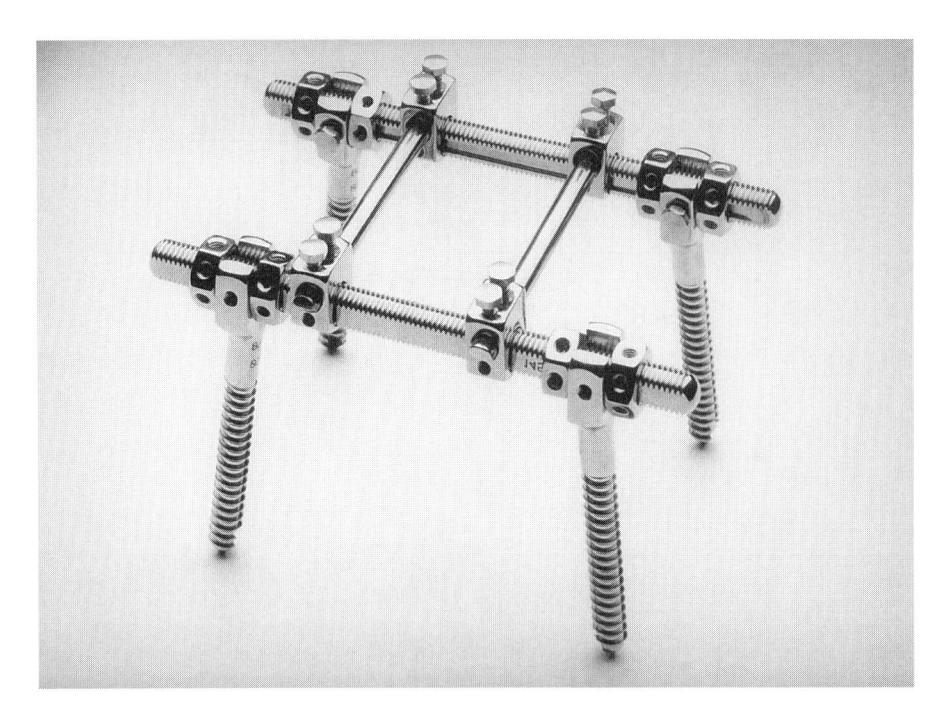

FIG. 32-1. The AMS reduction fixation system with transverse fixation assembly.

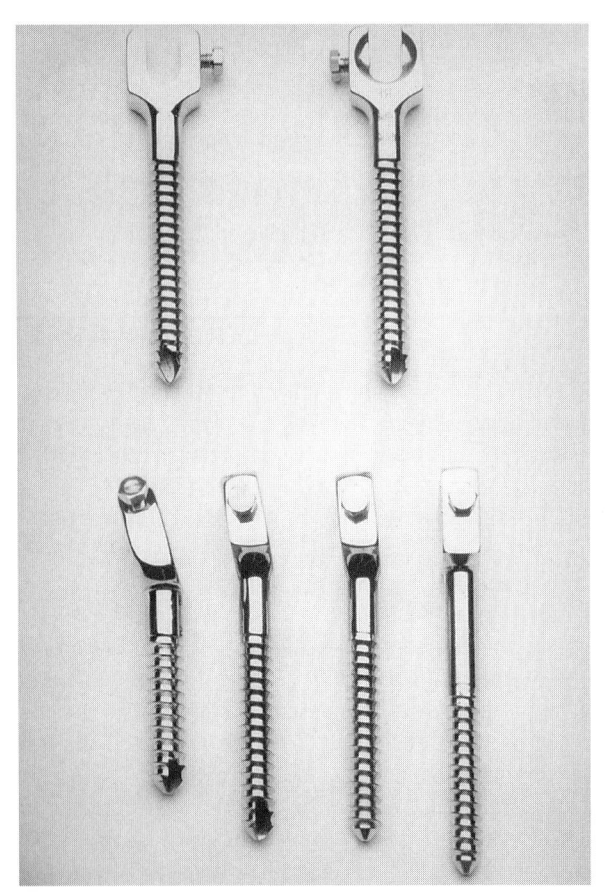

FIG. 32-2. RF self-tapping bone screws with U-shaped heads. Note variable angles and lengths.

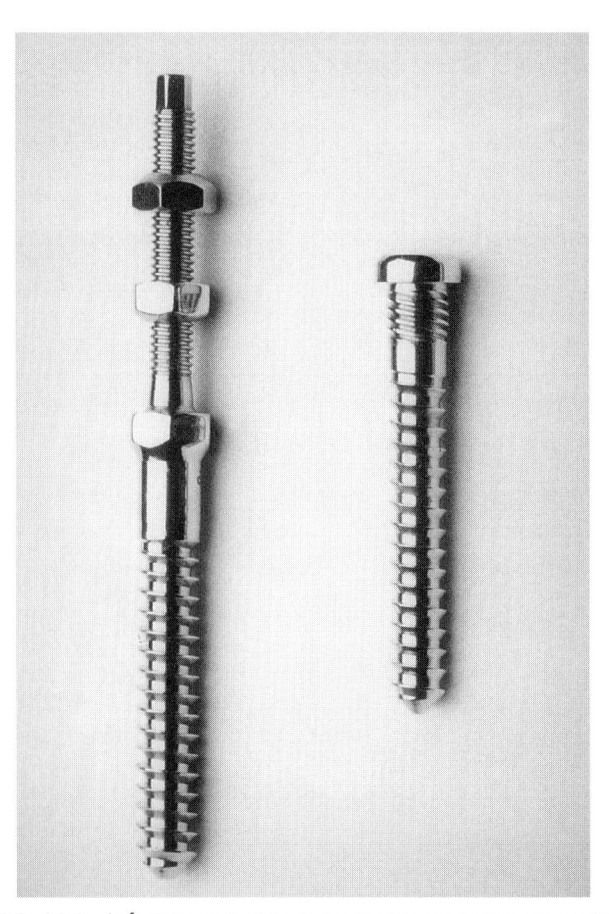

FIG. 32-3. *Left,* Transpedicular screws are used to reduce and stabilize in the anteroposterior plane, thereby avoiding the need to contour the rods. *Right,* Self-locking screws are used primarily to provide additional fixation in the sacrum.

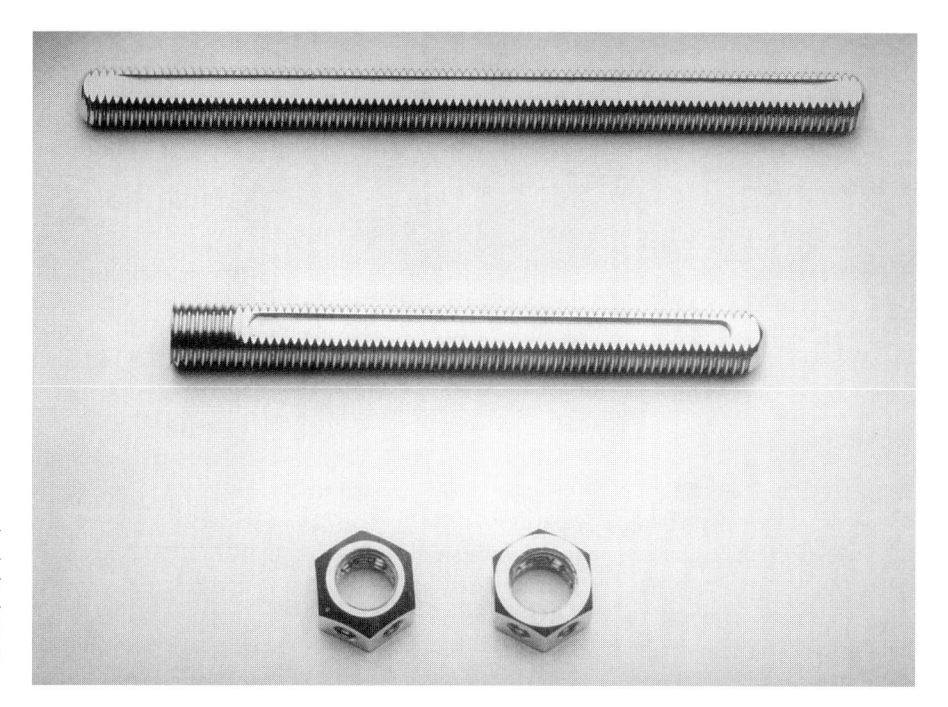

FIG. 32-4. Threaded rods allow for the application of controlled compression or distraction. Traction nuts allow for the controlled movement of the angled screws and blocks along the rod and firm attachment of the screws to the rod.

the screw into the sacral block at the desired angle. The application of the self-locking screw/sacral block component provides the option of double sacral fixation when L5-S1 deformities are being treated.

RF Threaded Rods

The RF threaded longitudinal rods are 8 mm in diameter and are offered in 10 lengths, ranging from 35 to 150 mm (Fig. 32-4). One side of the rod is flat; the other side of the rod is slotted to accommodate a set screw. When applied to the U-shaped screw heads, the rods prevent the screws from rotating within the pedicles and the U-shaped head of the screws prevent the rod from rotating about the screws. The fully threaded rod permits controlled movement in both directions for segmental compression, distraction or neutralization. Though not required in the majority of cases, the rods can be contoured in axial and sagittal planes up to 26 degrees without destruction of the threads.

Two RF traction nuts are used to secure the U-shaped head screws to the threaded rods. A convex-sided traction nut is threaded onto the rod to engage the concave side of the U-shaped head screw. The flat-sided traction nut is threaded onto the rod to abut the flat side of the U-shaped head screw. Each traction nut is designed to accept 3-mm set screws, which prevent loosening of the traction nuts along the rod.

RF Spondylolisthesis Reduction Block

The RF spondylolisthesis block is used in conjunction with the threaded transpedicular screw to reduce gradually kyphosis, lateral spondylolisthesis, or retrospondylolisthesis. The spondylolisthesis block is designed to slide onto the threaded rod and be secured in place by a set screw (Fig. 32-5).

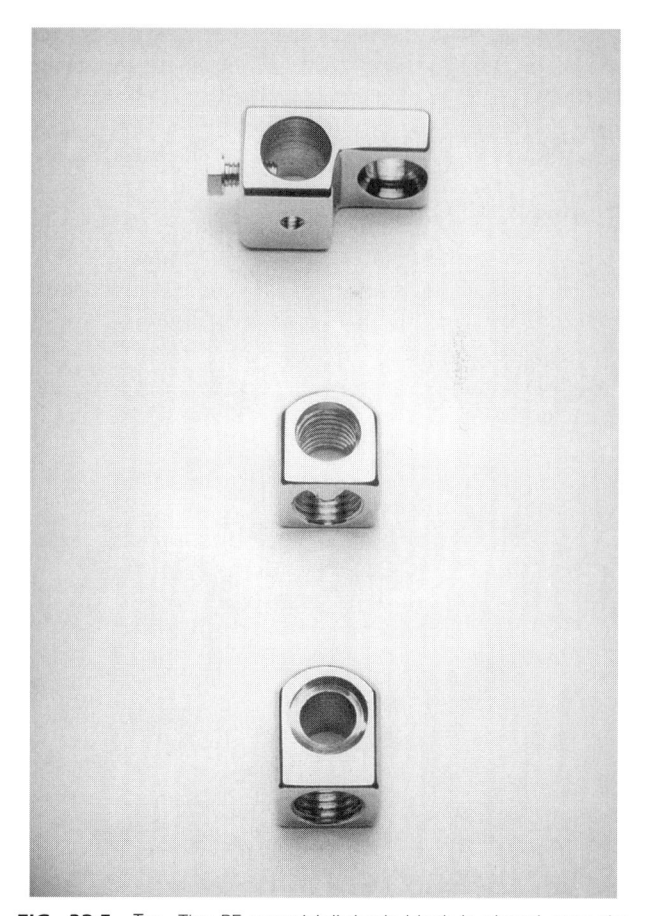

FIG. 32-5. *Top,* The RF spondylolisthesis block is placed onto the threaded rod and can be positioned to accept a screw placement that is more lateral or medial than superior or inferior screws. *Middle,* The sacral block allows for the application of double sacral fixation, when additional points of fixation are desired. *Bottom,* The pullback block can be used when a single-level reduction of Grade 1 or Grade 2 spondylolisthesis is to be completed. The use of the pullback block allows for application of the construct even at the lowest lumbar level.

This block allows for the secure connection of the threaded transpedicular screw to the rod when lateral or medial insertion of the screw within the pedicle is required, due to anatomic anomalies.

RF Sacral Block

The RF sacral block is used when double sacral fixation is desired (see Fig. 32-5). The block is threaded onto the end of the rod to abut the flat side to the 15-degree screw used in the S1 pedicle. It can be rotated to the desired angle to provide medial or lateral placement of the self-locking screw.

RF Pullback Block

The RF pullback block is used for short segment reduction and stabilization when one disk space is being bridged (see Fig. 32-5). Used in conjunction with the threaded transpedicular screw, the pullback block is threaded onto the end of the appropriate length rod (35, 40, or 50 mm). The pullback block is then placed over the threaded transpedicular screw and secured in place by tightening the hexagonal nuts on the threaded transpedicular screw. The rod is inserted into the U-shaped screw at the lower level and secured by use of the traction nuts. The use of this construct configuration provides the capability to stabilize and reduce a Grade I or II spondylolisthesis, yet minimize the number of levels included in the fusion.

RF Transverse Fixation Assembly

The RF transverse fixation assembly is applied to the threaded rods to add strength to the total construct and to resist translational forces (Fig. 32-6). Two transverse fixation assemblies are recommended for use in fracture-deformities above the L3 level. One assembly is recommended for use in nonfracture cases that span three levels above S1. They serve to improve the reduction of coronal plane deformity and to enhance construct stability.

INDICATIONS

The RF system can be employed in the treatment of unstable thoracic or lumbar spine fractures from the T10 through L5 vertebral levels. The RF system is indicated for the treatment of degenerative instability of the distal thoracic and lumbosacral spinal segments and as an adjunct to fusion in the treatment of unstable spondylolisthesis of the lumbosacral spine (Chang, 1990; Chang & McAfee, 1989, Fredrickson et al., 1992). The RF system is a bone screw–rod construct only, not an integrated system to be used in conjunction with laminar, transverse process or pedicle hook (claw) constructs. It provides excellent rigid control over two- to three-level spinal segment instability and is the only internal fixation system that provides lordotic distraction to reduce deformities and restore anatomic alignment (Chang, 1990; Chang & McAfee, 1989, Fredrickson et al., 1992) (Figs. 32-7 to 32-13) (Table 32-1).

TECHNIQUES

Preoperatively the segments to be included in the stabilization and fusion procedure (with or without decompression) are determined and mapped out on preoperative radiographs.

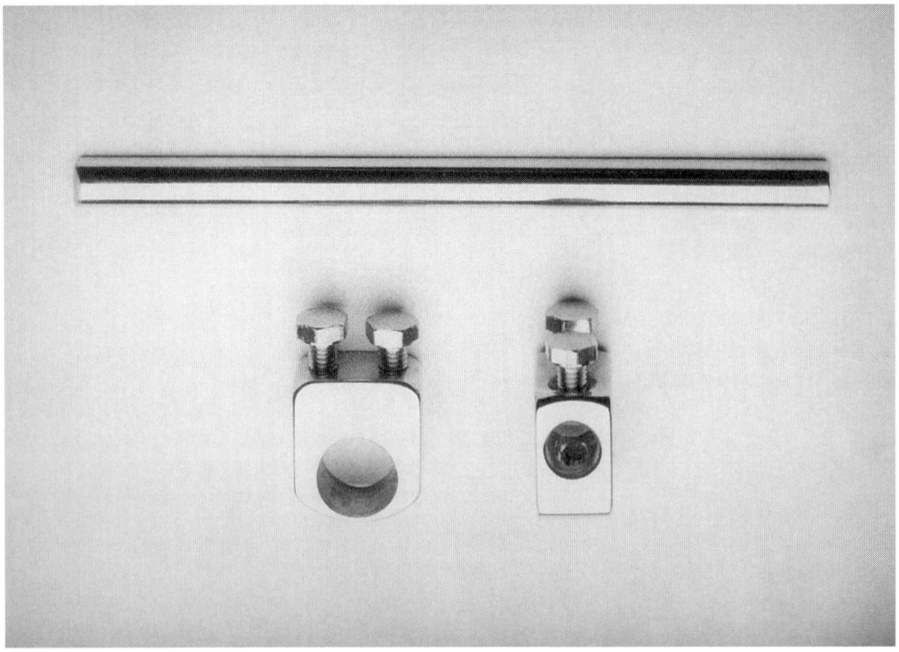

FIG. 32-6. The transverse fixation assembly is routinely used in the treatment of unstable burst fractures or when three levels are to be fused.

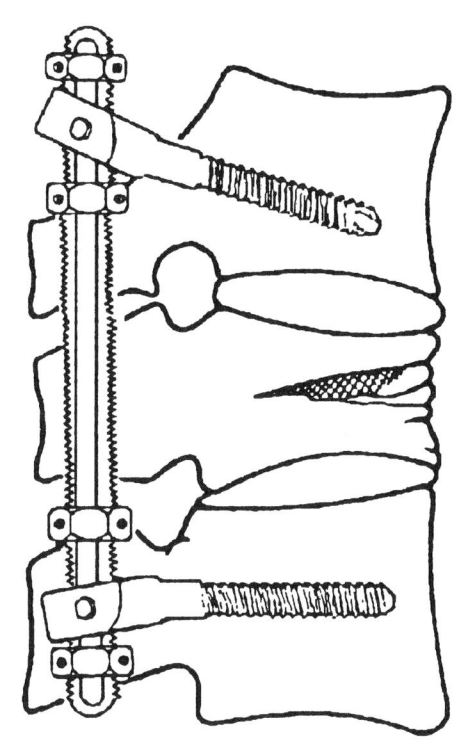

FIG. 32-7. Initial location of RF screws within the pedicle canal prior to tightening of the traction nuts.

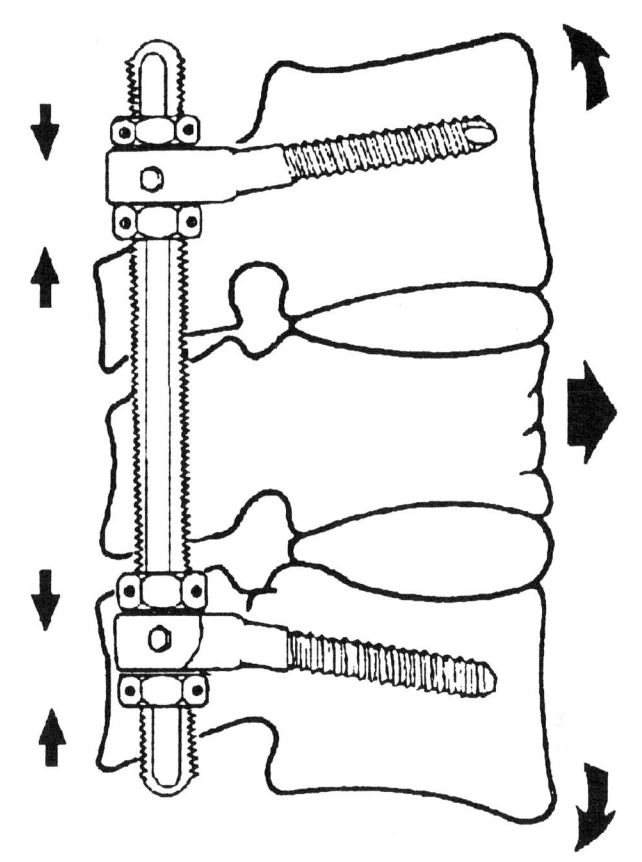

FIG. 32-8. Tightening of the traction nuts against the angled heads of the screws places the vertebral body in the desired lordosis.

The degree of "ideal" lordosis or premorbid lordosis is determined (sometimes only estimated) from the lateral spine radiograph using the modified segmental Cobb angle technique (Batzdorf & Batzdorff, 1988; Chang, 1990; Chang & McAfee, 1989). The normal thoracic kyphosis is measured and used as a reference. The "ideal" (reconstructed) lordosis is created equal to, or slightly larger than, this measurement. In general, for T12 and L1 vertebral bodies, RF screws with 0 degrees of angulation are used to create a straight thoracolumbar junction. For vertebral bodies below L1 (L2 to L5), screws with 5 or 10 degrees of angulation are used to create lumbar lordosis, gradually increasing the degree of angulation at each level caudally. RF screws with 15 degrees of angulation are used for sacral fixation.

Preoperative computed tomographic (CT) studies allow determination of pedicle diameter, inclination angle and an estimation of the depth of the pedicle-vertebral body complex for screw length determination (Krag, Weaver, Beynnon, & Haugh, 1988). Congenital anomalies, fracture deformities, and so forth are noted on these studies and are incorporated into the treatment schemes.

Through a standard dorsal midline approach the desired vertebral segments are exposed. The subperiosteal dissection is carried out laterally, bilaterally to expose the transverse processes and rib heads (thoracic vertebrae), transverse processes (lumbar vertebrae) and/or proximal sacrum (lateral to the S1 facet complex), as indicated. Great care should be exercised to avoid dissection of facet complexes that are not to be included in the stabilization and fusion procedure. Ligamentous attachments in and around such a facet capsule must be preserved to avoid delayed instability at an "untreated" level (typically proximal but occasionally distal) adjacent to the levels to be fused.

Decompression of the thecal sac and exiting nerve roots is next accomplished if indicated, being careful to decom-

Table 32-1
Indications and Contraindications for Use of RF System

Indications
  Two- to three-level segmental instability, T10 through S1
  Thoracolumbar fracture instability, T10 through L5
  Degenerative lumbosacral instability, L2 through S1 (including postoperative)
  Instability associated with spondylolisthesis
  Dorsal internal fixation/stabilization as an adjunct to ventral-lateral cord canal decompression-vertebrectomy, T10 through L5, (trauma, neoplasm, infection)
Contraindications
  Application in the absence of spinal instability
  Pediatric patient; immature, underdeveloped spine
  Use above T10 level
  Application without bone fusion substrate
  Application in patients with "soft bone" diseases/disorders
    Metabolic bone disorders
    Longstanding renal dialysis
    Advanced osteoporosis
    Widespread spinal metastatic neoplastic disease
    Advanced rheumatoid arthritis

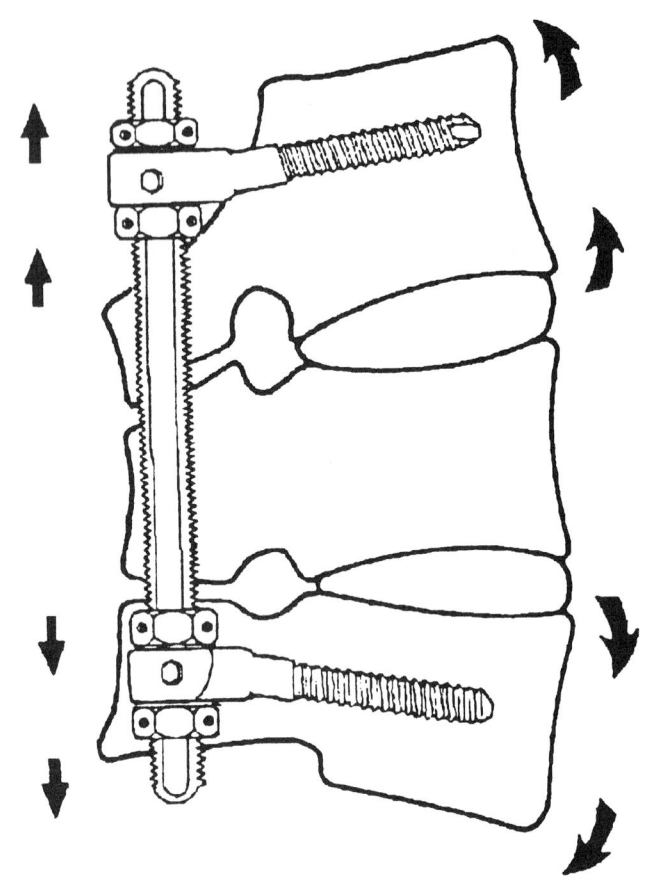

FIG. 32-9. Compression or distraction of the vertebral bodies is achieved by moving the traction nuts toward or away from the end of the rod.

decorticate the dorsal and dorsolateral surfaces of the vertebrae to be instrumented and fused, including the transverse processes (plus rib heads at T10, T11, and T12). Threaded rods of appropriate length are then loaded with two RF traction nuts for each screw, one convex, one flat-sided in appropriate orientation for the orientation of the screw they will span. The threaded rods are then placed into the U-shaped screw heads bilaterally (see Fig. 32-7). The traction nuts are then rotated along the threaded rods with wrenches to provide distraction, realignment, and the desired anatomic lordosis (see Figs. 32-8 and 32-9). Position is confirmed with intraoperative fluoroscopy. Slight overdistraction is accomplished to allow packing of the decorticated facet complexes with autograft bone, careful not to compromise the adjacent nerve root, which lies inferior and medial to the facet complex. The overdistraction is released to place the intrafacet graft in modest compression. Once the screw-rod construct is in optimal position, 3-mm set screws are tightened into position on each screw and traction nut to prevent movement and loosening. A transverse fixation assembly is applied if indicated (see Fig. 32-10). The remaining autograft bone is packed in, over, and around the remaining exposed dorsolateral decorticated surfaces of

press the lateral recesses bilaterally. The facet complexes to be fused are stripped of their cartilaginous capsules and decorticated with a high-speed drill. We use intraoperative fluoroscopy to assist in pedicle localization and bone screw placement. Using standard pedicle localization landmarks, cues dictated by the individual patient's anatomy and data provided by intraoperative fluoroscopy, a bone awl is used to sound the pedicle. A probe confirms pedicle localization and the lack of medial or lateral pedicle cortical disruption. The RF system screws are self-tapping, therefore we use a gearshift device to enter the vertebral body via the pedicle. After again probing each insertion site, self-tapping screws of the desired angulation are advanced into the vertebral bodies to be fused via the pedicles with the use of fluoroscopy to align each screw parallel to the vertebral end plate, to the desired depth (ideally, 60–80% of the vertebral body) (Krag, 1991). At S1 we aim medially into the sacral promontory rather than laterally toward the ala and generally attempt to achieve bicortical purchase for improved fixation.

Once the internal fixation screws are in place we harvest autologous iliac crest bone from the medial dorsal posterior iliae crest through a separate skin incision (Kirkpatrick & Hadley, 1993). On returning to the spinal fusion site we

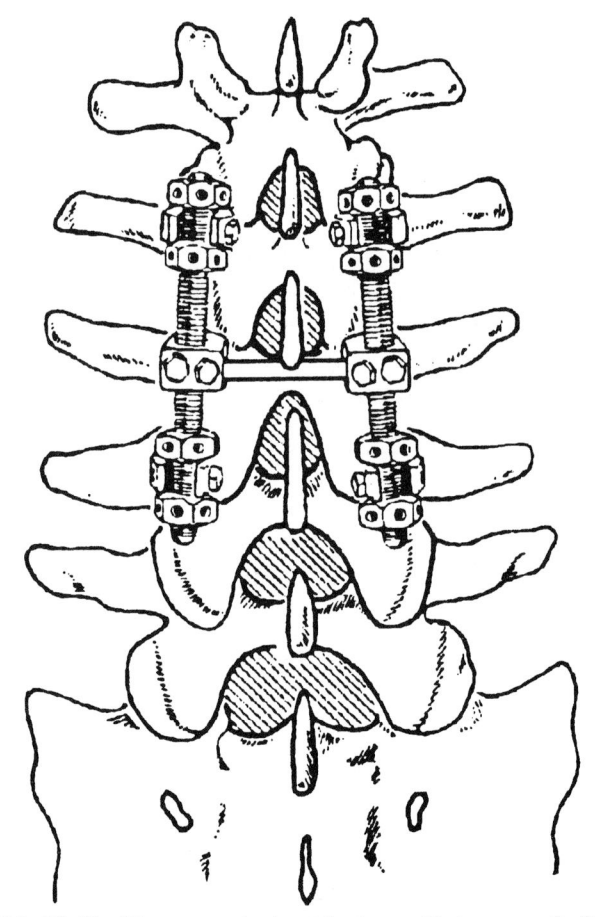

FIG. 32-10. RF construct for burst fractures with transverse fixation assembly in place. *Note:* Screws are not applied to the fractured vertebral body.

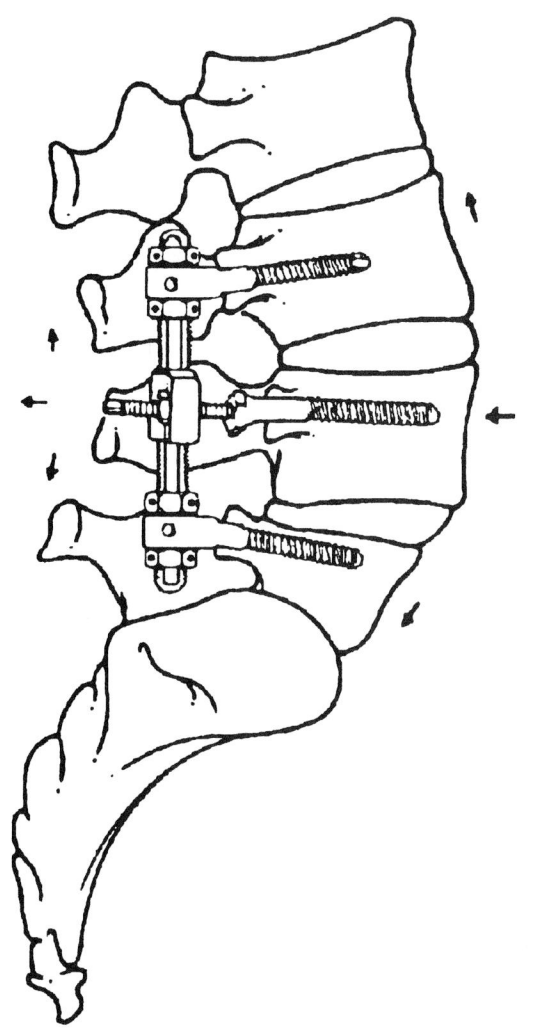

FIG. 32-11. RF construct for treatment of spondylolisthesis in which block and threaded transpedicular screws are used to reduce deformity to anatomical alignment.

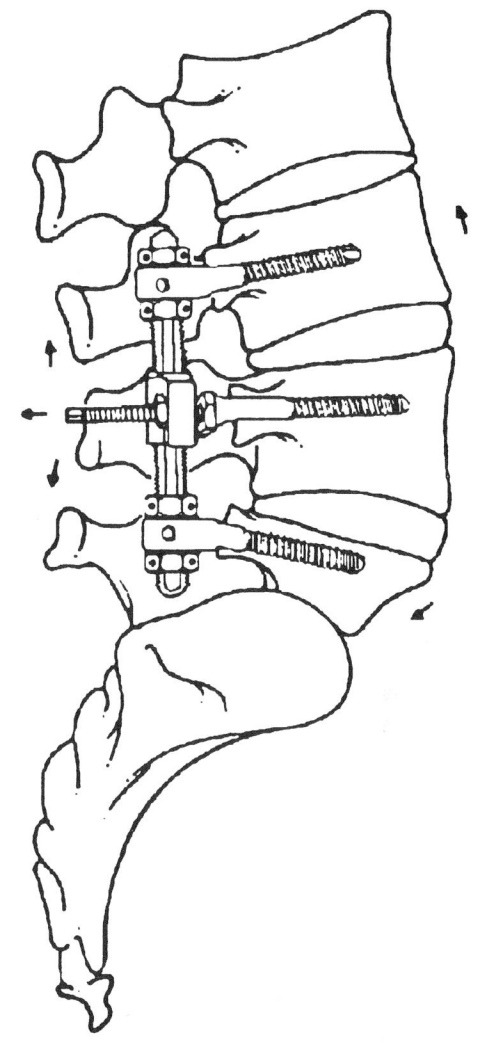

FIG. 32-12. When the traction nut of the threaded transpedicular screw is tightened to the block, the deformity is uniformly reduced.

the vertebrae to be fused (including the transverse processes), completing the stabilization and fusion procedure. Both surgical wounds are closed in standard fashion after irrigation with antibiotic solution and percutaneous drain placement.

CLINICAL RESULTS

We have used the AMS reduction fixation system six times, in the treatment of fracture deformities (one case), degenerative lumbar instability (two), and unstable L5-S1 spondylolisthesis (three) (Figs. 32-14 to 32-17). We performed these operations during a period of 4 months in 1992 after analyzing the system carefully and working with it in a cadaver-applied anatomy laboratory. Our team had extensive experience with bone screw and rod-plate fixation (a variety of systems) before using the RF system. Our clinical results and experience with the system have been favorable. We have thus far had no patient with a postoperative deficit, misplaced bone screw, postoperative infection, hardware failure or pseudoarthrosis. One patient died 13 months after surgery from a massive myocardial infarction. One patient has been lost to follow-up. No other patient has required a second surgery (mean follow-up, 14 months). One patient has intermittent symptoms suggestive of pseudarthrosis, but we cannot prove this clinically or radiographically and he has only intermittent complaints. One patient states he can "feel" his hardware when sitting for a long period. His radicular symptoms and signs and his symptoms of spinal instability have been relieved, but he gets a focal numbness-ache at his distal sacral screw insertion sites with prolonged sitting. These four patients demonstrate evidence of spinal stability clinically and radiographically and are being followed in the outpatient setting. The results of our limited clinical experience with the RF system has been similar to that of other investigators (Chang, 1990; Chang & McAfee, 1989, Fredrickson et al., 1992; Krag, 1991).

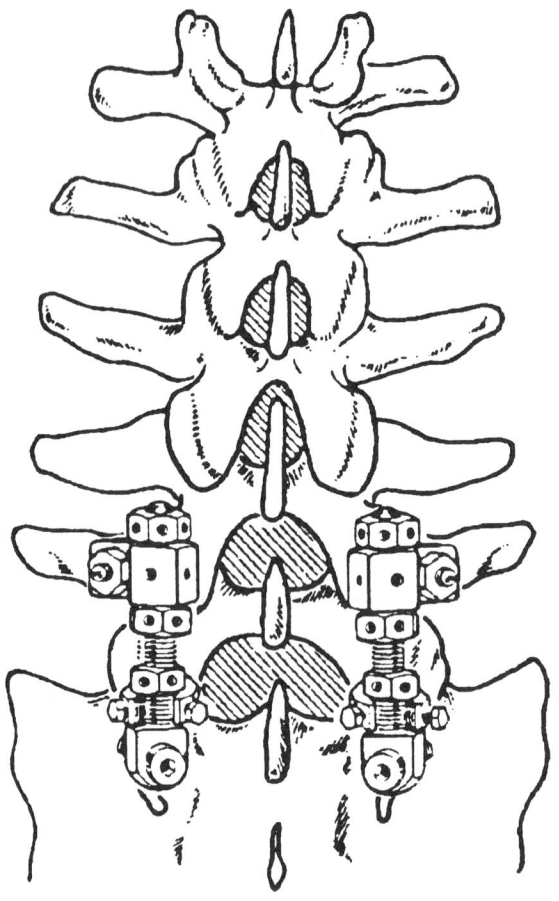

FIG. 32-13. Application of the spondylolisthesis block to treat an L5 spondylolisthesis with a construct that incorporates only the L5 and S1 levels.

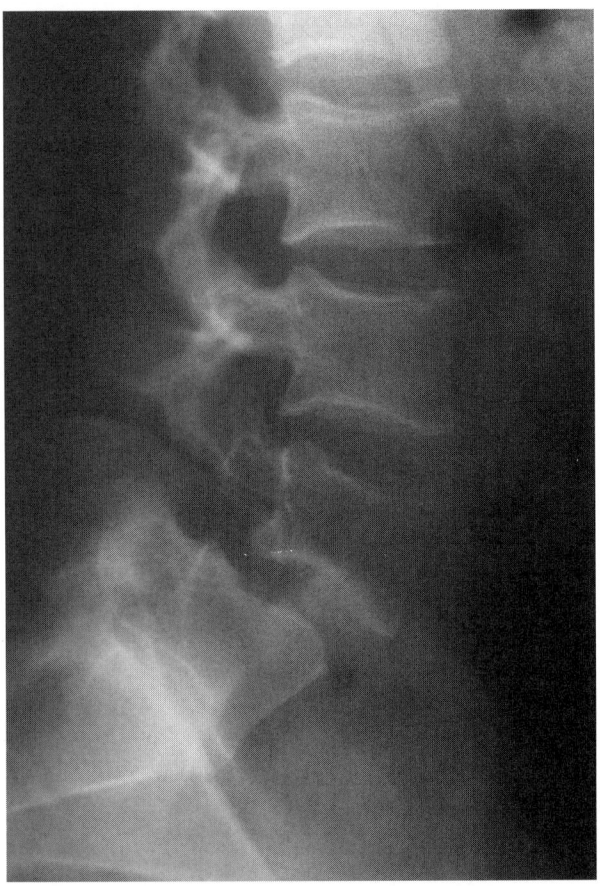

FIG. 32-14. Congenital Grade I L5-S1 spondylolisthesis with instability.

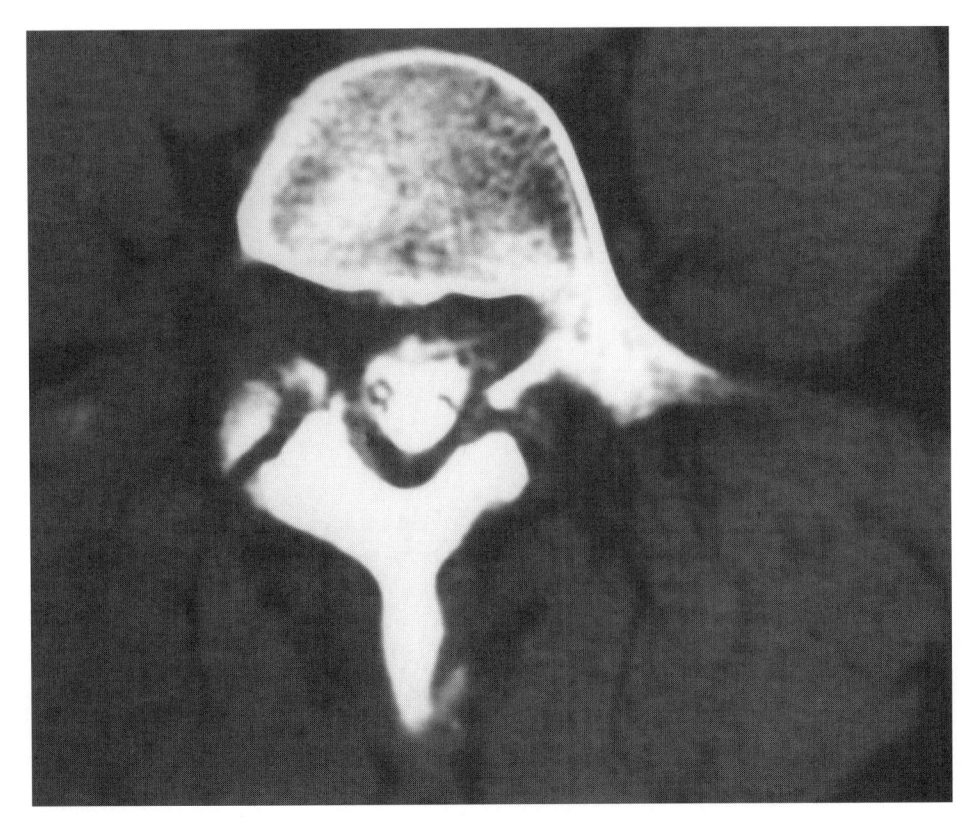

FIG. 32-15. Myelography CT study of patient in Fig. 32-14 with nerve-root compromise due to L5-S1 (unstable) spondylolisthesis.

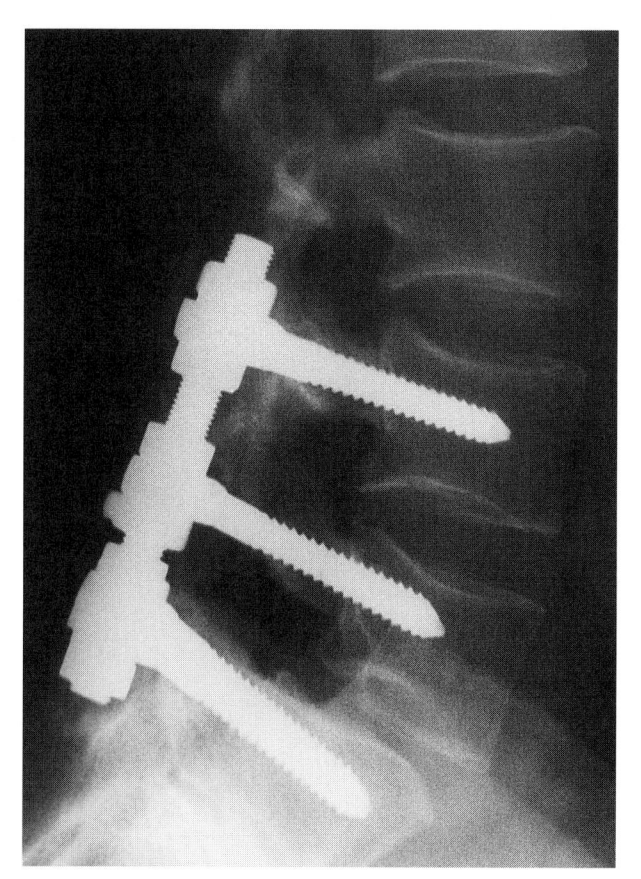

FIG. 32-16. Postoperative lateral view reveals L4-L5 and S1 internal fixation with RF system (12 months).

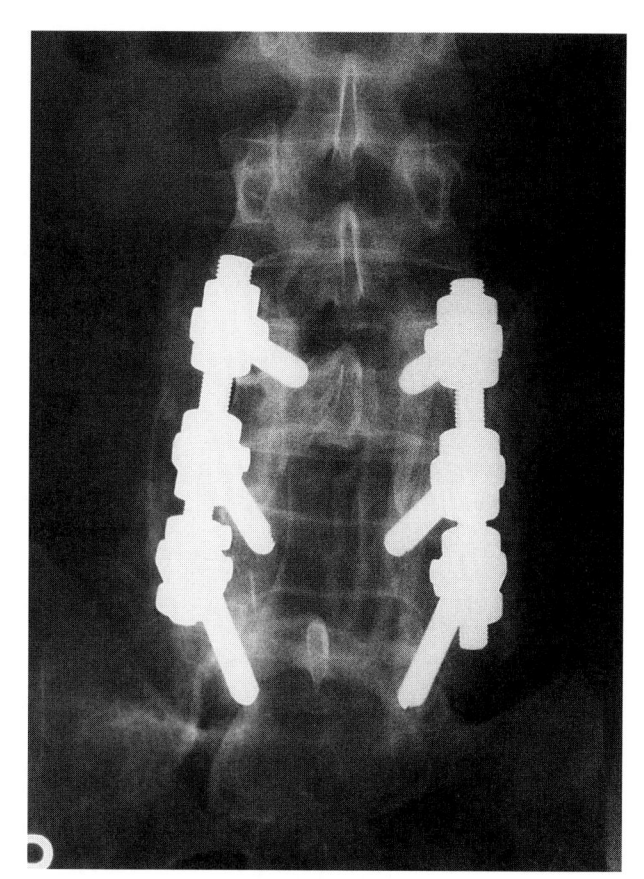

FIG. 32-17. Postoperative anteroposterior view of L4-L5-S1 internal fixation with bone fusion substrate (12 months).

The preliminary data provided by the protocol-directed multicenter clinical investigation of the RF device confirms that this is a safe, useful internal fixation system as an adjunct to bone healing for the appropriate indications (Table 32-2). Detailed analysis of this instrumentation system in comparison with other internal fixation systems is not available. Meaningful long-term follow-up of the RF system is being compiled by a number of investigators and is forthcoming but is not yet available at the time of this publication.

Table 32-2
Advantages and Disadvantages of the RF System

Advantages
  Applicable for fracture deformity, degernative instability, unstable spondylolisthesis
  Rigid internal fixation top-loading construct
  Angled screws with double washer rod construct for lordotic distraction
  Multiple diameters and lengths of self-tapping screws
  Sacral block for multiple sacral contact

Disadvantages
  Rod-screw construct only, not applicable to long segment deformity or use above T10
  Rod cannot be contoured
  Top-loading construct but washers difficult to advance in deep wound
  Small locking set screws difficult to secure
  High-profile construct, bulky

DISCUSSION

The AMS RF system is an effective reduction and internal fixation system for use in the treatment of traumatic or degenerative spinal instability from the T10 level through the sacrum. It is unique in that it can be used to achieve lordotic reduction and realignment of the thoracolumbar spine. It is effective, safe and appears to be both beneficial in the long run and associated with few complications (Chang, 1990; Chang & McAfee, 1989; Fredrickson et al., 1992).

We have used this device in only a half dozen patients because despite its apparent good clinical results thus far in our patients, it is a bulky, relatively high profile device that can be difficult and tedious to apply. Therefore, it is associated with increased surgeon frustration (more frustration than that encountered with other thoracolumbosacral internal fixation systems we have used). It is a well-engineered and biomechanically sound system. The U-shaped angled screws are an excellent adaptation of biomechanical principles, but the ideal or "correct" angles needed for anatomic realignment and lordosis are sometimes difficult to discern without some trial and error. The traction nuts (convex and flat-sided) are difficult to advance in a deep tight wound, particularly at L5-S1, and the 3-mm set screws are tedious (rarely impossible) to tighten. These reservations aside, we were able to accomplish the desired goals in the patients in whom we employed the RF system. It is likely that with more experience we will become better, quicker, and less easily frustrated with its insertion and application.

REFERENCES

Aebi, M., Etter, C., Kehl, T., & Thalgott, J. (1987). Stabilization of the lower thoracic and lumbar spine with the internal spinal skeleton fixation system. *Spine, 12;* 544–551.

Bryant, C.E., & Sullivan, J.A. (1983). Management of thoracic and lumbar spine fractures with Harrington distraction rods supplemented with segmental wiring. *Spine, 8,* 532–537.

Batzdorf, U., & Batzdorff, A. (1988). Analysis of cervical spine curvature in patients with cervical spondylosis. *Neurosurgery, 22,* 827–836.

Chang, K.W. (1990). Degenerative spondylothesis treated with reduction fixation system. *Journal of Surgical Association, Republic of China, 23,* 102–127.

Chang, K.W., & McAfee, P.C. (1989). Degenerative spondylolisthesis and degenerative scoliosis treated with a combination segmental rod-plate and transpedicular screw instrumentation system: A preliminary report. *Journal of Spinal Disorders, 1,* 247–256.

Dick, W., Kluger, P., Magerl, F., Woesdorfer, O., & Zach, G. (1985). A new device for internal fixation of thoracolumbar and lumbar spine fractures: The "Fixateur Interne." *Paraplegia, 23,* 225–232.

Fredrickson, B.E., Edwards, W.T., Rauschning, W., Bayley, J.C., & Yuan, H.A. (1992). Vertebral burst fractures: An experimental, morphologic, and radiographic study. *Spine, 17,* 1012–1021.

Jacobs, R.R., Nordwall, A., Nachemson, A., & Perren, S.M. (1984). A locking hook spinal rod system for stabilization of fracture-dislocations and correction of deformities of the dorsolumbar spine: A biomechanical evaluation. *Clinical Orthopaedics and Related Research, 189,* 168–177.

Kirkpatrick, J.S., & Hadley, M.N. (1993). Autograft vs. alloimplant as substrate for spinal fusion. *Perspectives in Neurological Surgery, 4,* 38–48.

Krag, M.H. (1991). Spinal Fusion: Overview of options and posterior internal fixation devices. In: J.W. Frymoyer (Ed.), *The Adult Spine: Pinciples and Practice, 1919–1945.* New York: Raven Press.

Krag, M.H., Weaver, D.L., Beynnon, B.D., & Haugh, L.D. (1988). Morphometry of the thoracic and lumbar spine related to transpedicular screw placement for surgical spinal fixation. *Spine, 13,* 27–32.

Roy-Camille, R., Saillant, G., & Mazel, C. (1986). Internal fixation of the lumbar spine with pedicle screw plating. *Clinical Orthopaedics and Related Research, 203,* 7–17.

CHAPTER 33

Segmental Fixation of the Lumbosacral Spine Using the Isola/VSP System

Setti S. Rengachary
Eric Flores

HIGHLIGHTS

The Isola spinal system was initially designed by Asher and associates as a sacral fixation device, but further modifications of the device has allowed the system to evolve into an "universal" type of posterior spinal segmental fixation system (Asher, Carson, Heinig, et al., 1988; Asher, Strippgen, Heinig, & Carson, 1992). The term *Isola* draws its name from the fancied resemblance of the initial sacral construct to a native butterfly of the Isola species (Fig. 33-1). The variable screw placement (VSP) plating system for rigid fixation of the lumbosacral spine developed by Steffee has been integrated into the Isola system. The systems use identical pedicular and sacral screws, allowing versatility and flexibility. Lumbosacral instrumentation with the Isola system may be accomplished either with a rigid plate or rod depending on surgeon's preference (Table 33-1). Biomechanically, the strength of rod constructs with cross-link(s) parallels that of the plate construct. Therefore, one does not choose plate versus rod stabilization based on relative biomechanical strengths of the constructs. A rod system with slotted connectors (discussed below) allows very long constructs without the need for the pedicle screws to align in a straight line. The plate system, in contrast, does not permit more than a minor malalignment of the pedicle screws; thus, constructs longer than two motion segments do not lend themselves to easy plate stabilization. However, those who are adept and experienced in plate stabilization may not follow this rule. Another advantage of the rod system is the ease with which the rod may be bent in the sagittal and coronal planes. Bending a plate in the coronal plane is difficult if not impossible. Thus, complex deformities are easier to correct with the rod than with the plate system.

The basic philosophy behind Isola instrumentation design is to achieve the following goals: (1) the final construct should have the lowest profile possible; (2) the construct should be very rigid biomechanically; (3) the instrumentation should be user friendly and have the least "fiddle" factor; and (4) the instrumentation should be simple, with a minimal number of implant components necessary to complete a construct.

RATIONALE OF PEDICLE FIXATION

Since the initial use of pedicle screws by Cotrel and colleagues (Cotrel, Dubousset, & Guillaumat, 1988) and Steffee (Steffee, 1989; Steffee & Brantigam, 1993), the pedicle fixation system for the lumbar spine has turned out to be the biomechanically best system for segmental fixation. Unique pedicular anatomy explains this advantage. The pedicle is a very strong anatomical bridge between the posterior spinal elements and the vertebral body. It is a cylindrical structure containing a very strong cortical shell with a core of cancellous bone. The screw purchase is of the strong cortical bone. The pedicle is the only link between the posterior column and the middle and anterior columns. Thus, a screw transversing the pedicle into the vertebral body stabilizes all three columns (Zindrick, Wiltse, Widell, et al., 1986). In contrast the hook and rod system anchors only to the posterior elements and does not allow for as rigid stabilization of all three columns. The pedicle, in addition, has a fairly large cortical-to-cancelleous-bone ratio. This permits a good anchor of pedicle screws. Biomechanically, the pedicles represent a conduit by which muscular forces applied to the

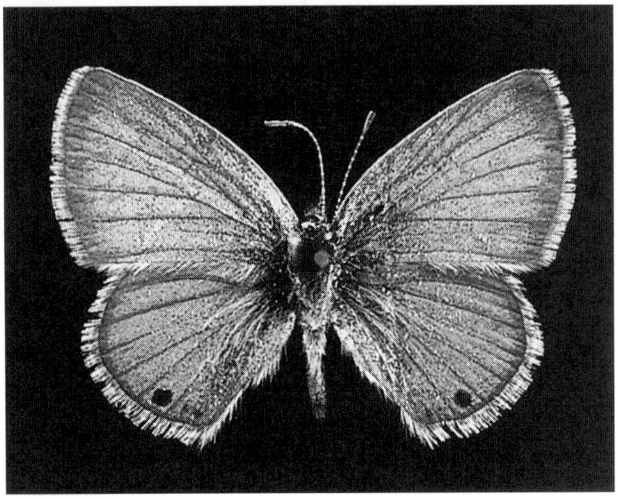

FIG. 33-1. Butterfly of the Isola species. (*Illustration courtesy of Abhay Sanan, M.D.*)

posterior spinal structures are transferred to the vertebral body. These anatomical and mechanical properties of the pedicle make it an ideal anchor site for spinal instrumentation. Pedicle screw fixation of the lumbar spine has virtually replaced older fixation systems, such as Luque rectangles and Harrington rods.

INDICATIONS FOR INTERNAL STABILIZATION OF THE LUMBOSACRAL SPINE

Considerable controversy exists among spine surgeons as to the indications for internal lumbosacral stabilization (Table 33-2). Controversy comes about because with the present state of knowledge, it is very difficult to define spinal instability. The conventional narrow definition to which neurosurgeons are accustomed is that there should be some sort of translational motion demonstrated in stress films. Although it is an extreme example of instability, it is no longer accepted as the only definition. Patients with chronic mechanical back pain with desiccated and degenerative

Table 33-1
Indications and Contraindications for Use of the Isola/VSP System

Indications
    Spondylolisthesis
    Traumatic instability
    Degenerative disease
        Spondylolisthesis
        Stenosis
        Diskogenic pain
    Infections—tuberculous
    Tumors

Contraindications
    Infections—pyogenic
    Osteoporosis

Table 33-2
Advantages and Disadvantages of the Isola/VSP System

Advantages
    "Universal" system
    Easy attachments of rods to plates
    Top-loading hooks and screws
    V-groove attachment design

Disadvantages
    Adaptors for plate/rod and plate/screw connections introduce possible points of movement in system

disks, collapse of disk height, sclerosis of the end plates, and foraminal narrowing may not show translational motions on stress films but may be considered to have instability that accounts for the pain. In a similar manner, patients with Grades I to II spondylolisthesis with a fixed dislocation may also be considered to have instability, but of a different sort, called "glacial instability," meaning that instability has occurred over time, not instantaneously. A patient with a grossly deformed lumbar spine with deformity in many planes, such as kyphoscoliosis due to advanced degenerative disease of the lumbar spine, may also be considered to have instability because of ligamentous failure. Although many such practical examples of instability may be cited, the term by itself lacks precise definition. Thus, from a pragmatic point of view we will discuss at this point the clinical indications for internal stabilization of the lumbar spine rather than dwelling on the scientific criteria for the definition of instability, because no satisfactory, universally accepted definition exists. There is also no consensus on the choice of techniques (e.g., rigid vs. semirigid constructs).

The Food and Drug Administration (FDA), at this point, has restricted the use of transpedicular screws in the lumbosacral region for high-grade spondylolisthesis. Approval for other indications is pending. Most spine surgeons, based on their personal experience and published reports, use pedicle screws for non-FDA-approved indications if they believe it is in the best interest of patient care. Certain safeguards are generally used. When the consent for surgery is obtained, the patient is informed that the device is not approved by the FDA for the indications for which it will be used. In addition, permission may be obtained from the institutional review board for the use of an investigational device. Although there are controversies with regard to indications for lumbosacral stabilization, the disorders discussed below are generally considered suitable for instrumented fusion by contemporary criteria.

Spondylolisthesis

Isthmic spondylolisthesis is perhaps the most common indication for internal stabilization of the lumbar spine. In all instances in which internal fixation is performed, it is intended as a temporary measure to stabilize the spine to facilitate optimal bone fusion. The hardware is in itself not sufficient to maintain the stability beyond a certain time frame, and all hardware will fail eventually. However strong the construct may appear to be, unless solid bony fusion occurs, patients' symptoms are likely to recur when the hardware loosens or breaks. It is therefore imperative that all measures be undertaken to promote good solid bony fusion. This may include use of generous amounts of autologous bone graft; use of bone-fusion-promoting agents, such as bone morphogenic protein (Grafton); use of external or internal electrical stimulators when specific indications for those exist; and use of bone extenders such as coral hydroxyapatite and collegraft (a mixture of bovine collagen and hydroxyapatite); however, efficacy of some of these measures has not been proven in spine fusion.

It is well known that the degree of isthmic spondylolisthesis is not necessarily related to the severity of symptoms. Thus, it is not uncommon to see patients with Grade III/IV spondylolisthesis go on for years and be completely asymptomatic. In contrast, patients with Grade I spondylolisthesis may have excruciating pain out of proportion to the degree of slip. This simply indicates that we still do not understand the physiologic mechanism by which pain is induced in patients with spondylolisthesis. Patients are selected after a trial of conservative treatment, which includes bracing, conditioning exercises of the back and abdominal muscles, nonsteroidal antiinflammatory drugs, and change in strenuous occupation when possible. If the above measures fail, then one should consider internal stabilization. The goals here are twofold. One, is to decompress the root that is impaired by pressure from the pseudarthrosis at the site of spondylolysis. This fibrous tissue around pseudarthrosis generally compresses the exiting rather than transiting root. For instance in the L5-S1 spondylolisthesis, it is not uncommon to find the L5 rather than the S1 root to be compressed. In order to decompress the root one should do a decompressive procedure that includes the excision of all the fibrous material around the pseudarthrosis and do a generous foraminotomy until the exiting root is completely decompressed. In patients with pure back pain without radicular symptoms such an aggressive maneuver may not be necessary. In planning internal fixation one should closely scrutinize the magnetic resonance imaging (MRI) scan in the sagittal plane. One should carefully look at the status of the disk, either above or below the olisthesis. If there is evidence of disk degeneration either immediately above or immediately below the olisthetic motion segment, one should seriously consider incorporating that segment in the fusion construct. Failure to do so will invite recurrence of back pain within months after the operation. The use of diskography as an adjunctive measure in this decision-making process has been controversial. The construct design will also depend on the degree of slip. It is wise to use one additional motion segment if the olisthesis is Grade II or higher.

There has been some debate as to whether one should be content with internal stabilization and in situ fusion or make an attempt to reduce the olisthesis before initiating fusion. The general tendency is to accept in situ fusion for low-grade (Grades I and II) spondylolisthesis because the long-term results for patients with in situ fusions are no different than for those in whom a reduction has been attempted. In fact there is a higher incidence of nerve-root impairment with attempts at reduction than with in situ fusion. Those who argue for reduction with fusion will cite improvement of body mechanics, due to improvement in anatomical alignment, greater stability, and better chance of long-term pain relief without recurrence as reasons for recommending reduction. For higher-grade (Grades III and IV) spondylolisthesis, however, attempted reduction and anatomical alignment is much more meaningful and more often carried out than with low-grade spondylolisthesis.

An additional area of controversy is whether to consider instrumented fusion or noninstrumented fusion for low-grade (Grades I and II) spondylolisthesis. There are those who argue that for one-level fusion, noninstrumented fusions carry as good a probability of solid fusion as instrumented fusions. Instrumentation is perhaps only indicated when more than one motion segment is fused. Emerging consensus, however, suggests that instrumented fusion ensures a higher rate of fusion, instant immobilization, and pain relief, and this is preferred.

Trauma—Burst Fracture of the Lumbar Spine

For unstable burst fractures of the lumbar spine, there is an option between posterior instrumentation and corpectomy with anterior stabilization (Gurwitz, Dawson, McNamara, et al., 1993; Sasso & Cotler, 1993). Patients with L5 burst fractures are best treated with posterior exploration, removal of the posteriorly protruding bone fragments, and internal stabilization from L4 through S1 (An, Vaccaro, Colter, et al., 1991). This is preferable to corpectomy and anterior fixation because it is not possible to fixate the L4 body to the sacrum without compromising the iliac vessels. For fractures at higher levels, either method is applicable. With posterior instrumentation and fusion there is a risk of delayed kyphosis because of lack of anterior load-sharing. Although the kyphosis may be inevitable, the degree of kyphosis that occurs over time may not be clinically significant. Resection of the vertebral body with strut grafting and anterior plating gives an esthetically and anatomically better construct than posterior approaches. The choice is left to the surgeon depending on his or her background and experience. If posterior instrumentation is decided on for burst fractures, one vertebral segmental level on each side of the burst fracture is incorporated in the construct. This is the least number of segments that one can fixate. With the currently available strong internal fixation devices there is usually very little justification or need for a 360-degree fusion in most patients with trauma.

If a posterior approach is decided on, the bone fragments retropulsed into the spinal canal from the vertebral body are either removed or tapped back into place. It is our experience that the fragments usually lie at the upper aspect of the vertebral body close to the pedicle rather than at the midbody or lower part of the body. In addition, there is usually some degree of annular rupture and disk protrusion. Usually a laminectomy is done followed by pedicular drilling. This gives access right up to the posterior surface of the vertebral body. The annulus fibrosus and disk are removed, as is the adjacent retropulsed fragment. Also, some verification of decompression may be necessary. Most often, however, mere palpation with angled curettes or dental instrument or a long nerve hook or a Murphy's probe will be sufficient to confirm the optimal decompression. Having removed the retropulsed fragments, one proceeds with instrumentation. There have been attempts to augment the bone of the vertebral body through the transpedicular approach by the use of a bone funnel. However, this technique has not gained popularity.

Degenerative Disease of the Lumbar Spine

Degenerative disease of the lumbar spine is a very common indication for decompression and internal stabilization. The clinical syndrome that results from degenerative disease can be classified into three major categories, as discussed below.

Degenerative Spondylolisthesis

Degenerative spondylolisthesis occurs generally at the L4-5 level, most commonly in women past the age of 65. This appears to be due to ligamentous instability as well as facet arthropathy. Because of the incompetence in the facet, the L4 vertebra migrates forward over L5. Ordinarily, the migration is limited to Grade I spondylolisthesis. High-grade spondylolisthesis is uncommon unless a facet had been removed during prior surgery. Because of facet interlocking, even if they have undergone advanced degenerative changes, forward translation of the vertebrae does not occur beyond Grade I. The sagittal rather than transverse orientation of facets further predisposes to anterior translation. The patient generally reports mechanical back pain, although there may be vague radiation of pain down the leg, but not in a typical radicular fashion. The hallmark of the disease is the aggravation of pain in sitting and standing positions, but relief lying down. Patients may have pain when they roll in bed from side to side. Bracing seldom gives enduring relief. These patients are best treated by decompressive laminectomy and internal stabilization. Lumbar myelography or MRI scan may show lumbar stenosis at the level of subluxation due to thickening of the ligamenta flavum, hypertrophy of facets, and subluxation. It would be a mistake to treat such patients merely with laminectomy because it would simply aggravate subluxation and aggravate the pain. One suggestion is just to reduce the subluxation and stabilize it without having to do a laminectomy. This will restore the canal dimension because of the alignment of the spine. However, long-term results of this mode of treatment are not available at this time.

Spinal Stenosis

Spinal stenosis is another manifestation of lumbar degenerative disease. It usually occurs from a combination of facet hypertrophy, thickening of the ligamentum flavum, and bulging annulus. There may be superimposed congenital narrowing of the spinal canal. There has been some controversy as to whether one should routinely stabilize the spine after decompressive laminectomy for straightforward lumbar stenosis. In coming to a decision in this regard several factors have to be taken into account. If the stenosis is extreme and the facet joints have to be removed to offer decompression, then internal stabilization is necessary. If one plans on a diskectomy, further destabilization of the motion segment occurs and therefore one would lean on internal stabilization. If there is a preexisting subluxation associated with tight stenosis, then one would consider internal stabilization as well.

Diskogenic Pain Related to Chronic Disk Disease at L5-S1 from Chronic Degenerative Changes in the Disk with Sclerosis of the Cortical End Plates with Narrowing of the Intervertebral Fragment

This syndrome occurs predominantly at L5-S1. The patients generally do not have radicular pain. Presumably this is related to old trauma that initiates degenerative change of the disk disease in a chronic fashion that results ultimately in decreased disk height, sclerosis of the end plates and narrowing of the foramina. Patients generally have intactable intermittent back pain that does not respond to conservative management. However, there is not always a direct correlation between the radiologic findings and the clinical syndrome. With the same degree of severity of disk narrowing, some patients tend to be totally asymptomatic and the findings turn out to be entirely incidental. Optimal treatment for this condition would be to perform a posterior lumbar interbody fusion, which will restore the height of the disk space, as well as open up the intervertebral foramen. Fusion should be followed by instrumentation.

Infections

Acute or chronic diskitis may lead to destruction of the disk cortical end plates and varying destruction of the vertebral body, resulting in instability. There has been some debate about whether one can implant metallic devices in the face of infection. It has been shown that with tuberculous infection there is no worsening of the infection with instrumentation. This same fact has been proven conclusively with pyogenic infections also, by Fessler and associates. Tuberculous infection, however, is common in the thoracic spine, but rarely occurs in the lumbar spine, so this discussion pertains only to pyogenic infections. A prudent approach would be to debride the disk space through a limited laminectomy, obtaining appropriate cultures, to pack the space with cancellous bone chips, and to follow the patient with bracing. If the patient shows continued instability, one can consider internal stabilization at a later stage, after 4 to 6 weeks of antibiotic therapy.

Tumors

The approach to lumbar or vertebral-body tumors depends on the location. Tumors located in the posterior elements are best resected through a posterior approach by a laminectomy. If the facets have to be removed and there is a question of destabilization through bone removal, then internal stabilization is indicated. However, tumors involving strictly the posterior column are quite rare. Most tumors occur in the vertebral body and may involve the pedicle. If that is the case, the anterior approach is preferred. The lateral extracavitary approach is an alternative. If the lesion involves both anterior and posterior elements then a 360-degree total vertebrectomy may be needed with both anterior strut grafting and posterior instrumentation.

ISOLA IMPLANTS

Pedicle Screws

As indicated earlier, the pedicle screws in the Isola system can be used with the VSP plate system as well. The pedicle screws have a bolt-type structure and share the biomechanical properties of the Isola sacral and iliac screws (Fig. 33-2). Typically, the pedicle screw consist of a tapered, threaded cancellous bolt with an integral hex nut from which a machine-threaded shank protrudes. The integral nut provides a seat for slotted connectors of plates, which are held in place by a tapered nut. Alternatively, a simple Isola hex nut can be used. Biomechanically the integral bolt-type construct allows for translation forces to be contained within the construct, resulting in a higher pullout strength and a lowering of shearing forces in the screw osseous interface. (Fig. 33-3).

Isola/VSP bone screws come in both stainless steel and titanium. The screws come in three standard diameters: 7, 6.25, and 5.5 mm. The cancellous threaded portions range from 25 to 50 mm at 5-mm increments. In the lumbar spine

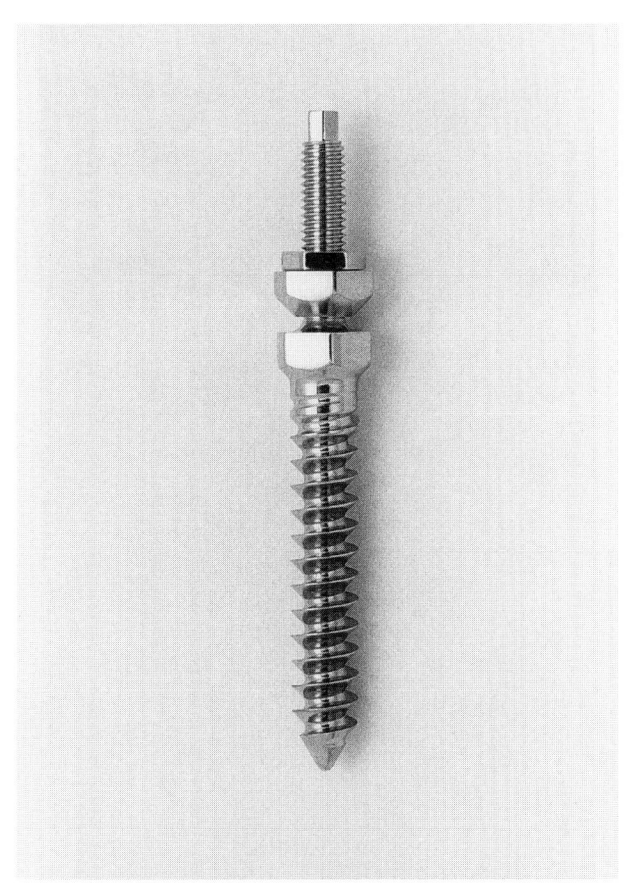

FIG. 33-2. Standard VSP/Isola pedicle screw. It has three components: a screw with integral hex nut, a tapered nut, and a locking nut.

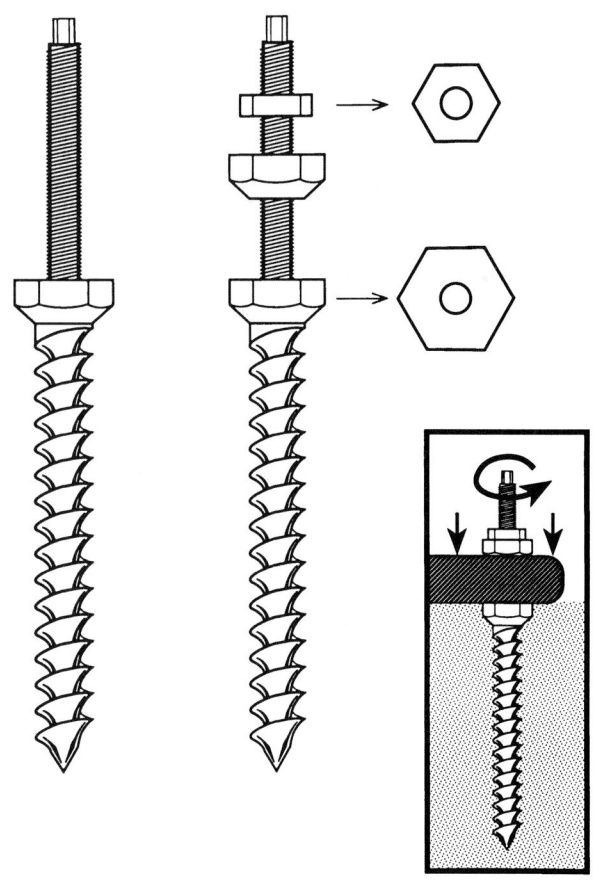

FIG. 33-3. Illustration of components of a pedicle screw. Note the bolt-type construct with VSP plate sandwiched between the integral hex nut below and the tapered nut above.

in an average adult, a 40-mm screw is most often used. The machine-threaded portion comes in three sizes: 16, 19, and 30 mm. The 30-mm machine-threaded screws are particularly useful for reduction of olisthesis. The use of 16-mm machine threaded screws obviates the need for cutting the machine-threaded portion when the construct is completed. The 19-mm machine-threaded screws allows for washers and yet does not need to be cut at the end of the procedure. These screws may be used as anchors either for attachment of a rod or a VSP plate. If a rod is used in the construct then one needs Isola slotted connectors for rod attachment. Slotted connectors allow some latitude in the coronal and sagittal planes for connection with rods. A hex nut holds the slotted connectors on the threaded portion of the screw. A hex nut may also be used to anchor the plate on the nested portion. A locking nut is available, but is not thought to be essential.

Iliac screws are designed for placement in the iliac bone for use as anchors. Iliac screws or the Galveston constructs are seldom needed for short segment lumbosacral spine stabilization. They are generally reserved for long thoracolumbar constructs. They are not discussed further in this chapter.

The sacral screws come in only one diameter, 8.5 mm. They are very sturdy screws and come in three lengths: 30, 35, and 40 mm. The 30-mm screw is generally used for fixation in the S2 segment, and the 35- or 40-mm screw for fixation in the S1 segment. The screws are to be used with a special 8.5-mm sacral tap. Sacral screws have a 23-mm machine-threaded length connector segment.

Plates

The VSP plates, as the name indicates, have nested slots that allow for variable screw placement. They come in two formats, standard and Asian. The Asian plates are thinner to allow for low profile when used in thin individuals. The plates are available in either titanium (plate width, 13 mm; height, 5.3 mm) or stainless steel (plate width, 13 or 16 mm; height, 4–6 mm). Plate lengths range from a 41-mm single-slot plate to a 141-mm four-slot plate. The wider plate is available in a 41-mm single-slot plate to a 197-mm five-slot plate. Longer plates can be obtained by special order. Special plate benders are available to contour the plates to conform to the curvature of the spine.

Rods

Isola rods are smooth and come in two diameters: $\frac{3}{16}$ and $\frac{1}{4}$ in. The standard rod length is 18 in. The rods can be easily contoured by either bending irons (Fig. 33-4) or in situ benders. There is some controversy about whether one should use $\frac{3}{16}$- or $\frac{1}{4}$-in. rods for lumbosacral fixation. Most agree that the $\frac{1}{4}$-in. rod is optimal and allows for a solid, rigid construct. However, others argue that the $\frac{3}{16}$-in. rod is better because it allows for some give and bounce, which facilitates early bone fusion.

Nuts and Washers

Titanium or stainless steel locking nuts are 8 mm in diameter and tapered nuts are 9.5 mm in diameter. Washers come in two configurations, cylindrical (in two sizes, 3 and 5 mm)

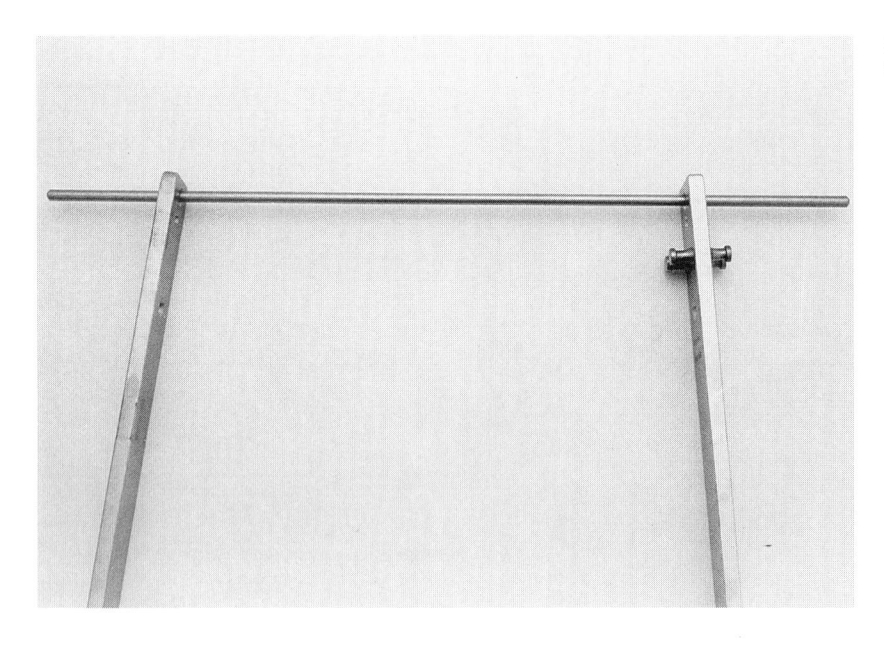

FIG. 33-4. Bending of an Isola rod using bending irons.

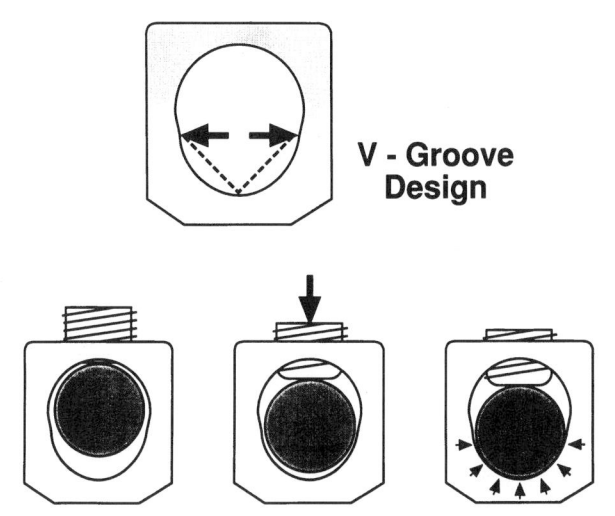

FIG. 33-5. V-groove hollow ground design (VHG) of the rod holes in the Isola slotted connectors. Note that as the set screw is tightened the rod moves from the roomier upper half of the hole into the snug-fitting lower half.

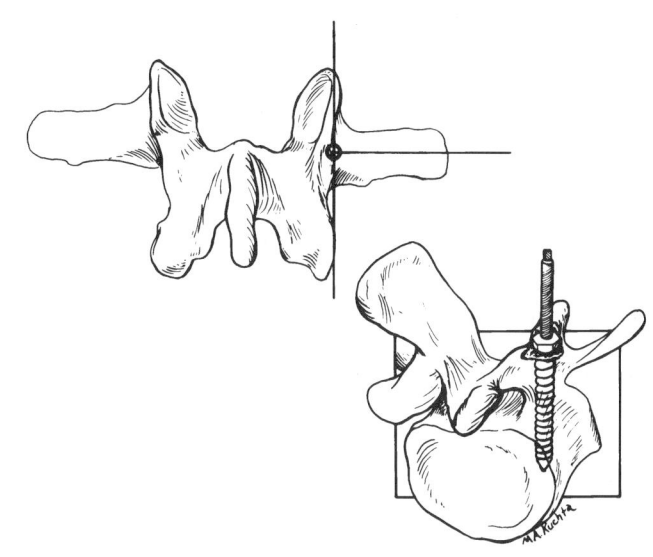

FIG. 33-6. Optimal entry point for the pedicle screw.

or tapered. The tapered washers are generally used over the sacral screw to correct the angulation. The cylindrical washers are used over the lumbar pedicular screws to lift the longitudinal member (rod or plate). This allows more room for bone graft to be placed under the construct over the facet joint and the transverse processes.

Slotted Connectors

Closed slotted connectors bridge the longitudinal members—the rod—to the screw anchors. A V-groove hollow ground (VHG) design is used to allow maximal rod contact within the hole for the rod. (Fig. 33-5) The hole for the rod is in two dimensions. When the rod is sliding through the connector, it glides easily in the upper, roomier part of the hole. Once the rod is placed optimally it is driven down into the snug-fitting lower half of the hole. This increases the area of contact with the rod and increases the biomechanical stability of the construct. The set screw drives the rod against the V-groove to maximize the contact. The set screw has the advantage of being loaded from the top yet giving a low profile.

Surgical Technique

Instrumentation and spinal fusion are virtually always done under general anesthesia. If the patient is too ill to tolerate general anesthesia, he or she is probably too ill to have a major surgical procedure. A cell-saver device is almost always used, although often there may not be enough blood loss to justify its use. More blood is generally lost from the graft harvest site than from the lumbosacral spine exposure. Our policy has been to use muscle relaxants rather than withholding them. We would depend on anatomical landmarks and radiologic guidance in locating the pedicle and root rather than muscle twitching as an indicator of root proximity. Preoperative autologous blood donation is encouraged, although some studies have suggested that it is not highly cost effective. The patient is positioned prone on rolls, a four-poster frame, a radiolucent Wilson frame, or an Andrews frame. The Wilson frame is most commonly used and is easier to use than the four-poster frame. In obese individuals the Andrews frame is preferred. With the use of the Andrews frame one forgoes the x-ray capability in the anteroposterior (AP) projection, but it may be a tradeoff to allow less venous bleeding.

A vertical midline incision is used to expose the lumbosacral spine. The incision should be generous and should extend one or two segments above and below the proposed fusion segments. The muscle separation is generally carried out with monopolar cautery to minimize blood loss, and the separation should be carried out over the facets and transverse processes bilaterally. Care should be taken to prevent damage to the facet capsule of the unfused motion segments. Should decompression be necessary, this should be done before instrumentation. The removed spinous processes of the laminae are cleared of soft tissue, crushed in a bone mill, and saved for later fusion.

As the first step in pedicle screw fixation, one should identify the entry point for the pedicle screw (Weinstein, Spratt, Spengler, et al., 1988). This is the junction of the transecting line of the transverse process with the superior articular process and the pars interarticularis (Zindrick, Wiltse, Doornick, et al., 1987) (Fig. 33-6). There is usually a small bony projection called the "mammary process" at this point. The mammary process is penetrated with a sharp awl. A Leksell rongeur may be used to remove cortical bone prior to the use of awl, but we prefer to leave as much

FIG. 33-7. (a) Gearshift. (b) Gearshift being used to penetrate the pedicle.

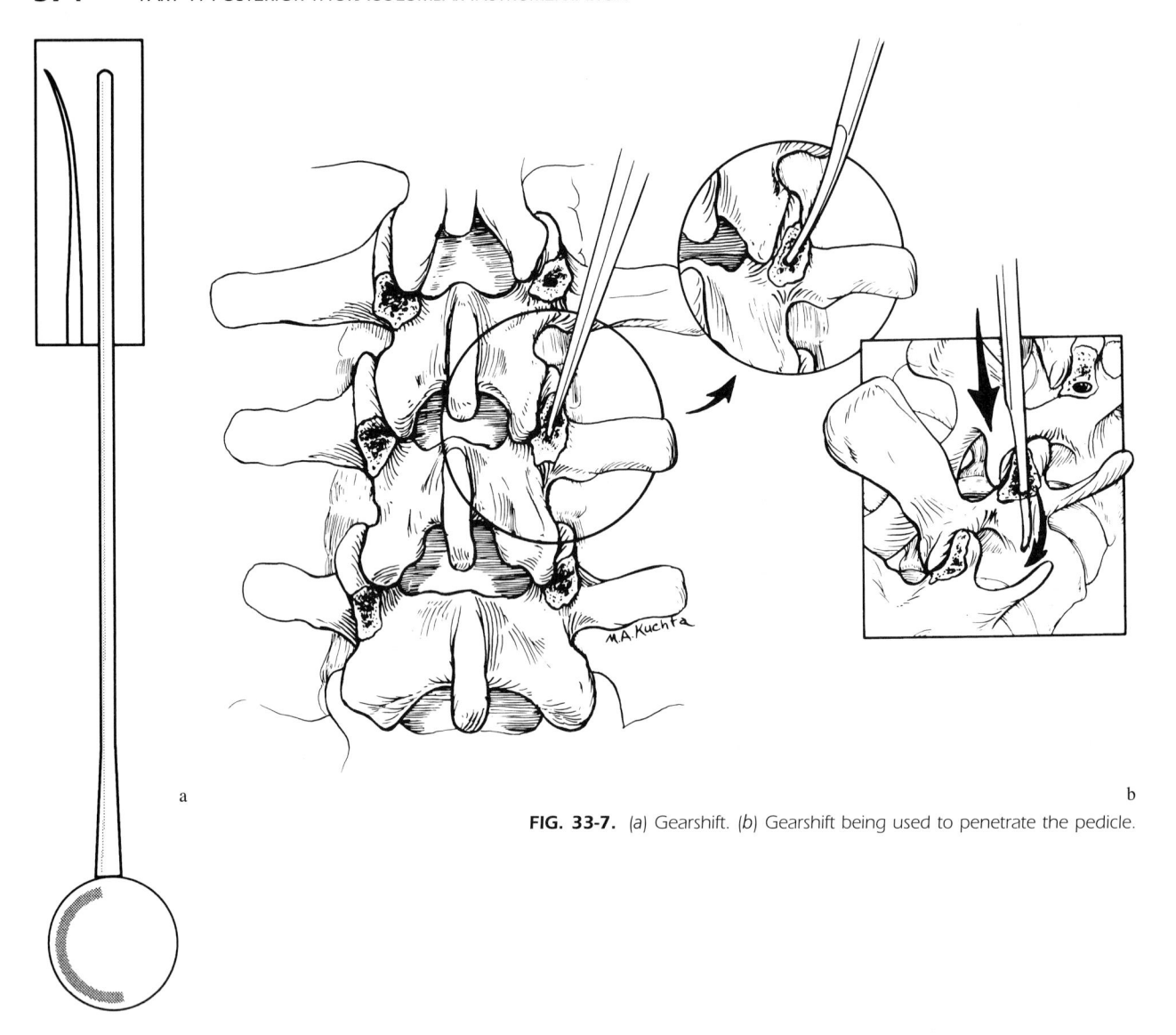

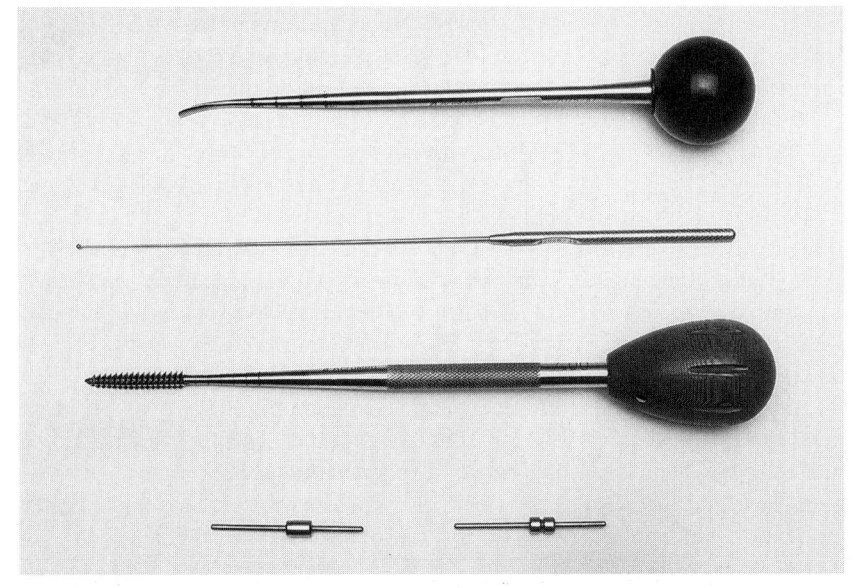

FIG. 33-8. Instrumentation useful in application of pedicle screw. *From top to bottom,* Gearshift, ball-tipped pedicle feeler, pedicle tap, and smooth and grooved markers.

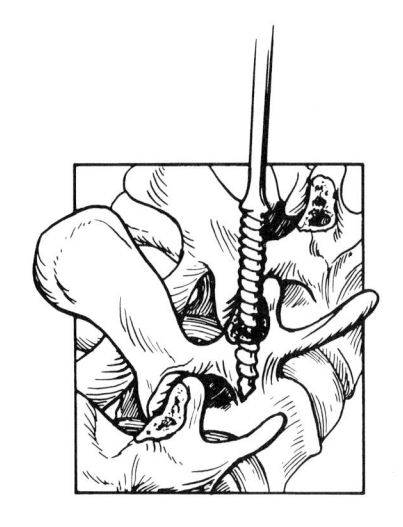

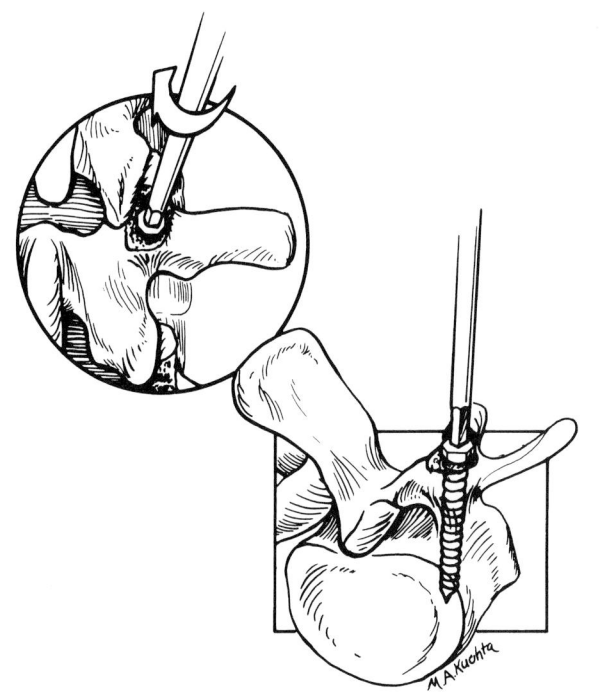

FIG. 33-9. Application of pedicle screw using the screw wrench.

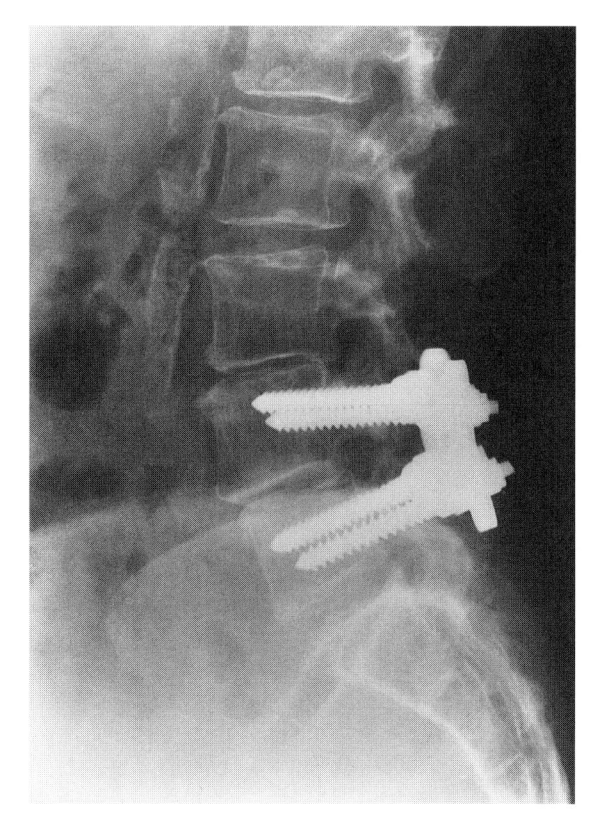

FIG. 33-10. Optimal length of penetration of pedicle screws.

intact cortical bone as possible around the screw entry site, which gives a better anchor. In individuals with heavy cortical bone, a small 3-mm olive-shaped cutting bur is preferred. After 4 or 5 mm of bone has been penetrated, a ballpoint probe is used to make sure that the cortex of the pedicle has not been violated. A dull "gearshift" is then used with the gentle curve winding medially to conform to the pedicular configuration with a gentle side-to-side rocking motion to penetrate the cancellous bone of the pedicle (Fig. 33-7). The ballpoint probe is again used to make sure that the cortex of the pedicle has not been violated. (Fig. 33-8) If a laminectomy has been carried out, the pedicle may be directly visualized or palpated with Murphy probe or a Penfield freer to make sure that the pedicle has not been violated. A marker is then placed into the hole created and lateral and AP radiographs are taken to confirm optimal trajectory. Grooved markers are placed on one side and smooth markers on the other. If the trajectory is not optimal, minor adjustments are made. The hole is then tapped with a tap of the appropriate size. We generally use taps slightly smaller than the intended pedicle screw. Bone bleeding is controlled either with a small amount of Gelfoam or bone wax. Methylmethacrylate may be used to improve the anchor in patients with severe osteoporosis, but this should be used with caution because even if there are minor holes in the walls of the pedicle, methacrylate may leak out into the spinal canal and cause root compression. The pedicle screw is then applied using a screw wrench (Fig. 33-9). When all the screws have been applied, lateral and AP radiographs are taken for final confirmation of optimal placement of the screws. Care should be exercised to avoid penetration of the disk space superiorly as this provides suboptimal screw purchase, as well as avoiding penetrating the ventral pedicular surface to avoid root injury. Appropriate screw length may be determined by a depth sounder, but we often guess the appropriate length of the screw from the depth of penetration of pedicle markers in the lateral radiographs and extrapolate the desired length of the screw (Fig. 33-10).

The screw length should allow the tip of the screw to penetrate one third to one half of the vertebral body. The screws are aligned as much as possible to prevent torque or bending moments if a plate construct is intended.

Implantation of Longitudinal Member

Isola Rod

If rods are used, the appropriate rod of the proper diameter is chosen. The rod of appropriate length is cut using a bench-top rod cutter (Fig. 33-11). In choosing the length one should make sure that the rod does not have an impact on unfused motion segments. Rod length measures from the last caudal instrumented facet to the facet of the motion segment immediately above the top of the construct. The rods are then bent using a bending iron to conform to the contour of the lumbar lordosis. In situations in which correction of a deformity is needed, the rod is contoured to the final desired configuration of the lumbar spine rather than to the lumbar spine in the deformed state. Slanted washers are then slipped over the threaded portion to sit on the integral hex nut in the sacral screw. Cylindrical washers may be used over other screws. Slotted connectors are then slipped on the rods and fixed to the machine-threaded portion of the bone screws with hex nuts (Fig. 33-12). It is important to loosen the hex nut used to anchor the slotted connector by one turn to allow for motion when the set screws are tightened. When the set screws have all been tightened, then one goes back and retightens the hex nut, securing the slotted connectors. The same procedure is repeated on the opposite side, and the transverse connector is then secured as a final step. For short-segment instrumentation, a single connector may be sufficient. For long-segment fusions, one at each end may be appropriate.

Plates

If plates are used, a template is initially applied over the pedicle screws to gauge appropriate contouring of the plate before fixation. Care should be exercised to avoid excessive plate length, which may impinge on the facet motion segments above the construct, resulting in postoperative discomfort during extension. Appropriate washers are then placed over the hex nuts and the contoured plate is placed over the washers. Bone graft material is then applied over the transverse processes and facets before the plate is put in place. A tapered hex nut, with the taper facing the plate is then tightened using the nut wrenches or the side-handled wrenches. Locking nuts are then applied and the excess machine-threaded portion is cut off with a cannulated screw cutter. Additional crushed bone graft is applied around the construct (Brantigan, Steffee, Keppler, et al., 1988; Henstorf, Gaines, & Steffee, 1987). Transverse connectors are generally not used if plates are used (Fig. 33-13).

Complications

Potential complications include root injury, dural tears, infection, and bleeding (Davne & Myers, 1992; West, Ogilvie, & Bradford, 1991). The best method of dealing with these complications is avoiding them in the first place. Bleeding is kept to a minimum by the use of meticulous surgical technique using monopolar electrocautery kept at a high setting whenever possible to dissect the muscle away from the bone. Infection is prevented by meticulous aspectic technique, use of plastic adhesive drapes, use of preoperative single-dose broad-spectrum antibiotic, copious irrigation of the wound after every step of the procedure with antibiotic solution, use of multiple-layer closure to avoid dead space, and use of a suction drain to avoid accumulation of blood in the epidural

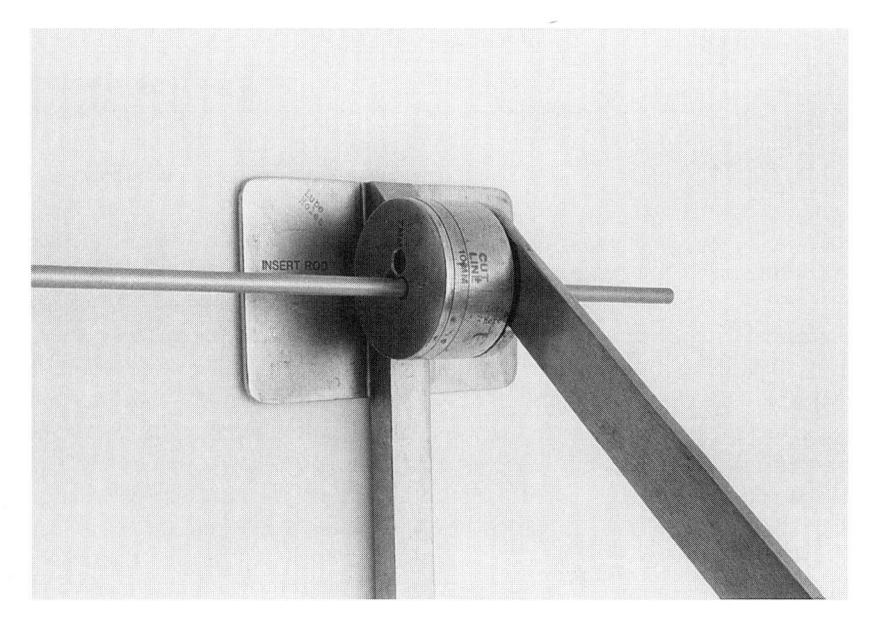

FIG. 33-11. Use of bench-top rod cutter.

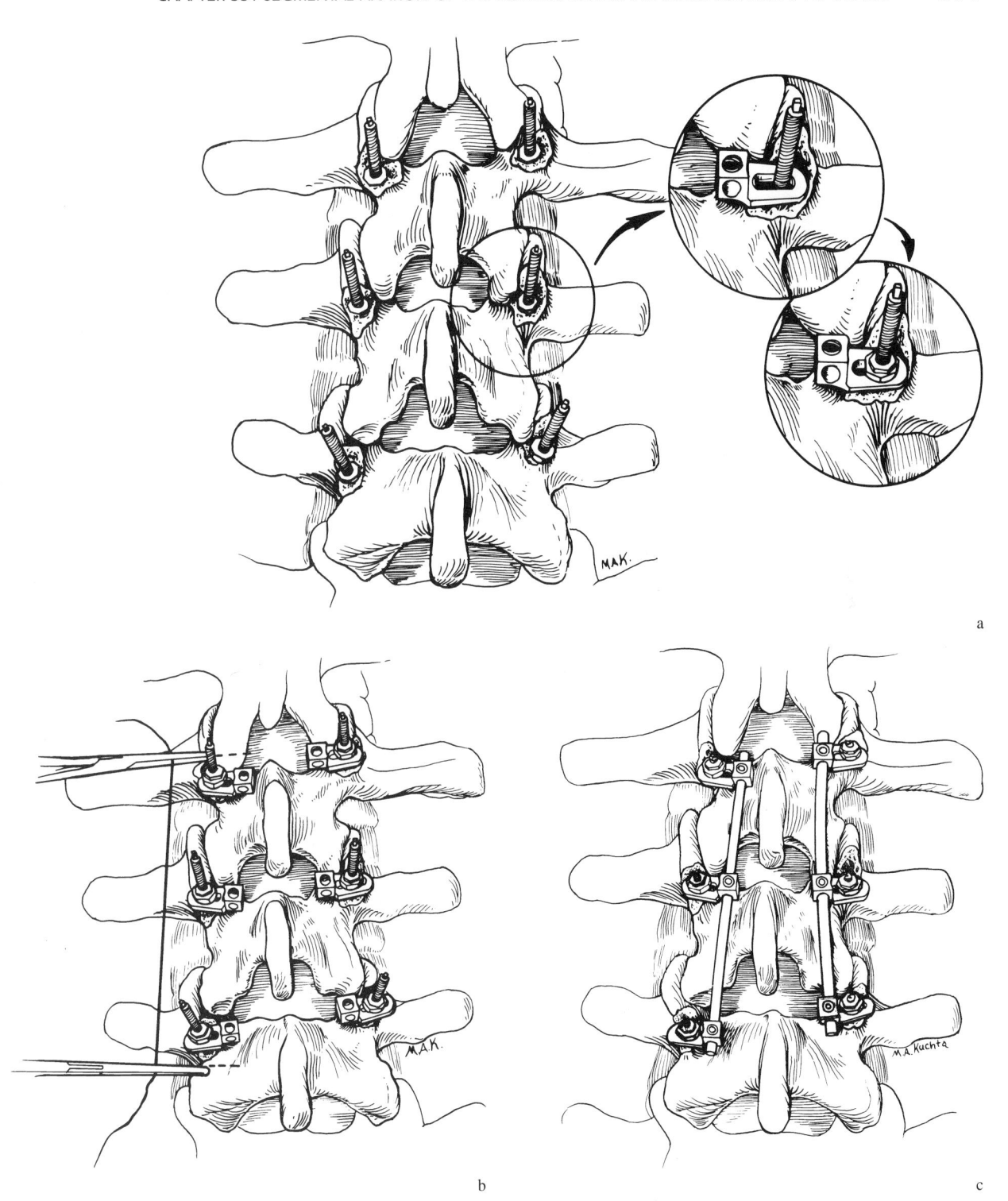

FIG. 33-12. (a) Slotted connectors in place. (b) Rod length is measured. (c) Rod has been threaded through slotted connectors.

and submuscular spaces. Dural tear is prevented by separating the dura from the ligamentum flavum and depressing it with a cotton pledget before using bone instruments. If a tear does occur, it should then be repaired promptly using 4-0 Neuralon. Fibrin glue may be applied, and a spinal drain may be necessary. Every effort must be made to make sure that the pedicle screw is not impinging on the root either medially or inferiorly. If such occurs, the screws should be redirected. It is not prudent to implant hardware in the face of acute infection, but when the infection is under reason-

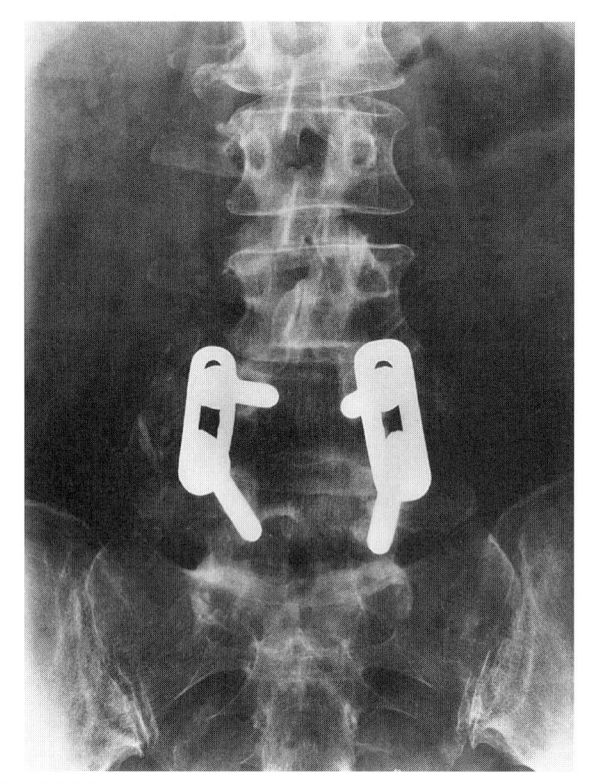

FIG. 33-13. VSP plate construct for lower lumbar fixation.

able control with antibiotics, it is permissible to consider debridement followed by internal stabilization. Appropriate antibiotic therapy should be continued for several weeks to months.

REFERENCES

An, H.S., Vaccaro, A., Colter, J.M., et al. (1991). Low lumbar burst fractures: Comparison among body cast, Harrington rod, Luque rod and Steffee plate. *Spine, 16,* S440–S444.

Asher, M., Carson, W., Heinig, C., et al. (1988). A modular spinal rod linkage system to provide rotational stability. *Spine, 13,* 272–277.

Asher, M.A., Strippgen, W.E., Heinig, C.F., & Carson, W.L. (1992). Isola spinal implant system: principles, design and application. In: H.S. An & J.M. Cotler (Eds.), *Spinal Instrumentation* (pp. 325–351). Baltimore, MD: Williams & Wilkins.

Brantigan, J.W., Steffee, A.D., Keppler, L., et al. (1992). Posterior lumbar interbody fusion technique using the variable screw placement spinal fixation system. *Spine, 6,* 175–200.

Cotrel, Y., Dubousset, J., & Guillaumat, M. (1988). New universal instrumentation for spinal surgery. *Clinical Orthopaedics and Related Research, 227,* 10–23.

Davne, S.H., & Myers, D.L. (1992). Complications of lumbar spinal fusion with transpedicular instrumentation. *Spine, 17,* S184–S189.

Gurwitz, G.S., Dawson, J.M., McNamara, M.J., et al. (1993). Biomechanical analysis of three surgical approaches for lumbar burst fractures using short-segment instrumentation. *Spine, 18,* 977–982.

Henstorf, J.E., Gaines, R.W., & Steffee, A.D. (1987). Transpedicular fixation of spinal disorders with Steffee plates. *Surgical Rounds in Orthopedics,* 35–43.

Sasso, R.C., & Cotler, H.B. (1993). Posterior instrumentation and fusion for unstable fractures and fracture-dislocations of the thoracic and lumbar spine. *Spine, 18,* 450–460.

Steffee, A.D. (1989). The variable screw placement system with posterior lumbar interbody fusion. In: P.M. Lin & K. Gill (Eds.), *Lumbar Interbody Fusion: Principles and Techniques in Spine Surgery* (pp. 81–93). Gaithersburg, MD: Aspen.

Steffee, A.D., & Brantigam, J.W. (1993). The variable screw placement spinal fixation system. *Spine, 19,* 1160–1172.

Weinstein, J.N., Spratt, K.F., Spengler, D., et al. (1988). Spinal pedicle fixation: reliability and validity of roentgenogram-based assessment and surgical factors on successful screw placement. *Spine, 13,* 1012–1018.

West, J.L., Ogilvie, J.W., & Bradford, D.S. (1991). Complications of the variable screw plate pedicle screw fixation. *Spine, 16,* 576–579.

Zindrick, M.R., Wiltse, L.L., Doornick, A., et al. (1987). Analysis of the morphometric characteristics of the thoracic and lumbar pedicles. *Spine, 12,* 160–166.

Zindrick, M.R., Wiltse, L.L., Widell, E.H., et al. (1986). A biomechanical study of intrapedicular screw fixation in the lumbosacral spine. *Clinical Orthopaedics and Related Research, 203,* 99–122.

CHAPTER 34

Fixateur Interne

Ronald W. Lindsey
Markus Rittmeister

HIGHLIGHTS

The fixateur interne (F.I.) was developed in Switzerland in 1984 by Walter Dick as a device for posterior reduction and fixation of the thoracolumbar spine (Dick, 1987; Dick, Kluger, Magerl, Woersdoerfer, & Zach, 1985). The F.I. evolved from the external spine fixation system (ESFS) created by Magerl (1984) as a temporary thoracolumbar spine stabilizing device (Figs. 34-1 and 34-2). However, the protruding external frame of the ESFS was cumbersome and therefore incompatible with the activities of daily living. Dick (1989, 1987) used the same pins but modified the external frame to clamps and threaded longitudinal rods, permitting internal placement of the entire apparatus (Fig. 34-3).

The standard F.I. construct consists of four Schanz screws that are placed bilaterally through the pedicles and into the intact vertebral bodies on either side of a fractured or compromised motion segment. The Schanz screws are connected to threaded longitudinal rods by mobile clamps, which allows for independent reduction and fixation of angular, axial, and rotatory malalignment (Figs. 34-4 and 34-5). On restoration of spinal alignment, the clamps can be fixed to achieve spinal stability over a more limited number of motion segments than with previously employed fixation systems. This extremely versatile implant can be applied in the treatment of a variety of thoracolumbar spine conditions, including fractures, spondylolisthesis, segmental instability, and neoplasms.

The standard for thoracolumbar spine fracture stabilization prior to the F.I. was the Harrington system, which required sublaminar hooks connected by longitudinal ratcheted rods over several normal segments above and below the level of instability to effect reduction and fixation (Dickson, Harrington, & Erwin, 1978). The F.I. achieves a similar effect, yet preserves normal motion segments (Aebi, Etter, Kehl, & Thalgott, 1987; Lindsey, Dick, Nunchuch, & Zach, 1993) (Fig. 34-6). The construct is simple, with only three components. Finally, the F.I. is as much a tool for reduction as a fixation device, permitting independent correction of angular, axial, and rotatory malalignment.

Therefore, the objective of this chapter on the F.I. will be (1) discuss the theory behind its development and technique philosophy, (2) present the implant system and its instrumentation, (3) demonstrate the technique of implantation, reduction and fixation, and (4) review the reported early clinical experience with this device.

THEORY AND DEVELOPMENT PHILOSOPHY

The principles behind the development of the F.I. reflects the progress that has been made in spinal instrumentation for instability, especially as it relates to fractures (Denis, 1983; Holdsworth, 1970). It has been established that the stabilization of unstable spine fractures, with or without neurologic deficit, facilitates rapid patient mobilization and rehabilitation (Dick, 1989; Dickson et al., 1978; Lindsey & Dick, 1991). The Harrington rod instrumentation, originally designed for the treatment of scoliosis, was first adapted for spine fracture fixation (Dickson et al., 1978). However, Harrington fixation requires sublaminar hook placement at the ends of the instrumented segment, long multisegment immobilization, and loss of physiologic lordosis due to its four-point bending reduction maneuver and is unable to

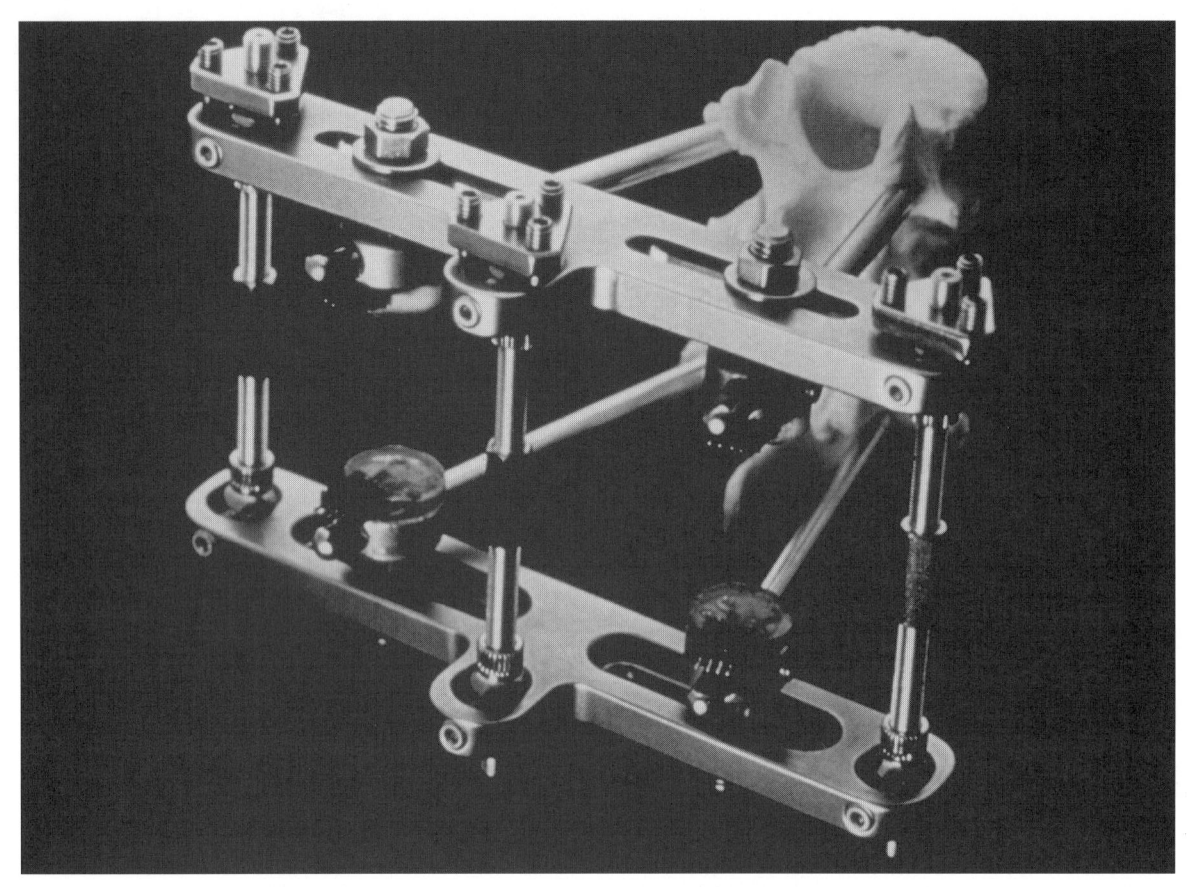

FIG. 34-1. The external spine fixation system (ESFS) design by Magerl to provide temporary thoracolumbar spine stabilization by means of transpedicular fixation.

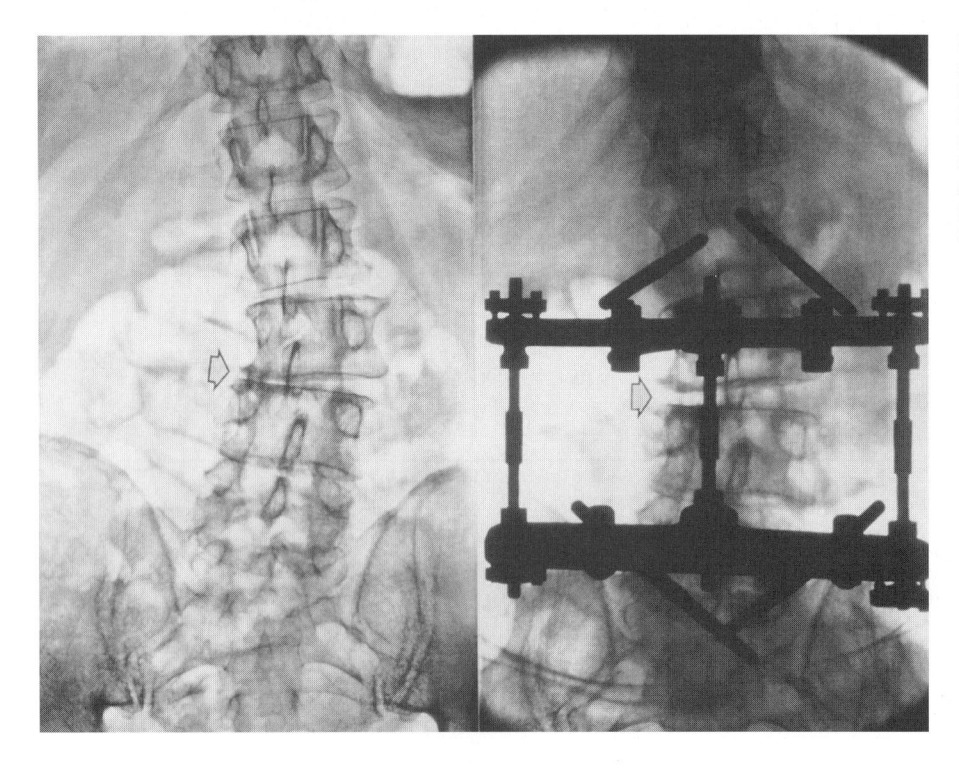

FIG. 34-2. Mid-lumbar degenerative scoliosis in a patient with foraminal stenosis, radiculopathy, and back pains. Following application of the ESFS, the spine is stabilized and the foraminal stenosis has been proved by distraction along the curves' concavity. The patient experienced resolution of both back and leg symptoms.

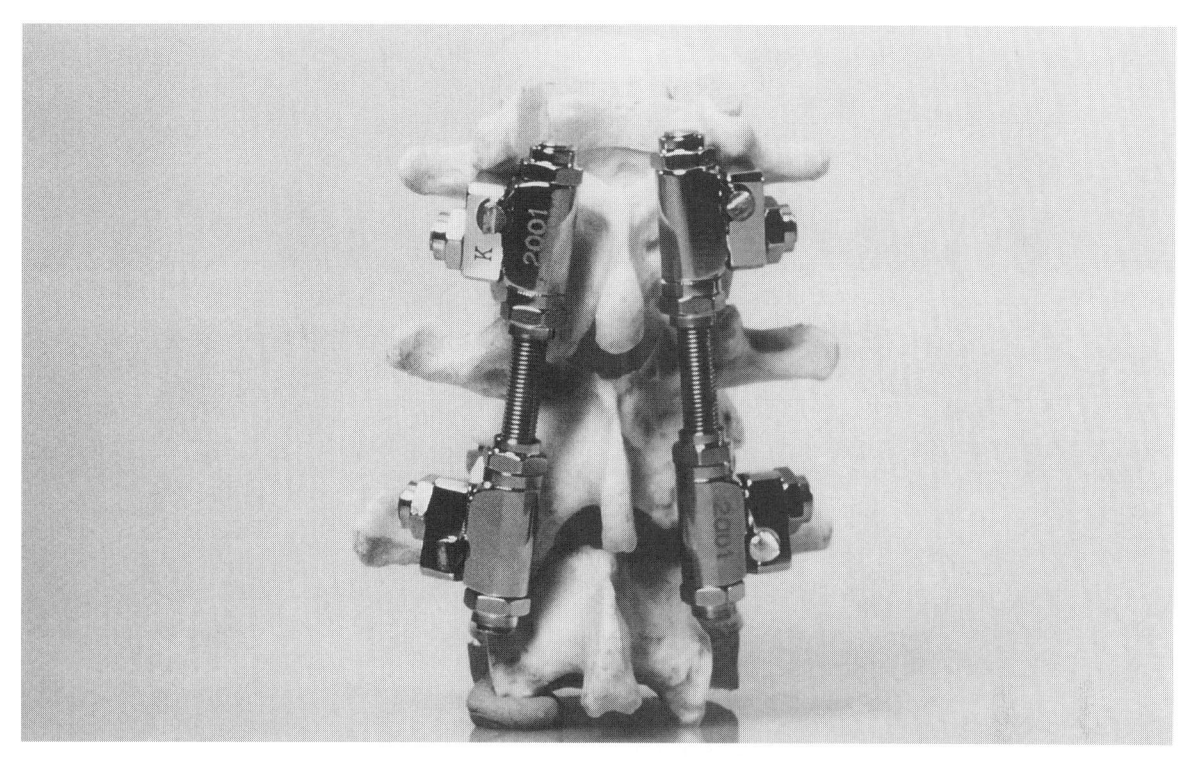

FIG. 34-3. The original fixateur interne, as designed by Dick, employs the same transpedicular fixation Schanz screw as the ESFS, but achieves correction and stability by means of an internal longitudinal connecting apparatus.

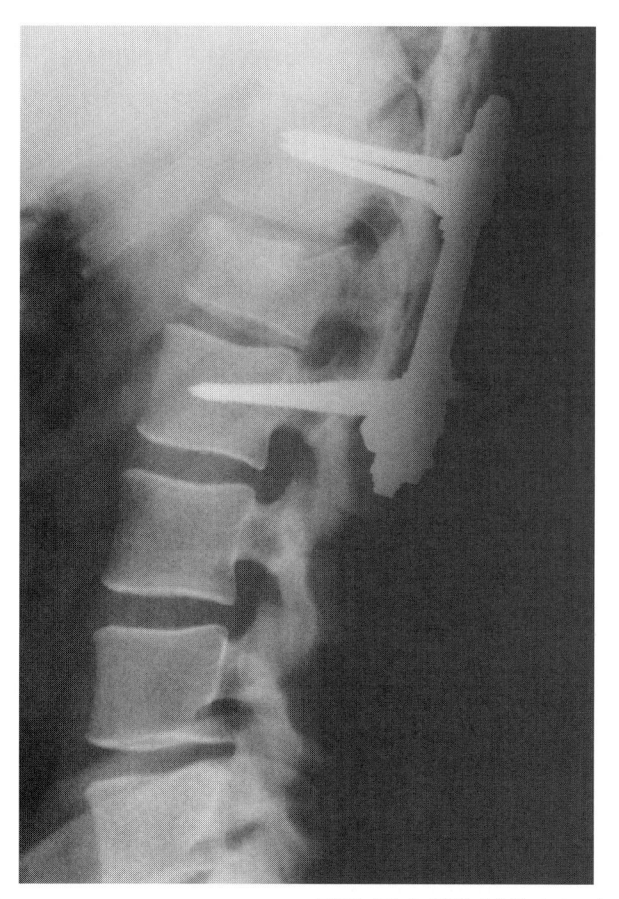

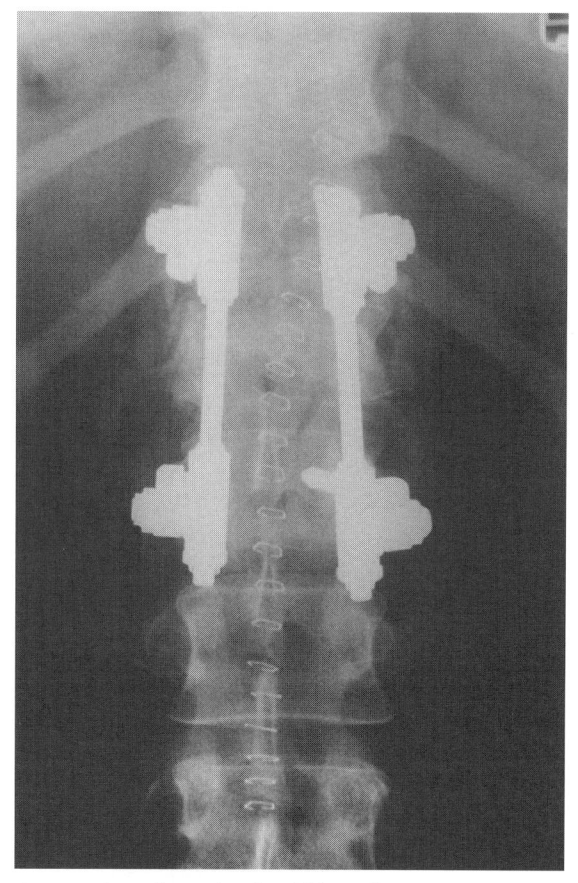

FIGS. 34-4 AND 34-5. Lateral and anterior posterior radiographs of an L1 burst fracture stabilized with the fixateur interne.

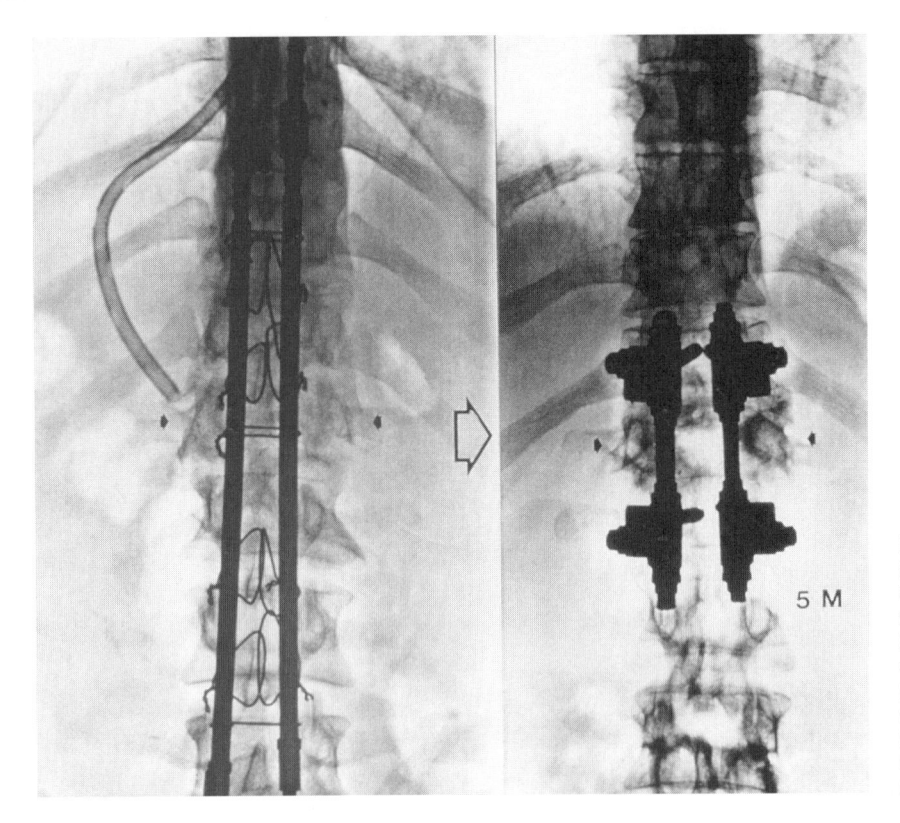

FIG. 34-6. An L1 burst fracture initially stabilized with Harrington rods extending over multiple segments with sublaminar wiring. The patient noted loss of lumbar lordosis and experienced significant limitation of sagittal plane function. At 5 months the patient was converted to the fixateur interne which provided adequate stability yet preserved motion in the uninjured motion segments.

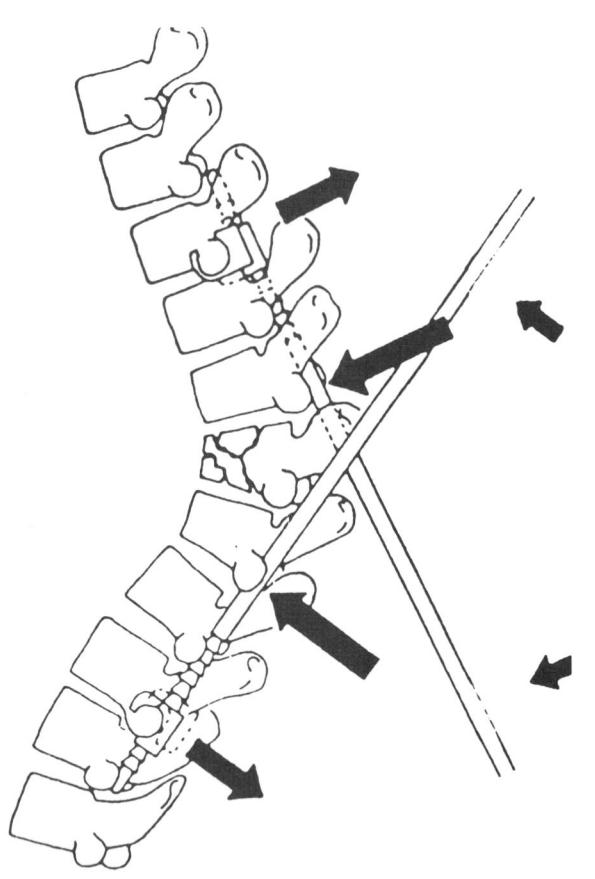

FIG. 34-7. The Harrington rod achieves sagittal plane correction by means of four-point bending which requires instrumentation over several normal segments above and below the injured level to establish an adequate lever for a reduction.

concentrate the corrective forces created at the injured, malaligned segment (Fig. 34-7). Therefore, spinal reduction was often suboptimal, fixation was tenuous, and many normal motion segments were needlessly compromised (Dick, 1987) (Fig. 34-8).

Roy-Camille has been credited with rediscovering the use of the pedicles for three-column spine fixation in 1963 (Roy-Camille, Saillant, Berteaux, & Salgado, 1976). Screws were passed across the posterior elements, through the pedicle, and into the vertebral body, and this mode of fixation has since proven superior to the hooks alone. Based on this principle of transpedicular fixation, Magerl (1984) developed an external fixation device (ESFS) for the treatment of spine fractures in 1977. By attaching an external frame to pins placed in a limited number of vertebral bodies and minimizing the motion segment compromised, he could extrinsically manipulate or realign the spine and maintain reduction until the healing had been achieved. Denis (1983) noted that realignment and stabilization were performed more effectively with the ESFS across all three columns without the need for three-point or four-point fixation. However, the disadvantages of the system included pin tract infections and the bulky, impractical presence of the external apparatus, which significantly limited activities of daily living (Magerl, 1984).

The F.I. as a modification of the Magerl external fixation, also employs long Schanz screws embedded in the pedicles of vertebral bodies adjacent to the unstable segment to restore spinal alignment. After reduction has been achieved, the stabilizing device is entirely implantable, thereby eliminating the bulky ESFS frame while maintaining many of

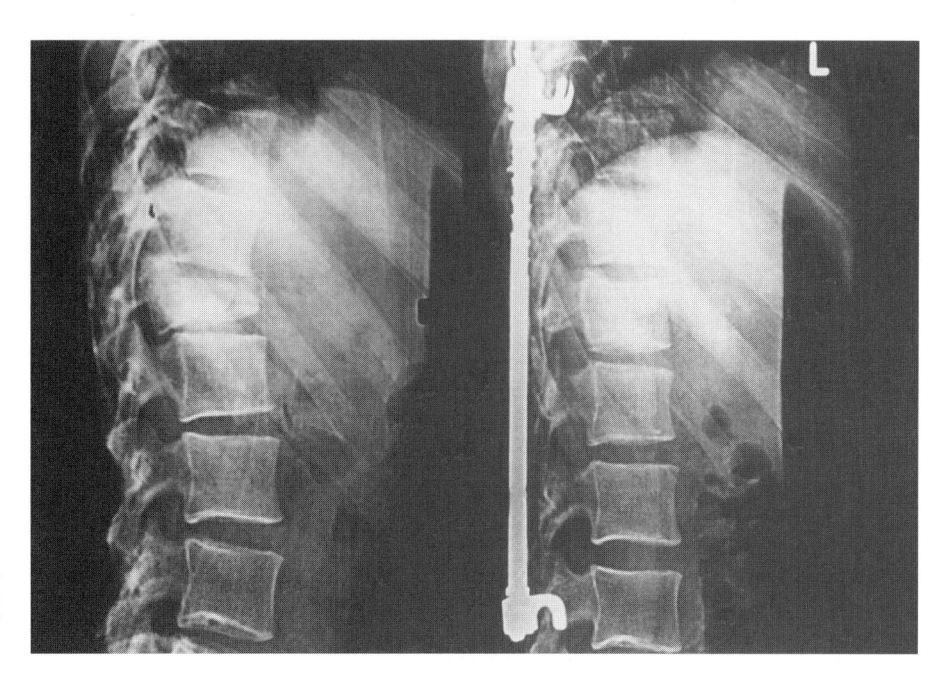

FIG. 34-8. The four-point bending maneuver required to effect with fracture and spinal canal reduction, the Harrington rod often results in loss of normal lumbar lordosis.

its favorable biomechanical features (Dick, 1987) (Figs. 34-9 and 34-10).

In summary, the major advantage of the F.I. concept over previous implants for posterior spinal instrumentation is the short fixation length with minimal compromise of normal motion segments (Aebi et al., 1987; Dick, 1987; Dick et al., 1985; Esses, 1989; Lindsey & Dick, 1991). The benefits of a shorter fixation length were readily appreciated by several authors using the long multisegment Harrington or Luque systems, with subsequent bone grafting for spine fusion limited to a short area about the injured spinal segments (Armstrong, 1976; Casey, Jacobs, & Asher, 1984). Theoretically, the unfused but rodded segments, would remain functional with rod removal. But the "rod long, fuse short" concept would still comprise the transiently stabilized motion segments with facet joint arthrosis and decreased mobility (Kahanovitz, Arnoczky, Levine, & Otis, 1984).

Pedicle screws placement with the F.I. construct has distinct advantages over many plate systems. Screw insertion site and angle are unrestricted and not determined by the position of the plate holes (Krag, Beynnon, Pope, et al., 1986; Marchese, Thalgott, & Aebi, 1991). The F.I., similar to its

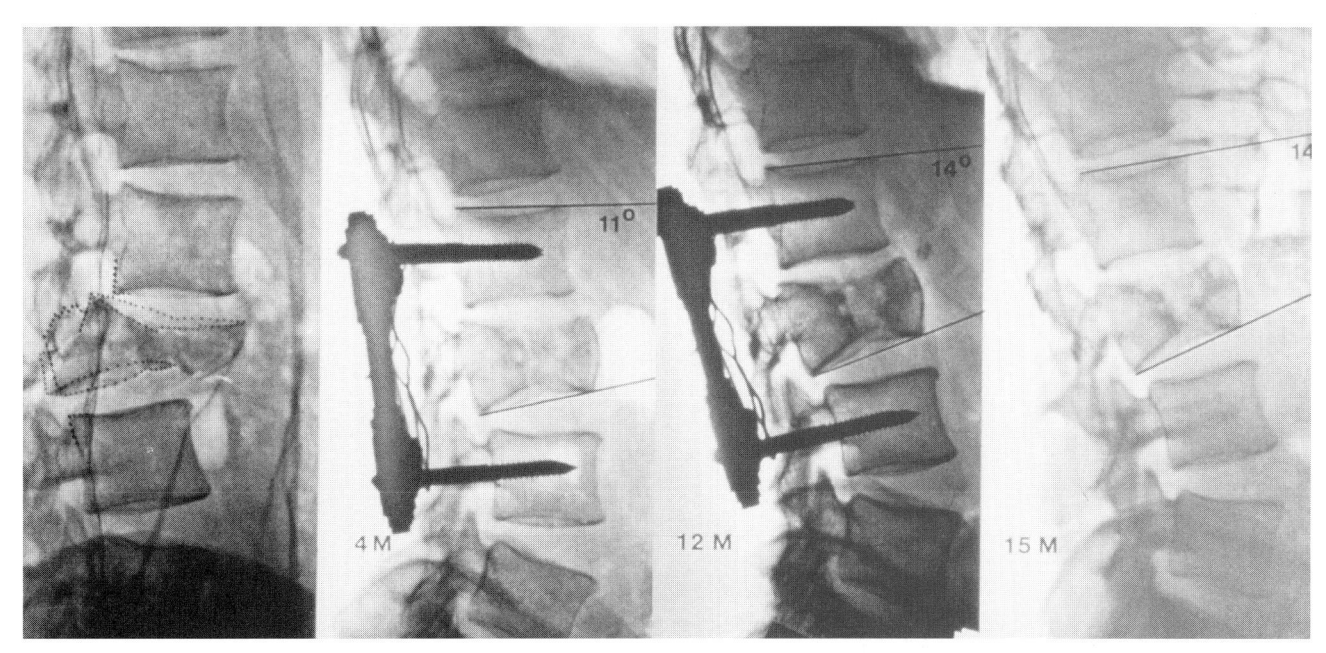

FIG. 34-9. Lumbar burst fracture with significant sagittal plane translation reduced with the fixateur interne, with stability maintained at twelve months and at fifteen months following implant removal.

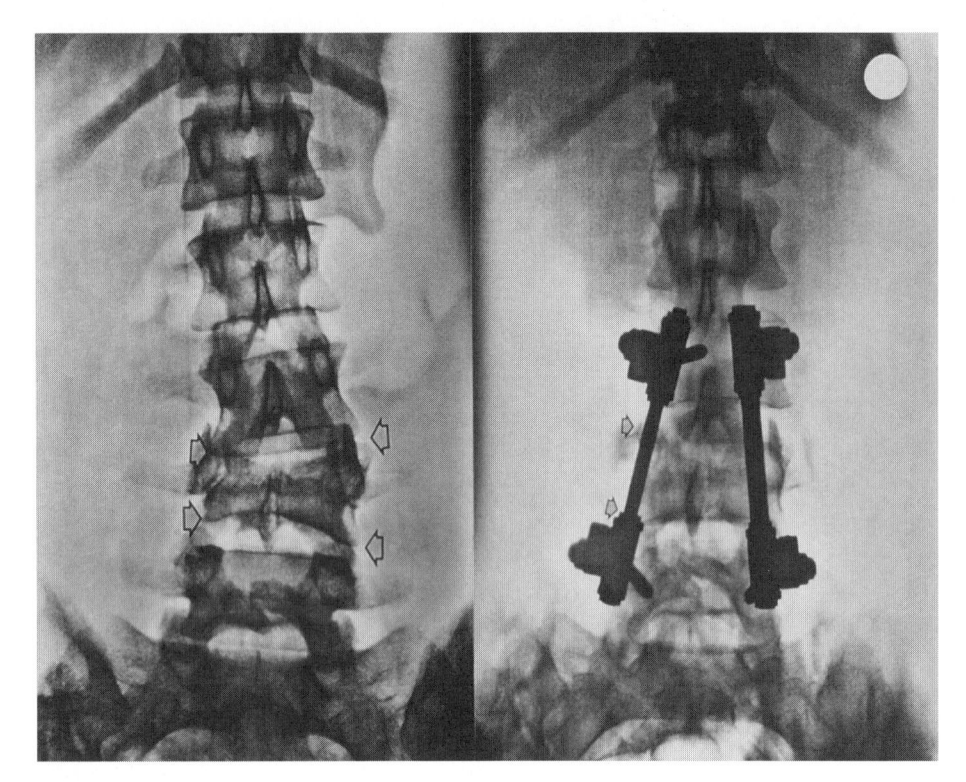

FIG. 34-10. Coronal plane correction of degenerative scoliosis utilizing the fixateur interne.

external fixation counterpart, is considered to be as much a reduction tool as a stabilizing implant (Aebi et al., 1987). This spine manipulation capacity is facilitated by both the pedicle position of the Schanz screws and their long lever arm. Unlike other implant systems (i.e., Harrington hooks, Luque sublaminar wires), the F.I. seeks to avoid penetration of the spinal canal. In this respect, F.I. removal is even safer than its placement, and safer than the removal of the previously noted systems (Nicastro, Traina, Hartjen, & Lancaster, 1984).

Finally, the Dick F.I. is a "fixateur" in the true sense, as stability is provided solely by the implant without relying on intact soft tissue. Loss of reduction due to alteration of the soft-tissue envelope, as with Harrington rod systems, is not a consideration (Dickson et al., 1978).

IMPLANTS AND INSTRUMENTS

The basic F.I. construct consists of symmetrical sets of two Schanz screws placed above and below the compromised spinal segments and connected to a longitudinal rod by a clamp that has axial, rotatory, and angular reduction potential (Dick, 1987) (Figs. 34-11 and 34-12). After obtaining the desired Schanz screw-longitudinal rod orientation, the clamp can be fixed independently to secure final spinal alignment. The original system (Modular Spine System, Synthes, Paoli, PA) was composed of stainless steel and used a threaded rod with a clamp secured by a lateral nut and superior/inferior nuts along the rod (Figs. 34-13 and 34-14). The new F.I. design consists of a titanium alloy with a smooth rod and a less bulky clamp secured by a single top-tightening set screw (Surgical Technique Guide, 1994). Because both systems are available, the authors will present both designs.

In the original F.I., Schanz screws have a 5-mm core diameter, 5- and 6-mm thread diameters, and thread lengths of 25 or 35 mm. Schanz screws lengths are 180 mm (5-mm diameter with either 25- or 35-mm thread) or 145 mm (6.0-mm diameter with 35-mm thread). Schanz screws for the new F.I. have a 5-mm core diameter, with either 6- or 7-mm thread diameters, a 35-mm thread length, and a 180-mm screw length (Fig. 34-15).

The original longitudinal connector was a threaded 7-mm-diameter rod available in lengths of 70, 100, 200, or 300 mm. The new rod is smooth, 6 mm in diameter, with lengths of 50, 75, 100, 125, 150, 200, 250, 300, 350, 400, 450, and 500 mm. The original clamp required superior and inferior washers and nuts to fix its axial and rotational position along the threaded rod. A separate lateral nut could be tightened to fix the Schanz screw to the clamp and control angular reduction (Figs. 34-16 and 34-17). The new clamp controls axial and rotational alignment on a smooth rod with a single set screw, while angular alignment of the Schanz screw is secured with a top-tightening nut (Fig. 34-18). Whereas the original clamp could be compressed or distracted along the threaded rod by tightening or distracting nuts superior and/or inferior to the clamp, the new clamp can be shifted along the smooth rod more rapidly by a device that compresses or distracts against a C-clamp that can be attached to the rod (Fig. 34-19).

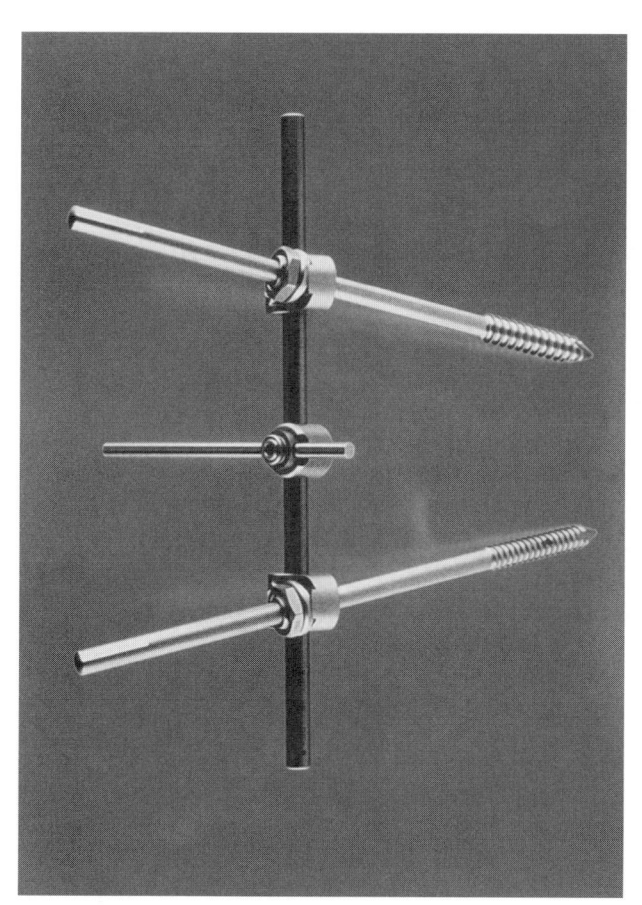

FIG. 34-11. The basic fixateur interne construct consists of a longitudinal rod which captures Shantz screws placed above and below the fractured segment. The clamp of fixing the Shantz screw to the rod has axial, rotatory, and angular reduction abilities which may be employed separately or in unison.

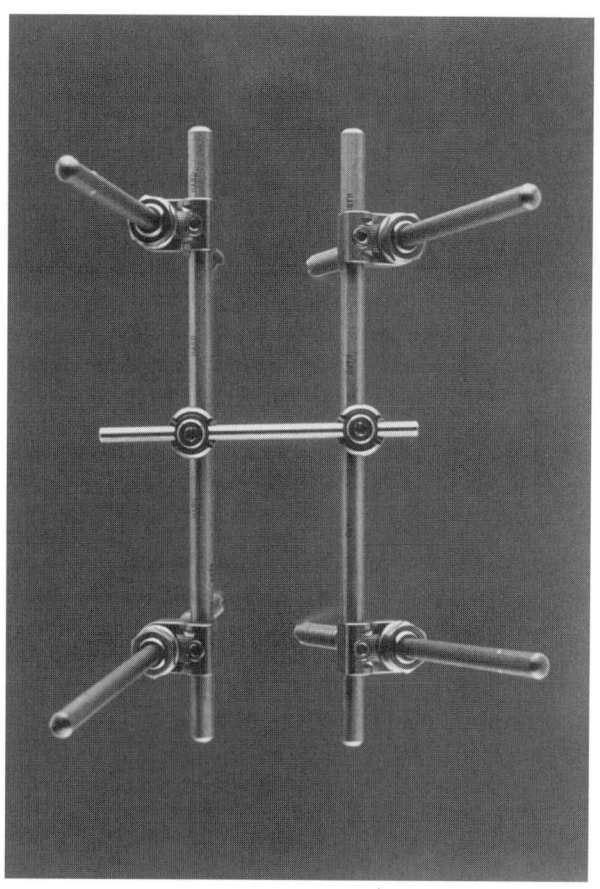

FIG. 34-12. The posterio-anteral view of the fixateur interne construct with cross linking.

FIG. 34-13. The original threaded longitudinal connecting rods for the fixateur interne which allowed controlled distraction and compression.

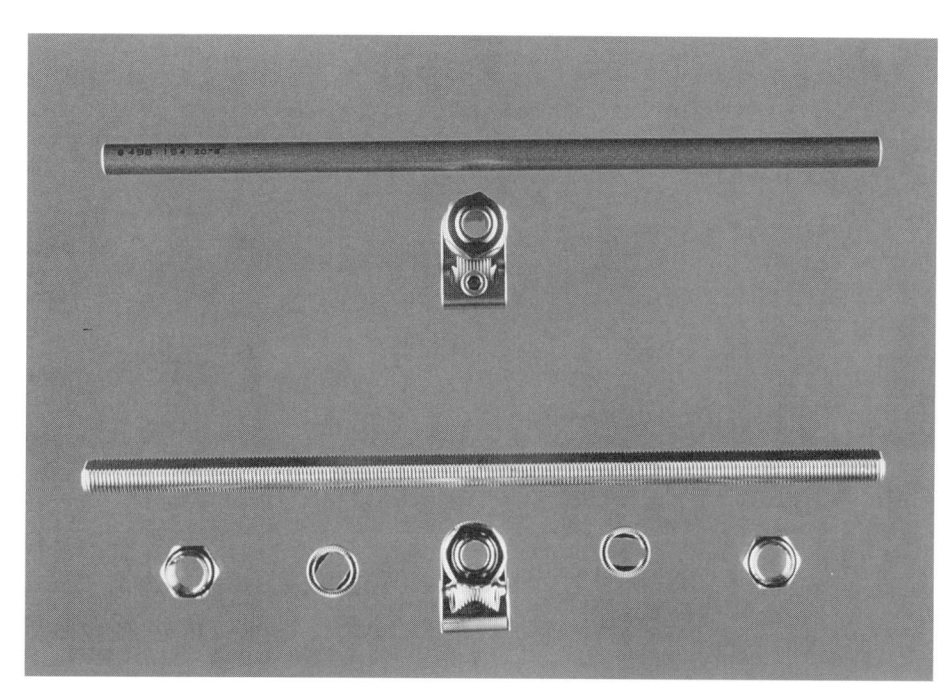

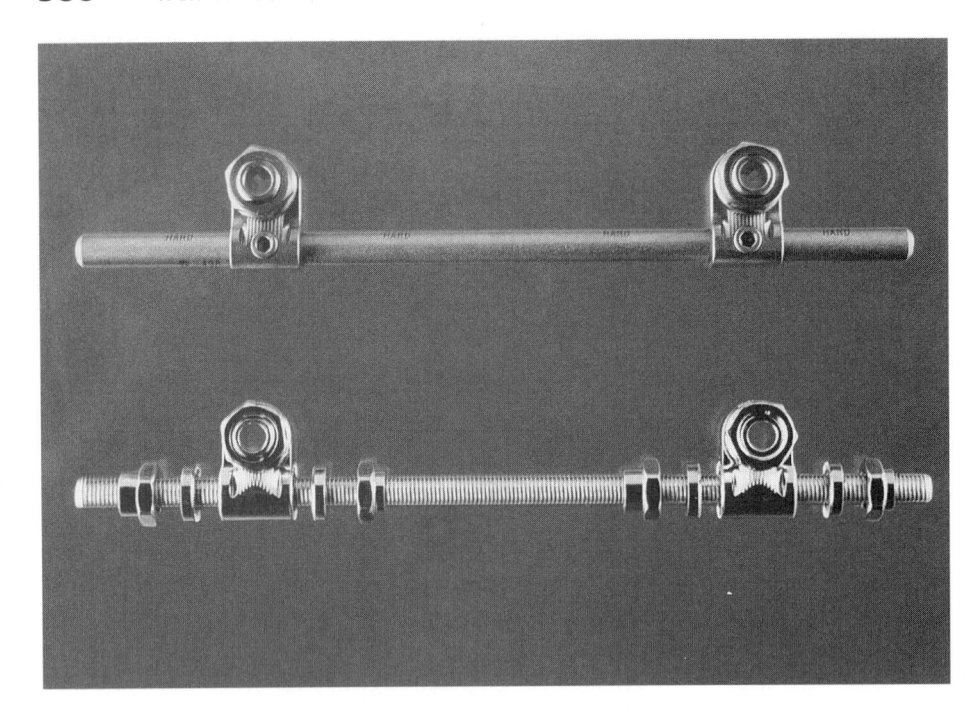

386 PART 4 / POSTERIOR THORACOLUMBAR INSTRUMENTATION

FIG. 34-14. Demonstrates the original and the revised fixateur interne design and their basic design differences.

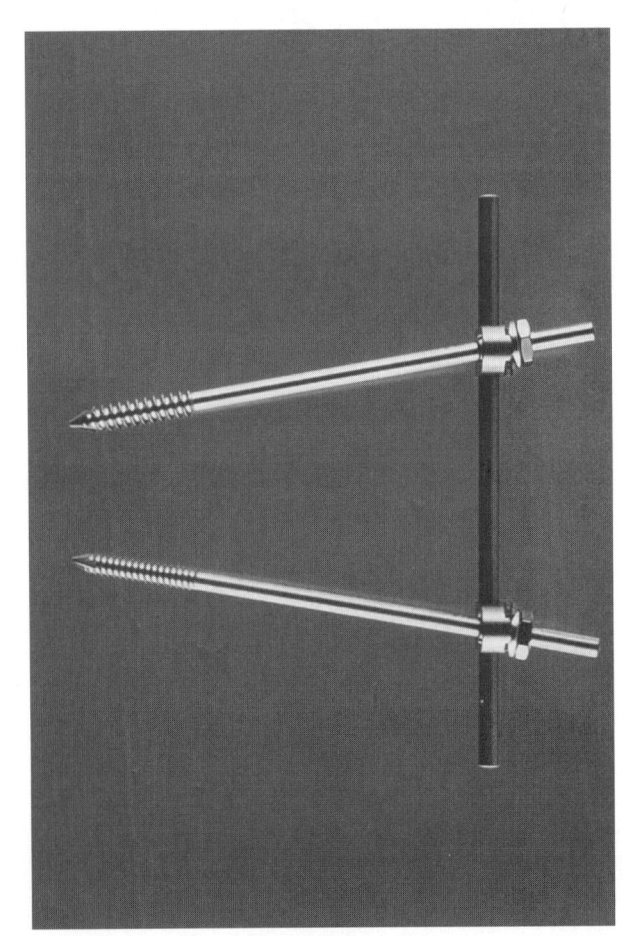

FIG. 34-15. A lateral projection of the longitudinal rod with the revised articulating clamps. This figure also depicts both the 6 mm and 7 mm thread diameters Schanz screws.

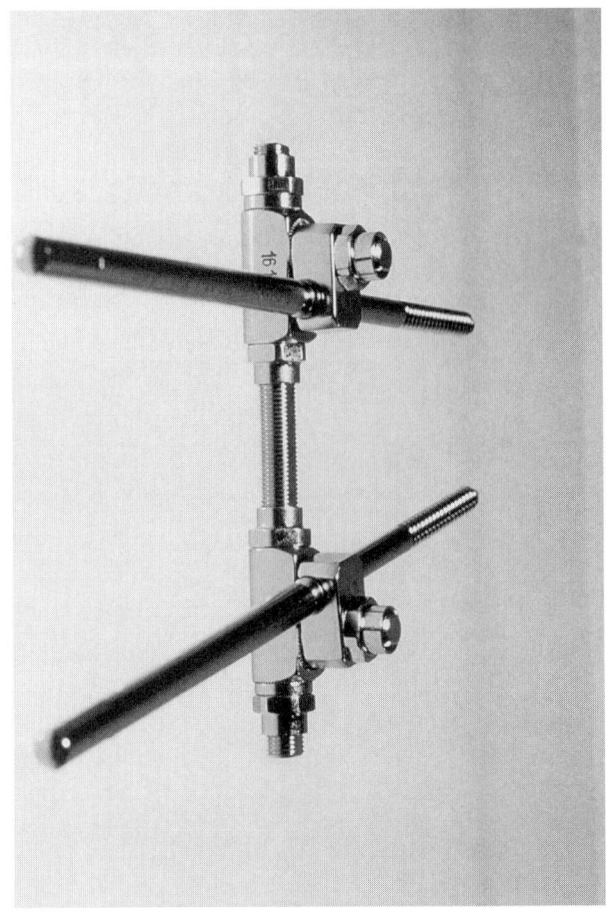

FIG. 34-16. Demonstrates the bulkier nature of the original fixateur interne design which required that the lateral nut in each clamp be tightened before sagittal plane reduction could be maintained.

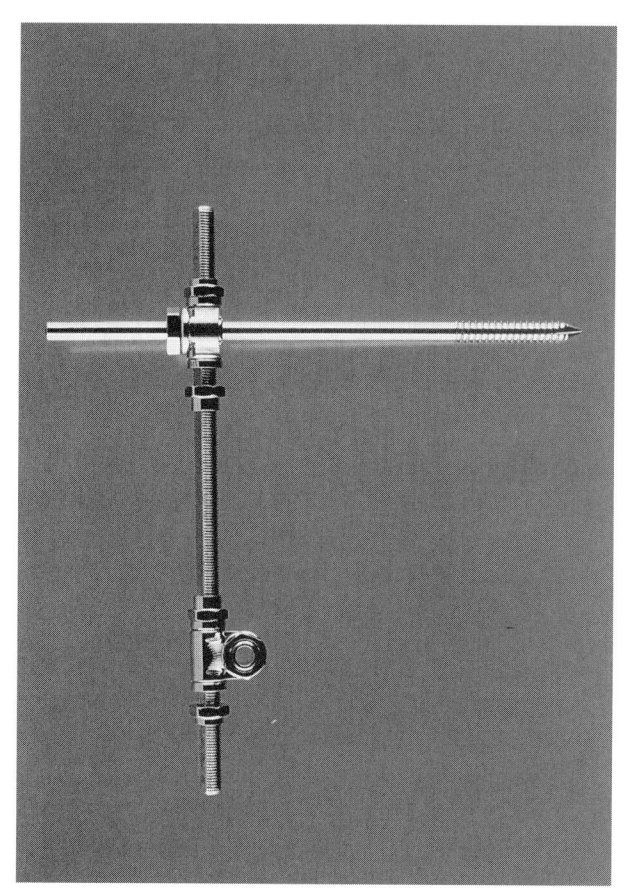

FIG. 34-17. *A lateral and a posterior view of the new fixateur interne clamp which has a single top-tightening nut to control the sagittal alignment of the Schanz screw.*

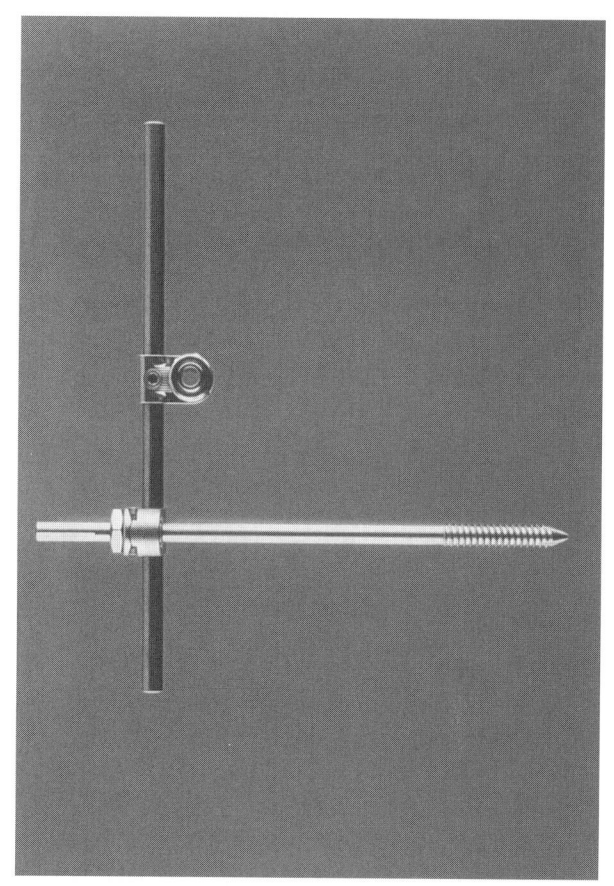

FIG. 34-18. *Another simple clamp design which also controls sagittal plane alignment from a single top tightening nut.*

The materials and dimensions of the components of both the Modular Spine System (original design) and the Universal Spine System (new design) are listed in Fig. 34-19. The instruments necessary for the application of the fixateur interne are depicted in Fig. 34-20 and include an awl, pedicle probe, universal chuck, long small hex screwdriver, cannulated socket wrench, distractor forceps, compressor forceps, rod-holding forceps (6 mm), bar-holding forceps (3.5 mm), bolt cutter head (5 mm long), handle for bolt cutter (13 mm), and handle for bolt cutter (24 mm).

TECHNIQUE OF IMPLANTATION (FRACTURE INSTRUMENTATION)

The F.I. surgical technique demands that the surgeon clearly understands both the normal and pathologic spinal anatomy and the implants and their associated instrumentation. The implant has a significant learning curve and the clinician is advised to perform the necessary maneuvers in vitro prior to actual in vivo utilization (Dick, 1987; Esses, 1989; Gertzbein & Robbins, 1990).

Anteroposterior and lateral plane radiographs will provide essential preoperative information on the type of injury, the spinal level, and the extent of spine malalignment necessary to plan the instrumentation. Computed tomography (CT) of the injured segment and the adjacent vertebral bodies to be instrumented is also a critical aspect of preoperative planning. The CT scan provides even more precise information on the vertebral bodies fractured, pedicle size and orientation, and posterior elements injured. In addition, CT scan data on the nature and extent of canal compromise can assist in planning axial distraction and canal realignment.

The patient should be positioned prone in a standard fashion to perform a posterior surgical exposure to the spine. Chest rolls or a spine frame are employed to allow the chest and abdomen to be free of ventral pressure. The spine is exposed through a posterior midline surgical approach with exposure of the laminae, facets, and transverse processes of the injured segment and in the adjacent segments one level above and below the level of injury. The recommended inferior limits of Schanz screw placement extends to the sacrum, while the superior limit is usually the lower thoracic segment but is most dependent on the size of the patient's pedicle (Dick, 1987; Esses & Bednar, 1991; Krag, Beynnon, Pope, et al., 1986).

Pedicle Anatomy

The pedicle is a tubular bone that connects the anterior and posterior column of the spine at each vertebral segment. On the lateral projection, the pedicle lies in the superior

	Modular Spine System (original)	Universal Spinal System (recent)
RODS: Material	Stainless Steel	Pure Titanium
Surface	Fully threaded	Smooth
Length (mm)	70, 100, 155, 200, 300	50, 75, 100, 125, 150, 200, 250, 300, 350, 400, 450, 500
Diameters (mm)	7	6
SCHANZ SCREWS: Material	Stainless Steel	Aluminum niobium alloy
Length (mm)	145, 180	180
Core Diameter (mm)	5	5
Thread diameter/ thread length/ screw length (mm)	5 / 25 / 180 5 / 35 / 180 6 / 35 / 145	6 / 25 / 180 7 / 35 / 180
CLAMPS: Design	Clamp with posterior nut, clamp with lateral nut, nut for 7mm threaded rod, washer for 7mm threaded rod	Clamp with posterior nut and top tightening set screw

FIG. 34-19. The table demonstrates the design and inventory differences between the modular spine system (original) and the universal spinal system (recent).

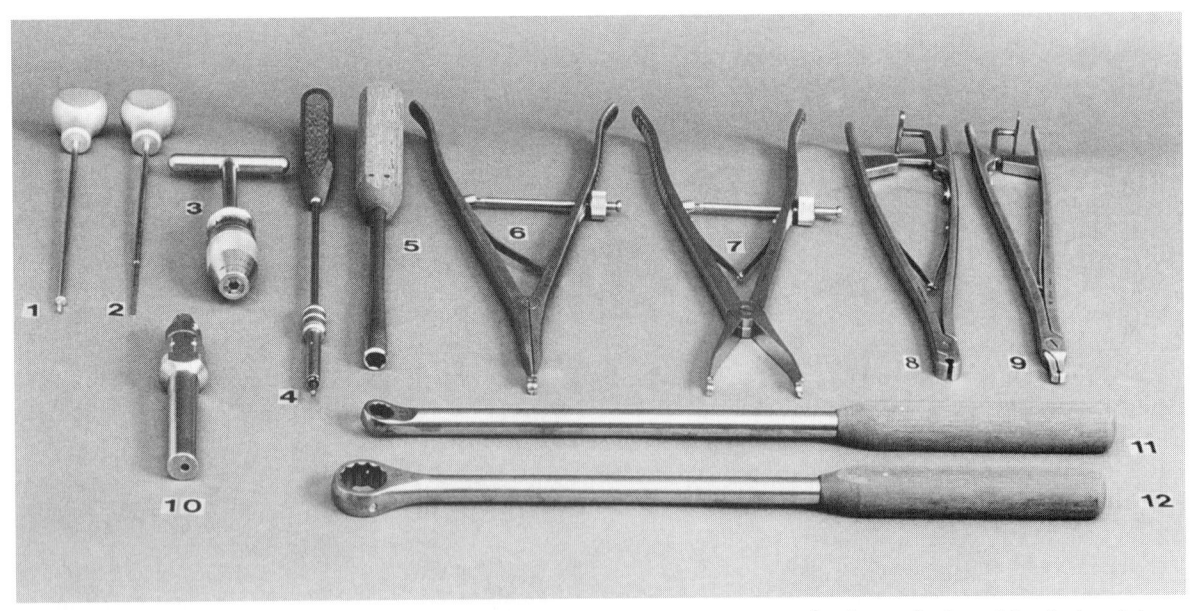

FIG. 34-20. The instruments necessary for the application of the fixateur interne.

one third of the vertebral body and on the anteroposterior (AP) radiographs it is in the superior lateral aspect of the body. It is oval in shape, with the vertical diameter greater than the horizontal diameter. At the first lumbar vertebra this vertical diameter is generally about 7 mm, while at L5 it is approximately 10 mm (Esses & Bednar, 1991). Krag et al. (1986) studied pedicle morphometry and rarely encountered pedicle diameters less than 5 mm below T10, with most being greater than or equal to 8 mm. In the axial projection, the pedicle is oriented directly sagittal in the thoracic spine, with progressively increasing convergence up to 20 to 30 degrees at L5. Pertinent anatomic structures to be avoided lie medial to the pedicle (the spinal canal and the dural sac) and inferior to the pedicle (the nerve root in the intervertebral foramen). The nerve root lies in the superior aspect of the invertebral foramen, often immediately adjacent to the inferior pedicle and is particularly susceptible to perforation.

Localization of the Pedicle

Several techniques have been recommended for pedicle localization, and all require both a radiographic and a clinical appreciation of the pedicle and spine anatomy. In the lateral projection, imaging permits proper screw drill starting position and orientation. To a lesser extent, AP images can assist in pedicle localization, but is possible only with a radiolucent operating room table or frame, progressively increasing obliquity of the x-ray beam in the lumbar spine as pedicle convergence increases, and high-quality imaging equipment (Fig. 34-21). A reasonable estimate of the convergence and subsequent beam obliquity needed can be determined on preoperative CT scans.

The most reliable techniques for frontal plane screw positions/orientation are (1) the intersection technique, in which the entry point for the Schanz screw is the intersection of two lines representing the midline of the transverse process extending lateral to medial and the lateral border of the upper facet extending cephalad to caudal; (2) the pars technique, in which the pars is described as the region of bone at the junction of the pedicle with the lamina. This junction can be decorticated and the presence of bleeding bone will assist in localizing the pedicle; or (3) the accessory process technique, involving the small bony prominence at the base of the transverse process. This process is the most lateral of all the starting points and would dictate that a convergent path be taken to secure fixation of the pedicle. Regardless of which technique is selected by the surgeon, it is important to appreciate that optimal Schanz screw placement requires screw convergence (Dick, 1987; Esses, 1989; Gertzbein & Robbins, 1990; Krag et al., 1986) (Fig. 34-22).

Once the entry point of the pedicle screw has been localized, the overlying cortical bone can be flattened with a rongeur. A blunt probe is placed over the entry site and manually inserted while converging up to 15 degrees. It is important to feel some resistance, suggesting bony contact, at all times. The probe is removed and the pilot hole sounded with a K-wire. If the K-wire plunges without an end point, the tract is likely to be out of the pedicle. If bone can be palpated throughout the tract, the K-wire is advanced parallel to the end plates. Once the K-wires have been positioned in pairs cephalad as well as caudal to the site of injury the result is checked with image intensification. The acceptable entry point is then drilled 1 cm deep using a 3.2-mm drill, and the Schanz screws manually are inserted without tapping. The Schanz screw is advanced into the vertebral body at least half of the lateral body width but not to exceed 80 percent (Krag et al., 1986) (Fig. 34-23). Krag et al. demonstrated that a screw depth of 80% versus 50% of the lateral body width improves pullout strength by approximately 33%. However, Krag et al. also noted that, depending on the convergence of the screw and the contour of the anterior vertebral-body cortex, reliable screw placement

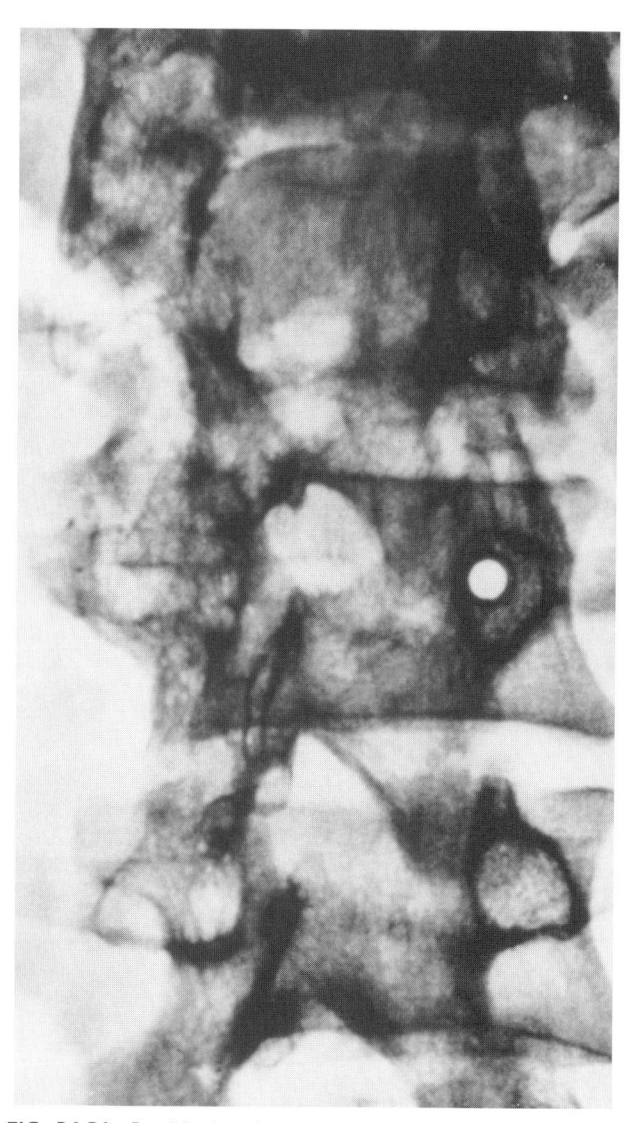

FIG. 34-21. By obliquing the x-ray beam from the sagittal plane toward the pedicle being targeted out of the sagittal plane and an excellent end on view of the pedicle is obtained. Note the "bulls-eye" pilot hole still visible following removal of a Schanz screw.

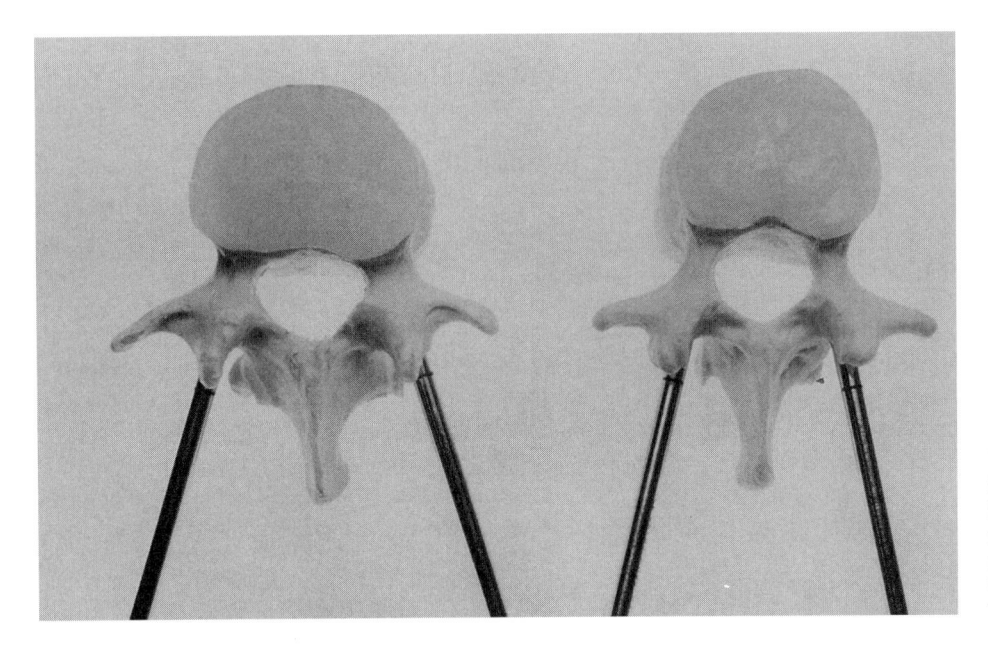

FIG. 34-22. Axial projection of saw bones instrumented with Schanz screws demonstrates the difference in pedicle size and convergence between the lumbar spine (on the left) and the thoracic spine (right).

without anterior cortex perforation can be achieved only up to 50% of lateral vertebral-body width. Therefore, depending on the convergence and body contour, the surgeon may feel more comfortable with extending purchase beyond 50% but should not exceed 80%. It is important to appreciate that Schanz screw perforation of the anterior cortex may not be easily felt by the surgeon.

Once Schanz screw placement is complete, bilateral longitudinal rods are positioned medial to the Schanz screws just adjacent to the spinous processes. The rods are connected to the Schanz screws by mobile clamps, which are not secured until reduction has been completed. Following this assembly, the reduction maneuver consists of independent correction of kyphosis and vertebral height and canal clearing. Kyphosis correction is accomplished first by approximating the dorsal ends of the Schanz screws (Fig. 34-24). The nuts securing the Schanz screws are tightened to secure a stable sagittal angle between the Schanz screws and the rods (Fig. 34-25). Next, the clamp and Schanz screw are distracted along the rod until the fractured body vertebral height is reconstituted (Fig. 34-26). The nuts securing the clamp to the rod are then tightened to stabilize both rotation and distraction (Fig. 34-27). The ends of the Schanz screws are then cut flush with the clamp using the bolt cutter (Fig. 34-28). Because of the enormous distraction loads that can be applied, it is important to emphasize that a distraction end point is often not easily appreciated, especially in situations in which the anterior longitudinal ligament is disrupted. As both the original modular version of the F.I. as well as the updated design are available for clinical use, their differences in technique of implantation are outlined below:

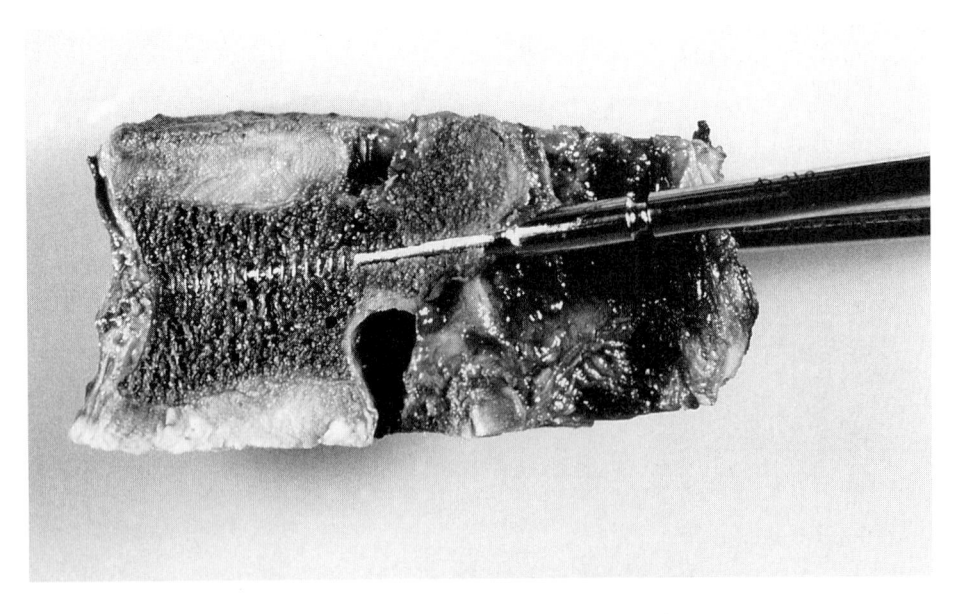

FIG. 34-23. This sagittally cut cadaver spinal segment demonstrates the proper placement of the Schanz screw from the lateral projection (i.e. adequate depth without anterior cortex perforation).

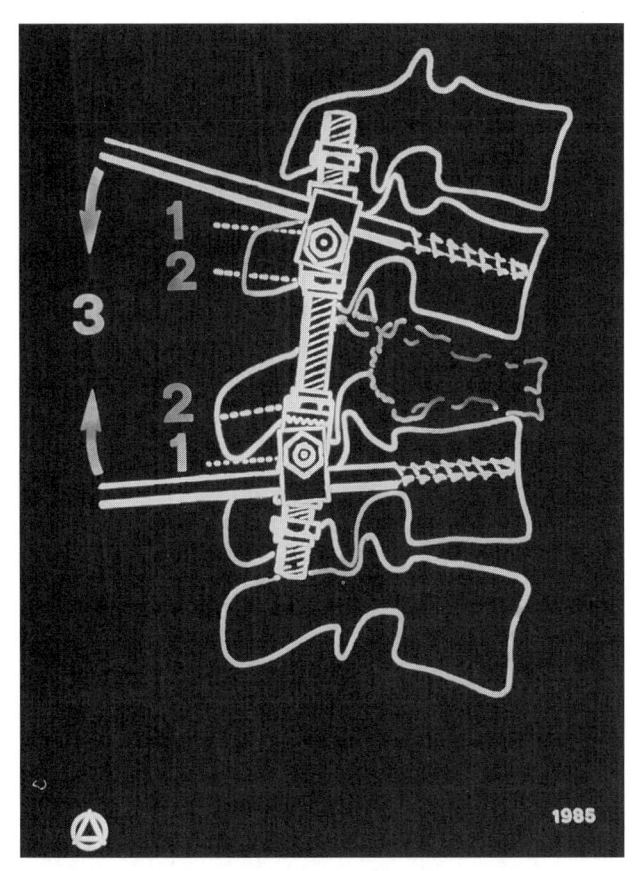

FIG. 34-24. To effect reduction, the Shanz screw rotates through the articulating clamp (1), which is supported by a distracting nut (2). Correction is initiated by approximating the posterior ends of the Schanz screws (3) to achieve sagittal plane correction.

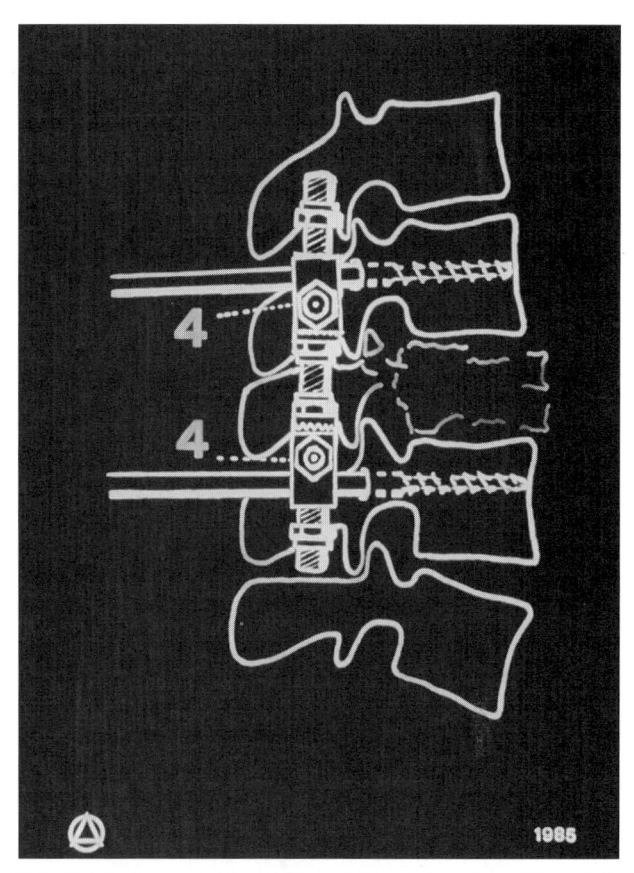

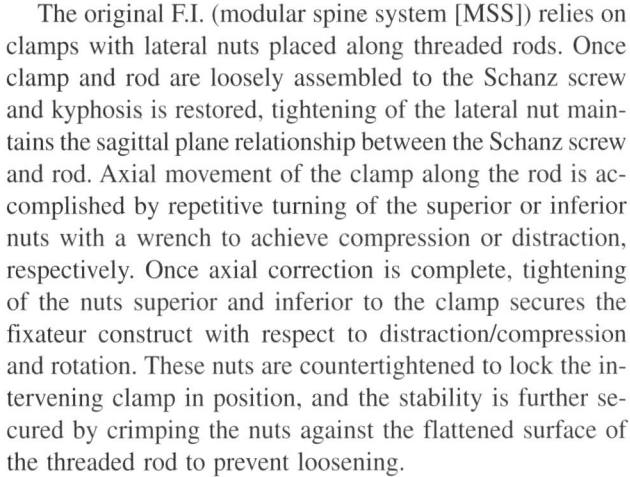

FIG. 34-25. The nuts lateral to the original design clamp (4) are tightened to secure sagittal plane correction.

The original F.I. (modular spine system [MSS]) relies on clamps with lateral nuts placed along threaded rods. Once clamp and rod are loosely assembled to the Schanz screw and kyphosis is restored, tightening of the lateral nut maintains the sagittal plane relationship between the Schanz screw and rod. Axial movement of the clamp along the rod is accomplished by repetitive turning of the superior or inferior nuts with a wrench to achieve compression or distraction, respectively. Once axial correction is complete, tightening of the nuts superior and inferior to the clamp secures the fixateur construct with respect to distraction/compression and rotation. These nuts are countertightened to lock the intervening clamp in position, and the stability is further secured by crimping the nuts against the flattened surface of the threaded rod to prevent loosening.

The newer F.I. design (universal spinal system [USS]) also facilitates the reduction maneuver as well as securing the spine stability. Again, a stable angle between Schanz screw and rod is provided first by tightening the top nut. The new rod is smooth, and superior and interior nuts have been eliminated in favor of a single top-tightening set screw. Specially designed distraction/compression forceps are applied along the smooth rod laterally and medially to the clamps (Figs. 34-29 and 34-30). Axial manipulation is effected by sliding the clamp along the smooth rod, substituting for the fiddle factor associated with the original implant.

Placement of the single top-tightening set screw secures rotation and distraction without countertightening or crimping superior and inferior nuts.

Patients can be mobilized immediately and, although the implant is stable itself, a light orthosis is usually recommended on mobilization of the patient (Dick, 1987; Lindsey & Dick, 1991). The orthosis is generally applied to support the muscles and soft tissue, not to assist with spinal alignment or stability. As minimal motion segments are compromised, more spinal motion can be recovered quite early. In general, paraplegic patients are able to sit in a wheelchair by 2 weeks, while neurologically intact patients can be ambulatory by day five. For select extremely stable fractures (i.e., the fixateur interne used in a tension band mode for a Chance fracture) postoperative external support is not essential (Dick, 1987).

BIOMECHANICAL ANALYSIS

The stability characteristics of the original fixateur interne (MSS) have been established in several in vitro studies (Dick,

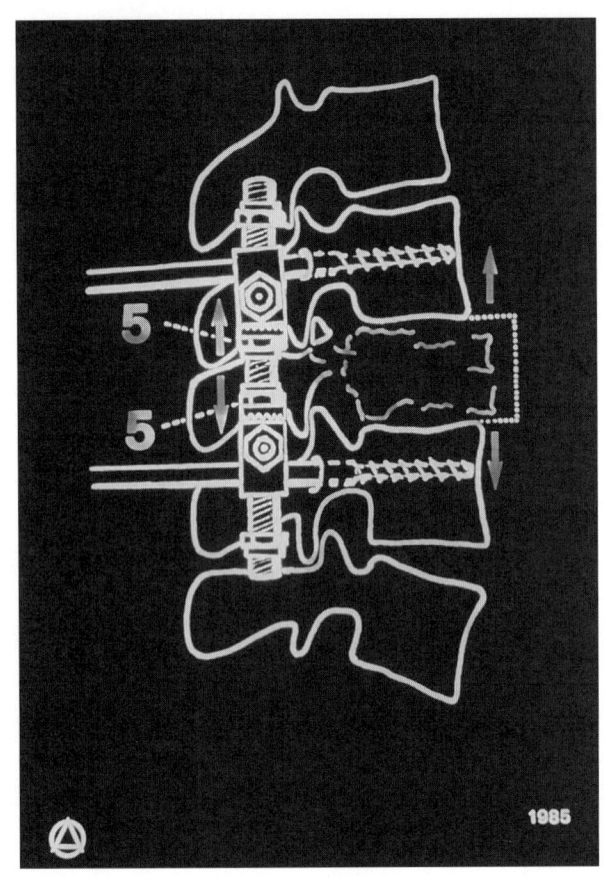

FIG. 34-26. The innermost nuts (5); (original design) are then tightened against their adjacent clamps to effect distraction and reconstitute vertebral body height.

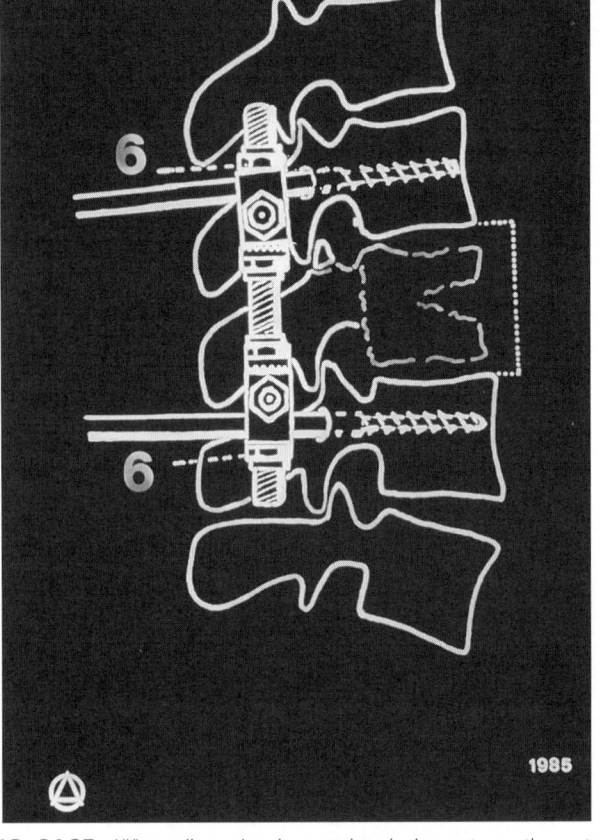

FIG. 34-27. When distraction is completed, the nuts on the outer aspect of the clamp (6) are tightened to stabilize both rotation and distraction.

1989; Dick, Woersdoerfer, & Magerl, 1985; Nolte, Steffen, Kramer, & Jergas, 1993; Panjabi, Abumi, Duranceau, & Crisco, 1988). Dick et al. attached the F.I. to polyethylene blocks to which axial and bending loading forces were applied. Loads up to 40 N were obtained in anterior bending and produced only elastic deformation. At 40-N loads the Schanz screw tips demonstrated linear deflection of up to 5 mm. Plastic deformation of the device occurred with loads greater than 40 N up to 70 N, resulting in a permanent linear deflection of 3 mm of the screw tips at 70 N. Despite the slight plastic deformation of the Schanz screws with excessive loads, disassembly of the clamp and its hinges did not occur (Dick et al., 1985). Excessive nonphysiologic loading, however will cause resorption of the cancellous bone around the Schanz screws. Therefore, the ultimate limiting factor in maintaining stability is postulated to be the bone purchase and quality, not the implant (Dick, Woersdoerfer, & Magerl, 1985) (Fig. 34-31).

Further in vitro biomechanical testing of the F.I. was performed on human cadaver spines destabilized anteriorly and posteriorly. Using historical controls, the F.I. proved superior to the Harrington rod system in withstanding bending moments. Two of the seven spines tested demonstrated migration of the Schanz screw within cancellous bone at 12 N and 20 N, respectively; however, this was thought to be due to the osteoporotic nature of the specimens, which had a mean age of 78 years. In vitro testing of a younger fresh spine in anterior bending up to a load of 47 N demonstrated elastic deformation of the instrumentation without screw migration within cancellous bone (Dick, Woersdoerfer, & Magerl, 1985).

In vitro three-dimensional testing of the Harrington instrumentation in combination load application has only demonstrated acceptable stability in flexion and extension, with less stability in lateral bending or rotation (Panjabi et al., 1988). However, three-dimensional stability was noted with the F.I. (Dick, 1987). In a separate F.I. in vitro model, L2-4 instrumented spines demonstrated good stability in flexion and lateral bending forces, while only moderate stability was established with rotational loads (Nolte, Steffen, Kramer, & Jergas, 1993).

INDICATIONS/CLINICAL FOLLOW-UP DATA/COMPLICATIONS

The F.I. has been widely used for more than a decade by a number of surgeons and institutions who have reported generally favorable results (Aebi et al., 1987; Dick, 1987; Esses,

Table 34-1
Indications and Contraindications for Use of the Fixateur Interne

Indications
  Fractures
  Spondylolisthesis
  Segmental instability
  Tumors

Contraindications
  Infections
  Osteoporosis
  Neoplasm within instrumented segment
  Morbid obesity

1989; Lindsey & Dick, 1991; Marchese et al., 1991) (Table 34-1). The largest reported clinical experience has been in fracture management in which the reduction potential of the implant of both kyphosis and canal compromise has been repeatedly emphasized (Aebi et al., 1987; Dick, 1987) (Fig. 34-32). Most of the problems or complications noted were technical and usually due to poor pedicle screw placement or nut loosening due to improper tightening (Aebi et al., 1987; Esses, 1989). Mechanical failure has occurred predominantly with Schanz screw bending or breakage in patients with significant loss of anterior or middle spinal column support (Dick, 1989; Esses, 1989).

The applications for the F.I. in the spine are numerous, and especially include all situations best addressed with spine manipulation, reduction, and stability over limited segments (Dick, 1989, 1987; Esses, 1989; Marchese et al., 1991; Ye, 1993). The most prevalent diagnosis to meet this criteria would be acute fractures of the thoracolumbar and lumbar spine. Congenital or degenerative segment instability or malalignment (i.e., spondylolisthesis) can also be managed with the F.I. Finally, late posttraumatic instability or

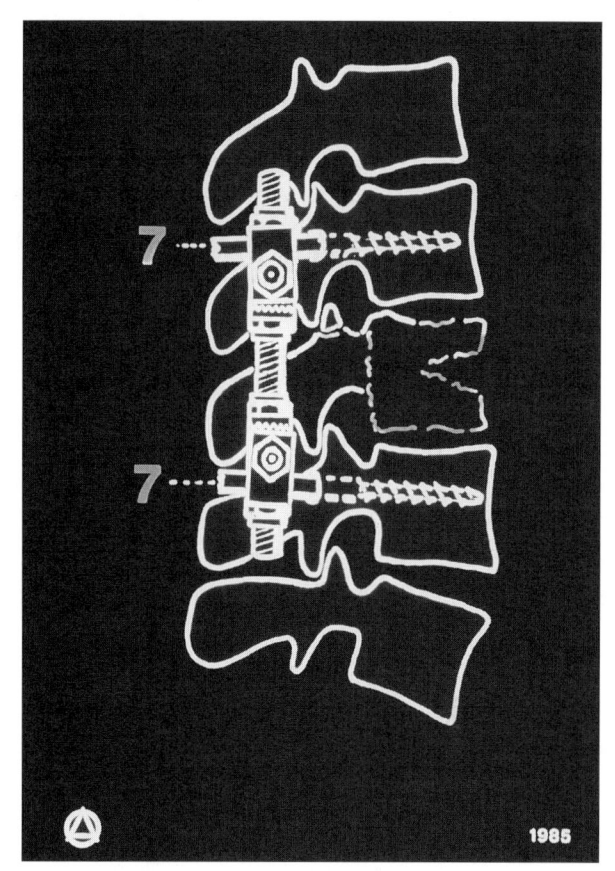

FIG. 34-28. The excess Schanz screw ends are cut (7) with a special resecting instrument.

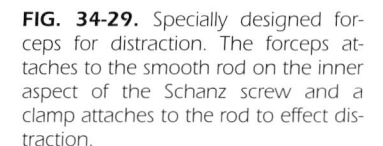

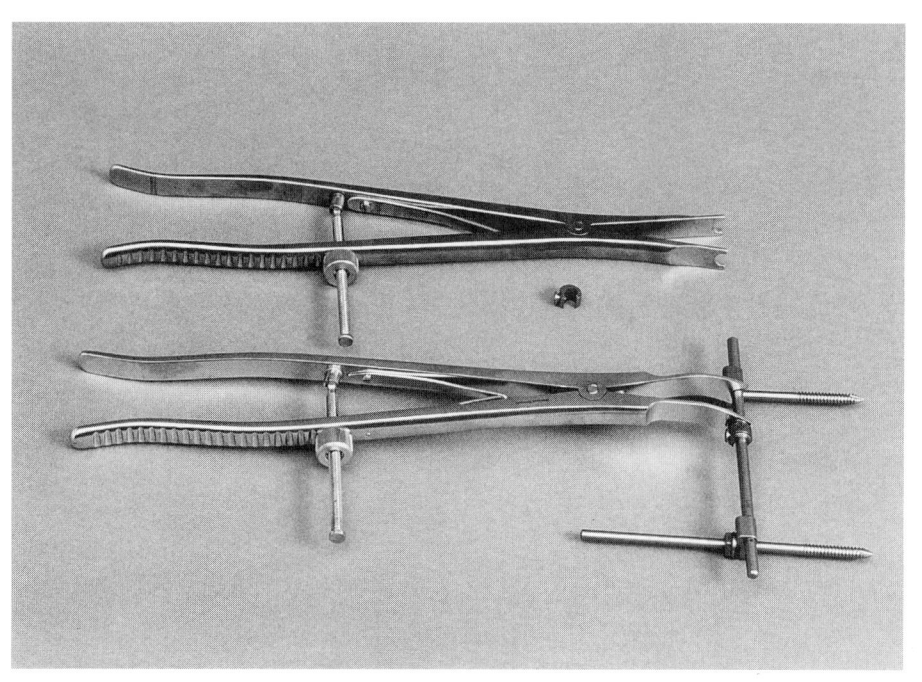

FIG. 34-29. Specially designed forceps for distraction. The forceps attaches to the smooth rod on the inner aspect of the Schanz screw and a clamp attaches to the rod to effect distraction.

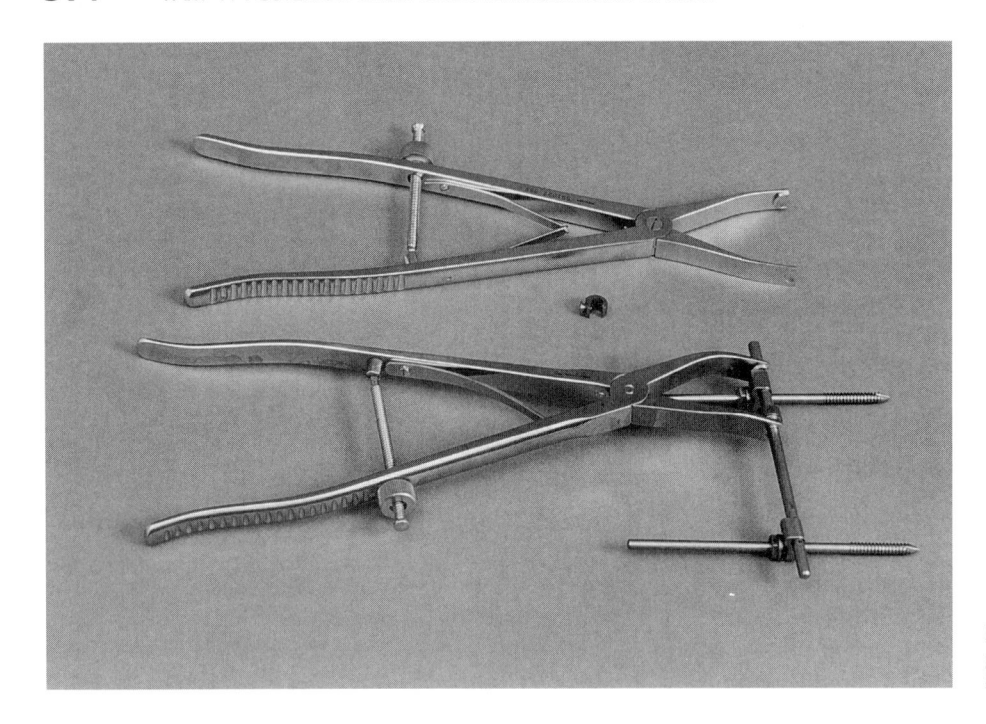

FIG. 34-30. Compression forceps are placed lateral to the Schanz screw and rod to apply compression.

deformity, degenerative disease, and instability following decompression or with pathologic lesions involving limited portions of the spine would be suitable F.I. candidates.

Several authors have reported their F.I. clinical experience for diverse spine pathologic conditions have yielded good to excellent results. Dick's (1987) original series of 180 F.I. patients from 1982 to 1986 included 111 fractures of this group, of which 110 healed. The one case of pseudarthrosis proved to be deficient in anterior and medial column bony support and was subsequently augmented with an anterior fusion to establish stability. In Dick's group, mean preoperative kyphosis of 20.4 degrees was corrected to 5.1 degrees postoperatively. Twenty patients were instrumented for posttraumatic instability after failure of either conservative management or another fixation system. These patients were reinstrumented with the F.I. and all went on to fusion with acceptable alignment and fixation. The remainder of the cases consisted of 7 successful stabilizations for degenerative disease, 16 cases of spondylolisthesis with anterior slip reduction from 71 to 31%, and 11 with tumor, in which 8 patients regained their independence and ambulatory potential (Dick, 1987).

Aebi et al. (1987) reported 32 cases of thoracolumbar spine burst fracture instrumented acutely with the F.I. The

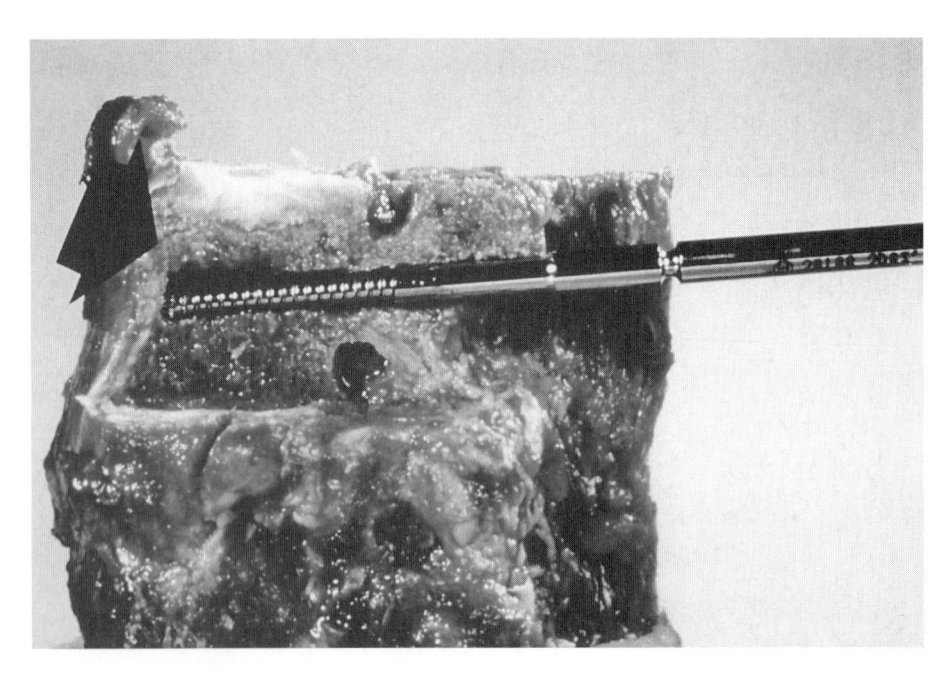

FIG. 34-31. A cadaver specimen demonstrating cancellous bone resorption about the Shantz screw following repetitive cyclic loading in-vitro. Fixation of the construct is not dependent on thread purchase within the body, but on the fixed angle that is maintained on the lordosed Schanz screw within the pedicle upon stabilization.

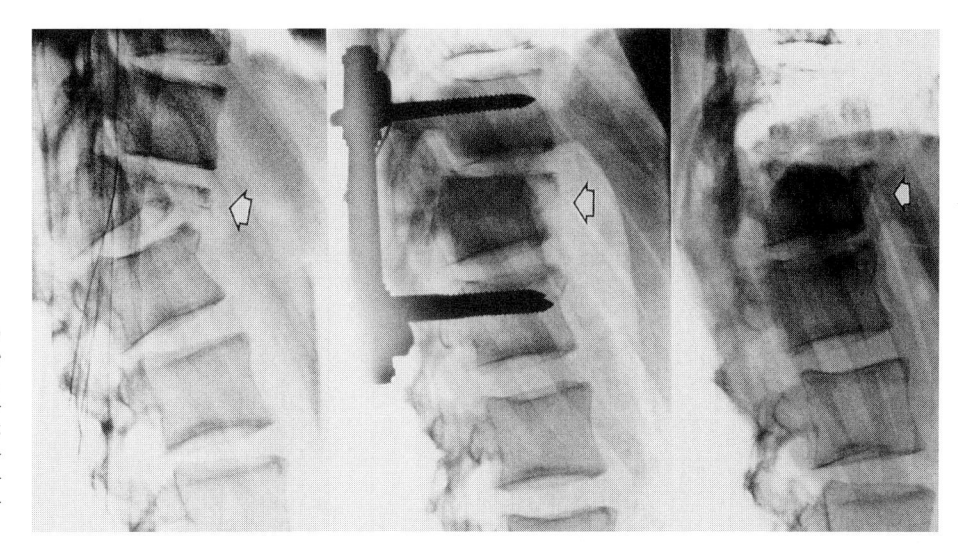

FIG. 34-32. An L1 burst fracture with severe kyphosis and retrolysthesis of the injured body into the spinal canal. Following instrumentation with the fixateur interne, the retrolysthesis has been reduced, and much of the vertebral height has been restored. After removal of the implant, the spinal alignment is well maintained.

authors emphasized the reduction potential of this system, especially in the middle column, by ligamentotaxis across the posterior longitudinal ligaments (Figs. 34-33 and 34-34). The patients were studied intraoperatively with myelography, which demonstrated acceptable reconstitution of the spinal canal in more than 95% (Fig. 34-35). After 1 year of follow-up, fracture reduction was well maintained without Schanz screw pullout or failure or neurologic deterioration. Two cases of nut loosening occurred early in their series and were thought by the authors to be due to a technical error from faulty wrench design.

Esses (1989) reviewed the cases of 48 patients treated with the F.I. for a variety of pathologic conditions. Their best results occurred in the patients treated for fractures in which significant postoperative canal reconstitution and kyphosis correction could be achieved. Spondylolisthesis, treated in six cases, could be reduced by one grade and held with posterior instrumentation alone. Excellent results occurred when the F.I. was used for multiple-level lumbar instability in 11 cases, pseudoarthrosis in 3 cases, and a single case of decompression for metastatic disease (Esses, 1989).

Ye (1993) reported on 24 cases instrumented with the F.I.; again, fresh fractures provided the best results, as acceptable reduction was achieved in all cases. Only partial reduction of kyphosis was possible in the late fracture group, and the authors emphasized the benefits of early F.I. application. In addition, good results were experienced in the treatment of spinal stenosis and ankylosing spondylitis.

Finally, Lindsey and Dick (1991) reported on 80 consecutive patients treated with the F.I. for unstable thoracolumbar spine fractures with neurologic deficit. Mean vertebral-body wedge angle was corrected from 17.4 to 7.9

FIG. 34-33. Lateral x-ray of an L1 burst fracture with kyphosis and retropulsion of the middle column. Instrumentation with the fixateur interne has restored a middle and an anterior vertebral height and has corrected kyphosis. Canal decompression is confirmed with an intraoperative myelogram.

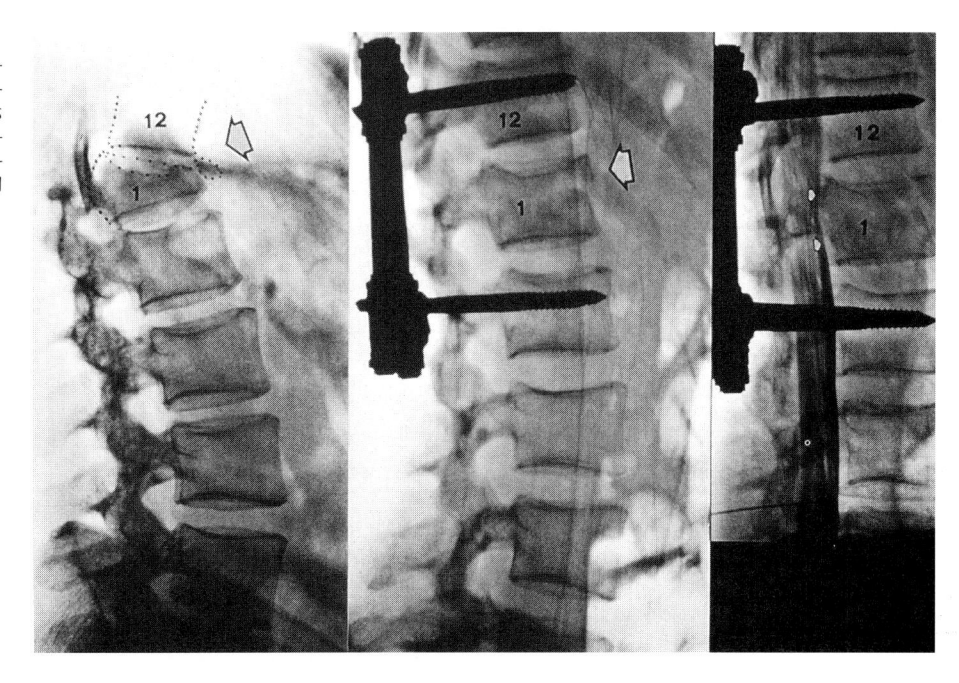

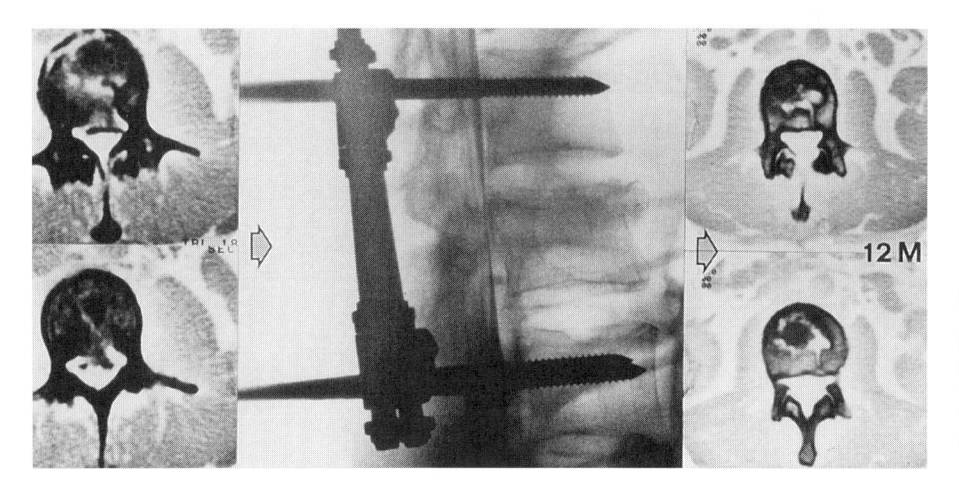

FIG. 34-34. CT scans of another burst fracture demonstrate preoperative middle column bony retropulsion into the canal. Indirect reduction of the middle column is achieved by instrumentation with the fixateur interne and confirmed by intraoperative myelogram and follow-up CT scan.

degrees. This reduction was maintained after 1- and 2-year follow-up and implant removal. However, an increase in kyphosis from the postoperative correction averaged about 5 degrees following implant removal. This was attributed to disk space collapse at the level of the fractured vertebral end plate with otherwise adequate maintenance of vertebral-body height and canal clearance.

Strict contraindications for use of the fixateur interne would include all situations whereby adequate pedicular screw fixation is not possible as in significant osteoporosis, infection, neoplasm, or absence of pedicles. Due to the limited actual points of implant articulation with the spine, and the normally high loads supported by the Schanz screws, morbid obesity would be a relative contraindication. The principle indication for the F.I. appears to be in the treatment of localized instability, especially thoracolumbar spine unstable fractures, requiring both sagittal and axial reduction (Aebi et al., 1987; Esses, 1989; Lindsey & Dick, 1991).

Advantages and Disadvantages

Most of the complications that occur with the F.I. are the result of technical errors, although there are inherent weaknesses in the system of which the clinician must be well aware (Table 34-2). The most common errors involve pedicle instrumentation and include missing the pedicle with the Schanz screw, inadequate screw depth in the pedicle, and too distal screw depth with possible perforation in the anterior cortex (Dick, 1987; Esses, 1989; Krag et al., 1986) (Figs. 34-36 and 34-37). Early loss of lordosis was often due to inadequate tightening or crimping of the nuts (with the old clamp system) (Aebi et al., 1987; Esses, 1989). Inadequate reduction was frequently the result of applying distraction to the system prior to sagittal plane correction; this creates tension in the anterior longitudinal ligament, which then resist attempts at kyphosis correction.

The complications that appear to be inherent in the system include the reported loss of some lordosis despite the system's maintaining its integrity over time (Dick, 1989; Lindsey & Dick, 1991). Also torsional instability has been cited with rotationally unstable fractures treated with the F.I. without cross-linking. However, the development of a cross-link system has greatly increased the torsional effectiveness

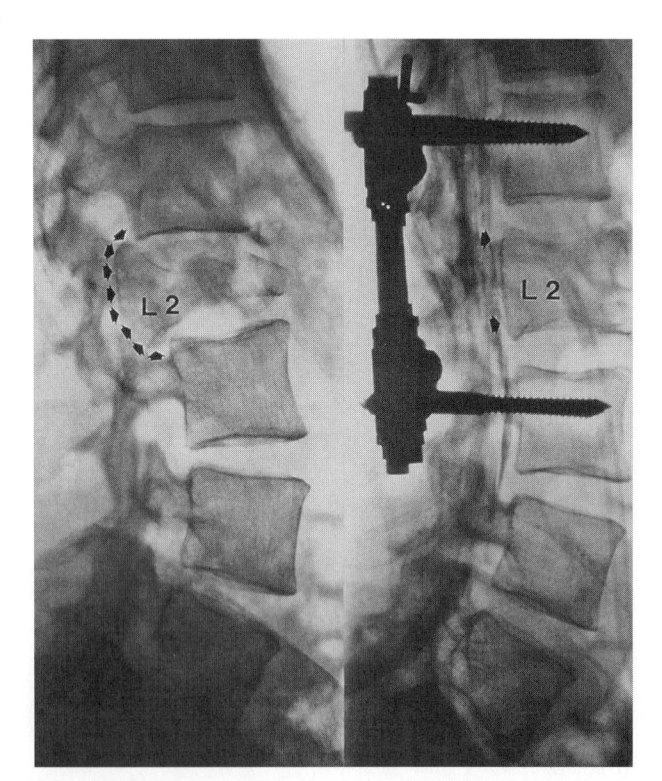

FIG. 34-35. An L2 burst fracture reduced with the fixateur interne; canal reconstitution is depicted by intraoperative myelography.

Table 34-2
Advantages and Disadvantages of the Fixateur Interne

Advantages
  Preserves normal motion segments
  Enables reduction of angular, axial, and rotatory malalignment
  Entirely implantable

Disadvantages
  Breakage and bending of poorly placed Schanz screws
  Torsional instability if system is not cross-linked
  Symptomatic pain from hardware following fusion

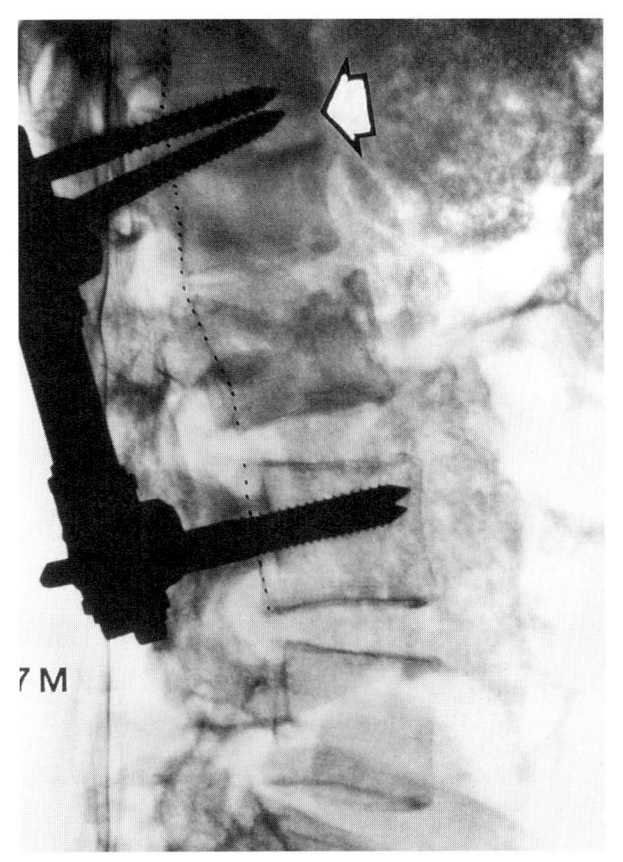

FIG. 34-36. Radiographs of the lumbar spine demonstrate poor Schanz screw placement of the upper portion of the construct. This patient experienced kyphosis progression which warranted revision surgery.

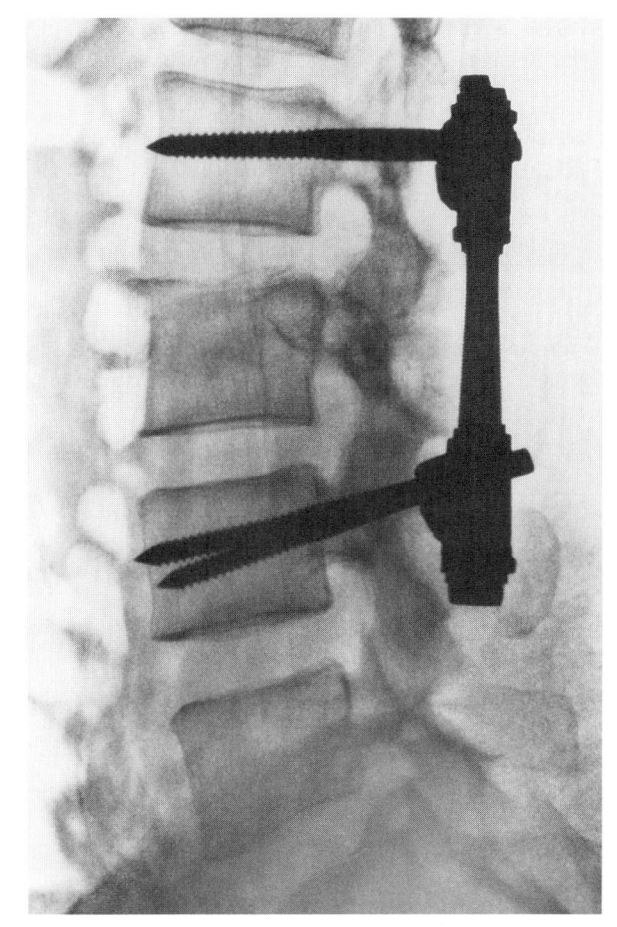

FIG. 34-37. The vertebral body anterior cortex has been penetrated at L2 and L4 by excessive depth of screw placement.

of the implant. Bending or breakage of Schanz screws has been noted and is perhaps caused by several factors (Dick, 1987; Esses, 1989). Inadequate depth of Schanz screw placement increases the load on the screw (Fig. 34-38). The Schanz screw design revision has moved the thread-smooth shaft junction, a potential stress riser, from the rotational center in the pedicle. Finally, retained F.I. hardware causing symptoms is usually reported following fusion and adequate fracture healing and is perhaps the result of otherwise unrestricted spinal mobility. It has also been suggested that many

FIG. 34-38. An L3 burst fracture has been adequately realigned with indirect spinal canal decompression using the fixateur interne instrumentation. However, early unrestricted functional activity without additional brace support resulted in a broken Schanz screw in ten months.

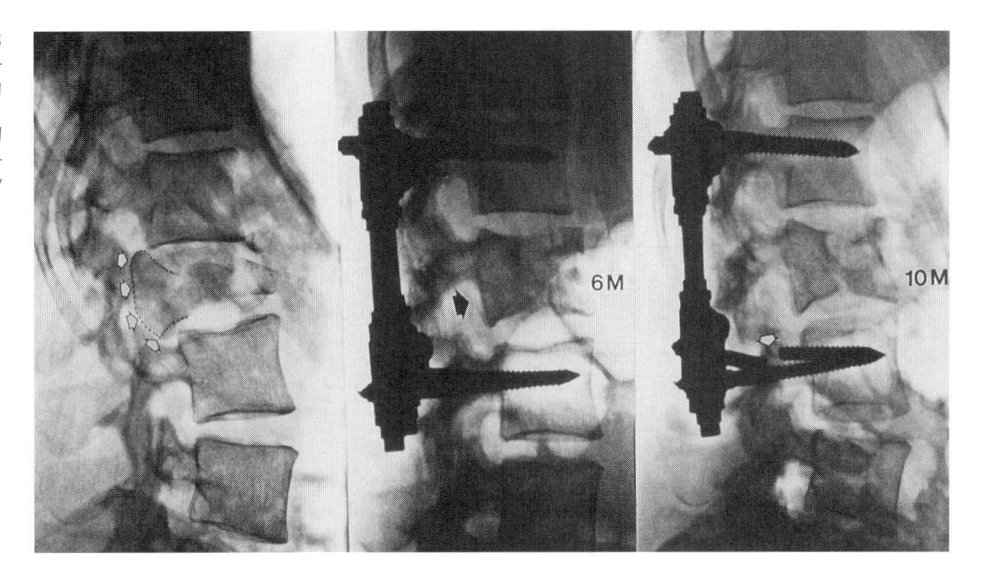

hardware-related symptoms were due to the bulkiness of the implant especially in the hypermobile thoracolumbar spine.

SUMMARY

The F.I. is a posterior pedicle instrumentation device that has the ability both to reduce and to establish spinal fixation over limited motion segments. The implant was designed to maximize reduction potential, especially sagittal realignment and spinal canal clearance, by concentrating reduction forces on only compromised spine regions. The use of pedicle for fixation also enhances sagittal, frontal, and axial reduction by means of its three-column purchase of the spine. The implants and the instruments are, themselves, few in number and easily applied. The technique, although simple, has a learning curve that can be quickly mastered by most surgeons familiar with spine anatomy and other routine spine surgical procedures.

REFERENCES

Aebi, M., Etter, C. Kehl, T., & Thalgott, J. (1987). Stabilization of the lower thoracic and lumbar spine with the internal spinal skeletal fixation system: Indication, techniques, and first results of treatment. *Spine, 12,* 544–551.

Armstrong, G.W.D. (1976). Harrington instrumentation for spinal fractures. *Proceedings of the Scoliosis Research Society.*

Casey, M.P., Jacobs, R.R., & Asher, M. (1984). The rod long-fuse short technique in the treatment of thoracolumbar and lumbar spine fractures. *Proceedings of the Scoliosis Research Society.*

Denis, F. (1983). The three-column spine and its significance in the classification of acute thoracolumbar spinal injuries. *Spine, 8,* 817–831.

Dick, W. (1989). *Internal Fixation of Thoracic and Lumbar Spine Fractures* (pp. 53–64). Stuttgart: Hans Huber.

Dick, W. (1987). The "fixateur interne" as a versatile implant for spine surgery. *Spine, 12,* 882–900.

Dick, W., Kluger, P., Magerl, F., Woersdoerfer, O., & Zach, G. (1985). A new device for internal fixation of thoracolumbar and lumbar spine fracture: the "Fixateur Interne." *Paraplegia, 23,* 225–232.

Dick, W., Woersdoerfer, O., & Magerl, T. (1985). Mechanical properties of a new device for internal fixation of spine fractures: The "fixateur interne" In: S.M. Perren & E. Schneider (Eds.), *Development of Biomechanics* (pp. 501–512). The Hague: Martinus Nijhoff.

Dickson, J.H., Harrington, P.R., & Erwin, W.D. (1978). Results of reduction and stability of the severely fractured thoracic and lumbar spine. *Journal of Bone and Joint Surgery, American Volume, 60,* 799–885.

Esses, S. (1989). The AO Spinal Internal Fixateur. *Spine, 14,* 373–378.

Esses, S., & Bednar, D. (1991). Posterior pedicular screw techniques. In: T. Errico, D. Bauer, & T. Waugh (Eds.), *Spinal Trauma* (pp. 301–307). Philadelphia.

Gertzbein, S., & Robbins, S. (1990). Accuracy of pedicular screw placement in vivo. *Spine, 15,* 11–14.

Holdsworth, F. (1970). Dislocations of spine. *Journal of Bone and Joint Surgery, American Volume, 52,* 1534–1551.

Kahanovitz, N., Arnoczky, S.P., Levine, D.B., & Otis, J.P. (1984). The effects of internal fixation on the articular cartilage of unfused canine facet joint cartilage. *Spine, 9,* 268–272.

Krag, M.H., Beynnon, B.D., Pope, M.H., et al. (1986). An internal fixator for posterior application to short segments of the thoracic, lumbar, lumbosacral spine. *Clinical Orthopaedics and Related Research, 203,* 75–98.

Lindsey, R., & Dick, W. (1991). The fixateur interne in the reduction and stabilization of thoracolumbar spine fractures in patients with neurologic deficit. *Spine, 16,* S140–S145.

Lindsey, R., Dick, W., Nunchuck, S., & Zach, G. (1993). Residual intersegmental spinal mobility following limited pedicle fixation of thoracolumbar spine fractures with the Fixateur Interne. *Spine, 18,* 478–479.

Marchese, D., Thalgott, J., & Aebi, M. (1991). Application and results of the AO Internal Fixation System in nontraumatic indications. *Spine, 16,* 162–169.

Magerl, F.P. (1984). Stabilization of the lower thoracic and lumbar spine with external skeletal fixation. *Clinical Orthopaedics and Related Research, 189,* 125–141.

Nicastro, J.F., Traina, J., Hartjen, C.A., & Lancaster, J.M. (1984). Intraspinal pathways of sublaminar wires during surgical removal. *Proceedings of the Scoliosis Research Society.*

Nolte, L., Steffen, R., Kramer, J., & Jergas, M. (1993). Fixateur Interne: a comparative biomechanical study of various systems. *Aktuell-Traumatol, 23*(1), 20–26.

Panjabi, M., Abumi, W., Duranceau, J., & Crisco, J. (1988). Biomechanical evaluation of spinal fixation devices: Stability provided by eight internal fixation devices. *Spine, 13,* 35–40.

Roy-Camille, R., Saillant, G., Berteaux, D., & Salgado, V. (1976). Osteosynthesis of thoracolumbar spine fractures with metal plates screwed through the vertebral pedicles. *Reconst Surg Trauma, 15,* 2.

Surgical Technique Guide for Correction of Scoliosis. (1994) Paoli, PA: Synthes.

Ye, Q. (1993). The application of Dick instrumentation in the field of spine surgery. *Acta Academiae Medicinae Sinicae, 15*(1), 39–44.

CHAPTER 35

Application of the Louis System for Thoracolumbar and Lumbosacral Spine Stabilization

René Louis

HIGHLIGHTS

Roy-Camille introduced the pedicular screw principle in 1971, which we have since adapted (1970). Decreasing the interval between holes from 13 to 9 mm allowed improved placement of pedicle screws throughout the thoracic and lumbar spine. Paired and symmetric plates with preestablished lengths are capable of satisfying most needs of the thoracic and lumbar spine. In addition, if necessary, these plates can be shortened intraoperatively for shorter spinal constructs. A specially designed "butterfly" plate has been precontoured to fit the lumbosacral junction to allow improved lumbosacral stabilization. These plates have been specifically designed to enable alar screw placement of the sacrum, but can also be used for anterior vertebral stabilization. Screws are available in 4.5- and 5.5-mm diameters.

Fusion techniques have been modified to allow transarticular posterior vertebral fusion rather than the classical intertransverse fusion. For this, corticocancellous bone chips from the spinous processes are used, thus eliminating the necessity to harvest bone from the iliac crest.

Reduction is achieved through two methods. The first method consists of triangulation used preoperatively and intraoperatively. The forces are placed on the head, the feet, and one perpendicular to the first and second applied behind the convexity of the deformity. If this method is not effective in reducing the defect, reductive instrumentation is used. This consists of a pair of distractive or compressive reducers used posteriorly, or anterior instrumentation of two types. The first is an elevator designed to lift the olisthetic vertebra above the sacrum. The second is a vertebral transverse displacement reducer that pushes the vertebral body of the olisthetic vertebra back into position. This instrumentation system is designed and marketed by Cremascoli-France, Toulon, France (An & Cotler, 1992; Louis, 1985a).

INDICATIONS AND CONTRAINDICATIONS

The indications for use of this instrumentation system are those of all vertebral osteosynthesis for provisional or permanent vertebral stabilization (Table 35-1). Provisional stabilization has two indications. First, fracture dislocation of the cervical articular masses can be reduced and stabilized by a 6-month osteosynthesis, after which the instrumentation can be removed with no underlying fusion of the mobile segments. Second, isthmic reconstruction for bilateral spondylolysis with a normal disk also is an indication for provisional stabilization (Louis, 1985a). Following fusion of the isthmic defect, instrumentation can be removed with completely normal mobility of the joint. All other indications for use of the stabilization construct require fusion of the corresponding mobile segments (Fig. 35-1). This includes fusion for a painful mobile segment resulting from a degenerative or previous infectious process (Louis & Maresca, 1976). Arthrodesis may be required for instability that results in secondary displacements or neurologic damage from traumatic injuries such as burst fractures, fractures with diskoligamentous rupture, or neurologic compression (Louis, Maresca, & Bel, 1977). Finally, fusion may be helpful in all situations in which it is necessary to repair either pathologic or iatrogenic instabilities (Fig. 35-2). These can result from reduction of a wedge fracture, tumor, or infection.

Table 35-1
Indications and Contraindications for Use of the Louis System for Thoracolumbar and Lumbosacral Stabilization

Indications
    Provisional
        Cervical facet fracture-dislocations
        Isthmic spondylolysis
    Permanent
        Degenerative disease
        Instability due to past infections
        Burst fractures
        Fractures with diskoligamentous disruptions
        Neurologic compression
        Tumor

Contraindications
    Scoliosis >30 degrees
    Ongoing infections
    Previous radiation therapy
    Osteoporosis (relative)

Contraindications to use of this instrumentation are those situations in which major surgical procedures should be avoided. This system is not well adapted to correction of lateral deformities of the spine; therefore, scoliosis above 30 degrees should not be managed with this instrumentation. In addition, patients with infectious complications from previous surgical procedures, or who previously have undergone radiation therapy, are not good candidates for vertebral fusion. Osteoporosis is a relative contraindication for this instrumentation, but this instrumentation can be used provided longer constructs are put into place.

ADVANTAGES AND DISADVANTAGES

There are numerous advantages to this instrumentation system (Table 35-2). The semirigid nature of this system decreases the onset of osteolysis around implanted screws. This instrumentation is rapidly implanted, usually in less than 1 hour. Fusion rates over the past 25 years of use of this instrumentation are close to 98%. The instrumentation is inexpensive. Landmarks are well defined, and position can be verified by use of an image intensifier. Because the transverse processes are not exposed in this technique, blood loss is minimal and the neurovascular bundles of the erector spinal muscles are not interrupted. The equipment is low-profile, which enables mobility of the overlying spinal muscles. Finally, this method, which induces intraarticular fusion, requires no massive bone harvesting and develops fusion sites directly on the intervertebral contact points.

Disadvantages of this system are those of a semirigid arthrodesis, which allows micromotion between the screw heads and the plate. To minimize complications resulting from this, patients are required to wear a back brace postoperatively for 4 months. This instrumentation is made of stainless steel and has had minimal problems of fracture or

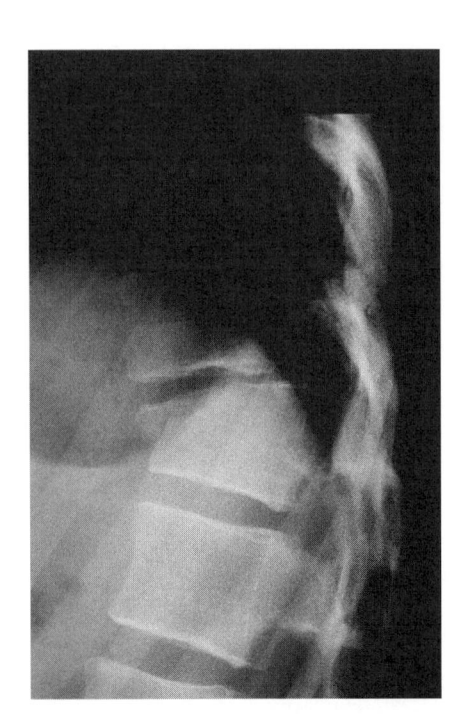

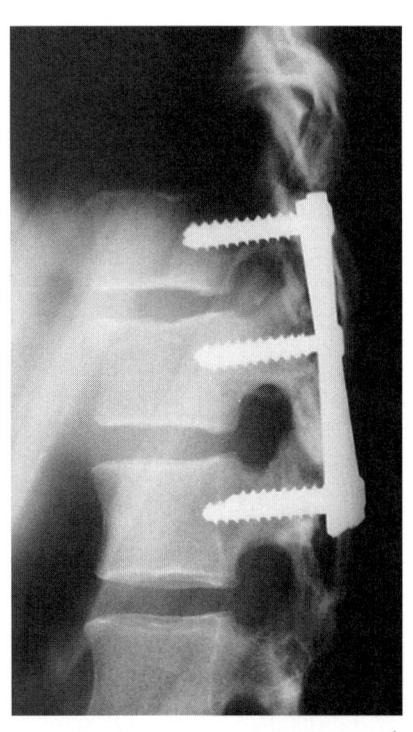

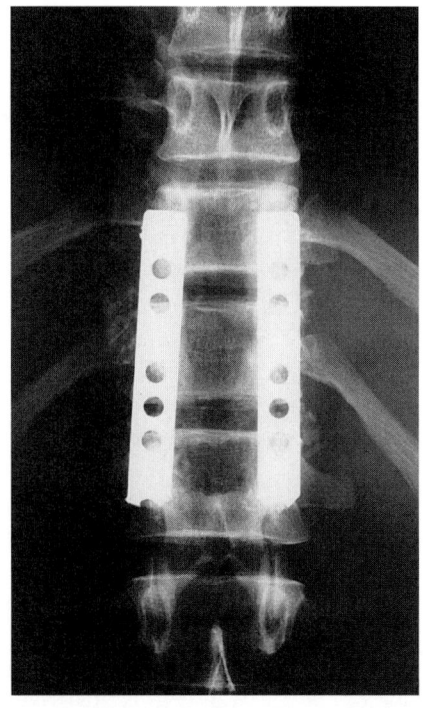

FIG. 35-1. (a to c) T12 fracture-dislocation with incomplete neural deficit treated with orthopedic reduction in a scoliosis frame and posterior surgery with decompression and stabilization the following day. Excellent results on functional, stability, and neurologic grounds.

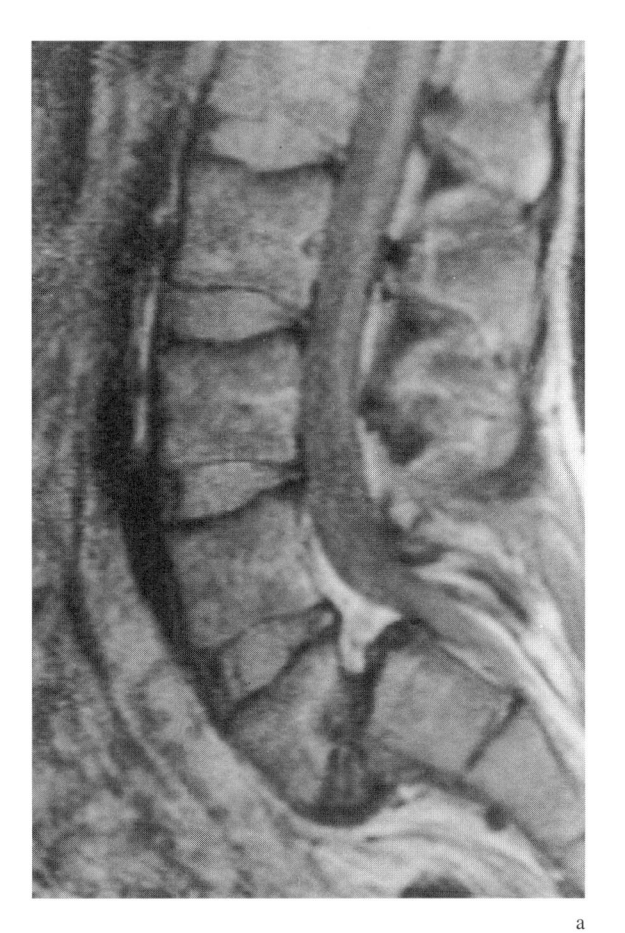

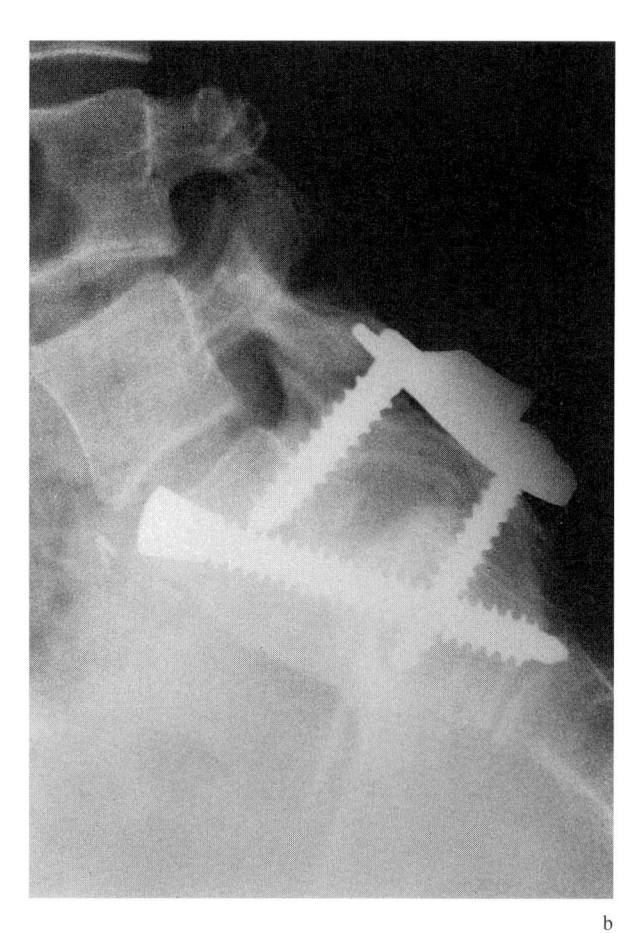

FIG. 35-2. (a and b) Severe L5 spondylolisthesis with low back pain irradiating to the thighs. We performed a combined approach with anterior reduction by our method. Excellent morphologic and functional results.

torsion of the screws. Because of the micromotion between screw heads and plates, this instrumentation system is not available in titanium. Finally, this method is poorly adapted to reduction and arthrodesis of scoliosis greater than 30 degrees.

Table 35-2
Advantages and Disadvantages of the Louis System for Thoracolumbar and Lumbosacral Stabilization

Advantages
  Semirigidity decreases osteolysis
  Rapid implantation
  Inexpensive
  High fusion rates
  Easily identified landmarks
  Minimal blood loss
  Relative sparing of erector spinal neurovascular bundles
  Low profile
  Intraarticular fusion

Disadvantages
  Semirigidity allows micromotion
  Not available in titanium
  Poorly adapted for scoliosis >30 degrees

TECHNIQUES

Stabilization of the thoracic and/or lumbar spine can be accomplished in a posterior, anterior, or a combined anterior and posterior approach. These approaches can be carried out either with or without the reduction of deformity.

Posterior Stabilization

Advantages

Insertion of pedicle screws in the sagittal plane is advantageous to oblique insertion. Sagittal insertion allows the screw to pass through thick and solid cortex, which is not found at the base of the transverse process. Sagittal insertion also has the advantage of passing through the medial and lateral cortex of the pedicles, also not possible when placing screws through the base of the transverse process.

Disadvantages

One disadvantage of inserting pedicle screws through the sagittal plane is that it requires the resection of the inferior portion of the overlying articular facet. This has not resulted in a problem in over 25 years of experience.

Screw-Insertion Landmarks

T1 to T3. The penetration point of pedicular screws in this region is located at the cross point of two lines (Fig. 35-3). One line is drawn 3 mm from the lateral edge of the articular facet. The other line is drawn 3 mm from the inferior edge of the articular facet. Screw directions should be angled medially 15 to 20 degrees. Screw length would be in the range of 25 to 30 mm and 4.5 mm in diameter.

T4 to T10. The penetration point of pedicular screws in this region is located at the cross point of a vertical line drawn 5 mm from the lateral edge of the articular facet and 3 mm from the inferior edge. This will fall on a crest involving the medial prolongation of the superior edge of the transverse process. The screw length will be 30 to 35 mm and diameter will be 4.5 mm.

T11 to L2. Pedicular penetration points are identical to those of T4-10 with an additional landmark represented by a curved line drawn 4 mm above and medial to the pars interarticularis. Screw length will be 35 to 40 mm and diameter will range from 4.5 to 5.5 mm depending on the patient's pedicular size.

L3 to L5. For insertion into these pedicles several landmarks are available. The most useful is at the cross point of two lines. The vertical line is parallel to the bottom of the pars interarticularis notch, and the horizontal one is drawn 4 mm above the inferior edge of the pars interarticularis notch. This crossing point will correspond to another one, which is identified as the cross point between a line running vertically through the lateral part of the joint line underlying the pedicle, and a horizontal line passing 1 mm above the lower extreme of this joint. Finally, the center of the pedicle approximately corresponds to the middle of the transverse process base. The L5 pedicle is slightly inclined caudally by 5 to 10 degrees. Therefore, screw penetration into the L5 pedicle should be slightly caudally directed. Screw lengths will range from 40 to 45 mm, and diameter will be 5.5 mm.

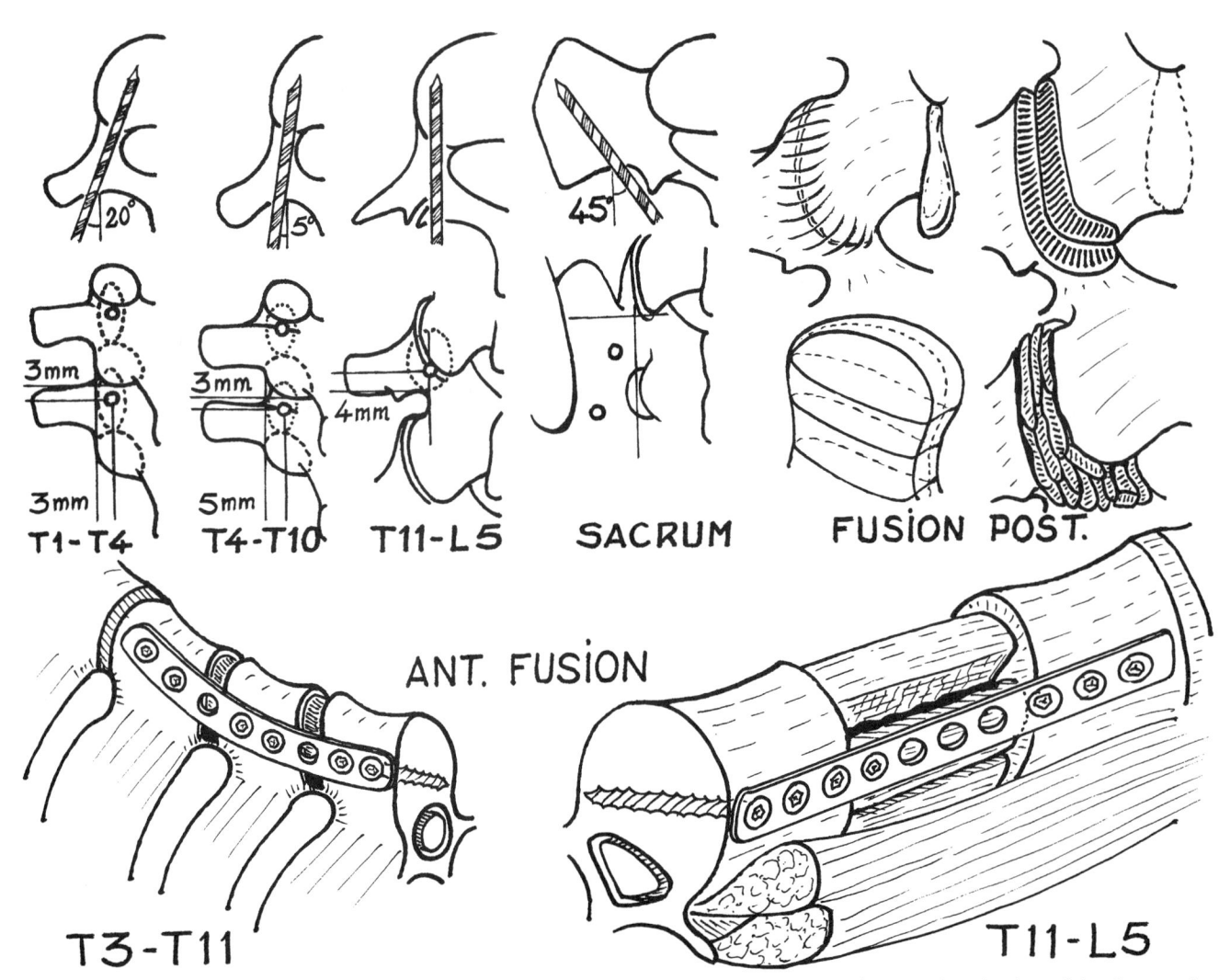

FIG. 35-3. Drawings of our technique with the landmarks for screw insertion in pedicles, for posterior fusion into facet joints with bone grafting cut from spinous processes and anterior interbody fusion with fibular struts and anterolateral screw plate.

Sacral Screw Insertion. In this method, placement of sacral screws is carried out into the sacral alae. Therefore, a 45-degree lateral and a 45-degree caudal angle are used. Screw length averages 45 mm, and diameter is 5.5 mm. The screw penetration point should be inferior and lateral to the posterior L5-S1 joint. Usually, the position of the plate allows a direct use of its inferior oblique holes for screw placement, with no further landmark necessary for placement of the screw. In fact, anatomical studies have enabled us to determine accurately the position of the inferior holes on the basis of the plate when the lumbar pedicle screws have been placed. However, it is always advisable to use small Kirschner pins provisionally to check the location by image intensification and correct it if necessary. Both anteroposterior (AP) and lateral views will be necessary for this verification.

Positioning of the Paired and Symmetric Plates

Except for stabilization of L5-S1, all constructs are paired symmetrical plates the length of which are chosen on the basis of the number of levels to be stabilized. Our preference is to use short constructs, except for totally paralyzed or osteoporotic patients, who require longer stabilization. Once the landmarks have been correctly identified with Kirschner pins, one can put the plates directly into place by sliding them over the pins. Extra holes, which are located inferiorly, can be cut off using a cutting forceps before permanent fixation. Prior to final fixation it is necessary to prepare the intermediate facet joints. This is done by resecting a portion of each intermediate facet joint and its articular cartilage and packing them with corticocancellous bone chips that have previously been cut off from spinous processes. To augment rapid incorporation of the spinous processes into the fusion mass, each spinous process should be sectioned into "match sticks," which have been cleared of all cartilaginous and fibrous elements. Because of the relatively minimal muscle dissection, the availability of additional blood supply will augment the fusion. All screws are then tightened. Complete hemostasis is ensured, resulting in wound closure requiring no drainage.

L5-S1 Plate Placement

L5-S1 stabilization is achieved using a "butterfly" plate, which is available in small, medium, and large sizes. The size of the plate to be used is chosen on the basis of the L5 interpedicular distance. After locating and drilling the L5 pedicles, two bayonet-shaped pedicular landmarks are positioned within them. The selected "butterfly" plate is slid along these landmarks, which are then removed and replaced with pedicular screws. Sacral fixation is performed by drilling directly through the sacral insertion holes at an angle 45 degrees lateral and 45 degrees caudal to the horizontal plane. Sacral screws are then placed directly into these holes. The four screws are then alternately tightened. Occasionally it is necessary to resect a small portion of the L5 lamina to obtain thorough contact of the plate to the L5 bony elements.

When this arthrodesis is used for bilateral spondylolysis, both the isthmic defects are decorticated and filled with corticocancellous bone chips obtained from the two spinous processes. When arthrodesis of L5-S1 posterior joints is necessary, the capsule of the L5-S1 joints is resected bilaterally, the synovial lining is removed and the joint is packed with bone chips.

Stabilization after Reduction

To avoid intraoperative reduction maneuvers, fresh spinal fractures are operated on in "lordotic traction." This is done by fixing the feet to orthopedic shoes attached to the caudal end of the table and placing traction on the head using a leather helmet. The amount of traction applied is controlled by a dynamometer. Finally, the operating table is angulated as required at the site of the vertebral fracture.

This maneuver has eliminated the necessity to incorporate a reduction device within our system (Fig. 35-4). For example, to perform a posterior vertebral osteotomy for spinal nonunion, reduction and stabilization must be performed following the osteotomy. To perform this procedure, prepared symmetric plates are placed but screwed in only at their upper end. Paired reducing instruments are then used with the cranial hook fixed to one screw hole of the plate and the caudal hook fixed to the lower edge of a lamina beneath the osteotomy. The osteotomy is then gradually closed and the caudal screws are inserted and tightened.

Pitfalls of This Method

The first possible mistake in any such operation is to misplace the pedicle screws. This can lead to damage of neural structures or to prevertebral large vessels. To avoid such complications, one should thoroughly locate anatomically and radiologically the necessary landmarks and avoid drilling further than 1 cm into the bone. Since the screws are self-tapping, further drilling is unnecessary. In addition, it is not necessary to reach the anterior cortex of the vertebral bodies with these screws. The tip of the screws should sit in the middle of the vertebral body when viewed on lateral imaging to avoid extraspinal positioning. When drilling pedicles, an assistant should feel the involved metameric territories to alert the surgeon to stop drilling immediately if any jumping movements are felt. If a pedicle screw is positioned incorrectly, repeated placement of screws into the same pedicle can result in an orifice too large to hold the screw solidly. In this case, this pedicle should be filled with bone chips before further screws are positioned. The structure of the plates enables easy adaptation to spinal curvatures in either kyphotic or lordotic shapes by bending the plates through use of a three-tipped forceps. Occasionally when performing posterior screw placement in an irreducible spondylolisthesis, it is necessary to mold the lumbosacral plate into a "bayonet" shape.

Long lumbosacral arthrodesis, stretching from above L2 to the sacrum, can be performed with paired symmetrical plates without the predesigned oblique sacral holes. This is

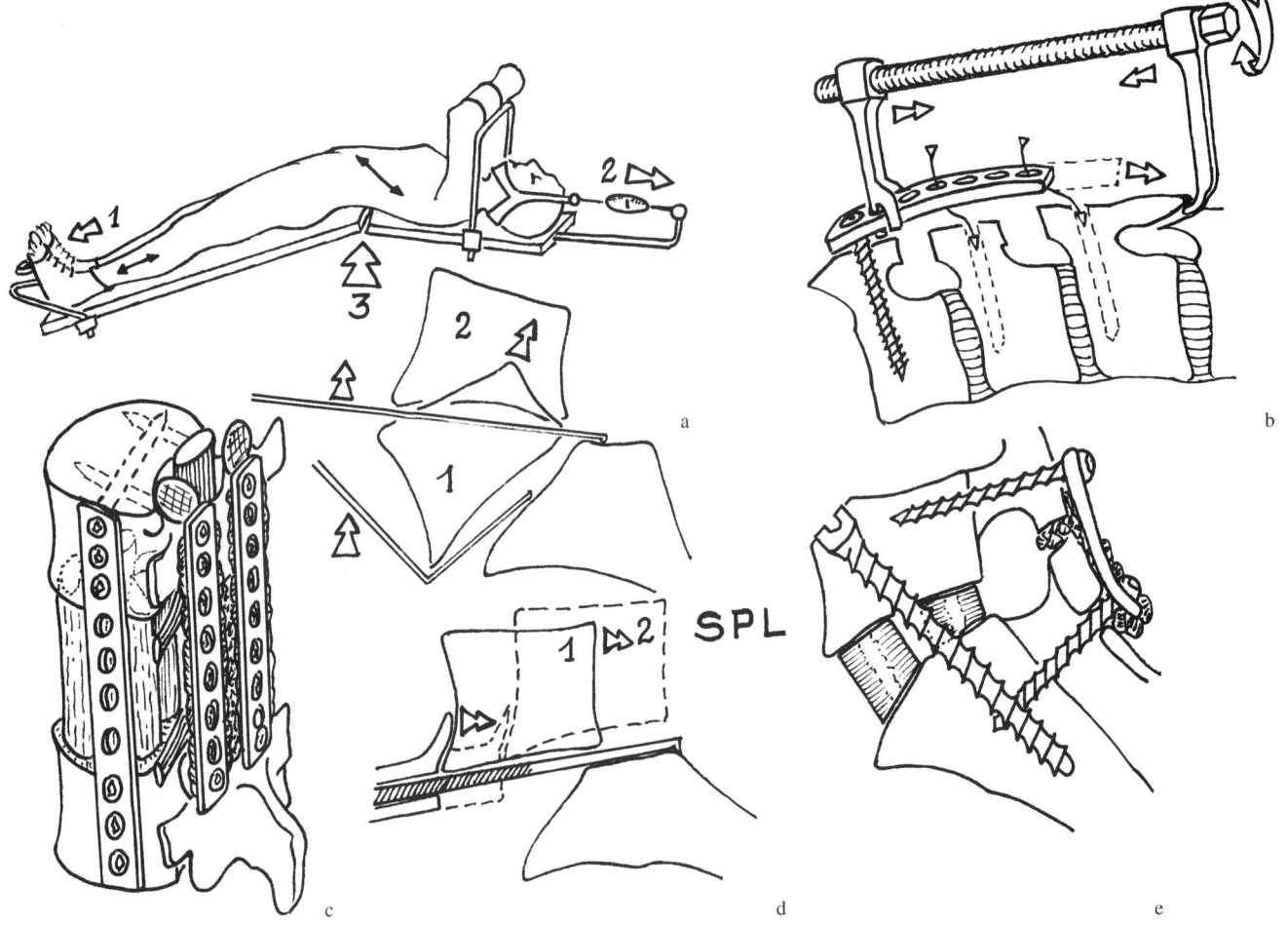

FIG. 35-4. Means for reduction of spinal deformities. (a) Operative spinal traction. (b) Compressive perioperative devices. (c) Combined approach using posterior and lateral plates for repair of the three spinal columns for vertebrectomy. (d) Anterior instrumental reduction for severe spondylolisthesis. (e) Combined approach using posterior plates and anterior intervertebral screw for repair of spondylolisthesis.

done by twisting the lower extremity of the plate and orienting them laterally to enable insertion of the screws into the oblique sacral holes.

Anterior Stabilization

To reach the thoracic and/or lumbar vertebral bodies, we use one of the approaches detailed in our textbook *Spinal Surgery* (Louis, 1982). For the thoracic vertebrae we prefer to use the right anterior approach. For the thoracolumbar junction we prefer the left thoracophrenolumbar approach (Fig. 35-5). With the patient in the supine position, for the lumbar spine, we use the left retroperitoneal approach. On the other hand, for lumbosacral anterior arthrodesis, we use the anterior midline transperitoneal approach. These various approaches enable us to have good exposure of the anterior and lateral sides of the vertebrae and disks on the ipsilateral side of the approach. These exposures require ligation of the intercostal or radicular branches of the aorta and vena cava, and mobilization of the major vessels. All of these anterior osteosyntheses should necessarily be performed together with an arthrodesis by an interbody fusion. The disks in between the osteosyntheses can be resected completely, if the dura needs to be decompressed, or partially leaving a posterior band, if no decompression is necessary. The vertebral end plates should be thoroughly curetted to remove cartilage and soft tissue but without damaging their cortices. For short arthrodesis between two vertebrae, we use tricorticoiliac grafts for the intervertebral space. For arthrodesis following the resection of one or more vertebral bodies, we use sagittal grafts from the fibular diaphysis. In the superior thoracic spine, one graft is sufficient, while for the inferior thoracic spine two fibular struts are used. Three are occasionally necessary for the lumbar spine. Each graft should have a straight transverse section to maximize fit into each of the prepared vertebral end plates. Osteosynthesis is carried out by selecting the appropriate plate length to span the resected vertebral bodies. In the thoracic spine two screws should be used in each vertebral body. Three screws are generally used in the lumbar spine. The plates are positioned in the anterolateral aspect of each vertebral body. Screw direction is nearly transverse, but has a slight oblique angle posteriorly. It is not necessary to reach the opposite cortex.

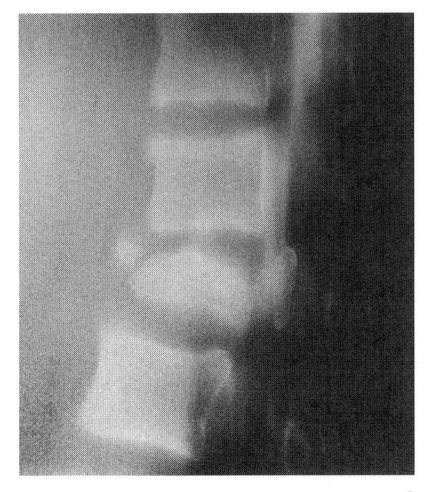

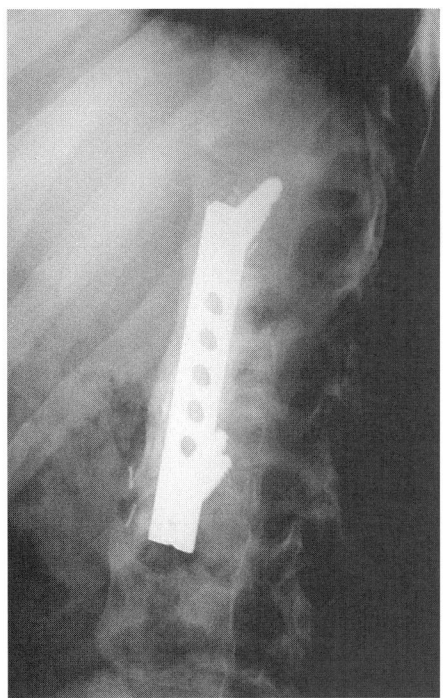

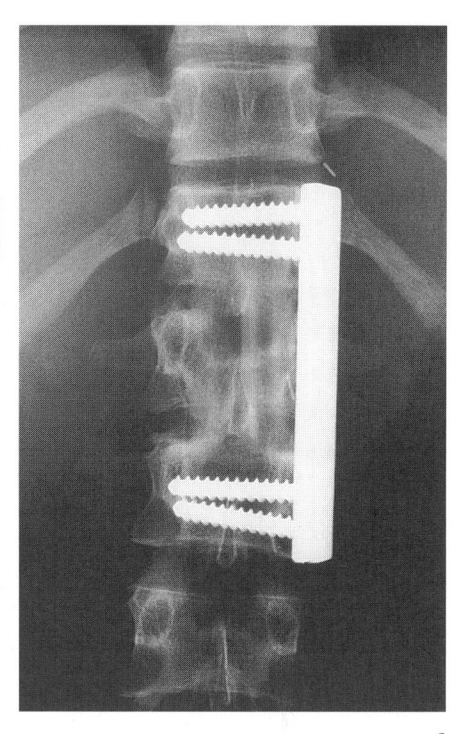

FIG. 35-5. (a to c) L1 burst fracture with incomplete paraplegia treated by anterior approach with perioperative spinal traction for reduction, anterior decompression of the vertebral canal, and reconstitution of the anterior pillar with fibular struts and anterolateral screw plate. Excellent results on neurologic and vertebral grounds.

Drilling is performed with a 2.8-mm-diameter drill and 4.5-mm screws are used in the thoracic spine. In the lumbar spine a 3.2-mm drill and 5.5-mm screws are used. Once again, drills should penetrate the vertebral body to only 1 cm. A curved plate is available for the thoracic spine to match its kyphosis. Plates can be shortened intraoperatively if necessary. Placement of screws and plates in the above described position has been chosen to avoid damage to major vessels in the event of screw backout. In addition, the inserted screws remain in front of the vertebral canal, minimizing the risk of spinal cord injuries. If it is necessary to perform intraoperative reduction of a kyphotic deformity, this can be achieved following vertebral-body resection by the traction apparatus previously described. By angling the operating table below the kyphotic deformity under image intensification, the deformity can be reduced. Following placement of the fibular strut grafts, traction is released, resulting in compression of the grafts. Finally, the plate is placed.

Combined Approach

We use combined approaches for three principal arthrodeses: severe fractures, vertebrectomies, and severe spondylolisthesis. Generally these procedures are staged at 8-day intervals to minimize blood loss.

Severe Spinal Fractures

For severe burst fractures with neurologic compromise, anterior decompression is performed first by extracting all vertebral fragments and restoring bony continuity with fibular grafting (Fig. 35-6). This is stabilized laterally with a plate as described above. Eight days later, posterior stabilization is carried out with optional further decompression. Posterior fusion followed by placement of symmetric plates completes the procedure.

Total Vertebrectomy

For primary spinal tumors, or isolated metastasis, a two-stage vertebrectomy is performed. The posterior stage is performed first by a laminectomy and bilateral pediculectomy. Bony continuity is restored with iliac grafts stabilized by posterior plates attached to the cephalad and caudal vertebrae. The intraspinal venous plexuses are cauterized to prepare for the anterior stage. Eight days later the anterior vertebrectomy is performed, followed by fibular vertical strut grafting and stabilization by an anterolateral plate.

Severe Spondylolisthesis

Severe spondylolisthesis is approached first through an anterior reduction. Through an anterior midline transperitoneal approach, the last two lumbar disks are exposed and completely resected. A series of elevators, with angulations ranging from 90 to 180 degrees, are inserted into the intervertebral space and used to lift the olisthetic vertebrae above the sacrum. When the L5 vertebra has reached sufficient height, the posterior longitudinal ligament is excised, exposing the dura. Continued distraction to 8 to 10 mm is per-

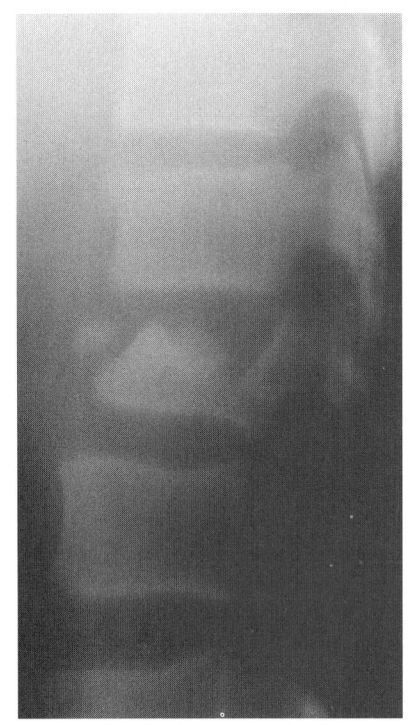

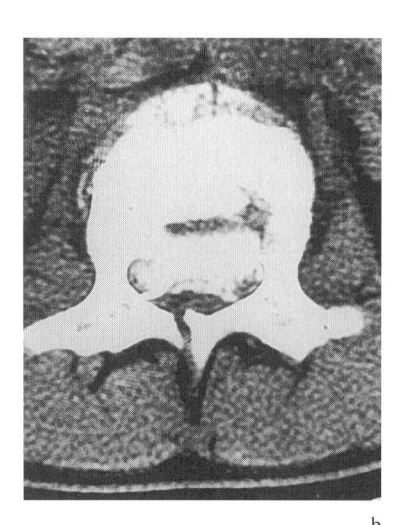

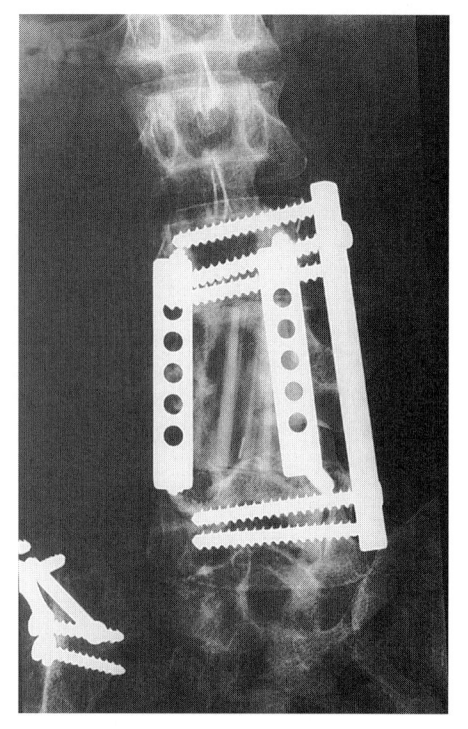

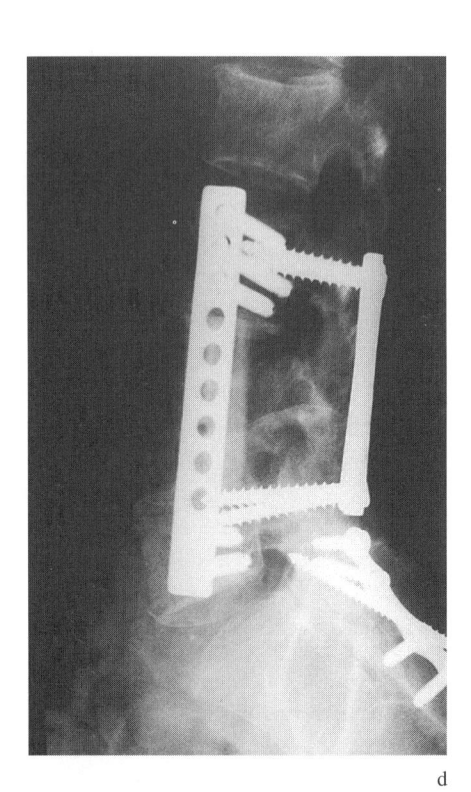

FIG. 35-6. *(a to d)* Severe burst fracture with incomplete cauda equina syndrome treated by combined approach. The vertebral canal has been decompressed, and the three pillars of the spine reconstituted with bone grafting and screw plates. Excellent results were achieved. An osteosynthesis of the pelvis has been necessary for pelvic lesions.

formed, and a reducing device made of axial and peripheral components is inserted. The axial component is hooked to the posterior edge of the sacral plate and the peripheral component screws onto the axial one. This pushes against the anterior aspect of the L5 vertebral body. This then enables reduction of L5 onto S1 under image intensification. The vertebral body is then locked into this position by inserting two Steinmann pins along the anterior edge of the L5 vertebral body and into the sacral plate. Osteosynthesis is performed using four fragments of fibular grafts positioned in the intervertebral space. A large transcorporeal screw is then introduced at the level of the superior L5 end plate and inserted to penetrate 3 to 4 cm into the midline of the sacral plate.

CLINICAL RESULTS

For analysis, the results have been divided into two periods of 10 years each: 1972 to 1982 and 1983 to 1993.

Results of Patients Operated on Between 1972 and 1982

Four hundred fifty-five patients were operated on in our department between 1972 and 1982. Four hundred forty could be assessed at the time of follow-up examination. Forty-one percent of the patients were female, 59% were male. The mean age was 47 years, ranging from 13 to 72 years. Two hundred ninety-three were sole posterior fusions, while 145 were combined fusions. Three patients who had previously undergone triple approach for revision of incorrect fusion performed in other hospitals underwent two-stage procedures. The arthrodesis level was L5-S1 for 216 cases (49%), L4 to S1 for 165 cases (38%), L3 to S1 for 44 cases (10%), L2 to S1 for 11 cases (2.5%), and L3 to L5 two cases (0.5%).

Two hundred sixty-six posterior fusions were performed in 218 patients for degenerative instability, 21 patients for failed disk surgery, 18 patients for nonunion for a former fusion, and 9 patients for metastatic nonunion or osteoarthritic sequelae. Twenty-seven patients underwent isthmic reconstruction, and 142 patients with spondylolisthesis were treated by two-step surgical procedure with reduction. Two total vertebrectomies were performed for L4 myeloma.

Mean follow-up was 3.6 months. Complications encountered in this first series were two subocclusive postoperative syndromes, one dehiscence of the abdominal wound, and one deep venous thrombosis of the left common iliac vein. We had one case of injury to the left iliac vein requiring three stitches, and two patients presented with clauda equina syndrome resulting from insufficient resection of the disk in one case and penetration of sacral wall debris into the canal in the other case. All patients recovered completely within a 3-month period. Three patients suffered from transient L5 root deficit. Two patients reported transient sexual difficulty.

The earliest screws were made out of chrome-cobalt alloy. In these screws, two anterior screw fractures and eight cases of posterior screw fractures were noted. The fusion rate of posterior fusions alone was 97.4%. On the other hand, combined approaches reached a fusion rate of 100%. For patients who underwent only posterior fusion, 78% reported satisfactory improvement of pain, and 22% were dissatisfied with the results. On the other hand, patients operated on by a combined approach reached 94% of satisfactory results, and 6% of dissatisfactory results on pain. Among the patients who were heavy laborers before the procedure, 56.5% returned to the same work, 29.5% went back to lighter work, while only 14% did not return to work.

Results of Patients Operated on between 1983 and 1993

Three hundred forty-eight patients underwent surgery during the period from 1983 to 1993. Three hundred twelve patients were available for evaluation. One hundred sixty-five were male (53%), and 147 were female (47%). The mean age was 49 years, ranging from 11 to 83 years. Two hundred three posterior fusions were performed and 109 combined anterior and posterior fusions were performed. Of these, 42 were for isthmic reconstruction, 63 for severe spondylolisthesis, and 4 for total vertebrectomy. The osteosynthesis rates were close to those of the first series. Mean follow-up was 25.2 months. The complications encountered were less significant due to the improved fixation using stainless steel material, larger-diameter screws, and an improved thread design. Three transient L5 deficits were noted, one iliac deep venous thrombosis, and one palsy of the crural nerve. Three patients had screw backout of a few millimeters, one patient had a broken screw noted 2 years later. In this series, no sexual difficulties and no subocclusive postoperative syndromes occurred. One deep wound infection occurred in a patient initially operated on with the Harrington technique in previously radiated tissue. The posterior fusion rate reached 98.6%, and the combined fusion rate was 100%. Results concerning pain and work recovery were approximately the same as those of the first series.

SUMMARY

We have presented a spinal stabilization technique using the posterior approach with pedicle screws and plates and an anterior approach in which screws are placed into the vertebral body. The construct is semirigid and requires the use of a back brace postoperatively. This technique enables intraarticular fusion using graft harvested directly from the spinous processes. Anterior approaches require intrabody fusion with the use of fibular struts. Indications for the procedure are the same as all vertebral osteosyntheses, with provisional constructs being used for spondylolysis, isthmic reconstruction, and cervical fracture. For all other indications, the fusion is permanent and instrumentation is not removed. When significant bony defects are created, either of pathologic or iatrogenic origin, this stabilization enables the restoration of continuity of all three vertebral columns, the anterior vertebral disk column and the two posterior zygapophyseal columns, secondary to autogenous grafts and one screwed plate for each pillar. This type of construct is particularly indicated for total vertebrectomy, severe spondylolisthesis reduced by anterior approaches, and most unstable fractures with neurologic lesions. The reduction of a kyphotic deformity is carried out either with intraoperative lordotic traction or by using a compressive posterior device or a spondylolisthesis anterior reduction device.

REFERENCES

An, H.S., & Cotler, J.M. (1992). Spinal internal fixation with Louis instrumentation. *Spinal Instrumentation.* Baltimore: William & Wilkins.

Louis R. (1985a). Lumbo-sacral fusion by internal fixation. *Clinical Orthopaedics and Related Research, 203,* 18–33.

Louis R. (1985b). Spinal stability as defined by our three column spine concept. *Anatomia Clinica 7,* 33–42.

Louis R. (1982). Surgery of the spine. Berlin, Paris, New York, Tokyo: Springer–Verlag, 328.

Louis, R., & Maresca C. (1976). Les arthrodèses stables de la charnière lombo-sacrée. *Revue de Chirurgie Orthopédique Supplements II, 62,* 70–79.

Louis, R., Maresca, C., & Bel P. (1977). Les fractures instables, la réduction orthopédique. *Revue de Chirurgie Orthopédique, 65,* 449–451.

Roy-Camille R. (1970). Ostéosynthèse du rachis dorsal, lombaire et lombosacré par plaques métalliques vissées dans les pédicules vertébraux et les apophyses articulaires. *Presse Medicole, 78,* 1447.

CHAPTER 36

Puno-Winter-Byrd (PWB) Transpedicular Spine Fixation System

J. Abbott Byrd, III
Rolando M. Puno

HIGHLIGHTS

The lumbar spine has been a source of pain since the beginning of humankind. Stories of patients with low back pain and sciatica have been recounted in the Bible and the works of Hippocrates (Cox, 1985). Elaborate treatments of this affliction have developed through the ages, though fortunately, for most patients, low back pain is self-limiting and will "cure itself." However, there is a patient population with significant pain that persists despite exhaustive nonoperative treatment attempts. This century has seen enthusiasm on the part of some physicians for the surgical treatment of this select group of patients (Chow, Leong, Yau, 1980; Cloward, 1953; Currant & McGaw, 1968; De Palma & Prabhakar, 1966; Freebody, Bendall, & Taylor, 1971; Graham, 1979; Lange, 1910; Shaw & Taylor, 1956; Stauffer & Coventry, 1972; Tanturi, Kataja, Keski-Nisula, et al., 1979).

The surgical treatment of the lumbar spine involves two basic elements: neural decompression and lumbar fusion. In general, neural decompression is relatively straightforward. On the other hand, surgeons have struggled with attempting to obtain better and more reliable fusions since Russell Hibbs (1911) first reported his fusion surgery for spinal deformities. It was recognized early that immobilization of the spine resulted in improved fusion rates. This led to the use of prolonged bed rest for patients following fusion surgery, which was often followed by extensive casting for prolonged periods. Not only was the medical treatment of these patients difficult and patient acceptance poor, but in addition, the fusion rates were low, often requiring several procedures to obtain successful fusion. The desire to produce more reliable fusion rates and improve patient care led spinal surgeons to seek improved techniques. The concept of internal fixation of the spine developed as a method to hold the spine still more reliably while fusion occurred. This both improved fusion rates and allowed earlier mobilization of the patient who underwent fusion.

In 1910, Lange reported his technique for spinal fusion using steel bars attached to the vertebrae, while King in 1944 reported his technique for spinal fixation using facet screws. Harrington published his classic work on the development of a hook and rod system to immobilize the spine in 1962. This was a giant leap forward in spinal instrumentation and has become the standard against which other systems are measured. Unfortunately, the use of Harrington instrumentation in the lumbar spine is not optimal primarily for two reasons. First, the distraction instrumentation leads to the loss of normal lumbar lordosis and the problems associated with this. Secondly, an intact lamina is necessary for instrumentation placement, which often precludes adequate decompression of the neural elements when necessary. In an attempt to avoid these problems, Roy-Camille began to instrument the lumbar spine with plates attached to the spine by screws placed through the plate and into the pedicles (Roy-Camille, Roy-Camille, & Demeulenaere, 1970). The advantage of this technique was readily apparent. Extensive decompressions could be performed, yet the spine could still be instrumented and lumbar lordosis preserved. However, the technique was limited by the use of plates with fixed holes, which markedly limited the variability with which the screws could be placed. Steffee began the modern era of pedicle screw fixation of the lumbar spine with his slotted plate, which allowed variable screw placement and enabled the surgeon to fit the instrumentation to the patient and not vice versa (Steffee, Biscup, & Sitkowski, 1986). However, limitations do exist with the Steffee plate instrumentation. While the instrumentation allows contouring in the sagittal plane it is not possible to contour the plate in the frontal or coronal plane, limiting its use in scoliosis. Also of concern is the limited area for bone grafting due to the size of the plate. Lastly, extension of a plate and screw system into the thoracic spine is difficult. Recognizing these limitations, we began in 1984 to develop a pedicle screw system to address these problems.

DEVELOPMENT OF THE PWB TRANSPEDICULAR SPINE FIXATION SYSTEM

Several guiding principles shaped the development of the initial PWB Transpedicular Spine Fixation System and its subsequent modifications. The initial desire was to produce a system that was applicable to scoliosis as well as to degenerative lumbar disease. This led to the use of a rod-screw construct rather than the popular plate-screw construct because the rod allowed contouring both in the sagittal and coronal planes (Figs. 36-1 and 36-2). Secondly, the system was designed to be entirely top-loading, which allowed placement of the rod on top of the screw rather than on the side of the screw, which greatly facilitates implantation. Lastly, it was our intent to develop a system that did not require any type of bushing or bearing to be placed on the rod because this increases both system complexity and implantation difficulty. These goals required the development of a unique rod-screw connector, which at the time had not been seen in the industry (Table 36-1).

The PWB rod-screw connector consists of a seat or channel in which the rod sits. The rod is secured by a cap and external nut, both of which are placed from the top after the rod is in place (Fig. 36-3). In an attempt to minimize the size of the implant, a threaded plug with internal threads on the seat was initially considered to secure the rod. However, there was concern that the plug would dislodge with tightening because of spreading of the wings on the seat. Thus, this design concept was abandoned in favor of the nut with external threads on the seat.

Initially, there was concern for stress-shielding of the spine by a totally rigid implant system as well as the high screw failure rate seen with other totally rigid pedicle screw systems. This led to the development of a semirigid system in which the seat and screw were two pieces (Fig. 36-4).

Table 36-1
Advantages of the PWB Transpedicular Spine Fixation System

Feature	Advantage
Rod-screw construct	Allows coronal and sagittal plane contouring
Rod-screw construct	Maximizes bone graft area
Top-loading	Facilitates implantation
No rod bushings	Facilitates implantation

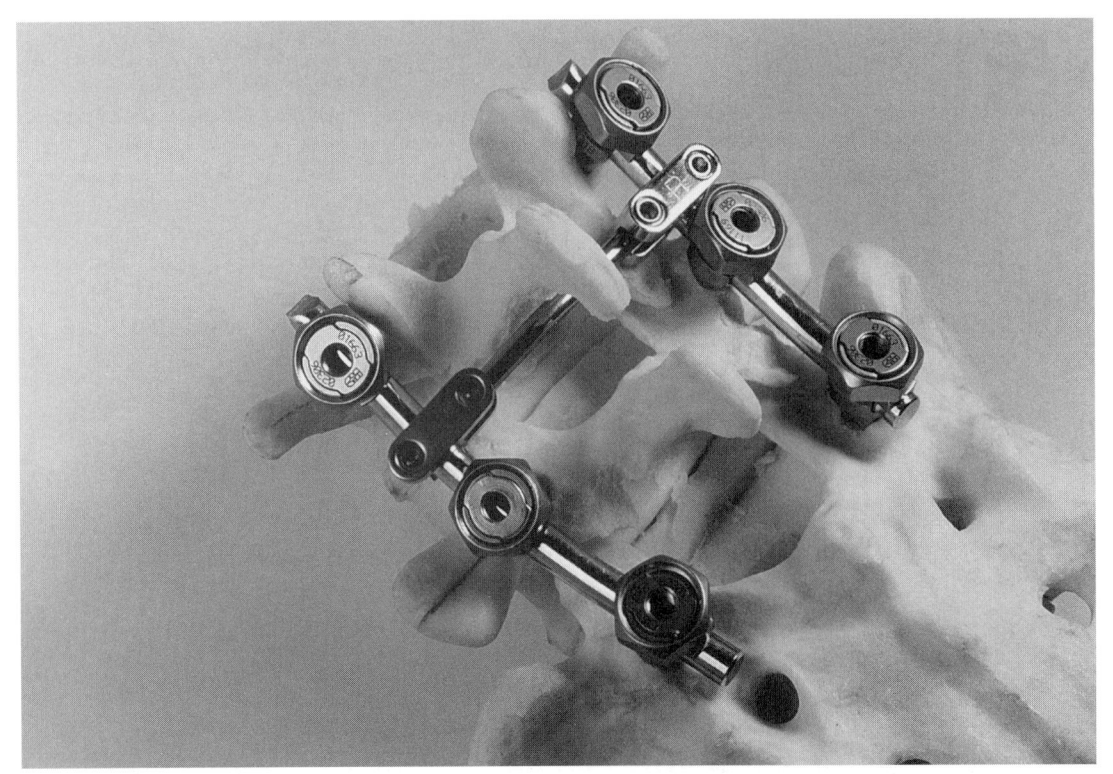

FIG. 36-1. Posterior view of a two-level integral PWB construct with cross-linking device in place.

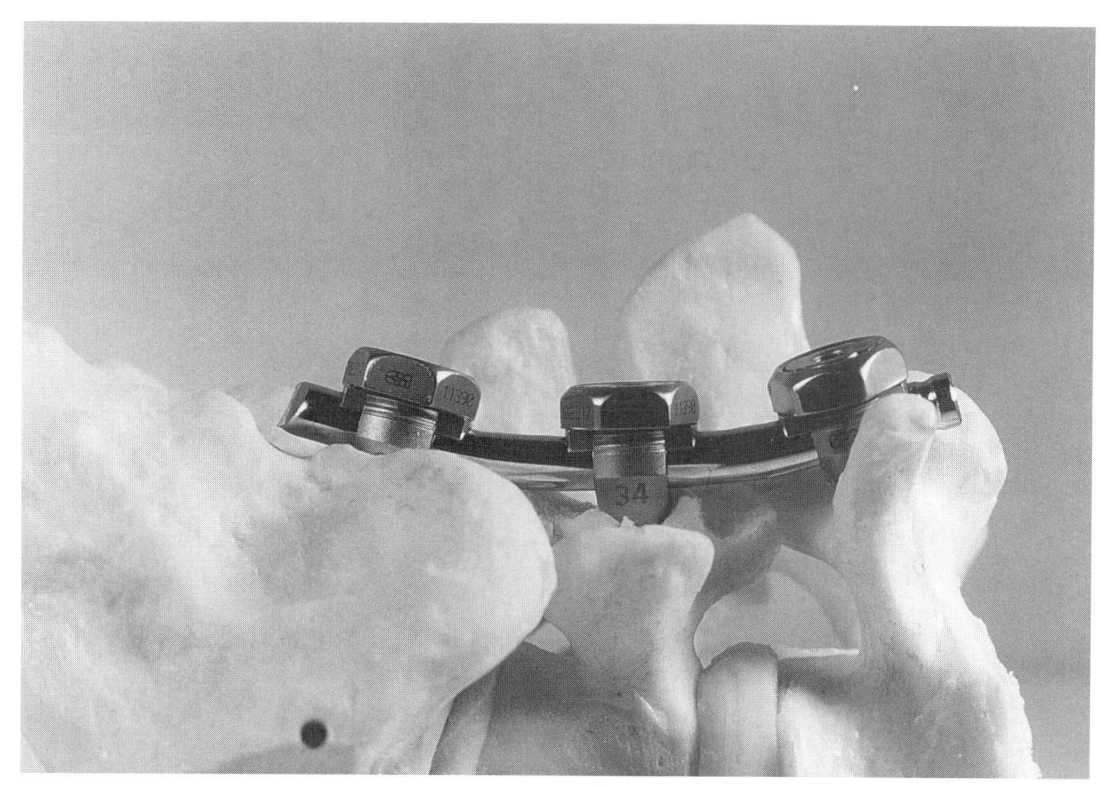

FIG. 36-2. Lateral view of a two-level integral PWB construct.

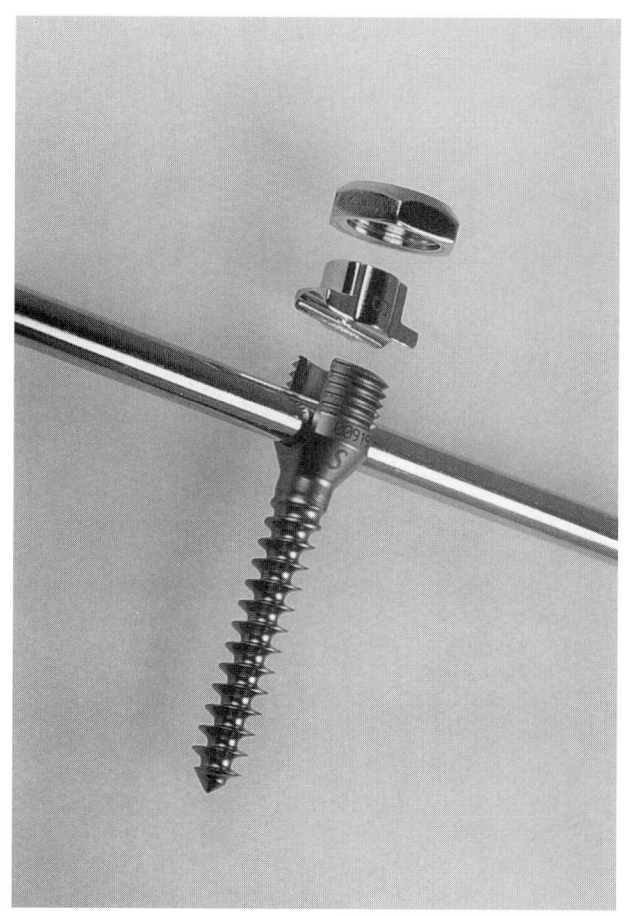

FIG. 36-3. Integral PWB assembly showing the screw, rod, cap, and nut.

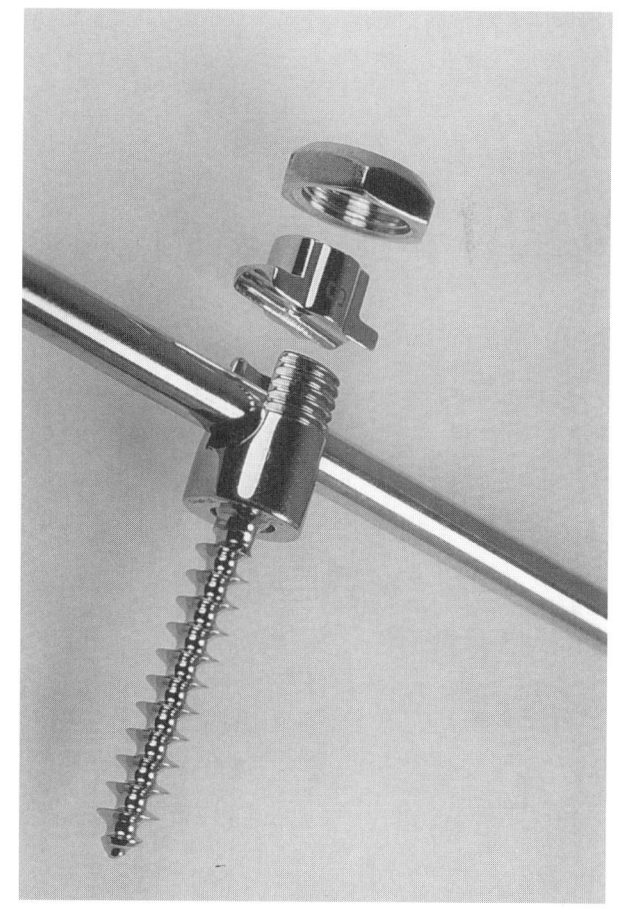

FIG. 36-4. PWB II semirigid assembly showing the screw, seat, rod, cap, and nut.

Tightening of the screw secures the seat to the spine but still allows micromotion at the screw-seat interface. This acts as shock absorber decreasing the stress on the implant.

Extensive biomechanical testing was done on the original implant design (Puno, Bechtold, Byrd, Winter, Ogilvie, & Bradford, 1991) and was submitted to the Food and Drug Administration for an Investigational Device Exemption, which was obtained in 1988. The first clinical trials with the PWB I began later that year with the two-piece seat-and-screw design, which was tightened with a nut from beneath the rod. It proved difficult to place this nut, leading to a design revision in which the nut was placed from the top, although the semirigid two-piece screw-and-seat design was still used. Implantation of this PWB II design began in 1989. The system was further modified in 1992 with the development of a rigid construct using a one-piece screw and seat and the addition of hooks to be used in the upper lumbar or lower thoracic spine. Implantation of this PWB III or Integral PWB began in 1992. Both the PWB II and the Integral PWB are available (Cross Medical Products, Inc., Columbus, OH), but the latter is the authors' choice at this time.

INDICATIONS AND CONTRAINDICATIONS

The use of the PWB Transpedicular Spine Fixation System is indicated whenever the surgeon desires to provide immediate stabilization to the lumbar spine by internal fixation while awaiting maturation of a solid fusion. The surgeon must remember, however, that no instrumentation can compensate for a faulty fusion technique. Attention to detail must be given when performing the fusion or increased instrumentation failure and poor patient outcomes will result.

Specific indications for which the PWB system has been successfully used since 1988 include lumbar scoliosis, spondylolisthesis, degenerative lumbar disk disease, fractures, tumors, failed-back syndromes, and repair of pseudarthrosis.

There are no contraindications for usage specific to the PWB system itself. However, contraindications to pedicle screw fixation in general include the presence of infection, morbid obesity, severe osteopenia, and abnormal spinal morphology, which prevents safe placement of the screws in the pedicles (Table 36-2).

IMPLANTS

The PWB system has both semirigid (PWB II) and rigid (Integral PWB) constructs, which may be used separately or mixed as the situation demands. The PWB II screw is made from 316 L stainless steel and has a 6.5-mm diameter with lengths from 35 to 50 mm in 5-mm increments. The screws are placed through seats that are available in four heights, the use of which will be described later in the "Surgical Technique" section. The material for the PWB integral screw is 22-13-5 stainless steel, selected because of the concerns for increased implant stress on a rigid system. This particular alloy of stainless steel has a 10 to 15% increased fatigue limit compared to 316 L stainless steel. In addition, the minor diameter is tapered to the third thread to provide increased fatigue strength to the screw. The PWB integral screw is available in diameters of 5.5, 6.5, 7.0, and 7.5 mm with the same lengths as the PWB II screws.

Table 36-2
Indications and Contraindications for Use of PWB Transpedicular Spine Fixation System

Indications
    Lumbar scoliosis
    Spondylolisthesis
    Degenerative disk disease
    Failed-back syndrome
    Repair pseudarthrosis
    Fractures
    Tumors

Contraindications
    Infection
    Morbid obesity
    Severe osteopenia
    Inadequate pedicles

Rods for both constructs are 6.35 mm in diameter, made from 316 L stainless steel and come in precut lengths from 5 to 38 cm. The rods are annealed, which increases their malleability and facilitates rod contouring.

The uniqueness of the PWB system lies with the clamping mechanism by which the rod is secured to the pedicle screw (Fig. 36-5). The rod is placed in the open channel of either the seat or the integral screw. A cap is then placed in the channel over the rod, thus capturing the rod. A nut is then screwed on either the seat or integral screw and tightened, thereby securing the cap and rod in place.

The PWB system may be cross-linked as desired by the surgeon using the modular cross-link assembly (Fig. 36-6). This consists of left and right couplers that fit onto the 6.35-mm-longitudinal rod and are secured with a set screw. The couplers are then interconnected with a 4-mm cross-link rod, which again is secured with a set screw. This design allows placement of the cross-link without any preplacement of a connector on the rod.

IMPLANT INSTRUMENTATION

As with the implant itself, much attention during the design phase has been given to keeping the instrumentation as simple as possible. Few instruments are required for implantation; they include an awl, a blunt probe, seat reamer, seat holder, screwdriver, hook holder, rod holder, cap-nut alignment guide, T-handle wrench, torque wrench, and torque stabilizer. Once in place, the construct may be manipulated using a spreader, compressor, or in situ bender. If the cross-link assembly is placed then an additional cross-link holder as well as a smaller rod holder and screwdriver are used.

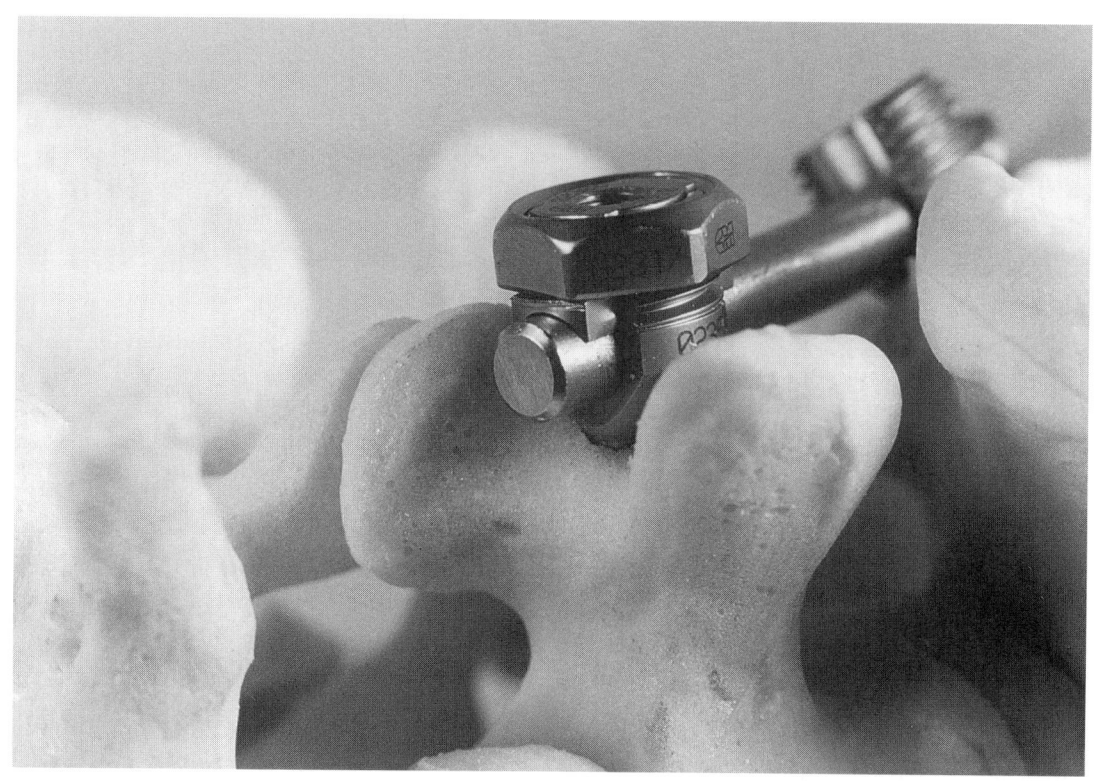

CHAPTER 36 / PUNO-WINTER-BYRD (PWB) TRANSPEDICULAR SPINE FIXATION SYSTEM   **413**

FIG. 36-5. Close-up view of the integral PWB clamping assembly showing the rod secured in the screw by the cap and nut.

SURGICAL TECHNIQUE

The implantation of any pedicle screw system involves two basic phases. The first is that of spinal exposure and pedicle-hole creation. The second involves implantation of the system itself. While detailed instruction regarding the first phase is outside the scope of this chapter, the authors have found the following to be of benefit when performing pedicle-screw fixation of the lumbar spine. In addition, numerous articles have been written that detail pedicle anatomy and screw placement (Asher & Strippgen, 1986; Banta, King, Dabezies, & Liljeberg, 1989; Berry, Moran, Berg, & Steffee, 1987; Esses, Botsford, Huler, & Rausching, 1990; Zindrick, Wiltse, Doornik, et al., 1987).

FIG. 36-6. Modular cross-linking assembly.

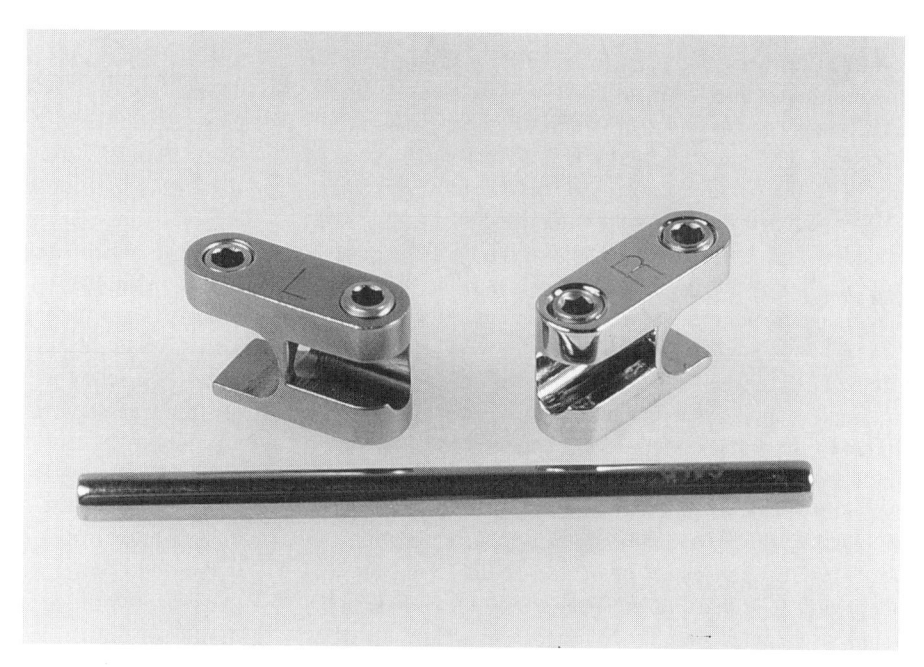

The surgeon must remember that the ease with which a system is implanted begins not only when the first screw is inserted but also with meticulous attention to detail for every step preceding implant placement. Bleeding must be kept to a minimum to allow accurate landmark identification for pedicle-hole placement. This is best accomplished by proper patient positioning to avoid abdominal compression followed by careful subperiosteal dissection with electrocautery coagulation to stop bleeding as it occurs. Care must be taken to preserve the facet capsules and interspinous ligaments above and below the levels to be fused. Once the spine is exposed laterally to the transverse processes the site for starting the pedicle holes must be identified. Before making any pedicle holes, the surgeon should survey the entire length of spine to be instrumented and attempt to visualize where the holes should be placed to create a smooth curve, as this will ease implantation of any instrumentation system. Identification of the insertion site is facilitated by removing all soft tissue from the lateral side of the superior facet, transverse process, and lateral side of the pars interarticularis with electrocautery. This step is crucial because there is minimal room for error, and if the hole does not start correctly it will not finish properly. In general, the entrance site to the pedicle is at the intersection of a transverse line through the middle of the transverse process with a second line drawn vertically along the lateral border of the superior articular facet. However, patient variation does occur, and the surgeon should review the plain films prior to hole placement, making special note of the medial-lateral relationship of the pedicle to the pars interarticularis and the superior-inferior relationship to the superior articular facet. This allows the surgeon to key off of these structures during surgery and make minor adjustments in the starting position for the pedicle hole, which will greatly facilitate pedicle hole creation. If any question exists concerning the starting point, the surgeon should not hesitate to perform a laminotomy to identify the medial border of the pedicle. The pedicle awl or a motorized drill may be used to make the starting hole by penetrating the outer cortical layer.

Once the starting point for the pedicle hole is identified, the pedicle hole must be created by cannulating the pedicle canal with the pedicle probe. The surgeon must remember that the pedicles progressively angle medially as one proceeds down the lumbar spine. The first lumbar pedicle is almost parallel to the sagittal plane, while each subsequent pedicle angles 5 degrees more medially, ending with the L5 pedicle, which angles 20 to 30 degrees toward the midline. With regard to cranial-caudal angulation of the pedicle hole, the surgeon should remember that this is usually perpendicular to the transverse process. Thus, the pedicle probe should usually be kept perpendicular to the transverse process in this plane. If this step is followed, the pedicle holes will usually point to a common central point, much like the spokes on a wagon wheel point to a central axis, and this will greatly facilitate implant placement. All pedicle holes should be palpated with a depth gauge to ensure that they are in bone; metallic markers should be placed and radiographs obtained to make sure that the holes are where the surgeon desires them to be. Both the PWB pedicle probe, which is calibrated for screw length, and the depth gauge should be left in place during lateral radiography, as this will allow accurate selection of proper screw length.

Once the pedicle holes have been created, the second phase of pedicle screw fixation or implant placement is ready to begin. If the PWB II (semirigid) is to be implanted, the pedicle reamer is used to plane or flatten the site where the seat will be. This allows the surgeon to orient the seats so that they define a smooth curve that is independent of screw angulation in the pedicle. Proper seat sizes are then selected from the four different seat heights available (I—1.68 mm, II—1.83 mm, III—1.98 mm, and IV—2.13 mm) to produce alignment of the bottom of the rod channel in the sagittal plane. These different seat heights allow the surgeon to compensate for the variation in sagittal position that exists in the vertebral segments. Trial seats are available to aid the surgeon in the selection of the permanent seats. The use of the Integral PWB (rigid) eliminates this step, which in combination with the fact that it is more rigid than the PWB II makes the Integral PWB the choice of the authors. Screw placement is now ready to begin. Screw length is selected to allow 60 to 70% penetration of the vertebral body. No attempt should be made to engage the anterior cortex because of the risk this presents to the retroperitoneal soft-tissue structures. In general, screw lengths of 40 to 45 mm are sufficient in the lumbar spine. Screw diameter should obviously be selected based on pedicle size which the preoperative computed tomographic (CT) or magnetic resonance imaging (MRI) scan should reveal. The surgeon should remember that screw strength and rigidity increase exponentially with increased diameter; thus, the largest-diameter screw that can be safely placed should be selected. Usual screw diameters are 5.5 to 6.5 mm for L1 and L2 and 7.0 to 7.5 mm for L3, L4, and L5. Though the screws will tap themselves, it is often helpful to tap the outer cortex, as this will make it easier to start the screws without their slipping from the pedicle hole. Taps are provided for all screw sizes. The PWB II screw is placed through the appropriate-sized seat and tightened with the hex screwdriver, drawing the seat down securely on the prepared seat bed. A seat holder may be used to guide the seat into place (Fig. 36-7). The Integral PWB screw is placed using the internal drive screwdriver, which fits securely in the channel of the screw. This screwdriver design provides the surgeon excellent control of the screw without fear that the screwdriver will slip off of the screw (Fig. 36-8). The screws are inserted so that the bottom of the rod channels are aligned in the sagittal plane. After screw placement, it is occasionally necessary to advance one screw half a turn or back a screw out half a turn, or both, to align the bottom of the rod channels. Careful attention to this step will greatly facilitate rod, cap, and nut placement. Proper screw placement should be confirmed by intraoperative PA and lateral radiographs.

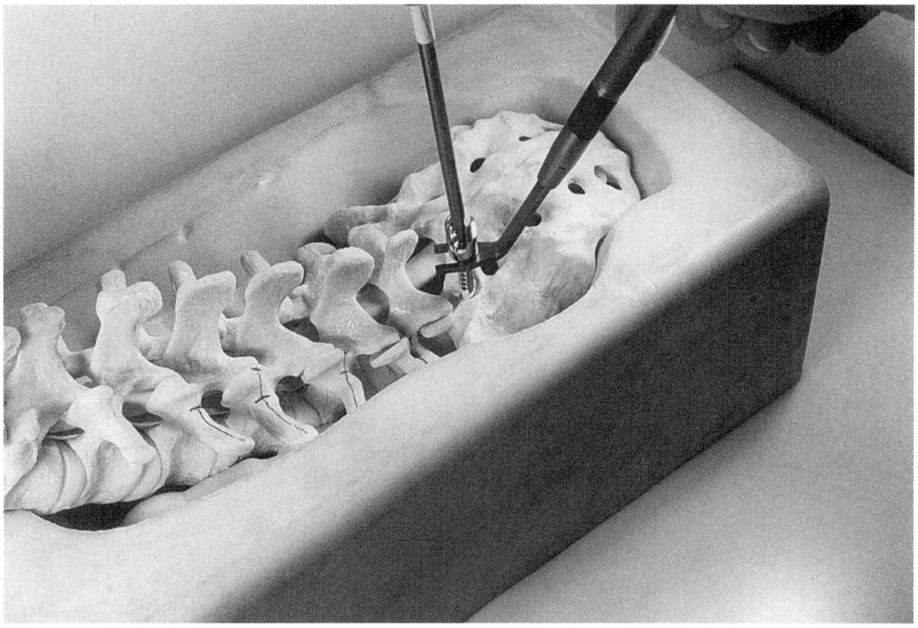

FIG. 36-7. Placement of the semirigid PWB II using the screwdriver and seat holder.

Screw placement in the sacrum is different than in the lumbar spine primarily because the anatomy of the sacrum is different from that of the lumbar spine. Since there is no transverse process present on the sacrum, the surgeon must use the caudal portion of the sacral articular facet to identify the entrance point for screw placement. In addition, because of sacral size the screw may be directed either medially or laterally, though medial insertion toward the sacral promontory is preferred because of the increased pullout strength that this yields. Lastly, safe purchase of the anterior sacral cortex is possible due to the fact that the great vessels bifurcate proximal to this level. The surgeon must remember, however, that the L5 nerve root passes just anterior to the sacral ala, and this area must be avoided if anterior cortical purchase is desired. Use of either 7.0- or 7.5-mm diameter screws is recommended in the sacrum due to the large size of the sacral pedicle.

After the pedicle screws have been placed, it is necessary to select the proper length 6.35-mm-diameter rod and contour it using the French rod bender to fit into the seats. A rod of sufficient length to extend 5 mm beyond the end screws should be selected. In general, if the screws are properly placed, only a gentle bend is required in the rod for proper fit in the screw channels. If radical rod bends appear

FIG. 36-8. Placement of the rigid integral PWB using the screwdriver.

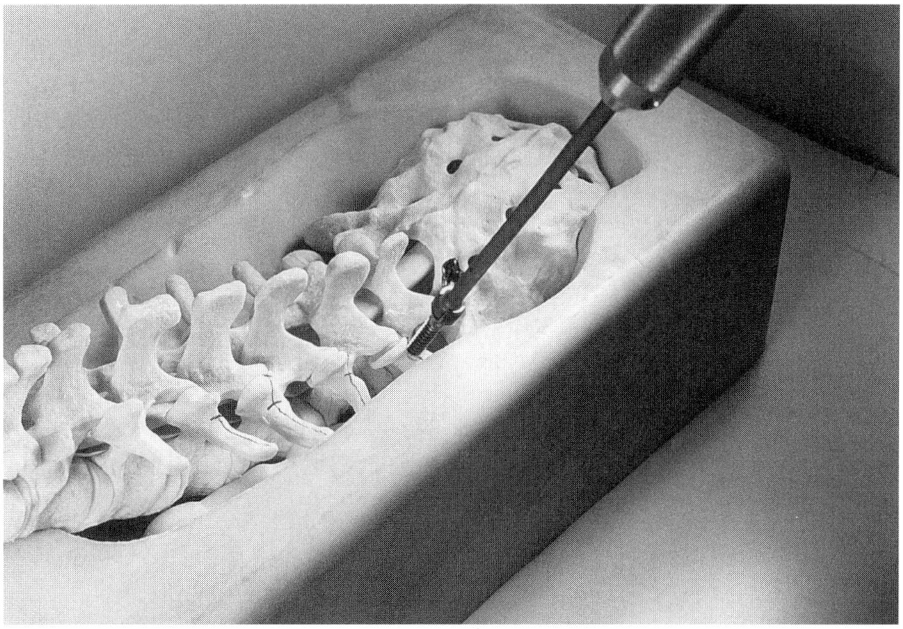

necessary the surgeon should reevaluate screw or seat placement and adjust these as necessary. However, with proper planning of screw or seat placement, adjustment is usually not required for rod placement. The rod holder is used to place the rod in the seats and if necessary an impactor or the integral screwdriver may be used to tap the rod into place. If properly placed, the rod will lay in the bottom of the rod channels and the wings or sides of the rod channels will be perpendicular to the rod. If this is the case, cap and nut placement will be readily accomplished. However, if the rod does not lay flat in the bottom of the rod channel then cap and nut placement may be somewhat difficult, depending on the degree of tilt that exists between the rod and the screw channel. In extreme cases it may be necessary to either adjust the screw/seat or recontour the rod.

Once satisfactory rod placement has been accomplished, the cap and nut are placed to secure the rod in either the PWB II seat or Integral PWB screw. This is accomplished using the cap-nut alignment guide, which was developed to minimize cross-threading of the nut. The scrub nurse first places the nut on the guide so that the flat side of the nut will face the rod. The cap is then placed on the guide and held in place with the small threaded rod that runs down the middle of the guide. Using the guide, the cap-nut assembly is placed into the PWB II seat or Integral PWB screw (Fig. 36-9). Though the fit of the cap in the seat or screw provides alignment of the nut, it is still possible to cross-thread the nut because of the necessary clearance tolerances that must exist. Because of this the surgeon must make certain by visual inspection that the cap-nut alignment guide is aligned with the seat or screw in both the coronal and sagittal planes. Once alignment is confirmed, the surgeon turns the outer barrel of the guide, thereby advancing the nut, which falls from the guide threads onto the threads of the seat or screw (Fig. 36-10). As this step is one of "touch and feel" and not force, the surgeon should turn the guide barrel with the thumb and fingertips and not use a power grip with the guide barrel in the palm. If the nut is started properly it will thread smoothly with little force required. If the nut cross-threads, the surgeon should back the nut up until a click is heard, signaling that the crossed threads have disengaged, realign the guide, and then advance the nut. Alternatively, the cap-nut alignment guide may be removed from the cap by turning the small central threaded rod counterclockwise. The T-handled socket wrench may then be used to back up the nut, realign it, and advance it properly (Table 36-3).

The nuts on one rod should not be tightened until all nuts have been placed. Once this has been accomplished, the T-handled socket wrench is used to tighten all nuts sequentially. At this stage, the distractor or compressor may be used to manipulate the spine as indicated. The nuts are then tightened to hold the spine in place. Final tightening of the nuts to 120 in.-lb is accomplished with the torque wrench, using the torque stabilizer to prevent the rod from twisting.

Once both the left and right sides of the spine have been instrumented the surgeon may cross-link the construct if ad-

Table 36-3
Troubleshooting the Integral PWB Transpedicular Spine Fixation System

Problem	Cause	Solution
Rod does not contact bottom of screw channel	Poor screw alignment in sagittal plane	Back out or advance screws as necessary
Rod angled in bottom of screw channel	Poor rod contouring or screws angled improperly	Recontour rod or, as a last resort, adjust screws
Nut cross-threaded	Malalignment of cap-nut alignment guide	Back nut off, realign guide, advance nut

ditional torsional stability is desired. In general, the longer the construct the more important it is to place cross-links, and for constructs involving more than three levels cross-linking should strongly be considered. If possible, two cross-links should be used, as this provides increased rotational stability (Asher, Carson, & Heinig, 1988; Puno, Bechtold, Kim, Sun, & Bradford, 1986).

It is recommended that final PA and lateral radiographs be obtained in the operating room prior to wound closure to make certain that instrumentation placement is as desired by the surgeon.

While the subject of bone grafting is outside the scope of this chapter, it is the authors' preference to use autogenous iliac crest graft whenever possible. Thorough decortication of the posterior elements is required and the authors prefer to place the bone graft after pedicle-hole creation and prior to instrumentation placement. Cottonoid strips may be placed in the pedicle holes to act as markers and prevent them from being covered up by the bone graft. After instrumentation placement, additional bone graft may be placed under the rods in the facet region as necessary.

CLINICAL EXPERIENCE

The first author (J.A.B.) began implantation of the PWB system in 1988, and to date 145 patients implanted with the PWB I/II system have at least 2 years of follow-up. A second group of 57 patients have been implanted with the Integral PWB beginning in late 1992 and reached 2-year follow-up in December 1994. The PWB I/II group consists of 59% women and 41% men, with a mean age of 52 years and a range of 20 to 81 years. The Integral PWB group consists of 49% women and 51% men, with a mean age of 49 years and a range of 26 to 75 years. Diagnoses for the PWB I/II group includes spondylolisthesis (69 patients), degenerative disk disease (37), failed-back syndrome (32), lumbar stenosis (6), and tumor (1). The Integral PWB group includes patients with spondylolisthesis (20 patients), degenerative disk disease (20), failed-back syndrome (9), lumbar stenosis (6), and fracture (2). Previous surgery had been per-

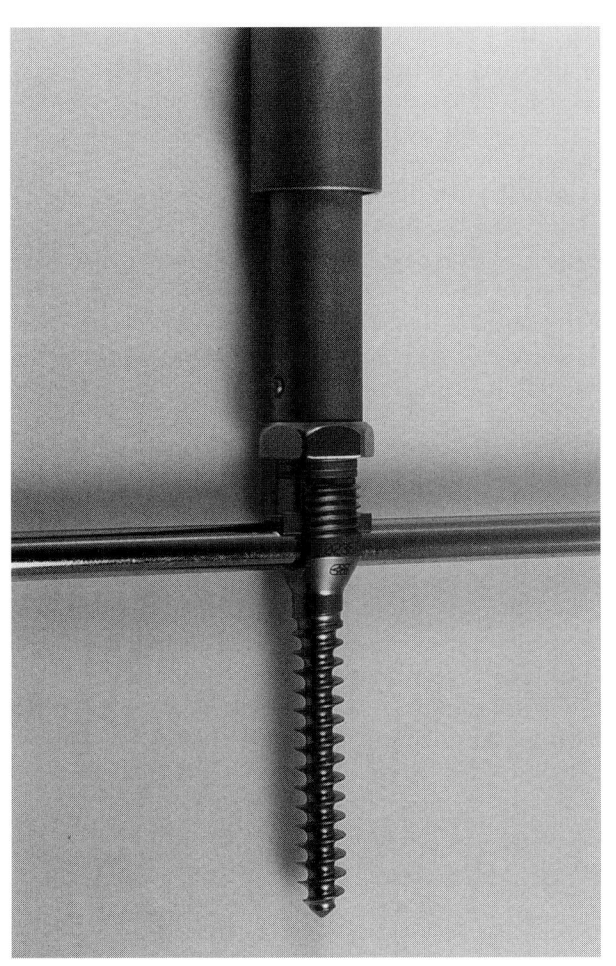

FIG. 36-9. Cap and nut in place on the cap-nut alignment guide, with the cap placed in the screw properly aligned and ready for nut advancement. Note the outer barrel in the raised position.

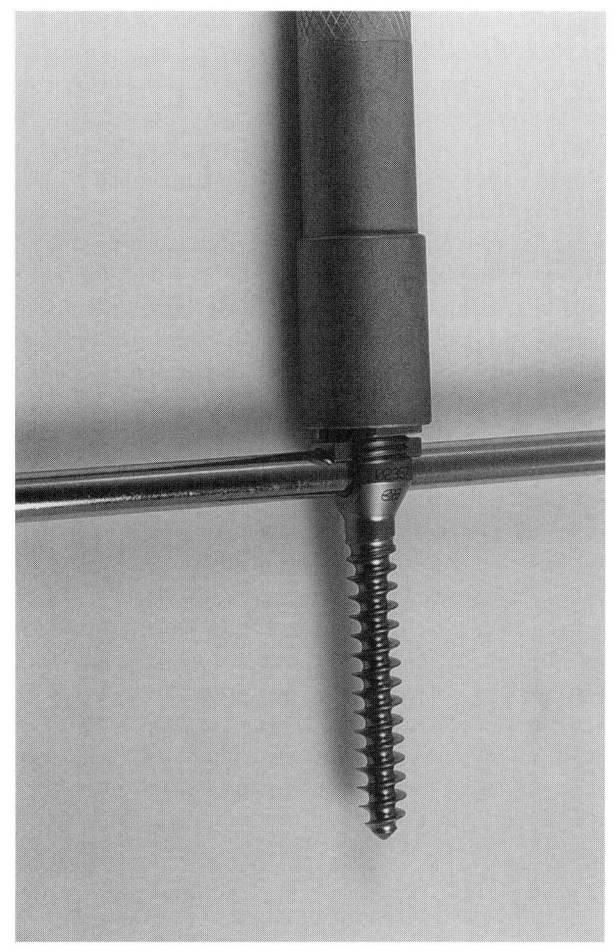

FIG. 36-10. The outer barrel has been lowered over the nut and used to advance the nut off of the threads on the cap-nut alignment guide and onto the threads of the integral PWB screw.

formed in 76 of the 145 PWB I/II patients and in 29 of the 57 Integral PWB patients. All patients in both groups underwent posterior lateral spinal fusion, while 45 patients in the PWB I/II group and 38 patients in the Integral PWB group underwent an additional interbody fusion either anteriorly or posteriorly. Instrumented segments for the PWB I/II groups include one in 58 patients, two in 66 patients, three in 15 patients, four in 5 patients and five or more in 1 patient. Instrumented segments for the Integral PWB include one in 23 patients, two in 23 patients, three in 6 patients, four in 3 patients, and five or more in 2 patients. In these study groups, a total of 810 screws have been implanted for the PWB I/II group and 334 screws for the Integral PWB. The average operating time is 322 minutes for the PWB I/II group and 308 minutes for the Integral PWB group. The average blood loss for the two groups is 727 and 688 ml, respectively.

The results of these two study groups have been evaluated from two perspectives. The first is the clinical result, which deals with patient outcome, and the second is the implant result, which deals with intrinsic implant issues. Clinical results have been determined by evaluating fusion rates, return-to-work status, and pain relief. The determination of accurate fusion rates using radiography is somewhat difficult if not impossible. However, because exploration of every fusion to determine solidity is not feasible, practicality requires the use of radiography to determine the status of the fusion. Radiographic criteria for a solid fusion include the absence of a visible defect in the fusion mass, a smooth border on the fusion mass that flows either into the vertebral bodies anteriorly or the transverse processes and facet joints posteriorly, trabeculation in the fusion mass crossing the area to be fused, or the absence of motion on flexion-extension films. Using these criteria, the fusion rate for the PWB I/II group at 2 years is 82%. This was a worst-case calculation because seven patients were lost to follow-up, all of whom were considered to have fusion failures. The Integral PWB group has reached the 2-year follow-up with a fusion rate that will be in the 85 to 90% range. Return-to-work data were obtained for both worker's compensation and non–worker's compensation patients. In the PWB I/II group, 27 of 41 worker's compensation patients (66%) returned to work, whereas in the Integral PWB group, 12 of 19 worker's compensation patients (63%) returned to work.

All 40 non–worker's compensation patients in both groups returned to work. Pain relief again is difficult to assess, but this was attempted using patient questionnaires during routine follow-up. In general, the average patient received 60 to 70% pain relief in both groups.

Intrinsic PWB implant results were determined by evaluating hardware failure rates and failure rates at the coupling site between the screw and the rod. Of the 810 PWB I/II screws implanted in this series, 8 (1%) have broken. In addition, 3 (1%) of the 334 Integral PWB screws implanted have broken. The rod has pulled out of the coupling device only twice with the PWB I/II, and this has not occurred with the Integral PWB. These two failures occurred early in the experience and were probably the result of inadequate tightening of the nut. This problem has been addressed through the use of a beam-type torque wrench to standardize tightening torque.

Other complications not intrinsically related to the PWB system include screw pullout in one patient, misplaced screw in one patient, and two superficial infections in each of the PWB I/II and Integral PWB groups. No deep infections occurred in either of the groups. In addition, three late deaths were experienced in the PWB I/II group, though none were specifically related to the lumbar surgery itself. Also, one patient in the PWB I/II group suffered a postoperative cerebrovascular accident, from which he has partially recovered. Otherwise no complications have occurred in these two study groups.

Reoperations have been necessary in 22 of the PWB I/II patients. One patient each has required replacement of a broken screw, redirection of a screw, excision of a disk herniation above previous fusion, removal of a retropulsed Posterior Lumbar Interbody Fusion (PLIF) fragment and debridement of a superficial wound infection. Two patients each have required reinsertion of a rod pullout and exploration of the fusion for pseudarthrosis with repeat bone grafting and reinstrumentation. It has been necessary to extend the fusion in three patients and decompress above the level of instrumentation in four patients. Six patients have undergone exploration of their fusion, which was found to be solid, and the hardware was removed. Only one patient in the Integral PWB group has required reoperation and that was to debride a superficial wound.

DISCUSSION

The PWB system has evolved over a 10-year period from a set of drawings to a refined system that is being implanted both domestically and internationally. Through the use of a rod-screw construct, the instrumentation affords the surgeon the greatest freedom available in implantation in both the sagittal and coronal planes. Its uniqueness is found in the coupling device that secures the rod to the screw. This clamping mechanism is top loading, which greatly facilitates rod contouring and implantation. In addition, once the rod is in place the top-loading feature greatly eases nut placement, instrumentation and spinal manipulation, and nut tightening. Though implant modifications have occurred in response to the clinical experience, the basic rod clamping mechanism has remained the same, withstanding the test of time. The rod clamping mechanism is quite secure and if the nuts are properly tightened there should not be a failure at the rod-screw interface. The Integral PWB screws have been designed through the use of the tapered minor diameter to maximize both intrinsic screw strength and bone pullout strength. The clinical results have validated the PWB design as intrinsic instrumentation failures have been few since implantation began in 1988. The surgeon must remember, however, that implant strength is not a substitute for meticulous fusion technique and one must not get "carried away" with the instrumentation and forget that the purpose of the operation is to obtain a solid arthrodesis.

The PWB system allows the placement of both semirigid and rigid constructs through the use of the PWB II and Integral PWB, respectively. However, during the past several years the authors have implanted the rigid or Integral PWB almost exclusively for several reasons. First, it appears that the fusion rates are improved through the use of a rigid system as compared with a semirigid system. Secondly, implantation of the Integral PWB is easier than the PWB II in that the surgeon does not need to prepare the seat bed, which is so crucial to the accurate placement of the PWB II. Rather, once the pedicle hole is created, the Integral PWB screw is inserted to the proper depth, which allows alignment of the screws in the sagittal plane. Lastly, the use of a rigid system eliminates the concern for small shifts in spinal position that may occur with the use of a semirigid system.

SUMMARY

The PWB Transpedicular Spine Fixation System is a carefully designed rod-screw spinal fixation device. When properly implanted it safely provides excellent immobilization and fusion rates of the instrumented spine.

REFERENCES

Asher, M., Carson, W., & Heinig, C. (1988). A modular spinal rod linkage system to provide rotational stability. *Spine, 13,* 272–277.

Asher, M.A., & Strippgen, W.E. (1986). Anthropometric study of the human sacrum relating to dorsal transsacral implant design. *Clinical Orthopaedics and Related Research, 203,* 58–62.

Banta, C.J., King, A.G., Dabezies, E.J., & Liljeberg, R.L. (1989). Measurement of the effective pedicle diameter in the human spine. *Orthopedics, 12,* 939–942.

Berry, J.L., Moran, J.M., Berg, W.S., & Steffee, A.D. (1987). A morphometric study of human lumbar and selected thoracic vertebrae. *Spine, 12,* 362–367.

Chow, S.P., Leong, J.C.Y., & Yau, A.C. (1980). Anterior spinal fusion for deranged lumbar intervertebral disc. *Spine,* 452–458.

Cloward, R.B. (1953). Treatment of ruptured intervertebral disc by vertebral body fusion—indication, operative technique, and after care. *Journal of Neurosurgery, 10,* 154–168.

Cox, J.M. (1985). *Low Back Pain* (4th ed.) (p. 1). Baltimore: Williams & Wilkins.

Curran, J.P., & McGaw, W.H. (1968). Posterolateral spinal fusion with pedicle grafts. *Clinical Orthopaedics and Related Research, 59,* 125–129.

De Palma, A.F., & Prabhakar, M. (1966). Posterior-posterobilateral fusion of the lumbosacral spine. *Clinical Orthopaedics and Related Research, 47,* 165–171.

Esses, S.I., Botsford, D.J., Huler, R.J., & Rausching, W. (1990). Surgical anatomy of the sacrum—A guide to rational screw fixation. Presented at the North American Spine Society annual meeting, Montery, CA.

Freebody, D., Bendall, R., & Taylor, R.D. (1971). Anterior transperitoneal lumbar fusion. *Journal of Bone and Joint Surgery, British Volume, 53,* 617–627.

Graham, C.E. (1979). Lumbosacral fusion using internal fixation with a spinous process for the graft. *Clinical Orthopaedics and Related Research, 140,* 72–77.

Harrington, P.R. (1962). Treatment of scoliosis: Correction and internal fixation by spine instrumentation. *Journal of Bone and Joint Surgery, American Volume, 44,* 591–610.

Hibbs, R.A. (1911). An operation for progressive spinal deformities. *New York Journal of Medicine, 93,* 1013–1016.

King, D. (1944). Internal fixation for lumbosacral fusion. *American Journal of Surgery, 66,* 357–361.

Lange, F. (1910). Support of the spondylitic spine by means of buried steel bars attached to the vertebrae. *American Journal of Orthopedic Surgery, 8,* 344–361.

Puno, R.M., Bechtold, J.E., Byrd, J.A., Winter, R.B., Ogilvie, J.W., & Bradford, D.S. (1991). Biomechanical analysis of transpedicular rod systems—A preliminary report. *Spine, 16,* 973–980.

Puno, R.M., Bechtold, J.E., Kim, A.B., Sun, B.N., & Bradford, D.S. (1986). Anterior spinal fixation—Clinical and biomechanical analysis. Presented at the Orthopaedic Research Society annual meeting, New Orleans.

Roy-Camille, R., Roy-Camille, M., & Demeulenaere, C. (1970). Osteosynthese du rachis dorsal, lombaire et lombo-sacre. *La Presse Medicale, 78,* 1447–1448.

Shaw, E.G., & Taylor, J.G. (1956). The results of lumbosacral fusion for low back pain. *Journal of Bone and Joint Surgery, British Volume, 38,* 484–497.

Stauffer, R.N., & Coventry, M.B. (1972). Posterolateral lumbar spine fusion. *Journal of Bone and Joint Surgery, American Volume, 54,* 756–768.

Steffee, A.D., Biscup, R.S., & Sitkowski, D.J. (1986). Segmental spine plates with pedicle screw fixation—A new internal fixation device for disorders of the lumbar and thoracolumbar spine. *Clinical Orthopaedics and Related Research, 203,* 45–53.

Tanturi, T., Kataja, M., Keski-Nisula, L., et al. (1979). Posterior fusion of the lumbosacral spine. *Acta Orthopedica Scandanavica, 50,* 415–425.

Zindrick, M.R., Wiltse, L.L., Doornik, A., et al. (1987). Analysis of the morphometric characteristics of the thoracic and lumbar pedicles. *Spine, 12,* 160–166.

CHAPTER 37

Correction of Spinal Deformity and Instability Using the Edwards Modular System

Charles C. Edwards

HIGHLIGHTS

The Edwards Modular Spinal System (Scientific Spinal Ltd., Baltimore, MD) combines the axial adjustability of Harrington instrumentation with the advantages of segmental screw fixation, and introduces the concept of transverse adjustability. The result is a highly versatile spinal system that is adjustable in all planes of motion to correct spinal deformity and provide segmental fixation.

DEVELOPMENT

The Edwards Modular Spinal System (EMSS) has evolved over the past 15 years. By 1982, Edwards rod-sleeves and anatomic hooks were developed for use with conventional Harrington instrumentation in the treatment of lumbar fractures. Rod-sleeves restore full lordosis and generate a dynamic extension moment for improved late alignment (Edwards & Levine, 1986). The hooks introduced the anatomic L-shape for better load distribution to minimize both hook dislodgment and laminar resorption with late loss of correction (Edwards & Levine, 1986). In 1983, the Edwards Modular Spinal System contributed the first sacral screw and sacral fixation device designed for attachment of spinal rods to the sacrum (Edwards, 1984). Thus, Edwards instrumentation became the first "modular" system offering both hook and screw fixation alternatives for the lumbosacral spine (Edwards, Levine, et al., 1987). The fully ratcheted universal rod was introduced in 1985 and evolved to provide bidirectional ratcheting and segmental fixation. The adjustable connectors were developed in 1985 to permit transverse control of vertebral position (Edwards, Levine, et al., 1987). The uniquely adjustable yet rigid cross-locks were perfected in 1992 to complete the six components that compose the EMSS.

The ability to move individual vertebrae gradually in all three dimensions gave rise to a new approach to deformity correction. By applying corrective forces to stretch contracted anterior collagen structures gradually, it became possible to correct spondylolisthesis, kyphosis, scoliosis, and other deformities more completely than in the past and usually without the need for anterior release operations (Edwards, 1990).

RESEARCH AND EDUCATION

Continuing advancement of the EMSS arises from a unique academic-industrial partnership organized under the Spinal Research Foundation. The research and educational program as well as the manufacturer, Scientific Spinal Ltd., are directed by the Spinal Fixation Study Group (SFSG). The study group was formed in 1986 and consists of selected surgeons who meet regularly and send radiographs and clinical data to the Spinal Research Center of the University of Maryland. Through the ongoing analysis of the 4500 cases contributed by study group surgeons and rigorous biomechanical testing, the author and associates were able to perfect the instrumentation steadily, develop new surgical techniques, and define their indications.

The favorable clinical results achieved with the EMSS are due, in part, to surgeon selection and education. During the first 8 years of the program implants have been restricted to surgeons accepted into the SFSG who complete a sequential workshop training program and who submit cases to document competence. The implants, constructs, and their indications are now refined and the system is available to more spinal surgeons. However, formal workshop training and progressive experience with the instrumentation and techniques are strongly recommended before embarking on correction of complex or major deformities.

BIOMECHANICS

The author's surgical goal is to achieve better decompression of neural tissues and greater correction of deformity with less invasive surgery than prior alternatives. To accomplish this goal, Edwards instrumentation and techniques incorporate five biomechanical principles.

Versatility of Attachment

Laminar hooks are provided for upper lumbar and thoracic attachment and screws for lumbosacral fixation. Linkages (i.e., anatomic hooks or adjustable connectors) between the screws and rods act as universal joints to allow optimal positioning of all screws, regardless of the type or severity of deformity.

Three-Dimensional Control

The position of individual vertebrae in all planes of motion is adjusted and controlled with the implants themselves and without the need for external outriggers or manual manipulations. Segmental axial control is obtained with ratcheted universal rods. Independent control of vertebral translation, angulation, and rotation is provided by rod-sleeve spacers and adjustable connectors.

Stress Relaxation

Independent axial and transverse adjustability makes it possible to move individual vertebrae slowly in any direction. The ability to apply corrective forces in small gradations over time allows the surgeon to stretch out contracted tissues gradually, even after many years of deformity (Edwards, 1990; Edwards & Levine, 1986; Edwards & Rosenthal, 1988). By using intraoperative viscoelastic stress relaxation, there is less dependence on anterior or transcanal releases.

Indirect Decompression

Cord decompression can be accomplished by direct removal of the offending bone or fragments, but this usually requires anterior surgery and corpectomy or pediculectomy. Alternatively, neural structures can be decompressed indirectly by applying corrective forces to improve vertebral or fragment alignment (Edwards & Levine, 1986). Edwards techniques are designed to maximize indirect decompression so as to minimize the need for and extent of direct decompression.

Dynamic Loading

After reduction of rigid deformities, the wedge effect of sleeves or connectors slightly bow the rods within their elastic range to generate continuing corrective forces. The result is improved late maintenance of correction (Edwards & Levine, 1986).

Load Sharing

The instrumentation, combined with the vertebrae and ligaments, provides sufficient stiffness to stop unwanted gross motion and initiate union, but without so much rigidity as to stress-shield bone or overly stiffen instrumented motion segments. After reduction, most constructs direct axial loads through the posterior elements to promote fusion maturation. Accordingly, instrumentation removal is rarely necessary.

SYSTEM COMPONENTS AND TECHNIQUES

The EMSS is composed of six basic components that are assembled into a variety of "constructs" depending on the biomechanical needs of each case. These six components or "modules" include: (1) anatomic hooks for laminar attachment; (2) spinal screws for secure fixation to the sacrum or lumbar pedicles (FDA Investigational); (3) universal rods for bidirectional axial control; (4) rod-sleeves as fixed transverse spacers; (5) adjustable connectors for transverse control in all directions; and (6) cross-locks to fix relative rod position and enhance construct stiffness.

Anatomic Hooks

Design

These patented L-shaped hooks are designed to make contact with both the edge and undersurface of the proximal lamina. This improves stress distribution to minimize resorption, loosening, and dislodgment (Edwards & Levine, 1986). The L-shape also directs the straight hook-shoe against the undersurface of the lamina to minimize canal protrusion; hence, the anatomic hooks can be placed safely around either the inferior or superior laminar edge. Low, medium, and high anatomic hooks are available to ensure a snug fit around the lamina and to minimize rod prominence (Fig. 37-1, a). New open top hooks make it possible to lay a rod into the hook bodies when multiple hooks are used on a rod. In addition to attaching to lamina or mamillary processes, the hooks serve as a fixed linkage between the screws and rods.

Proximal (Cephalad-Facing) Hook Insertion

1. Detach the ligamentum flavum and medial aspect of the facet capsule from the undersurface of the proximal lamina with a small curette.
2. Bur any prominence from the proximal edge of the adjacent inferior lamina to facilitate hook insertion. Square off the lamina medial to the facet-laminar junction to provide a flat contact surface for the hook.
3. Clean the underside of the proximal lamina with a no. 3 Penfield elevator.
4. Select the lowest anatomic hook that will fit around the lamina. Low hooks provide 4 mm of clearance, medium 7 mm, and high 10 mm. Mount the hook on the two-pronged Edwards pusher, angle and rotate it 15 degrees toward the midline, and insert the hook under the facet-laminar junction facing cephalad (Fig. 37-1, b).

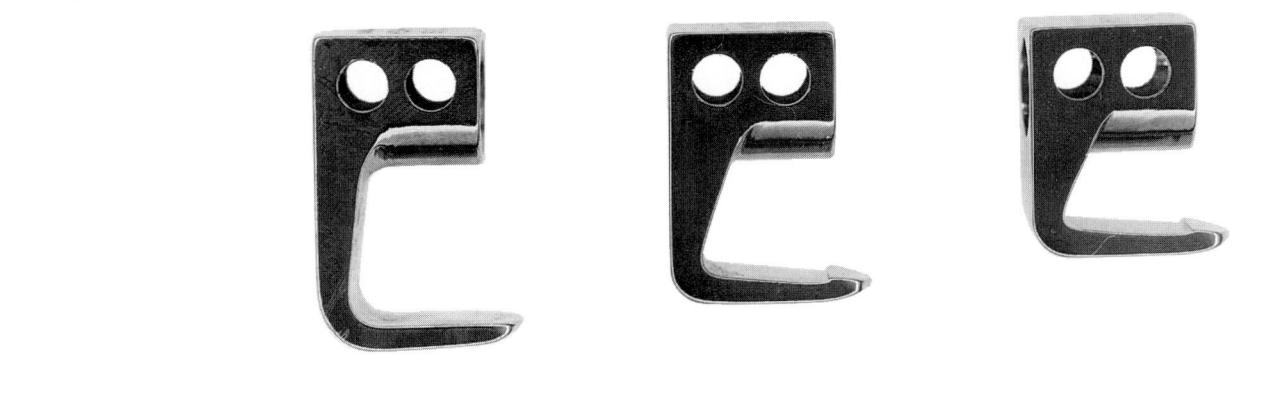

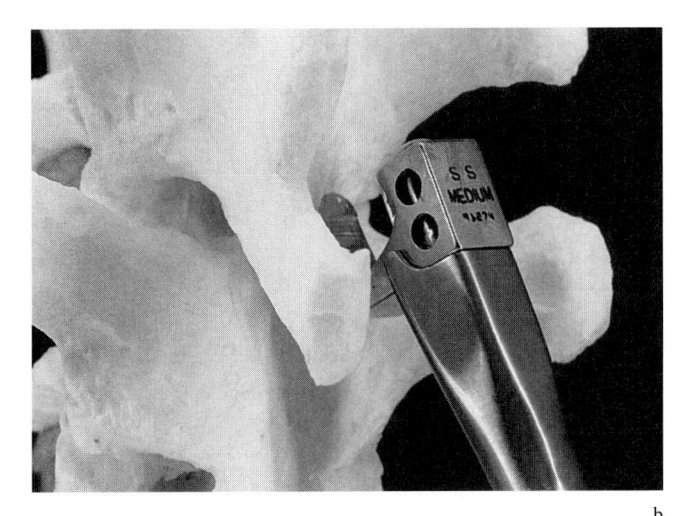

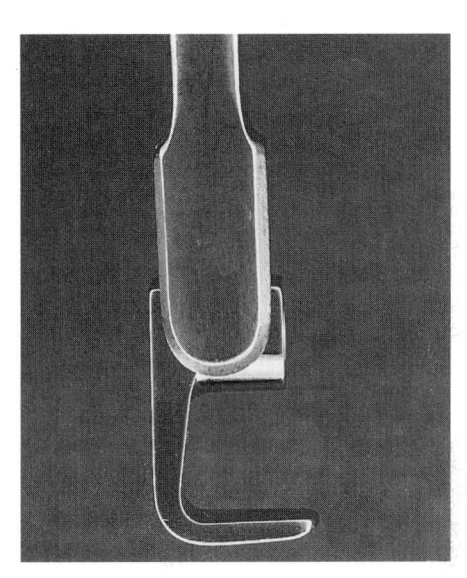

FIG. 37-1. Anatomic spinal hooks. (a) Anatomic hooks attach rods directly to the lamina and also provide a linkage between spinal screws and rods. The hooks have a patented L-shape for maximal laminar stress distribution and minimum canal penetration. The three sizes (low, medium, high) ensure a snug fit about the lamina for maximum stability and minimum instrumentation prominence. (b) Proximal facing anatomic hook loaded on the Edwards hook pusher in preparation for insertion under the inferior edge of a thoracic lamina. (c) Distal facing high anatomic hook loaded on the Edwards hook holder prior to placement over the superior aspect of a lumbar lamina.

Distal (Caudad-Facing) Hook Insertion

1. Using a large Kerrison rongeur, remove any overhanging bone from the adjacent proximal lamina to expose the ligamentum flavum fully.
2. Detach the ligamentum flavum from the superior aspect of the distal lamina with a 15-in. blade scalpel or small angled curette and remove it with a rongeur.
3. Using a Kerrison rongeur, form an 8-mm-wide seat for the hook at the laminar ridge where the ligamentum flavum inserts on the distal lamina.
4. Mount the lowest hook that will fit around the lamina on the anatomic hook holder (Fig. 37-1, c). Lower the hook into the laminotomy and direct it caudally until it is fully seated.

Open Hook Application

Open hooks facilitate assembly for bilaminar claws or anytime more than two hooks are placed on a rod. A closed hook is used at the end(s) of the rod while open hooks are used in between. To lock an open hook to the rod, simply screw the removable hook top (door) onto the doorholder, and slide the door into the grooves from the rear of the open hook. The washer that sets final hook position on the rod also holds the sliding door in place. No set screw is required.

Sacral/Spinal Screws

Design

Edwards sacral screws have recessed, self-tapping flutes to minimize risks of insertion and a ball tip to guide the screw down a predrilled hole and push away any soft tissues encountered should the screw exit the anterior cortex. Deep screw threads help prevent loosening and pullout when reducing resistant deformities. Screws are provided in various lengths from 30 to 55 mm for unicortical pedicle or bicortical sacral fixation. (Fig. 37-2)

Several features to minimize breakage were first introduced by the Edwards screw. These include a tapered proximal diameter to eliminate the stress-riser effect at the shank-head junction (Edwards et al., 1987), a screw seating reamer to provide lateral head support (Edwards et al., 1987), and use of a hook or connector linkage between the screw and rod to absorb peak impact loading (Edwards, 1984).

The screws are available in four head configurations: the standard screw has a double-bevel opening to accommodate the shoe of an anatomic hook or adjustable connector. Its geometry facilitates assembly, but then locks the lumbosacral angle during the application of compression (Edwards, 1984). The distraction screw head has a fixed-angle slot that preserves lumbosacral lordosis during distraction. Angled- and straight-hole screws articulate directly with spinal rods for low-profile instrumentation on the posterior surface of the sacrum or anterolateral surface of the vertebral bodies (Edwards, 1992b).

Lateral S1 Insertion

1. Expose the bony dimple immediately caudal to the L5-S1 facet and in line with the dorsal S1 foramina.
2. Drill through the posterior cortex dimple with 2-mm bits directed 35 degrees laterally and approximately 25 degrees caudally and perpendicular to the posterior canal cortex (Fig. 37-3, *a* and *b*). The drill bits will usually rest on the caudal tip of the L5 spinous process, but it may be necessary to remove the top of this process for sufficiently lateral inclination. Push the 2-mm bits anteriorly until they abut the anterior cortex.
3. Obtain a lateral x-ray film. The bits should be 1 to 2 cm distal (caudal) and parallel to the S1 end plate (Fig. 37-3, *b*).
4. Enlarge each 2-mm hole to 3.5 mm and carefully drill just through the anterior cortex of the lateral-sacral ala. Stay within the medial reflection of the sacroiliac ligament to avoid injury to the adjacent L5 root.
5. Mount the seating reamer on an air driver and ream past the L5-S1 facet to the lowest point of fully intact cortical bone.
6. Use a depth gauge (with the foot oriented medially) to select a screw that will just engage the anterior cortex and insert it tightly against the posterior cortex using the hex-wedge screwdriver.

Medial S1 Insertion

Medially directed S1 screws should be considered for fixation to first sacral vertebrae with poorly developed ala, for one level L5-S1 fixation, and for lumbosacral scoliosis.

1. Enter through the midpoint of the lateral wall of the superior S1 facet (Fig. 37-3, *a*).
2. Direct a T-handled probe 25 degrees medially while converging 10 degrees with the sacral end plate toward the anterosuperior corner of the vertebral body (Fig. 37-3, *a* and *b*).
3. Place K-wires in the probe holes to confirm position radiographically and determine screw length.

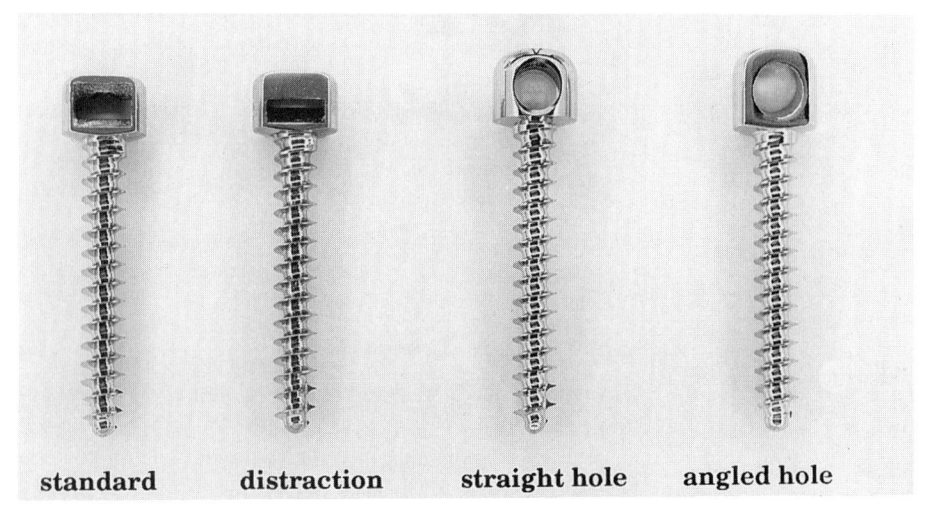

FIG. 37-2. Sacral screws. Edwards sacral screws have four head configurations: Standard and distraction screws articulate with spinal rods via adjustable connectors or anatomic hooks. Straight-hole and angled-hole screws articulate directly with spinal rods. All screws feature blunt tips and recessed flutes to reduce insertion risk and a tapered minor diameter to enhance fatigue strength. Screws are available in thread lengths ranging from 35 to 55 mm.

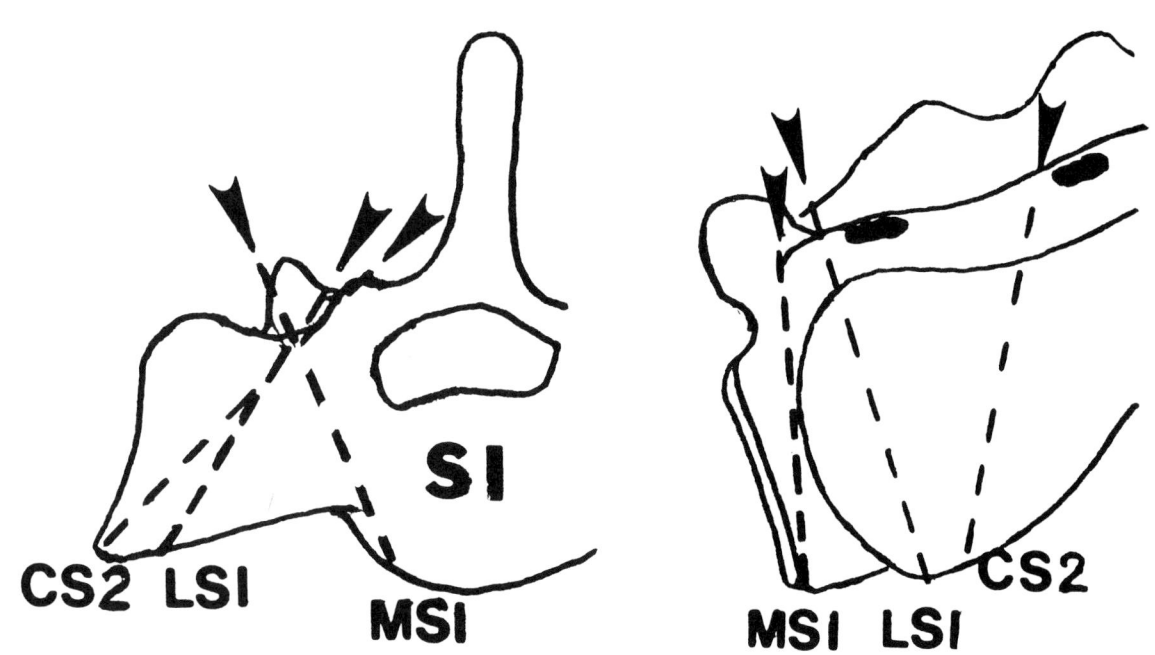

FIG. 37-3. Sacral fixation. Biomechanical testing has demonstrated three sacral screw positions for maximal stable fixation: lateral S1 (L-S1), cephalo medial S1 (MS1), and converging S2 (CS2).

4. To facilitate medial screw placement, use the Edwards screw inserter. First, slit the lumbosacral fascia overlying the paraspinous muscles; then insert the bullet-tipped trochar and sleeve over one of the K-wire markers. Hold the sleeve in place and remove the trochar and wire;
5. Pass the seating reamer through the inserter sleeve to prepare the bed for the screw
6. Attach a sacral screw to the hex-wedge screwdriver and pass it through the inserter sleeve to place the screw into the sacrum.

Midsacral Insertion

Biomechanical testing has shown the Edwards converging S2 screw position to be more secure than other midsacral alternatives (Edwards, 1990; Edwards, Curcin, Turner, & Topeleski, 1995).

1. Identify the S2 pedicle by palpating the inferior edge of the S1 foramina and the superior edge of the S2 foramina.
2. Bur through the posterior cortex at the point two thirds of the distance from true midline to a line that bisects the midposition of S1-S2 foramina and just proximal to the S2 foramen (Fig. 37-3, *a*).
3. Advance the T-handled probe directed 40 to 45 degrees laterally and converging 20 to 25 degrees toward the lateral S1 screw and S1 end plate (Fig. 37-3, *a* and *b*). The midsacral screw tip should ultimately lodge into the anterolateral beak of the S1-S2 ala (Fig. 37-3, *a* and *b*).
4. Once the correct position is confirmed radiographically, use the seating reamer to create a half-moon screw bed, and insert the appropriate length straight- or angled-hole Edwards sacral screw.

Posterior Lumbar Screw Insertion (FDA Investigational)

When central stenosis, laminectomy, or translational deformity require posterior screw fixation, the following technique is recommended:

1. To determine pedicle orientation, take intraoperative x-rays and thoroughly clean the transverse process and pars. The pedicle center approximates the intersection of the line crossing the middle of the transverse process with the lateral margin of the facet joints
2. Open the posterior cortex with a 3-mm bur. For pedicles within the fusion, enter through the superior facet, just lateral to the center of the pedicle. For proximal screws, adjacent to unfused facets, the entry point should be 3 to 4 mm caudal and lateral to the center of the pedicle, near the intersection of the transverse process and pars. This will avoid injury to the proximal unfused facet.
3. Use the T-handled probe to find the isthmus of the pedicle. For the midposition pedicles the probe should parallel the superior vertebral end plate and angle medially along the axis of the pedicles as follows: L1—0 degrees, L2-3—5 degrees, L4—10 degrees, and L5—20 degrees. For the most cephalad vertebra, the probe should be directed 10 degrees more cephalad and medial than usual to avoid the proximal facet. It should pass across the middle of the isthmus and terminate at the anterior-superior corner of the vertebral body adjacent to the end plate.
4. Insert 2-mm drill bits in the probe holes and obtain anteroposterior (AP) and lateral films to confirm position.
5. Check all four quadrants of each hole with a depth gauge to be sure you remain within the cortex of the pedicle.

6. Use the Edwards seating reamer to create a flat surface for the screw head just above the level of the transverse process.
7. Determine screw length with a depth gauge advanced to the anterior cortex and insert the self-tapping screw.

Universal Rods

Design

Universal rods permit ratcheting in both directions for segmental compression or distraction (Fig. 37-4, *a*). The fine ($\frac{1}{16}$ in.) ratcheting allows precise positioning, which is maintained with wide or narrow C-washers. The rods have an octagon at one end for rotational control. They have the same $\frac{1}{4}$ in. outside diameter as earlier rods, but their larger minor diameter and the lack of a discrete stress-riser make the Edwards universal rods less susceptible to fatigue failure. Terminal lock washers prevent hook-rod disengagement. Fully ratcheted universal rods range in length from $2\frac{1}{2}$ in. for one-level fusions to 18 in.

Rod Assembly

1. Pass the octagonal end of the rod through a hook at one end of the construct and apply the primary C-washer: for compression—in the groove between the octagon and end of the rod; for distraction—in the last groove within the ratcheted portion of the rod.
2. Add any additional hooks, sleeves, or ring connectors to the rod.
3. Insert the hook at the opposite end of the rod into the screw slot or under the lamina and gently load into compression or distraction with the spreader (Fig. 37-4, *a*). The side of the spreader with the hole in the handle faces the hook, sleeve, or connector to be moved.
4. Always limit spreader force to 20 kg (only on finger or thumb on each arm of the spreader). Allow at least 20 minutes to elapse between the beginning of load application and final ratcheting to permit stress-relaxation. Temporary rod clips are available to fix hook or connector position until final reduction is achieved.
5. Apply stop C-washers to hold the final position of all axially loaded hooks or connectors. Select a narrow or wide washer that completely fills the space between the hook and next ratchet on the rod (see "Washer Application").
6. Cut off excess rod length with side-biting bolt cutter. If a bolt cutter will not fit, use a side-cutting bur.
7. If less than 1 cm of rod projects beyond the upper hook in distraction, add terminal washers (wide or narrow) to prevent hook-rod disengagement.

Washer Application

Both narrow and wide washers are applied with a special crimper. A small ridge at the outside of the washer articulates with a groove in the jaws of the crimper for precise washer positioning and crimping. The crimper can be loaded from either side to facilitate approaching a rod or connector stem from either the right or left. To add a washer:

1. Orient the C-washer so its opening is symmetric with the opening of the jaws (Fig. 37-4, *b*).
2. Place the edge of the washer flush with the face of the crimper jaws to articulate the washer ridge with the crimper groove.
3. Press the washer over the rod with the washer flush against the hook and connector.
4. Slowly squeeze the crimper jaws with a one-handed moderate grip and rotate the crimper back and forth once on the rod. If there is less than full crimping of the washer, complete crimping with a "power grip" clamp.

The Edwards Modular Spinal System includes a washer remover instrument to rapidly open washers for removal. First, insert the blade side (pointed end) of the washer remover and pry the washer about $\frac{1}{8}$ in. apart. Then, reverse (rotate) the remover and insert the small feet flush onto the rod to open the C-washer fully for removal from the rod.

Rotational control of rod position is achieved with either a cross-lock or a rotation-stop. The rotation-stop slides over the octagon at the end of the rod to articulate with the rod and hook so as to lock rod rotation. It is held in place with a narrow C-washer at the end of the rod.

Spinal Rod-Sleeves

Edwards rod-sleeves (Zimmer, Warsaw, IN) serve as a fulcrum for the correction of angular deformity and also provide both translational and rotational control by wedging between the rods, facets, and spinous processes (Edwards & Levine, 1986). The polyethylene spacers are available in four sizes to accommodate various anatomic levels (Fig. 37-5) and can be sculpted with a bur to match the geometry of the posterior elements. Sleeves contain barium sulfate for x-ray visualization. For assembly, slide a rod sleeve over the end of a universal rod prior to insertion. Advance the sleeve along the rod with a spreader. The spring effect of the rod sleeve will keep it in place on the rod.

Adjustable Connectors

Design

Connectors between the rods and standard screws act as universal joints to facilitate screw fixation of malpositioned vertebrae (Fig. 37-6). By extending or shortening the connectors, the surgeon can gradually reduce kyphosis, lateral spondylolisthesis, or retrospondylolisthesis and actively derotate scoliotic vertebrae. After reduction, connectors are locked to stabilize the spine.

Two types of connectors attach spinal rods to standard screws. Ring connectors (Fig. 37-6) are placed during rod assembly and can be ratcheted up or down to facilitate reduction of complex deformities. Open connectors can be added following rod assembly. The original open connectors snapped onto the ratcheted rod, while new open connectors feature a door that slides in place to lock the connector onto a rod. Both types feature 90- and 105-degree stems to facilitate screw attachment.

Rod-rod connectors extend between rods and serve two functions: They will approximate two spinal rods, for

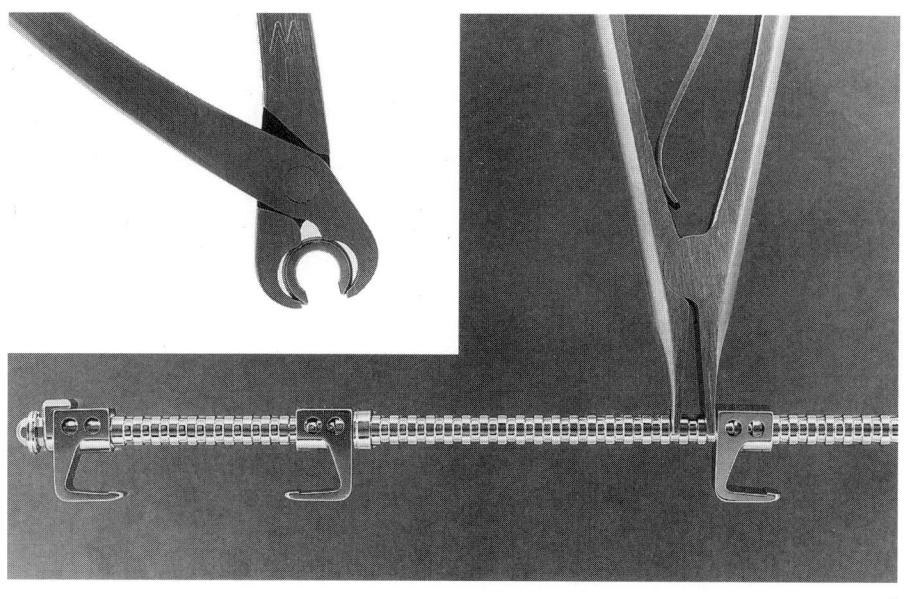

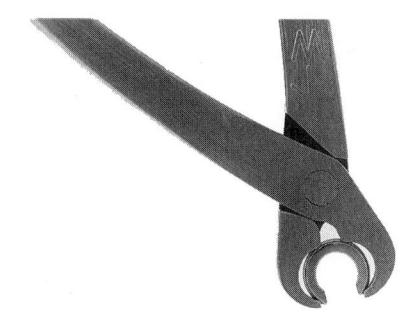

FIG. 37-4. Universal spinal rods. (a) The rods permit bidirectional ratcheting of hooks or connectors in small gradations. Final hook position is set with wide or narrow C-washers. (b) Washers are applied and formed about the rod in one step with a special washer crimper.

example, to pull an independent claw toward a long rod. Secondly, a pair of rod-rod connectors will rigidly join one rod to another to extend the length of a spinal construct.

Connector Assembly

1. Slide an assembled ring connector over the end of the rod or snap an open connector onto the rod.
2. Screw the threaded stem of an adjustable connector onto the connector driver instrument.
3. Set the length of the stem with the socket wrench portion of the driver and control the rotation of the stem shoe with the cap of the driver.
4. Direct the connector shoe through the slot of a standard Edwards screw.
5. Fix the shoe to the screw by crimping a narrow C-washer into the groove near the end of the shoe.
6. Gradually adjust the length of the connector stem using only two fingers on the handle of the socket wrench. If resistance is encountered, wait 5 minutes and turn again.
7. To lock a connector after reduction, first align a flat washer on the nut with the side of the connector body. Drop the square lock washer over the nut and connector pin. Bend the pin against the nut and cut off all protruding stems with an end-cutting bolt shear.

Cross-Locks

Design

Cross-locks serve to fix one spinal rod to another so as to enhance the rigidity of a construct and divide loads across multiple points of spinal attachment. The Edwards cross-lock consists of two jaws that attach to a slotted plate by means of threaded stems and nuts. They are designed for simple application after rod placement and construct assembly. They adjust for length to speed selection and minimize inventory requirements. They feature a radial joint to accommodate any angulation between rods so contour-

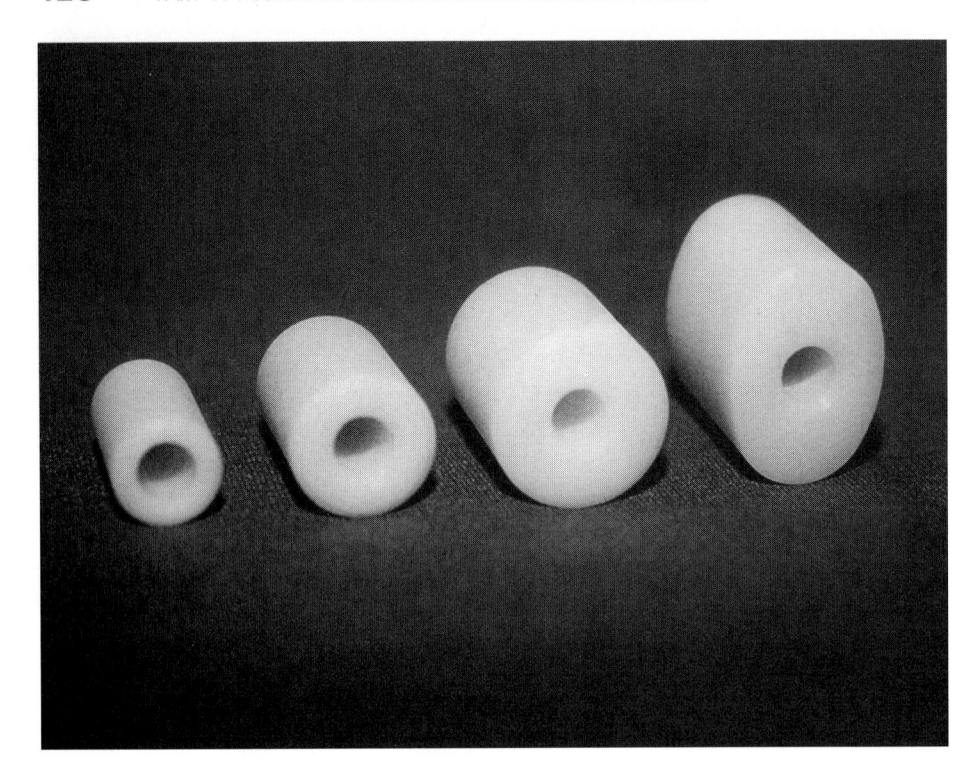

FIG. 37-5. Spinal rod-sleeves. Polyethylene sleeves slide over the universal rods and are available in four sizes: small (thoracic), medium (thoracolumbar), large (upper lumbar), and elliptical (low lumbar).

ing is unnecessary. Despite their versatility and relatively small size, mechanical testing has suggested that cross-locks provide more overall rod-to-cross-link rigidity than any other system tested to date (Turner, Topoleski, & Edwards, 1993).

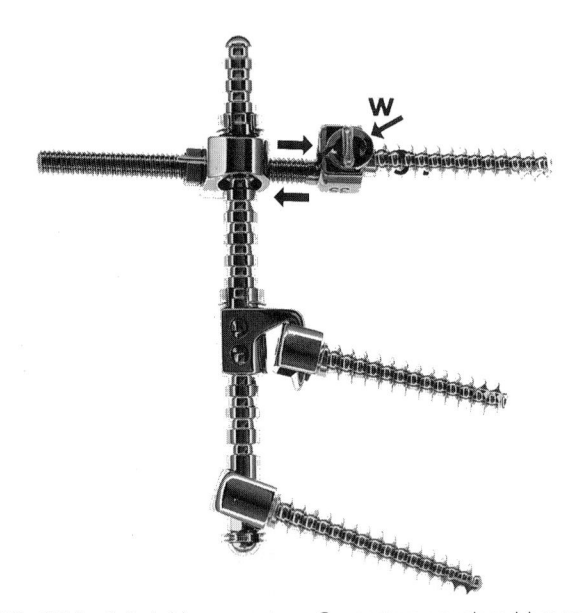

FIG. 37-6. Adjustable connectors. Connectors are placed between the rods and screws to correct spinal deformity. The connector shoe is affixed to a standard screw with a narrow C-washer (w). Connectors can be lengthened or shortened with a socket wrench to change the position of individual vertebra in the transverse plane.

Assembly

1. Disassemble a cross-lock and screw the two jaw stems onto the jaw holders.
2. Slip the cross-lock jaws under the medial side of the universal rods, matching the grooves on each the jaw with the ratchets on the rod (Fig. 37-7, *a*).
3. Lift upward on the jaw holder to wedge the jaws opposite one another on the spinal rods. Untwist the jaw holder; the jaws should remain wedged in place on the spinal rods (Fig. 37-7, *a*).
4. Select the appropriate length cross-lock plate. Pass the slot over the threaded stem of the length adjustable jaw (with transverse grooves) and the hole over the angle-adjustable jaw (radial grooves) (Fig. 37-7, *b*).
5. Place a nut in the end of the socket wrench, screw it onto each jaw stem, and tighten the two nuts until maximum grip strength is reached.
6. Finally, retract the socket wrench just above the nuts and angulate it to break off the threaded stem just above the nuts (Fig. 37-7, *c*).

SURGICAL CONSTRUCTS

Preoperative Planning

Before embarking on a reconstructive spinal procedure, the author recommends the following planning sequence:

1. Analyze bending films and neuroradiographic studies to determine sites of neural impingement, anterior bony bridges, or posterior blocks to reduction that must be resected before

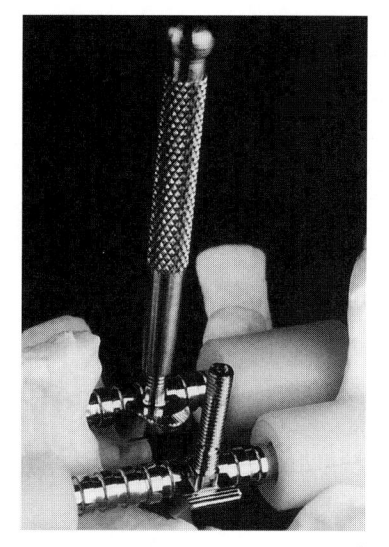

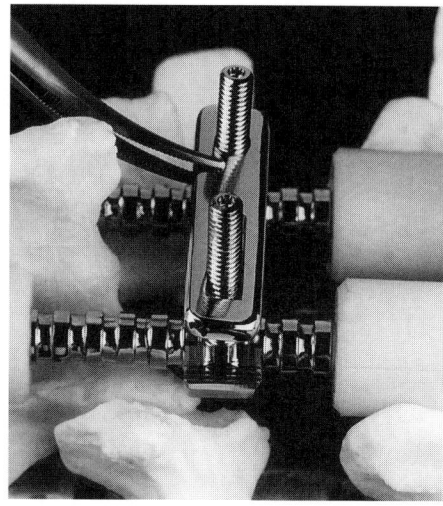

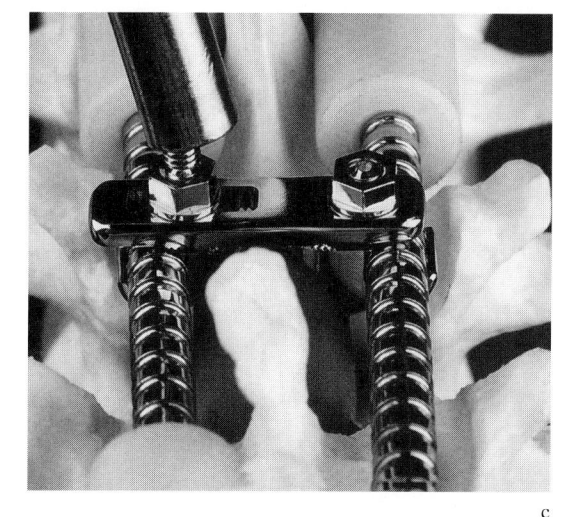

FIG. 37-7. Cross-lock application. (a) Radial and length-adjustable jaws are wedged onto the universal rods by pulling upward with a jaw holder. (b) The cross-lock plate slides over the threaded stems of the two jaws. (c) Nuts are tightened with a socket wrench to lock the assembly. The threaded stems are then removed by undulating the socket wrench.

spinal instrumentation. Anterior bony bridging or fixed anterior bony impingement on the cord will require preliminary anterior surgery.
2. From radiographs determine the direction of forces causing spinal deformity and/or instability. Diagram the necessary opposite corrective forces on radiographs and select or design the construct to apply the needed corrective forces.
3. Determine the order of reduction when treating deformities. For most translational deformities first distract, then translate, and finally compress. Remember, the gradual application of optimal corrective forces will reduce most deformities without anterior release.

Construct Selection

The six components of the EMSS described above are assembled in various ways to form seven basic constructs and numerous variations depending on the biomechanical needs of each case. The posterior compression construct, used in cases with intact facets or interbody grafts, provides both stability and physiologic axial loading to promote fusion. The anterior neutralization construct works in conjunction with an anterior strut graft to reconstruct vertebral bodies after reduction of acute kyphosis or corpectomy.

Other constructs are designed to apply optimal corrective forces. The rod-sleeve construct restores anatomic alignment and provides stable fixation for thoracolumbar and upper lumbar fractures. The D-L construct uses pedicle screws for short-segment distraction and lordosis to reduce and fix either low lumbar fractures or degenerative listhesis.

Chronic deformities are corrected with the kyphoreduction, spondylo, and scoliosis constructs. These constructs apply corrective forces very gradually to facilitate stress relaxation and limit the need for anterior or transcanal release procedures. The kyphoreduction construct provides three-point loading followed by posterior column shortening for chronic posttraumatic or other kyphotic deformities. The spondylo construct achieves full reduction of spondylolisthesis and spondyloptosis without anterior surgery. The various scoliosis constructs facilitate reduction for an array of deformities ranging from idiopathic thoracic scoliosis to degenerative lumbar kyphoscoliosis with lateral listhesis.

COMPRESSION CONSTRUCT FOR PRIMARY FUSION WITH INTACT FACETS OR INTERBODY GRAFT, PSEUDARTHROSIS REPAIR, AND DISLOCATIONS AND DISTRACTION INJURIES

Indications and Biomechanics

The compression construct provides in situ fixation in compression across the facets of just one or multiple motion segments (Fig. 37-8). It combines either hook or screw fixation with universal rods. The compression construct achieves considerable stability by locking the facet joints and tensioning on the anterior longitudinal ligament. Hook linkages between the rod and spinal screws permit physiologic axial loading across the posterior bony elements, yet block tension and shear (Edwards, 1984). Stability with axial loading creates an ideal environment for bony union. Accordingly, the compression construct is useful in the repair of nonunions and for primary fusion with either intact facets or an interbody graft. The compression construct also provides an extension moment to oppose residual flexion instability after flexion-distraction injuries. Hence, it is used to stabilize posterior ligamentous ruptures, Chance fractures, and facet dislocations (Edwards, 1993) (Table 37-1).

Precautions

Absent Facets

The compression construct requires intact facets or lateral fusion masses against which to compress and maintain foraminal height. Without facets, an interbody graft should be used in conjunction with the compression construct (Table 37-2).

Table 37-1
Indications and Contraindications for Use of the Edwards Modular System

Indications
  Compression construct
    Posterior ligmentous ruptures
    Chance fractures
    Facet dislocations
    Primary fusion with intact facets or interbody graft
    Pseudarthrosis repair
  Anterior neutralization construct
    Acute mild kyphosis
    T6-L4 corpectomy
  Spinal rod-sleeve method
    T6-L3 burst fractures or fracture dislocations
    Bilateral facet dislocations
  Distraction-lordosis construct
    Low lumbar burst fractures
    Degenerative spondylolisthesis
  Kyphoreduction construct
    Chronic posttraumatic kyphosis
    Vertebral collapse from tumor or infection
    Scheuermann's disease
  Spondylo construct
    Isthmic L5-S1 spondylolisthesis, all grades
    Severe, grade 2+, degenerative spondylolisthesis
  Scoliosis construct
    Idiopathic thoracic and lumbar scoliosis
    Kyphoscoliosis
    Degenerative lumbar/L5 scoliosis with lateral spondylolisthesis
Contraindications
  Acute spinal infection
  Severe osteoporosis

Table 37-2
Advantages and Disadvantages of the Edwards Modular System

Advantages
  Versatility of attachment
  Three-dimensional control
  Gradual correction allows stress relaxation
  Dynamic loading
  Load sharing

Disadvantages
  Multiple components to assemble
  Use of complex constructs for rigid correction of deformities require instrument experience

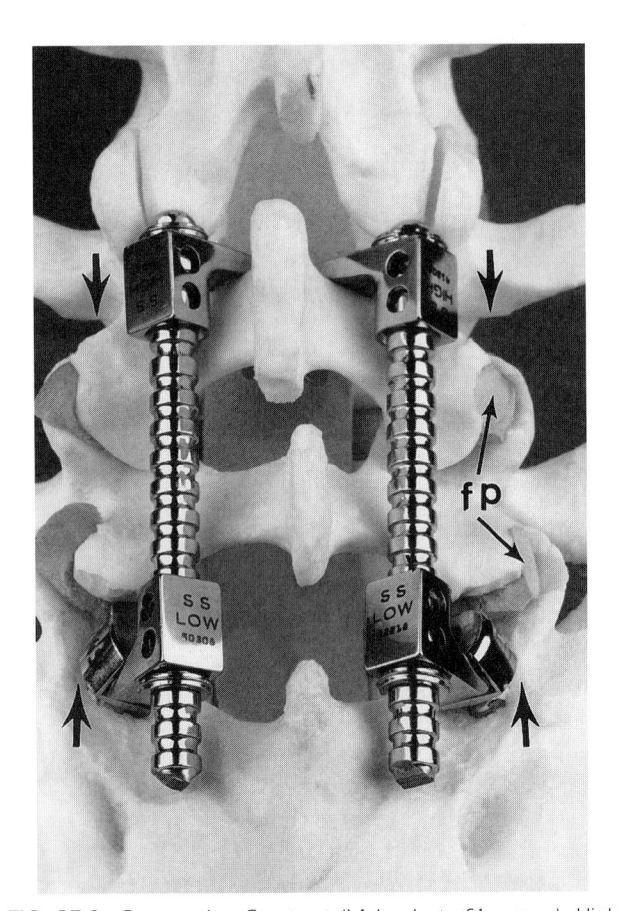

FIG. 37-8. Compression Construct (L4 hooks to S1 screws). High anatomic hooks fit over the superior aspect of the L4 lamina while bicortical lateral S1 screws attach to the sacrum via a low hook linkage. Facets plugs (fP) maintain foraminal height and speed facet fusion.

Foraminal Stenosis

When using the compression construct, foraminal space is usually preserved with facet bone graft plugs (see Fig. 37-8). Nevertheless, narrowing of the foramen and disk bulging can occur with compression to some extent. Therefore, foraminotomy is advised prior to instrumentation in patients with known or borderline stenosis.

Surgical Technique

Preinstrumentation

Laminar hooks should be used in situations in which there is adequate space in the central canal. Screw-to-screw compression should be used when central canal stenosis exists or for single level L4-5, or L5-S1 fixation. Lateral sacral screw orientation is generally used since lateral screws are easier to insert and have equal fixation strength to medially directed screws. Medial sacral screws are used for single-level L5-S1 constructs to achieve parallel rod alignment for optimal compression.

After placing hook and/or screws, we recommend lateral decortication and insertion of a bone plug across each facet joint. The cancellous facet plug will help maintain foraminal height and encourage fusion. To plug a facet joint, first bur a $\frac{1}{4}$-in. hole thru the middle of each facet joint with a large pineapple burr. Obtain corticocancellous plugs from the posterior iliac crest with a Craig biopsy set and tamp them directly into the facet holes with the Craig pusher using the Craig biopsy tube as a guide (see Fig. 37-8).

Hook-to-Screw Construct Assembly (i.e., L4-S1)

1. Place caudal facing hooks over the top of the L4 lamina. First resect the overhanging distal edge of the adjacent L3 lamina, then detach the ligamentum flavum and notch the cephalad edge of the L4 lamina about 5 mm to a ridge formed by the insertion of the ligamentum flavum. Finally, insert the shortest hook that can be accommodated into the laminotomy with a hook holder (Fig. 37-9, *a*).
2. Insert laterally directed standard sacral screws as shown in Fig. 37-3.
3. Contour universal rods into lordosis to prevent sacral abutment during compression.
4. Seat the proximal primary hook with a hook holder and pass the octagonal end of the rod cephalad through the hook body (Fig. 37-9, *b*). If the end of the rod impinges on the adjacent L3 lamina, extend the laminotomy to seat the hook more distally.
5. Attach a narrow washer in the groove at the end of the rod so as to fix the rod to the hook (Fig. 37-9, *b*).
6. Pass a low hook over the distal end of the rod with a hook holder and lower it until its shoe is opposite the S1 screw slot (Fig. 37-9, *c*).
7. Place a spreader between the distal hook and the end of the rod and advance the hook shoe into the screw slot (Fig. 37-9, *d*).
8. Position the operating table to restore normal lordosis and balance the compressive loads between the rods with only one finger about the spreader handle.
9. Apply stop washers (narrow or wide) to fix distal hook position (Fig. 37-8).

Screw-to-Screw Construct Assembly

When standard screws are used for proximal attachment, the octagonal end of the rod is articulated first with a low hook in the distal screw (typically S1) (Fig. 37-10). Compression is applied with a spreader above the proximal screw low hook linkage. If the rod is too short to accommodate a spreader, initial compression can be applied with a Gaines Compressor (Zimmer). Excess rod length projecting beyond the proximal stop washer should be removed with bolt shears or a side cutting bur.

Segmental Compression Construct

When treating multiple nonunions, I recommend screw fixation on both sides of each nonunion. When fusing four vertebrae I recommend fixation at three or more levels. In both cases the segmental compression construct is indicated. The segmental compression construct consists of a compression construct with midposition standard screws attached to the rods with adjustable connectors (Fig. 37-11). To complete a segmental compression construct:

1. Assemble the screw-to-screw construct as described above and attach ring or snap connectors to midpoint screws.
2. Sequentially shorten midposition connectors to prevent excess lordosis and enhance rotational stability. Balance connector shortening and axial compression under x-ray control to set the desired lordosis. Decrease lordosis by shortening connectors; increase lordosis by additional rod compression.
3. Set two-finger tightness with both the connector driver (socket wrench) and spreader for optimal construct stiffness and apply lock washers.

360-Degree Fusions

For recurrent lumbar nonunions or for cases at high risk for nonunion, such as lumbosacral fusion in complete paraplegia we combine a posterior compression construct with an anterior interbody graft. The interbody graft consists of one or two autogenous tricortical iliac crest grafts or a fresh-frozen femur or cage packed with autogenous cancellous graft. The graft(s) are centered just posterior to the midpoint of the vertebral body. Application of posterior compression tensions the residual anterior ligament–annulus complex and locks the facets to provide great stability, anterior and posterior axial loading, and a large graft contact surface to create the ideal environment for successful fusion.

Clinical Results

The compression construct is the construct most frequently used by members of the SFSG. In a study of 148 cases with lumbosacral pseudarthrosis, surgeons found the construct easy to master and associated with an 87% union rate (Edwards, 1991a). When an interbody graft was added to the construct, the union rate exceeded 95%.

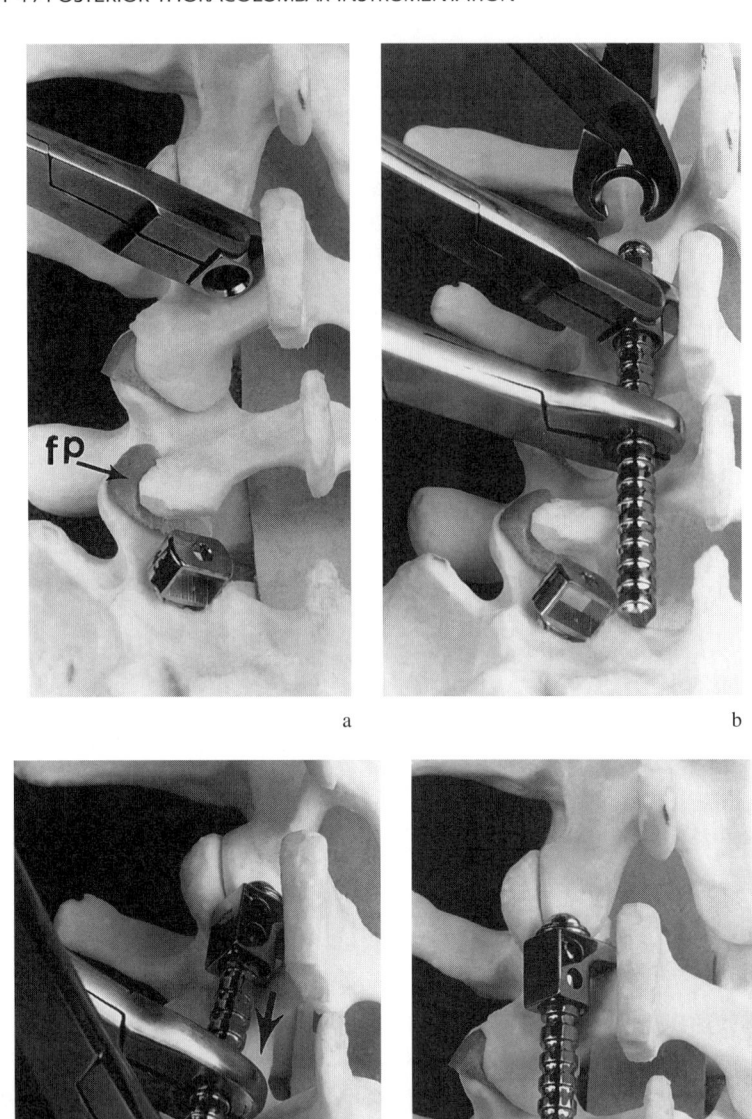

FIG. 37-9. Compression Construct Assembly (L4-S1). (a) After placement of facet plugs and a laterally directed sacral screw, a high anatomic hook is placed over the superior margin of L4. (b) The octagonal end of a slightly contoured universal rod is passed cephalad through the L4 hook and a narrow washer is applied to the washer at the end of the rod with a washer crimper. (c) A low hook is passed over the distal end of the rod and into the slot of the sacral screw while caudal pressure is maintained on the hook holder to keep the proximal hook in place. (d) Compression is applied with the spreader positioned between the distal hook and the end of the ratcheted rod.

Edwards & Weigel (1988) conducted a prospective study of 65 nonunions between L3 and the sacrum. All were treated with the compression construct, iliac grafting, and postoperative bracing. Patients were followed for 2 to 10 years (average, 5 years); union was assessed with quantitative flexion-extension films. Overall, 86% of the pseudarthroses were successfully repaired after one operation, whereas 95% of the single-level repairs united.

A similar study was conducted on 42 patients by McCutcheon and Cohen (1991). They experienced a comparable fusion success rate of 86%; complications were confined to transient radiculopathy in one patient, and infection in one. Michelson and associates have reported 58 patients treated with noninstrumented fusions compared with 71 treated with the Edwards compression construct for degenerative lumbosacral disease. After a minimum follow-up of

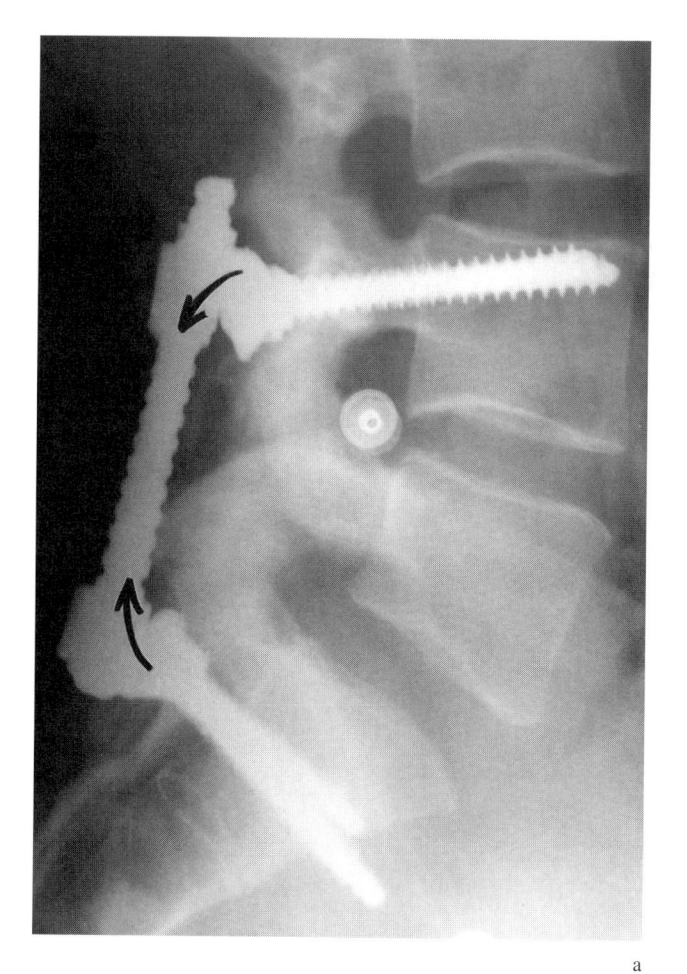

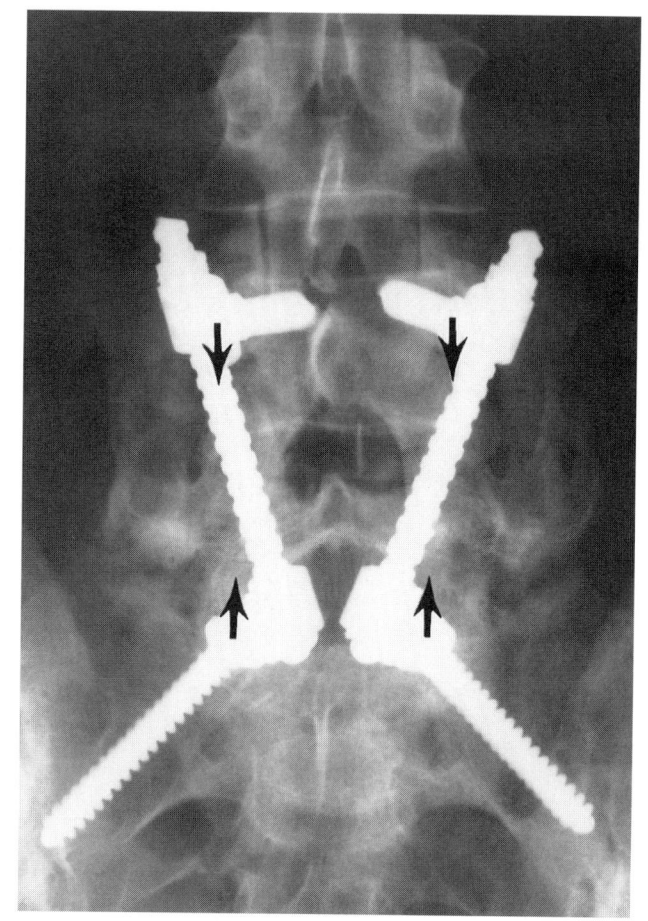

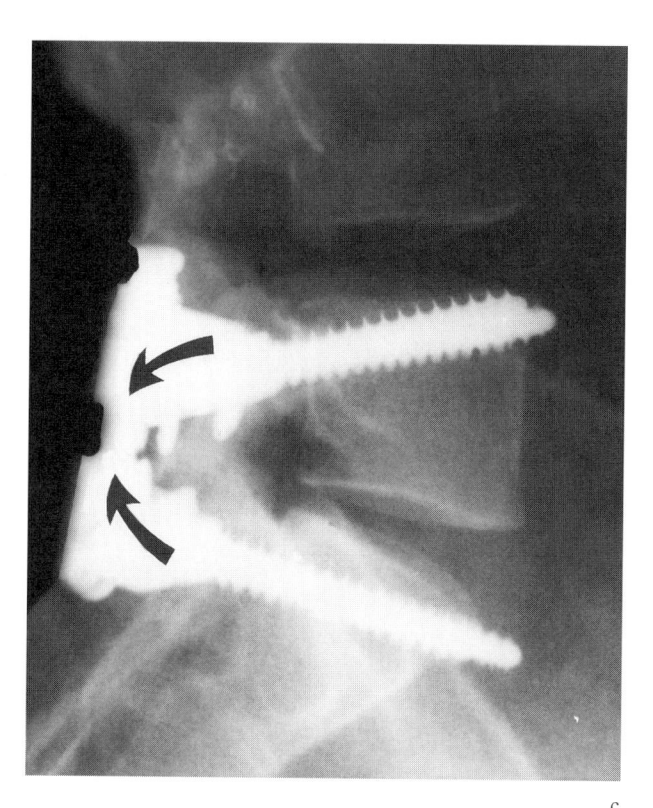

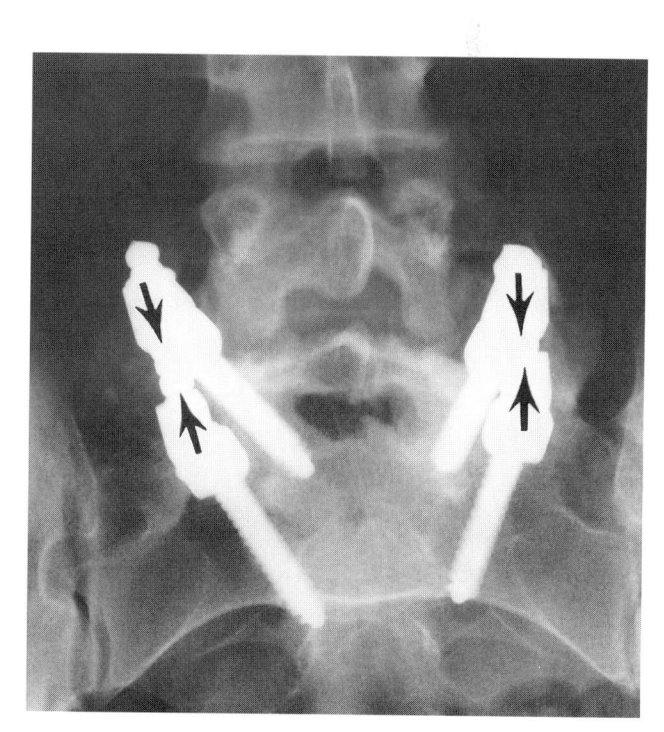

FIG. 37-10. Screw-to-Screw Compression Constructs. (a and b) L4 to S1 construct using laterally directed bicortical sacral screws. (c and d) L5-S1 construct using cephalomedial sacral screw orientation.

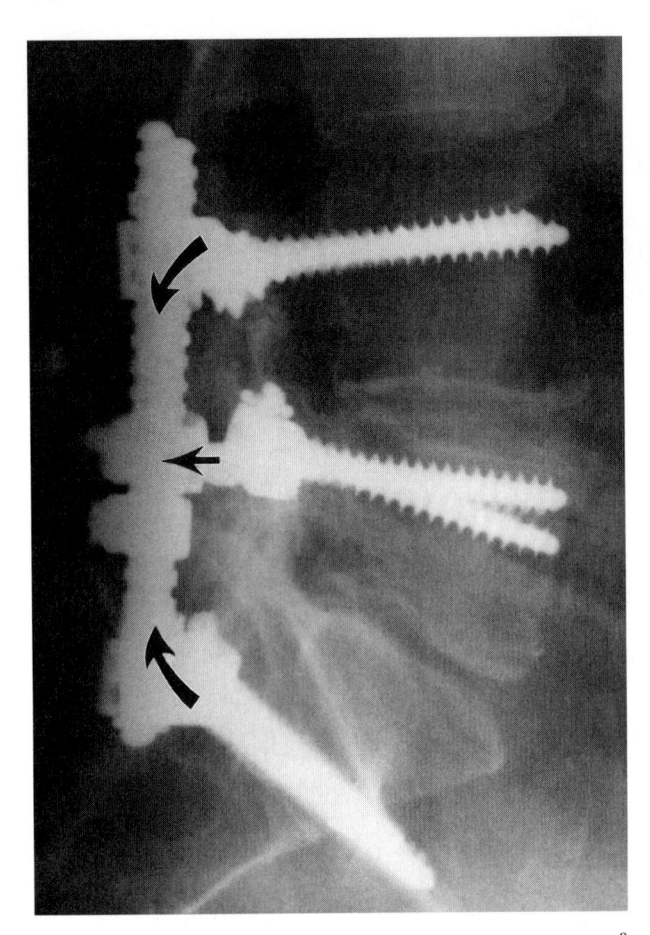

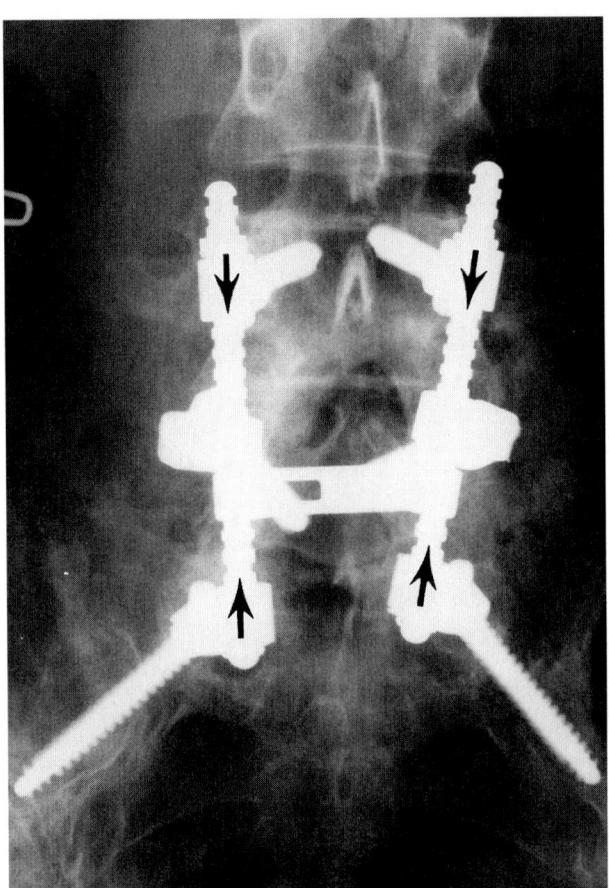

FIG. 37-11. Segmental compression construct. Intermediate screws attached to rods with adjustable connectors to provide segmental fixation for the treatment of nonunions and for long instrumentations. The segmental compression construct provides extremely stable fixation without impairing physiologic axial loading.

2 years they found that the addition of the compression construct increased the union rate from 68 to 92%—a statistically significant difference (Schwab, Nazarian, Higgs, Mahmud, & Michelson, 1994).

Dislocations tested with a short-segment compression construct fixation have been reviewed by several authors. Edwards and Levine (1986) noted that the compression construct maintained excellent reduction after bilateral facet dislocation and promoted early union in all cases. However, late reduction of dislocation or excessive compression without use of facet bone plugs was found to accentuate bulging of the disrupted disk in some cases (Levine, Bosse, et al., 1988).

ANTERIOR NEUTRALIZATION CONSTRUCT FOR CORRECTION OF ACUTE MILD KYPHOSIS AND VERTEBRAL-BODY RECONSTRUCTION AFTER CORPECTOMY (T6-L4)

Biomechanics

The anterior neutralization construct consists of a universal rod directly attached to the vertebral body above and below a fracture or corpectomy with spinal screws. It is used in conjunction with a compressible bone graft (Fig. 37-11, *a*). The ratcheted universal rod is first distracted to reduce deformity and facilitate corpectomy decompression. Compression is then applied across a bone graft spacer to stabilize the segment until fusion (Levine et al., 1988) (Fig. 37-12, *a*).

Precaution

When there is posterior ligamentous and facet disruption from trauma or surgery, the anterior neutralization construct should be combined with appropriate posterior instrumentation.

Surgical Technique

Straight-hole screws are placed anterolateral to posterolateral across the vertebral bodies above and below the fracture or corpectomy. Washer spacers are placed under the screw heads as needed. Distraction is applied with a temporary outrigger to provide access for partial corpectomy and cord decompression. To assemble the outrigger, insert the shoes of high anatomic hooks in the spinal screw holes and then slide a universal rod through the hooks oriented

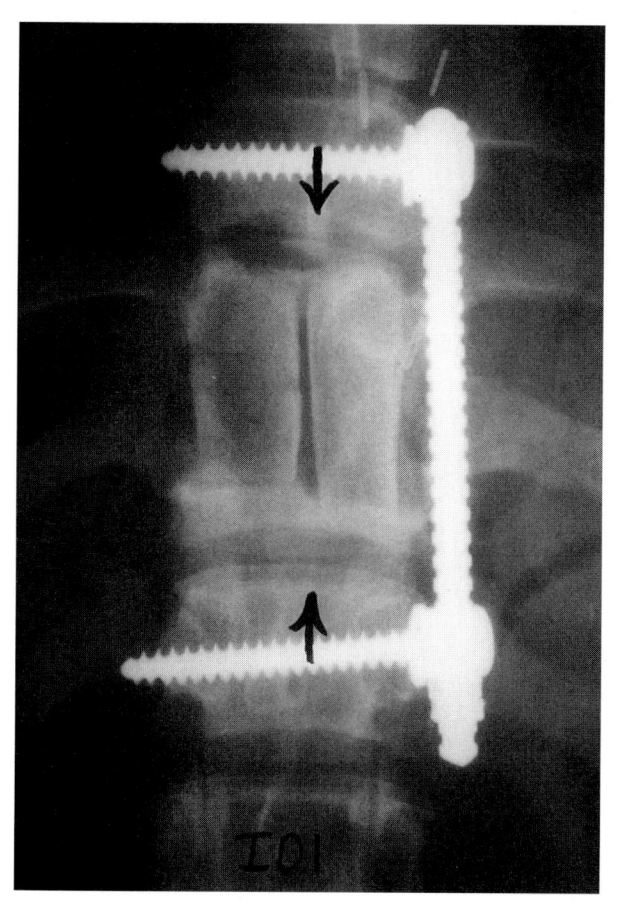

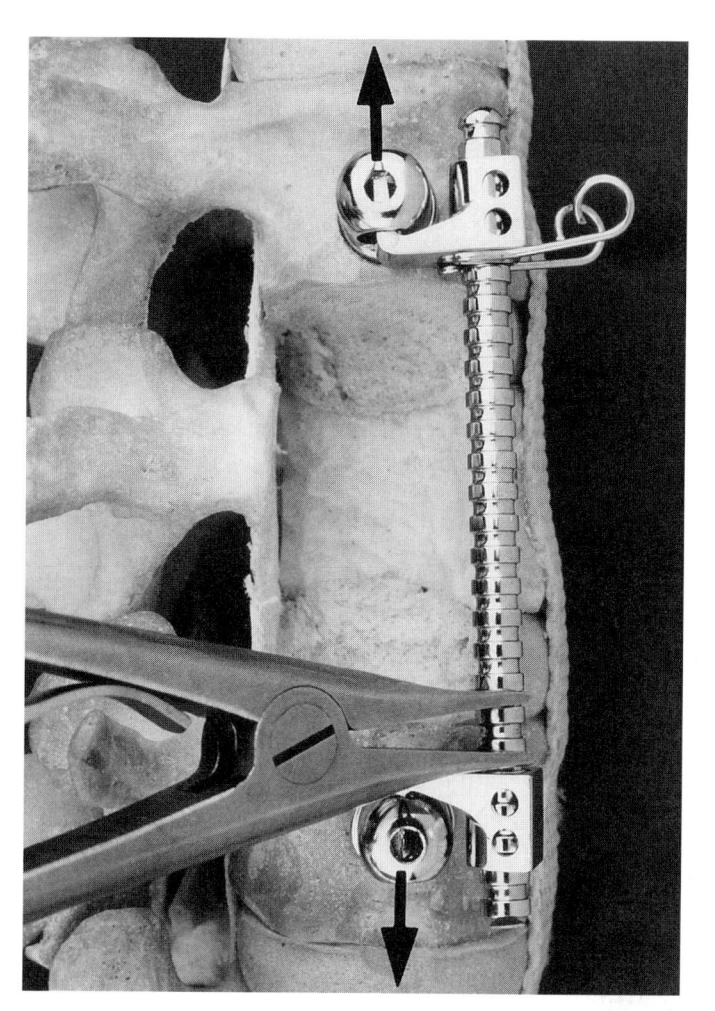

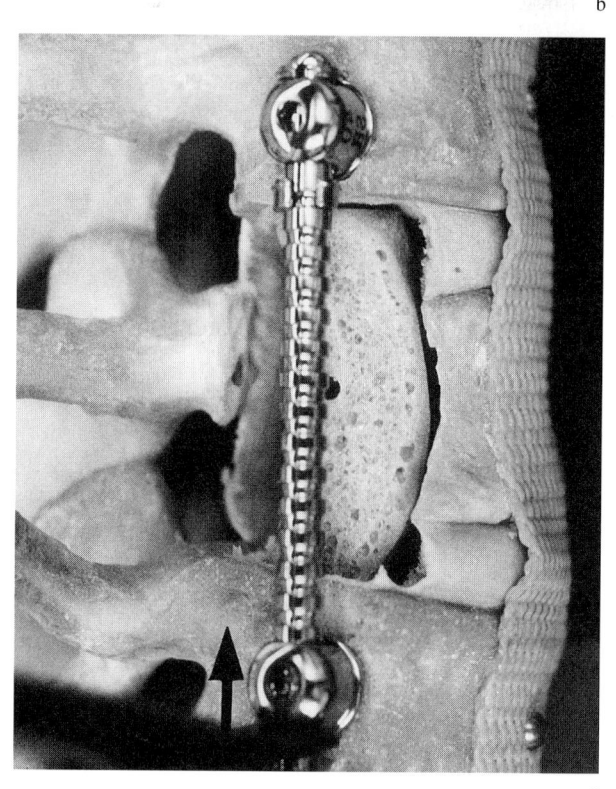

FIG. 37-12. Anterior Neutralization. (a) Universal rods connect straight-hole screws above and below the partial corpectomy. Stability is achieved by compressing across two iliac tricortical grafts. (b) Kyphosis is corrected by gradually distracting between spinal screws with an outrigger composed of two medium hooks and a universal rod. (c) After placement of a graft or cage filled with cancellous bone, a universal rod is placed through the screws and compression is applied with a spreader to lock the graft in place.

into distraction. Apply distraction with the universal rod to eliminate any kyphosis and facilitate placement of a large anterior graft (Fig. 37-12, b). A fresh-frozen femoral allograft or cage packed with autologous cancellous bone has worked well as an anterior graft spacer. After placing the graft, the outrigger is removed and the universal rod is inserted directly through the straight-hole screws. Gentle compression is then applied across the graft using a spreader on the outside of the distal screw (Fig. 37-12, c). Compression is maintained by crimping washers on the outside of the spinal screws. When additional stability is required, two rods are used and joined with short-rod cross-locks. Stop washers can be added one ratchet below the screws to allow axial loading yet limit late anterior collapse from graft settling.

SPINAL ROD-SLEEVE METHOD FOR T6-L3 BURST FRACTURES OR FRACTURE DISLOCATIONS AND BILATERAL FACET DISLOCATIONS WITH INCOMPLETE DEFICIT

Indications and Biomechanics

The rod-sleeve construct combines anatomic laminar hooks with straight universal rods and polyethylene sleeves. It is highly effective in the reduction and fixation of unstable burst fractures and fracture dislocations with an intact anterior ligament. It also provides stable fixation after manual reduction of bilateral facet dislocations, since the anterior ligament is preserved in these injuries as well. Polyethylene sleeves are generally centered directly over the superior facets of the fractured vertebrae, where they span the spinous processes above and below the traumatic disruption (Fig. 37-13). In the sagittal plane, the sleeves wedge between the rods and facets to restore maximum lordosis and correct any anterior-posterior translational deformity. In the coronal plane, sleeves wedge between the facets and spinous processes to correct medial-lateral translation (Fig. 37-13, a). The sagittal plus coronal wedge effects provide rotational alignment and stability as well (Edwards, 1991b; Edwards & Levine, 1986; Panjabi, Abumi, Duranceau, & Crisco, 1988). The result is anatomic alignment for most thoracic and lumbar injuries.

If surgery is performed within several days of injury, sleeves facilitate indirect decompression of retropulsed fragments. Sleeves wedge the superior facets and pedicles apart to untrap central retropulsed fragments, which are then reduced by distraction ligamentotaxis. Sleeves also generate localized hyperlordosis to translate the fractured vertebral body and any residual retropulsed fragments anteriorly away from the cord and roots (Edwards & Levine, 1986).

Other features of the rod-sleeve construct are responsible for superior late maintenance of alignment (Edwards, Rhyne, Weigel, & Levine, 1991; Hanley & Starr, 1991). First, anatomic hooks have broad laminar contact area, which results in less laminar resorption and hook loosening. Second, laminar resorption from the rod is eliminated by the large contact area and similar stiffness between the polyethylene sleeve and laminar bone (Fig. 37-13, a). Third, sleeves of the appropriate size bow the rods within their elastic range. This dynamic lordotic force compensates for anterior ligament relaxation to maintain full lordosis and stable fixation until fusion (Edwards, 1991b).

Because the rod-sleeve method generates considerable corrective force, length of instrumentation can be much shorter than with previous rod techniques. The standard sleeve construct spans only three interspaces for lumbar injuries and four interspaces for thoracic injuries. It typically extends to only one vertebra below the fracture and therefore instruments no more distal motion segments than a short pedicle screw fixator.

Precautions

The rod-sleeve method should not be used for shear injuries with rupture of the anterior ligament since the ligament helps prevent over distraction and plays an important role in construct stability (Edwards, 1993).

Surgical Techniques

Standard Rod-Sleeve Technique

The standard (short) sleeve construct is selected when the preoperative computed tomography (CT) scan demonstrates a stable posterior arch, such that anterior pressure against the superior facet will be transmitted through the pedicles to major vertebral-body fragments (Fig. 37-13, b).

In surgery, the patient is placed over two transverse rolls to facilitate postural reduction. The surgeon identifies the facets opposite the fractured end plate and selects the largest sleeve that will fit comfortably between the superior facet and adjacent spinous processes, generally small (2 mm) for midthoracic, medium (4 mm) for thoracolumbar, large (6 mm) for upper lumbar, and elliptical (8 mm) for midlumbar placement. A bur is used to remove any bony prominences and/or to narrow the sleeves as needed for a snug fit between the facets and spinous processes.

Anatomic hooks are inserted into the first interspace, 3 to 4 cm on either side of the sleeves. The shortest hook that will fit around the lamina is selected. Proximal hooks are inserted at the junction of the lamina and medial edge of the facet as described in the section on the compression construct.

Distal hooks are placed 3 to 4 cm below the sleeve, typically on the first lamina below the fracture, also as outlined in the section on the compression construct. Right and left distal hooks are seated concurrently to make sure the laminotomies are sufficiently lateral to accommodate both hooks under the lamina, but not so wide as to compromise the pars.

To assemble the standard rod-sleeve construct, first press a sleeve over the universal rod. Crimp a narrow washer into the groove $\frac{1}{2}$ in. from the octagonal end of the rod. Slide the

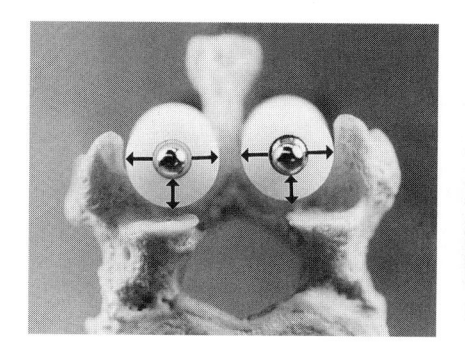

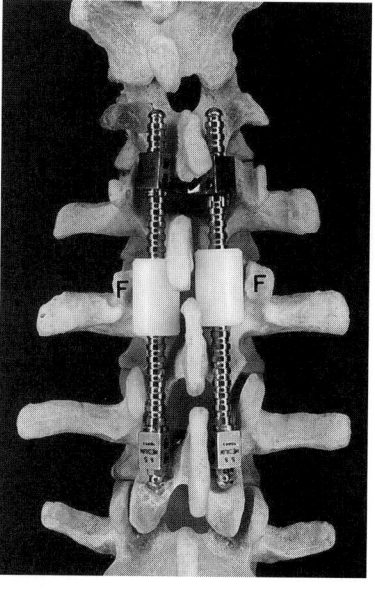

FIG. 37-13. Rod-sleeve constructs. (a) Sleeves provide an anterior-posterior wedge effect to restore lordosis and bow the rods. They also generate medial and lateral forces to restore alignment and spread pedicles to facilitate indirect decompression of posterior cortical fragments. (b) Standard sleeve construct. Sleeves are centered on the superior facets (f) of the fractured end plate; instrumentation crosses three interspaces in the lumbar spine and four in the thoracic spine. (c) Tandem-sleeve construct. Sleeves are centered over adjacent facets when both superior and inferior end plates are comminuted (Denis type-A fractures). (d) Bridging-sleeve construct. Sleeves are placed over facets on either side of an unstable posterior arch or laminectomy. The resultant four-point loading provides effective reduction and fixation for severe burst fractures and fracture dislocations.

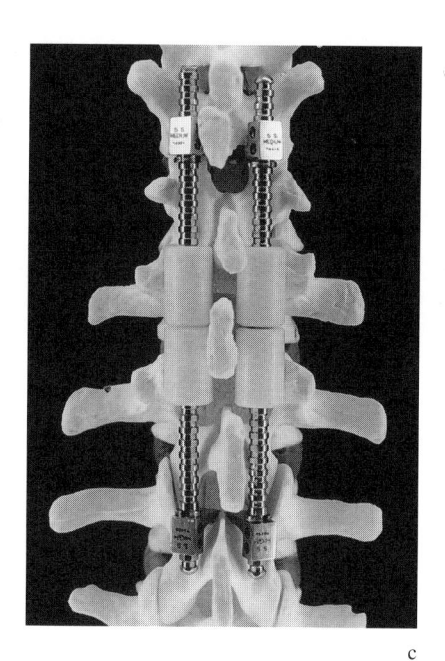

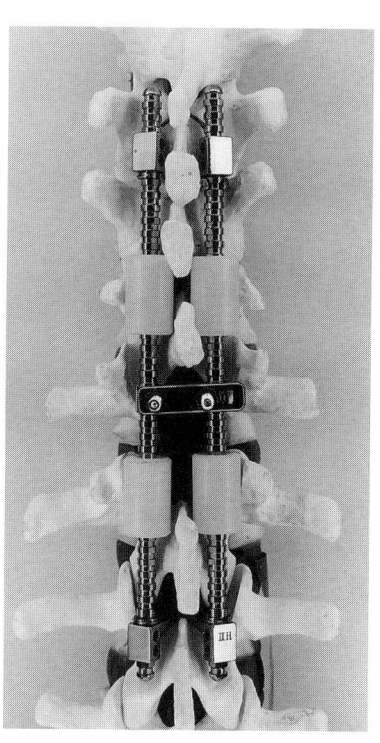

rod through the upper hook while gently rocking the hook back and forth with a hook holder. Position the sleeve just proximal to the apical facet.

To reduce a kyphotic deformity, grasp the distal end of the rod adjacent to the washer with a rod holder. Gradually push down (anteriorly) with about 50 lb of force on the rod while pulling up posteriorly on the distal hook until the octagonal end of the rod is opposite the hole in the distal hook (Fig. 37-14, c). Using a spreader against the proximal hook, advance the rod into the lower hook while rocking the hook until it engages the washer. Assemble the second rod in the same manner, then move the sleeves with a spreader until they are centered directly over the superior facet of the fractured vertebrae (Fig. 37-14, d). This will complete reduction and should produce a slight bow in the rod. Finally, apply incremental distraction over 20 minutes. This should be limited to one finger on either side of the spreader. Apply narrow or wide washers to fix the final

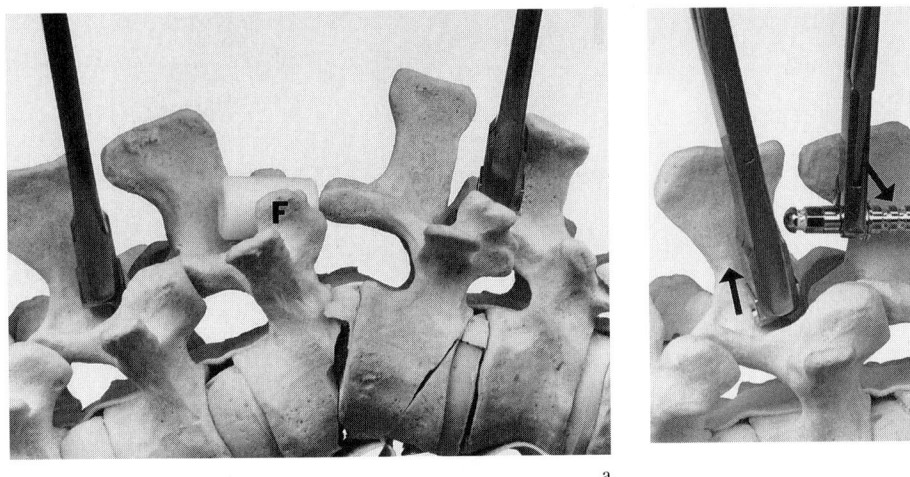

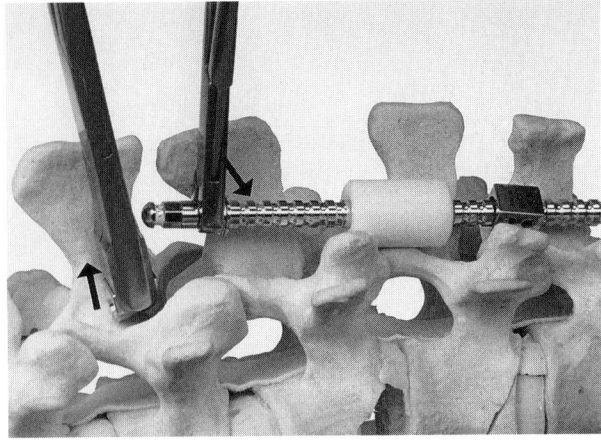

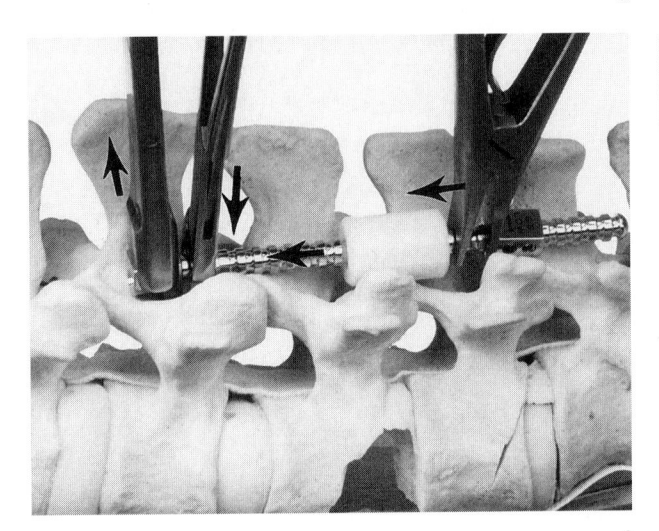

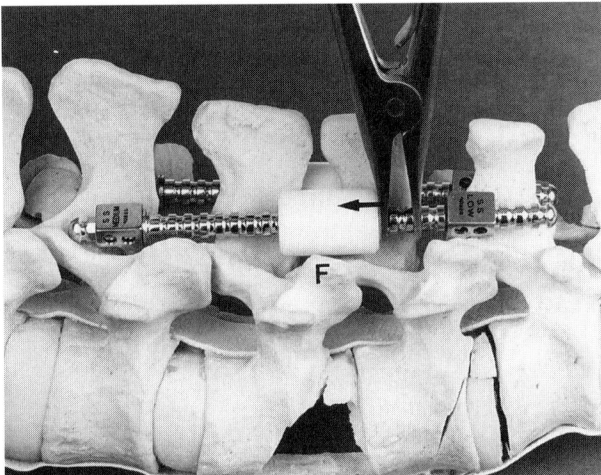

FIG. 37-14. Rod-sleeve reduction. (a) Sleeves are centered over the superior facets (F) of the fractured end plate. Hooks are inserted 3 to 4 cm from each edge of the sleeves. (b) A universal rod with sleeve has been passed proximally through the upper hook. Initial reduction is accomplished by pushing down on the distal end of the rod while pulling up on the distal hook. (c) The distal hook is engaged by advancing the rod with a spreader, while holding the reduction. (d) The spreader is reversed to move the sleeves down the rod until they are centered on the superior facets (F) of the disrupted interspace.

hook positions precisely (Edwards, 1991a; Edwards & Curcin, 1994a, 1993) (Fig. 37-13).

After instrumentation, obtain a lateral radiograph or image to confirm reduction. For incomplete paraplegics, document indirect decompression with myelography or ultrasound. Perform a posterolateral fusion with fresh iliac bone. Patients can be ambulated after drains are removed in a total contact polypropylene orthosis. When bracing is not possible or when treating patients with osteoporotic bone, consider supplemental fixation with a proximal bilaminar claw as described in the section on the kyphoreduction construct.

Tandem-Sleeve Technique

Both the superior and inferior end plates are disrupted in Denis type A fractures (Fig. 37-13, c). These burst fractures are best treated with the tandem-sleeve construct. One pair of sleeves is centered over the facets opposite the superior end plate, while a second pair is centered over the facets opposite the fractured inferior end plate. Hooks are placed in their usual position approximately 3 cm from sleeve edges. The four-point loading provided by the tandem-sleeve construct will maintain alignment to fusion for even the most unstable burst fractures.

Bridging-Sleeve Technique

The bridging-sleeve construct (Fig. 37-13, d) is selected when the preoperative CT scan shows an unstable arch or when pedicle resection has been performed to permit posterolateral decompression. An unstable arch is characterized by major pedicle comminution, widely displaced pedicles that are discontinuous with major body fragments or depressed laminar fractures (Edwards, 1993, 1991b). When the posterior arch is unstable, two pairs of sleeves are centered over the facets of the first intact posterior arch above and below the fractured vertebrae. Sleeve position and the fracture reduction sequence is the same as for the standard and tandem-sleeve techniques. After both rods are inserted and sleeve position is adjusted, a rod cross-lock can be added between the sleeve pairs for enhanced stability.

Clinical Results

Excellent clinical results are consistently reported for the rod-sleeve method. It has been found effective for thoracic and lumbar burst fractures, fracture dislocations, and bilateral facet dislocations (Edwards & Levine, 1986; Edwards et al., 1991; Garfin, Mowery, Guerra, et al., 1990; Hanley & Starr, 1991; Kurz, Hurkowitz, & Samberg, 1989; Levine, Friedman, & Edwards, 1990). The largest spinal injury series published used the rod-sleeve method for 135 thoracic fractures. Surgery was performed early, averaging 19 hours from injury. The method successfully corrected all kyphosis and provided sufficient indirect decompression of the canal in 96% of patients with incomplete paraplegia. There were few complications and no patient sustained neurologic worsening. At 3-year follow-up, average kyphosis was less than 2 degrees, substantially better than reported for alternative techniques (Edwards & Levine, 1986) (Fig. 37-15).

Hanley and Starr (1991) conducted a prospective series of 22 thoracolumbar junction fractures treated with the rod-sleeve method. They reported restoration of canal area to 86% of normal via indirect decompression, late kyphosis of only 3 degrees, and no major complications.

Patel, Brown, and Donaldson (1994) compared the incidence of surgical failures between two treatment groups: (1) rod-hook (usually rod-sleeve) constructs and (2) various pedicle screw or multiple hook systems. They noted statistically significant better results and fewer complications with the rod-sleeve group.

Results of 44 severe burst fractures with the rod-sleeve method and no anterior grafting documented excellent long-term results after 5 to 10 years of follow-up. There was average reconstitution of 91% of the crushed vertebral-body area without anterior surgery or grafting. Average kyphosis across the fractured vertebrae and disk space was limited to only 3 degrees (Edwards et al., 1991). Considering these results, there seems to be little reason for accepting the increased difficulty and risk of pedicle screw fixation for thoracolumbar spinal injuries.

DISTRACTION-LORDOSIS (D-L) CONSTRUCT FOR LOW LUMBAR BURST FRACTURES AND DEGENERATIVE SPONDYLOLISTHESIS

The D-L construct applies distraction and lordosis across two lumbar motion segments—L4 to S1. Low hook linkages connect the proximal and distal screws to universal rods. Fixed-angle distraction screws are used proximally to maintain lordosis during distraction. Midposition connectors are extended to apply lordosis (Edwards et al., 1987) (Fig. 37-16). The D-L Construct is used in the treatment of low lumbar fractures and degenerative spondylolisthesis.

Low Lumbar Fracture

Biomechanics

For L4 or L5 burst fractures, screws are inserted into the vertebrae on either side of the fractured body. Screws are also placed into the pedicles of the fractured vertebrae, since the stout L4 or L5 pedicles almost always remain intact. After construct assembly, the proximal hooks are ratcheted to restore vertebral height, and the midposition connectors are extended to provide lordosis and translate the fractured vertebral body anteriorly away from the cauda equina (Fig. 37-16, *b* and *c*). When necessary, a laminectomy can be performed to further decompress roots (Edwards, 1993, 1991b).

Precaution

The D-L construct is not appropriate for many L3 and upper lumbar fractures since the pedicles are usually comminuted or discontinuous with the vertebral body.

Surgical Technique

To reduce an L5 burst fracture, for example, screws are placed into the pedicle of L4, L5, and across the sacral ala at S1. The L5 screws are seated deeply and directed caudally, because vertebral-body comminution is usually limited to the proximal one third of the body (Rosenthal, Levine, & Edwards, 1988). Fixed-angled distraction screws are used both proximally and distally to maintain lordosis during distraction (Fig. 37-16, *c*).

Straight universal rods are attached to the screws via low anatomic hook linkages at L4 and S1. Adjustable connectors are snapped onto the rods and attached to the L5 screws. The proximal hooks are distracted and the L5 connectors lengthened under image control to restore height and lordosis (Edwards, 1993; Edwards & Curcin, 1993).

Clinical Results

The first 16 low lumbar fractures treated with the D-L construct were presented in 1989. The D-L restored good alignment and provided sufficiently stable fixation to permit early patient ambulation. At 1 year of follow-up, 89% vertebral height was maintained and lordosis at the fracture level was restored to 6 degrees. Fusion occurred in 94% of the cases. Complications were limited to one hook dislodgment and one radiculopathy (Levine, Garfin, et al., 1989). In a SFSG report on 40 cases with more than 1 year of follow-up, reduction was maintained and primary union was achieved in 90% (Edwards, 1991a).

Degenerative Olisthesis

Biomechanics

The D-L construct is used most often for reduction, indirect canal decompression, and fixation of degenerative L3-4 or L4-5 olisthesis. Screws are placed in the slipped and adjacent two distal vertebrae to provide a firm base. Universal rods are distracted to restore normal intervertebral height, flatten bulging disks, and enlarge stenotic

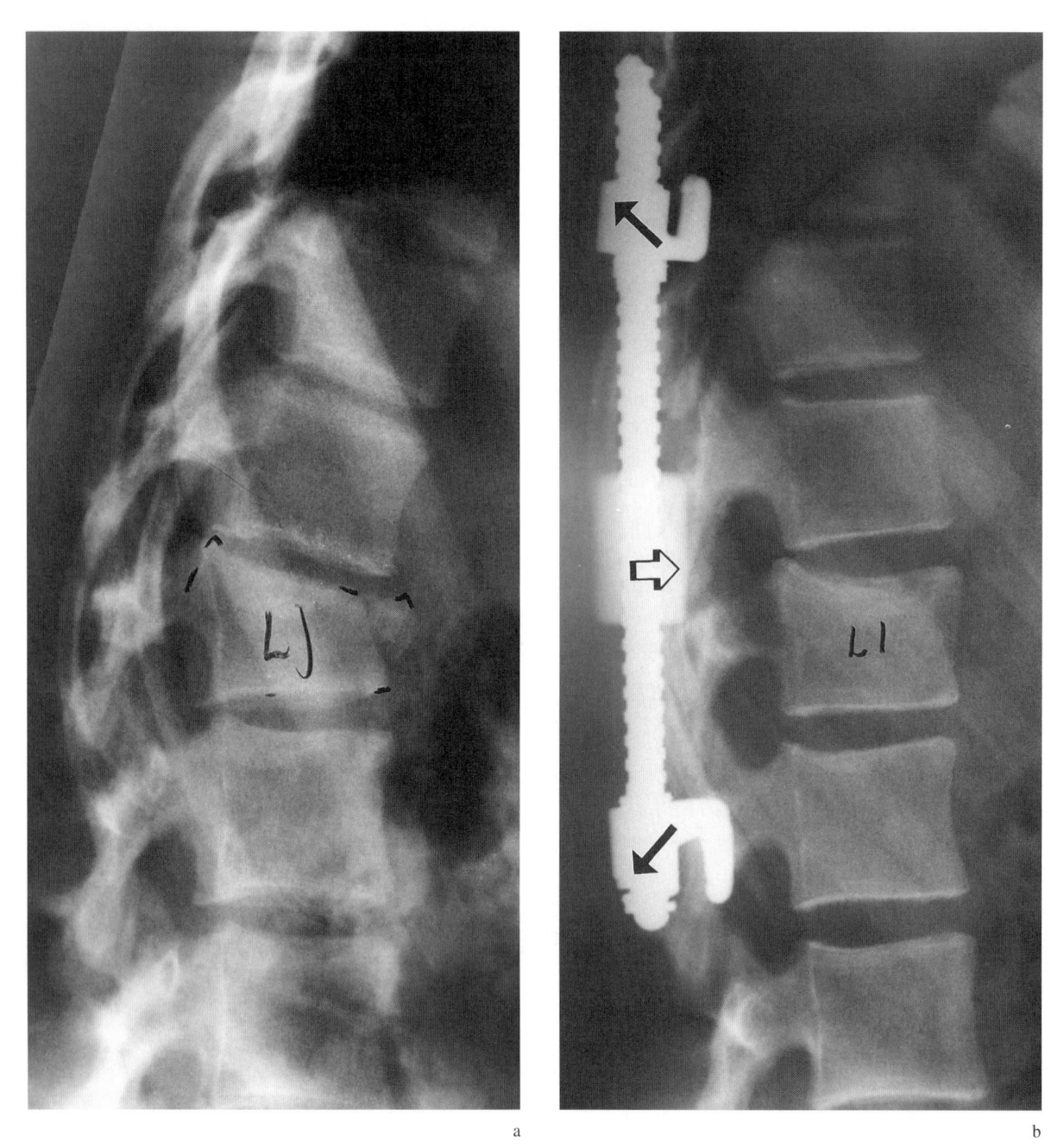

FIG. 37-15. Rod-sleeve examples. (a) Preoperative x-ray film of burst fracture with retropulsed posterosuperior fragment causing incomplete paraplegia. (b) Rod-sleeve reduction on second day restored anatomic alignment and achieved indirect decompression of the retropulsed fragment. (c) Preoperative x-ray film of L1 pathologic compression fracture with posterior extension of tumor into the canal. (d) Bridging-sleeve construct restored height, alignment, and stability after laminectomy and posterolateral decompressions to remove tumor from the canal.

foramina. Lengthening the midposition (L5) connectors rotates the lower two vertebrae into flexion underneath the slipped proximal (i.e. L4) vertebra. This reduces the olisthesis and counteracts translational instability (Edwards, 1992b; Edwards & Curcin, 1993; Edwards & McConnell, 1992) (Fig. 37-17, a and b). After reduction the aligned spine can be left in gentle compression to enhance lordosis and facilitate union.

The D-L construct can be extended across multiple levels when necessary. Proximal and distal vertebrae attach to contoured universal rods via hook linkages while midposition connectors are either lengthened or shortened to reduce retrolisthesis, spondylolisthesis, or lateral olisthesis deformation.

Technique

Most patients with degenerative olisthesis have hypertrophic superior facets and lateral stenosis. Prior to instrumentation, a laminotomy is performed to remove the anteromedial osteophytes from the superior facets (i.e., L5) and enlarge the foramen at the olisthetic level. For L4-5 spondylolisthesis, screws are placed in L4-5 and S1 to cross both the olisthetic L4-5 and typically degenerative L5-S1 joint. To assemble the D-L construct (Edwards & McConnell, 1992):

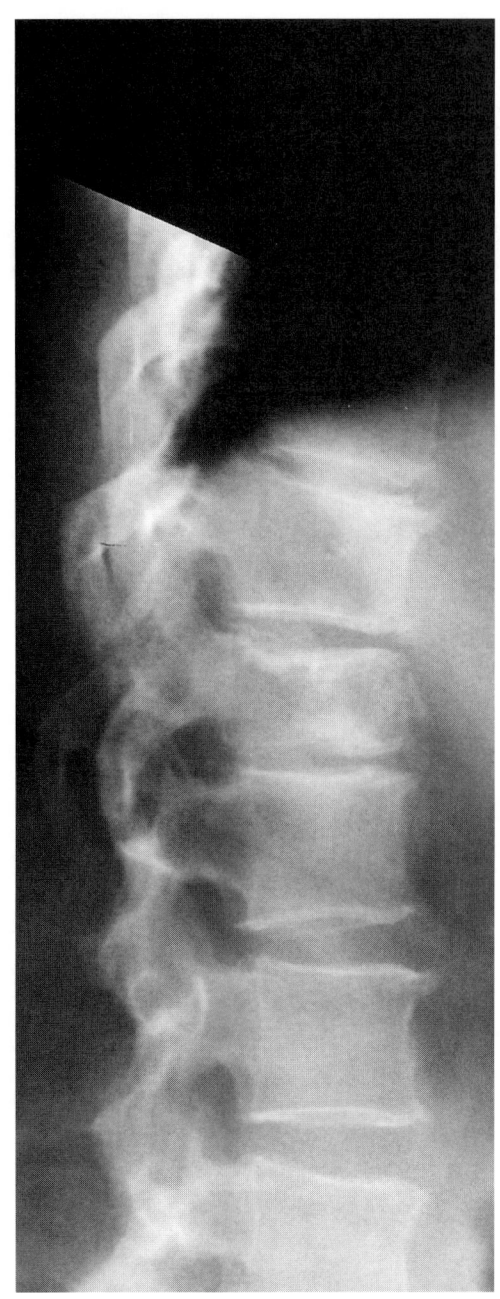

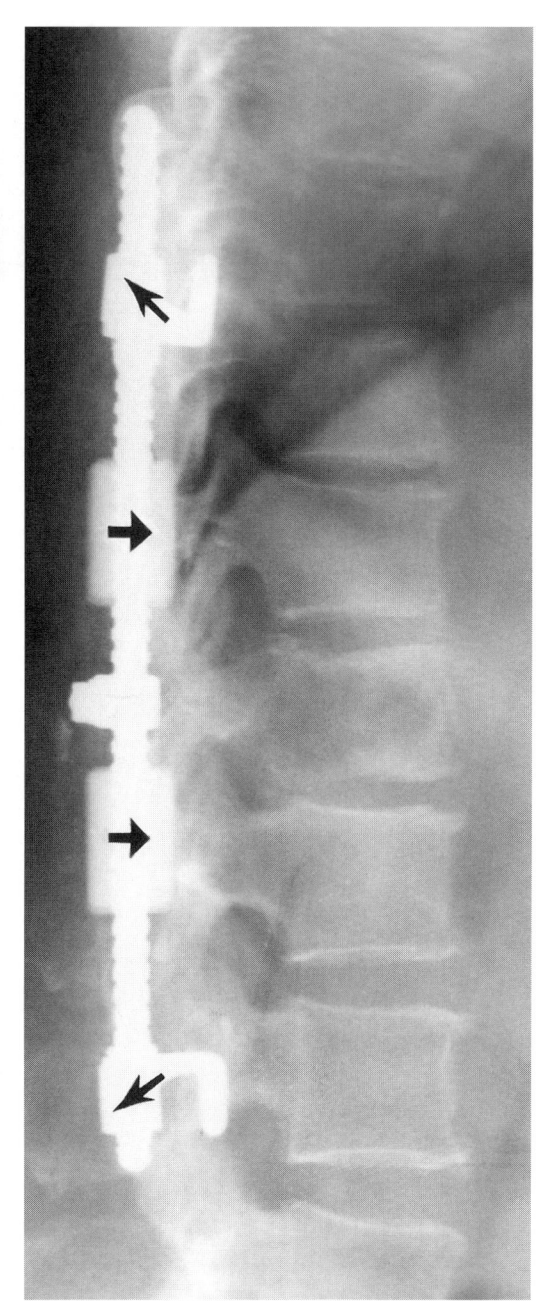

1. Use distraction screws at L4, angled 15 degrees cephalad to maintain lordosis during distraction.
2. Use standard screws distally to allow L5-S1 to rotate into flexion about the screw slot during L4-5 slip reduction.
3. Seat the middle screw deeply to provide room for placement of an adjustable connector.
4. Assemble straight universal rods with the octagon facing distally using low hook linkages in distraction.
5. Snap midpoint connectors onto the rods and hold their stems perpendicular to the rods with clips or washers.
6. Under image control, slightly distract to restore disk height and lengthen the midpoint connector(s) to rotate L5 under L4 to reduce the olisthesis.
7. Apply a cross-lock to enhance stability.

Precaution

When treating spondylolisthesis nonunions, very large or active patients, or those otherwise at risk for nonunion, leave the construct in compression. First, temporarily assemble the D-L instrumentation using rod clips. After olisthesis reduction, remove one rod at a time and reorient the terminal hook linkages to compression. Reextend the mid-

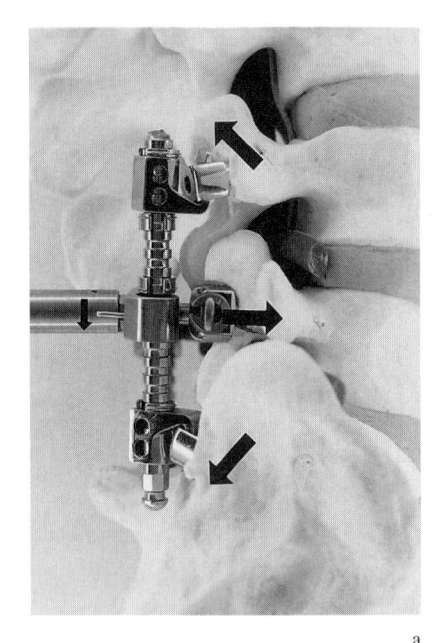

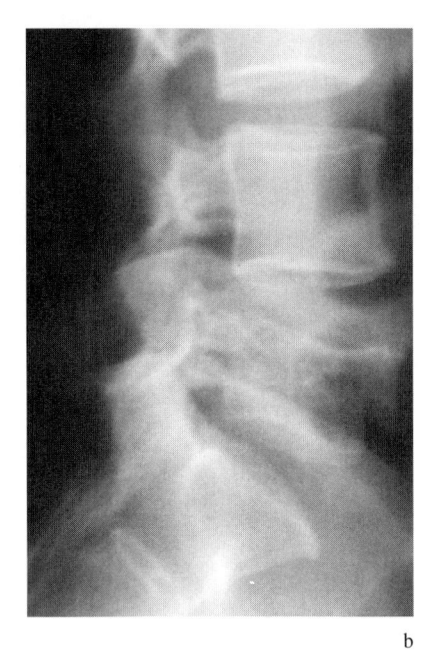

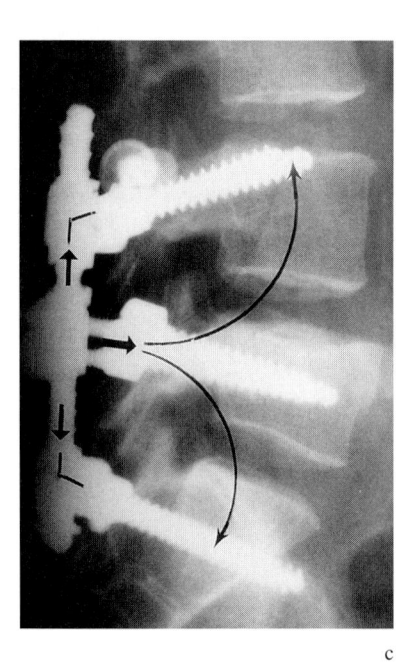

FIG. 37-16. D-L construct for low lumbar fractures. (a) D-L construct on a model. A socket wrench is used to lengthen an adjustable connector. (b and c) L5 burst fracture reduced and stabilized with L4 to S1 D-L construct. Lordosis is maintained with fixed-angled distraction screws at L4 and S1 while L5 screws into the stable inferior portion of the burst vertebra are translated anteriorly by extending the adjustable connectors. The resulting extension moment counteracts flexion forces to maintain reduction.

point connectors to maintain olisthesis reduction and apply a cross-lock.

Clinical Results

Eighty-seven cases of degenerative L4-5 olisthesis treated with the D-L construct left in distraction were reported by the SFSG. All had more than 1 year of follow-up. Ninety-four percent maintained reduction of slippage and 85% achieved primary union. The SFSG also reported late results on 146 patients with spinal stenosis and instability. They were treated with the D-L and extended D-L constructs across multiple lumbar levels usually including the sacrum to reduce various olistheses, open foramen, and stabilize the spine until fusion. Fixation was maintained in 98% and primary union occurred in 82% (Edwards, 1991a).

KYPHOREDUCTION CONSTRUCT FOR CHRONIC POSTTRAUMATIC KYPHOSIS, VERTEBRAL-BODY COLLAPSE FROM TUMOR OR INFECTION, AND SCHEUERMANN'S DISEASE

Biomechanics

The kyphoreduction construct attaches to the spine proximally with bilaminar hook-claws, and distally with screws or an independent claw. Rod sleeves at the apex provide the fulcrum. Adjustable connectors between the rods and distal screws are shortened every 5 minutes for sequential three-point loading to achieve use of viscoelastic stress relaxation of contracted anterior ligament or scar (Fig. 37-18, *a*). Full correction is usually possible without either anterior release or vertebrectomy where anterior autofusion has not occurred. After angular correction, connectors are ratcheted up the rods into compression to shorten the posterior column. This will further reduce any kyphosis and encourage fusion by permitting physiologic axial loading across the posterior elements. (Fig. 37-18, *b*). Following reduction, universal rods are generally bowed within their elastic range to provide a continuing extension moment to counteract flexion and prevent recurrent kyphosis (Edwards & Rosenthal, 1988; Edwards & Rhyne, 1990) (Fig. 37-18, *c* and *d*).

Precautions

1. When confronted with rigid deformity or porotic bone, stress at the bone-implant interfaces should be reduced by adding an additional pair of caudal facing hooks proximally and an additional pair of screws distally.
2. If normal sagittal alignment cannot be achieved with posterior surgery alone, then anterior release grafting at the apex should be performed.

Surgical Technique

Prior to surgery, flexion-extension films and sagittal tomograms are obtained to rule out either an anterior bridge or substantial retropulsion causing cord impingement (Edwards & Rosenthal, 1988; Kurz, Hurkowitz, & Samberg, 1989). At surgery, the patient is placed on transverse rolls. Multiple partial facetectomies and a chevron osteotomy are performed at the apex to permit the posterior column shortening nec-

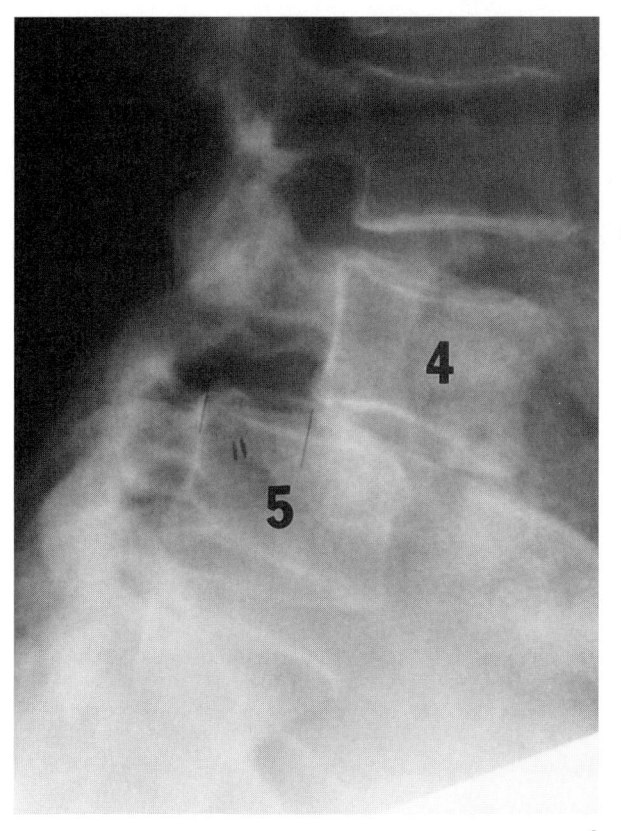

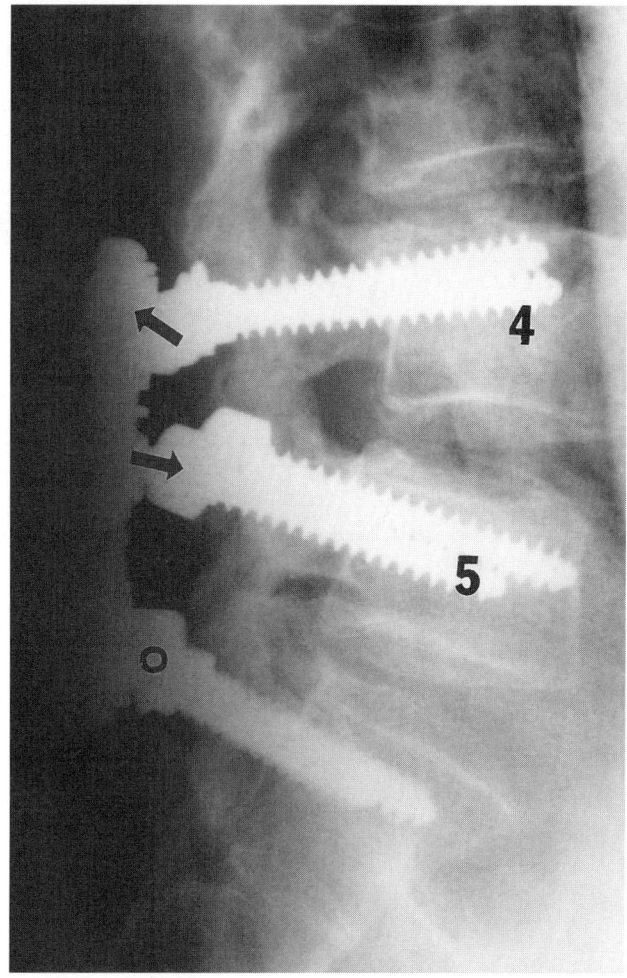

FIG. 37-17. D-L construct for degenerative olisthesis. (a) Severe L4-5 degenerative olisthesis following decompressive surgery. (b) Reduction and fixation with a D-L construct used to rotate L5 back under L4.

essary for restoration of anatomic alignment. Proximal hook claws and distal screws are centered at least 5 cm from the apex. Independent bilaminar claws are used instead of screws for distal attachment in the midthoracic spine.

To assemble the proximal claw and kyphoreduction construct (Edwards & Curcin, 1993):

1. Place caudal facing (usually medium) hooks over the top of the most proximal lamina to be instrumented as described in the section on distal (caudal facing) anatomic hook insertion. Insert cephalad facing low or medium open hooks under the adjacent lamina as in the section on cephalad facing anatomic hook insertion.
2. Contour a universal rod into normal sagittal alignment and pass the octagonal end through the proximal hook body. Crimp a narrow washer in the groove at the end of the rod to secure the hook.
3. Lower the rods into the body of the inferior open hook pair, replace the hook doors, use a spreader to compress each hook pair together, and apply C-washers to complete the proximal bilaminar claws.
4. For distal fixation insert standard screws or center an independent hook claw approximately 5 cm below the apex.
5. Attach 90-degree ring connectors between the distal screws and rods as described in the section on adjustable connector assembly. Orient standard screws with slot openings facing cephalad to facilitate articulation with connector shoes. Position connector stems lateral to the universal rods. When using claws for distal fixation, attach the claws and primary rods with rod-rod connectors (Fig. 37-18, b).
6. Gradually shorten the connectors every 5 minutes until the rods abut the spinal screws. Limit force application by turning the socket wrench with only two fingers. Harvest graft and decorticate during the 1 to 3 hours required for stress relaxation of chronic deformities.
7. Gradually apply compression with the spreader to shorten the posterior column and cross-lock the construct.

Clinical Results

A prospective study of 15 cases of posttraumatic kyphosis reduced with the kyphoreduction construct has been reported. The average patient was 44 years old and presented 4 years after spinal injury. Three patients had anterior bony

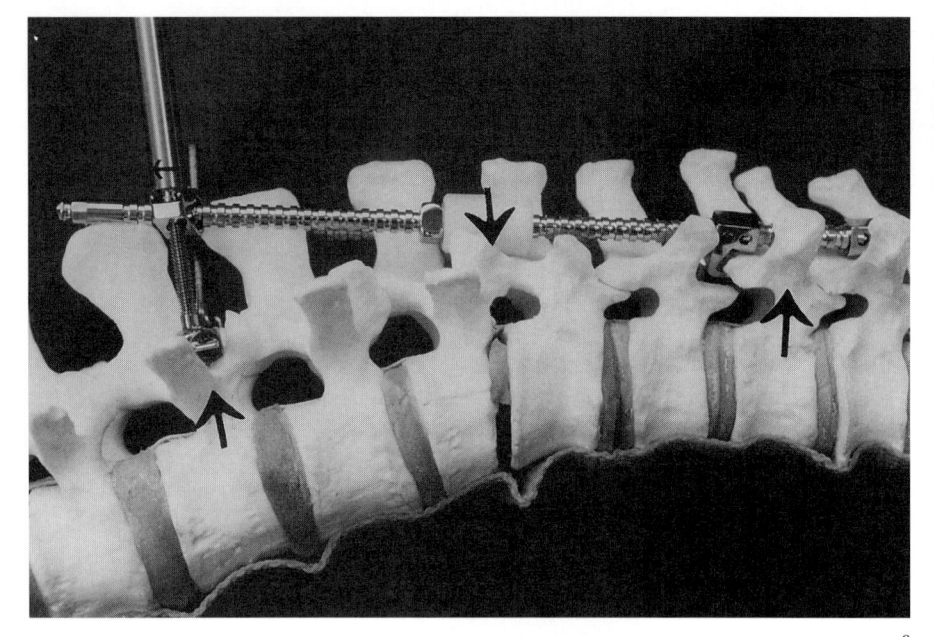

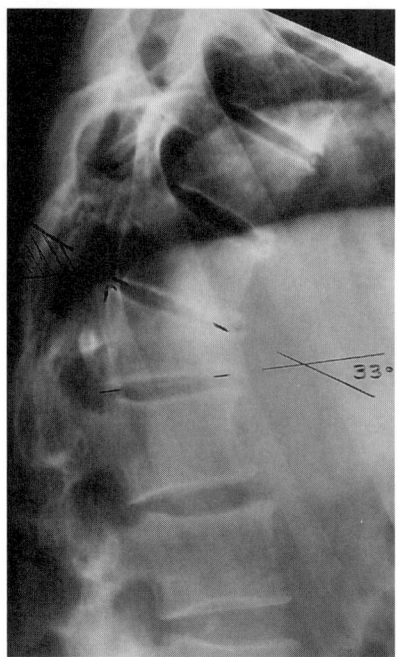

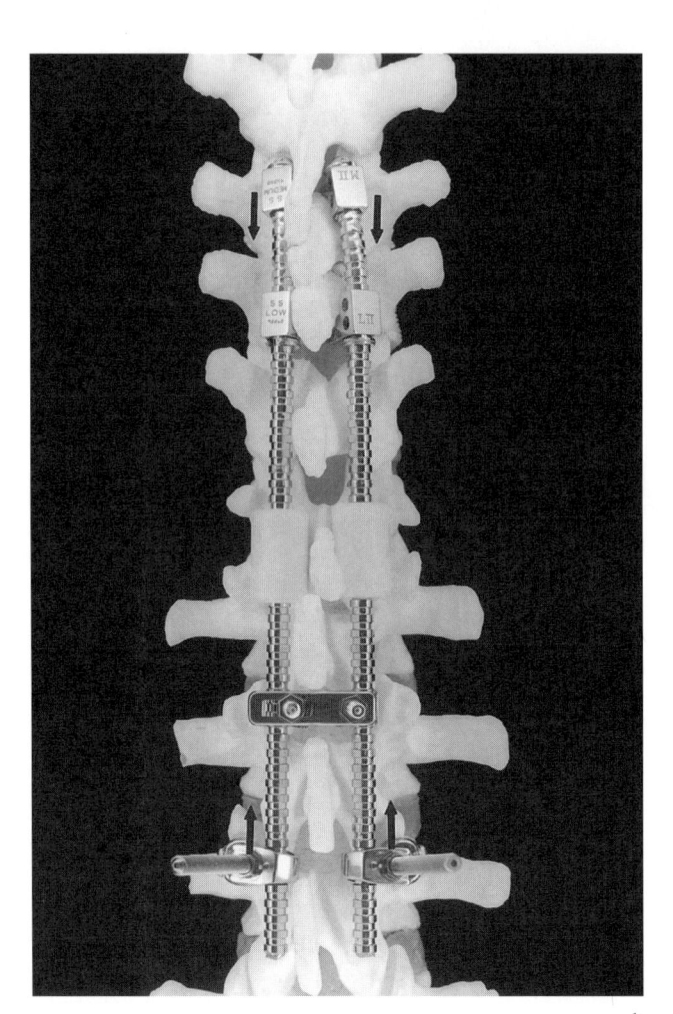

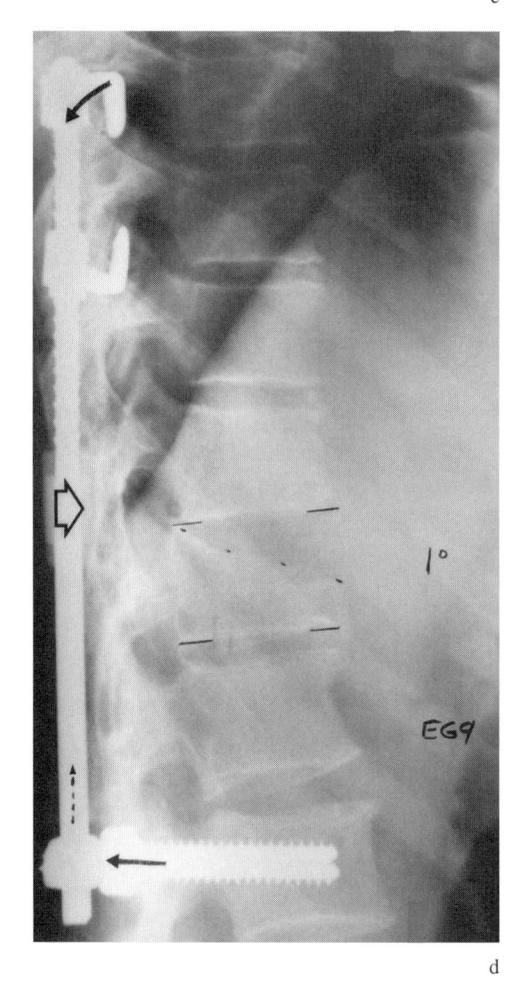

FIG. 37-18. Kyphoreduction construct. (a) Proximal fixation is achieved with a bilaminar claw. Sleeves centered over the kyphotic apex serve as the fulcrum. Distal fixation is provided by screws attached to rods with adjustable connectors. The connectors are gradually shortened by turning a socket wrench for three-point loading to correct the kyphosis. (b) The connectors are ratcheted proximally with a spreader to shorten the posterior column and load the posterior fusion mass. A cross-lock enhances the stability of fixation. (c) Fixed 33-degree T12 kyphosis in a 51-year-old man who presented with deformity and severe low back pain 15 years after fracture and posterior fusion. (d) Complete reduction and pain relief was obtained using the kyphoreduction construct alone without the need for either anterior release or low back surgery.

bridges or retropulsed bone that required preliminary anterior surgery. The 12 remaining cases were reduced using the principle of intraoperative stress relaxation via the kyphoreduction construct. Thirty-seven degrees of average preoperative kyphosis was corrected 88% to 6 degrees and held at 11 degrees long-term. At 4 years' average follow-up, 94% of patients had achieved solid fusion with no clinically significant complications (Edwards & Osborne, 1994) (Fig. 37-18, c and d).

The SFSG reported 26 cases with over 1 year of follow-up. There was 94% maintenance of reduction-fixation and a primary union rate of 96% (Edwards, 1991a). Results to date suggest the kyphoreduction construct is consistently able to reduce posttraumatic, post-tumor, degenerative, Scheuermann's, and even osteoporotic kyphosis. Anterior surgery and grafting is rarely necessary when full anatomic alignment is achieved with posterior kyphoreduction construct at surgery.

SPONDYLO CONSTRUCT FOR ISTHMIC L5-S1 SPONDYLOLISTHESIS, ALL GRADES, AND SEVERE, GRADE 2+ DEGENERATIVE SPONDYLOLISTHESIS

Indications

Spondylo construct fixation is indicated for low-grade slips to permit full root decompression, stop slip progression, lessen postoperative pain, and negate anterior shear forces and, thus, promote union. Spondylo construct reduction and fixation is indicated for high-grade deformities to also restore lumbosacral lordosis and normal spine alignment, improve the patient's appearance and self-image, and provide anterior column support for L5 so as to maintain reduction over time. Finally, for spondyloptosis, the spondylo construct and associated techniques are indicated to decompress the sacral roots and reconstruct the spine without the need for L5 vertebrectomy or anterior pelvic surgery (Amundson, Edwards, & Garfin, 1991).

Biomechanics

The concept of gradual instrumented reduction for spondylolisthesis without anterior release or diskectomy was developed by the author in the mid-1980s (Edwards, 1986). The goal was to achieve full anatomic correction of the deformity with less surgery and morbidity than former methods. Four principals were combined to accomplish this goal: (1) Simultaneous application of distraction, posterior translation of the lumbar spine, and sacral flexion (lordosis). (2) Sacral fixation at two well-separated proximal and midsacral points that could provide a sufficient extension moment to achieve and maintain spondylolisthesis reduction. (3) Use of viscoelastic stress relaxation to gradually lengthen contracted anterior structures. (4) Full correction of sagittal alignment and placement of L5 directly over the sacrum to promote union and long-term maintenance of correction.

Precautions

Successful reconstruction of spondylolisthesis requires careful preoperative planning and attention to such technical details as L5 root dissection, precise placement of midsacral screws, and patience. Whereas reduction of spondylolisthesis carries a relatively low risk of root deficit, this risk rises for grade 4 slips when the slip angle (inferior L5) exceeds 40 degrees.

Reduction of the more severe grade 4 slips or spondyloptosis requires prior experience correcting lower-grade slips and attendance at the Intermediate Spinal Fixation Study Group Workshop for instruction in the use of staged reduction, posterior osteotomies, somatosensory evoked potential (SSEP)/wake-up test monitoring, and other specialized surgical techniques that are beyond the scope of this chapter.

Surgical Technique

Spondylolisthesis (Grades I to IV)

Grades I to IV spondylolisthesis is reduced in a single-stage posterior operation (Edwards, 1991c; Edwards & Curcin, 1993). After L5 laminectomy, the fibrocartilage and osteophytes overlying the L5 roots are removed to expose the L5 roots and pedicles fully. Instrumentation usually crosses only the L5-S1 interspace (Fig. 37-19, a and c). Fixation to L4 is only required for Grade IV slips with significant L4-5 retrolisthesis or known L4-5 diskdegeneration. SSEP or electromyographic (EMG) monitoring is recommended for Grade III or greater slip reductions, combined with a wake-up test for Grade IV or greater slips.

To assemble the spondylo construct (Edwards & Curcin, 1993):

1. Insert standard screws under direct vision from the lateral aspect of the superior L5 facet directed, parallel with the superior end plate and across the L5 body.
2. Insert standard screws at S1 just lateral to the dimple below the L5-S1 facet, perpendicular to the cortex in the sagittal plane and 30 degrees laterally across the anterior ala as outlined in the section on lateral S1 screw placement.
3. Carefully insert angled-hole screws in the converging midsacral position as discussed in the section on lateral screw placement.
4. Slide a low or medium hook facing caudally over the rod into the S1 screw slot. The hook linkage should hold the rod at a 30-degree angle with the long axis of the proximal sacrum.
5. Cross-lock the rods (use an angled jaw) between the S1 and S2 screws to negate the lateral pullout load on the midsacral screws during reduction (Fig. 37-19, c).
6. Place ring connectors over the proximal end of the rods with the stems positioned lateral to the universal rods and lock the connector shoes to the L5 screws with washers (Fig. 37-19, a).
7. Sequentially distract the L5 ring connectors up the rods to restore disk space height. Shorten the L5 connectors with the socket wrench to "two-finger" tightness every 5 minutes (Fig. 37-19, a).
8. In the final stage of reduction, progressively release all distraction and further shorten the L5 connectors until normal alignment is achieved and connectors are "bottomed-out" (Fig. 37-19, b).

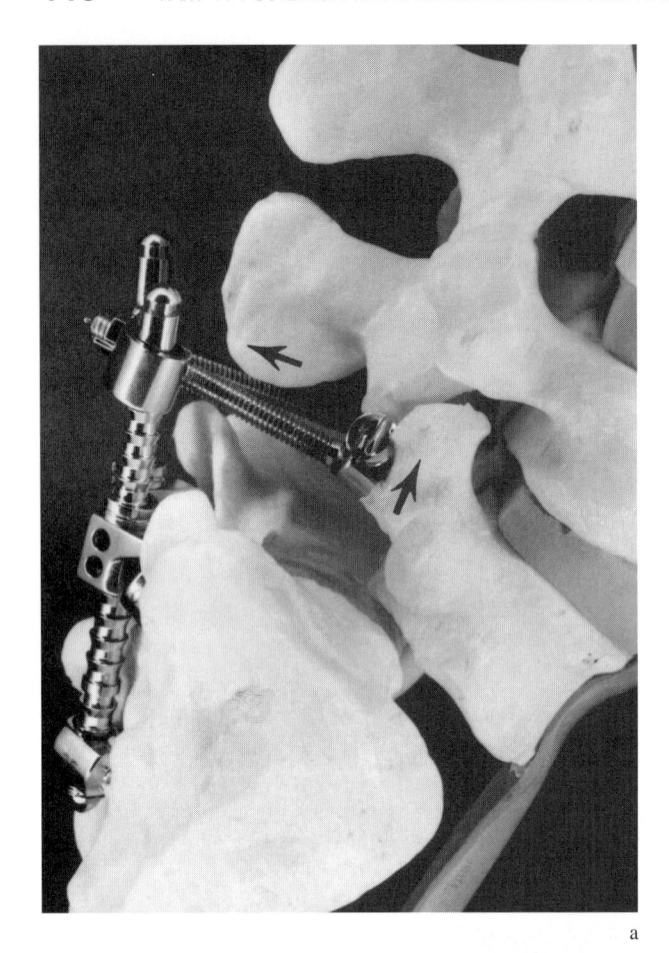

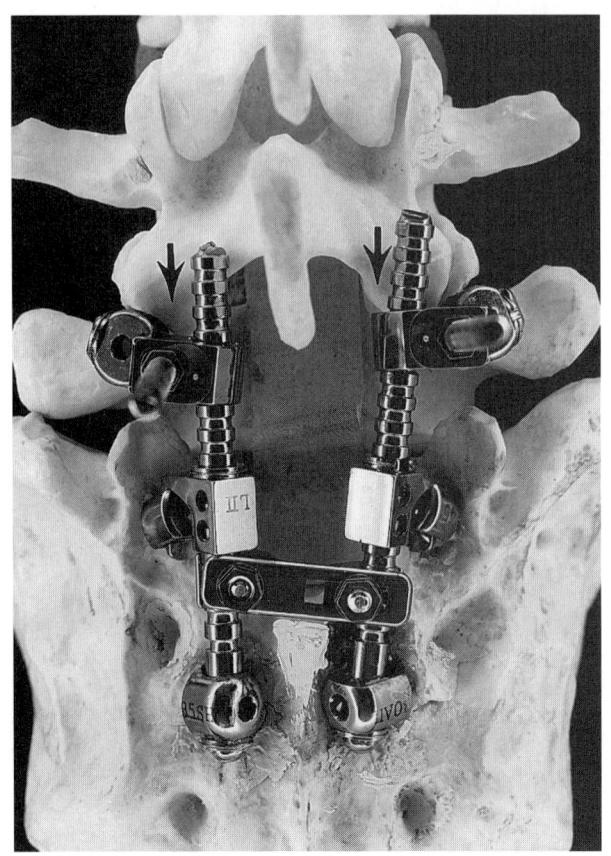

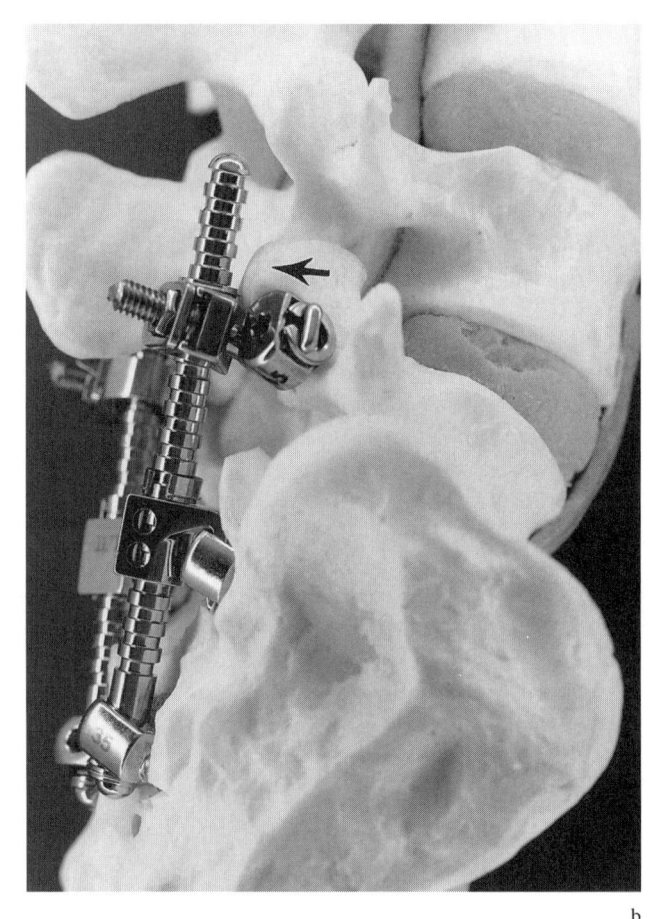

FIG. 37-19. Spondylo construct. (a) Lateral view of Grade IV spondylolisthesis deformity on model fixed with spondylo construct prior to reduction. Distraction is applied by ratcheting connectors on the universal rods with a spreader while posterior translation is effected by shortening the adjustable connectors. (b) Connectors are shortened incrementally to facilitate stress relaxation. As spine length approaches normal, distraction is steadily released until anatomic alignment is restored. (c) Gentle compression is then applied with a spreader to enhance lordosis and axial loading.

9. Apply very gentle axial compression with the spreader to promote anterior column axial loading and confirm unobstructed egress of the L5 nerve roots.

Spondyloptosis

When the entire L5 vertebral body resides below the sacral dome on standing films, the deformity is known as "spondyloptosis" (Edwards & Curcin, 1994a). Surgical reconstruction of these cases is particularly challenging, but the results are often dramatic in terms of patient appearance, pain relief, and satisfaction. When embarking on correction of spondyloptosis, careful preoperative analysis and special surgical techniques are required to avoid excessive L4 and L5 root stretch. Before surgery, we use five risk determinants to calculate the permissible amount of spinal lengthening at any one procedure that is compatible with normal root function (Edwards & Curcin, 1994a). Typically, spondyloptosis is reduced in two posterior stages scheduled 1 week apart. Severe spondyloptosis deformities also require posterior sacral dome osteotomy and occasional inferior L5 body osteotomy from the posterior approach to shorten the spine (Edwards, 1991c). To extend the time for reduction, alar rods and overhead traction wires attached to L4 screws are applied early in the case to begin lifting L5 out of the pelvis for L5 root decompression and screw placement. Final reduction is accomplished under image control with an L4 to S2 spondylo construct as described in the section on spondylolisthesis. Neurologic function is monitored with both SSEPs using dural leads and periodic wake-up tests (Edwards, 1991c; Edwards & Curcin, 1994a). Using these new techniques, full reduction of spondylolisthesis and spondyloptosis is now routinely accomplished without the need for anterior surgery.

Clinical Results

Spondylolisthesis

The author has reported the long-term results following reduction for 18 cases of Grade II to IV spondylolisthesis (Edwards, 1990). Ninety-one percent of the olisthetic deformity was permanently corrected. Final kyphosis averaged 4 degrees, and 32 mm of (L5-S1) trunk height was restored (Fig. 37-19). Solid arthrodesis was achieved in 94% of cases; the only pseudarthrosis and implant failure occurred in a patient who refused postoperative bracing. One patient (5.5%) with borderline spondyloptosis experienced unilateral L4-5 weakness.

Similar results are reported for the SFSG's first 134 patients with over 1 year of follow-up (Edwards, 1991a) (Fig. 37-20). Reduction was maintained in 96%, and primary fusion was achieved in 87%. Infection occurred in 1.5%. Six percent had transient postoperative L4 or L5 root symptoms, but only 1% had lasting unilateral dorsiflexion weakness. Hence, gradual instrumented reduction performed by well-trained spine surgeons corrects the deformity with a higher union rate and no more complications than standard in situ fusion with reduction.

Spondyloptosis

Early patients who underwent spondyloptosis reduction experienced a moderate rate of nonunion, midsacral fixation failure, and unilateral dorsiflexion weakness (Amundson et al., 1991). With continued refinement of methods, complications have been reduced to an acceptable level. In a prospective study of 20 consecutive optosis patients treated by the author with over 2 years' follow-up, the 100% preoperative slip was reduced 86% and maintained at 80% following union. Lumbo sacral kyphosis of 36 degrees was corrected to 17 degrees of lordosis, and 5 cm of trunk height was restored in the average optosis patient. Some degree of lumbar root deficit occurred in 25%, but only two patients (10%) had functionally significant ankle dorsiflexion weakness. None required bracing or suffered sacral-root dysfunction (Edwards & Curcin, 1994b).

Long-term results were excellent. Union occurred in 80% of the patients after the initial procedure and 100% after one repair. All remained in atomic alignment. Back pain was eliminated in 50% of cases and was significantly reduced in another 40%. Ninety-five percent of the patients expressed overall satisfaction (Edwards & Curcin, 1994b).

Similar results have been reported for a series of 14 high-grade spondylolisthesis and optosis patients treated by Hu, Bradford, and colleagues (1994) with Edwards instrumentation and spondylo reduction techniques. Hence, with steady refinement in both preoperative planning and surgical technique, reconstruction of spondyloptosis by gradual instrumented reduction and selective posterior osteotomies has become a consistently effective procedure with a lower rate of major complications than alternative methods.

SCOLIOSIS CONSTRUCT FOR IDIOPATHIC THORACIC AND LUMBAR SCOLIOSIS, KYPHOSCOLIOSIS, AND DEGENERATIVE LUMBAR AND LUMBOSACRAL SCOLIOSIS WITH LATERAL LISTHESIS

Biomechanics

The versatility of fixation, modularity and three-dimensional adjustability of the EMSS simplify correction of scoliosis. In order to achieve greater correction of deformity with less extensive surgery we employ several biomechanical principles, as discussed below.

Direct Reduction of Deformity

Universal rods are contoured into normal anatomic alignment. Deformities are reduced through the application of corrective forces until the spine is fixed to the precontoured rods. Rotated and olisthetic vertebrae are directly reduced by adjustable connectors attached to the rods (Fig. 37-21).

Lateral Attachment Sites

To maximize the corrective moments (rotational forces) required for reduction of scoliotic (coronal plane) deformity,

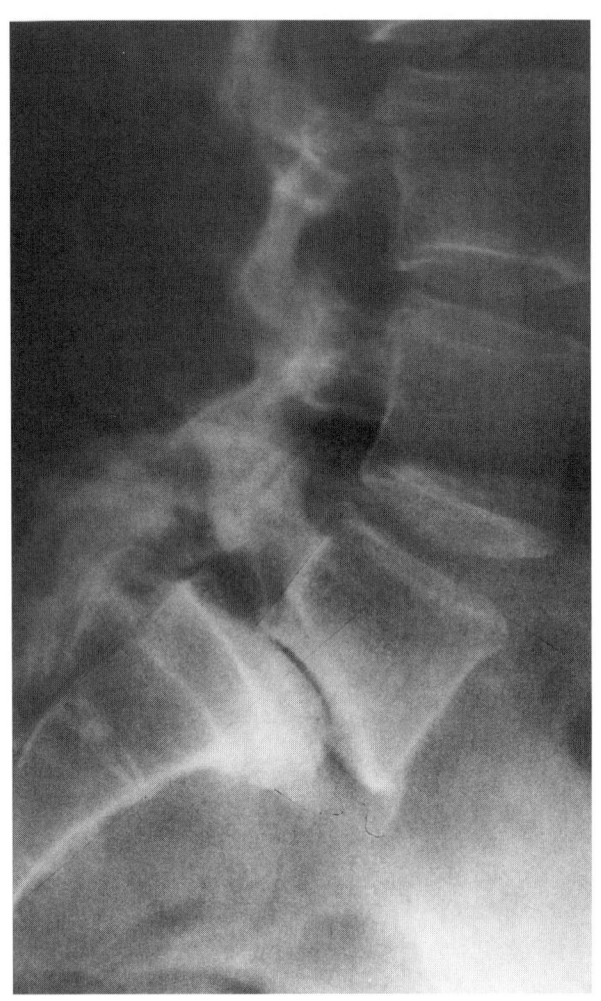

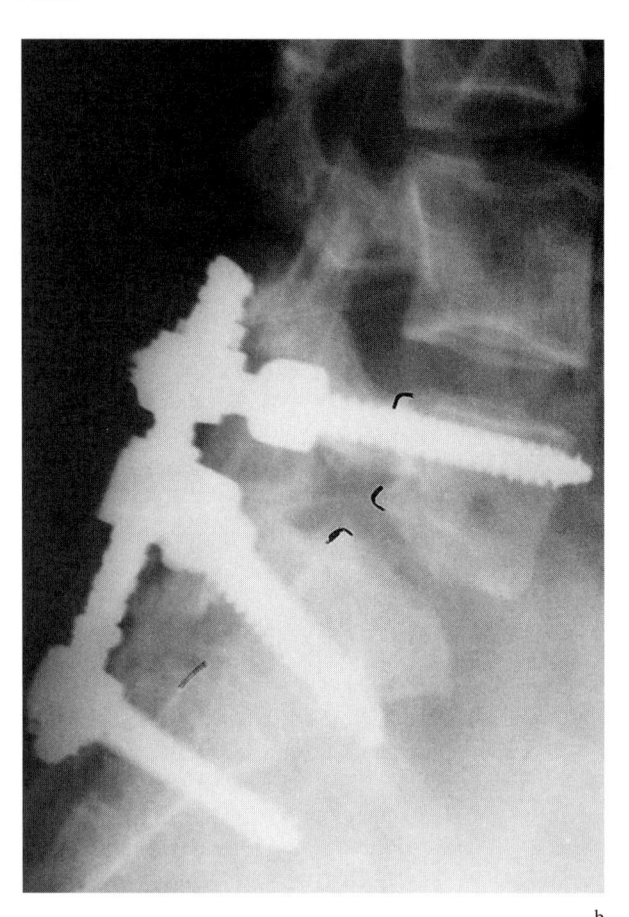

FIG. 37-20. Grade II spondylolisthesis. (a) Preoperative radiographs of Grade II spondylolisthesis and nonunion after failed in situ fusion. (b) Correction of slippage and negation of anterior shear instability to promote union.

we attach compression and distraction rods as far as possible from the midline. Hence, pedicles, rather than lamina, are often used for distal attachment (Fig. 37-21). Medially directed sacral screws with heads lateral to the S1 facet joint are used when compressing or distracting from the sacrum. Proximal hook attachment to a stout mamillary process, when available is preferred over lamina attachment for thoracic compression.

Stable Base for Olisthesis

For lasting correction of unstable olisthesis, we attach spinal rods at two or more vertebral levels distal to an olisthesis so as to create a stable base for universal rod fixation if anterior grafting is not anticipated.

Multiple Sacral Attachments

For long lumbosacral instrumentations several well-separated points of sacral fixation (as described in the section on sacral screw insertion) are employed to prevent the late loss of fixation that has plagued this type of surgery in the past.

Multiple Rods

When a greater number of corrective forces are required in one region of the spine than can be accomplished with one pair of rods, we add supplemental rods. Our aim is the most efficient point of application for each corrective force and the ideal sequence for reduction (Fig. 37-22).

Stress Relaxation

In order to achieve maximum correction of deformity and lessen dependence on anterior release operations, the Edwards scoliosis constructs provide incremental adjustability in all planes of motion so as to facilitate stress relaxation of contracted tissues.

Reduction Sequence

Correction of deformity is accomplished by the gradual application of initial distraction on concavities, partial reduction of any kyphosis with three-point loading, lateral translation of olisthesis and active derotation of malrotated

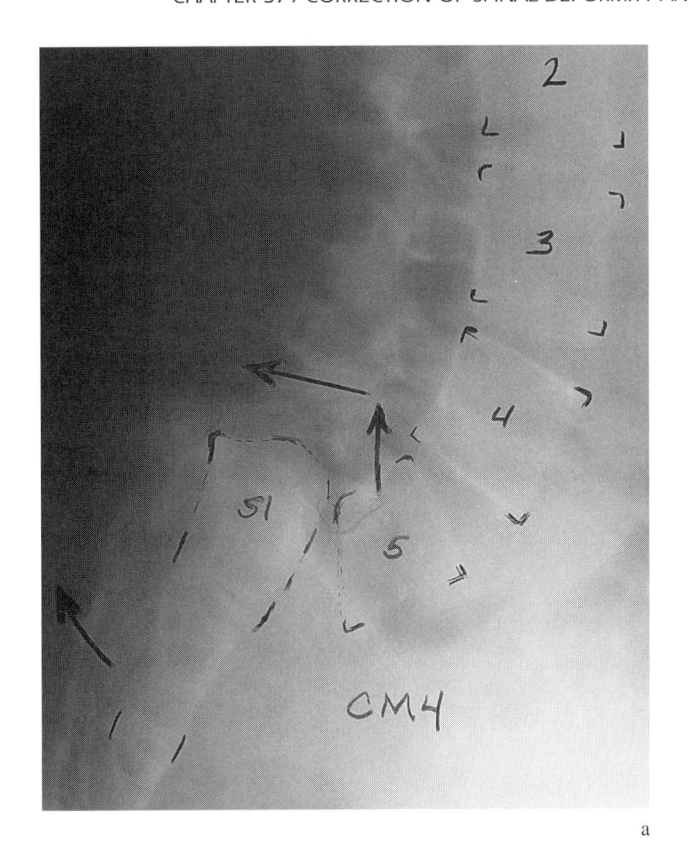

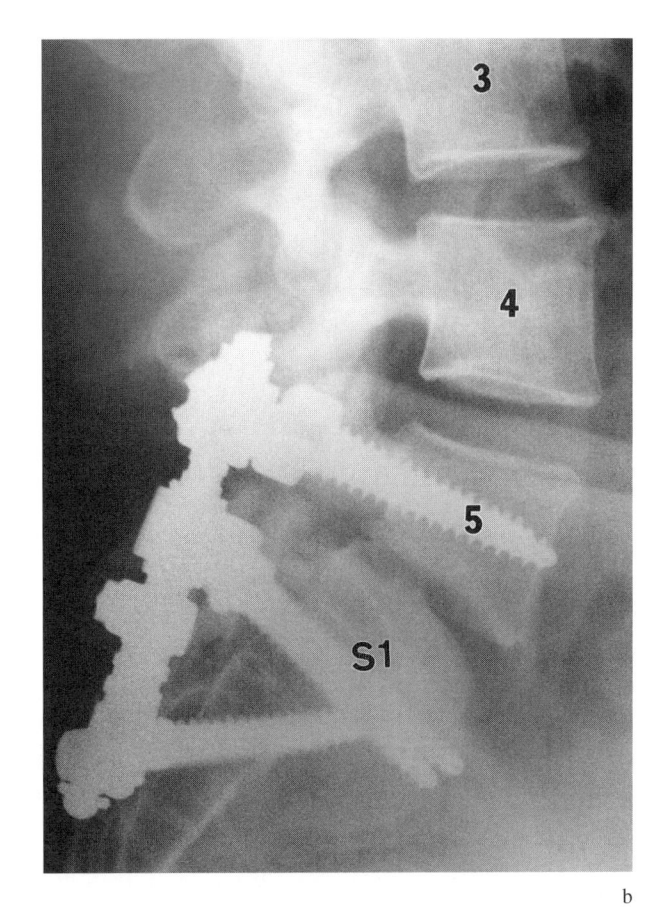

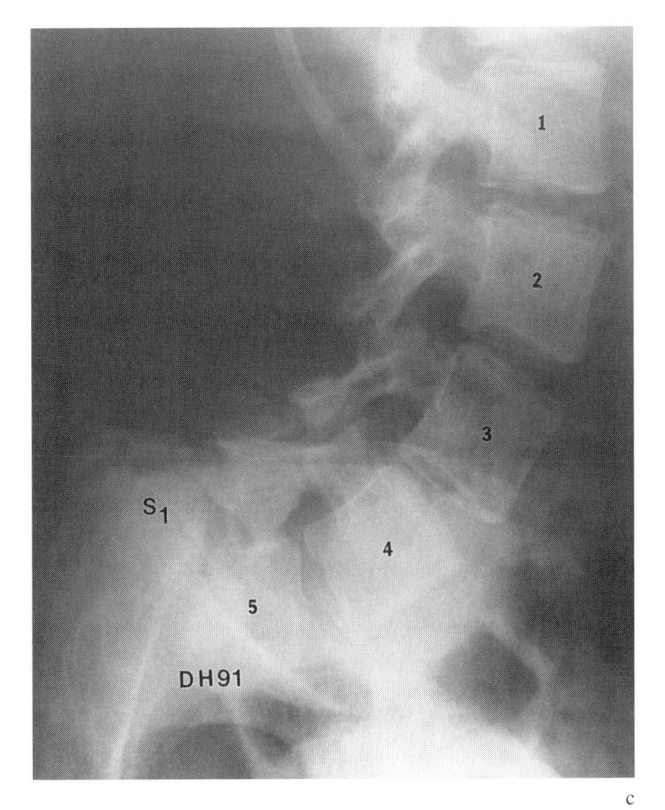

CHAPTER 37 / CORRECTION OF SPINAL DEFORMITY AND INSTABILITY USING THE EDWARDS MODULAR SYSTEM / **449**

FIG. 37-21. Spondyloptosis. (a) Progressive spondyloptosis in an 11-year-old girl. (b) Full correction was achieved with gradual posterior instrumented reduction. (c) Severe spondyloptosis in a 12-year-old girl. (d) Restoration of normal spinal alignment following posterior sacral dome osteotomy and gradually posterior instrumented reduction alone.

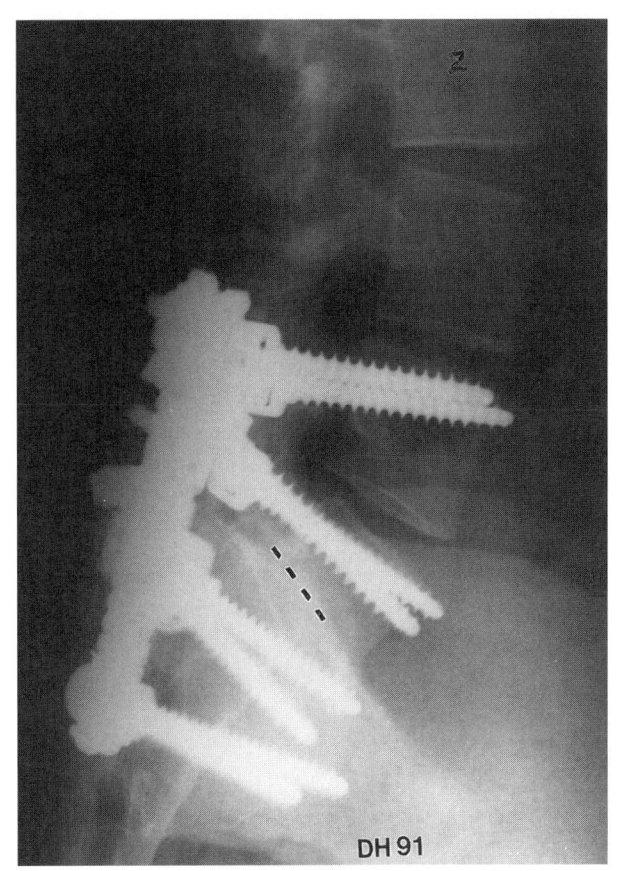

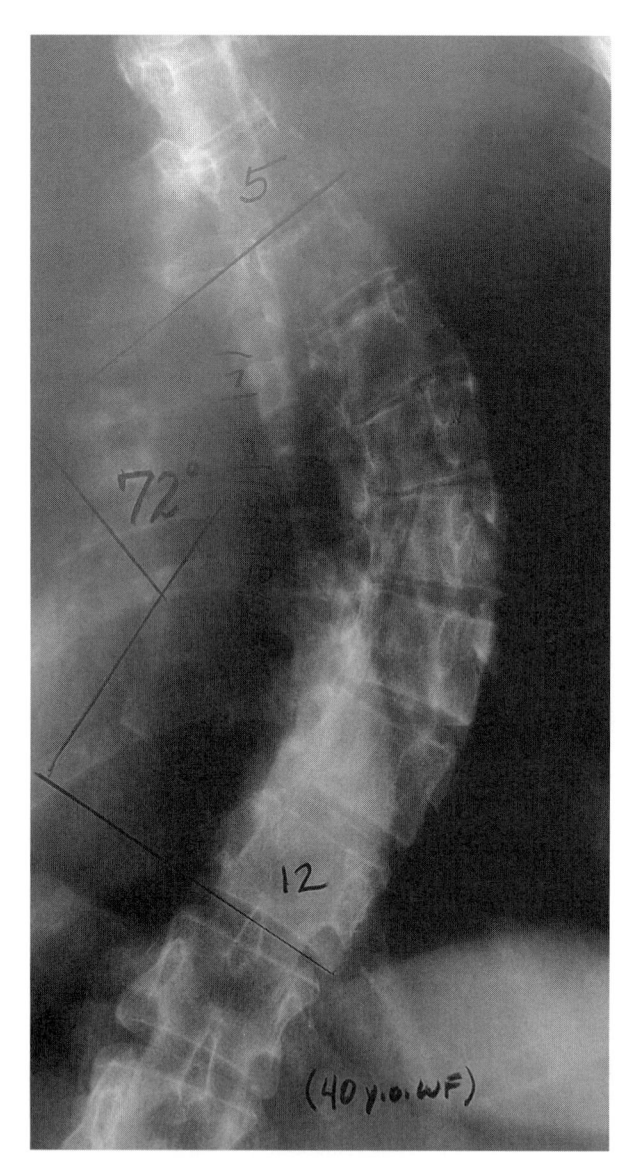

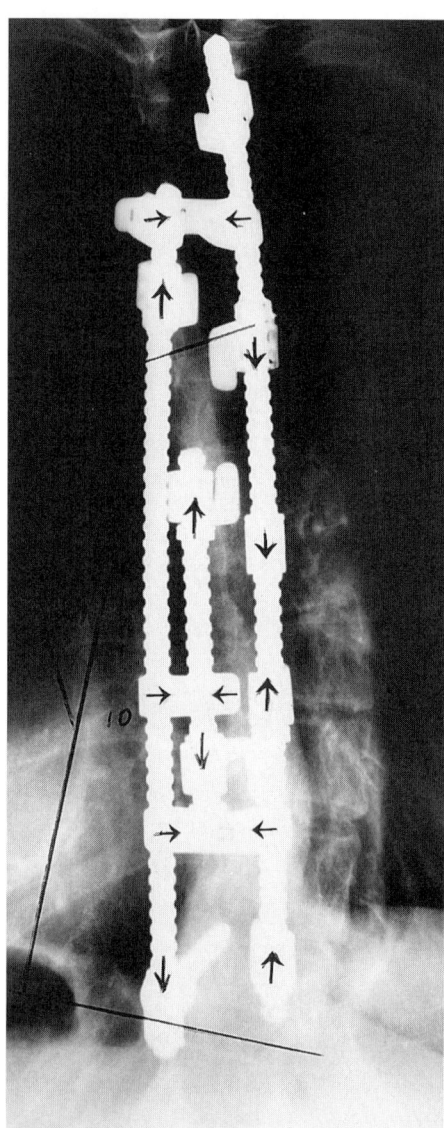

FIG. 37-22. Thoracic scoliosis construct. (a) 72-degree rigid T5-12 curve in a 40-year-old woman. (b) 43-degree correction achieved by incrementally moving the scoliotic vertebrae toward the contoured rods. The distraction rod on the concavity extends from a laminar hook proximally to a screw distally. Derotation is achieved with a short distraction rod at the apex, which is progressively pulled posteriorly and laterally with a rod-rod connector. Compression is applied on the convexity of the apex with the central bilaminar claw on the convex compression rod. Finally, the primary distraction and compression rods are approximated with transverse loaders to complete the reduction. Final rod position is maintained with three cross-locks.

vertebra with connectors, and finally segmental compression on the convexities.

Cross-Locking

After reduction, cross-locks are applied to interconnect the various rods. The cross-locks serve to fix laterally translated apical vertebrae in place, divide the bone-metal interface stresses among the multiple points of fixation and to enhance overall construct stability (see Figs. 37-21 and 37-22).

Precautions

1. Apical screws. Pedicles near the apex of deformity are not only rotated with the vertebrae but also typically curved in a windswept pattern. Therefore, safe insertion of screws requires a laminotomy for direct visualization.
2. Lumbar instrumentation. The incidence of late failure rises with the length of instrumentation. Since surgery for degenerative lumbar scoliosis is usually to relieve low lumbar pain and radiculopathy, it is best to refrain from instrumenting more

proximal asymptomatic curves unless it is required to correct decompensation.

Preoperative Planning

1. From standing and bending films, determine and mark on the x-ray films the corrective forces to apply in order to counteract directly the forces causing the deformity.
2. Calculate the amount of correction that must be achieved and the limits of correction for each curve so as to leave the patient with normal coronal and sagittal compensation.
3. Identify and label foci of symptomatic nerve-root impingement due to structures such as facet osteophytes that will not be relieved by reduction of the deformity alone. Plan appropriate direct decompression of these structures prior to instrumentation.
4. Determine the presence of anterior bony bridges or posterior blocks to reduction and plan the appropriate anterior resection or posterior partial facectomies and/or closing wedge osteotomies.
5. Select the optimal surgical construct and sites of spinal attachment.
6. Determine the order of reduction.

Surgical Technique

Thoracic and Thoracolumbar Scoliosis

Flexible lordotic-scoliosis idiopathic curves can be corrected by rotation of a contoured universal rod with four hooks (closed end and open central hooks) to convert scoliosis to kyphosis as taught by Cotrel (1988). A wrench on the octagon at one end of the universal rod and a rod holder will accomplish the derotation maneuver, while the application of a rotation-stop will hold the rod's rotational position. After both rods are in place, cross-locks are added for additional rotational stability.

For more severe or rigid thoracic or thoracolumbar deformities, consider mobilizing concave rib articulations and performing convex posterior facectomies or osteotomies near the apex. The scoliosis is reduced by sequentially bringing the spine to a long universal rod contoured into physiologic kyphosis. The initial rod is placed on the concave side of the deformity, attached proximally with an anatomic hook and rotation-stop and distally to a spinal screw. A second short two- to three-level distraction rod attached with laminar hooks (distraction claw) is centered on the concavity of the apex. A rod-rod connector or transversly positioned universal rod attached with two medium hooks is used to approximate the long distraction rod and short distraction claw. This will help derotate and partially reduce the scoliosis. A third long rod is placed on the convexity and assembled in compression. Its closed proximal hook is usually attached to a mamillary process; the midposition open hooks form a claw about the apical convexity, and the distal closed hook fits under a lamina. The two long rods are pulled together near the top and bottom of the construct with short transverse rods and hooks or rod connectors; once approximated, the rods are cross-locked (see Fig. 37-21).

Lumbar Scoliosis

Lumbar curves are reduced with segmental concave distraction and convex compression on universal rods attached to standard screws via hooks and connectors. The adjustable connectors attached to apical screws are lengthened on one side and shortened on the other to deteriorate apical vertebrae actively. The most laterally displaced rods are transversely approximated and cross-locked.

Kyphoscoliosis

For correction of a kyphoscoliotic deformity, one half of a kyphoreduction construct is assembled on the convexity with a distraction rod on the concavity. An apical derotation connector is attached via a screw or short distraction claw on the concavity. Distal connectors are shortened on the kyphoreduction side to correct kyphotic deformity. The distraction rod and claw are lengthened to straighten the concavity. Apical connectors are shortened for derotation. Short transverse rods further approximate the spinal rods to complete scoliosis reduction and are replaced with rod cross-locks to stabilize the completed construct.

Degenerative Lumbar and Lumbosacral Scoliosis with Lateral Olisthesis

These complex deformities typically occur in older patients and are associated with rigidity and osteoporosis. Restoration of normal overall spine alignment is essential for lasting clinical success. Achieving this goal without anterior surgery in the elderly population requires a combination of surgical techniques (Crandall & Edwards, 1994b; Edwards & McConnell, 1992).

The first step in degenerative scoliosis repair is the decompression of symptomatic roots and resection of hypertrophied facets blocking reduction. For severe lumbosacral scoliosis with lateral olisthesis, we initiate correction with a highly efficient iliac strut rod. This temporary device consists of a universal rod affixed to the posterior ilium with a cancellous washer on one end with a low hook articulating with a screw in the most laterally displaced vertebra on the other end. Ratcheting the hook up the rod applies an optimally directed force to reduce partially both the lumbosacral scoliosis and lateral listhesis before the application of the spinal rods (Crandall & Edwards, 1994a).

Reduction of the lumbosacral obliquity is completed and stabilized with short, laterally positioned rods based on medially directed S1 screws (Edwards & Curcin, 1993; Edwards & McConnell, 1992). When there is significant lateral listhesis, longer central rods are added (Crandall & Edwards, 1994b). They are often based on laterally directed S1 or midsacral screws to achieve the necessary two or more well-separated points distal to the slip. They are cross-locked to the short lateral rods for added support. Adjustable connectors attach the central rods to screws in the slipped vertebrae. The ring connectors are oriented with their stems opposite the direction of slip so as to pull the slipped vertebrae back into alignment when they are shortened (Fig. 37-23).

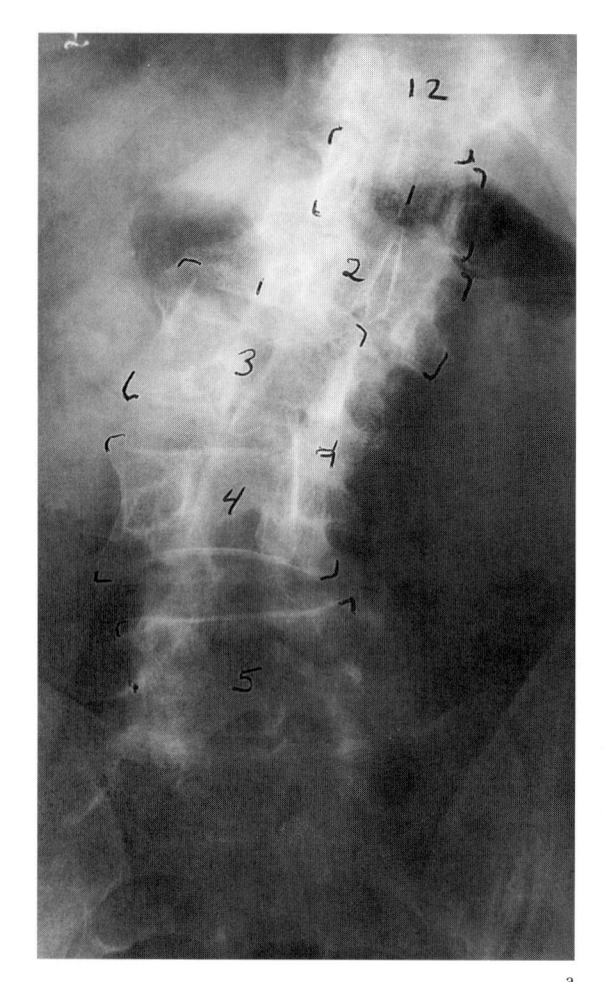

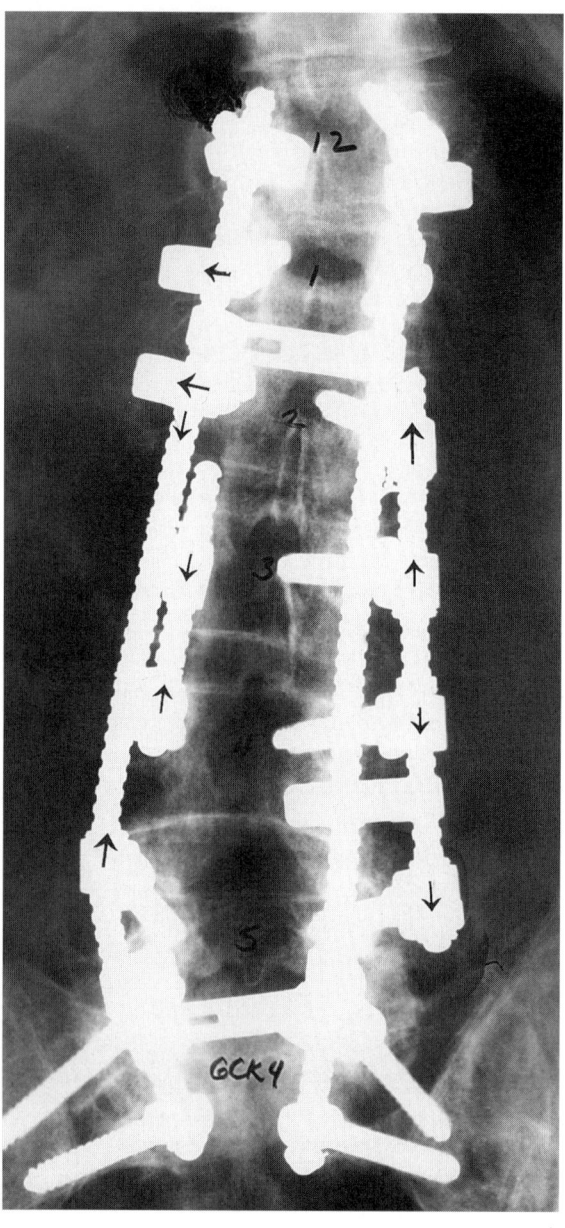

FIG. 37-23. Degenerative lumbar scoliosis construct. (a) Lateral olisthesis and kyphosis in a 66-year-old man. (b) After appropriate decompressions and posterior osteotomies, short rods were used to reduce the severe olisthetic-scoliotic-kyphotic deformity between L2-4. L3-4 was compressed on the convexity while distraction was applied on the concavity between L2-3 and L4. Panlumbar alignment and fixation was achieved with long (T12 to S2) primary rods precontoured into appropriate lumbar lordosis. The rods were securely anchored distally with screws in L5, S1, S2 cross-locked together. Adjustable connectors to T12, L1, and L2 were then sequentially shortened to correct the upper lumbar lateral olisthesis and kyphosis. The various rods were cross-locked to divide fixation loads and increase the rigidity of the construct.

Many panlumbar degenerative deformities present with hypolordosis or actual upper lumbar kyphosis. To maximize lordosis, the central rods become a kyphoreduction construct. The rods, contoured into lumbar lordosis, are anchored proximally with a bilaminar claw, have sleeves on the apex, and distal connectors that attach to low lumbar or sacral screws.

When it is necessary to instrument from the sacrum to L2 or more proximally, distal fixation should extend to the midsacrum and incorporate four to six sacral screws (Fig. 37-23, b). The number of screws depends on the correction forces required, the rigidity of the deformity, and the degree of osteoporosis. Cross-locks are placed between the various rods to divide stress among the various screws and enhance scoliosis construct rigidity.

Clinical Results

In a series of 82 cases of scoliosis reported by the SFSG, 88% maintained reduction and fixation, and primary union occurred in 84% (Edwards, 1991a). Crandall and Edwards

(1994b) have completed a small prospective series of rigid lumbosacral deformities with lateral olisthesis in older patients (median age, 64). Correction was accomplished with the temporary iliac strut rod and the new multirod construct. Results showed greater percentage correction of deformity and overall spine alignment without anterior surgery than previously reported. There were no losses of sacral fixation or neurologic complications.

SUMMARY

The Edwards Modular Spinal System and surgical techniques have steadily grown from the research program of the Spinal Fixation Study Group. The system now affords the surgeon unmatched versatility of attachment and construct design together with the ability to adjust the position of individual vertebra in all three dimensions. Hence, it is well suited for the full range of thoracolumbar and lumbosacral disorders. The same six components can provide quick, biocompatible fixation for single-level lumbosacral fusions, on one hand, or have the ability to correct spondyloptosis or severe lumbosacral scoliosis/olisthesis without anterior surgery on the other. Through continued analysis of clinical data provided by the Spinal Fixation Study Group, the instrumentation and techniques will continue to evolve in an ongoing effort to overcome the many problems and limitations we still face in reconstructive spinal surgery.

REFERENCES

Amundson, G., Edwards, C.C., & Garfin, S.R. (1991). Spondylolisthesis. In: R.H. Rothman & F.A. Simeone (Eds.), *The Spine* (3rd ed.) (pp. 913–969). Philadelphia: W.B. Saunders.

Cotrel, Y., Dubousset, J., Guillaumat, M. (1988). New universal instrumentation in spinal surgery. *Clinical Orthopedics, 227*, 10–21.

Crandall, D.G., & Edwards, C.C. (September 1994a). A temporary iliac strut rod for treatment of degenerate lumbar scoliosis with lateral listhesis. Presented at the Scoliosis Research Society annual meeting, Portland, OR.

Crandall, D.G., & Edwards, C.C. (September 1994b). Reduction of degenerative lumbar scoliosis and lateral listhesis with a multi-rod construct. Presented at the Scoliosis Research Society annual meeting, Portland, OR.

Edwards, C.C. (1993). Edwards instrumentation for spinal injuries. In: S. Garfin & B. Northrup (Eds.), *Principles and Techniques in Spine Surgery* (pp. 187–208). New York: Raven Press.

Edwards, C.C. (January 1992a). Adjustable cross-locks for the Edwards Modular Spinal System. FDA 510K #915672 Amendment.

Edwards, C.C. (1992b). The Edwards Modular System for three-dimensional control of the lumbar spine. *Spine: State of the Art Reviews, 6*, 235.

Edwards, C.C. (December 1991a). Edwards Modular Spinal System. FDA IDE #G900219 Amendment.

Edwards, C.C. (1991b). Reconstruction of acute lumbar injury. *Operative Techniques in Orthopedics, 1*, 106.

Edwards, C.C. (1991c). Reduction of spondylolisthesis. In: R. Dewald & K. Bridwell (Eds.), *Spinal Disorders* (pp. 605–634). Philadelphia: J.B. Lippincott.

Edwards, C.C. (1990). Prospective evaluation of a new method for complete reduction of L5-S1 spondylolisthesis using corrective forces alone. *Orthopedic Transactions, 14*, 549.

Edwards, C.C. (1986). Reduction of spondylolisthesis: Biomechanics and fixation. *Orthopedic Transactions, 10*, 543.

Edwards, C.C. (1984). The sacral fixation device: Design & preliminary results. *Proceedings of the Scoliosis Research Society, 135*.

Edwards, C.C., & Curcin, A. (1993). The Edwards Modular Spinal System. In: C. Brown (Ed.), *Techniques of Instrumentation*. Chicago: Scoliosis Research Society.

Edwards, C.C., & Curcin, A. (1994a). Instrumented reduction of high-grade spondyloptosis. *Seminars in Spine Surgery, 6*(1), 34.

Edwards, C.C., & Curcin, A. (September 1994b). Spondyloptosis: Definition and long term results of reduction and fusion. Presented at the Scoliosis Research Society annual meeting, Portland, OR.

Edwards, C.C., Curcin, A., Turner, P.J.F., & Topeleski, L.D.T. (1995). New alternatives for secure sacral screw fixation: Biomechanical testing and clinical trials. *Orthopedic Transactions, 17*.

Edwards, C.C., & Levine, A.M. (1986). Early rod-sleeve stabilization of the injured thoracic and lumbar spine. *Orthopedic Clinics of North America, 17*, 121.

Edwards, C.C., Levine, A.M., et al. (1987). A modular system for 3-dimensional correction of lumbosacral deformities. *Orthopedic Transactions, 11*, 19.

Edwards, C.C., & McConnell, J.R. (1992). The surgical reconstruction of degenerative lumbar stenosis and listhesis. In: G. Anderson & T. McNeill (Eds.), *Spinal Stenosis* (pp. 373–392). St. Louis: Mosby.

Edwards, C.C., & Novak, V. (1995). Comparative mechanical testing of crosslink alternatives for posterior spinal instrumentation. *Orthopedic Transactions*.

Edwards, C.C., & Osborne, V.A. (1994). Correction of post-traumatic kyphosis with a new kyphoreduction construct and stress relaxation. *Orthopedic Transactions 18*, 1037.

Edwards, C.C., & Rhyne, A. (1990). Late treatment of post-traumatic kyphosis. *Seminars in Spine Surgery, 2*, 63–69.

Edwards, C.C., Rhyne, A.L., Weigel, M.C., & Levine, A.M. (1991). 5-10 year results treating burst fractures with rod-sleeve instrumentation and fusion. *Orthopedic Transactions, 15*, 728.

Edwards, C.C., & Rosenthal, M.S. (1988). A new method for correcting late post-traumatic kyphosis. *Orthopedic Transactions, 12*, 257.

Edwards, C.C., & Weigel, M.C. (1988). A prospective study of 51 low lumbar nonunions. *Orthopedic Transactions, 12*, 608.

Garfin, S.R., Mowery, C.A., Guerra, J., et al. (1990). Thoracolumbar spine trauma. In: *Orthopaedic Knowledge Update* (pp. 425–440). Park Ridge, IL: American Academy of Orthopedic Surgeons.

Hanley, E.N., & Starr, J.K. (1992). Junctional burst fractures. *Spine, 17*, 551–557.

Hu, S.S., Bradford, D.S., et al. (1994). Reduction of high-grade spondylolisthesis using Edwards instrumentation. *Orthopedic Transactions, 18*, 1035.

Kurz, T.L., Hurkowitz, H.N., & Samberg, L.C. (1989). Management of major thoracic and thoracolumbar spinal injuries. *Spine: State of the Art Review, 3*, 243.

Levine, A.M., Bosse, M., et al. (1988). Bilateral facet dislocations in the thoracolumbar spine. *Spine, 13*, 630.

Levine, A.M., Friedman, C., & Edwards, C.C. (1990). The use of a short rod-sleeve construct for fixation of thoracolumbar spine trauma. *Orthopedic Transactions, 14*, 264.

Levine, A.M., Garfin, S., et al. (1989). The operative treatment of L4 and L5 burst fractures. *Orthopedic Transactions, 13*, 753.

McCutcheon, M.E., & Cohen, M. (1991). Early clinical results for painful nonunions of the lumbar spine treated with Edwards Modular Spinal Fixation. *Orthopedic Transactions, 15*, 254.

Panjabi, M.M., Abumi, K., Duranceau, J., & Crisco, J.D. (1988). Biomechanical evaluation of spinal fixation devices: Stability provided by eight internal fixation devices. *Spine, 13*, 1135.

Patel, A.I., Brown, C.W., & Donaldson, D.H. (October 1994). Failure of spinal instrumentation in the treatment of thoracic fractures with a neurologic deficit. Presented at the annual meeting of the North American Spine Society, Minneapolis, MN.

Rosenthal, M.R., Levine, A.M., & Edwards, C.C. (1988). Burst fractures in the low lumbar spine. *Orthopedic Transactions, 12,* 231.

Schwab, F.J., Nazarian, D.G., Higgs, G.B., Mahmud, F., & Michelson, C.B. (October 1994). Effects of spinal instrumentation on lumbosacral fusion. Presented at the ninth annual meeting of the North American Spine Society, Minneapolis, MN.

Turner, P.J.F., Topoleski, L.D.T., & Edwards, C.C. (1993). Sacral screw fixation strength under surgically relevant loads. *Transactions of the Orthopedic Research Society, 18,* 405.

INDEX

A

Accessory process technique for screw orientation, 389
ACDF (*See* Anterior diskectomy and interbody fusion)
Acroplate system, 23
Acute rigid kyphosis, 171
   anterior fixation for, 182, 184, *185–187*
   iliac crest grafts preferred for, 184
Adjacent-level degeneration, 332
Adjustable connectors, 422
   assembly of, 427
   design of, 426–427, *428*
Adson-Beckman retractors, 319
Alar hooks, *253*, 254
ALIF (*See* Anterior lumbar interbody fusion)
Alignment loss, 137
Allen's classification of fractures and dislocations, 108
Allograft bone, 42

Page numbers in italics indicate illustrations; page numbers followed by t indicate tables.

All-screw construct (Simmons), 325, *326, 330*
ALPS (*See* Anterior locking plate system)
AMS reduction fixation (RF) system
   advantages and disadvantages of, 365t, 365–366
   background and development of, 357
   clinical results, 363, *364,* 365, 365t
   contraindications to use, 361t
   indications for use, 360, 361t, *361–364*
   system components
      pullback block, *359,* 360
      sacral block, *359,* 360
      screws, 357, *358,* 359
      spondylolisthesis reduction block, *349,* 359–360
      threaded rods, 359, *359*
      transverse fixation assembly, 360, *360*
   techniques of application, 360–363, *361, 362*
Anatomic hooks
   in Edwards modular system
      design of, 422, *423*
      distal hook insertion, 423, *423,* 436

      open hook application, 423–424
      proximal hook insertion, 422, *423,* 436
   for Harrington rod system, 251
Anchor screws, 26–27, *27*
Andrews frame, 336, 373
Angled-hole screws, 424, *424*
Ankylosing spondylitis
   lateral mass plating contraindicated with, 130
   Luque segmental fixation of, 258, 269
Anterior buttress plate fixation, 146, *146*
Anterior cervical fusion
   Caspar system for (*See* Caspar system)
   cervical plates (*See* Anterior cervical plate fixation)
   odontoid screw fixation (*See* Odontoid screw fixation)
   Orion system (*See* Orion Anterior Cervical Plate System)
Anterior cervical plate fixation, 25–33
   cable for supplemental fixation of, 115, *116*
   compared with posterior wiring methods, 111–112

Anterior cervical plate fixation (*Cont.*)
  CSLP system for (*See* Cervical spine locking plate (CSLP) system)
  techniques of, 25–26, 30–32
Anterior column deficiencies, 35
Anterior column instability, 289–290
Anterior compression, 130
Anterior decompression, 172
  Rezaian spinal fixator for, 195, 195t
  surgical approaches to, 176
  techniques, 25
  in two-stage procedure, 212
Anterior diskectomy
  in Caspar instrumentation, 19, *20*
  CSLP system used following, 29, *30*
Anterior diskectomy and interbody fusion (ACDF), 42
Anterior distractive devices, 172
Anterior lateral rod, *178*
Anterior locking plate system (ALPS), description and surgical technique, 205–206, *206, 207*
Anterior lumbar interbody fusion (ALIF), 325, 331
Anterior neutralization construct, 429
  biomechanics of, 434, *434, 435*
  indications and contraindications for use, 430t
  precaution, 434
  surgical technique, 434, *435*, 436
Anterior release grafting, 442
Anterior spinal fixation
  advantages and disadvantages of, 209, 209t
  anterior locking plate system (ALPS), 205–206, *206, 207*
  background and development of, 201
  biomechanical data, 206–207, 207t
  clinical results, 207, 208, 209
  complications with, 209, 209t
  history of, 201–202
  indications for, 202, 202t
  instrumentation systems for, 204–206, *205–207*
  surgical technique, 202–204, *204*
  Syracuse I-plate system (*See* Syracuse I-plate system)

Anterior stabilization
  failure of, Roy-Camille system used for, 152
  Louis system used for, 404–405, *405*
Anterior strut grafting, 211–212
Anterior thoracolumbar instrumentation
  bench-top testing of, 212–213
  Kaneda system, 159–167
Anterior vertebrectomy, 240
  methylmethacrylate and Steinmann pin fixation following, 238t, 238–240, *239*, 239t, 246
Anterior wedge compression fracture, 160
Anterolateral approach to thoracolumbar spine, 211
Antibiotic-impregnated cement, 236, 240
AO/ASIF Spinal Instruments for Anterior Surgery, 226, 227
AO DCP plate, 225
AO internal fixator, 178, *191*
AO pedicle fixation, 269
AO posterior hook plate fixation, 112
AO titanium anterior thoracolumbar locking plate (ATLP) system
  advantages of, 227, 227t, 233
  background and development of, 225–226, *226*
  contraindications to, 226–227, 227t
  indications for, 226, 227t
  results of use, 229, 232
  technique, 227–229, *228–232*
Apfelbaum drill guide, *6, 8*
Apfelbaum instrumentation system, *6, 7, 8, 9*
Apfelbaum retraction system, *4, 6*
Apical screws, 450
Apofix fixation system
  advantages and disadvantages of, 82, 83t
  components of system, 79, 82, *82*
  technique of application
    at C1-2 level, 84–85
    at subaxial levels, 85
Armstrong CASP plates, 212, 213
Articular mass
  implanting screws in, *148*, 148–149, *149*
  separation-fracture of, 152, *153, 154*

Articulated rod pusher, *300*, 301, 303
ASIF T-plate, 212
Atlantoaxial cervical fusion
  occipitocervical plate fixation for, 106
  using Songer cable system
    Brooks fusion, 65–66, *67*, 68
    Gallie fusion, 68, *69*
Atlantoaxial instability
  Luque rectangle fixation for, 89, *90*, 90t, *91*, 91–92, 92t
  occipital-cervical fusion in, 68
  of posterior cervical spine, 77–87
  posterior interfacet screw used for (*See* Posterior interfacet screw)
  wiring techniques for, 45–55
Atlantoaxial screw fixation, *103*, 103–104, 104t
  transfacet, 77
Atlas cable system, 142–143
ATLP system (*See* AO titanium anterior thoracolumbar locking plate system)
Axial compression, biomechanics of Luque fixation and, 258–259
Axial load injuries, systems contraindicated with, 257–258, 259
Axial loads, methylmethacrylate and, 237
AXIS fixation system, 139–146
  AXIS templates, 140, *140*
  case report, 145–146, *146*
  comparison with other methods, 145, 145t
  indications and contraindications, 139, 144t, 144–145, 145t
  posterior cervical fixation with
    exposure, 140
    patient positioning, 140
    preoperative plan, 139
  postoperative care with, 144
  supplemental fixation techniques
    atlantoaxial stabilization, 143
    lateral mass fixation, 142–143
    vertebral pedicle strengthening, 143–144, 146, *146*
  surgical technique
    bone graft placement, 142, *143*
    depth gauge use, 141, *141*
    drilling screw holes, 141, *141*

AXIS fixation system (*Cont.*)
  plate contouring, 142, *142*
  plate holder use, 142, *142*
  starter hole placement, 140–141, *141*
  tapping drill holes, 141, *141*
  template use, 140, *140*

B

Bacteriologic infection, 60, 62t
Ballpoint pedicle probe, *374,* 375
Barrel chests, 4, 10
Basilar invagination, 68, *70*
Bending irons, 300, *300, 301,* 376
  See also Customized bending
Bilaminar claw, 442, *444*
Bilateral clamping, 126, *127*
Bilateral dislocations, 151
Bioactive ceramic vertebral prosthesis, 160, *167*
Biomechanical considerations
  advantages of lateral mass plates, 116
  in anterior spinal fixation, 206–207, 207t
  characteristics of fixateur interne, 391–392, *394*
  in Edwards modular system, 422
  in kyphotic deformities, 172–174
  in lower cervical spinal wiring, 111–112
  in occipitocervical plate fixation, 105
  in PIS fixation, 93
  in Songer cable system, 59
Biomechanical criteria in radiography, 108, 108t
Bleeding, 30, 376
Blockers, *289,* 296
Blocking forceps, *300,* 301–302
Body cast
  with anterior fixation, 177, 190
  with posterior instrumentation, 198
Bohlman triple wire technique, 109t, 110, 110t, 111
Bolt-and-plate construct, 325, *326, 327, 330*
  bolt-plate interface, 320, 322, *322*
Bolt cutters, 390, *393*
Bolt placement
  in Dynalok Fixation System, 320
  in Simmons plating system, 331, 333
  in Z-plate system, 216, *216, 217*
Bolts
  diameter *vs.* strength, 310, *311*
  in Dynalok system, 311, *313, 314*
  in Z-plate instrumentation, *214,* 214–215
  tightening procedure, 217, *219,* 220, *221*
Bone awl
  for bolt placement, 216, *216*
  use in AXIS fixation system, 140–141, *141*
  use in spinous process wiring, 46, *47*
Bone chips
  in PIS fixation, 97–98, *98*
  use in PLIF with instrumentation, 329, *330*
  use with Louis system, 399, 403
Bone grafts
  with anterior buttress plate fixation, 146, *146*
  compression of, 213, *219,* 220, *220*
  cortical-cancellous (*See* Cortical-cancellous bone grafts)
  dangers of excessive pressure, 32
  decompressive procedures and, 25
  fibular, 30, 172, 184
  harvesting
    instrumentation for, *14,* 18–19
    for use with interlaminar clamping systems, 82–83, *84*
  iliac crest grafts (*See* Iliac crest grafts)
  interbody grafting, 35
  in interspinous fusion, 49, *50*
  intervertebral-body grafting, 26
  lateral mass plating and, 133
  measuring for, 217, *218*
  in occipital-cervical fusion, 68, *71*
  pathomechanics of fusion and, 174
  to promote bony fusion, 369
  site preparation for, 30–31
  strut grafting (*See* Strut grafting)
  systems used in
    AXIS plate fixation, 142, *143*
    Caspar plate system (*See* Caspar system)
    Edwards modular system, *430,* 431, *435,* 436
    Halifax interlaminar clamp system, 126
    Isola/VSP instrumentation, 376
    Kaneda system, 160, 165
    Louis system, 404, 405, 406
    PIS fixation, *94,* 97–98, *98*
    Rezaian spinal fixator, 194, *195*
    Simmons plating system, 325, 331
    TSRH instrumentation, 282
  in thoracolumbar fixation, 348
  used in posterior wiring techniques, 110, 111
  without instrumentation, 206–207, 207t
Bone morphogenic protein (Grafton), 369
Bone quality, importance of, 60, 62t, 240
Bone resection, in corpectomy, 30
Braces (*See* Halo brace; Orthosis; Postoperative bracing)
Broad compression plates, 212–213
Brooks fusion, 50, 52, *52,* 77, 87
  Songer cable system used in, 65–66, *67,* 68
Bull's eye sign, 279, *280,* 389
Burst fractures, 171, 172, 175
  AMS reduction fixation for, *362*
  anatomical considerations in, 173
  bone graft placement in, 176
  cervical, 115
  collapsed vertebral body due to, 195, 195t
  distraction for, 211
  Edwards D-L construct for, 439–442, *442*
  Edwards tandem-sleeve method for, *437,* 438, 439
  Isola/VSP fixation system for, 369–370
  Kostuik-Harrington instrumentation used
    results of, 178, 186, 187, 190
    surgical technique, 177–178, *177–181*
  types of fractures, 159, 176
  Louis system instrumentation for, 405, *406*
  neurologic injury with, 176
  posterior splinting of, 194
  thoracolumbar (*See* Thoracolumbar burst fractures)
  treated with fixateur interne, *381, 382*
"Butterfly" plate, 399, 403

C

Cables
- in Codman Sof'wire system, 113
- double (*See* Double cable)
- Dwyer, 185, *190*
- ease of use, 57
- failure of, 90° bend and, 118, *120*
- Isola cable, 61, *63*, 73
- kinds of, 61, *63*
- made of titanium, 60, 61, 113
- in PIS fixation, *94*, 96, 97
- postoperative breakages of, 73
- safety of, 57
- sequential tightening complicated by, 263–264
- single, 61, *63*
- stainless steel in, 60, 113
- strength of, 57, *58*, *59*, 75, 75t
- tensile strength of, 57, *58*, *59*, 75, 75t
- used with implants, 116, *117*
- used with plate fixation devices, 116, *119*
- use in anterior fixation, 201
- use in rod and wire systems, 257, 263
- *See also* Sublaminar cabling; specific cable systems

Cancellous screws, 36, 36t, 132, *132*
Cancer (*See* Tumors)
Cannulated screw systems, 9, *9*
Capener gouges, 338
Cap-nut alignment guide, 416, *417*
C-arms, positioning for odontoid screw fixation, 4, *5*
Caspar caliper, 18, *19*
Caspar head holder, 4, 13, *16*
Caspar plate system, 26
- advantages of, 23
- background and development of, 13, 14t, *14–15*, 15t
- biomechanics of, 23
- bone graft harvesting instrumentation, *14*, 18–19
- compared with other systems, 23–24, 24t, 111, 112
- complications, 24, 24t
- disadvantages of, 24, 24t
- grafting with
  - harvesting graft, *14*, 18–19
  - site preparation, 18
  - sizing, 18, *19*
- patient positioning, 13, *16*
- plating techniques, 19
  - corpectomy, 19, *21*
  - multiple-level diskectomy, 19, *20*
  - partial corpectomy, 19, *21*
  - single-level diskectomy, 19, *20*
  - surgical procedure, 20, *22*, 22–23, *23*
- results of use, 23
- soft-tissue retractors, 13–14, *14*
- vertebral-body distractors, *14*, 14–15, *17*, *18*, *18*

"Catheter method" of sublaminar cabling, 119
Caudad screws, locking, 35–36, 36t
CCD (*See* Compact Cotrel-Dubousset system)
C-configuration of Luque L-rods, 259–260, 263
CD instrumentation (*See* Cotrel-Dubousset instrumentation system)
Cell saver, 195, 240
Cemented arthroplasties, methylmethacrylate in, 235, 237
Central wire passage, advantages of, 261
Cephalad screws, locking, 35–36, 36t
Cerebellar tonsils, displacement of, 95, *96*
Cerebral palsy, 68
Cervical burst fractures, supplemental fixation of, 115
Cervical collar, 55
- in atlantoaxial fixation, 53, 55
- with AXIS fixation system, 144
- in Brooks fusion, 52
- in facet wiring, 47
- failed treatment with, 3
- in Gallie fusion, 49
- in interspinous fusion, 49
- for non-surgical alignment of fractures/dislocations, 109
- in occipitocervical fixation, 53, 55
- in odontoid screw fixation, 3, 9, 10, 11
- for postoperative immobility, 89, 92, 107
- soft, 105, 144
- used with Halifax system, 126
- use following lateral mass plating, 137
- use in PIS fixation, 98
- use with Caspar system, 22, 23
- use with Roy-Camille system, 152

Cervical hooks, specialized, 290
Cervical hyperlordosis, PIS fixation contraindicated with, 95, 95t
Cervical spine fractures, sublaminar fixation for, 114
Cervical spine locking plate (CSLP) system
- advantages and disadvantages of, 32t, 33
- description of, *26–28*, 26–30, 27t
- development of, 26
- indications and contraindications, 28t, 28–30, *29–31*, 30t
- locking plates
  - description of, 26, *26*
  - selection and positioning, 31–32
- surgical technique, 30–32

Cervical spine stabilization
- clinical results, 40, 42
- Codman Sof'wire system for (*See* Codman Sof'wire system)
- Orion system for (*See* Orion Anterior Cervical Plate System)

Cervical spondylosis, 42
Cervical subluxation
- CSLP system contraindicated for, 30
- lateral mass plating for, 133, 134, *135*

Cervical traction, 89
Cervical trauma, CSLP system restricted in, 29–30, 30t, *31*
Cervicothoracic junction, plate and screw positioning at, 32
Cervicothoracic segment, methylmethacrylate contraindicated in, 239
Chiari malformation (Type I), PIS fixation for, 95, *96*
Chopin block, 298, *298*, 302, 305
Chronic pain
- caused by sacral fixation techniques, 265
- as indication for surgery, 274–275, 275t, 368, 370
- relief of
  - methylmethacrylate and Steinmann pin fixation, 243
  - PWB system and, 418

INDEX **459**

Chronic pain (*Cont.*)
    Rogozinski spinal rod system for, 335, 335t, 336, 346
    Simmons plating system for, 328
    with TSRH instrumentation, 243
Cinch, 113, *114*, 118
Clamping mechanism, 412, *413*, 418
Clamps
    displacement of, 126
    failure of, screw loosening and, 118
    in Halifax system
        color-coding of, 123, *124*
        placement of, 125, *126*, 126t
    in MSS and F.I. construct, 384, *386, 387*
Clamp system for intraoperative skull fixation, 102, *102*
Codman interlaminar clamp
    advantages and disadvantages of, 82, 83t
    complications of use, 86
    components of system, 78, *78*
    results of use, 85
    technique of application, *78–79*, 83–84, 85
Codman Sof'wire system
    background and instrumentation, 113, *114, 115*
    indications for use, 114–116, 115t, *115–120*, 118
    sequential tightening complicated by, 263–264
    technique of use, *115*, 118–120, *120*
Cold-rolled metal, advantages of, 298, 303
Collapsed vertebrae, following CSLP application, 33
Collar-ended screws, 174, *174*, 178
Compact Cotrel-Dubousset system (CCD)
    advantages and disadvantages of, 306–307, 307t
    background and development of, 297
    clinical experience
        degenerative spine, 305, *306*
        Pott's disease, 305
        spondylolysis, 303–305, *304, 305*
        trauma cases, *301*, 303
        tumors of spine, 305–306, *307*
    components of system, 297–299

hooks, 298, *298, 299*
lumbar and sacral pedicle screws, 298, *298, 299*
rod-implant locking devices, 299, *299*
rods, 297–298, *298*
sacral Chopin block, 298, *298*
transverse linking device (TLD), 299, *301*
instruments in, 299–302, *300*
    correction instruments, *300*, 300–301
    locking wrenches, *299*, 300
    miscellaneous instruments, *300*, 301–302
    rod holder and rod gripper, 299, *300*
    screwdrivers, 299, *300*
    universal implant holder, 299, *300*
introduction of CCD2 instrumentation, 307
placement of devices
    hooks, 302
    pedicle screws, 302
    rod-implant blocking devices, 303
    rod placement and correction of deformities, 302
    sacral screws and Chopin blocks, 302
    transverse linking devices, *301*, 303
Compression construct, 429
    indications and biomechanics, 430, *430*, 430t
    precautions
        absent facets, 430, 430t
        foraminal stenosis, *430*, 431
    results of use, 431–432, 434
    surgical technique
        360-degree fusions, 431
        hook-to-screw construct assembly, *425, 430*, 431, *432*
        preinstrumentation, *430*, 431
        screw-to-screw construct assembly, 431, *433*
        segmental compression construct, 431, *434*
Compression forceps, *300*, 300–301
Compression rod, 251–252
Computed tomography (CT)
    advantages of titanium, 36, 36t, 106, 314, *316, 317*

anatomical considerations in, 173
for preoperative assessment
    of cervical spine injuries, 108
    of neural compression, 89, *90*
    of posttraumatic kyphosis, 178
    of trauma of lower cervical spine, 129
for preoperative planning, 195
    with AMS reduction fixation system, 361
    with AXIS fixation system, 139, 143
    for F.I. instrumentation, 387
    with Halifax system, 123–124
    with Kaneda system, 161
    for methylmethacrylate and Steinmann pin fixation, 240
    for odontoid screw fixation, 3–4
    for PIS fixation, 95, *95*
    for posterior lumbosacral fusion, 336
    for PWB system instrumentation, 414
    for spinal rod-sleeve method, 436
stainless steel and, 226
Congenital anomalies, 89
Congenital disorders, 60, *62*
Constructs
    assembly of, 282
    cross-linking in, *385*, 396
    design of, 290
    hybrid, 278, 639
    multiple-level, 320, 321–322
    quadrangular, 161
    rigid, 412
    screw-rod (*See* AMS reduction fixation system)
Contact dermatitis, 236
Contoured anterior spinal plate, 225
Cord compression
    atlantoaxial instability and, 93, *96*
    as indication for surgery, 109, 109t
Corpectomy
    bleeding caused by, 30
    CSLP system used with, 28, *29*
    decompression and, 162–163
    fluoroscopy used in, 30
    multiple-level, 115
    partial, 19, *21*
    with strut reconstruction, 42
    trough corpectomies, 19, *21*
Correction instruments, *300*, 300–301

Corrosion resistance of titanium alloy, 315
Cortical-cancellous bone grafts
  in Brooks fusion, *67, 68*
  in Gallie fusion, 68
  in interspinous posterior cervical fusion, 70
  in Luque rectangle fixation, 92
  in occipital-cervical fusion, 68, *71*
  in sublaminar cabling fusion technique, *67, 73, 75*
Cortical screws, 143
Cotrel-Dubousset (CD) instrumentation system, 273
  background and development of, 287
  compact version (*See* Compact Cotrel-Dubousset system)
  components of
    device for transverse traction (DTT), 287, *288*
    hooks and screw anchors, 287, *288, 289*
    rods, 287, *288*
  contraindications to use, 289t, 289–290
  eight-hook universal fixation, 259
  indications for use, 289, 290t
  techniques of application
    anchor site selection and preparation, 292, *292*
    facet (pedicle) hooks, 292, *293*
    general considerations, 289–290, *290, 291*
    pedicle screw placement, 293–294, *295*
    rod placement, 294, 296, *296*
    transverse process hook placement, 292–293, *294*
  use for flat-back syndrome, 185, *190*
  See also Compact Cotrel-Dubousset system
Creep, spinal deformities and, 174
Crimpers, 174, 221, *222*, 426, *427*
Crimper-tension device, 62, *64–66*, 68
Cross-bars
  in ladder configuration, 340, *341*
  torsional stresses and, 333, *334, 335*
Cross-linking, 177, *181*, 314
  bolt-to-bolt, 320

development of, 273
in F.I. construct, *385*, 396
in PWB system, 412, *413*, 416
Cross-locking, 422
  assembly of cross-locks, 428, *429*
  design, 427–428
  kyphoreduction construct, *444*
  scoliosis construct, *449*, 450, *450*, 451
Cross-threading, correction of, 416, 416t
Customized bending French rod bender, 415–416

D

Danek transverse connectors, 267
Decompression, for acute rigid kyphosis, 184
Decompressive laminectomy, 276
Decortication of bone
  in pedicle screw instrumentation, 337, *338*, 338–339
  surgical technique for, *319*, 319–320
Deformities, correction of, 59, 60
Degenerative disorders
  anterior fixation for, 201
  AXIS fixation system used for, 139
  CCD used for, 305, *306*
  CD instrumentation for, 287
  degenerative arthrosis, 93, 95t
  degenerative olisthesis, 439–442, *443*
  disk degeneration, 195, 195t
  disk disease, 412, 412t, 416
  Edwards modular system used for, 432, 434, 451, *452*
  fixateur interne indicated for, 394
  instability caused by
    ATLP system for, 226, 227t, 232
    lateral mass plating for (*See* Lateral mass plating)
    interlaminar clamping systems used for, 85
    Kaneda instrumentation used for, 160, 167
    Louis system for stabilization of, 399, 407
    lumbar and lumbosacral, 370
    lumbar instability
      AMS reduction fixation for, 360, 363, 365

short-segment pedicle fixation for, 290
  of lumbar spine, 370
  posttraumatic, 68–69
  scoliosis (*See* Scoliosis)
  Songer cable system for
    occipital-cervical fusion, 68, *70, 71*
    posterior cervical fusion, 60, *62*
  spondylolisthesis (*See* Spondylolisthesis)
  TSRH system indicated for, 275t, 275–276
Dens, upward migration of, 105, 106
Depth gauges
  in AXIS fixation system, 141, *141, 144*
  in Dynalok system, 311, *313*
  in implanting screws, 39, *41*
  in PWB system instrumentation, 414
  in Z-plate anterior thoracolumbar system, 215, *215*
Depth of wire penetration (DOWP), 261
Device for transverse traction (DTT), 287, *288*
Dewar posterior fusion, 109t, 110, 110t, 111, *112*
Diaphragm, dissection and repair of, 196, 198
Direct reduction, 447, *450*
Disk degeneration, 195, 195t
Diskectomy, 42
  anterior, 19, *20*, 29, *30*
    with interbody fusion (ACDF), 42
  grafting and, 215
  multiple-level, 19, *20*
  radical, 329
  single-level, 19, *20*
Disk herniation, 137
Diskitis, acute or chronic, 370
Diskogenic disease, 328, 328t
Diskogenic pain, 370
Diskography, preoperative, 178, *183*, 336, 369
Disk spacer, placement of, 329
Dislocations
  cervical orthosis for alignment of, 109
  classification of, 108–109
  Edwards compression construct for, 434

Dislocations (*Cont.*)
  of facets (*See* Facet dislocations)
  with fracture (*See* Fracture dislocations)
  Roy-Camille system used for
    bilateral dislocations, 151
    unilateral dislocations, 149–151, *150, 151*
  transversal, 302
Dissection
  of diaphragm, 196, 198
  for posterior lumbosacral fusion, 336
Distraction
  for burst fractures, 211
  using Schanz screws, 390, *392*
  See also Distraction-lordosis construct; Kostuik-Harrington systems
Distraction/compression forceps, 391, *393, 394*
Distraction forceps, *300,* 300–301
Distraction hooks, *253*
Distraction instrumentation, 259
Distraction-lordosis (D-L) construct, 429
  for degenerative olisthesis
    biomechanics, 439–440, *443*
    precaution, 441–442
    results of use, 442
    surgical technique, 440–441
  indications and contraindications for use, 430t
  for low lumbar fracture, 439, *442*
Distraction rods
  in Edwards modular system, 451
  in Harrington system, 251, *252,* 255
Distraction screws, 174, *174, 424, 424*
Distractors, 311, *313*
Double cable
  in Brooks fusion, 66
  in Gallie fusion, 68, *69*
  in interspinous fixation, *115,* 118
  in posterior cervical fusion, 70, 72, *72, 74*
  in Songer cable system, 61, *63*
  use in occipital-cervical fusion, 68, *71*
Double pass/double cable method, *115,* 118, 120, *120*
Down's syndrome, 85
DOWP (depth of wire penetration), 261

Drains, 22, 198, 329
Drill bit, 141, *141*
Drill guides
  Apfelbaum, *6, 8*
  in ATLP system, 228, *229, 230*
  in Caspar instrumentation, 15, 22
  inserting, 38, *39*
  use in AXIS fixation system, 141, *141*
  use in fixation of occiput, 104
  use with ALPS system, 206
Drilling direction
  in lateral mass plating, 132–133, *134*
  for PIS fixation, *94,* 96–97, *97*
Drilling techniques, 22
  for screw holes, 38–39, *39*
Drummond button fixation, 260
DTT (device for transverse traction), 287, *288*
Dual distraction fixation, 252
Duchenne's muscular dystrophy, 68
Dunn device, vascular complications of, 161, 209, 225
Dural injury
  Isola/VSP instrumentation and, 376, 377
  Luque instrumentation and, 268
  preventing, 331, 333
Dwyer system, 172
  for correction of scoliosis, 159
  urologic complications associated with, 209
Dynalok Fixation System
  advantages and disadvantages of, 316t
  background and development of, 309–310, 310t
  biomechanics of, 310–315, *311–313*
    implants, 311, 313–314, *313–315*
    instruments, 310–311, *313*
    titanium *versus* stainless steel, *313,* 314–315, *316,* 316t, *317*
  clinical experience with, *315,* 322, *322*
  indications and contraindications to, 310, 310t
  Offset Connector Set, 321–322
  postoperative care, 320–321
  surgical planning, 318
    screw insertion technique, 318
    surgical approach, 316

  surgical technique
    decortication, *319,* 319–320
    exposure, 318–319
    insertion of construct, *313,* 320, *321, 322*
    pedicle preparation, 319
    TSRH system crossover, 321–322
Dynamic loading, 422

E

Edwards Modular Spinal System (EMSS)
  advantages of, 453
  background and development of, 421
  biomechanics of, 422
  research and education in, 421–422
  surgical constructs using, 428–430
    anterior neutralization construct (*See* Anterior neutralization construct)
    compression construct (*See* Compression construct)
    construct selection, 429–430
    D-L construct (*See* Distraction-lordosis construct)
    kyphoreduction construct (*See* Kyphoreduction construct)
    preoperative planning, 428–429
    scoliosis construct (*See* Scoliosis construct)
    spinal rod-sleeve method (*See* Spinal rod-sleeve method)
    spondylo construct (*See* Spondylo construct)
  system components
    adjustable connectors, 426–427, *428*
    anatomic hooks, 422–424, *423*
    sacral/spinal screws, *424,* 424–426
    spinal rod-sleeves, 426, *428*
    universal rods, 426, *427*
Edwards sacral fixation device, 251, 254
Electrocautery, used with Roy-Camille system, 148
Elevator, in Louis system, 399
Emergency treatment of cervical spine injuries, 107–108
"Empty facet" sign, 346, *348*
EMSS (*See* Edwards Modular Spinal System)

Endotracheal intubation, 131
End plate preparation, 329
Epidural scarring, 332
ESFS (external spine fixation system), 379, *380*, 382
External spine fixation system (ESFS), 379, *380*, 382
Eyebolts, 276, *276*, 277, *277*

F

Facet arthrosis, 85
Facet cabling technique, 72–73, *75*
Facet dislocations
  associated with Hangman's fracture, 153
  with fracture, 114, *115*, 130
  interspinous fixation for, 114
  overreducing, 73, *75*
  reducing, 70, 73, *75*
  two-hole lateral mass plates used for, 134, *135*
  See also Dislocations; Fracture dislocations
Facet fracture, 116
Facet hooks (*See* Pedicle hooks)
Facet-joint fracture/dislocations, Roy-Camille system used for, *151*, 151–152
Facet joint fusion, clamps used in, 123, *126*
Facet plugs, *430*, 431
Facet wiring, 47, *47*
Failed-back syndromes, repair of, 412, 412t, 416
Fat graft, 329
Ferguson-Allen fracture/dislocation classification, 108–109
F.I. (*See* Fixateur interne)
Fibular bone grafts, 30, 172, 184
Fine adjustment wrench, 123, *125*
Fixateur interne (F.I.)
  advantages of, 382–383, *383*, *384*
  background of, 379, *380*–382
  biomechanical analysis of, 391–392, *394*
  clinical follow-up data, 392–397, 393t, *395*, *396*
    advantages and disadvantages, 396t, 397, *397*
    complications, 393, 394, 396, 396t, 397
    indications and contraindications, 393t, 393–396, *395*, *396*
  fracture instrumentation technique, 387, 389–391
    pedicle anatomy and, 387, 389
    pedicle localization, 389–391, *389–394*
  implants and instruments in, 384, *385–388*, 387
  technique of application, 391, *393*, *394*
  theory and development philosophy, 379, 382–384, *382–384*
Fixation failure
  at lumbosacral junction, 260
  with methylmethacrylate, 246
  reducing, 325
Fixed angle screws, 276, *276*
Flat-back syndrome, 171, 175, 273
  anterior fixation indicated for, 202
  as complication of Harrington rod system, 255
  Kostuik-Harrington instrumentation for, 184–185
    materials, 185
    results of surgery, 185
    surgical technique, 185, *188–191*
Flex bar connector, 68, *69*
Flexion/distraction injury, 114, *115*, 115t
Flexion instability
  interspinous fixation for, 114, 115t, 115–116, *117*
  Rezaian spinal fixator for, 194
Fluoroscopy
  intraoperative
    in Caspar instrumentation, 13, *16*
    for children, 32
    in methylmethacrylate and Steinmann pin fixation, 241
    in odontoid screw fixation, 4, 7
    in PLIF with instrumentation, 328
  study of sublaminar passage, 57, 66
  use in corpectomy, 30
Foramen magnum region, Luque rectangle fixation and, *91*, 91–92
Foraminotomy, 29
Foreign-body reaction to methylmethacrylate, 237
"Four quadrant" test, 337
Fracture dislocations
  of articular masses, 147
  of cervical articular masses, 399, *400*
  "empty facet" sign of, 346, *348*
  Luque devices indicated for, 258
  thoracolumbar fixation for, 346, *347–349*
  See also Dislocations; Facet dislocations
Fractures
  classification of
    lower cervical spine, 108–109
    odontoid fractures, 3, *4*
  reduction of
    AMS reduction fixation system for, 360, 361t, *361–364*, 363
    ATLP system for, 225
    closed, 108–109
    CSLP system used to stabilize, 28
    determining pattern of, 108
    F.I. construct for, 379, 393, 393t, 394–396, *395*, *396*
    lateral mass plating for (*See* Lateral mass plating)
    lower cervical spinal injuries, 109
    in odontoid screw fixation, 4
    prior to placement of ATLP system, 226
    PWB system indicated for, 412, 412t, 416
    Rogozinski system for, 335, 335t, 336t
    Roy-Camille system used for (*See* Roy-Camille posterior screw plate fixation system)
    of spinous process, 73
    thoracic and thoracolumbar, 290, *291*
    with Z-plate system, 216–217, *218*
    Z-plate system for, 215
Fractures in situ, 344, *344–349*, 346
French rod bender, 300, *300*, 415–416
Fully constrained instrumentation systems, 309, 310, *315*
Fusion failure
  anterior fixation indicated for, 202
  following decompression and stabilization, 25
  in methylmethacrylate fixation, 237

Fusion failure (*Cont.*)
  in posterior lumbosacral fusion, 343
Fusion rates, for instrumentation systems, 309–310
  anterior instrumentation, 212
  PWB system, 417, 418
  Simmons plating system, 333
  TSRH instrumentation, *283*, 283–284, *284*
Fusion site preparation and wound closure, 282

G

Gaines compressor, 431
Gallie fusion, 49, *51*, 77
  using Songer cable system, 68, *69*
Galveston Luque technique, 258
Galveston pelvic fixation technique, 265–267, *268, 269*
  HSC unit rods for, 257
  for sacral fixation, 263
  security of, 260
Galveston unit rods, 266–267, *269*
Gardner-Wells tongs, 82–83, 109, 129, 140
Gearshift, *374,* 375
Gelfoam, uses of, 241, *242,* 329, *374,* 375
Gill procedure, 303
"Glacial instability," 368
Goniometer, 347, *350*
Graft dislodgement, 207
Grafton (bone morphogenic protein), 369
Graft retropulsion, 332
Granulomatous infections, 160
Grooved markers, *374,* 375

H

Haid Universal Bone Plates, 131, *131*
Halifax interlaminar clamp, 123–127
  advantages and disadvantages of, 127
  background and development of, 123
  biomechanics of, 123
  bone grafting with, 126
  clamps and screws, 123, *124, 125*
  complications of use, 86–87, 126
  indications and contraindications, 123–124, 125t
  postoperative care with, 126
  surgical technique, 124–126
    clamp placement, 125, *126,* 126t
    closure, 126
    exposure, 125
    preparation, 125
    unilateral or bilateral clamping, 126–127
Halifax PLUS interlaminar clamp
  advantages and disadvantages of, 82, 83t
  components of system, 78–79, *80*
  technique of application, *80–81,* 84
Halo brace, 55
  intolerance of, 3
  MRI-compatibility of, 109
  for noncompliant patients, 73
  uses of, 23, 32, 87
Halo system intraoperative skull fixation, 102, *102*
Halo vest
  for hangman's fracture, 133
  use with AXIS fixation system, 144
Halter traction, 31, 140
Hangman's fracture
  management with halo vest, 133
  Roy-Camille system used for, 153–154
Harms cage, 240
Harri-Luque technique, 252, 254, 255, *255*
Harrington rod system, 198, 225, 250
  advantages and disadvantages of, 253, 253t
  complications of, 254–255, *255*
  compression rods, *178,* 251
    Kaneda anterior device compared to, 213
  disadvantages of, 379, 382, *382*
  distraction rods, 211, 238
    for posttraumatic kyphosis, 253
    use of, 171–172
  Edwards modifications of, 249, 252, 421
  fixateur interne compared with, 379, *382,* 392
  Harri-Luque technique, 254, 255
  indications and contraindications, 252t, 252–253, 255–256
  limitations of, 343–344
  Luque segmental fixation compared to, 269
  modifications of, 251–252, *253, 254*
  standard application of, *252–255,* 253–254
  for thoracolumbar burst fractures, 159, 225, 343
Harrington spreader, 254
Heavy wire twister, 263, *264*
Hematoma, TSRH instrumentation and, 284
Hemovac drains, 198, 329
Hibbs fusion, 152
High-speed bur, 337, *338*
Holt probes, 319
Hook and rod systems, 367, 409
  cable used in combination with, 116, *118*
  disadvantages of, 343–344
  universal, 257
Hook-bars, 333, *334,* 348, *351*
Hook holders, 254, 277–278, *279, 423*
Hook pushers, *300,* 301, *423*
Hooks, 333, *334*
  in CD instrumentation, 287, *288, 289*
  cervical, 289
  claw configuration of, 282, 290, *291,* 451
  distraction hooks, *253*
  facet hooks (*See* Pedicle hooks)
  in Harrington rod instrumentation, 251, 252
  infralaminar, *290–292,* 292
  loosening of, 85, 86
  offset, *298, 298, 299, 299,* 302
  sacro-alar, *253*
  site preparation and placement
    in CD instrumentation, 292–293, *293, 294*
    in Harrington rod instrumentation, 254, *255*
    in TSRH instrumentation, *281,* 281–282, *282*
  supralaminar, 292, *292*
  thoracic, 282
  in TSRH instrumentation, 276–277, *278*
  See also Laminar hooks; Pedicle hooks; Transverse process hooks
HSC unit rods, 257

Hybrid constructs, 278, 639
Hyperlordosed rod, 347–348, *351*

I

Iatrogenic disorders
    AXIS fixation system used for, 139
    Louis system for stabilization of, 399
    lumbar kyphosis (*See* Flat-back syndrome)
Iliac crest bone plugs, 329, *330*
Iliac crest grafts, 30
    in atlantoaxial wiring techniques, 49, 50, *50–52*, 52
    for burst fractures, *178*
    insufficient in posttraumatic kyphosis, 172, 187
    with Kaneda stabilization, 163
    in occipitocervical plate fixation, 104–105, *105*
    in PIS fixation, *94*, 97
    in posterior lumbosacral fusion, 339, 343
    preferred for acute rigid kyphosis, 184
    for Scheuermann's kyphosis, 180, *183*
    in sublaminar fusion, *67, 73, 75*
    use with Caspar system, *14*, 18–19, *19*
    use with PWB system, 416
Iliac screws, 372
Iliac strut rod, 451, 453
Iliac vein laceration, 209
Image intensifier, uses of, *94*, 97, *97*, 104, 104t, 240, 403
Implant removal
    with CCD system, 303, 304, 305
    with fixateur interne, 384
    with Simmons plating system, 333
    surgery for, 343, 344
Indirect decompression, 341, 422
Infections
    bacteriologic, 60, 62t
    as contraindication
        to anterior plate fixation, 35
        to CD instrumentation, 289
        to CSLP system, 29
        to F.I. instrumentation, 396
        to Louis system, 400
        to methylmethacrylate and Steinmann pin fixation, 240
        to PLIF with instrumentation, 328, 329t
        to Rezaian spinal fixator, 195
        to Rogozinski spinal rod system, 335, 335t
    granulomatous, 160
    as indication for surgery
        interlaminar clamping systems, 85
        Isola/VSP fixation system, 370–371
        Kaneda stabilization system, 160, 167
        lateral mass plating (*See* Lateral mass plating)
        Louis system for stabilization, 399
        occipital-cervical fusion in, 68
        TSRH system, 274, 275t
    pyogenic, 370
Infectious complications
    of CCD system, 305
    of Halifax interlaminar clamp system, 126
    of Isola/VSP instrumentation, 376–378
    of Louis system instrumentation, 407
    of PWB system, 418
    of TSRH instrumentation, 284
Inflammatory disease, 89
Informed consent, 95, 368
Infralaminar hooks, *290–292*, 292
In situ fusion, 369
Instrumentation failure
    cables, 90° bend and, 118, *120*
    caused by trauma, 284
    clamp failure, 118
    in Harrington rod system, 254–255
    hook and clamp loosening, 85, 86
    of Isola Galveston configuration, 260
    in PIS fixation, 99
    plate placement and, 134
    preoperative planning to avoid, 255
    rates of, 309
    with TSRH system, 284–285
    wire failure, 45, 46, 116, 264
    See also Screw failure
Instruments
    in cervical spine locking plate system, 27, 27t
    in Codman Sof'wire system, 113, *114*
    for F.I. construct application, 387, *388*
    for PIS fixation, 95
    required for PWB system assembly, 412
Interbody fusion
    CSLP system used following, 29, *30*
    methylmethacrylate used in, 239–240
    Rogozinski spinal rod system used with, 333
Interbody grafting, 35
Interfacet fixation, 113, 114, *115*, 118
Interlaminar clamps (*See* Interlaminar fixation of posterior cervical spine)
Interlaminar fixation of posterior cervical spine, 77–87
    advantages and disadvantages of, 82, 83t, 87
    background and history of, 77
    clinical results, 85–87
    indications and contraindications for, 77, 82, 83t, 87
    similarities to Codman Sof'wire, 116, 118
    systems for
        Apofix fixation device (*See* Apofix fixation system)
        Codman interlaminar clamp (*See* Codman interlaminar clamp)
        Halifax PLUS interlaminar clamp (*See* Halifax PLUS interlaminar clamp)
    techniques of, 82–85
        bone-graft harvesting, 82–83, *84*
Intersection technique of screw orientation, 389
Interspinous fixation, 113, *115*, 118
    for facet dislocations, 114
    for flexion/distraction injury, 114, *115*, 118
    for flexion instability, 114, 115t, 115–116, *117*
    for rotational injury, 114
Interspinous fusion
    bone grafts in, 49, *50*
    lateral mass plates in, 73
    posterior cervical fusion, 69–70, 72, *72, 74*

Intertransverse fusion, 325, 331
Intervertebral-body bone grafting, 26
Intraoperative skull fixation
  Caspar head holder, 13, *16*
  Mayfield skull clamp, 4
  for occipitocervical plate fixation, 102, *102*
  See also Patient positioning
"Introducer," 198
I-plate system (*See* Syracuse I-plate system)
Irreducible fractures, 10
Isola cable (Songer cable system), 61, *63*, 73
Isola Galveston configuration, 260
Isola iliac screws, 260
Isola/VSP fixation system
  background and development of, 367, *368*, 368t
  complications, 376–378
  implantation of longitudinal member
    plates, 376, *378*
    rods, 376, *376*, *377*
  implant components
    nuts and washers, 372
    pedicle screws, *371*, 371–372
    plates, 372
    rods, 372
    slotted connectors, 373, *373*
  indications for, 368t, 368–371
    degenerative disease of lumbar spine, 370
    infections, 370–371
    spondylolisthesis, 368–369
    traumatic burst fracture, 369–370
    tumors, 371
  rationale of pedicle fixation, 367–368
  surgical technique for, 373, *373–375*, 375–376
Isthmic reconstruction, 303–304
  Louis system instrumentation for, 407
  provisional stabilization of, 399, *401*
Isthmic spondylolisthesis, 368–369

J

Jet twister, 263, *264*
Jewett brace, 303

K

Kaneda anterior spinal stabilization system, 159–167, 174
  application of device, 161–166
    closure, 165–166
    components, 161, *161*
    exposure of spine, 162
    graft placement and, 163–164, *163–168*
    multisegmental fixation, 164–165
    patient positioning, 161–162, *162*
    postoperative care, 166
    preoperative imaging, 161
    preparation for grafting and instrumentation, 162–163
    surgical approach, 161
  biomechanics of, 161, 207, 207t
  complications of use, 167
  contraindications to use, 161
  cross-linking in, 161, 212
  development and design of, 159, 225
  indications for use of, 159–160, 160t
    for degenerative disease, 160, 167
    for infections, 160
    for posttraumatic kyphosis, 160
    for scoliosis, 160, 165
    thoracolumbar fractures, 159–160
    for tumors, 160, 167
  multisegmental fixation device, 164–165
  results of use, 166–167
  stability of, 213
Kaneda distractor, 163
Kaneda gouge, 163, *164*
"Keystone" approach to graft site preparation, 30
Kirschner wire (K-wires)
  in implanting Dynalok system, 310, 311, 319
  in odontoid screw fixation, 6, 7, 9, *9*
  in PIS fixation, 98, *98*
  in Schanz screw placement, 389
Knodt rods, 238, 242
Kostuik device, biomechanics of, 207, 207t
Kostuik-Harrington systems, 212
  bench-top testing of, 212, 213
  biomedical considerations in, 173–174
  clinical studies of, 175
  complications related to, 171, 175
  discussion of results, 186–187, 190–191
  history of, 171–172
  indications for use, 175, 175t
    acute burst fractures, 176–178, *177–181*
    acute rigid kyphosis, 182, 184, *185–187*
    loss of lumbar lordosis (flat back syndrome), 184–185, *188–191*
    posttraumatic kyphosis, 175, 178, 180, *182*, *183*
    Scheuermann's kyphosis, 180–182, *183*, *184*
    thoracolumbar burst fractures, 159
  instrumentation of, 174, *174*, 175, 175t
  pathomechanics of fusion, 174
  surgical approaches for use, 176
  technical points, 176
K-wire inserter, 311, *313*, 319
Kyphoreduction construct, 429
  biomechanics of, 442, *444*
  indications and contraindications for use, 430t
  precautions, 442
  results of use, 443, *444*, 445
  surgical technique, 442–443, *444*
Kyphoscoliosis, 451
Kyphosis/kyphotic deformities
  acute rigid kyphosis (*See* Acute rigid kyphosis)
  anatomical considerations in, 173, *173*
  biomechanical considerations, 172–174
  burst fractures (*See* Burst fractures)
  correction of
    anterior neutralization construct for, 434, *435*, 436
    with CCD system, 302
    with F.I. construct, 390, *391–393*
    with Kaneda system, 163, *165*
    Kostuik-Harrington systems for (*See* Kostuik-Harrington systems)
    Luque L-rods for, 263
    with MSS, 391

Kyphosis/kyphotic deformities (*Cont.*)
   Rezaian fixator for (*See* Rezaian anterior fixation system)
   rod placement for, 294
   with Schanz screws, 390, *391–393*
   flat-back syndrome (*See* Flat-back syndrome)
   iatrogenic kyphosis (*See* Flat-back syndrome)
   lateral mass plating ineffective for, 130
   postlaminectomy, 28, 35, 171, 175
   posttraumatic (*See* Posttraumatic kyphosis)
   reduction of, *178,* 227, 437–438, *438*
   rigid round backs, 171
   Scheuermann's kyphosis (*See* Scheuermann's kyphosis)
   screw breakage following correction, 187
   secondary to osteoporosis, 171, 173, 175
   secondary to tumors, 171, 175
   with two-column fractures, 346, *350*
   of upper thoracic spine, 95, 95t

L

Ladder-shaped configuration, 333, *335,* 340
Lag effect, 9, *10*
Laminar elevator, *300,* 301
Laminar hooks
   as alternative to sublaminar wire, 266, *268*
   in Apofix fixation device, 79, 82, *82*
   in CD instrumentation, 287
   contraindications to, 254
   in Edwards modular system, 422
   hazards of, 258
   lumbar, 277, 282
   in TSRH instrumentation, 277
Laminectomy
   CSLP system used following, 29, *30*
   decompressive, 276
   kyphotic deformities following, 28, 35, 171, 175
   neurologic deficit and, 171
   in PLIF with instrumentation, 328
   with Roy-Camille system, 152
   spinous process wiring contraindicated following, 47
   in thoracolumbar fixation, 347, *350*
   use of facet wiring following, 47
Laminotomy
   in pedicle screw instrumentation, 337, *337*
   screw placement and, 143, 144
   sublaminar wire placement and, 262, *262*
Lateral attachment sites, 447–448, *450*
Lateral gutter fusion, 333
Lateral mass plating
   advantages of, 116
   anterior buttress plate fixation, 146, *146*
   background and advantages of, 129, 130t, 137
   cable for supplemental fixation of, 115–116, *117*
   complications of, 137, 137t
   contraindications to, 130, 131t
   imaging for evaluation, 129–130
   indications for, 130, 130t
   initial assessment and management, 129
   operative management
     perioperative management, 130–131
     techniques used, 131–137
     timing of operation, 130
   outcome of procedure, 137–138, 138t
   postoperative management, 137
   techniques for
     bone grafting, 133
     choice of plating system, 132
     Haid Universal Bone Plates, 131, *131*
     plate length and placement site, 134–135, *135, 136,* 137
     screw and plate placement, 132–133, *133–135*
     small notched titanium reconstruction plates, 131–132, *132,* 137
   use in interspinous fusion, 73
Lateral wire passage, disadvantages of, 261
Lewin clamp, 46, *47*

Ligamentous injuries
   facet dislocations caused by, 130
   unrecognized, 137
Ligation of vessels, 209
Line of gravity, restoration of, 193–194
Load-bearing instrumentation, 309, 310, *315*
Load-sharing instrumentation, 309, *315,* 422
Locking screws
   inserting, 40, *42*
   stability and, 35–36
Locking wrenches
   in CCD system, 300, *300*
   in Halifax system, 123, *125*
Lock screwdriver, 40, *42*
Longitudinal connectors, 384, *386, 387,* 390
Lordosis, loss of (*See* Flat-back syndrome)
Lordotic curvature, adjusting, 37
Lordotic posture, 35, 36t
Lordotic traction, 403, *404,* 407
Louis system, 399–407
   advantages and disadvantages of, 400–401, 401t
   anterior stabilization with, 404–405, *405*
   background and development of, 399
   combined surgical approach
     for severe fractures, 405, *406*
     for severe spondylolisthesis, 405–406
     with total vertebrectomy, 405
   indications and contraindications, 399–400, *400,* 400t, *401,* 407
   posterior stabilization with, 401–404
     advantages and disadvantages of, 401
     following reduction, 403, *404*
     pitfalls of method, 403–404
     plate positioning, 403
     screw insertion landmarks for, *402,* 402–403
   results of use, 406–407
   surgical techniques, 401–406, 407
Lower cervical fixation
   lateral mass plates for (*See* Lateral mass plating)
   occipitocervical plate fixation, 104, *104*

Lower cervical fusion
  indications for, 68–69
  interspinous posterior cervical
    fusion, 69–70, 72, *72, 74*
  postoperative care, 73
  sublaminar cabling fusion, *67,* 73, *75*
  wiring techniques for, 107–112
Lower cervical spine, Roy-Camille system used in (*See* Roy-Camille posterior screw plate fixation system)
Lower lumbar fixation
  Harrington rod system contraindicated for, 255
  Isola/VSP instrumentation for, 376, *378*
Low lumbar burst fractures, 439–442, *442*
Lumbar instrumentation, 450–451
Lumbar laminar hooks, 277, 282
Lumbar pedicle screws, 298, *298, 299*
Lumbar spine
  CCD system for (*See* Compact Cotrel-Dubousset system)
  degenerative disease of, 370
  screw placement in, 414, *415*
  transpedicular fixation of (*See* Puno-Winter-Byrd transpedicular fixation system)
Lumbar stenosis, 416
Lumbar tumors, 371
Lumbosacral arthrodesis, 403–404
Lumbosacral instrumentation, 367, 368t
Lumbosacral junction, fixation across, 260
Lumbosacral segment, methylmethacrylate contraindicated in, 239
Lumbosacral spine
  indications for internal stabilization of, 368t, 368–371
    burst fracture, 369–370
    degenerative disease, 370
    infections, 370–371
    isthmic spondylolisthesis, 368–369
    tumors, 371
  stabilization of
    AMS reduction fixation system for, 357, 360
    Isola system segmental fixation (*See* Isola/VSP fixation system)

Louis system for (*See* Louis system)
  using Rogozinski system (*See* Rogozinski spinal rod system)
Luque-Galveston fusion, 73
Luque L-rods, 198, 257, *258*
  cable used in combination with, 116, *117*
  cross-links developed for use with, 273
  techniques of use, 263
  used with Harrington rod system, 252, *254*
  use for flat-back syndrome, 185
  use in occipital-cervical fusion, 68, *71*
Luque plate-screw system, 309
Luque rectangle fixation, 89, *90,* 90t, *91,* 91–92, 92t
Luque rectangles, 91, *91,* 257, *258*
  techniques of use, 263
Luque segmental fixation
  advantages and disadvantages of, 258, 259t
  applications of, 269
  background and development of, 257–258, *258,* 259t
  biomechanics of, 258–260
  clinical results and complications of, 267–269
  Galveston technique of pelvic fixation, 265–267, *268, 269*
  techniques of, 260–264, *261–267*
Luque wire twister (potato hook), 263, *264*

M

Magerl atlantoaxial fixation technique, 141, 143
Magerl posterior hook plate, 111
Magerl/Seemann technique, 133
Magnetic resonance imaging (MRI)
  for injury assessment
    cervical spine injuries, 108
    neural compression, 89, *90*
    trauma of lower cervical spine, 129
  instrumentation compatibility
    advantages of titanium, 27, *28,* 36, 36t, 61, 106, 214, 314, *317*
    disadvantages of stainless steel, 226
    halo, 109

interlaminar clamps, 79, 82, 123
postoperative
  advantages of methylmethacrylate and Steinmann pin fixation, 243, *245*
  to detect syringomyelia, 213
  for preoperative planning, 195
  with Halifax system, 123–124
  with Kaneda system, 161
  in lumbosacral fixation, 369
  in methylmethacrylate and Steinmann pin fixation, 240
  in occipitocervical fixation, 53
  in odontoid screw fixation, 4
  for PIS fixation, 95, *96*
  in posterior lumbosacral fusion, 336
  in PWB system instrumentation, 414
Malformations
  occipitocervical plate fixation contraindicated with, 102
  use of PIS fixation for, 93, 95t
Manual in-line traction, 31
Mayfield frame, 68
Mayfield skull clamp, 4
Mechanical instability, 335, 335t
Metabolic diseases, fixation contraindicated with, 130, 137, 335, 335t
Metal sensitivity
  as contraindication to use
    anterior plate fixation, 35
    Rezaian spinal fixator, 195, 195t
    Rogozinski spinal rod system, 335, 335t
  nickel allergy, 226
Methylmethacrylate
  antibiotic-impregnated, 236, 240
  background and development of, 235–236, *236*
  failure of cement fixation, 246
  fiber reinforcement of, 238
  in Kaneda anterior spinal stabilization, 164, 166
  in Luque rectangle fixation, *91,* 92
  modifications of, 238
  for osteoporotic bone, 175, 181, 375
  physical characteristics of, *236,* 236–238
  for stabilization of Galveston unit rods, 267

Methylmethacrylate *(Cont.)*
　use in osteopenic individuals, 190, 205
　use with Caspar system, 22
Methylmethacrylate and Steinmann pin stabilization, 235–246
　advantages of, 246
　background and development of, 235–236, *236*
　indications for, 238t, 238–240, *239,* 239t
　instruments designed for, 239, *239*
　physical characteristics of PMMA monomer, *236,* 236–238
　results of use, 241–243, *244–246,* 246
　technique of, 240–241, *241–243*
Miami collar, 73
Micromotion, 400, 401, 412
Midposterior approach, with Roy-Camille system, 148, *148*
Minerva brace, 55
Minerva jacket, 152
Mixed implants, 306
Modular cross-link assembly, 412, *413,* 416
Modular Spine System (MSS)
　biomechanical characteristics of, 391–392, *394*
　composition and components of, 384, *385–388*
　technique of application, 391
　See also Fixateur interne (F.I.)
Moe spinal instrumentation set, 249, *253,* 254
Molded brace, 296
Moss titanium cage system, 227–228
Motion segments, instability of, 134, 135, 137
MSS (*See* Modular Spine System (MSS))
Multidirectional stability, 105, 106
Multiple-level clamping, 127
Multiple-level constructs, 320, 321–322
Multisegmental fixation, 164–165
Muscle disorders, occipital-cervical fusion in, 68
Myelography
　intraoperative, 212, 394, *396,* 445
　for preoperative planning, 109, 178, 195
　use with computed tomography, 89, 129

N

Neck extension, fluoroscopic guidance for, 4
Neoplasms (*See* Tumors)
Nerve-root injury, 332, 376, 377
　caused by screw penetration, 137
Neural compression, signs and symptoms of, 89, *90*
Neural decompression
　of lumbar spine, 409
　in occipital-cervical fusion, 89
Neurologic complications
　of Harri-Luque technique, 255, *255*
　of TSRH instrumentation, 284
Neurologic deficit
　fracture of thoracolumbar spine and, 166–167, 348
　improvement of
　　following TSRH instrumentation, 283
　　with Kaneda system, 160, 166–167
　　with occipitocervical plate fixation, 106
　　with Z-plate instrumentation, 213
　increase in, 137, 171
　prevention of deterioration, 343
　in trauma of lower cervical spine, 129, 130
Neurologic disorders, occipital-cervical fusion in, 68
Neurologic injury
　with burst injuries, 176
　cervical plating systems and, 26
　as complication of surgery for flat-back syndrome, 185
　with Halifax interlaminar clamp system, 126
　role of decompression in, 191
　sublaminar wiring and, *48,* 48–49, 52, 77, 114, 261–262
　　advantages of Songer cable system and, 57, 73
　　in placement and removal, 258
　　from wire passage, 260–261, 267–268
Neurovascular injury, avoiding, 199
Noncannulated screws, 9, *10*
Noncompliant patients
　halo brace for, 73
　Rogozinski spinal rod system contraindicated for, 335, 335t
　Songer cable system and, 69, 73
　sublaminar cabling fusion technique for, 73
Nonunion
　with CCD system, 305
　due to rheumatoid arthritis, 73
　Edwards compression construct for, 431–432
　Louis system instrumentation for, 407
　treating with odontoid screw fixation, 10, *10,* 11
Nuts and washers, 372–373, 426, *427*
Nylon and Mersilene bands, 264

O

Oberhill retractors, 319
Obese patients
　F.I. instrumentation contraindicated, 396
　Luque instrumentation for, 258
　occipitocervical plate fixation for, 102, 103
Occipital-cervical fusion
　neural decompression in, 89
　using Songer cable system
　　indications for use, 59–60, 60t
　　techniques of, 68, *70, 71*
Occipital-cervical instability, 89, *90,* 90t, *91,* 91–92, 92t
Occipitocervical dislocation, 154
Occipitocervical fusion, 154
Occipitocervical plate fixation
　advantages and disadvantages of, 101, 106, 106t
　complications of, 106
　contraindications for, 102
　indications for, 101, 102t
　patients, 105
　results of, 106
　surgical procedure
　　atlantoaxial screw fixation in, *103,* 103–104, 104t
　　biomechanical considerations in, 105
　　fixation in lower cervical spine, 104, *104*
　　fixation of occiput, 104–105, *105*
　　patient positioning, *102,* 102–103
　　surgical approach, 103, *103*

INDEX **469**

Odontoid fractures
 classification of, 3, *4*
 See also Odontoid screw fixation
Odontoid screw fixation, 3–11, 77
 advantages and disadvantages of, 10–11, 11t
 complications associated with, 10, *10, 11*
 contraindications to use, 4, 4t, 10
 exposure for, 5–6, *6*
 indications for, 3, *4,* 4t
 preparation and positioning for, 3–4, *5*
 screw insertion techniques, 6, *7*
  Apfelbaum system, *6,* 7, *8,* 9
  cannulated screw systems, 9, *9*
  mechanisms of screw failure, 10, *11*
  noncannulated screws, 9, *10*
  postoperative care, 9–10
Offset bolt, *326,* 331
Offset Connector Set, 321–322
Offset hooks, 298, *298,* 299, *299,* 302
Offset introducer forceps, *300,* 301
Open pedicle technique, for posterior lumbosacral fusion, 337
Orion Anterior Cervical Plate System
 clinical results of use, 40, 42
 development and features of, 35–36, 36t, 37t
 surgical techniques using, 37–40, *37–42,* 41t
Orthosis
 braces (See Halo brace; Postoperative bracing)
 cervical (See Cervical collar)
 molded plastic, 177, 182, 190, 349
 thoracic or thoracolumbar, 282
 thoracolumbar, 349
  with ATLP system, 229
  following CCD instrumentation, 303
 thoracolumbosacral
  in Dynalok fixation, 321
  in Kaneda anterior spinal stabilization, 166
  in Z-plate instrumentation, 221
 total contact, 438
 use following F.I. instrumentation, 391
Os odontoideum
 interlaminar clamping systems used for, 85, 87

posterior cervical fusion in, 60, *62*
Osteomyelitis
 CD instrumentation used for, 289, *290*
 CSLP system contraindicated with, 29
 spinal stabilization for, 274, 275t
 thoracolumbar
  ATLP system for, 226, 227t
  Kaneda system used for, 160
Osteopenia
 as contraindication
  with ATLP system, 226, 227t
  to PLIF with instrumentation, 328, 329t
 Dynalok fixation and, 319, 322
 methylmethacrylate for, 190
 rigid arthrodesis systems and, 334
 use of I-plate system for, 204
Osteophytes in bone graft site, 31
Osteoporosis
 additional orthosis needed with Caspar system, 23
 anterior plate fixation and, 40
 intraoperative vertebral-body fracture and, 175
 kyphosis secondary to, 171
 processes contraindicated with
  anterior plate fixation, 35
  CD instrumentation, 289
  CSLP system, 29
  F.I. instrumentation, 396
  lateral mass plating, 130, 137
  Louis system, 400
  odontoid screw fixation, 10
  PIS fixation, 95, 95t
  Rezaian spinal fixator, 195
  Rogozinski spinal rod system, 335, 335t
  Roy-Camille system, 152
 sublaminar cabling fusion technique for, 73
 sublaminar fixation for flexion/distraction injury with, 114
Osteoporotic bone
 kyphoreduction construct and, 442
 methylmethacrylate and Steinmann pin fixation and, 240
 methylmethacrylate used with, 235
Osteoporotic fractures
 compression fracture, 160
 kyphosis secondary to, 173, 175

Osteotomy
 anterior fixation indicated for, 202
 ATLP system for support following, 226, 227t
 posterior, 403, 445
 in surgery for flat-back syndrome, 185, *186, 190*
Outrigger, temporary, 434, *435,* 436

P

Pain, postoperative control of, 166, 320, 341
Palacos R methylmethacrylate, 236
Pannus, *90*
Paraspinal rods, 161, *161,* 164, *165*
Pars technique of screw orientation, 389
Patient-controlled analgesia system, 166, 320
Patient positioning
 for anterior fixation, 202
  Caspar plating, 13, *16*
  Louis system instrumentation, 404, *405*
  odontoid screw fixation, 3–4, *5*
  Rezaian spinal fixation, 196
  for use of Kaneda system, 162, *162*
 for posterior fixation
  Dynalok Fixation System, 318
  F.I. instrumentation, 387
  Halifax system, 124
  interlaminar clamping systems, 82–83
  Isola/VSP instrumentation, 373
  Louis system instrumentation, 403, *404,* 407
  lumbosacral fusion, 336
  PIS fixation, 96, *97*
  PLIF with instrumentation, 328
  posterior wiring techniques, 110
  PWB system instrumentation, 414
  Roy-Camille system, 148, 149
  for TSRH instrumentation, 279
  for use of AXIS fixation system, 140
Pedicle fixation, rationale of, 367–368
Pedicle hooks
 in CD instrumentation, 287, 292, *293*
 hazards of, 258

Pedicle hooks (*Cont.*)
  site preparation and placement of, 281, *281*
  in TSRH instrumentation, 277
Pedicle localization
  for F.I. instrumentation, 389–391, *389–394*
  landmarks for, 279–280, *280*
Pedicle preparation
  for hook placement, 281, *281*
  for PWB system instrumentation, 414
  for TSRH instrumentation, 279–280, *280*
Pedicles
  absence of, 396
  anatomy of, 387, 389
  biomechanics of, 367–368
  facet hooks placement, 292, *293*
  general preparation of, 319
  sizes and shapes of, 322, *338*, 347
  tapping, 331, 333
Pedicle screw fixation, 255
  contraindications to, 412, 412t
  with Isola/VSP instrumentation, 373, *373*, 375, 375–376
  with Kostuik-Harrington system, 175, 190
  results of, 282–283
  with Rogozinski spinal rod system, 333, *334*
  technique of, 337–341, *337–342*
Pedicle screws, 333, *334*
  alignment of, 340, *340*
  in all-screw attachment, 341, *342*, 343, 343t
  as alternative to sublaminar wire, 266, *268*
  angled, 357, *358*, 365
  in CCD system, 298, *298*, 299, *299*, 302
  in CD instrumentation, 290, *290*, *291*
  in Isola/VSP system, *371*, 371–372
  in Louis system, *402*, 402–403
  malpositioned, 284, 403
  placement of, 143–144, 146, *146*
    in CD instrumentation, 293–294, *295*
    in F.I. construct, 383–384
  preparation for insertion, *339*, 339–340
  size selection, 281
  transpedicular screws, 357, *358*, 360
Pedicular sounds, 311, *313*, 319, 329
Pelvic fixation, 269
Percutaneous vertebroplasty, 235
Philadelphia collar (*See* Cervical collar)
Physical therapy, 321
Pin driver, *239*, 241, *241*
Pin holder, *239*, 241, *241*
PIS fixation (*See* Posterior interfacet screw fixation)
Placement forceps, 123, *125*
Plate and screw systems for posterior fixation, 198
Plate bender, 142, *142*
Plate cross-linking devices, 257
Plate dislodgment, 33, 42
Plate failure, placement and, 134
Plate fixation devices
  cable used with, 116, *119*
  development of, 25–26
Plate holders
  attaching to Orion plate, 37–38, *38*
  in AXIS fixation system, 142, *142*
  use with ALPS system, 206, *206*
Plate ring, 311, *313*, 320
Plates
  bench-top testing of, 212–213
  cervical spine locking plates, 26, *26*, 31–32
  compared to distractive devices, 172
  cross-link, 264
  determining sizes of
    in AXIS fixation system, 140, *140*
    in Z-plate anterior thoracolumbar system, 217, *218*
    in Dynalok system, 311, *313*, 314
    in Isola/VSP system, 372, 376, *378*
  lengths of, 36, 36t, 37, *37*
  Orion plates, 38
  placement of
    in ATLP system, 228, *228*
    in lateral mass plating, 134–135, *135*, *136*, 137
    in Louis system stabilization, 403
    plate failure and, 134
  selecting
    in ATLP system, 228
    in Caspar system, 20, *22*
  slotted, 409
  two-hole, 133, 134, *135*
  use in Isola/VSP instrumentation, 376, *378*
  vertebral-body plates, 161, *161*, 163, *163*
  Yuan I-plates, 212
  Z-plates, 214, *214*
  See also Lateral mass plating; Plating systems
Plating systems, 367, 409
  for anterior fixation, 201–202
  for anterior thoracolumbar fixation, 204
  Caspar system
    advantages of, 13, 15t
    with corpectomy, 19, *21*
    with diskectomy, 19, *20*
    techniques of, 20, *22*, 22–23, *23*
  for pedicular arthrodesis, 333
  Simmons system (*See* Simmons plating system)
PLIF (*See* Simmons plating system)
PMMA (*See* Methylmethacrylate)
Polyethylene tubes, 240
Polymethylmethacrylate (*See* Methylmethacrylate)
Porosity reduction, in methylmethacrylate, 238
Porte-manteau procedure, *151*, 152, *154*
Posterior cervical fixation
  AXIS fixation system for (*See* AXIS fixation system)
  interlaminar, 77–87
  Songer cable system used for (*See* Songer cable system)
  wiring techniques for, 45–55
Posterior column disruption, 161
Posterior column instability
  Caspar system contraindicated in, 23
  Halifax interlaminar clamp system for, 123–124, 125t
  lower cervical fusion for, 68–73
Posterior decompression, two-stage, 212
Posterior distraction instrumentation, 198, 211, 212
Posterior fusions
  complications of, 174
  pseudarthrosis rates following, 174, 180, 184, 185
  stress fractures following, 180

Posterior fusions (*Cont.*)
   to supplement Kostuik-Harrington instrumentation, 186–187, 190
Posterior interfacet screw (PIS) fixation
   biomechanics of, 93
   bone graft used in, *94,* 97–98, *98*
   closure, 98
   complications of use
      instrumentation failure, 99
      pseudarthrosis, 98, 98t, *99*
      screw length and, 98
   contraindications for use, 95, 95t
   drilling direction for, *94,* 96–97, *97*
   indications for use, 93, 95t
   informed consent, 95
   positioning for use, 96, *97*
   postoperative treatment, 98
   preoperative evaluations, 95, *95, 96*
   preparation for, 96
   principles of use, 93, *94*
   special instruments used, 95
   surgical approach, 96
Posterior lumbar interbody fusion (*See* Simmons plating system)
Posterior pedicle screw systems, 212
Posterior stabilization and fusion
   Louis system used for (*See* Louis system)
   secondary to anterior distraction, 172, 178
   Songer cable system used for, 59–60, 60t
Posterolateral fusion
   Rogozinski system used in, 333
   Simmons plating system in, 325, 331
Postlaminectomy kyphosis, 171, 175
   anterior fixation for stability of, 35
   CSLP system used for, 28
Postoperative bracing
   with CD instrumentation, 296
   Jewett brace, 303
   with Louis instrumentation, 400, 407
   with Luque segmental fixation, 264
   Minerva brace, 55
   Minerva jacket, 152
   molded brace, 296
   SOMI brace, 32, 89
   See also Orthosis

Postoperative breakages
   associated with Caspar system, 24, 24t
   in ATLP system, 232
   of cable in Luque-Galveston fusion, 73
   with CCD system, 304
   with Kaneda instrumentation, 167
   with Kostuik-Harrington instrumentation, 175, 178, 187
   with Louis system instrumentation, 407
   in PLIF with instrumentation, 332
   with PWB system, 418
   of Schanz screws, 393, 396t, 397, *397*
   of screws in PIS fixation, 99
   with Simmons plating system, 326
   of Steinmann pins, 53, 243, *245*
   with TSRH instrumentation, 284–285
   of Y-plate, 106
Postoperative care
   with AXIS fixation system, 144
   with Dynalok Fixation System, 320–321
   with Halifax interlaminar clamp, 126
   with Kaneda system, 166
   with lateral mass plating, 137
   for lower cervical fusion, 73
   in methylmethacrylate and Steinmann pin fixation, 241
   for odontoid screw fixation, 9–10
   pain control, 168, 324, 341
   for PIS fixation, 98
   with Rezaian anterior fixation system, 198
Posttraumatic kyphosis
   Harrington distraction system for, 253
   iliac crest grafts insufficient for, 172, 187
   Kaneda system used for, 160, 163, *165*
   Kostuik-Harrington systems for, 175, 178, *182*
      results of use, 180, *183,* 187
      preoperative assessment of, 178, *183*
Potato hook (Luque wire twister), 263, *264*

Pott's disease, 201, 305
Pregnant patients, 258
Premolded plates, 147, *148*
Preoperative planning
   to avoid instrumentation failure, 255
   for Edwards modular instrumentation, 428–429, 451
   for F.I. instrumentation, 387
Provisional stabilization, indications for, 399, 400, *401,* 407
Pseudarthrosis, 276
   caused by wires or clamps, 93
   as complication
      of anterior fixation, 182
      of interlaminar clamping, 86, 87
      of Kaneda instrumentation, 167
      of occipitocervical plate fixation, 106
      of PIS fixation, 98, 98t, *99*
      of TSRH instrumentation, 284
   following F.I. instrumentation, 394
   posterior fusion and, 203
   prevention with AXIS fixation system, 139
   rates following posterior fusions, 174, 180, 184, 185
   repair of, 412, 412t
Pseudocapsule, 243, 246, *246*
Psychiatric disorders, 335, 335t
Pullback block, *359,* 360
Puno-Winter-Byrd (PWB) transpedicular fixation system, 409–418
   advantages and disadvantages of, 418
   background of, 409–410
   clinical experience with, 416–418
   components of, 412, *413*
   development of, 410, *410,* 410t, *411,* 412
   indications and contraindications, 412, 412t
   instruments used, 412
   surgical technique, 413–416, *415,* 416t, *417*
Pyogenic infections, 370

Q

Quadrangular construct, 161

R

Radiography
  anteroposterior (AP) radiographs, 39–40
  in assessment of cervical spine injuries, 108, 108t
  assessment of neural compression by, 89, *90*
  intraoperative
    in anterior fixation, 204, *204*, 206
    in application of ATLP system, 229, *232*
    in implanting and tightening screws, 39–40
    in insertion of Dynalok Fixation System, 318, *319*
    with Kaneda system, 162
    in methylmethacrylate and Steinmann pin fixation, 241
    in posterior lumbosacral fusion, 336, 337, *339*
    in PWB system instrumentation, 414
    in Rezaian spinal fixation, 198
    in thoracolumbar fixation, 347
  postoperative
    advantages of titanium in, 27, *28*, 314
    following CSLP application, 32
    in preoperative planning, 195
    for F.I. instrumentation, 387
    with Halifax system, 123–124
    with Kaneda system, 161
    for methylmethacrylate and Steinmann pin fixation, 240
    for PIS fixation, 95
    in posterior lumbosacral fusion, 336, 346
    to verify cervical spine alignment, 83
  See also Computed tomography (CT); Magnetic resonance imaging (MRI); Myelography
Radiotherapy (RT), 238
Radius of curvature, 261, *261*
Ratchet screws (See Distraction screws)
Redlund-Johnell technique for preoperative evaluation, 105
Reduction
  direct, 447, *450*
  with hook-bars, 348, *351*
  of kyphotic deformities, *178*, 227, 437–438, *438*
  with pedicle screws, 383–384
  rod distractor for, 348, *351, 353*
  of spondylolisthesis, 319–320, 328, 331
  of spondyloptosis, *315*, 322
  See also AMS reduction fixation system; Fractures, reduction of
Reduction bolts, 311
Reduction sequence, 448, 450
Reductive instrumentation, 399
Relaxation of tissues, 174
Reoperations, with PWB system, 418
Respiratory therapy, 198
Retrolisthetic instability, 275, 275t
Retroperitoneal approach
  with Kaneda system, 162, 166, 167
  to thoracolumbar spine, 211
Revision, 237, 238
Rezaian anterior fixation system
  advantages and disadvantages of, 199, 199t
  anesthesia used, 196
  biomechanical considerations, 193–194
  contraindications to use, 195, 195t
  design of, 193, *194*, 195
  indications for use, 195, 195t
  patient positioning, 196
  postoperative management, 198
  prerequisites, 195
  review of medical literature, 198–199, 199t
  surgical technique, 196, *197*, 198
Rezaian spinal fixator, 193, *194*
Rheumatoid arthritis
  interlaminar clamping systems used for, 85, 86, 87
  neural compression caused by, *90*
  occipitocervical plate fixation for, 101, 105
  Songer cable system for
    nonunion with, 73
    in occipital-cervical fusion, 68, *70*
    in posterior cervical fusion, 60
  use of PIS fixation for, 93, 95t, *96*, 99
Rheumatologic disorders, 139, 143
Right-angle nerve hook, 337, *337*
Right anterior surgical approach, 404, *405*
Rigid constructs, 412
Rigid deformity, 442
Rigidity of instrumentation, 116, 213, 227
Rigid rod system, 334, *335*
Rigid round backs, 171, 175
Robinson wire twister, 46, *46*
Rod and TLD bar holder, *300*
Rod and wire systems, axial load injuries and, 257–258
Rod cutter, 376, *376*
Rod distractor, 348, *351, 353*
Rod fixation, wires used for, 260
Rod fracture, 268
Rodgers wiring technique, 109t, 110t, 110–111
Rod gripper, 299, *300*, 301
Rod holders, 299, *300*, 416
Rod-implant locking devices, 299, *299*
Rod introducer lever, *300*, 301
"Rod long and fuse short" technique, 264, 343
  liabilities of, 255, 383
Rod pusher, *300*, 301
Rods
  cable used in combination with, 116
  in CCD system, 297–298, *298*, 302
  in CD instrumentation, 287, *288*, 294, 296, *296*
  entry point for, 265
  importance in Galveston pelvic fixation, 266, *268*
  in Isola/VSP system, 372, *372*
  in posterior lumbosacral fusion, 340, *340*
  in PWB system instrumentation, 412, 415–416
  in TSRH system, 276, 284
Rod-screw connector, 410, *411*
Rod-screw constructs (See Puno-Winter-Byrd transpedicular fixation system)
Rod-sleeves, 422
Rod systems
  advantages of, 367
  for anterior fixation, 198–199, 201, 204
  disadvantages of, 101
  for pedicular arthrodesis, 333–335

Rod template, 294
Rogozinski spinal rod system
  benefits of, 349, 352
  biomechanical considerations, 333–335
  development of, 333
  operative techniques
    complications of, 343
    exposure, 336
    for pedicle screw instrumentation, 337–341, *337–342*
    results of, 341, 343, 343t
  system components, 333, *334, 335*
  use in lumbosacral spine
    contraindications to, 335t, 335–336
    indications for, 335, 335t, 336t
    operative technique, 336–343
    preoperative radiologic evaluation, 336
    surgical criteria and patient selection, 336
  use in thoracolumbar spine, 343–349
    acute fractures, 346–349, *350–353*
    conclusions, 349
    fractures in situ, 344, *344–349*, 346
Rotational control, 116, 259
Rotational injury, 114
Rotational stability, 213
Roy-Camille lateral mass plates, 131, *131*, 137
  technique, 132–133, 137
Roy-Camille posterior plate fixation, 112
Roy-Camille posterior screw plate fixation system
  approach, 148, *148*
  effectiveness of, 154
  indications for use of, 149–154, 152t, 154t
    for lower cervical spine, 149–152, 150t
      dislocations, 149–151, *150, 151*
      facet-joint fractures and dislocations, *151*, 151–152
      failure of anterior stabilization and, 152
      postoperative care and results, 152
      procedures complementary to, 152
      separation-fracture of articular mass, 152, *153, 154*
      severe sprains, 152
      surgical technique, 148–149, *149*
      preoperative radiologic evaluation, 336
      surgical criteria and patient selection, 336
  use in thoracolumbar spine, 343–349
    acute fractures, 346–349, *350–353*
    conclusions, 349
    fractures in situ, 344, *344–349*, 346
Rotational control, 116, 259
Rotational injury, 114
Rotational stability, 213
Roy-Camille lateral mass plates, 131, *131*, 137
  technique, 132–133, 137
Roy-Camille posterior plate fixation, 112
Roy-Camille posterior screw plate fixation system
  approach, 148, *148*
  effectiveness of, 154
  indications for use of, 149–154, 152t, 154t
    for lower cervical spine, 149–152, 150t
      dislocations, 149–151, *150, 151*
      facet-joint fractures and dislocations, *151*, 151–152
      failure of anterior stabilization and, 152
      postoperative care and results, 152
      procedures complementary to, 152
      separation-fracture of articular mass, 152, *153, 154*
      severe sprains, 152
      surgical technique, 148–149, *149*
      teardrop fractures, 152
    plates and screws in, 147, *148*
    for upper cervical spine, 153–154, 154t
      hangman's fracture, 153–154
      occipitocervical fusion, 154
      surgical technique, 149
Roy-Camille screw insertion technique, 141, 318, 319

S

Sacral attachments, 448
Sacral block, *359*, 360
Sacral fixation, Galveston technique, 263, 265–267, *268, 269*
Sacral screws
  in Edwards modular system
    design of, 424, *424*
    lateral insertion, 424, *425*
    medial insertion, 424–425, *425*
    midsacral insertion, 425, *425*
    posterior lumbar insertion, 425–426
  in Isola/VSP system, 372
  landmarks for insertion of, *402*, 403
  pedicle screws, 298, *298*, 299, *299*, 302
  preparation and placement of, 279–280, *280*, 415
Sacro-alar hook, *253*
Sagittal deformities, 315
Schanz screws, 379, *381*
  breakage or bending of, 393, 396t, 397, *397*
  kyphosis correction with, 390, *391–393*
  in MSS and F.I. construct, 384, *386*
  optimal placement of, 389–390, *390*
  in transpedicular fixation, 382–383
Scheuermann's kyphosis, 171, 172, 175
  complications of posterior fusions for, 174
  Iliac crest grafts for, 180, *183*
  Kostuik-Harrington instrumentation for, 180
    indications for use, 181
    results of use, 181–182, *184*, 187
    surgical technique, 180–181, *183*
  rod placement in, 176
Scoliosis
  anterior correction of, 172, 185
  anterolateral surgical approach, 211
  ATLP system contraindicated with fixed deformity, 226, 227, 227t
  correction with CCD system, 302

Scoliosis (Cont.)
   degenerative
      CCD system used for, *306*
      indications for fusion in, 275, 275t
   Dwyer system for correction, 159, 198
   Edwards scoliosis construct for. *See* Scoliosis construct
   Harrington rod system developed for, 251, 252, 255
   Kaneda system used for, 160, 165
   Louis system contraindicated for, 400, 401
   pediatric, 352
   PWB system indicated for, 412, 412t
   rod-hook-screw systems preferable for, 315
   rod placement for correction, 294
   segmental fixation for, 258
   sublaminar wire passage and, 267–268
   treated with ESFS, *380*
   Zielke system developed for correction of, 159
Scoliosis construct, 429–430
   biomechanics of, 447–448, *449, 450, 450*
   clinical results, 452–453
   indications and contraindications for use, 430t
   precautions, 450–451
   preoperative planning for, 451
   surgical technique
      for kyphoscoliosis, 451
      for lumbar and lumbosacral scoliosis, 451–452, *452*
      for lumbar scoliosis, 451
      for thoracic and thoracolumbar scoliosis, *450,* 451
Screw anchors, 287, *288, 289,* 289
Screw backout, 205
Screw breakage
   following correction of kyphotic deformity, 187
   with I-plate system, 207
   with Louis system instrumentation, 407
   in PIS fixation, 99
   with PWB system, 418
   with TSRH instrumentation, 285
   See also Postoperative breakages

Screwdrivers
   in CCD system, 299, *300*
   in Dynalok system, 311, *313*
   hexagonal in ALPS system, 206, *207*
   use in PWB system instrumentation, 414, *415*
Screw entry point, determining, 140, *140*
Screw failure, 10, *11,* 141, 262
   of Isola iliac screws, 260
Screw holes, drilling, 38–39, *39*
Screw insertion techniques, 39, *41*
   in lower cervical spinal fixation, 104, *104*
   See also Odontoid screw fixation
Screw length
   complications due to, 98
   determining, *375,* 375–376
   importance in PIS fixation, *94,* 97
   selection of, 22, 337–338, *339,* 339t
Screw loosening
   associated with Caspar system, 24, 24t
   associated with CCD system, 305
   clamp failure caused by, 118
   with Halifax interlaminar clamp system, 126
   with interlaminar clamping systems, 86–87
Screw migration, 32, 143, 418
Screw placement
   in anterior fixation systems, 204
   in atlantoaxial screw fixation, *103,* 103–104, 104t
   in ATLP system, 228, 229, *230–232*
   complications caused by, 137
   importance in PIS fixation, *94,* 97
   intraoperative skull fixation for, 102, *102*
   in lateral mass plating, 132–133, *133–135*
   in lumbar spine, 414, *415*
   in PWB system instrumentation, 414, *415*
   in Simmons plating system, 331, 333
   in TSRH instrumentation, 280–281
   variable, 409–410
   in Z-plate instrumentation, 221, *222*
Screw pullout, 143, 418

Screws
   in AMS reduction fixation system, 357, *358,* 359, 360, 365
   anchor, 26–27, *27*
   angled-hole, 424, *424*
   apical, 450
   cancellous, 36, 36t, 132, *132*
   cephalad, locking, 35–36, 36t
   collar-ended, 174, *174,* 178
   cortical, 143
   distraction screws, 174, *174,* 424, *424*
   in Dynalok system, 311, *313,* 313–314, *314*
   in Edwards modular system, 422
   fixed angle, 276, *276*
   in Halifax system, 123, *125*
   iliac, 372
   implanting in articular masses, *148,* 148–149, *149*
   Isola iliac, 260
   in Isola/VSP system, 371–372
   locking, 35–36, 40, *42*
   noncannulated, 9, *10*
   odontoid. *See* Odontoid screw fixation
   rescue screws, 22
   in Roy-Camille system, 147, *148*
   self-locking, 357, *358,* 359
   self-tapping, 9, 15, *17, 18*
   set screws, 294, *296*
   straight-hole, 424, *424*
   techniques for implanting. *See* Screw insertion techniques
   temporary, in ATLP system, 228, *229*
   tightening, 39–40
      torque wrench for, 341, *341*
      two-finger tightness, 22
   titanium, 132, *132,* 226, *226*
   transcortical, 239
   transpedicular, 357, *358,* 360
   in TSRH system, 276, *276,* 277
   variable-angle, 276, *276,* 277
   vertebral-body, 161, *161,* 163, *164*
   See also Pedicle screws; Sacral screws; Schanz screws
Seat holder, 414, *415*
"Sea urchin" reduction forceps, 150
Secondary instability, 275t, 275–276
Segmental axial control, 422
Segmental compression and distraction, 333

Segmental fixation
  in CD instrumentation, 287
  with Harrington rod system, 252, 254
  See also Luque segmental fixation
Segmental instability
  classification of, 275, 275t
  fixateur interne indicated for, 379, 393, 393t
  PLIF with instrumentation to correct, 328, 328t
Selective vertebral immobilization, 36
Self-locking screws, 357, *358*, 359
Self-retaining retractors, 318–319
Self-tapping screws
  distractor screws, 15, *17, 18*
  in odontoid screw fixation, 9
Semiconstrained instrumentation systems, 309, *315*
Semirigid assembly of PWB system, 410, *411,* 412, 414
Separation-fracture of articular mass, 147, 152, *153,* 154
Set screws, 294, *296*
SFSG. *See* Spinal Fixation Study Group
Shearing forces, odontoid screw fixation and, 10, *11*
Shear injuries, 436
Short neck
  as contraindication to fixation, 4, 10, 102
  use of Caspar system and, 13
Silastic tubing with methylmethacrylate, 163–164
Simmons plating system
  background and development of, 325–326, *326, 327*
  complications of use, 331–332
  contraindications and disadvantages, 328, 328t, 329t
  indications and advantages, 328, 328t, 329t
  PLIF technique used with, 328–329, *330*
  results of use, 333
  tips for successful use of, 331, 333
Simplex P methylmethacrylate, 236
Single cable, 61, *63*
Single-stage anterior decompression and instrumentation, 212
Slotted connectors, 372, 373, *373, 376, 377*

Slotted plates, 409
Small bone fixation, 113
Small notched titanium reconstruction plates, 131–132, *132,* 137
Soft collar. *See* Cervical collar
Soft-tissue retractors, 13–14, *14*
Sof'wire, 78, *78,* 84
Sof'wire system. *See* Codman Sof'wire system
Somatosensory evoked potentials (SSEPs), monitoring, 57
  in application of Halifax system, 124
  in Edwards modular instrumentation, 445, 447
  in Kaneda system instrumentation, 161
  in lateral mass plating, 130, 131
  in methylmethacrylate and Steinmann pin fixation, 240
  in posterior wiring techniques, 110
SOMI brace
  for postoperative immobility, 89
  use with CSLP system, 32
Songer cable system
  advantages of, 57, 59, 73, 75t
  biomechanical principles of fixation, 59
  contraindications for use, 60, 62t
  ease of use, 57
  indications for use of, 59–60, 60t
    congenital and degenerative disorders, 60, *62*
    deformities, 60
    trauma, 60, *61*
    tumors, 60
  posterior cervical fusion techniques using, 60–75
    atlantoaxial cervical fusion, 65–68
    general technique, 62, *64–66,* 66
    lower cervical fusion (C3 to T1), 68–73
    occipital-cervical fusion, 68, *70*
    principles of instrumentation, 60–65, *63*
    review of experience, *58, 59,* 73, 75, 75t
    sublaminar cabling fusion, 75
  safety of, 57
  sequential tightening complicated by, 263

  strength of, 57, *58, 59,* 75, 75t
Southwick wiring, 110
Spatula, in Roy-Camille system, 149–150, *150,* 151
Speed of fixation, Luque fixation techniques for, 262–263
Spinal abnormalities
  acquired, 89
  correction of, 328, 328t
Spinal canal, surgical remodeling of, 253, *255*
Spinal canal compromise
  with ATLP system, 232
  caused by burst fracture, *179, 180*
  inadvertent wire encroachment, 262, *262*
  Kaneda system used for, 160
  preventing, 20
  with three-column fracture, 348, *352*
  with two-column fracture, 344, *345, 346*
Spinal decompression, 203
Spinal Fixation Study Group (SFSG), 421, 431, 442, 445, 452–453
Spinal instability, classification schemes for, 274, 274t
Spinal muscular atrophy, 68
Spinal rod-sleeve method, 429
  contraindications to, 430t
  indications and biomechanics, 430t, 436, *437*
  precautions, 436
  results of use, 439, *440–441*
  sleeve design, 426, *428*
  surgical techniques
    bridging-sleeve technique, *437,* 438–439
    standard method, 436–438, *437, 438*
    tandem-sleeve method, *437,* 438
Spinal stenosis, 328, 328t, 370
Spinous process fixation
  with Luque instrumentation, 264, *266, 267*
  sublaminar cabling fusion technique for, 73
  wiring techniques, 46–47, *47*
    facet cabling technique as adjunct, *72,* 73
    in Luque rectangle fixation, 91, *91*
Spiralock Thread Form, 310, *312*

Spiralok nut, 325, *326*, 331
Spondylitis, segmental wire fixation of, 257
Spondylo construct, 429
  biomechanics of, 445
  indications and contraindications for use, 430t, 445
  precautions, 445
  for spondylolisthesis
    results of use, 447, *448*
    surgical technique, 445, *446*
  for spondyloptosis
    results of use, 447, *449*
    surgical technique, 447
Spondyloepiphyseal dysplasia, 85
Spondylolisthesis
  AMS reduction fixation for, 360, 363, *363–365*
  anterior fixation for, 201, 202, 204
  CCD system for, *300*, 301, 302, 303–305, *304, 305*
  degenerative
    Edwards D-L construct for, 439–442, *443*
    Isola/VSP fixation system for, 370
  Edwards spondylo construct for, 445, *446*
  fixateur interne indicated for, 379, 393, 393t, 394, 395
  fusion without correction of deformity, 284
  isthmic, 368–369
  Louis system instrumentation for, 403, 405–406, 407
  patient positioning for surgery, 328
  postoperative imaging of, 314, *317*
  PWB system indicated for, 412, 412t, 416
  reduction of
    using Dynalok Fixation System, 313–314, 322
    using PLIF with instrumentation, 333
  restriction on transpedicular screw fixation, 368
  sacral fixation for, 403
  TSRH instrumentation for, 274, 275t, 284
Spondylolisthesis reduction block, *359*, 359–360
Spondylolysis
  correction with CCD system, 303–305, *304, 305*

TSRH system indicated for, 274, 275t
Spondyloptosis
  anterior fixation of, 202
  Edwards spondylo construct for, 447
  reduction with Dynalok fixation, *315*, 322
Spondylosis, 28, 164–165
Sprains, severe, 152
SSEPs. *See* Somatosensory evoked potentials
Stabilization
  biomechanics of devices for, 111–112
  for osteomyelitis, 274, 275t
  provisional, 399, *400, 401*, 407
  using Schanz screws, 390, *392*
Stainless steel
  in ALPS system, 205
  in cables, 60, 113
  compared with titanium, *313*, 314–315, *316*, 316t, *317*
  disadvantages of, 215, 226
  Dynalok implants available in, 311
  in Isola/VSP system, 371, 372
  in Louis system, 400–401
  in Modular Spine System, 384
  monofilament wire, 45, 46t
  for PWB integral screw, 412
  in rod and wire systems, 257
Static posterior fixation, 225
Static strength, 325–326
Steffee pedicle fixation, 259
Steffee plate-screw system, 309
Steinmann pins
  asymptomatic fracture of, 243, *245*
  in Dewar posterior fusion, 111
  in Galveston pelvic fixation, 265
  methylmethacrylate and. *See* Methylmethacrylate and Steinmann pin stabilization
  in occipitocervical fixation, 53, *55*
  postoperative breakage of, 53
  selection of, 240–241, *241*
  with TSRH instrumentation, 279
Sternal-occipital-mandibular immobilizer. *See* SOMI brace
Straight-hole screws, 424, *424*
Stress fractures, postoperative, 180
Stress relaxation, 422, 445, 448
Stress risers, 57, 59
Stress-shielding, 332

Strut grafting
  for acute fracture, 211–212
  for acute rigid kyphosis, 184
  for anterior fusion, 203–204
  in Kaneda anterior spinal stabilization, 163–164, *165, 166*
  in occipitocervical fixation, 53, *54, 55*
Stryker frame, 69–70, 82, 110
Stylet, 91, *91*
Sublaminar cabling
  fluoroscopic study of, 57, 66
  Isola cable designed for, *63*
  methods of, 118–119
  pliability of Sof'wire and, 118
  techniques of, 66, *67, 68*
  See also Cables; Sublaminar wiring
Sublaminar cabling fusion technique, *67, 73, 75*, 75
Sublaminar fixation
  Codman Sof'wire system for, 113, 116
  compared to Drummond button fixation, 260
  segmental, 257
Sublaminar wiring, 109t, 110, 110t, 111
  cross-links developed for use with, 273
  depth of wire penetration in, 261, *261*
  facet cabling technique as adjunct, *72*, 73
  importance of radius of curvature in, 261, *261*
  included in Harri-Luque technique, 254, *255*
  in Luque rectangle fixation, 91, *91*
  placement or removal of
    neurologic injuries caused by, 260–261, 267–268
    penetration of spinal canal in, 261–262
    risks of neurologic injury, *48*, 48–49, 52, 57, 73, 77, 114, 258, 267–268
    techniques, 261–262
  standard techniques, *48*, 48–49, 52
  used with Harrington rod system, 252
  wire passer, *48*, 49
  See also Sublaminar cabling; Wire; Wiring techniques

Suboccipital-mandibular-
    immobilization brace. *See*
    SOMI brace
"Suck" test, 329, 337
Supplemental fixation
    Codman Sof'wire system for, 115
    with proximal bilaminar claw,
        438
    rods in scoliosis construct, 448,
        450, 451, 452
Supralaminar hooks, 292, *292*
Surgery, general complications of,
    331–332
Surgical approaches
    for anterior fixation, 202
    anterolateral, 211
    combined, 405–406, *406*
    complications associated with,
        167, 180
    retroperitoneal, 162, 166, 167,
        211
    right anterior, 404, *405*
    transthoracic retroperitoneal, 162,
        165, 167
    in use of ATLP system, 227
Surgical decompression, 89
Synthes plate-screw system, 309
Synthes plate system, 23–24, 24t
Synthes small notched titanium
    reconstruction plates, 131–132,
        132, 137
Syracuse I-plate system
    biomechanics of, 207, 207t
    description and surgical technique,
        204–205, *205*
    plate positioning, 204, *204*
    for thoracolumbar burst fracture,
        208, 209
Syringomyelia, postoperative, 213
Systemic toxicity, caused by
    methylmethacrylate, 236

T

Table head holder, for patient
    positioning, 149, 150
Tapping drill holes, in AXIS fixation
    system, 141, *141,* 144
Taps
    in CCD system, *300,* 301
    in Dynalok system, 311, *313,* 319
T-bolt, 311, *313,* 320
Teardrop fracture, 152, 154
Templates, 140, *140,* 320

Tensile strength
    of cable *vs.* wire, 57, *58, 59,* 75,
        75t
    of Codman Sof'wire system, 115
Tensile stress, 237
Tensioner, 113, *114*
Texas Scottish Rite Hospital (TSRH)
    Universal Instrumentation
    System, 212, 273–285
    advantages and disadvantages of,
        276, 276t
    background and development of,
        273
    complications, 284
    cross-link plates for stabilization of
        L-rods, 264
    Dynalok Fixation System crossover,
        321–322
    indications for use of, 273–276
        degenerative disorders, 275t,
            275–276
        infection, 274, 275t
        spondylolysis/spondylolisthesis,
            274–275, 275t
        trauma cases, 274, 274t
        tumors, 274, 275t
    instrumentation, 276t, 276–278
        application of, 277–278, *279*
        cross-links, 277, *278*
        hooks, 276–277, *278*
        rods, 276
        screws, 276, *276,* 277
    instrumentation failure, 284–285
    preferred for sagittal deformities,
        315
    results of use
        correction of deformity, 284
        fusion rate, *283,* 283–284, *284*
        neurologic function and back
            pain, 283
        patient population, 282–283
    stability of, 213
    surgical technique, 278–282
        construct assembly, 282
        fusion site preparation and
            wound closure, 282
        hook site preparation and
            placement, *281,* 281–282, *282*
        patient positioning and exposure,
            279
        pedicle preparation and screw
            placement, 279–281, *280*
Thoracic fractures, 439
Thoracic hooks, 282

Thoracic rods, 116, *118*
Thoracolumbar burst fractures
    ATLP system for, 226, 227t, 229,
        232
    F.I. instrumentation for, 394–395,
        395, 396
    fractures with neurologic deficit,
        395–396
    fixation for, 346–349, *350–353*
        anterior, 202, *208,* 209
    Harrington rod instrumentation for,
        159, 343, *382*
    Kaneda instrumentation for,
        166–167
    Kostuik-Harrington instrumentation
        for, 159
    Rogozinski spinal implant for,
        343
    Syracuse I-plate system for, *208,*
        209
    Z-plate instrumentation for (*See*
        Z-plate anterior thoracolumbar
        instrumentation)
Thoracolumbar fractures
    junction fractures, 439
    posttraumatic kyphosis following,
        160
Thoracolumbar spinal stabilization
    AMS reduction fixation system for,
        357, 360
    background and development of
        instrumentation, 251, *252*
    Harri-Luque system for (*See*
        Harri-Luque technique)
    Harrington system for (*See*
        Harrington rod system)
    Louis system for (*See* Louis
        system)
Thoracolumbosacral orthosis (TLSO),
    166, 221, 321
Threaded rods, 359, *359*
Three-column fracture, 348–349, *352,
    353*
Three-column stability, 328, 329t
Three-hole plates, 133, 134–135, *135,
    136,* 137
Three-point fixation, 93, *94,* 165,
    171
Three point shear clamp locking
    mechanism, 276, *278*
Tile plates, 147, *148,* 152
Titanium
    advantages of, 27, *28*
    brittleness of, 260

Titanium (Cont.)
  cables made of, 60, 61, 113
  cancellous bone screws made of, 132, *132*
  compared with stainless steel, *313*, 314–315, *316*, 316t, *317*
  CT- and MRI-compatibility of, 213
  in Dynalok implants, 310, 311, *313*
  fatigue fractures in pins, 239
  in Haid Universal Bone Plates, 131
  in Isola/VSP system, 371, 372
  "manufacturing sensitivity" of, 314, 315
  in Orion plate system, 36, 36t
  in plates and screws, 226, *226*
  Synthes reconstruction plates made of, 131–132, *132*, 137
  in Y-plate for occipitocervical plate fixation, 106
Titanium alloy, 314, 315
  in AXIS plates, 142
  in fixateur interne, 384
TLD (*See* Transverse linking device (TLD))
TLSO (*See* Thoracolumbosacral orthosis (TLSO))
Torque wrench
  cannulated, 333
  deflection beam, 311, *313*, 322
  for Rogozinski spinal rod system, 341, *341*
  for Songer cable system, 62, *66*
  for Z-plate instrumentation, 220, *221*
Toumy syringe, 241, *242*
Towel clip, 46, *47*
Traction
  for alignment of fractures/dislocations, 109
  in bone grafting, 31
  halter traction, 31, 140
  manual in-line, 31
Traction nuts, 359, *359*
  placement of, *361*, 362, *362*
  problems with, 365
Transarticular screw fixation, 105, *105*
Transcortical screws, 239
Translational instability, 275, 275t
Transpedicular fixation, 382, 399
  PWB system for (*See* Puno-Winter-Byrd transpedicular fixation system)

Transpedicular screws, 357, *358*, 360
Transthoracic retroperitoneal approach, 161
  closure, 165
  complications with, 167
  exposure of spine, 162
Transversal dislocations, 302
Transverse adjustability, 421
Transverse fixation assembly, *359*, 360, *360*, *362*, 362–363
Transverse fixators, in Kaneda system, 161, *161*
  application of, 164, *166–168*
  results of use, 167
Transverse linking device (TLD), 299, *301*
  placement of, *301*, 303
Transverse process hooks
  in CD instrumentation, 292–293, *294*
  site preparation and placement of, 281–282, *282*
  in TSRH instrumentation, 277
Trauma
  AXIS fixation system used for, 139, 143
  CD instrumentation for instability, 287
  to cervical spine, 107, 149
  Harrington rod fixation for, 252–253
  instrumentation failure caused by, 284
  interlaminar clamping systems used for, 85, 86
  lateral mass plating for (*See* Lateral mass plating)
  Louis system for stabilization of, 399
  posterior cervical fusion in, 60, *61*
  Rogozinski spinal rod system used for, 335, 335t, 336t
  TSRH system indicated for, 274, 274t
  use of CCD system in, *301*, 303
  use of PIS fixation for, 93, 95t
Triple cabling technique, 120, *120*
TSRH system (*See* Texas Scottish Rite Hospital Universal Instrumentation System)
Tuberculous abscesses, 211
Tuberculous infection
  Isola/VSP fixation system for, 370

  Kaneda system used for, 160
Tumors
  anterior fixation for, 202, 209
  AXIS fixation system used for, 139
  CD instrumentation for, 287
  of cervical vertebrae, 28, *29*
  destruction of atlas-axis interface by, 89, *91*, 92
  F.I. system for, 379, 393t, 396
  instability caused by
    ATLP system for, 226, 227t, 232
    CCD system used for, 305–306, *307*
    Kaneda system used for, 160, 167
    lateral mass plating for (*See* Lateral mass plating)
    methylmethacrylate and Steinmann pin fixation for, 238t, 238–240, *239*, 239t, 242
    interlaminar clamping systems used for, 85, 86
  Isola/VSP fixation system for, 371
  Kaneda system for, 160, 167
  kyphosis secondary to, 171, 175
  Louis system instrumentation for, 405, 407
  metastatic, 167, 195
  occipitocervical plate fixation for, 101
  PWB system indicated for, 412, 412t, 416
  replacement of vertebral body due to, 195, 195t
  Rogozinski system used following resection, 335, 335t, 336t
  Songer cable system for, 60, 68
  TSRH system indicated for, 274, 275t
  Z-plate anterior thoracolumbar system indicated for, 215
Tumors of spine, CCD system for, 305–306, *307*
Two-column fractures
  kyphotic deformity with, 346, *350*
  spinal canal compromise with, 344, *345*, *346*
Two-hole plates, 133, 134, *135*
Two-stage procedures for kyphotic malunion, 212

U

Ultrasonography, intraoperative, 212
Unilateral clamping, supplementation of, 126–127
Unilateral dislocations, 149–151, *150, 151*
Universal implant holder, 299, *300*
Universal rods (Edwards system), 422
   assembly of, 426, *427*
   design of, 426, *427*
   use in anterior neutralization construct, 434, *435*
   washer application, 426, *427*
Universal spinal system (*See* Fixateur interne)
Unstable arch, *437,* 438–439
Unstable olisthesis, 448
Upper lumbar fractures, 439
USS (*See* Fixateur interne)

V

Variable angle screws, 276, *276, 277*
Variable fixation devices, 225
Variable screw placement (VSP) plating system, 367, 371
Vascular complications, 159
Vertebral artery
   abnormality of, 95, *95,* 95t
   penetration during lateral mass plating, 137
Vertebral bodies
   intraoperative fracture in osteoporotic bone, 175
   replacement with methylmethacrylate, 235
   tapping, 39, *40*
Vertebral-body distractor, *14,* 14–15, *17,* 18, *18*
Vertebral-body plates, 161, *161,* 163, *163*
Vertebral-body reconstruction
   following corpectomy, 434–436
   following tumor resection (*See* Methylmethacrylate and Steinmann pin stabilization)
Vertebral-body screws, 161, *161,* 163, *164*
Vertebral-body spreader, 227, *228*
Vertebral-body tumors, 371
Vertebral osteomyelitis (*See* Osteomyelitis)
Vertebral osteoporosis (*See* Osteoporosis)
Vertebral transverse displacement reducer, 399
Vertebrectomy
   in anterior fixation procedures, 203
   total, 405, 407
V-groove hollow ground (VHG) design, 373, *373*
VSP plates, 372
VSP plating system (*See* Variable screw placement plating system)

W

Wake-up test, 445
Washer crimper, 426, *427*
Wedge compression method of C1-2 fixation, 50, 52, *52*
Weinstein screw insertion technique, 318, *319*
Wertheim-Bohlman fusion technique, *54*
Wilson frame, 373
"Wiper effect" of intrapelvic rod movement, 266, *268*
Wire
   beaded double, 261
   breakage with Luque instrumentation, 268–269
   double-stranded, 45–46
   failure of, 45, 46
      in Luque fixation, 264
      "wrapping" and asymmetric stress, 116
   K-wire (*See* Kirschner wire)
   limitations of, 113
   methods of twisting, 46, *46*
   monofilament stainless steel, 45, 46t, 257
   sublaminar passage of (*See* Sublaminar wiring)
   tensile strength of, 57, *58, 59,* 75, 75t
   tightening procedures, 263, *265*
   used for rod fixation, 260
Wire-holding forceps, 46, *46*
Wire passer, *48,* 49
Wire-twisting devices, 46, *46*
"Wire wrap" technique, avoiding, 260
Wiring techniques
   atlantoaxial
      Brooks fusion, 50, 52, *52*
      Gallie fusion, 49, *51*
      interspinous fusion, 49, *50*
   disadvantages in suboccipital instability, 101
   general considerations in, 45–46, *46,* 46t
   for lower cervical spine, 107–112
      background of, 107
      biomechanics of stabilization devices and, 111–112
      classification of fractures and dislocations, 108–109
      emergency resuscitation and, 107–108
      indications for, 109, 109t
      nonoperative treatment and, 109
      posterior techniques, 109–111, 110t
      preoperative radiography, 108, 108t
   occipitocervical, 52–53, *53–55*
   operative techniques in, 46
      facet wiring, 47, *47*
      spinous process wiring, 46–47, *47*
      sublaminar wiring, *48,* 48–49, 52
   posterior, 109–110, 110t
      Bohlman's triple-wire technique, 111
      Dewar fusion, 111, *112*
      Rodgers technique, 110–111
      sublaminar (*See* Sublaminar wiring)
   supplemental orthosis for, 53, 55
Wisconsin buttons, 264, *267*
Wisconsin spinal fixation techniques, 260
Wisconsin wiring, 264, *267*

X

X-rays (*See* Radiography)

Y

Y-plate
   atlantoaxial screw fixation and, 103
   biomechanics of, 105
   surgical procedure for, 102
   tailoring, 104
Yuan I-plates, 212

Z

Zielke-Slot system, 212
Zielke system
   for correction of scoliosis, 159
   for flat-back syndrome, 185
   Kaneda system compared to, 161
Zimmer C methylmethacrylate, 236
Z-plate anterior thoracolumbar instrumentation
   advantages and disadvantages of, 223, 223t
   design criteria, 213t, 213–215, *214*
   history and development of, 211–213
   indications for use, 213, 215
   methylmethacrylate and Steinmann pin fixation used with, 238
   surgical technique, 215–217, *215–222*, 220–221
Z-plate compressor, *219*, 220, *220*
Z-plate crimper, 221, *222*
Z-plate distractor, 217, *218*
Z-plates, 214, *214*

ISBN 0-07-020645-7